Handbook of Toxicologic Pathology

SECOND EDITION

Volume 1

EDITED BY

WANDA M. HASCHEK

Department of Veterinary Pathobiology
College of Veterinary Medicine
University of Illinois at Urbana-Champaign
Urbana, Illinois

COLIN G. ROUSSEAUX

Department of Cellular and Molecular Medicine
University of Ottawa
Ottawa, Canada

MATTHEW A. WALLIG

Department of Veterinary Pathobiology
College of Veterinary Medicine
University of Illinois at Urbana-Champaign
Urbana, Illinois

ACADEMIC PRESS

A Harcourt Science and Technology Company

San Diego   San Francisco   New York   Boston   London   Sydney   Tokyo

Copyright © 2002, 1991 by ACADEMIC PRESS

Academic Press
A division of Harcourt, Inc.
525 B Street, Suite 1900, San Diego, California 92101-4495, USA
http://www.academicpress.com

Academic Press
Harcourt Place, 32 Jamestown Road, London NW1 7BY, UK
http://www.academicpress.com

Library of Congress Catalog Card Number: 2001088191

International Standard Book Number: 0-12-330215-3 (set)
International Standard Book Number: 0-12-330216-1 (volume 1)
International Standard Book Number: 0-12-330217-X (volume 2)

PRINTED IN THE UNITED STATES OF AMERICA
01 02 03 04 05 06 MM 9 8 7 6 5 4 3 2 1

The editors dedicate this book to their parents,
Maria U. and Karol A. Haschek (deceased, 1999),
Francesca and Georges E. Rousseaux (deceased, 1993),
Marian B. and Thomas V. Wallig, and
all other individuals who have supported us in our life's endeavors,
encouraged us when needed, mentored us in our learning, and inspired us in
our educational pursuits for the betterment of society.

Contents

5. Carcinogenesis

Stephen Mastorides and
R. R. Maronpot

6. Applied Clinical Pathology in Preclinical Toxicology Testing

G. S. Smith, R. L. Hall, and
R. M. Walker

PART B

The Practice of Toxicologic Pathology

8. Basic Techniques
Thomas J. Bucci

9. Managing Pitfalls in Toxicologic Pathology
Peter C. Mann, Jerry F. Hardisty, and
Mary D. Parker

Contents

15. Use and Misuse of Statistics in the Design and Interpretation of Studies
Shayne C. Gad and
Colin G. Rousseaux

16. Preparation of the Report for a Toxicology/Pathology Study

Hugh E. Black

PART C

Selected Topics in Toxicologic Pathology

17. Risk Assessment: The Changing Paradigm

Stephen K. Durham and
James A. Swenberg

18. Principles of Risk Communication: Building Trust and Credibility with the Public

Ronald W. Brecher and Terry Flynn

Contents

Contents

26. Heavy Metals
Sharon M. Gwaltney-Brant

Contents

31. Liver
Russell C. Cattley and
James A. Popp

32. Pancreas
Daniel S. Longnecker and
Glenn L. Wilson

33. Kidney
Kanwar Nasir M. Khan and
Carl L. Alden

Contents

Contents

Contents

Contributors

Numbers in parentheses indicate the volume and pages on which the authors' contributions begin.

Carl L. Alden (2:255), Global Metabolism and Investigative Sciences, Pharmacia, St. Louis, Missouri 63167

Val R. Beasley (1:631; 1:645), Department of Veterinary Biosciences, University of Illinois at Urbana-Champaign, Urbana, Illinois 61802

Stephen A. Benjamin (1:529), Department of Pathology, Colorado State University, College of Veterinary Medicine and Biomedical Sciences, Fort Collins, Colorado 80523

T. A. Bertram (2:121), Central Research Division, Pfizer Inc., Groton, Connecticut 06340

Hugh E. Black (1:419), Hugh E. Black & Associates, Inc., Sparta, New Jersey 07871

Patricia M. Blakley (2:895), Kinsmen Children's Centre and Department of Pediatrics, College of Medicine, University of Saskatchewan, Saskatoon, Saskatchewan, Canada S7N 0W8

Brad Bolon (2:509), Amgen, Thousands Oaks, California 91320

Ronald W. Brecher (1:447), GlobalTox International Consultants Inc., Guelph, Ontario, Canada N1H 7K9

Karrie A. Brenneman (2:509), IDDEX, Portland, Oregon

Thomas J. Bucci (1:171), Pathology Associates International, National Center for Toxicological Research, Jefferson, Arkansas 72079

J. E. Burkhardt (2:457), Drug Safety Department, Pfizer, Inc., Global Research and Development, Groton, Connecticut 06348

Charles C. Capen (2:681), Department of Veterinary Biosciences, The Ohio State University, Columbus, Ohio 43210

Bruce D. Car (1:243), Department of Discovery Toxicology, DuPont Pharmaceuticals Company, Newark, Delaware 19714

Russell C. Cattley (2:187), Amgen Inc., Thousand Oaks, California 91320

C. Chan (1:207), Sierra Biomedical, A Division of Charles River Laboratories, Inc., Sparks, Nevada 89431

I. Chu (2:647), Environmental and Occupational Toxicology Division, Bureau of Chemical Hazards, Health and Welfare Canada, Ottawa, Ontario, Canada K1H 8M5

Paul J. Ciaccio (1:243), Department of Discovery Toxicology, DuPont Pharmaceuticals Company, Newark, Delaware 19714

Samuel M. Cohen (2:337), Department of Pathology/Microbiology and the Eppley Institute for Cancer Research, University of Nebraska Medical Center, Omaha, Nebraska 68198

Nancy R. Contel (1:243), Department of Discovery Toxicology, DuPont Pharmaceuticals Company, Newark, Delaware 19714

Claudio J. Conti (2:85), Department of Carcinogenesis, The University of Texas M.D. Anderson Cancer Center, Smithville, Texas 78957

Paul S. Cooke (1:501), Department of Veterinary Biosciences, University of Illinois at Urbana-Champaign, Urbana, Illinois 61802

Diane M. Creasy (2:785), Huntingdon Life Sciences, East Millstone, New Jersey 08875

Myrtle A. Davis (1:67), Department of Pathology, University of Maryland School of Medicine, Baltimore, Maryland 21201

Ronald A. DeLellis (2:681) Department of Pathology, New York Hospital, Cornell Medical Center, New York, New York

David C. Dorman (1:251; 2:509) CIIT Centers for Health Research, Research Triangle Park, North Carolina 27709

Stephen K. Durham (1:437), Discovery Safety Optimization, Bristol-Myers Squibb PRI, Princeton, New Jersey 08543

Jeffery I. Everitt (1:251) CIIT Centers for Health Research, Research Triangle Park, North Carolina 27709

C. Farman (1:207), Sierra Biomedical, A Division of Charles River Laboratories, Inc., Sparks, Nevada 89431

Victor J. Ferrans (2:363), Ultrastructure Section, Pathology Branch, National Heart, Lung, and Blood Institute, National Institutes of Health, Bethesda, Maryland 20892

Eugenia Floyd (1:269), Department of Drug Safety Evaluation, Pfizer Nagoya Laboratories, Taketoyo, Aichi 470–2393, Japan

Terry Flynn (1:447), Frontline Corporate Communications Inc., Kitchener, Ontario, Canada N2H 6M6

George L. Foley (2:847), Drug Safety Evaluation, Pfizer Global Research & Development, Groton, Connecticut 06348

Paul M. D. Foster (2:785), CIIT Centers for Health Research, Research Triangle Park, North Carolina 27709

Shoji Fukushima (2:337), First Department of Pathology, Osaka City University Medical School, Osaka 545, Japan

Shayne C. Gad (1:327), Gad Consulting Services, Raleigh, North Carolina 27511

N. Gillett (1:207), Sierra Biomedical, A Division of Charles River Laboratories, Inc., Sparks, Nevada 89431

Mary E. P. Goad (1:459), Department of Veterinary Pathology, Louisiana State University School of Veterinary Medicine, Baton Rouge, Louisiana 70803

Dale L. Goad (1:459), Department of Veterinary Anatomy and Cell Biology, Louisiana State University School of Veterinary Medicine, Baton Rouge, Louisiana 70803

Sharon M. Gwaltney-Brant (1:701), ASPCA, National Animal Poison Control Center, Urbana, Illinois 61802

Fletcher F. Hahn (1:529), Lovelace Respiratory Research Institute, Albuquerque, New Mexico 87185

James R. Hailey (1:157), National Institute of Environmental Health Sciences, Research Triangle Park, North Carolina 27709

R. L. Hall (1:123), Covance Laboratories, Madison, Wisconsin 53704

Jerry F. Hardisty (1:187), Experimental Pathology Laboratories, Inc., Research Triangle Park, North Carolina 27709

Wanda M. Haschek (1:3; 1:645; 2:1; 2:3), Department of Veterinary Pathobiology, College of Veterinary Medicine, University of Illinois at Urbana-Champaign, Urbana, Illinois 61802

Emile de Heer (2:585), Department of Pathology, Leiden University Medical Centre, 2300 RC Leiden, The Netherlands

Ronald A. Herbert (1:157), National Institute of Environmental Health Sciences, Research Triangle Park, North Carolina 27709

Eugene Herman (2:363), Division of Drug Biology, Food and Drug Administration, Washington, D.C. 20204

Rex A. Hess (1:501), Department of Veterinary Biosciences, University of Illinois at Urbana-Champaign, Urbana, Illinois 61802

Ronald D. Hood (2:895), Department of Biological Sciences, The University of Alabama, and Ronald D. Hood & Associates, Toxicology Consultants, Tuscaloosa, Alabama 35487

W. Jee (2:457), Division of Radiobiology, University of Utah, Salt Lake City, Utah 84108

Elizabeth H. Jeffery (1:15; 1:67; 1:595), Department of Food Science and Human Nutrition, Department of Veterinary Biosciences and College of Medicine, University of Illinois at Urbana-Champaign, Urbana, Illinois 61802

Michael P. Jokinen (1:157), Pathology Associates International, Durham, North Carolina

Kanwar Nasir M. Khan (2:255), Global Toxicology, Pharmacia, Skokie, Illinois 60077

Andres J. P. Klein-Szanto (2:85), Department of Pathology, Fox Chase Cancer Center, Philadelphia, Pennsylvania 19111

C. Frieke Kuper (2:585), TNO Nutrition and Food Research, 3704 HE Zeist, The Netherlands

Donna F. Kusewitt (1:529), Department of Veterinary Biosciences, The Ohio State University, Columbus, Ohio 43210

P. Lappin (1:207), Sierra Biomedical, A Division of Charles River Laboratories, Inc., Sparks, Nevada 89431

Daniel S. Longnecker (2:227), Department of Pathology, Dartmouth Medical School, Lebanon, New Hampshire 03756

Peter C. Mann (1:187), Experimental Pathology Laboratories, Inc., Research Triangle Park, North Carolina 27709

R. R. Maronpot (1:83), Laboratory of Experimental Pathology, National Institute of Environmental Health Sciences, National Institutes of Health, Research Triangle Park, North Carolina 27709

Stephen Mastorides (1:83), Department of Pathology, Division of Molecular Pathology, Memorial Sloan-Kettering Cancer Center, New York, New York 10021

J. P. McGrath (2:647), Lilly Research Laboratories, Eli Lilly and Company, Greenfield, Indiana 46140

Kristen J. Nikula (2:3), Global Investigative Toxicology, Pharmacia Corporation, St. Louis, Missouri 63167

Ricardo Ochoa (1:307), Drug Safety Evaluation, Pfizer Inc., Groton, Connecticut 06340

Mary D. Parker (1:187), Experimental Pathology Laboratories, Inc., Research Triangle Park, North Carolina 27709

Robert L Peiffer (2:539), Department of Ophthalmology, University of North Carolina, School of Medicine, Chapel Hill, North Carolina 27590

Richard E. Peterson (1:501), School of Pharmacy and Environmental Toxicology Center, University of Wisconsin, Madison, Wisconsin 53706

James A. Popp (2:187), Dupont Pharmaceutical Co., Newark, Delaware 19714

Barbara E. Powers (1:529), Department of Pathology, Colorado State University, College of Veterinary Medicine and Biomedical Sciences, Fort Collins, Colorado 80523

Colin G. Rousseaux (1:3; 1:327; 2:1; 2:895), Department of Cellular and Molecular Medicine, Faculty of Medicine, University of Ottawa, and Therapeutic Products Programme, Health Canada, Ottawa, Ontario, Canada K1H 8M5

Anne M. Ryan (1:479), Department of Pathology, Pfizer Global Research and Development, Groton, Connecticut 06349

John C. Seely (1:157), PATHCO Inc., Research Triangle Park, North Carolina 27709

Cynthia C. Shackelford (1:157), Experimental Pathology Laboratories, Durham, North Carolina

G. S. Smith (1:123), CanBioPharma Consulting Inc., Rockwood, Ontario, Canada N0B 2K0

Philip F. Solter (1:631), Department of Veterinary Pathobiology, University of Illinois at Urbana-Champaign, Urbana, Illinois 61801

James A. Swenberg (1:437), Laboratory of Molecular Carcinogenesis and Mutagenesis, University of North Carolina, Chapel Hill, North Carolina 27599

Timothy G. Terrell (1:479), VistaGen Inc., Burlingame, California

Gregory S. Travlos (1:157), National Institute of Environmental Health Sciences, Research Triangle Park, North Carolina 27709

M. E. Tumbleson (1:595), Department of Veterinary Biosciences, University of Illinois at Urbana-Champaign, Urbana, Illinois 61802

V. E. Valli (2:647), College of Veterinary Medicine, University of Illinois at Urbana-Champaign, Urbana, Illinois 61802

Henk Van Loveren (2:585), National Institute of Public Health and the Environment, 3720 BA Bilthoven, The Netherlands

John F. Van Vleet (2:363), Department of Veterinary Pathobiology, School of Veterinary Medicine, Purdue University, West Lafayette, Indiana 47907

Joseph G. Vos (2:585), National Institute of Public Health and the Environment, 3720 BA Bilthoven, The Netherlands

Kenneth A. Voss (1:645), Agricultural Research Service, U.S. Department of Agriculture, Athens, Georgia 30604

R. M. Walker (1:123), Pfizer Global Research and Development, Mississauga, Ontario, Canada L5K 1B4

Matthew A. Wallig (1:3; 1:39; 1:595; 2:1), Department of Veterinary Pathobiology, College of Veterinary Medicine, University of Illinois at Urbana-Champaign, Urbana, Illinois 61802

Hideaki Wanibuchi (2:337), First Department of Pathology, Osaka City University Medical School, Osaka 545, Japan

Herbert E. Whiteley (2:539), Department of Pathobiology, University of Connecticut, Storrs, Connecticut 06269

Glenn L. Wilson (2:227), Department of Structural and Cellular Biology, College of Medicine, University of South Alabama, Mobile, Alabama 36688

Hanspeter R. Witschi (2:3), Toxic Substances Research and Training Program, University of California at Davis, Davis, California 95616

Jeffrey C. Wolf (1:157), Experimental Pathology Laboratories, Durham, North Carolina

J. C. Woodard (2:457), College of Veterinary Medicine, University of Florida, Gainesville, Florida 32608

John T. Yarrington (2:681), WIL Research Laboratories, Inc., Ashland, Ohio 44085

Yang-Dar Yuan (2:847), Retinoid Research, Allergan Inc., Irvine, California 92612

Preface

Our original goal was to produce a unique textbook for those in the field of toxicologic pathology. These efforts resulted in the publication of the first edition of the *Handbook of Toxicologic Pathology*, which is now considered a reference text. Our goals for the second edition of the *Handbook of Toxicologic Pathology* have been to update the material found in the first edition and to expand the scope of the book to address additional and new needs of readers. This has resulted in a significant expansion of this edition to two volumes: Volume 1—General Toxicologic Pathology; and Volume 2—Organ-Specific Toxicologic Pathology.

Toxicologic pathology is the study of the adverse effects of drugs, chemicals, and other health-related products on cellular and organ structure and function. This interface between toxicology and pathology is becoming more and more important, as industry, academia, and governments look for solutions to problems for which an integration of toxicology and pathology is essential. In addition, this field is rapidly expanding because of the increasing regulatory emphasis on the interpretation of biological effects in the context of evaluation of risk of exposure to humans. And, as always, there have been rapid scientific and technological advances since the first edition.

The *Handbook of Toxicologic Patholog, Second Edition* addresses issues facing those who practice in the field of toxicologic pathology as well as those interacting with health professionals in this field. Although we briefly cover the subjects of toxicology and pathology in a general context, the reader is advised to seek further in-depth information concerning these basic disciplines from the numerous textbooks available. The field of toxicologic pathology continues to expand due to the rapid scientific advances in areas such as molecular biology, physiologically based pharmacokinetic modeling, biologically based dose–response modeling, genomics, and emerging fields such as proteomics and metabonomics. In addition, technological advances have provided new methodologies such as laser capture dissection and new imaging modalities. Therefore, we have included not only a number of new chapters that address the basic practice of the discipline but also chapters that address these new developments.

Since toxicologic pathology will continue to expand in this developing discipline, we hope that readers of this second edition will write to us with suggestions for chapter additions or areas that they wish to see included the next time this text is revised

We thank Ms. Natalie Marks, soon to be DVM, for her efforts in coordinating this project. We are also most grateful for the assistance of Drs. C. L. Alden (Pharmacia, St. Louis, MI, USA), A. M. Hayes (University of Guelph, ON, Canada), L. D. Morton (TAP Pharmaceuticals, Deerfield, IL, U.S.A), R. Ochoa (Pfizer Inc., Groton, CT, U.S.A), J. A. Popp (DuPont Pharmaceuticals, Newark, DE, U.S.A), R. A. Roth (Michigan State University, East Lansing, MI, U.S.A), L. L. Smith, (AstraZeneca, Alderley Park, UK), and B. Wagner (Short Hills, NJ, U.S.A.) of the advisory board, whose wisdom and assistance enabled us to bring this second edition to fruition. We are indebted to our chapter reviewers—a partial listing follows: C. L. Alden, V. R. Beasley, R. W. Brecher, T. J. Bucci, S. M. Cohen, D. M. Danilenko, R. R. Dubielzig, B. M. Francis, R. Gorman, R. L. Hall, R. R. Maronpot, G. L. Meerdink, D. G. Morton, L. D. Morton, V. W. Persky, J. A. Popp, G. S. Smith, L. L. Smith, G. Walker, and J. M. Ward.

Wanda M. Haschek
Colin G. Rousseaux
Matthew A. Wallig

PART A
Basics of Toxicologic Pathology

1

Toxicologic Pathology: An Introduction

Colin G. Rousseaux
Department of Cellular and
Molecular Medicine
Faculty of Medicine
University of Ottawa
and
Therapeutic Products Programme
Health Canada
Ottawa, Ontario
Canada

Wanda M. Haschek
Department of Veterinary
Pathobiology
College of Veterinary Medicine
University of Illinois
at Urbana-Champaign
Urbana, Illinois

Matthew A. Wallig
Department of Veterinary
Pathobiology
College of Veterinary Medicine
University of Illinois
at Urbana-Champaign
Urbana, Illinois

I. An Overview of Toxicologic Pathology

A. WHAT IS TOXICOLOGIC PATHOLOGY?

Toxicologic pathology integrates the disciplines of pathology and toxicology and is generally performed in an applied experimental setting. Pathologists study the nature of disease, evaluating changes produced in cells, tissues, or organs in response to a "challenge," whether it is it infectious, neoplastic, immune mediated, or toxic. These diseases leave significant visual "footprints" in cells and tissues. Toxicologists, however, tend to focus on the biochemical basis of the science of poisons. The discipline of toxicologic pathology requires knowledge of pathology and toxicology, as well as other related disciplines, so that integration of morphological, biochemical, and functional changes can be accomplished in a logical manner with respect to their biological significance.

Widespread interest in toxicology pathology grew with the advent of the National Toxicology Program (NTP) in the United States and similar programs in other countries created to address the concerns over pollution. Similarly, the increasing demand placed on industry to demonstrate that products are "safe" catalyzed widespread interest in toxicologic pathology. With exposure of fraud in laboratory testing occurring in the late 1970s, good laboratory practice regulations demanded procedures that are now central to the industrial toxicologic pathologist's work. Thus, the field of toxicologic pathology was born. Before this time, investigation of the effects of toxicants on body tissues was done on a case-by-case basis.

In the process of acquiring knowledge concerning the safety and efficacy of chemicals used by humans, or to which they are exposed, it became necessary (1) to describe the adverse effects caused by these compounds in a structural and functional manner and (2) to be able to predict the likelihood of these effects under various conditions. Thus, dose–response characterization of these effects has become an integral and important part of the field of toxicologic pathology. As understanding the biology of disease at the molecular level that is caused by poisons is necessary to be able to predict low-dose extrapolations of disease, a considerable amount of research has gone into developing appropriate models that will predict these adverse effects.

The toxicologic pathologist must have a mastery of both experimental and comparative pathology. A toxicologic pathologist differs from a diagnostic or forensic pathologist who interprets the pathological manifestations of spontaneous or maliciously induced toxicological disease. In contrast, main role of the toxicologic pathologist is to determine the biological significance of chemically induced alterations in form, function, or both, as manifested by the formation of lesions in tissues. In other words, toxicologic pathology is an essential part of hazard identification, dose–response data generation, and risk characterization essential for risk analysis and assessment and management of human and animal chemical exposure. In addition, toxicologic pathology is sometimes referred to as "industrial" pathology, as predicting risk following exposure to a xenobiotic, be it a pharmaceutical agent, a pesticide, a food additive, or a contaminant, is largely confined to the industrial setting.

B. THE PHILOSOPHY OF TOXICOLOGIC PATHOLOGY

Pathology can be defined as the study of the molecular, cellular, tissue, or organismal response of the living body when exposed to injurious agents or deprivations. It is central to the development of and progress in all of medicine, be it humans or animal. Pathology began as a science of observation. Descriptions of altered morphology were, and still are, an important basis for understanding normal versus diseased tissue. The quest for understanding the cause of disease resulted in efforts to associate morphological changes, i.e., lesions, with their cause(s). As the discipline grew, associations were made between lesions and etiologies resulting in the use of pathology as a diagnostic tool in medicine, initially for forensic purposes. Observations of altered morphology were initially done on a gross autopsy or necropsy level. With the development of the microscope and

then the electron microscope, observations could be made at the cellular and subcellular levels. More recent techniques have been applied to detect changes at molecular and gene levels.

Pathology: is it an art or science? This question often asked by other scientists is not new. Most practicing pathologists have discussed the difficulties of the "art of pathology" with their scientific colleagues and, therefore, are aware of the implications of such a statement. The "art" of pathology refers to the imagination, imitation, and interpretation associated with the skilled application of learned techniques to distinguishing "true" lesions from incidental, artifactual, or postmortem changes.

However, the "science" of pathology refers to an organized body of knowledge that has been accumulated on a subject, which is then used by the pathologist to draw conclusions from the observations and interpretations made while viewing a change in tissue or organ morphology. Therefore, pathology is both an art and a science, and as such is considered central to determining the biological significance of observed changes via the integration of molecular, biochemical, functional, and morphological data. Toxicologic pathology specifically addresses the art and science of alterations in form and function induced by toxicants by integrating two disciplines—toxicology and pathology (and sometimes others)—so that a better logical evaluation can be made using the best of both human traits.

One of the most important roles for toxicologic pathology is in the process of risk assessment. Risk assessment is not a truly stochastic process. Data gaps, perception of the importance of the data, and assumptions that must be made due to lack of the means to obtain data often make this science less predictive than is thought by the general public. For this reason, the judgment of the significance of lesions and judgment of how to fill the gaps in our knowledge is crucial to good risk management.

The control and logic used in science usually give precise accurate data regarding a specific question where few variables are evaluated.

4

However, this method leads to a "laser beam" approach to answering questions. In contrast, experience and judgment give the broadest view to a question of risk where numerous variables are evaluated concurrently. This method gives us a "flashlight" approach to answering questions and the interpretation of what is seen relies on the experience of the observer. By combining the precision of the laser beam approach of risk assessment with the flashlight judgmental approach to viewing disease, the public, industry, and government will be served better with respect to safety (risk) assessment. The integration of both the broad beam (flash light) and focused (laser beam) approach is core to the practice of toxicologic pathology.

II. The Need for Toxicologic Pathology in Modern Society

A. WHAT LED TO THE NEED FOR TOXICOLOGIC PATHOLOGY?

Most modern Western societies enjoy a standard of living that has never before been achieved in the history of human development. Associated with this rise in standards have been a decrease in life-threatening infectious diseases and an associated increase in the longevity of the population as a whole. The result has been a population boom that has also led to an increased desire for "the better things in life." As the industrial revolution became the petrochemical revolution, and the pharmaceutical industry developed, little thought was given to any other aspect of production other than efficacy of the product. The side effect of this newfound affluence (i.e., diseases of "lifestyle"), as well as the disposal of by-products and waste products, has plagued modern society practically from the inception of the industrial revolution.

For a long time pollution was only recognized as a "potential" problem, and the dogma for a long time was "The solution to pollution is dilution," in some ways a parody of Paracelsus's dictum that, *"All substances are poisons; there is none which is not a poison. The right dose differentiates a poison from a remedy."* It was

not until the automobile was beginning to make life in the city unbearable, rivers and lakes were no longer safe for recreation, songbirds were noted by their absence, and babies were born with grossly deformed limbs following exposure to thalidomide that the general public began to recognize the negative aspects of industrial development.

Democratic Western societies responded to issues raised by focus groups and to the concerns of the general public by introducing legislation to address a number of issues not only regarding the environment but also the safety of products for consumption. To address this requirement, pathologists were recruited to evaluate morphologic changes following exposure to xenobiotics of concern under controlled conditions (i.e., safety testing). Pathologists eventually became recognized for their abilities to work in a team setting with scientists in other disciplines and become critical to identification, interpretation, and integration of functional and morphological changes in safety assessment, where data from laboratory animals were extrapolated to potential risk of exposure in humans. The field of toxicologic pathology was born.

1. A North American Perspective

In 1984, five separate committees of experts from the National Research Council, under contract to the NTP, developed a strategy for evaluating the safety of chemicals intended for human use. The committee listed a "universe" of five million substances, under which several categories were identified. Of these, a "select universe" of 65,725 chemicals was considered to be of concern by the NTP.

All of these chemicals obviously could not be tested for toxicity, so it was decided to characterize the status of 100 substances on which at least minimal toxicity information was available. These 100 compounds were selected from seven categories defined by the committee. Classification based on use or function rather than on chemical structure resulted in chemicals appearing more than once in the groups selected. There were limitations to this approach. Approximately 20% of the examples in the "select universe" were duplicates, leaving 53,500 substances mutually exclusive among the groups. Of the "select universe" of 65,725 chemicals, 48,523 were used in commerce.

Most of these substances were produced in unknown amounts, and little information was available concerning their toxic effects because of the propriety nature of the compounds. The realization that obtaining complete health hazard assessments on each substance would require further testing of 82% of drugs and vehicles, 90% of pesticides and "inert" ingredients, 95% of food additives, and 98% of cosmetic ingredients highlighted the magnitude of this task. Furthermore, as a result of increasingly strict regulations for testing, more than 50% of previously completed chronic tests would need to be repeated. Testing all chemicals would represent a significant effort to address possible health risks so it became necessary to determine the extent of testing that should be conducted to minimize the risk of human exposure to hazardous chemicals.

Government agencies continue to struggle with the paradox of a society, which disposes of approximately 2 kg of waste per person per day, but does not clearly understand all risks associated with different manufacturing and disposal methods. The regulatory bodies responsible to the public for ensuring the "safety" that society demands often have difficulty reconciling perceived risk with true health risks. In addition, public acceptance of a specific risk is clouded by the view that all industrially based products must be "risk free." For this reason, risk communication has become central to appropriate risk management (Chapter 18).

North Americans are faced with thousands of leaking landfills and, at the same time, with an increasing sensitivity of citizens to "apparent risks." There is urgent need for professionals to interpret credibly such hazards as are found, for example, in water carried in an asbestos pipe, in high concentrations of SO_2 in stack effluent, in leaking underground storage tanks, or in contamination of a building with polychlorinated biphenyls (PCBs) from a ruptured transformer.

Who then must deal with this seemingly overwhelming number of issues for which society demands resolution? Those in the field of toxicologic pathology are ideally suited to this task.

A sentinel network of animal diagnostic laboratories in North America and other countries often can detect environmental risks before an effect is noted in the human population. The dioxin exposure in Times Beach horses in Missouri, the polybrominated biphenyl outbreak in Michigan cattle, and the DDT exposure of peregrine falcons are examples of animals serving as sentinels of environmental contamination. The routine flow of diagnostic material through such laboratories provides continuous surveillance of our chemical environment. Therefore, in many situations the toxicologic pathologist in the diagnostic laboratory is as valuable as the toxicologic pathologist in the industrial setting identifying potential problems and risk factors.

The thalidomide disaster in the 1960s emphasized the need to evaluate drugs in a rigorous way for safety. Although the field of teratology was born following recognition that infants born with phocomelia were from mothers who had taken thalidomide during the first trimester of pregnancy, the need for detailed safety assessment of pharmaceuticals was identified. The role of the toxicologic pathologist became pivotal to development programs in the pharmaceutical industry.

The largest number of toxicologic pathologists are employed by industry, be it pharmaceutical, agrochemical, chemical, or contract research organizations (CRO). Toxicologic pathologists are involved in the safety assessment of drugs, chemicals, biotechnology-derived products, and medical devices; laboratory animal disease surveillance; drug discovery, including identification of therapeutic targets and phenotypic determination of transgenic animals; validation of animal models; evaluation of drug efficacy, often using animals models; and investigation of mechanisms of toxicity. Toxicologic pathologists are also employed by regulatory agencies and as consultants to industry or contract organizations.

Toxicologic pathologists in academia practice their discipline in a diverse manner. These individuals participate in training residents (or graduate students) as well as veterinary or medical students in general and systemic pathology. Often, this training involves active practice in a diagnostic laboratory where many toxicologic pathologists have service appointments. Most academic toxicologic pathologists also have active research programs and often consult for industry needing their expertise.

2. The Challenges Facing Toxicologic Pathology

Toxicologic pathology requires additional working knowledge of disciplines other than pure morphology. In fact, those in the field of toxicologic pathology require a working knowledge of what the body does to a chemical (pharmacokinetics and toxicokinetics) (Chapter 2) and what the chemical does to the body (pharmacology, toxicology, and pathology) (Chapters 3 and 4).

Individuals may be exposed to toxic substances by a variety of routes, but dermal and inhalation exposures are the most common routes of unintentional exposure. Fat-soluble substances such as phenolic compounds, vitamins D and K, and steroid hormones are readily absorbed through the skin; thus, it is important to recognize the chemical characteristics of the compounds in question (Chapter 29). Widespread exposure to potentially toxic gases and particles occurs in the work place as well as in everyday life. In addition, exposures to gases are complicated by particles that may facilitate pulmonary exposure and add to the insult on the respiratory system (Chapter 28).

The oral route is the third common route by which a toxic substance may enter the body. Absorption of a substance across the gastrointestinal wall depends on its lipid solubility, pH, and ionization constant and the nature of the mucosal lining at the site of absorption. These issues are discussed in detail in Chapter 30.

The route of exposure to be used in toxicity testing is determined by considering the chemical and physical properties of the compound, the route for its intended use, and natural protective barriers such as hair or coat (Chapters 8 and 9). The route of administration may also be governed by special biological attributes of the test species and its environment (Chapter 12), which is particularly important for fishes and insects.

For many practicing toxicologic pathologists, the bioassay for determining the carcinogenicity of test articles is central to their day-to-day work. The general approach of conducting carcinogenicity and chronic toxicity tests involves treating male and female rats and mice. The bioassay for a test article comprises four experiments, the results of which are often equivocal or difficult to interpret. For example, a positive result in one treatment group and negative results in the other three treated groups may be seen. The mathematical methods used in clarifying issues such as these are discussed in Chapter 15.

A range of exposures, including low-level and slightly toxic doses, in more than one species is necessary, as the aim of these assays is to provide data for human health risk assessment. At the National Toxicology Program and the National Institutes of Health (NIH), bioassays usually include the maximum tolerated dose (MTD; established previously by experimental feeding) and two other dose levels, generally one-half and one-quarter MTD. The standard industrial design usually includes both rats and mice in groups of 100 males and 100 females, whereas the Food and Drug Administration (FDA) requires groups of 50. Additional animals are often included to allow more than one control group or to permit examination of specimens during the course of the experiment. For more details, see Chapter 14.

Species variation in the handling of test substances makes extrapolation of results from rodents to humans at best difficult and at worst a tenuous process as discussed in Chapter 9. It is doubtful whether a toxic response to a test substance administered at a high dose in a rat necessarily reflects the action of the same compound at a low dose in humans. However, given the state of our present knwoledge and

economic constraints, this method is the best we have on which to base social, political, legislative, and financial decisions.

Application of new technologies to examine, for instance, the mechanisms of chemical carcinogenesis (including the ability of a chemical to bind DNA), DNA repair mechanisms, mutagenicity studies, and impairment of cell–cell communication, may provide helpful information for use in the decision-making process (Chapters 5 and 13). Studies of DNA adduct formation have addressed some aspects of the pharmacokinetics of DNA damage and repair and how specific cell reactions to carcinogens may relate to mutagenesis, initiation, and progression. However, at present these techniques cannot replace whole animal studies.

The validity of rodent bioassays continues to be questioned. There have been questions concerning the relevance of rodent carcinogenesis experiments, the validity of linear extrapolation of data that has been obtained from inbred strains of animals exposed to high doses of substances to low-level human exposure, and the variable nomenclature to describe lesions. With the advent of mechanistic studies (Chapter 17), the use of special techniques (Chapter 10), new animal models (Chapter 13), new technological approaches (Chapter 11), consistent nomenclature (Chapter 7), and report writing (Chapter 16), progress has been made. Integration of clinical, clinical pathology data, and morphologic findings is also assisting the risk assessment risk management process (Chapter 6).

As one contemplates the dimensions of the problem of safety assessment and assessment of risk, one is reminded of Albert Einstein's remark, "*No amount of experimentation could ever prove me right; a single experiment can prove me wrong*". This comment epitomizes the dilemma of toxicologic pathology: results may indicate that a substance may be toxic or carcinogenic, but there is never the certainty to say that it is not.

3. Risk Assessment in Toxicologic Pathology

There appear to be two schools of thought concerning the best way to generate data for risk assessment: *in vitro* and *in vivo* testing. Both arguments have validity and both have their place in truly assessing risk. Mechanistic and quantitative assessment methods, such as proto-oncogene activation, have been touted as explaining the relationship of mutagenesis in animals to the pathogenesis of cancer in humans. However, these studies evaluate only one aspect of the process of carcinogenesis and its control, whereas *in vivo* methods using the whole animal approach allow for consideration of factors such as organ–organ interactions, pharmacokinetics, species variation in metabolism, and the complex process of carcinogenesis in its totality. For this reason, the use of animals as the best available approach has been vigorously defended. However, *in vitro* systems can be very useful in the investigation of basic mechanisms of toxicity at the cellular level. At present, both approaches have merit the more precise, quantifiable *in vitro* methods suit predictive analysis, whereas the whole animal bioassay addresses multiple toxicokinetic and toxicological effects. There are pragmatic consideration as well, which complicate the picture, including the high cost of animal studies and the ethical issues surrounding the use of animal in research.

Even though the whole animal bioassay continues to be the "gold standard" for assessing cancer risk, there are flaws in this approach, as used currently, to generalize from increased or accelerated tumor development in inbred rodents to a possible carcinogenic effect in humans. However, until we are able to establish quantifiable methods with a high positive predictive value, it is important to protect the most susceptible and most heavily exposed portion of the human population from chemicals that are reasonably likely to cause cancer.

Thorough discussion of bioassay design and interpretation of toxicologic experiments in rodents is addressed in Chapter 15. Extrapolation from high dose to low dose and from one species to another (from "mice to men") is fraught with uncertainties and difficulties; even the question of whether carcinogens and mutagens have a "threshold" below which there is no effect is still hotly debated.

The uses of risk assessment and risk management are now implemented in most regulatory situations (Chapter 17). Basically there are four steps: hazard identification, dose–response assessment, and exposure assessment and risk characterization. Hazard identification is purely scientific, ultimately resulting in a statement as to the consequences of exposure, e.g., explosive. Subjectivity enters the picture when judgment concerning the significance of the findings is required. The importance of recognizing where scientific logic ends and judgement begins has become an essential duty of the toxicologic pathologist in product development and risk management. As with all subjective assessment, application of science, current dogma, and judgement can vary widely, indicating the political nature of risk management. Risk management is intended to weigh adverse health risks with benefits and policy choices made that should be most beneficial to the public.

B. THE VALUE OF TOXICOLOGIC PATHOLOGY

The primary values that the field of toxicologic pathology brings to the scientific community are the ability to describe and interpret changes induced by chemicals, drugs, and biotechnology-derived products in the tissues and fluids of laboratory animals and to assess their significance for humans. However, the ability to integrate clinical observations, morphological changes, hematological aberrations, altered clinical chemistries, and other data is an exceedingly valuable asset. These skills enable the toxicologic pathologist to add value to discovery, research and development, regulatory approval, and postmarketing activities of many product lines. In addition to the integration of findings in the experimental and research world, the toxicologic pathologist may be able to solve specific pre-and postmarket problems by using diagnostic and experiential judgmental approaches.

Toxicologic pathology is central to risk analysis, risk assessment, and risk communication through the integration of toxicologic pathology with relevant disciplines and evolving new technologies. This approach to risk assess-

ment results in risk management that is based not only on broad input from the scientific side, but also reasoned judgement, where hard qualitative and quantitative data are not available.

III. The Future of Toxicologic Pathology

A. ANIMALS AND TOXICOLOGIC PATHOLOGY

Considerable pressure placed on researchers by animal rights groups to eliminate the use of animals in toxicologic studies has resulted in efforts to improve and develop new assays that use fewer animals or substitute *in vitro* or non-living systems for animals. These groups have gained widespread publicity and have even conducted "liberation raids" on animal laboratories throughout the world. Unfortunately, although there is considerable awareness and sensitivity to these issues on the part of the public, there is a lack of understanding of the importance of animal use in testing. The benefits of products that arise from medical research for all humans are numerous, but the cost in both fiscal and animal terms is not realized by all whom receive the benefit. The resulting paradox consists of great enthusiasm for the ultimate product that benefits human health with little willingness to consider the animal and environmental costs. For example, cholesterol-lowering drugs are now being taken by millions of patients; however, many recipients of this treatment do not support the extensive animal research that was necessary to test these compounds for toxicity and effectiveness before they were marketed.

Another paradox is prevalent: public concern over animal use in testing is increasing, but so is the public's concern for safety. Few would deny that elimination of the painful, and inexact, Draize rabbit eye irritancy test would be a step forward. In fact, various *in vitro* tests, including the use of a number of different cell lines, have been examined as alternative methods. Unfortunately, when attempts have been made to validate these tests with a broad spectrum of compounds, the correlation with the Draize test

9

has been, at best, equivocal. The assessment of long-term effects by *in vitro* methods is almost impossible given our present limited technological expertise. Despite such problems, alternative technology may be able to assist in safety assessment. Ironically, many do not recognize that many of the *in vitro* and *ex vivo* models developed rely on the initial collection of animal tissues for the model.

It was originally thought that extrapolation from *in vitro* studies to humans would not be difficult. However, just as extrapolation from high doses in rodents to low doses in humans requires nonvalidated assumptions in risk assessment, so does extrapolation from *in vitro* observations. For example, it was originally thought that rodent carcinogenicity assays and short-term genotoxic tests were in close agreement. An agreement of over 90% was observed between carcinogenicity in rodents and mutagenicity in the Ames *Salmonella* reverse mutation assay; thus the formation of promutagenic lesions in DNA was assumed to be a common mechanism of action for all carcinogens. Later it was found that of 44 chemicals that tested positive for rodent carcinogenicity, 24 were negative for mutagenicity in the *Salmonella* assay. This discordance complicates risk analysis greatly, and highlights the importance of evaluating pharmacokinetic and metabolic interactions of chemicals within living systems. In this case the *in vitro* method did not give clear-cut answers. It should be noted that this discordance did not invalidate either assay, but led to a better understanding of the limitations of each assay and to venture into the genetic and epigenetic pathogenesis of cancer.

The real advantage of using *in vitro* testing lies in the ability to control extraneous sources of variation and to decrease the number of animals used in research. Paradoxically, as these procedures become more powerful in establishing mechanisms, they often lose applicability to a multicellular multiorgan organism. Even though some *in vitro* tests have been shown to correlate well with their *in vivo* counterparts, *in vivo* testing still gives risk assessors the most applicable data (apart from human response and exposure data) for use in risk assessment.

Pressure to change standard methodology has had a visible impact on the practice of toxicologic pathology. Median lethal dose (LD_{50}) testing, Draize testing, animal bioassays, and the validity of some procedures continue to be strongly criticized. With the emergence of newer techniques of molecular biology, the role of the pathologist is moving away from classical anatomic pathology. It is not enough to design long-term toxicity tests based solely on the morphological examination of large numbers of organs. As much information as possible must be obtained from each animal. Target organ toxicologic pathology still is essential, but each organ cannot be treated as a separate entity—the animal must be viewed as a whole, not as a collection of organs. For details concerning system toxicologic pathology, see Chapter 27–44.

B. THE "PRACTITIONER" OF TOXICOLOGIC PATHOLOGY

A "Practitioner" of toxicological pathology utilizes toxicologic pathology in an applied manner on a daily basis, most often in an industrial setting. This does not preclude research in many cases but the research is usually specifically focused in an applied manner to solve a problem or meet a goal within the industrial setting. Because the toxicologic pathologist's vital role in risk assessment within the industrial setting, there will be continued participation in the product life cycle. As new methods become validated and implemented, such as molecular probes, a new dimension for morphologic evaluation will be established (Chapter 10). However, change is not limited to more sophisticated visualization of altered morphology in that toxicologic pathologists will be expected to provide more than unambiguous diagnoses and dose–response assessment via interpretation of hematoxylin and eosin-stained tissue sections. As the toxicologic pathologist assumes a greater role in product development, such as serving as study director for compounds under development as pharmaceutical agents, the impact of their observations, interpretations, and comments will become even greater. Therefore, issues such as consistency of terminology (Chapter 7), study design (Chapter 14), statistical interpretation (Chapter 15), integration of data into meaningful assessments of health risks (Chapter 17), and communication of risk (Chapter 18) will need to be familiar to the toxicologic pathologist. Another real value that a toxicologic pathologist can add to product development is the ability that the discipline has to solve problems, sometimes before they even begin.

In the diagnostic laboratory, toxicologic pathology will continue to be central to diagnosis and prevention of spontaneous chemically induced disease. New morphological manifestations of accidental poisonings are often first described in the diagnostic laboratory. The utility of naturally occurring chemically induced diseases should not be underestimated, as it is often these cases that add crucial information to understanding the mechanisms of similar chemical groups. It was thought that there would be an emerging role for the practitioner of toxicologic pathology in the evaluation of environmental issues. However, this role has not become a major source of employment for many practicing toxicologic pathologists. This situation may be due to the current training and experience of those involved in environmental toxicology and chemistry, which often result in efforts focused primarily at finding the quintessential biomarker for toxic disease rather than integration of observed morphologic changes with etiologic causes.

For those toxicologic pathologists who have assisted in evaluating environmental issues, there has been recognition that the practice of toxicologic pathology can add valuable information for diagnosing problems, detailing background disease prevalence and investigating toxicity where chemistry fails. Already there is awareness by some in the environmental toxicology field that clinical pathology can be a useful part of the investigative armamentarium, but the majority of clinical pathology work is presently done in preclinical toxicology and

diagnostic pathology. (Chapter 6) Perhaps when environmental toxicologists broaden their search for answers beyond the "magic bullet biomarker," the toxicologic pathologist will be sought after to help solve environmental problems.

C. THE "RESEARCHER" IN TOXICOLOGIC PATHOLOGY

Traditionally, those that have used morphology in research but were not certified pathologists have not always been recognized as belonging to the field of toxicologic pathology. As the discipline of toxicologic pathology has evolved, this is no longer the case. Research in toxicologic pathology is essential for understanding the mechanisms of toxic tissue injury and to fill data gaps that impeded risk assessment. In fact, by understanding the pathogenesis of altered morphology, normal bodily events have been elucidated. For example, the use of teratogenic substances has aided our understanding of embryonic and fetal development (Chapter 44).

Toxicologic pathologists participate in research in many settings, including industry, academia, and government. Descriptive research is still a necessary part of the field. With the synthesis of new compounds, or modification of old ones, a precise standardized definition of changes associated with exposure to these compounds is necessary (Chapters 21 and 22). Similarly, toxicologic pathology may involve simple associative types of research, including retrospective studies using archived tissues, cross-sectional surveys, and longitudinal studies of disease progression and remission (Chapter 15). However, it is new techniques, animal models, and controlled inferential research that will probably receive the most attention and effort in an attempt to understand the mechanisms of disease (Chapters 11, 13, 19 and 20).

The techniques of molecular biology are being used to probe the mechanisms of carcinogenesis (Chapter 10). Activated oncogenes have been found in both human and animal tumors. For example, tumorigenesis is associated with the expression of activated oncogenes in transgenic mice. Identification of an oncogene specifically activated by a given chemical in both species may aid in the extrapolation of data from bioassays conducted in rodents. In fact, the p53 knockout mouse is presently being used to aid in the identification of carcinogens (Chapters 5 and 13).

An example of how toxicologic pathology addresses mechanistic research is molecular dosimetry. Studies concerning the balance between DNA damage and repair add important quantitative data to the knowledge of molecular dosimetry. Molecular dosimetry is based on measurement of the molecular dose that reaches and forms adducts with the DNA molecule, a process dependent on the ability of the particular cell type to repair the damaged DNA. For example, hepatocytes are more capable of repairing DNA damage induced by dimethyl hydrazine than endothelial cells; following exposure to dimethyl hydrazine, 100% of animals will develop hemangiosarcomas and only 40% will develop hepatomas. Molecular dose bears a closer relationship to biological effects than external dose because many factors, such as absorption, distribution, and biotransformation, affect the ultimate dose to the DNA molecule. More details concerning molecular dosimetry and other mechanistic research can be found in Chapter 17. From such quantitative studies may emerge more rational and repeatable methods of extrapolating high doses in one species to low doses in another; these data may support risk characterization values derived from animal data, hence enhancing the risk assessment process.

Today's rapid pace of scientific advancement and the development of new technologies that can be exploited to address toxicological issues means that we will continue to see large strides made in understanding mechanisms of xenobiotic-induced alterations and diseases. The combination of morphological techniques, which provide topographic specificity, with novel technologies that permit large-scale assessments of metabolic intermediates, proteins, and mRNA, but generally lack topographic specificity, can be used to facilitate the study of

mechanisms of toxicity underlying xenobiotic-induced, microscopically detectable lesions. The combination of traditional lesion identification with laser capture microdissection, for example, will permit the direct molecular assessment of lesions by a variety of such new technologies.

D. THE "CONSULTANT" IN TOXICOLOGIC PATHOLOGY

The consultant is usually brought in on an "as needed" basis for solving a particular problem or as part of regularly scheduled program reviews that use independent outside expertise to validate findings. Again, it is the integrative nature of the discipline that aids consultants in adding value for their customers. Whether the consultant is employed as part of a pathology working group to address specific findings or to give advice regarding a product development plan, it is the diverse experience of a toxicologic pathology consultant that usually results in a value added judgment. The consultant may also act as a practitioner to read studies for smaller companies or to assist other toxicologic pathologists when work load exceeds staff capabilities. The comments made in the previous section concerning the practitioner hold true regarding the consultant who reads studies. However, with an ever-increasing need to shorten the time to getting a product on the shelf, the role of consulting in toxicologic pathology will most likely expand.

E. THE "MANAGER" IN TOXICOLOGIC PATHOLOGY

A number of scientists involved in product research and development find themselves moving toward more managerial roles. The toxicologic pathologist is well poised to fill such a position, as the management of scientific issues concerning product research and development is often best solved using the integration of a number of disciplines. However, a manager requires more than just a solid toxicologic pathology background to succeed in such a role. Those in managerial positions require strong communication skills to deal with upper management, regulators, lawyers, and external stakeholders. For this reason, skilled communication techniques are a prerequisite for success in a managerial role, particularly when it comes to risk management (Chapter 18).

F. TRAINING FUTURE TOXICOLOGIC PATHOLOGISTS

In Northern America, advanced training in pathology for veterinarians and physicians has generally been through residency programs that emphasize diagnostic pathology and/or research programs leading to a Ph.D. degree and certification in pathology. Biologists who enter the specialty of toxicologic pathology have generally completed a Ph.D. program in experimental pathology.

On completion of their training in comparative pathology, pathologists are often hired as toxicologic pathologists without any specific training in experimental design and other issues essential to the practice of toxicologic pathology. Classical comparative pathology programs typically do not have requirements for training in toxicology, pharmacokinetics, pharmacodynamics, and statistics. Several institutions now provide the opportunity for trainees to obtain training in these essential areas, as well as offering courses in the pathology of toxicant-induced disease. In addition, a number of pharmaceutical companies are offering summer externships for trainees to gain experience in toxicologic pathology.

The majority of toxicologic pathologists are veterinarians trained in veterinary (comparative) pathology, coming from training programs that generally reside in academic institutions, with most in veterinary schools. A typical residency program is 2 to 3 years with eligibility to take the certification examination given by the American College of Veterinary Pathologists (ACVP) after 3 years of approved training. On passing the examination, candidates become diplomates of the ACVP and are recognized as specialists in veterinary pathology by the American Veterinary Medical Association. Programs that combine the residency with a Ph.D. degree take 5 to 7 years to complete. In general, both ACVP certification and the Ph.D. degree are required for regular academic positions or for industry positions.

A Ph.D. degree is not essential, however, for employment in diagnostic laboratories or in toxicology contract organizations. Recruitment into pathology training programs is difficult because of the length of time required for completion of the programs; the traditionally low stipend that is paid during the training; the competition with recruitment by other veterinary medicine specialties that require less time for completion of training programs as well as paying lucrative salaries; and the high debt burden incurred by many veterinary students. In addition, academic institutions are faced with shortages of faculty responsible for training such candidates and lack of funding to support trainees.

At present, academic institutions hiring veterinary pathologists are faced with competition primarily from industry, which is causing difficulty for some programs. Academic institutions need qualified toxicologic pathologists for their programs, but suffer from an inability to offer competitive compensation in return for the multiple responsibilities of academic pathologists such as teaching, research, and service work through the diagnostic laboratories. Both the ACVP and the Society of Toxicologic Pathology have recognized these problems and are developing plans to address some of these issues.

Other countries may have different training requirements. For many years the toxicologic pathologist was trained on the job with a mentor or through a mentoring program. Although mentoring is an integral part of any training program, the knowledge gained by the student may be limited by the experience of a single mentor. For this reason more formal training is now in place in many countries, e.g., Royal College of Pathologists (United Kingdom). Because of the need for recognition of qualification of a veterinary pathologist for complying with GLP regulations in all countries, the creation of the International Academy of Toxicologic Pathologists (in July 2000) was given a mandate to accredit, but not certify, those who meet the criteria of a toxicologic pathologist.

IV. Summary

The toxicologic pathologist is well suited to play a pivotal role in decision making within the risk assessment framework because of a broad and deep understanding of most processes, which generate data for interpretation, and an understanding of the numerous limitations on the biological significance of such data. Because of their function in interpreting laboratory assays and because they also act as a link between epidemiologists and toxicologists, these pathologists are invaluable in the risk assessment process.

Most toxicologic pathologists are engaged in the conduct of bioassays in industry, toxicology, contract organizations, or government. Not to be overlooked, however, are the toxicologic pathologists employed by academic institutions and diagnostic laboratories. The field of toxicologic pathology will continue to expand in these institutions as well. The responsibility of training new toxicologic pathologists to meet the increasing demands of industry,

government, and academia will fall on academic institutions with training programs. Both private and public sectors will require the expertise of toxicologic pathologists to deal with issues of real and perceived health risks to their business, constituents, or populations. There is currently a shortage of toxicologic pathologists to fill positions in these various institutions. As the role of the toxicologic pathologist continues to expand, even more opportunities for employment and contribution to society will become available. However, the anticipated retirements of toxicologic pathologists in all sectors will exacerbate the already critical shortage of veterinary pathologists, let alone those to fill positions in toxicologic pathology.

SUGGESTED READING

Tryphonas, L., Schwartz, L. W., Levin, S., and Haschek, W. M. (1994). Toxicologic pathology: Modern challenges and the need for a new educational strategy. *Toxicol. Pathol.* **22**, 330–332.

2

Biochemical Basis of Toxicity

Elizabeth H. Jeffery

Department of Food Science and Human Nutrition
Department of Veterinary Biosciences and College of Medicine
University of Illinois at Urbana-Champaign
Urbana, Illinois

I. Introduction

Interaction between a toxic agent and an organism is a two-way process; both toxin and organism play a role in the final outcome of toxicity. This chapter is written for those not recently exposed to the discipline of toxicology as a review of the biochemical basis for toxicologic interactions. It aims to (1) define the effect that the organism has on the compound, in terms of absorption, distribution, metabolism, and excretion; (2) define the initial effect that the toxic agent has on the organism in terms of interacting with specific sites (receptors, enzymes, and so forth) or nonspecific sites (membranes, protein, and so forth); (3) identify factors that cause variation in these events; and (4) summarize the biochemical events that follow the initial insult, frequently preceding detectable morphologic change.

No compound is without the potential to cause a toxicologic effect. Even molecules that are too large or too highly ionized to cross membranes may exert an adverse effect from outside the organism, e.g., by altering uptake of a nutrient during passage through the lumen of the intestine. Alternatively, such compounds may gain entrance into the body by pulmonary macrophage ingestion following inhalation. For many xenobiotics that are readily absorbed, the body can metabolize and excrete them, thus avoiding accumulation to toxic levels, although even small changes in this balance between accumulation and excretion may prove fatal. A human readily metabolizes inhaled cyanide over the period of time that a cigarette is smoked. However, if several cigarettes are swallowed or if fresh cassava rich in cyanoglycosides is ingested, the body cannot metabolize the bolus of cyanide sufficiently rapidly to maintain subtoxic levels, and toxicity ensues.

The site of toxicity of a xenobiotic is strongly dependent on its distribution. The pulmonary toxicant paraquat concentrates in the lung, whereas its analog diquat concentrates in the

Handbook of Toxicologic Pathology, Second Edition
Volume 1
Copyright © 2002 by Academic Press
All rights of reproduction in any form reserved.

liver and is hepatotoxic. A second factor in determining the site of toxic action is the site specificity of the endogenous component(s) with which the xenobiotic interacts. For example, whole body radiation results in particularly severe damage to the crypt epithelial cells of the intestine because this is an area of highly active cell turnover. Another major determinant of site of toxicity is the site of enzymes of bioactivation. For example, acetaminophen toxicity is limited to those organs containing enzymes for bioactivation, which include liver, kidney, lung, and nasal epithelium. A fundamental principle of both pharmacology and toxicology is that the action or effect is proportional to the dose reaching the site of action. This dose–response relationship applies both to the individual (as the dose of acetaminophen is increased, so the extent of liver necrosis increases) and to the population (as the dose increases, so the frequency of fatalities among treated individuals increases). The dose at the critical organ site will vary not only with exposure of the whole organism, but also with factors affecting absorption, distribution, metabolism, and excretion. For example, if kidney function is impaired, many compounds normally excreted in the urine will accumulate to toxic levels. This includes normal body components such as uric acid (resulting in gout) as well as xenobiotics such as aluminum (resulting in dialysis dementia). Studying the effect of decreasing doses of a toxin, one frequently encounters a threshold dose below which there appears to be no toxicity. A xenobiotic will not necessarily exhibit the same threshold for all effects, and a lower threshold for pharmacologic effects than for toxic effects allows clinical use of a drug. An area of considerable controversy is whether there is a threshold for carcinogenicity. This is an important consideration in evaluation of safety in handling chemicals. In considering toxic but noncarcinogenic compounds, one can accept a low level of toxic insult (e.g., carbon monoxide interacting with 10% of blood hemoglobin) with no noticeable adverse effects. Even a low level of cell death due to the presence of a hepatotoxin may not

significantly compromise quality of life. Alternatively, if carcinogens do not exhibit the absolute threshold theorized, then even a single molecule may prove fatal.

II. Absorption

A. PASSAGE ACROSS MEMBRANES

1. Simple Diffusion

The process of simple diffusion shows no substrate specificity and no receptor requirements. It involves the entire membrane and depends solely on the lipid–water partition. Polar, or water soluble, compounds are in an equilibrium between ionized and nonionized forms. The ionized form has such a low lipid–water partition that it is essentially insoluble in lipid membranes, and only the nonionized portion is available for diffusion across the membrane. Ionization is dependent on the pK_a of the compound and the acidity of the environment. Due to the volume disparity between aqueous and lipid areas of the cell, diffusion is rate limited by lipid solubility, increasing with increasing lipid solubility. Once through the membrane, the substance will reequilibrate between ionized and nonionized forms, depending on the pH of the aqueous intracellular environment.

2. Passage through Pores

Plasma membranes contain pores that allow small ionized particles to pass through them. Typically the pore size is only 2–7 Å, and only 2 or 3% of the membrane is devoted to these pores. As the pressure rises on one side of the membrane, particles that are almost the same size as the pore (about 100 MW) are forced through these pores. Also, there are larger pores, or interendothelial gaps, between the endothelial cells of the capillary wall, allowing passage of larger water-soluble compounds from plasma to the extracellular space. The number and size of these interendothelial gaps vary widely; they are absent in the brain due to the tight junctions between cells and are about 40 Å in most other tissues. These gaps are a little larger (70 or 80 Å) at the renal glomerulus,

16

allowing molecules of less than 69,000 MW to filter into the urine.

3. Specialized Transport Systems

Substrate-specific carrier proteins allow rapid transport of polar compounds across membranes. Some carrier proteins facilitate diffusion, transporting compounds down a concentration gradient, whereas others are integrated into an energy-requiring active transport system for the transport of substances against a concentration gradient. Xenobiotics bearing structural or charge similarities to nutrients and endogenous substrates can interact with the specific carrier systems, competing with the endogenous substrate for uptake. For example, the active transport system for uracil and other pyrimidine bases is involved in the uptake of the chemotherapeutic agents 5-fluorouracil and 5-bromouracil. The facilitated transport systems for intestinal calcium and iron uptake facilitate the uptake of inorganic lead. Because these systems do not normally function at saturation, this additional uptake usually has little effect on transport of the true substrate. This is very different from the case in which a xenobiotic interacts irreversibly with a carrier, altering the normal transport process. For example, triethyl lead, the toxic metabolite of tetraethyl lead, is thought to interact with the mitochondrial transport system for chloride ions, enhancing the rate of chloride efflux greatly.

B. ABSORPTION ROUTES

Toxicologically significant routes of absorption are the gastrointestinal tract, the lungs, and the skin. During transport, some chemicals are modified through metabolism and/or binding. Because of this modification, correct modeling of absorption is essential in toxicological evaluations. For example, if a small dose of cadmium chloride is given orally, it distributes to the kidney. Given intravenously, it distributes to the liver. Although the reason for this has not yet been determined, it may be that orally administered cadmium leaves the mucosal cell bound to metallothionein, and that this complex is handled differently than the inorganic ion.

Although weak acids and neutral compounds can be absorbed by simple diffusion from the acid stomach, the small intestine is the major site for absorption of xenobiotics from the gastrointestinal tract. The intestinal surface area is far larger than that of the stomach, transit time is far longer, and intestinal pH is approximately neutral (6–8) so both weak acids and weak bases are partially nonionized and readily absorbed. Also, the intestine contains a large number of specialized uptake systems for nutrients that will transport xenobiotics with structural similarities to the endogenous substrates. Inside the intestinal mucosal cell, mixed function oxidases metabolize many xenobiotics (see Chapter 30). If metabolites are covalently bound to cellular macromolecules, or if xenobiotic metals bind cellular components, products may remain inside the mucosal cell and be sloughed into the lumen during normal cycling of the intestinal epithelium. In this way, binding to the intestinal mucosal cell acts as a major barrier to the dietary uptake of xenobiotic metals.

Because of the large surface area, the rapid blood flow, and the thin alveolar wall, pulmonary absorption is a rapid and effective route of uptake for gases, volatile compounds, and even some small particulates. Ionizable compounds are absorbed rapidly across the alveolar wall by passive diffusion. For compounds that are relatively poorly water soluble, such as ethylene, uptake is limited by blood flow. Metals do not accumulate in the lungs, but pass directly into plasma so that metal absorption is many times greater in the lungs, but pass directly into plasma so that metal absorption is many times greater in the lungs than in the intestine.

The skin is an excellent barrier to all but highly lipid-soluble compounds such as solvents (see Chapter 29). However, if the keratinized epidermal layer is removed by abrasion or hydrated by soaking the skin for a prolonged period of time, absorption is increased greatly. Dissolution of xenobiotics in amphipathic solvents such as dimethyl sulfoxide enhances their percutaneous absorption. The dissolved nonionized fraction increases and is said to undergo "solvent drag," i.e., the xenobiotic and solvent are absorbed together.

III. Distribution

A. VOLUME OF DISTRIBUTION

Body water may be divided into three compartments: the vascular, extracellular, and intracellular spaces. To pass from plasma to extracellular fluid, a compound must either be lipid soluble for diffusion across the endothelial membrane or sufficiently small to pass through an interendothelial pore. To pass on from the extra- to the intracellular space, a compound must either diffuse or pass through the very much smaller pores of the plasma membrane.

With no further refinements, the volume of distribution of a compound would be 3, 12, or 41 liters in the average adult male, depending on whether distribution was limited to the vascular space alone, the vascular and extracellular spaces, or freely diffusible throughout total body water, respectively. Two factors serve to add complexity to this distribution pattern. First, excretion is continuous, so that after an initial distribution period of a few minutes, even compounds totally confined to the plasma compartment (e.g., Evans Blue) slowly disappear as they are excreted from the body. Second, very few compounds are distributed evenly within each compartment. This simple three compartment model must therefore be refined to contain multiple compartments depending on the (1) variation in capillary interendothelial pore size, from very large in the liver to almost absent in the brain; (2) presence of transport systems that permit organ-specific concentration of toxic compounds, such as uptake of iodine in the thyroid; and (3) presence of intracellular storage sinks that shift the equilibrium toward the storage organ, e.g., the uptake of fluoride, lead, or strontium into the hydroxyapatite lattice of bone.

B. STORAGE

Storage of a toxic substance implies accumulation with no adverse effects. However, there is a fine line between storage of a toxic compound and subthreshold accumulation. For example, a physiological change may cause release from storage, such as the release of polychlorinated biphenyls or DDT from adipose tissue during starvation or weight loss. Alternatively, storage may interfere with the physiological function of the storage component, as postulated for vitamin B_{12} in tobacco amblyopia. Tobacco amblyopia is a chronic neural disorder seen in heavy smokers with marginal levels of vitamin B_{12}. Cyanide from cigarette smoke can be temporarily stored bound to vitamin B_{12}. As hepatic rhodanese metabolizes unbound cyanide, an equilibrium shift allows release of the vitamin. However, as long as the vitamin acts as a storage site for cyanide, it is unavailable for intermediary metabolism, resulting in B_{12} deficiency symptoms (see Chapter 23).

1. Identification of Storage Sinks

Removal of a xenobiotic from plasma into a storage sink will decrease the fraction available for detoxification or excretion, as both processes are concentration dependent. This in turn lengthens the biological half-life, which favors accumulation during multiple exposures. One clear indication that a compound has concentrated in a storage sink is a low plasma concentration and a long half-life. One exception to this occurs when a xenobiotic is stored in the blood, bound to plasma proteins such as albumin or ceruloplasmin. In this instance, when the plasma is sampled a very large proportion of the xenobiotic will be found in plasma, even though the compound exhibits an extended half-life. The reason for the extended half-life is that only unbound compounds are available for glomerular filtration by the kidney. Albumin, the major plasma protein involved in binding to xenobiotics, is too large to be filtered at the glomerulus. Dialysis of the plasma sample during routine plasma analysis separates protein-bound and protein-free forms of the xenobiotic. This allows determination of the low free plasma concentration, consistent with the presence of a storage site and with the long half-life found experimentally.

2. Plasma Proteins

Many endogenous and xenobiotic compounds bind plasma proteins. For example, the chlorinated hydrocarbon insecticide dieldrin, the organophosphate paration, and the carbamate, Sevin (carbaryl) are all bound in excess of 95% to plasma proteins. Two features are important to the toxicologist. First, protein-bound compounds are not filtered at the glomerulus and therefore tend to have a long half-life. Second, because binding is reversible, introduction of a second compound that binds plasma proteins can cause the sudden release and toxicity of a previously bound xenobiotic. This is particularly true for the wide variety of compounds that bind albumin, which alone makes up 50% of total plasma protein. Some proteins, such as transferrin, which binds iron and aluminum, are more specific, leading to less generalized competition between xenobiotics.

3. Liver and Kidney

Metabolism of xenobiotics causes changes in their physical and chemical characteristics, which can trap metabolites within the liver or kidney. Chromium(VI) passes easily into the liver where it is reduced to chromium(III), which cannot cross the membrane to reenter the extracellular space. Thus although environmental chromium(III) is not carcinogenic because it cannot gain entrance to the body, environmental chromium(VI) provides a source of intracellular chromium(III) that can bind DNA and initiate carcinogenesis. Liver and kidney bioactivate compounds to reactive electrophiles that bind covalently to tissue protein, lipid, or DNA. Whether reactive intermediates can escape from the cell in which they were formed is a point of controversy. Most are thought to be too reactive to travel from their site of formation and some, such as allylisopropyl acetamide, are so reactive that they bind to the cytochrome P450 enzyme (CYP) involved in their formation, destroying the enzyme. Thus loss of a specific *CYP* can indicate a role for that enzyme in bioactivation of a reactive intermediate. Discrete necrosis of only those pulmonary cells containing the enzymes for bioactivation, the Clara cells, following pulmonary intoxication by acetaminophen or low doses of ipomeanol argues against loss of reactive intermediates from the cell. However, as the dose of ipomeanol is increased, a few adjacent non-Clara cells exhibit necrosis. The reason for this is unclear. Some reactive intermediates are further metabolized to conjugates that can leave the cell, but may be subsequently broken down to release the toxic metabolite at a secondary site (see Section IV, A,2,a).

The cytosolic metal-binding protein metallothionein binds to the essential metals zinc and copper, as well as to several foreign metals, including mercury and cadmium. In humans, the half-life for hepatic cadmium-metallothionein is measured in months. However, upon leaving the liver, cadmium is seen to relocate to the kidney. Because the half-life for kidney cadmium-metallothionein is measured in decades, the body load of cadmium slowly concentrates in the kidney. Nephrotoxicity is seen when levels rise above a threshold of 200 μg/g kidney cortex.

4. Fat

Polycyclic organic xenobiotics are highly lipid soluble. They concentrate in fat depots, which results in low plasma levels and extended half-lives. For example, when cattle rations in Michigan were accidentally contaminated by polybrominated biphenyls (PBB) in 1973, these compounds became stored first in fat deposits of the cows and then, via milk fat, bioaccumulated in fat stores of the people of Michigan, where PBBs can still be detected. While there is no known effect of PBBs at the storage site, this store is a potential hazard, as mobilization during starvation or other stress could lead to efflux into the bloodstream with subsequent redistribution and toxicity. Similarly, patients treated for acute exposure to organophosphorus pesticides may be released from the hospital and later suffer a relapse due to mobilization of the insecticide from fat stores.

19

5. Bone

Several xenobiotic elements, including cadmium, aluminum, lead, strontium, and fluorine, accumulate in bone (see Chapter 36). Many of these elements have been found to interfere with bone chemistry so that normal turnover and replacement of bone matrix does not occur. Aluminum is thought to inhibit calcium uptake into bone, while having no effect on normal osteoclastic calcium loss from bone. This effect leads to an osteoporotic loss of calcium from bone. Cadmium can replace bone calcium in calcium-deficient mice, producing osteomalacia. Interestingly, although bone often stores more than 90% of body lead, the skeleton is not the major target for lead toxicity. Hwever, lead has been shown to adversely affect bone growth.

C. BARRIERS

1. Blood–Brain Barrier

The historical concept of an impenetrable blood-brain barrier, while comforting, is far from absolute. Although water-soluble compounds are effectively excluded, lipid-soluble substances can freely pass across this barrier to concentrate in the fatty nervous tissue (see Chapter 37). Exclusion of polar substances depends on the fact that junctions between capillary endothelial cells are far tighter in the brain than in the rest of the body, eliminating interendothelial pores. Glial cell end feet tightly abut the endothelium so that a compound must pass through, rather than around, two extra cell layers to pass into the cerebrospinal fluid. Furthermore, active transport systems similar to those found in kidney serve to transport organic acids and bases out of the brain. The blood–brain barrier is undeveloped in immature animals and develops incompletely in certain areas of the brain, such as the olfactory bulbs. Somewhat similar to the blood–brain barrier is the blood–testis barrier, protecting the male gamete from many xenobiotics (see Chapter 42). Strangely, there is no known corresponding barrier protecting the female gamete.

2. Placental Barrier

Lipid-soluble xenobiotics diffuse freely from maternal to fetal blood, and thus to the fetus. The less lipid soluble a compound, the more effectively it is excluded by the placenta. This barrier is equally effective from either direction; therefore any fetal metabolism of a xenobiotic to a more polar metabolite would tend to trap the metabolite in the fetus. Fortunately, most drug-metabolizing systems develop after birth so that this particular event is avoided.

IV. Biotransformation

Biotransformation, or metabolism, of a xenobiotic can alter its distribution and action dramatically, leading to detoxification and excretion or to bioactivation and toxicity. Compounds that are so physically similar to an endogeneous compound that they enter the body via its active transport mechanism may also share its sites for biochemical action and its route of metabolism, leading to eventual catabolism and excretion. For xenobiotics entering by diffusion, several organs, particularly the liver, contain enzymes with very broad substrate specificity that will metabolize a wide variety of lipid-soluble compounds. Biotransformation to a more water-soluble product usually enhances excretion, decreasing the likelihood of accumulation to toxic levels. However, these same enzymes can bioactivate a number of xenobiotics to reactive intermediates, producing cytotoxicity or carcinogenicity.

A. DETOXIFICATION AND BIOACTIVATION

Biotransformation has traditionally been divided into two phases. Phase I metabolism is degradative, involving oxidative, reductive, and hydrolytic reactions that cleave substrate molecules. Products may be more or less toxic than the parent compound. Phase II metabolism is synthetic, involving conjugation or addition of xenobiotics to endogenous molecules. While traditionally phases II metabolites have been considered as almost invariably nontoxic, exceptions are growing with our increasing knowledge base. Frequently phase I metabolism produces a suitable site on the metabolized molecule to allow phase II conjugation to occur. For example, benzene is not a substrate for any phase II reaction, but can undergo phase I oxidation to phenol. Phenol can undergo phase II glucuronidation, forming phenol-*O*-glucuronide, which is excreted.

1. Phase I Metabolism

a. Cytochrome P450. Cytochromes P450 are a family of enzymes involved in the oxidation and reduction of lipid-soluble compounds. In highest concentration in the liver, they are present in most tissues, including kidney, lung, gut, and nasal epithelium. Several CYP are dedicated to specific endogenous metabolic steps, such as kidney mitochondrial 1-a-hydroxylase, which is highly substrate specific and appears to metabolize 25-hydroxycholecalciferol and no xenobiotics. However, CYP in the hepatic endoplasmic reticulum show far less substrate specificity, catalyzing oxidation or reduction of many chemicals. Furthermore, a single substrate may be metabolized to the same product by several CYP, each with its own kinetic characteristics. In excess of 20 isozymes are now recognized. Substrate specificities, characteristic inducibilities, and amino acid sequences are highly conserved across species, confirming the use of animal models in biotransformation studies. CYP-dependent oxidation frequently leads to a decrease in the lipid–water partition, decreasing fat storage and increasing the fraction in body water, resulting in an increased rate of urinary excretion. Oxidative attack occurs at N, S, and C bonds, resulting in the insertion of one atom of oxygen. For example, the *N*-alkylated compound *N*-methylaniline is metabolized to an intermediate oxidation product that breaks down to formaldehyde and aniline.

Occasionally the oxidized products are highly toxic unstable electrophiles. Of the many mechanisms of oxidative attack, *N*-hydroxylation and aromatic C-oxidation (epoxide formation) are associated most frequently with bioactivation to toxic intermediates. Rather than aiding

excretion, this change traps the electrophile inside the cell. Excretion is dependent on further metabolism by epoxide hydration or glutathione (GSH) conjugation. When this does not occur, GSH stores are depleted, covalent binding to cellular components occurs, and excretion is inhibited.

b. Epoxide Hydrase. Epoxide hydrase (or hydrolase) hydrates epoxide products of CYP oxidation to form the corresponding dihydrodiols. The enzyme most studied is microsomal and forms *trans* diols. A cytosolic epoxide hydrase exists that may be more active toward lipid epoxides. Epoxide hydration is associated with the detoxification of reactive epoxides, increased water solubility, and increased excretion. For example, epoxide hydrase catalyzes the hydrolysis of the toxic 3,4-epoxide of bromobenzene to an excretable product, 3,4-dihydrodiol. For a few compounds, epoxide hydration is a step toward further metabolism to form a toxic product. Benzo[*a*]pyrene 7,8-dihydrodiol 9,10-epoxide. Naphthalene also undergoes P450-dependent epoxidation followed by epoxide hydrase-dependent dihydrodiol formation. In the eye, this product is reduced to the catechol by lenticular catechol reductase, and the catechol autooxidizes to 1,2-naphthoquinone with the release of peroxide. The naphthoquinone is then rereduced to the catechol at the expense of GSH. This cycle depletes orbital GSH, causing oxidative damage that results in catarct formation.

c. Other Phase I Reactions.

i. Hydrolysis Hydrolyzing enzymes are widespread throughout the body, including the plasma, and catalyze the hydrolysis of esters. Classification is ill-defined due to the wide substrate distribution and overlapping substrate specificity.

ii. Reduction A number of nitro and azo compounds undergo an NADPH-dependent reduction that is inhibitable by carbon monoxide, implicating cytochrome P450 in this reaction, although a separate flavin nitroreductase also exists. Carbon tetrachloride and halothane are metabolized both oxidatively and reductively by cytochrome P450. In both cases,

21

reduction causes bioactivation to a toxic intermediate, while oxidation is a detoxification step. The oxygen tension in the liver affects the route of metabolism, and reduction is favored as the oxygen tension falls. A number of aldehyde reductases, including alcohol dehydrogenase (named for the reverse reaction), are found throughout the body and may catalyze the reduction of toxic lipid-oxidation products.

iii. Non-CYP oxidation There is an FAD-containing monooxygenase that is a non-CYP, microsomal system able to oxidize secondary amines and several sulfur compounds, including sulfides, thiols, and thioesters. Another microsomal oxidation system, particularly prevalent in kidney, is prostaglandin synthetase, a glycoprotein with a heme center. This enzyme produces peroxide as a by-product during the synthesis of prostaglandins from arachidonic acid. A number of xenobiotics are cooxidized during this process by the peroxide. However, the *in vivo* significance of this cooxidation is unknown at present. There are also at least two other distinct groups of amine oxidases, both widely distributed. The monoamine oxidases are mitochondrial flavoproteins involved primarily in the catabolism of monoamine neurotransmitters and several xenobiotic amines. Diamine oxidases are vitamin B_6-dependent cytosolic enzymes that preferentially metabolize short chain aliphatic diamines.

Alcohol dehydrogenase is a cytosolic enzyme, present in liver and eye, that catalyzes the oxidation of a variety of alcohols, including methanol, ethanol, and ethylene glycol. In the reverse direction, it catalyzes the reduction of a number of xenobiotics, including chloral hydrate. There are also a large number of aldehyde dehydrogenases and oxidases with no metabolic role yet assigned to them.

2. Phase II Metabolism

Most frequently, products of phase II metabolism are more water soluble, more easily excretable, and less toxic than either parent compounds or phase I metabolites. Typically, conjugation involves the addition of an endogenous compound (e.g., glucuronic acid) to a xenobiotic in a two-step reaction, each step requiring an enzyme. Step 1 is the high-energy activation of either the conjugating agent (e.g., UDP-glucuronic acid formation for glucuronidation) or the xenobiotic (e.g., benzoyl-CoA formation for benzoic acid conjugation to glycine). Step 2 is the synthesis of the conjugate.

a. Glucuronidation. Glucose is readily available for glucuronidation, while the pool of sulfate or glycine available for conjugation is relatively small. This availability of endogenous substrate serves to increase the importance of glucuronidation relative to sulfation in endogenous and xenobiotic metabolism. The family of enzymes responsible for glucuronide conjugation, the glucuronosyl transferases, are present in the microsomal fraction of liver and other tissues. *N*-, *O*-, and *S*-glucuronides are formed and excreted into bile and urine.

In both the lumen of the colon and the bladder, bacterial -glucuronidase can release the xenobiotic from the glucuronide conjugate. While this deconjugation probably plays a physiological role in the metabolism and enterohepatic circulation of estrogen, it may also be responsible for the release of certain carcinogens. For example, 2-acetylaminofluorene undergoes *N*-hydroxylation and glucuronidation in the liver, but is deconjugated to an ultimate carcinogen in the bladder. Thus conjugation permits travel to a site distant from that of initial metabolism, where a compound may undergo reactivation through deconjugation.

b. Glutathione Conjugation. Glutathione (GSH), either spontaneously or with the aid of transferase enzymes, conjugates electrophiles, allaying the potential toxicity of reactive metabolites. The resultant conjugate is metabolized further to the cysteinyl conjugate by removal of glutamine and glycine. The cysteinyl conjugate is acetylated, and the product formed, termed mercapturic acid, is excreted readily in the urine. The hepatic synthesis of GSH, limited by cysteine availability, is frequently slower than conjugation. For this reason, GSH stores can fall during conjugation, leading to a temporary inability to conjugate electrophiles, loss of redox potential, and inability to quench peroxidation via GSH peroxidase. Because GSH levels exhibit a distinct diurnal variation, xenobiotics that only exert their toxicity after GSH has been depleted exhibit the greatest potency at approximately 6 PM in rodents, the nadir in their diurnal variation in hepatic GSH levels. A number of GSH conjugates, including many allylic compounds, have been found to undergo further metabolism to reactive thionocompounds, producing nephrotoxicity.

c. Metal Metabolism. Like reactive intermediates, inorganic metal ions can bind to a wide variety of cellular components, altering charges and inhibiting normal function. While relatively little is known at this time about the metabolism of metals, several metals form excretable complexes with GSH. Metallothionein can bind a number of metals (Cd, Hg, Cu, Au, Ag, Zn, Pt), but may serve solely to divert the metal from binding elsewhere. No role for metallothionein in the excretion of metals has been found. Indeed, hepatic metallothionein actually inhibits the biliary excretion of metals. A few metals, most notably the oxyanions of chromium and arsenic, undergo reduction to ions that cannot penetrate the cell membrane, causing accumulation and toxicity. Organic compounds of metals are highly lipid soluble, allowing access to the brain where they cause a number of toxic responses.

B. ROLE OF ENZYME LOCATION IN TOXICITY

When a reactive intermediate is formed during metabolism, often it will exert its toxicity in the immediate vicinity. Many xenobiotics bioactivated by hepatic CYP cause centrilobular necrosis (see Chapter 31). Upon examination, one finds that the highest concentration of CYP is in the centrilobular region. The centrilobular region is also rich in conjugating enzymes. The oxygen-rich periportal region contains mostly enzymes of intermediary metabolism for plasma protein synthesis and lipid and carbohydrate metabolism. Necrosis of the periportal region is associated with direct-acting hepatotoxic agents that enter the liver at the portal triad

via the portal vein and do not require bioactivation. Examples are hepatotoxic metals such as iron, manganese, and arsenic, and also phosphorus. Because the biliary tree drains from this region, bile salt damage and hepatic necrosis resulting from the accumulation of biliary excretory products during cholestasis is first seen in the periportal region.

The kidney contains many of the same metabolizing enzymes as the liver, but at lower concentrations. Also, depending on the route of exposure, the kidney receives a smaller dose of xenobiotic than the liver because of the first-pass effect. The enzymes for bioactivation are located in the straight portion of the proximal tubule, resulting in necrosis at this site following bioactivation of a xenobiotic (see Chapter 34). The kidney also contains the enzyme cysteine β-lyase, which deconjugates cysteinyl conjugates formed in the liver or kidney, producing reactive sulfur intermediates. This pathway is responsible for the nephrotoxicity of vinyl halides. A similar intestinal pathway exists whereby intestinal microflora deconjugate biliary metabolites of aromatic halides. This is followed by portal uptake of the sulfur metabolite and transport to the liver for hepatic S-methylation and S-oxidation. The toxicologic consequences of this intestinal pathway have yet to be determined.

V. Excretion

A. URINARY EXCRETION

1. Urinary Filtration

Excretion of xenobiotics into urine depends on filtration without reabsorption and/or active secretion through the renal cell. The renal artery is short and wide, producing a high hydrostatic pressure for the ultrafiltration of components that are almost too large to pass through the 80-Å interendothelial pores into the renal tubules. Components greater than 69,000 MW, such as those bound to plasma proteins, are too large and therefore not available for filtration. In addition, active secretory systems catalyze excretion through the proximal tubule cell into the tubular lumen, regardless of plasma protein binding. Because proximal tubule cells contain many of the drug-metabolizing enzymes found in the liver, xenobiotics often undergo metabolism during passage through these cells.

Once filtered, nutrients such as glucose are reabsorbed in the proximal tubule. This is also the site for reabsorption of a number of xenobiotics, leading to recirculation or accumulation in the kidney. Both passive and active reabsorption processes exist.

2. Passive Reabsorption of Xenobiotics

Of the 100–150 ml plasma filtered per minute, 80% of the water is reabsorbed passively at the proximal tubule due to an osmotic gradient established by the active uptake of sodium ions. Further reabsorption at the loop of Henle and the distal tubule results eventually in the production of approximately 1 ml urine/min. During this reabsorption process, both lipid-soluble and neutral compounds are freely reabsorbed. Reabsorption of ionizable compounds depends on the pH of the urine, which varies between 4.5 and 8. As the pH increases, acids become more ionized and are therefore unable to cross the membrane for reabsorption. Manipulation of urinary pH is commonly used to improve the excretion of toxic substances. Oral sodium bicarbonate increases the pH of the filtrate so that acids ionize and their excretion improves. Conversely, bases are ionized at low pH and excretion is effected by ammonium chloride acidification.

3. Active Reabsorption of Xenobiotics

Xenobiotics are reabsorbed by the carrier systems that exist for the reabsorption of filtered nutrients. The major system for the reabsorption of amino acids is γ-glutamyl transpeptidase, particularly involved in preventing the urinary loss of cysteine and glutathione. When γ-glutamyl transpeptidase is inhibited, xenobiotic conjugates of GSH and cysteine appear in urine, indicating that these conjugates are normally reabsorbed. Several metals are also reabsorbed, although to date little is known of the mechanisms of absorption. Lead accumulates within the nucleus as a microscopically visible nuclear inclusion body and cadmium accumulates bound to cytosolic metallothionein. Neither lead nor cadmium appears to reenter the circulation, chronically accumulating in the kidney and eventually producing nephrotoxicity.

4. Active Secretion of Xenobiotics

There are at least two separate systems for active secretion, one for organic acids and the other for organic bases. The physiologic role for the acid system is the clearance of uric acid and the glucuronide and sulfate conjugates of endogenous compounds such as steroids. That this is a single carrier-mediated transport system is shown by competition between acids. Probenecid is an acid transport inhibitor that was developed during World War II to competitively prolong the half-life of penicillin. Today, probenecid is used as a tool to study the excretion of acids. A similar but separate transport system exists for the excretion of organic bases, such as morphine.

B. MECHANISMS OF URINARY SYSTEM TOXICITY

Disturbance of nutrient reabsorption at the brush border of the proximal tubule is the first sign of toxicity for many nephrotoxic substances. The lost nutrients can be identified and quantified in the urine. For example, an early sign of cadmium nephrotoxicity is the appearance of microglobulins in the urine. A second group of nephrotoxic substances, of which puromycin is an example, increase glomerular permeability by altering the glomerular membrane charge. Clinically, this is identified by albuminuria. A few sulfonamides exhibit decreased water solubility after hepatic metabolism. Acetyl sulfathiazole is 10-fold less soluble than sulfathiazole. Although not noticeable in the systemic circulation, as the urine concentrates during water reabsorption, these metabolites may crystallize out, causing necrosis of the tubule. Other mechanisms of nephrotoxicity include accumulation following reabsorption, particularly of metals and of compounds undergoing bioactivation in the proximal tubule. A number of chemicals that are bioactivated by the mixed function oxidase system in the liver, such as acetaminophen and CCl_4, also undergo bioactivation in the kidney. Whether they produce hepatotoxicity, nephrotoxicity, or both depends on conditions that modulate the site of greatest metabolism. For a few halogenated organic mercapturic acids formed in the liver, deacetylation is followed by metabolism by cysteine β-lyase in the kidney, which catalyzes the loss of the cysteine moiety except for the sulfur atom, which remains bound to the xenobiotic. This cleavage of the cysteine conjugate produces a highly reactive species that covalently binds proteins, and nephrotoxicity ensues.

A secondary effect of nephrotoxicity is that renal failure, due to toxicity or disease, will extend the half-life of any compound normally excreted in the urine, causing accumulation and toxicity of otherwise subtoxic doses. The effect of renal insufficiency on disposition and toxicity of xenobiotics is of significant clinical importance. While biliary excretion may increase during renal failure, the magnitude of this effect is seldom sufficient to compensate for the loss of urinary excretory pathways. Dialysis, while clearing the blood of excretory products that are normally filtered into urine by the kidney glomerulus, does not have the capacity to remove the protein-bound xenobiotics that the kidney normally secretes into urine. For example, transferrin-bound aluminum, normally excreted in the urine, is not removed by dialysis and accumulates in bone and brain of dialysis patients.

Like the large intestine, the bladder houses bacteria that can reactivate conjugated xenobiotics. The enzyme β-glucuronidase causes the loss of the glucuronide moiety, frequently leaving an electrophilic species that can covalently bind to protein or DNA in the bladder wall. This mechanism is thought responsible for the bladder carcinogenicity of 2-acetylaminofluorene. This aromatic amine undergoes *N*-hydroxylation followed by acetylation, sulfa-

tion, or glucuronidation. Deconjugation of the acetylated and sulfated products gives rise to liver or kidney tumors, depending on the site of breakdown. The more stable glucuronide travels to the bladder, where it gives rise to cancer following removal of the glucuronide moiety.

C. BILIARY EXCRETION

Biliary excretion is not easily studied clinically. Fecal collections reflect unabsorbed ingesta and intestinal secretory products as well as bile products, and some biliary products may be reabsorbed during transit through the intestine prior to fecal elimination. Animal models involving cannulation of the bile duct overcome some of these problems, but lead to nonphysiologic conditions due to interruption of the enterohepatic circulation of bile acids and other components. Unlike urinary excretion, biliary excretion is relatively independent of hydrostatic pressure. Rather, biliary excretion depends on the hepatic concentration of the xenobiotic. Substances passing into the bile have been grouped according to their plasma:bile ratios. Group A, those with a plasma:bile ratio approximating 1.0, are thought to pass into bile passively down a concentration gradient. Substances in group A are mostly small molecules in equilibrium with total body water. Group B substances, those that are concentrated in the bile, constitute a growing number of compounds known to be actively secreted into the biliary canaliculi. Group C, those with a plasma: bile ratio greater than 1.0, tend to be bulky polar molecules such as inulin and mannitol that cannot cross membranes readily. Compounds of less than a certain molecular weight (325 in rats; 500–700 in humans) are thought to be excreted mainly in urine, whereas larger compounds are excreted into bile. However, this generalization is not accurate for highly polar substances. As in the kidney, there appear to be two separate carrier-mediated biliary transport systems for the excretion of organic acids and bases; sulfobromophthalein (BSP) excretion by the organic acid system is commonly used as a measure of liver function.

25

A third transport system is responsible for the excretion of steroids. Unless biliary metabolites are ionized at intestinal pH, excretion is thwarted by reabsorption, termed enterohepatic recirculation. Glucuronides are often deconjugated by intestinal microflora, which increases lipid solubility, permitting reabsorption and recirculation. This enterohepatic circulation can increase the biological half-life of a xenobiotic greatly, prolonging toxicity by producing chronic exposure. Oral administration of polythiol resins to specifically bind mercury, or of activated charcoal to absorb a number of other xenobiotics, can block reuptake by the intestine and alleviate toxicity. Colon cancer, thought to be promoted by bile acids, can be initiated by a carcinogen that has been bioactivated and conjugated in the liver, excreted in the bile, deconjugated by intestinal microflora, and finally reabsorbed into the colonic mucosa.

Glutathione conjugates are excreted into the biliary canaliculi where γ-glutamyl transpeptidase and a dipeptidase on the luminal surface remove first glutamate and then glycine, leaving the xenobiotic conjugated only to cysteine. All three products are reabsorbed into the liver, from where the cysteinyl conjugate travels to the kidney for acetylation and excretion as a mercapturic acid.

Cholestasis, the slowing or cessation of bile flow, is caused by a number of steroid derivatives, including anabolic and contraceptive steroids. This results in the retention of compounds normally excreted in the bile, with consequent accumulation to toxic levels. For example, diethylstilbestrol is solely excreted via the bile, and experimental cholestasis increases the half-life of the xenobiotic, causing accumulation to toxic levels. Conversely, an increased bile flow is seen with phenobarbital and the steroids pregnenolone 16-α carbonitrile and spironolactone, inducers of hepatic mixed function oxidation.

D. PULMONARY EXCRETION

The lungs are an important site for absorption and excretion of volatile substances, including solvents, alcohols, anesthetic gases, pesticide fumigants, and cyanide. Excretion is passive, and hyperventilation improves excretion of these substances by maximizing the concentration gradient. Because oxygen must competitively remove carbon monoxide from hemoglobin, hyperbaric oxygen is recommended in treating carbon monoxide poisoning. At 1 atm pressure, replacing air with pure oxygen decreases the half-life of carboxyhemoglobin fourfold, from 320 min to little more than 1 hr. The Clara cell, present within the bronchiolar epithelial lining, contains an active drug-metabolizing system and can therefore bioactivate certain xenobiotics, causing necrosis.

Ipomeanol and acetaminophen can both produce necrosis of Clara cells. Other lung cell types may contain metabolizing enzymes, but in far lesser amounts. With such a ready source of oxygen for the production of free radicals, alveolar cells are particularly susceptible to compounds that produce oxidative stress, such as bleomycin and paraquat.

E. OTHER EXCRETORY MECHANISMS

Many metals are excreted by binding and incorporation into sulfhydryl-rich hair and nails. The term excretion is used here only to denote irreversible storage in a form that has no noticeable adverse or toxic effect. Excretion of metals into hair or nails has been used to confirm exposure and even to determine, by measuring the distance from site of deposition to scalp, when the exposure may have occurred. The analysis of hair samples was used to confirm the suggestion that the violent mood changes suffered by Sir Isaac Newton in his later years were most likely connected with mercury poisoning. Possibly President Andrew Jackson also suffered neurotoxicity from the metals of the bullet lodged in his shoulder for a significant portion of his life. This too could be determined by hair analysis. Storage of xenobiotics, such as selenium in horse hooves, can adversely affect hoof function and therefore cannot be termed excretion. Similarly, "excretion" of PCBs into milk is of questionable service, as it serves to intoxicate the neonate even though it clears the mother. Awareness of excretion into milk has led to growing concern for the passage of social drugs and environmental pollutants from mother to child. Milk, made up partly of lipids, has a pH slightly lower than that of blood and therefore tends to transport both fat-soluble and basic xenobiotics.

VI. Factors Causing Variation in Handling of Toxic Compounds

A. GENETIC FACTORS

1. Species Variation

The use of animal models in drug metabolism and toxicity testing relies on the assumption that while the relative importance of a single metabolic pathway may vary among species, that pathway is nevertheless present in most species. The formation of particular metabolites and their subsequent specific toxic effects on the body are repeated across many species. Across the animal kingdom, there is striking homology in enzymes and storage proteins involved in handling xenobiotics. For example, metallothioneins, present in such diverse species as clams and humans, can be induced successfully in Chinese hamster ovary cell lines for the study of tolerance to metals. Ethanol-inducible CYP 2E1 exhibits both a similar amino acid sequence and a similar substrate specificity in mouse, rat, rabbit, baboon, and humans.

Genetic differences frequently appear to involve the loss of, or change in, a gene otherwise common across many species rather than the development of completely different systems in different species. Species variation is therefore often due to lack of a particular enzyme or changes in relative importance of a particular route of metabolism. The cat has the enzymes required for glucuronidation of endogeneous estrogens, but not for the nonspecific glucuronidation of many xenobiotics, causing species-specific sensitivity to a number of compounds that are normally excreted as glucuronides, such as acetaminophen. The Gunn strain of rats similarly lacks the enzymes for glucuronidation.

A species difference is responsible for the relative lack of sensitivity to malathion in humans compared with insects. Humans exhibit relatively greater esterase activity than insects. Therefore, in humans, malathion is deesterified to a metabolite that is only a poor substrate for bioactivation to malaoxon, the toxic metabolite.

2. Variation within a Species

In utero, the embryo and fetus have little ability to metabolize xenobiotics. Hence few xenobiotics are bioactivated by the fetus. Although the fetus has high metallothionein levels, thought to reflect the need for zinc during DNA replication, metal exposure is limited due to the placental barrier, as is the entrance of polar xenobiotics. At birth there is a dramatic change, and the neonate becomes uniquely susceptible to xenobiotics. Both the intestinal wall and the hepatic metabolizing systems are undergoing development, allowing for high absorption of xenobiotics, but poor metabolism and excretion. Metal uptake at the intestinal wall is at least threefold higher in the neonate than in the adult. Pregnant and lactating women absorb a greater fraction of essential and xenobiotic dietary metals than nonpregnant women, a reflection of their increased requirement for essential metals. In this regard, iron or calcium deficiency is found to increase the intestinal absorption of xenobiotic metals even in nonpregnant females or male adults. It should also be noted that, in the adult rat, females exhibit considerably slower hepatic mixed function oxidation than males. However, sexual differences are not consistent in mice, varying with the strain, and are absent in humans. As the adult ages, there is a slow decrease in basal drug-metabolizing activity and a pronounced decrease in inducibility of the drug-metabolizing system. The effect of aging on the inducibility of metallothionein has not been studied.

Inhibition of drug-metabolizing enzymes has practical biological implications in the development of economically useful poisons. The inhibition of mixed function oxidation by piperonyl butoxide has been used to magnify the effect of the pesticide carbaryl, an inhibitor of acetylcholinesterase that is detoxified by CYP. A subset of insects, tolerant to carbaryl because of a high rate of CYP-dependent oxidation of carbaryl, can be sensitized by piperonyl butoxide coadministration.

B. ENVIRONMENTAL FACTORS

1. Induction of Defense Systems

Enzymatic systems that defend the body against toxic insult exhibit a remarkable ability to increase when required. Specific CYP enzymes can be induced by their substrates so that many drugs and xenobiotics enhance their own metabolism. Due to the lack of substrate specificity between these enzymes, this also has the effect of enhancing the metabolism of other xenobiotics. The action of phenobarbital has been studied in great detail and has been shown to cause the induction of at least two CYP, as well as epoxide hydrase and glucuronosyl transferase. Phenobarbital also causes a generalized proliferation of the smooth endoplasmic reticulum. Superoxide dismutase has been found to increase under conditions of prolonged oxidative stress. Metallothionein increases in response to starvation and cold stress as well as exposure to metals.

Induction can serve to increase the relative importance of one metabolic route over another, thus altering the site or extent of toxicity. For example, phenobarbital induces the bioactivation of bromobenzene to the toxic 3,4-epoxide, lowering the threshold for hepatotoxicity. Conversely, 3-methylcholanthrene decreases hepatotoxicity by inducing the enzyme that causes formation of the 2,3-epoxide at the expense of the 3,4-epoxide, as well as inducing epoxide hydrase, which is able to detoxify any 3,4-epoxide formed. Induction is not limited to the effect of pharmacologic doses of xenobiotics, but appears to be an integral part of human interaction with the environment.

Cigarette smokers metabolize many foreign chemicals at three or four times the rate of nonsmokers. By increasing enzymes involved in the bioactivation of carcinogens, induction may play a role in the synergistic effect of certain environmental factors such as cigarette smoking on cancer incidence. Enzyme induction is probably protective in many other instances, resulting in the enhanced elimination of xenobiotics. For example, cold, starvation, endotoxin release, and a number of other environmental stresses have a significant effect on the toxicity of xenobiotics, variably inducing oxidative drug metabolism and increasing GSH and metallothionein levels. It is this complexity of response that makes theoretical modeling, with our present knowledge, an unacceptable alternative to using animal models for toxicity testing.

2. Inhibition of Metabolism

Because the mixed function oxidase system has a broad substrate specificity, many compounds inhibit each other's in vitro metabolism. Under normal in vivo conditions, mixed function oxidase enzymes are rarely saturated so that competition for metabolism is of little importance. This is in contrast to competition between xenobiotics for binding to plasma proteins or metallothionein, both of which are frequently saturated and therefore greatly affected by relative concentrations of competing xenobiotics. Xenobiotics that decrease the amount of P450 enzyme available for metabolism, either by forming an intermediate complex (piperonyl butoxide and SKF 525A) or by destroying the enzyme (metals and allyl compounds), significantly inhibit in vivo drug metabolism.

Inhibition of drug-metabolizing enzymes has practical biological implications in the development of economically useful poisons. The inhibition of mixed function oxidation by piperonyl butoxide has been used to magnify the effect of the pesticide carbaryl, an inhibitor of acetylcholinesterase that is detoxified by cytochrome P450. A subset of insects, tolerant to, carbaryl P450-dependent oxidation of carbaryl because of a high rate of cytochrome, can be sensitized by piperonyl butoxide coadministration.

VII. Interaction of Agent and Organism

A. SITE SPECIFICITY

Frequently, the interaction between toxic agent and organism is site specific, and the xenobiotic exhibits a high affinity for a single subcellular site. An example is the specific interaction of aminotriazole with the enzyme catalase, causing inhibition of catalatic activity. Even xenobiotics that appear to exert a generalized toxicity throughout the body may do so by interacting with a single endogenous component present at many sites in the body. More frequently, a xenobiotic will interact with several subcellular components and only the component interacting at the lowest dose is recognized as the site of action. A series of structurally similar xenobiotics may be compared for their relative affinities at two or more sites, where interaction at some sites will produce wanted effects and at others, unwanted effects. Such structure–activity relationships are used to develop drugs and economically useful poisons. The analogue causing the wanted effect, but having least affinity for the site responsible for the unwanted effect(s), becomes the drug of choice.

Many xenobiotics interact with particular chemical groupings such as sulfhydryl or amino groups, common to many subcellular components. These nonspecific interactions permit the xenobiotic to interact with a wide variety of cellular components. For example, metals interact with sulfhydryl, amino, imino, carboxyl, and hydroxyl groups, disturbing the normal function of multiple intermediary metabolic pathways. However, because some metals have a greater affinity for sulfhydryl than for hydroxyl groups (e.g., cadmium) while others show the reverse (e.g., calcium), overall responses of the body to the different metals differ dramatically.

Ethanol, general anesthetics, and a large number of solvents dissolve in membranes, altering membrane fluidity and producing central nervous system depression because of their lipid solubility. In response to the constant presence of addictive quantities of ethanol or the solvent toluene, the body incorporates a larger proportion of unsaturated fats into the plasma membrane in an attempt to normalize membrane fluidity and regain normal physiologic function in the presence of the xenobiotic. A larger dose of ethanol or general anesthetic will again disrupt membrane function, and alcoholics have been found to require not only more alcohol than normal to become overtly drunk, but also more general anesthetic to maintain unconsciousness during surgery.

Only a few compounds, of which caustics are a good example, are completely nonspecific in their site of action, independent of any chemical characteristics of the organism under attack. Necrosis due to caustic substances at the two extremes of the pH scale is due to a corrosive attack on the surface of a cell without requiring absorption; therefore, caustics are effective topically. For example, after accidental ingestion of household cleansing agents, necrosis can be seen around the mouth and esophagus. Ingested aspirin tablets cause a localized drop in pH during dissolution, resulting in necrosis of the stomach wall.

B. DOSE DEPENDENCY AND SITE OF ACTION

Interaction between a toxic agent and an organism depends on the dose arriving at a particular site and the affinity of the xenobiotic for that site. If a xenobiotic or nutrient interacts with more than one site in the organism, each site will have its own peculiar affinity for the xenobiotic, measurable as the dissociation constant K_d, or K_m if the site is an enzyme. As the dose of a xenobiotic is increased, the xenobiotic will interact with an ever-increasing number of different sites with ever-decreasing affinities. In the test tube or cell culture, and to a lesser degree even in whole animal studies, it is possible to reach concentrations seldom reached in the environment. Thus, while the interaction of a biological ligand with very high concentrations of a xenobiotic may be a useful tool for mechanistic studies, it does not necessarily

29

portray the site of toxicity of that same xeno-biotic at lower concentrations. For example, 10 mg/kg of cadmium administered intra-pertoneally to rats as cadmium chloride causes encephalopathy with hemorrhage into the gray matter. However, 6 mg/kg is also fatal, but without significant neuropathology. Many compounds incubated with a single cellular component such as DNA may interact with that component in the test tube, but may either never reach sufficient concentration to do so in the living organism or may interact at alterna-tive sites and never reach the component in question at all. It is possible that some of the lack of substrate specificity seen experimentally with drug-metabolizing enzymes is due to the use of abnormally high concentrations of xeno-biotics and that drug metabolism in the pres-ence of environmentally significant xenobiotic concentrations is relatively more specific.

C. CRITICAL ORGAN FOR TOXICITY

Site specificity, as described in the preceding sections, refers to a particular intracellular site due to specificity of a chemical interaction. Often a xenobiotic may interact at that same subcellular site in several organs, although a particular organ is always the first to exhibit toxicity. This organ specificity, termed the crit-ical organ, is due to a variety of causes. In toxicities causing a generalized loss of energy metabolism, such as cyanide inhibition of cyto-chrome oxidase, the critical organ is the central nervous system (CNS), and death due to respiratory arrest occurs because of the greater oxygen sensitivity of the respiratory center, even though cytochrome oxidase is inhibited in all tissues. Similarly, radiation and the antimetabolites that interfere with purine and pyrimidine metabolism first affect organs undergoing most rapid turnover, such as bone marrow, intestinal mucosa, and actively grow-ing tumors. In mice, acetaminophen bioactiva-tion occurs to a greater extent in liver than in other tissues, making liver the critical organ for acetaminophen toxicity. If liver metabolism is inhibited, then pulmonary or renal toxicity becomes critical.

D. TEMPORAL OUTCOME OF INTERACTION

In animals given a sublethal dose of a com-pound that destroys an enzyme (e.g., allyliso-propyl acetamide destruction of CYP) or that depletes other cellular components (e.g., ex-ample, bromobenzene depletion of GSH), the pattern of recovery is not just a slow return to normal values. Rather, a rapid resynthesis of the depleted component results in an overshoot that is followed by a slow return to normal values. For example, mouse hepatic GSH values fall to a nadir 2–4 hr after a sublethal dose of acetaminophen and then rise to approximately 200% by 12 hr before reaching normal values again by 24–36 hr. Because of this, only a temporal study will reveal the effect that a xenobiotic has on the content of the component with which it interacts. Further, while ultrastructural changes may be observed within the same time frame as the initial bio-chemical changes, histological changes may not be readily visible until considerably later, when the depleted component may have already returned to normal levels. Disruption of the cell, leading to the release of characteristic cyto-solic enzymes into the plasma, will also be delayed, as this is a result of cell death rather than a cause of cell death. Thus experimental design should include a consideration of the time after exposure to which the measurement of specific end points is best suited.

VIII. Site-Specific Interactions

A. RECEPTORS AND ENZYMES

1. Substrate Binding Site: Competition, Suicide Substrates, and Antimetabolites

The more site specific a toxic agent, the more likely that its action depends on physically mimicking the natural component that interacts at that site. Once at the site, its difference from the natural component produces the character-istic toxic action. A xenobiotic may interact with a receptor, either causing (as an agonist) or preventing (as an antagonist) the effect evoked by the endogenous substrate for this receptor. For example, atropine is a muscarinic antagonist, interacting with the acetylcholine-binding site at nerve terminals, but eliciting no signal. If a xenobiotic is only able to evoke a submaximal response, the term "partial agonist" may be applied.

A number of xenobiotics can inhibit the normal action of an enzyme by competing as substrates. Often these are not very potent *in vivo* inhibitors because neither the xenobiotic nor the natural substrate is present at a sufficiently high concentration for the enzyme to become rate limiting. Conversely, xenobiotics that form a stable substrate–enzyme complex that dissociates only very slowly are potent *in vivo* inhibitors. For example, organophosphate pesticides and related chemical warfare agents form a lasting complex with acetylcholine esterase, which, when involving greater than 50% of the enzyme, cause accumulation of the natural substrate, acetylcholine, to toxic levels. Treatment of organophosphate poisoning relies on competitively replacing the organophosphate with pralidoxime. While pralidoxime is by definition also in competition with acetylcholine, it forms only a temporary complex before releasing the enzyme for normal hydrolysis of acetylcholine. Carbamate pesticides also act by inhibiting acetylcholine esterase, but the complex formed is short-lived in comparison with the organophosphate complex, and recommended treatment is to stimulate excretion rather than administer pralidoxime. Some xenobiotics, while still interacting at the substrate-binding site, are termed suicide substrates because they destroy the enzyme during metabolism, affecting a long-lasting noncompetitive inhibition that requires synthesis of new enzyme to reverse the inhibition. Many xenobiotics containing allyl groups, such as allylisopropyl acetamide, are bioactivated to such highly reactive intermediates that, immediately upon formation, they covalently bind to cytochrome P450, causing breakdown of the heme center of CYP, often to characteristic green pigments. Carbon tetrachloride and carbon disulfide are also suicide substrates for cytochrome P450.

Some xenobiotics, termed antimetabolites, successfully replace the normal enzyme substrate, forming an abnormal product that then disturbs metabolism at a later point in intermediary metabolism. Fluoroacetate, galactosamine, and ethionine are examples. Incorporated into the citric acid cycle, fluoroacetate forms fluorocitrate, which inhibits the next step, aconitase-dependent conversion to isocitrate. This results in a generalized loss of energy metabolism, manifested clinically as fatal effects on the heart and the respiratory center. Galactosamine depletes UTP by forming UDP-galactosamine in place of UDP-glucuronic acid and ethionine replaces methionine, causing a depletion of ATP due to S-adenosyl ethionine formation. This latter antimetabolite then ethylates DNA, inhibiting protein synthesis. A number of antimetabolites have been developed as anticarcinogenic drugs, becoming incorporated into the pathways of purine and pyrimidine biosynthesis. Chemotherapeutic efficacy relies on sensitivity being greatest in cells that are replicating most actively. For example, the antifolate methotrexate, while nonspecifically inhibiting all DNA synthesis, is most toxic to those cells in the logarithmic growth phase, including cells of growing tumors.

2. Activation, Induction, or Synergism

Interaction of xenobiotics with enzymes at sites other than the substrate-binding site can either increase or decrease enzyme activity. An increase in maximal velocity of an enzyme with no concomitant increase in amount of that enzyme is termed activation and, for example, may be caused by allosteric addition of a cofactor such as magnesium, which might aid in bringing substrates into juxtaposition at the site of action of an enzyme. In contrast, chelation and removal of magnesium could inhibit the enzyme.

While activation/deactivation causes no change in the absolute amount of enzyme, many xenobiotics can cause the induction of enzyme, resulting in increased flux due to an increased amount of enzyme. Commonly, xenobiotics cause the increased synthesis of the enzymes specifically involved in their own metabolism. Due to lack of substrate specificity of the drug-metabolizing enzymes, this induction also increases the rate of metabolism of other xenobiotics. While xenobiotics can be grouped according to which of several different isozymes they induce, the mechanism of induction of drug-metabolizing systems remains unknown for all but a select few xenobiotics. A cytosolic carrier has been identified that binds a number of polycyclic hydrocarbons such as dioxin and 3-methyl cholanthrene, traveling with them into the nucleus, where DNA-directed synthesis of new cytochrome P450 occurs. This carrier does not bind phenobarbital, and a search for a cytosolic protein binding to phenobarbital or to any xenobiotic that induce, the same CYP enzymes as phenobarbital has been unsuccessful.

Synergism is an increase in the activity or toxicity of two or more components over and above the added effects of the individual components, regardless of mechanism. Ethanol and carbon tetrachloride, both hepatotoxins, produce unexpectedly severe hepatotoxicity when administered together. Cigarette smoking and occupational carcinogen exposure in miners and steel workers appear to be synergistic with relation to induction of lung cancers. Similar to synergism is potentiation, where the potentiator alone appears to have no adverse effect, but increases the toxicity of another xenobiotic greatly. Glutathione depletors potentiate the toxic effect of many xenobiotics normally removed harmlessly by GSH conjugation. Diethylmaleate removes GSH by conjugation, and buthionine sulfoximine by inhibition of GSH synthesis. Both potentiate the toxicities of acetaminophen and bromobenzene. The area of synergism and potentiation of toxicities deserves a great deal of attention if our knowledge of toxicology is to be more than academic, as exposure to a polluted environment seldom consists of exposure to a single chemical.

B. MECHANISMS OF SITE-SPECIFIC TOXICITIES

1. Direct and Cascade Effects

Many elegant descriptions of xenobiotic inhibition of individual enzymes have been made by the bench scientist, e.g., the action of cyanide on cytochrome oxidase or of lead on aminolevulinic acid dehydratase. However, the initial insult may be one or two steps removed from the final physiological change that overwhelms the body. Organophosphates inhibit the hydrolysis of acetylcholine, and toxicity is due to the adverse effects of the accumulated acetylcholine. Cyanide inhibits cytochrome oxidase in the respiratory center of the CNS, which then no longer governs respiration, and death ensues due to the cessation of respiration.

The effect of intoxication on the whole animal often encompasses a wide range of effects. For many chemicals the initial insult causes a sequence, or cascade, of several effects by, for example, switching on a cAMP-dependent pathway or causing the slow accumulation of an endogenous metabolite. Thus the normal balance of intermediary metabolism is disrupted. Triglyceride accumulation is a common response to a number of hepatotoxic agents, resulting from a disruption of the balance among uptake, synthesis, and release of triglycerides. However, individual xenobiotics vary in the mechanisms by which they cause this imbalance. For example, ethanol is thought to inhibit the mitochondrial utilization of lipids, hydrazine to increase the uptake and synthesis of lipids, and carbon tetrachloride to inhibit the release of triglycerides by the inhibition of lipoprotein synthesis.

The hemorrhagic effect of aspirin is due to aspirin acetylation of cyclooxygenase. In the platelet, cyclooxygenase forms prostaglandin H, which is further converted to thromboxane A_2 by thromboxane synthetase, which product is responsible for enhancing platelet aggregation. In a similar pathway in the endothelial cell wall of the circulatory system, prostaglandin H is formed by cyclooxygenase and then converted to prostaglandin PGI_2, which inhibits platelet aggregation. While this causes irreversible inhibition of prostaglandin synthesis in both the platelet and the capillary endothelium, a new enzyme can be synthesized in the endothelial cell, but not in the anuclear

of cells to DNA damage and evaluate carcinogenic potential by measurement of increased rates of DNA repair. To date, all chemicals that have been shown to enhance DNA repair in hepatocyte culture have been found to be carcinogenic.

SUGGESTED READING

Klaassen, C., Amdur, M. O., and Doull, J. (1996). "Casarett and Doull's Toxicology," 5th Ed. McGraw-Hill, New York.

Lewis, D. F., Watson, E., and Lake, B. G. (1998). Evolution of the cytochrome P450 superfamily: Sequence alignments and pharmacogenetics. *Mutat. Res* **410**; 245–270.

Lu, F. C. (1985). "Basic Toxicology. Fundamentals, Target Organs, and Risk Assessment." Hemisphere, Washington.

Pelkonen, O., and Raunio, H. (1997). Metabolic activation of toxins: Tissue-specific expression and metabolism in target organs. *Environ. Health Perspect.* **105** (Suppl. 4), 767–774.

Pratt, W. B., and Taylor, P. (1990). "Principles of Drug Action: The Basis of Pharmacology," 3rd Ed. Churchill Livingstone, New York.

Timbrell, J. A. (1982). "Principles of Biochemical Toxicology." Taylor and Francis, London.

—————————— *3* ——————————

Morphologic Manifestations of Toxic Cell Injury

Matthew A. Wallig
Department of Veterinary Pathobiology
College of Veterinary Medicine
University of Illinois at Urbana-Champaign
Urbana, Illinois

I. Introduction

Whatever the cause of injury to a cell, toxic or otherwise, and whatever the biochemical events, simple or complex, that lead to the injury or death of the cell, the pathologist must rely on a visible morphological change as a means of detecting when a disruption of homeostasis has occurred. This visible manifestation of disrupted function, whether at the ultrastructural, microscopic, or macroscopic level, is a lesion. The lesion is still the primary means by which a toxicologic pathologist arrives at a diagnosis, hopefully one that includes the etiology as well as a description of the underlying morphologic alterations.

The basic unit of life is the cell; therefore, any morphologic alterations to a tissue as a result of injury must begin with the response of the cell itself to the injurious situation. A thorough evaluation (and understanding) of a lesion must logically begin at this level. The development of a lesion at the cellular level is dependent on a variety of factors that influence how the cell responds to the disruption in homeostasis forced upon it.

Handbook of Toxicologic Pathology, Second Edition
Volume 1

A. KEY CELLULAR COMPONENTS IN CELL INJURY

Although alteration or damage to any one organelle or structure in a cell can ultimately result in injury to the cell as a whole, there are several critical cell systems that are of prime importance in the process of lethal cell injury. It is in these structures where disruptions, if severe enough, will almost without question result in the death of the cell. These structures are the plasma membrane, site of osmotic, electrolyte, and water regulation (as well as signal transduction); the mitochondrion, site of aerobic respiration; the endoplasmic reticulum, site of much protein synthesis as well as calcium storage in some cases; and the nucleus, where the genetic material of the cell is sequestered and in which transcription of the genetic code takes place. The biochemical consequences of damage to these structures were discussed in Chapter 2.

B. FACTORS INFLUENCING INJURY

One of the most obvious factors influencing the development of a lesion is the severity of the damage itself. If the damage to the cell is mild, with rapid recovery, a lesion may never manifest itself morphologically, although a functional disruption may occur or a biochemical alteration may become detectable. Greater or more prolonged damage may severely alter tissue structure to the point that it is impossible to determine a pathogenesis or etiology. Another possibility is that the damage is so profound that not only the cell but the entire individual dies before the injury can become morphologically manifest. Acute cyanide intoxication is a classic example.

Cells with high metabolic activity tend to suffer injury more easily and quickly than those with lower metabolic requirements. Metabolically active cells, such as neurons, myocardial cells, and renal proximal convoluted tubule (PCT) epithelial cells, are absolutely dependent on a continuous oxygen supply for normal function. Uninterrupted and high concentrations of O_2 for aerobic metabolism are necessary to provide the ATP for maintenance of membrane polarity and membrane integrity (neurons), for continual muscular contraction/relaxation and Ca^{2+} transport (myocardium), and for transport of fluids, electrolytes, and metabolites (renal PCT). Even small changes in O_2 tension leading to mildly decreased ATP production may seriously alter the essential functions of these cell types and potentially impact the survival of the individual. In contrast, cells with low metabolic activity, such as fibroblasts and adipocytes, are less affected by low O_2 supply and can tolerate a very low oxygen environment—hence their prominent role in regeneration and scarring. Related to this, the degree of specialization can be an important determinant of cellular response to injury. Functionally "plastic" (i.e., relatively undifferentiated) cells, such as fibroblasts, adapt to a variety of conditions, assume an assortment of different roles, and can also tolerate almost totally anaerobic conditions and a variety of toxic insults. Retinal rods and cones, however, which must expend a great deal of energy to maintain their highly specialized membrane structures for trapping photons of light, can only tolerate an absolute minimum of disruption of homeostasis before degeneration or death ensues.

The "biochemical phenotype" of a particular cell, including its membrane receptor complement, may protect or predispose it to injury. For example, a cell with a *fas* receptor on its surface respond to *fas* ligand binding by undergoing apoptotic necrosis (i.e., apoptosis), whereas a cell without this receptor will be totally unaffected. In a similar fashion, certain cells may accumulate toxic concentrations of xenobiotics because they have specific uptake systems that allow the cell to "mistakenly" accumulate a substance that it either cannot metabolize or that it bioactivates. Gentamicin toxicity in the PCT epithelium is an example of such a situation. Gentamicin is taken up by the PCT organic transport system, accumulates in the lysosomes, and eventually interferes with lipid metabolism and lysosomal function to the point where the lysosome malfunctions and kills the cell. Cells having certain phase I metabolizing enzymes, especially certain members of the cytochrome P450 family, may bioactivate, rather than detoxify, certain xenobiotics. This manifests itself as an enhanced or selective susceptibility to damage by a particular xenobiotic. For example, the presence of CYP 2E1 in hepatocytes makes them uniquely susceptible to damage by acetaminophen, which is bioactivated to a highly reactive quinone imine by this P450 isozyme.

The "innate" capacity of a cell to respond to the injurious stimulus (e.g., a high concentration of antioxidant enzymes) can have a substantial impact on its ability to handle injury. The hepatocyte, for example, which receives 60% of its blood supply directly from the gastrointestinal tract, can tolerate a high degree of "toxic" insult entering from that source. This is due to its tremendous complement of phase I and phase II detoxification enzymes, as well as its high concentrations of the antioxidants glutathione, vitamin E, and vitamin C. Cells lacking high concentrations of endogenous antioxidants, antioxidant enzymes, or phase I and phase II enzymes can be especially prone to toxic injury.

All these factors and many more contribute to a variation in susceptibility to injury among the different cells within the tissues and organs of an organism. Regardless of the type of injury or the factors present that mitigate or exacerbate that injury, the cell has only a limited number of responses available to it for survival.

C. REACTION OF THE BODY TO INJURY

The reaction (or overreaction) of the rest of the organism to the injured or dead cell has a key role in the morphologic manifestation of toxic cell injury. In some cases, it is the exuberance of the inflammatory cells attracted into the affected area, rather than the injury itself, that leads to the development of an overt and even severe lesion. The inflammatory reaction is generally an essential component in the elimination of damaged tissue, but it can be a "two-edged sword" that converts a relatively mild injury into a severe one that may even hinder resolution of a lesion. Much of the severe necrotizing damage in acute toxic pancreatitis, for example, arises not from the zymogen granules released from dying acinar cells, but rather from the activated neutrophils attracted into the lesion by the granule contents. Such a reaction is typically associated with the type of cell death that recently has been termed "oncotic necrosis," whereas the inflammatory reaction is much more likely to be muted or even absent with the type of cell death described as "apoptotic necrosis." The difference in response to these two types of cell death has been linked to the observation that cells dying by oncotic necrosis leak intracellular materials and produce substances that are likely to attract neutrophils. Apoptotic necrosis, with its orderly sequence of disintegration and preservation of membrane integrity, produces virtually no factors attractive to neutrophils.

D. ADAPTATION

A cell typically exists within a very narrow range of physiochemical conditions necessary for life and will exert much of its metabolic energy and resources toward maintaining these conditions. This is termed homeostasis. Ion gradients, intracellular pH, and cytosolic osmolarity, for example, are vigorously maintained by the cell even at the cost of its own specialized functions. A cell threatened with a loss of homeostasis will often jettison its specialized structures and cut back on its specialized functions, no matter how important they may be to the rest of the organism. Substantial deviations from homeostasis may lead to death of the cell. Less substantial deviations can lead to a new level of function or metabolic activity that is the cell's attempt to maintain its internal environment. This is called adaptation.

1. Atrophy

One form of adaptation is atrophy, which, simply put, is a reduction of mass in a cell, tissue, or organ. At the cellular level, atrophy is often a response to decreased demand for the specialized functions of a particular cell. For example, decreased workload on a muscle attached to a limb that is immobilized by a cast will lead to a decrease in the myocytic content of actin, myosin, and other proteins associated with muscle contraction. This will be reflected as decreased diameter and volume of the myofibers within that muscle (Fig. 1). Loss of the appropriate stimulation needed for the specialized function of a particular cell may result not only in a decrease in the metabolic activity, but in loss of its organellar structure and content as well. Examples of this are loss of innervation to a muscle or lack of hormonal stimulation to an endocrine-dependent tissue such as a thyroid follicular cell. Other examples of atrophy include a reduction in nutrient or oxygen supply due to inadequate or reduced blood flow and direct pressure from adjacent cells or stroma.

At the most basic level, an atrophied cell has undergone catabolism. This is often reflected ultrastructurally by an overt breakdown of cellular organelles, including mitochondria, endoplasmic reticulum, microtubules, and microfilaments, among others. Atrophied cells typically contain decreased numbers of organelles and increased numbers of autophagic vacuoles within the cell, often fused with lysosomes. Specialized structures, such as cilia, contractile apparatuses, secretory granules, and microvilli, may be much reduced in number or

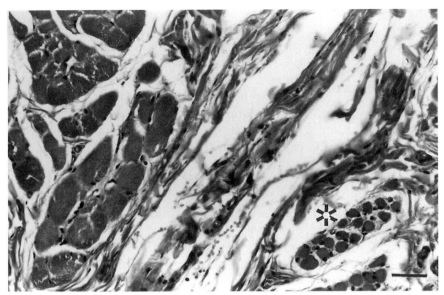

Figure 1. Atrophy. Skeletal muscle from the tongue of a young horse that atrophied secondary to impairment of blood supply to that portion of the tongue. Affected muscle bundles (*) are reduced in size, as are individual myofibers. There is also increased space between fibers. Hematoxylin and eosin. Bar: 25 μm.

even absent. In severe cases, loss of specialized structures may be so extensive that the cell may no longer be phenotypically recognizable (Fig. 2). Metabolically active cells that have a high turnover of membrane components, such as myocytes, neurons, and hepatocytes, may accumulate lysosomes filled with solid precipitates of partially degraded complex lipids and lipoproteins, forming golden brown lipofuscin and ceroid, the "wear and tear" pigments. Histologically, the atrophied cell may be obviously reduced in size, have decreased staining affinity with hematoxylin and eosin, have an altered shape, or be less differentiated in morphology. Grossly, one may only see a reduction in the overall size or mass of the tissue or organ in which the affected cell type is found, with perhaps a softer texture or paler color.

Atrophy at the tissue or organ level, however, can reflect more than just a reduction in cellular mass. A decrease in cell number can also result in a reduction in mass at the gross level. Atrophy in this case is the result of cell death, either by apoptotic necrosis or by oncotic necrosis (depending on the nature and the

severity of the toxic insult), leaving behind a tissue that may not only be smaller, but may have a variety of differing characteristics depending on the cause of the atrophy (Fig. 3). In cases where the loss of cells has occurred via apoptotic necrosis, one may observe within surviving cells, or within nearby tissue macrophages, "vacuoles" that represent phagolysosomes containing portions of the dead cells in various stages of degradation. Histologically, these may appear as hyalin droplets. Apoptotic bodies may be observed, but inflammation usually is not present. The gross appearance of these changes is generally not different from that seen in cases where there is a reduction in cell mass without cell death. In more subtle cases, tissue mass may have to be determined by weighing the affected organ and calculating organ-to-body weight ratios.

In cases where oncotic necrosis is the cause of the reduction in tissue or organ size, one typically observes not only swollen and burst cells, with spillage of cell content, but also some degree of inflammation, often with resultant scarring. In these cases, the reduction in tissue

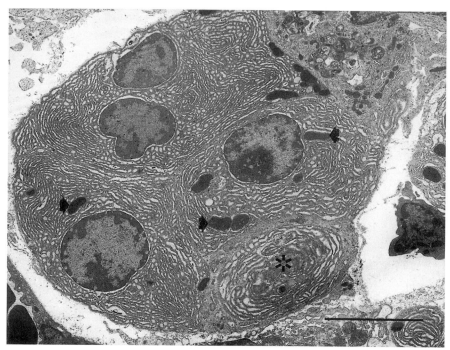

Figure 2. An atrophic pancreatic acinus from a male Fischer 344 rat after a bout of edematous pancreatitis induced by the phytochemical crambene. Acinar cells are reduced in size, lack polarity, are devoid of granules, and have few mitochondria (small arrows). An autophagic vacuole containing acinar cell cytoplasm (*) is present in one cell. Bar: 10 μm.

or organ size may be uneven, depending on the degree of scar tissue present, and the tissue or organ firmer than normal and grayish or whitish (as a reflection of the scarring).

2. Hypertrophy

Hypertrophy is an increase in mass of a cell, tissue, or organ without cellular proliferation. Classically, hypertrophy is a response to increased metabolic demand for the specialized function provided by the particular cell. At ultrastructural and histological levels, this translates into an increase in the volume of cytoplasm and an increase in the number of cell organelles, microfilaments, microtubules, and other specialized structures. Hypertrophy is usually difficult to quantify at ultrastructural and light microscopic levels without specialized morphometric techniques, but is usually evident grossly. As with atrophy, weighing an organ and calculating organ-to-body weight ratios may be the only

way to detect subtle forms of hypertrophy. The consequences of hypertrophy are often benign and merely reflect a physiologic response to an increased demand on a tissue for its specialized function. However, there are situations where the increased mass exceeds physiologic limits and dysfunction of the hypertrophied tissue occurs. An example of "pathologic" hypertrophy in response to a toxic stimulus is the tremendous hypertrophy of smooth endoplasmic reticulum in the hepatocyte in individuals treated with phenobarbital and other anticonvulsant drugs, which in severe cases can lead to loss of other hepatocytic functions.

II. Reversible Cell Injury

Cell injury is any disruption that results in the loss of a cell's or tissue's ability to maintain homeostasis, whether at normal or adapted levels. In other words, the cell can no longer

43

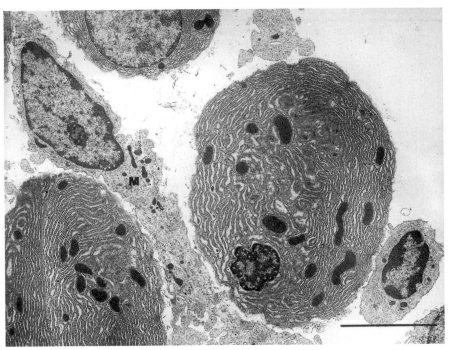

Figure 3. A single remaining atrophied pancreatic acinar cell from a Fischer 344 rat treated with crambene, which causes extensive apoptotic necrosis of most acinar cells in the pancreas. A tissue macrophage (M) is present near the atrophied cell. Bar: 10 μm.

regulate its environment within physiologic limits. The inability of a cell to regulate its internal environment may not result necessarily in the death of the cell, even if there is a loss of specialized function. Reversible injury is sometimes referred to as degeneration, although this term has been used in the past to describe other conditions that may not be reflective of injury. The disruption or injury, ranging from mild to severe, is not enough to kill the cell even if its specialized function in the body is impaired. It must be remembered, however, that even though a cell may be reversibly injured, if the loss of function is one that is vital for the survival of the individual as a whole, death of the individual may occur even though a single cell has not died.

The biochemical "point of no return" for an injured cell has been much debated and researched over recent years. It now appears that the mitochondrial permeability transition, leading to leakage of the electron transport chain enzyme cytochrome c into the cytosol, may be the final step in both oncotic and apoptotic necrosis. This event represents the transition from a cell that can repair itself and recover to a cell that will progress inexorably toward death, but it has no definitive morphologic correlate, unfortunately at the light microscopic level. A variety of other clinical, biochemical, and light microscopic features may be considered when trying to assess the reversibility of a lesion, including such things as the presence of obviously dead cells adjacent to less severely injured cells, the presence of an inflammatory reaction, the duration of the injurious stimulus (if known), clinical signs in the animals, and clinical pathology parameters (if available), even the type of cell involved and the tissue affected.

There are two cellular morphologic changes commonly recognized as reflecting reversible injury, although in either case these changes may progress further to those characteristic of cell death. These are cell swelling and fatty change.

A. CELL SWELLING

Cell swelling is an early change that occurs in most types of acute injury and which can be a prelude to more drastic changes. Cell swelling results when the cell loses its ability to precisely control the movement of ions and water into and out of the cytosol. For the most part, this reflects the influx of sodium (followed by water) across the membrane into the cell due to defective function or insufficient capacity on the part of $Na^+ - K^+$ ATPases. Direct damage to these "pumps," inadequate supplies of the essential substrate, ATP, or an inability to keep up with the influx of sodium due to direct damage to the plasma membrane itself may all contribute to cell swelling.

Cell swelling is characterized histologically by cells that are typically swollen or enlarged in size, with compression or displacement of adjacent structures. Staining affinity is often diminished, giving the cells a pale or "cloudy" appearance. Vacuoles, usually manifestations of dilated endoplasmic reticulum or Golgi (Fig. 4), may form if the $Na^+ - K^+$ ATPases in the endoplasmic reticulum are sufficiently functional to pump at least some of the excess sodium (followed by water) into its lumenal spaces.

Contributing to the morphologic changes associated with cell swelling is the loss of normal shape, due not only to the influx of water, but also to the influx of calcium into the cell via the diminished capacity or function of the $Na^+ - Ca^{2+}$ exchange pumps, which are also dependent on ATP. The dissociation of cytoskeletal elements and the loss of intercellular connections that result from excessively high free cytosolic calcium levels lead to additional shape distortion and a tendency for the cell to assume a spherical shape if anatomically possible. Nuclear changes are often mild or minimal, at least in the early stages, and the nucleus generally occupies a location that is typical for the particular cell type (Fig. 5).

Cell swelling is not lethal *per se* and may indicate relatively mild injury; however, cells that are injured severely or lethally will go through a phase of swelling as well. Therefore, it must be remembered that lethally injured cells

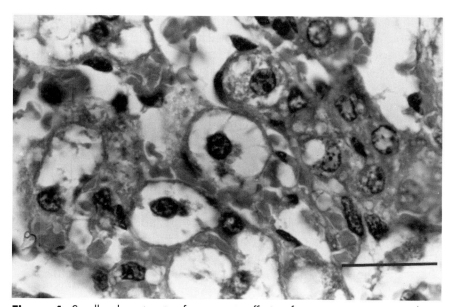

Figure 4. Swollen hepatocytes from a cat suffering from severe anemia and systemic hypoxia. Cells are rounded and contain numerous clear vacuoles. Nuclei, however, still appear viable. Hematoxylin and eosin. Bar: 25 μm.

45

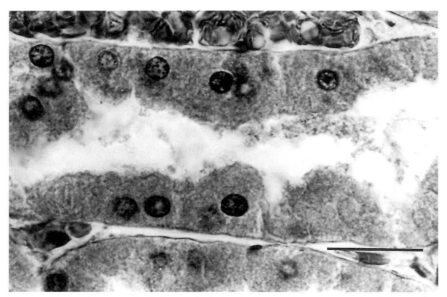

Figure 5. Swollen renal tubular epithelial cells from a dog in septic shock. Note the bulging of the apical portions of the cells, loss of brush border, and elevation of nuclei from the basal portions of cells. Hematoxylin and eosin. Bar: 25 μm.

that were fixed in the early stages of swelling can be interpreted as only being mildly injured. The location of the cell swelling must also be considered when assessing the consequences of cell swelling. Cell swelling in the myocardium secondary to poor vascular perfusion will at some point lead to separation of actin–myosin microfilaments, altered contraction, and ion shifts that affect depolarization—events with serious clinical consequences even if the cells are reversibly injured (Fig. 6). Swelling of astrocytes in the brain during hyperammonemia after liver failure can have tremendous functional consequences, even if no lethal injury has occurred. In contrast, cell swelling in the liver can be quite marked but have long-term consequences if the injurious stimulus is removed.

B. FATTY CHANGE

Fatty change is another manifestation of reversible injury that is often observable in cells that metabolize large quantities of fat, e.g., hepatocytes, myocardial cells, and renal tubular cells. Pathologic accumulations of intracellular fat may occur as a result of damage to several different cellular compoenents. Direct damage

to membranes of cells with a high flux of triglycerides passing through them can lead to an excessive buildup of triglyceride within the cytoplasm due to an impaired capability to export triglycerides. Hypoxia or damage to mitochondria within a cell can lead to insufficient β-oxidation of triglycerides and accumulation of unmetabolized triglycerides within the damaged mitochondrion and cytoplasm. Damage to protein synthetic machinery by the direct action of toxins or hypoxia can result in decreased synthesis of apoprotein for lipid transport and decreased synthesis of oxidative enzymes for β-oxidation of fatty acids, with the resultant storage of unmetabolized and/or untransported lipids within the cytoplasm. Fatty change is seen most often in hepatocytes, which must deal with large-scale fluxes in lipid. Swelling of fat-laden cells can progress to the point of occluding blood supply or crowding out other organelles needed for normal cellular function, resulting in lethal cell injury, even if the initial inciting stimulus was mild.

Ultrastructurally, fatty change is characterized by the accumulation of amorphous,

46

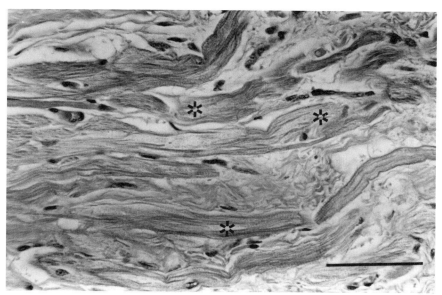

Figure 6. Cell swelling with loss of striations in the myocardium of a horse. Myofibers are swollen (*) and rarefied, and there is separation of myofibrils. Hematoxylin and eosin. Bar: 25 μm.

moderately electron-dense cytoplasmic inclusions, free within the cytosol but often associated with a proliferative or mildly dilated endoplasmic reticulum. The inclusions can be small and dispersed, often associated with acute, rapidly developing injury (Fig. 7), or quite large, occupying the entire central area of the cell and pushing organelles peripherally. This type of "macrovesicular" fatty change has been linked to more slowly developing toxic

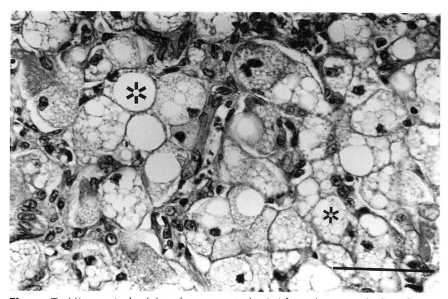

Figure 7. Microvesicular (*) and macrovesicular (*) fatty change in the liver from a cat suffering from acute hepatic lipidosis. In most hepatocytes, vacuoles are small and dispersed throughout the cytoplasm. Hematoxylin and eosin. Bar: 25 μm.

injury. Microscopically, fat-laden cells are swollen and clear, with numerous round, clearly defined spaces that appear as vacuoles or one large central vacuole compressing cytosol and nucleus around the periphery of the cell (Fig. 8). Due to conventional processing techniques that wash out triglycerides and other lipids, frozen sections must be used to preserve the fat in place, followed by special stains such as Oil Red O, Sudan Black, or osmium tetroxide to stain lipids orange or black. This is occasionally done to distinguish lipid-filled vacuoles from other types of vacuoles, particularly those filled with water due to cell injury. The gross appearance of fatty liver is a classic lesion in pathology, with its orange or yellow coloration, reticulated pattern, and friable, often greasy texture. Lipid accumulations in nonhepatic tissues are less visible, but can be noted occasionally in the myocardium under conditions of hypoxia, usually in myocytes bordering an infarct. This is due to damage to the β-oxidation pathways in the mitochondria. It must be remembered, however, that not all fatty change is due to toxic injury. The kidney, for example, will accumulate triglycerides when there is

hyperlipidemia, e.g., during the course of diabetes mellitus. Macrophages will often accumulate lipids when involved in inflammatory lesions where large amounts of lipid must be taken up, digested, and metabolized, e.g., in conditions where there is degeneration or death of white matter in the central nervous system (CNS). This does not generally represent injury to the macrophage, however.

III. Irreversible Cell Injury

Irreversible injury results from a severe disruption in homeostasis that leads to a point where normal function can no longer be restored and the cell begins an inexorable slide toward death, whether by an uncontrolled process (i.e., "oncotic" or "accidental" necrosis) or in a tightly regulated, orderly manner ("apoptotic" necrosis). In either case, the dead cell will ultimately be degraded and dissolved, disappearing permanently. In both forms of death, the exact point of "death" is often disputed, but the morphologic changes that precede or follow the "point of no return" often can be identified and may suggest a mechanism

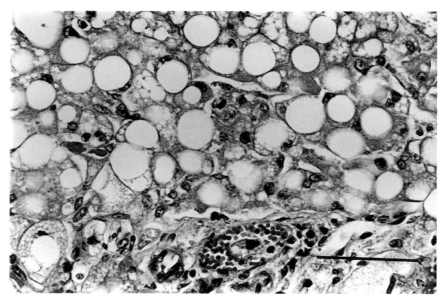

Figure 8. Macrovesicular fatty change in the liver from a goat with pregnancy toxemia. The vacuoles are large and displace other cellular structures to the periphery of the cell. Hematoxylin and eosin. Bar: 25 μm.

or etiology (Table I). It must be kept in mind that the term "necrosis" encompasses not only the primary event of cell death in the living organism, but also the secondary cellular changes that follow the actual death process. The degradative changes that follow death of the cell are often the most important part of identifying cell injury morphologically, especially in cases of oncotic necrosis. It must also be remembered that these change occur in all cells after death of the entire organism (postmortem autolysis). It is the reaction of the surrounding viable tissue to the dead cells that allows the pathologist to distinguish antemortem cell death from postmortem autolytic changes.

A. ONCOTIC NECROSIS

The ultrastructural changes that occur in oncotic necrosis are frequently the same as those that follow those of reversible cell injury, i.e., cell swelling with rarefaction of the cytosol due to the influx of water, dilation of the cisternae of the endoplasmic reticulum, loss or deformation of specialized surface features, and rounding of the cell. The ultrastructural changes that are associated with oncotic necrosis, however, generally precede the histologic manifestations of injury by hours and occasionally days, resulting in a "lag" between when the cell has actually died and the time when this death can be observed microscopically by the pathologist.

TABLE I
Necrosis vs Apoptosis

Characteristic	Necrosis	Apoptosis
Gross changes	Grossly evident with disruption of normal tissue structure and detail, scarring if long-term	Minimal or atrophy without scarring
Histologic changes	Whole fields of cells affected	Individual cells scattered throughout the affected tissue
	Hypereosinophilia	Hyperbasophilia or hypereosinophilia
	Loss of cell borders with irregular fragmentation	Formation of round bodies, often within a "halo"
	Irregular chromatin clumping, pyknosis, karyorhexis, and/or karyolysis; rupture of nuclear envelope	Chromatin condensation into "caps" or "crescents," within round nuclear bodies; preservation of nuclear envelope
Ultrastructural changes	Swelling and loss of surface structures with "blebbing" and loss of apical portions of cytoplasm	Condensation followed by rapid "zeiosis" (budding)
	Rarefaction of cytoplasm followed by condensation after death	Condensation of cytoplasm followed by rarefaction after ingestion by phagocytes
	Swelling and loss of organellar integrity	Preservation of organellar integrity
	Low-amplitude swelling of mitochondria followed by high-amplitude swelling and rupture	Preservation of mitochondrial ultrastructure
	Rupture and degradation of internal and external membranes with bursting of the cell	Preservation of internal and external membranes with preservation of membrane around apoptotic bodies
	Irregular clumping and degradation of chromatin; rupture of nuclear envelope	Migration of uniformly degraded chromatin to margins of nuclear envelope; preservation of nuclear envelope
Sequelae	Release of intracellular enzymes into extracellular millieu	Retention of intracellular enzymes within the apoptotic bodies
	Release of proinflammatory cell breakdown products	No release of proinflammatory products
	Ingress of neutrophils followed by macrophages	Ingestion by adjacent cells or by tissue macrophages
	Active inflammation with scarring	Atrophy with stromal collapse but *no* scarring

49

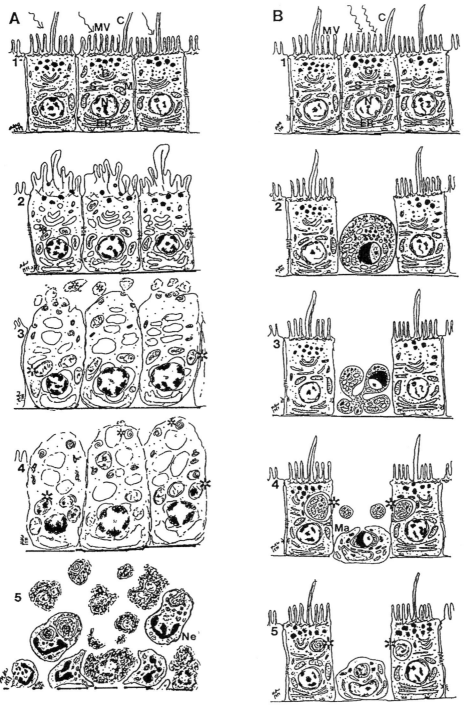

Figure 9. Morphologic changes associated with oncotic (A) and apoptotic (B) necrosis in a "prototypical" secretory epithelial cell. C, cilium; ER, rough endoplasmic reticulum; G, Golgi apparatus; M, mitochondrion; Ma, macrophage; MV, microvillous brush border; N, nucleus; Ne, neutrophil; and S, smooth endoplasmic reticulum. Changes represented in A: 1, toxic stimulus affecting the entire population of cells; 2, initial swelling with swelling of microvilli and cilia, low-amplitude swelling of mitochondria (*) clumping of chromatin

Plasma membrane changes are among the first changes observed after injury and are characterized by loss of surface specialization, including the disappearance of microvilli and swelling of cilia (Fig. 9A-1). Intercellular attachments break down (Fig. 10), and the injured cell may detach from neighbors because of separation of gap junctions, dissolution of the terminal web, and degradation of maculae densae and zonulae adherentes. Cytoplasmic "blebs" or outpocketings may form on the surfaces of injured cells. These may actually detach from the surface of the swollen cells and float away into the lumen (if present) or interstitial space to eventually lyse and release their contents (Fig. 9A-2). Swelling continues, due to changes in membrane permeability, as the result of membrane pump failure, direct free radical damage to membrane proteins and phospholipids, breakdown by activated phospholipases (as a result of unrestricted calcium influx), or a host of other membrane damaging reactions. The plasma membrane will ultimately rupture (Fig. 11). Portions of partially degraded, insoluble membranes will eventually aggregate into laminated structures termed myelin whorls (Fig. 9A-3).

Mitochondria are perhaps the most dramatically affected organelles during the process of oncotic necrosis, first undergoing a form of swelling termed "low-amplitude" swelling as ATP is progressively depleted (Fig. 9A-1). This change is typified by swelling of the outer compartment as water and electrolytes are lost from the inner compartment and pass into the intermembranous space. The result is early condensation of the inner compartment, but this does not necessarily indicate irreversible injury. Small or large mitochondrial inclusions may form. Small inclusions result from the precipitation of small, very electron-dense calcium phosphate crystals due to the loss of internal calcium homeostasis. Larger, more electron-dense "flocculent densities" are accumulations of partially degraded protein and membrane elements (Fig. 12). If the injury is severe or persistent, mitochondria will undergo high-amplitude swelling (Fig. 10–12), with massive swelling of both inner and outer compartments and large-scale accumulation of precipitated mineral and protein, a sure sign of impending doom for both the organelle and the cell (Fig. 9A-3 and 4). It is at the point where the inner compartment swells and the outer compartment swells to the point of bursting that the mitochondrial permeability transition, considered by many to be the "point of no return" in the process of cell death, occurs. In the transition, particles on the inner membrane responsible for ATP production become detached, preventing any further ATP production. Prominent accumulation and precipitation of Ca^{2+} salts occur if some degree of blood flow is present or subsequently restored and Ca^{2+} enters the cell unimpeded. Soon after the transition, the mitochondrial outer membrane ruptures.

As mitochondria undergo the changes that ultimately lead to the death of the cell, the efflux

and dilation of endoplasmic reticulum cisternae; 3, continued swelling of cells, with loss of microvilli and cilia, "blebbing" with loss of bits of superficial cytoplasm (*), high-amplitude swelling of mitochondria (*), further clumping of chromatin, further dilation of endoplasmic reticulum cisternae, and detachment of ribosomes; 4, rupture of plasma membrane and internal membranes, including the nuclear membrane, further condensation of chromatin, myelin whorls (*), and flocculent densities within burst mitochondria (*); 5, condensation of cellular remnants and ingestion of cellular debris by neutrophils. Changes represented in B: 1, reception of an apoptotic stimulus by a single cell in the population; 2, abrupt condensation of cytoplasm, shrinkage and rounding of the cell with preservation of organellar morphology, and the condensation of chromatin into a homogeneous cap at one pole of the nucleus; 3, budding of the cell into membrane-bound bodies containing intact organelles; 4, ingestion of apoptotic bodies by tissue macrophage and adjacent epithelial cells (*); and 5, digestion of apoptotic bodies by the macrophage and adjacent epithelial cells (*).

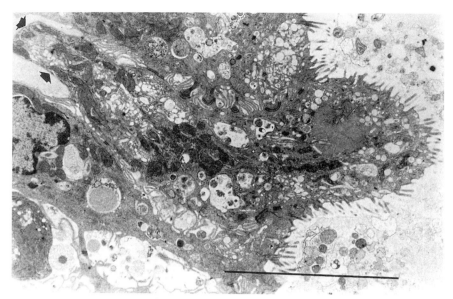

Figure 10. An equine colonocyte in the early stages of oncotic necrosis after exposure to phenylbutazone. Note the swelling of the apical cytoplasm, swelling of mitochondria, and the detachment of the cell from adjacent cells and the basement membrane (arrows). Bar: 10 μm. Courtesy of Dr. David Freeman, Department of Veterinary Clinical Medicine, University of Illinois at Urbana-Champaign.

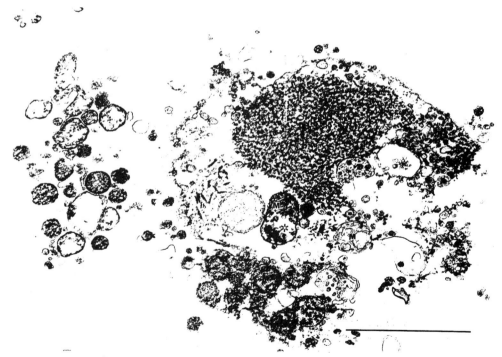

Figure 11. A culture NRK SLE rat renal epithelial cell exposed to $1.0\,\mu M$ okadaic acid for 48 hr, resulting in oncotic necrosis. Note swollen mitochondria, flocculent densities within one of the swollen mitochondria, loss of nuclear membrane, partial dispersion of chromatin, and rupture of the plasma membrane. Bar: 5 μm. Courtesy of Dr. Myrtle Davis, Department of Pathology, University of Maryland at Baltimore.

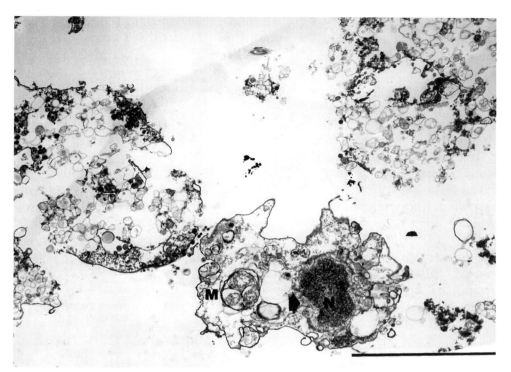

Figure 12. Culture NRK SLE rat renal epithelial cells undergoing oncotic necrosis after treatment with 1.0 µ*M* okadaic acid for 48 hr. Two of the cells have burst and released their contents. The cell in the middle of the field has an intact but convoluted plasma membrane, rarefied cytoplasm, a mitochondrion (M) undergoing high-amplitude swelling, and a pyknotic nucleus (N). Bar: 10 µm. Courtesy of Dr. Myrtle Davis, Department of Pathology, University of Maryland at Baltimore.

of water into the cytosol continues and the endoplasmic reticulum dilates and fragments in an attempt to eliminate the excessive accumulation of water from the cytosol. The endoplasmic reticulum often dilates so much that it forms water and ion-filled electron-lucent cisternae that appear as vacuoles by light microscopy. As injury progresses, ribosomes detach from the rough endoplasmic reticulum and protein synthesis shuts down. After rupture of the cell membranes (both external and internal), protein degradation begins in earnest, especially after lysosomes begin to release their enzyme contents. At this point, the remnants of cytoplasm become denser and actually shrink (Fig. 9A-5). This pattern of swelling during the process of death followed by condensation afterward is characteristic of oncotic necrosis. It is the mirror image of apoptotic necrosis, in which the opposite pattern is observed.

Nuclear morphologic changes associated with irreversible cell injury are primarily changes in the morphology of chromatin. Nuclear chromatin clumps along the nuclear membrane (Fig. 9A-1), and the distinction between euchromatin and heterochromatin is lost because of the drop in pH that typically occurs during the progression of oncotic necrosis. The nucleus and its chromatin may initially shrink and condense as the swollen cytosol and enlarged perinuclear space impinge on it, creating the morphologic change known as pyknosis (Figs. 9A-4 and 12). Eventually the nuclear membrane will break down and rupture, and the nucleus itself will swell. Nuclear swelling is accompanied by rarefaction of the nucleoplasm and dispersion of aggregated bits of chromatin attached to the fragmented membranes (Fig. 11), leading to the changes characteristic of karyorrhexis. Eventually the entire mass of chromatin, nucleoplasm, and nuclear membrane become sufficiently degraded to fade from view, a morphologic change that has been termed karyolysis.

After the cell is functionally "dead," lysosomes begin to swell and release enzymes into the cytoso. "Autolysis," as traditionally described, begins at this point. Lysosomal membranes are relatively resistant to damage and degradation, and in most cases of toxic injury release their contents late in the process of oncotic necrosis. Cases where the activation of lysosomes is the primary trigger in oncotic necrosis are relatively few. In copper toxicity, for example, the large amounts of copper that accumulate in lysosomes eventually cause their rupture, releasing enzymes and highly oxidative forms of copper into the cell.

Once the point of no return in the process of oncotic necrosis has been reached, and release of lysosomal enzymes has occurred, the degradation of cell components becomes widespread, and the lesion that is easily recognized as "necrosis" becomes manifest via the light microscope (Table 1). The morphologic changes are relatively stereotypical, although there is much variation among the various tissues in the body due to their numerous biochemical, functional, and morphological peculiarities. In most cases, the cytoplasm becomes hypereosinophilic and hyalinized due to the degradation of proteins, releasing reactive groups that can interact with eosin, and due to the degradation of ribosomal RNA. Occasionally, eosinophilic or basophilic cytoplasmic granules representing swollen mitochondria may be observed. As degradation progresses, the cytoplasm becomes "moth-eaten" and fragmented. In some tissues, especially where there is a large flux of calcium in and out of the tissue, there may be a very marked degree of calcification. These tissues may be replete with basophilic crystals, giving the dead cells a bluish, stippled, fragmented, or even crystalline appearance (Fig. 13). As mentioned earlier, there are nuclear changes that are characteristic of oncotic necrosis: pyknosis, where nuclear chromatin has condensed into an irregular deeply basophilic mass (Fig. 14); karyorhexis, where the chromatin has fragmented and drifted away from the nuclear membrane (Fig. 15); or karyolysis, where dissolution of chromatin is the primary feature (Fig. 16). These changes do not necessarily follow in sequence, and one or all can be observed in a necrotic tissue.

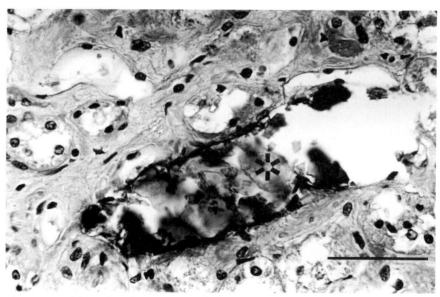

Figure 13. Mineralized necrotic renal tubular epithelium (∗) from a cat intoxicated by ethylene glycol. Hematoxylin and eosin. Bar: 25 μm.

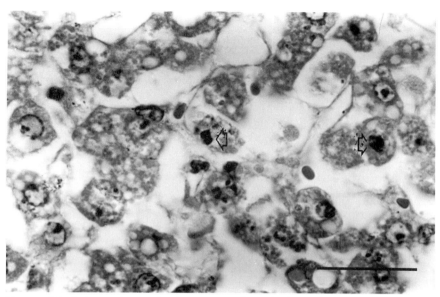

Figure 14. Pyknosis (arrows) in hepatocytes from the liver of a dog with clostridial sepsis. Hematoxylin and eosin. Bar: 25 μm.

Gross changes associated with oncotic necrosis are variable and very much dependent on the tissue in which the injury has occurred, the etiology of the injury, and the response of surrounding tissues. In some cases, the affected tissue may be paler than surrounding tissue and somewhat reduced in volume, especially if blood flow to the affected area has been compromised or cut off completely. If the blood supply is still intact or has been restored after the lethal insult, the tissue may be swollen, engorged with blood, darker than normal, and

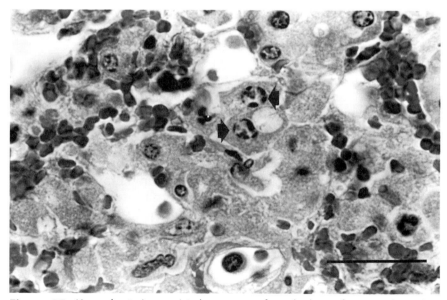

Figure 15. Karyorhexis (arrows) in hepatocytes from the liver of a cat with cardiomyopathy with congestive heart failure and subsequent hypoxia. Hematoxylin and eosin. Bar: 25 μm.

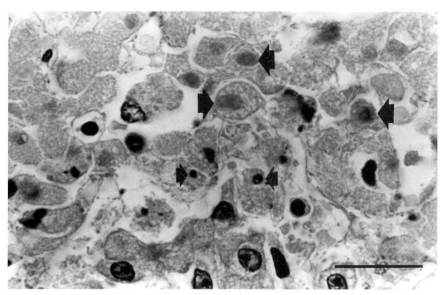

Figure 16. Karyolysis (large arrows) in hepatocytes from a dog with severe hypovolemic shock. Pyknosis (small arrows) is also present. Hematoxylin and eosin. Bar: 25 μm.

soft. On occasion, there is a central pale area surrounded by a zone of red tissue—a vascular response to the dead tissue. The gross and histologic manifestations of oncotic necrosis have in the past been classified into several categories, three of which will be briefly described. With "coagulation necrosis," the general structural organization of the tissue is still discernible, although specific details are lost. Histologically, "shadows" of dead cells can be ascertained. This type of change is observed most often when the blood supply is completely cut off and inflammatory cells have not had a chance to move in and clean up the mess, but it can also be seen in tissues where cells contain few lysosomes and the autodegradation of dead cells proceeds at a slower pace. Liquefaction necrosis is seen more often where infectious, rather than toxic, agents have caused the injury, and is often associated with a severe acute inflammatory response with large numbers of neutrophils. The neutrophils characteristically spill out their lysosomal enzymes into the affected tissues, creating a lesion that is typically soft and semiliquified in consistency. Some tissues, particularly the CNS, undergo liquefactive necrosis as a matter of course whenever

there is large-scale oncotic necrosis. Caseous necrosis is confined almost entirely to situations where infectious agents or occasionally foreign material is involved. In this case, the necrotic tissue is whitish, pale yellow or pale green, soft, and pasty.

B. APOPTOTIC NECROSIS

Apoptotic necrosis is a common but until recently underappreciated type of cell death that has had a variety of names in the past, including "single cell necrosis," "programmed cell death," "cell suicide," "necrobiosis," and "apoptosis," to name just a few. Morphologically, apoptotic necrosis is usually much harder to detect than oncotic necrosis due its rapid progression once triggered, the rapid disposition of dead cells via ingestion by adjacent cells or resident macrophages, and the participation of only small numbers of cells at any one time during the process.

Ultrastructurally, apoptotic necrosis has unique features that are quite distinct from oncotic necrosis (Table I). The first and most obvious change is the detachment of the dying cell from its neighbors and its rapid transformation into a "round" (i.e., spherical) morphology with a loss of specialized surface structures (Fig. 9B-2). If the cell is a secretory cell, it will degranulate prior to assuming a rounded configuration. Initial dilation of the endoplasmic reticulum may be observed, but this is indicative of pumping of ions and water into the cisternae as a prelude to condensation of the cytoplasm. As the cytosol becomes denser and organelles cluster closer together, "zeiosis," or pinching off of the cell into round (i.e., spherical) membrane-bound fragments, occurs frequently (Fig. 9B-3). However, it must be emphasized that the integrity of the plasma membrane is preserved, even after cellular fragmentation. Organelles within the rounded apoptotic body or cell fragments are well preserved and even functional in many cases. Nuclear changes unique to apoptotic necrosis can occur prior to, during, or even some time after the cytoplasmic changes have occurred and are characterized by preservation of the nuclear envelope, segregation of the nucleolus from chromatin, and the uniform condensation of chromatin into crescents or smooth-edged clusters along the intact nuclear envelope (Fig. 9B-2 and 3). The nucleus may also undergo zeiosis and, as with the cell membrane, the nuclear membrane remains intact. It is only after ingestion by adjacent tissue cells or resident macrophages that changes that are more typical of oncotic necrosis are observed (Fig. 9B-5). Thus, in contrast to oncotic necrosis, condensation rather than swelling is the key feature during the death process, to be followed by swelling once the cell has fragmented and been ingested by adjacent tissue cells or macrophages.

The actual histologic changes associated with apoptotic necrosis are relatively unique and easy to discern. The most obvious change is a "rounding up" shrinkage and fragmentation of individual cells within a tissue rather than the loss of whole fields of cells. Rounded up cells or their fragments are most often shrunken, condensed, and either hyperbasophilic or hypereosinophilic. The bodies are round in profile and have clearly defined cell boundaries. They are often surrounded by a clear space or "halo,"

which in most cases represents a phagocytic vacuole within an adjacent tissue cell or macrophage that has ingested the dead cell or its fragments (Fig. 17). Dense condensation of chromatin within an intact nuclear membrane is prominent, with the chromatin forming a "cap" or "crescent" along one edge of the nuclear envelope. The number of cells undergoing apoptotic necrosis that can be observed in a tissue at any one time is in most cases relatively low, and only 1–2% of the total cell population may have the characteristic morphology even in a tissue in which widespread and massive apoptotic necrosis is occurring. The rapidity of formation and degradation of the bodies by adjacent cells or phagocytes are major factors behind the low number of identifiable apoptotic bodies in a histologic section.

Apoptotic necrosis can be triggered by a huge variety of stimuli, many of them having nothing to do directly with toxic injury. Mild toxic injury that is insufficient to lead outright to oncotic necrosis can trigger apoptotic necrosis. This is especially true for toxic insults that injure the genome such that DNA repair systems are overwhelmed, triggering the *p53*-related pathways to initiate the cell death process. It should also be emphasized that mild injury not involving the genome can trigger apoptotic necrosis in cells that are capable of utilizing this pathway and that apoptotic necrosis is in some respects a "preferred" way for a cell to die.

Some investigators have seen sufficient variability in the morphologic manifestations of apoptotic necrosis to further subdivide it into at least two types based less on the ultimate morphology and more on the differences in the sequence of cytosolic and nuclear changes that occur among various cell types. "Type I" apoptotic necrosis, also known as "heterophagic" or "classic" apoptosis, is seen most commonly in cell types with high mitotic activity or the potential for high mitotic activity. In this form, nuclear condensation of chromatin is an early event, and ingestion by resident macrophages is a prominent feature (Fig. 18). Cells undergoing this form of apoptotic cell

57

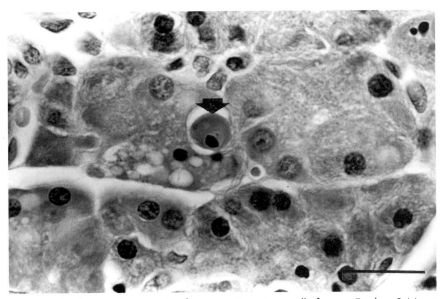

Figure 17. Apoptotic necrosis of pancreatic acinar cells from a Fischer 344 rat after exposure to the phytochemical crambene. An apoptotic body (arrow) within an autophagic vacuole is present at the center of the field. Hematoxylin and eosin. Bar: 25 μm.

death tend to have a low lysosomal content as well and the apoptotic fragments are more stable. In "type II" apoptosis, however, nuclear condensation of chromatin is often considerably delayed, sometimes until after fragmentation of the cell as a whole has occurred. Vacuolation is much more prominent, and the internal lysosomal release of enzymes often begins before fragmentation has begun, even though external membrane integrity is preserved throughout the process (Fig. 19). Phagocytosis of the apoptotic fragments is a prominent feature of this type of apoptotic necrosis. Apoptotic necrosis in thymocytes is considered to be typical of the type I form. Apoptotic necrosis in the renal tubules caused by okadaic acid would be more typical of the type II form. It has become apparent, however, that a mixture of the two types can be observed, e.g., in the prostate gland undergoing involution after castration.

Both types of cell death can and do occur simultaneously in an injured tissue, with those cells that are sufficiently uninjured to retain control of their osmoregulatory apparatus, energy production, and protein synthetic machinery taking the option of an orderly, controlled cell death rather than the willy-nilly, unregulated and disorderly process that typifies oncotic necrosis. Their more severely injured neighbors may not have that option, and therefore a combination of both processes may occur. This is a common feature, when looked for, in many cases of toxic cell injury, where cells most directly and severely injured by the toxic agent will express features typical of oncotic necrosis, whereas cells further removed from the site of injury or exposed to lower concentrations will have changes typical of apoptotic necrosis or a mixture of both features (Fig. 20).

C. SEQUELAE

1. Clinicopathological Considerations

The clinicopathological consequences of cell injury or death are often evident before the animal dies because cytoplasmic blebs can break off an injured cell and release cytoplasmic enzymes into the interstitial space to eventually find their way into the plasma. A lethally injured cell will also spill its contents into

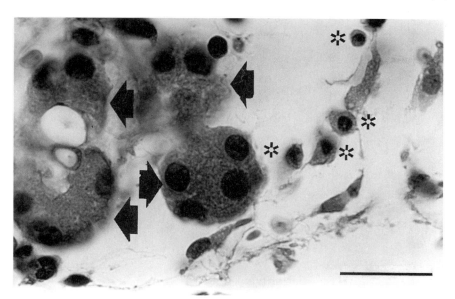

Figure 18. Macrophages (∗) in a portion of exocrine pancreas where there has been extensive apoptotic necrosis of acinar cells. Acini (arrows) containing atrophied acinar cells are scattered throughout the section. Hematoxylin and eosin. Bar: 25 μm.

tissue fluids. The site where tissue injury may be occurring can often be identified based on the type of enzyme, isoenzyme, or constituent released. In general, free cytosolic enzymes will leak out first from an injured cell, followed by mitochondrial membrane-bound and ultimately lysosomal enzymes, as cell injury becomes progressively more severe.

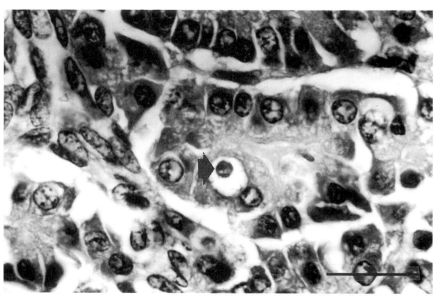

Figure 19. Apoptotic necrosis (arrow) of a hepatocyte in a dog that had undergone prolonged inanition. Note that the apoptotic body has been ingested by a neighboring hepatocyte. Hematoxylin and eosin. Bar: 25 μm.

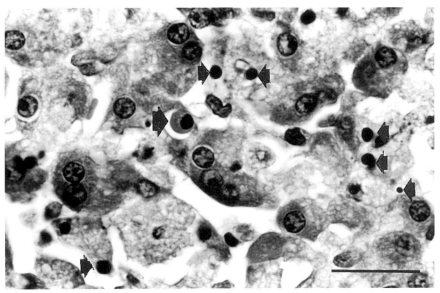

Figure 20. Oncotic and apoptotic necrosis occurring simultaneously in the exocrine pancreas of a Fischer 344 rat. Cells undergoing oncotic necrosis are present in clusters or groups and contain pyknotic nuclei (small arrows), while the cell undergoing apoptotic necrosis (large arrow) has discrete cell borders and the typical chromatin "cap." Hematoxylin and eosin. Bar: 25 μm.

2. Sequelae to Oncotic Necrosis

An inflammatory response of some sort is an almost universal sequela to oncotic necrosis, regardless of cause, provided the organism survives the initial insult long enough to mount a response that is evident. Membrane fragments and partially degraded cellular contents released when the dying cells burst are in large part responsible for eliciting the inflammatory reaction. Lipid fragments released from dying cells are especially biologically active and very chemoattractive to neutrophils and macrophages. Endothelial cells in the vicinity of the dying cells, if injured themselves or activated by contact with the spilled cellular contents, will also release soluble mediators of inflammation such as interleukin-1. Some lethally injured cells have the capability to make their own mediators, such as leukotrienes, which then act as chemoattractants for neutrophils. The initial influx of inflammatory cells into an area where oncotic necrosis is occurring is generally neutrophilic. Neutrophils will also produce mediators that attract more neutrophils and eventually macrophages to the site of injury. It is the influx of neutrophils that is important from a pathophysiologic viewpoint, as neutrophils are often indiscriminate in the manner in which they scavenging cellular material, releasing their lysosomal degradative enzymes as they do.

The somewhat nondiscriminate degradative activity of neutrophil often results in significant damage to the supporting stroma that is far out of proportion to the initial damage by the toxic agent. This in turn leads to replacement of the damaged stroma and parenchyma with nonfunctional fibrous scar tissue that serves as "filler" to replace the missing supportive tissues. In tissues in which oncotic necrosis has occurred there is usually some scar tissue present, which in general is proportional not only to the amount of damage to the parenchyma, but also to a large extent of the degree of inflammation that has been elicited by the toxic event. Fibrous scar tissue is composed predominantly of type I collagen and contains little elastin, laminin, type IV collagen, or other types of stromal proteins that maintain parenchymal cells in proper arrangement with one another.

As such it is a poor environment in which to support functional parenchymal tissues. For this reason, parenchymal regeneration is frequently incomplete or even nonexistent if the damage is extensive (Fig. 21). This implies at least some degree of permanent loss of function in the affected tissue. In tissues with substantial reserve capacity, this may not lead to overt or serious dysfunction of the affected organ until another insult occurs that exceeds the reserve capacity of the organ.

A variety of factors determine the degree of inflammation that occurs after toxic injury. The type of tissue affected may predispose it to an exuberant influx of neutrophils. Exocrine pancreas, for example, with its rich supply of proteases when undergoing oncotic necrosis, stimulates a dramatic influx of neutrophils that in turn causes even more damage, often convering a mild lesion into a fulminating one. Another factor is the extent of damage caused by the toxic insult. A renal infarct, with its extensive loss of parenchymal tissue, will elicit a more intense inflammatory response than a localized lesion only part of a nephron. The

degree of blood flow to the injured tissue has an important impact on the degree of inflammation. An area of oncotic necrosis with intact blood flow is far more likely to have a massive influx of inflammatory cells than an ischemic lesion. The extent of damage to supporting stroma by the toxic insult is still another factor in determining the degree of inflammation that will result. Damage to epithelium that leaves the basement membrane and underlying stromal tissue intact, e.g., an erosive lesion of the gastrointestinal tract or the skin, usually results in a far less florid inflammatory response than an insult that penetrates the basement membrane and damages the underlying stroma. Finally, the response of adjacent or neighboring cells, especially if these cells are part of the fixed macrophage system, may have a substantial effect on the degree of inflammation that occurs after a bout of oncotic necrosis. Activation of Kupfer cells in the liver after a toxic insult to hepatocytes has been found to cause a much greater degree of inflammation and ongoing damage than situations where these cells remain quiescent.

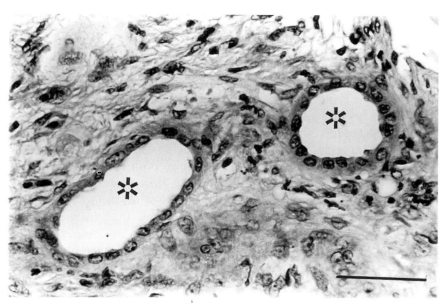

Figure 21. Extensive fibrosis in the kidney following a bout of severe widespread oncotic necrosis. Tubules (*) are lined by flattened, incompletely differentiated tubular epithelium that is trapped within the scar tissue. Hematoxylin and eosin. Bar: 25 μm.

Although fibrous scar tissue may be well vascularized in its early stages, this neovascularization is not orderly with regards to providing an environment favorable for the regeneration of parenchymal cells but rather an environment favorable for the proliferation of fibroblasts and deposition of collagen. Contraction of the affected area occurs due to the "myofibroblast" function of the reparative stromal cells migrating into the area in response to signals from macrophages that have entered the site to scavenge cellular and stromal debris. The shrinkage of the affected area that results from the contractile activity of these cells serves to draw the adjacent tissues out of alignment. Whereas this may allow for quicker resolution of the defect and decrease the area that must be filled with connective tissue, this may have an adverse effect on adjacent viable tissues within the organ, possibly altering function. With the regression of capillaries and further deposition of dense type I collagen, which condenses over time, tissues are further pulled out of alignment by tough, inelastic, white (grossly) connective tissue that can serve as a permanent barrier to any future regeneration.

3. Sequelae to Apoptosis

The feature that distingushes sequelae of apoptotic necrosis and oncotic necrosis from each other is the lack of inflammatory response, in the classic sense of the word, in tissues in which apoptotic necrosis has occurred. In typical apoptotic necrosis, neutrophil chemoattractants are not generated so neutrophils are usually not observed even when widespread, massive apoptosis is present. Release of intracellular enzymes into surrounding tissue fluids or into the bloodstream is also generally minimal and insufficient to trigger an endothelial reaction, activate inflammatory cells (in particular neutrophils), or elevate the usual biochemical indices used to assess cell death in a particular tissue. Transglutaminase-mediated cross-linking of the cell membrane, stabilizing it into a rigid shell, is partly responsible for this. However, there are changes in the membranes of the apoptotic bodies that make them quite

attractive to adjacent cells and macrophages (Fig. 22). Phosphatidyl serine on the outer membrane of an apoptotic cell or cell fragment, everted during the cytoskeletal derangement that occurs during the process of zeiosis and the "immature" glycans that are exposed on the surface of an apoptotic cell, is especially attractive to macrophages.

As might be expected, atrophy is a common sequela to apoptosis (Fig. 19). Although this is unfavorable in the short term, due to loss of function, the atrophied tissue has the potential to completely regenerate, if the apoptotic stimulus is removed, as the supporting stroma is intact and unaffected by lytic enzymes from neutrophils. Furthermore, scarring does not take place and therefore there are no bands of dense fibrous tissue to inhibit regeneration. Finally, because apoptosis affects individual cells in "shotgun" fashion, and generally does not completely eliminate every single cell in an area, there are usually healthy, undamaged cells nearby that can replace the lost cells if the apoptotic stimulus is removed. However, in socalled "permanent" cell populations, where mitosis is no longer possible (e.g., neurons and retinal rods and cones), apoptotic necrosis may result in permanent loss of function.

4. Hyperplasia

Hyperplasia can be elicited by a variety of stimuli, both physiologic and pathologic, and can create a favorable environment for initiated cells to "fix" genetic mutations that can lead to cancer. In the context of cell injury, however, compensatory hyperplasia can be an important and visible response to both reversible and irreversible cell injury. This type of hyperplasia occurs when a portion of an organ or tissue is removed or damaged and the remaining portion undergoes hyperplasia to compensate for the loss and to regenerate the lost tissue. Hyperplasia of this sort can only occur in labile or stable cell populations with the capacity to undergo mitosis. Tissues such as liver or bone marrow are typical examples of tissues that readily undergo such reparative processes. The hyperplastic response may result in resolution

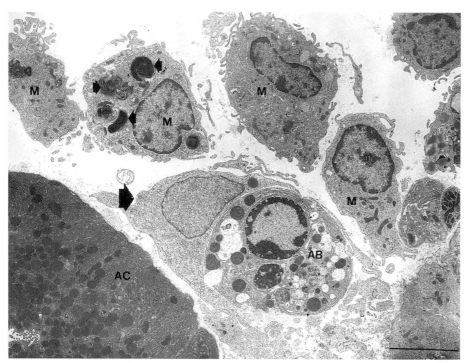

Figure 22. A macrophage (large arrow) ingesting an apoptotic body (AB) within the pancreas of a Fischer 344 rat in which extensive apoptotic necrosis has occurred. Tissue macrophages (M) containing ingested apoptotic bodies (small arrows) appearing as inclusions are present as well. Intact pancreatic acinar cells (AC) are also present. Bar: 15 μm.

of the lesion if the conditions are appropriate for orderly regeneration, e.g., intact stromal support, adequate vascular supply, and a suitable milieu of hormones or growth factors. Hyperplasia may also be inappropriately exuberant, unorganized, or even harmful if these factors are not present. Furthermore, the increase in mitotic activity increases the chances that genetic alterations that may have occurred during the toxic insult are propagated within a new cell population.

5. Metaplasia

Metaplasia, the reversible substitution of one type of fully differentiated cell for another type within a given adult tissue, can also be a sequela to cell injury. Metaplasia occurs when there is abnormal stimulation of tissue growth, generally because of faulty wound healing from a persistent toxic insult or constant mechanical disruption of the injured area. Metaplastic cells have a selective advantage over normal parenchymal cells in the area under the pressure of persistent toxic insult, but function of the affected tissue will be impaired because the original population of specialized cells has been replaced by less specialized cells. As with hyperplasia, metaplasia can predispose a tissue to neoplastic changes, as alternative biochemical pathways, inactive in the original cell population, are now expressed, possibly predisposing the tissue to further preneoplastic changes if oncogenes happen to be in those pathways.

IV. Concluding Comments

The descriptive information provided in the preceding paragraphs is in many ways "generic" in nature, portraying events as they should occur in all cells that are injured regardless of the insult that initiated the injury. It is a synopsis of numerous *in vivo* and *in vitro* observations made in countless studies over a large span of years. However, even though the morphologic manifestations of cell injury and death are in many ways stereotypical, especially at the ultrastructural level, there are nevertheless many minor and major variations that can occur at all levels—ultrastructurally, histologically, and grossly—that make each situation in which cell injury occurs unique. This is due to a seemingly endless variety of factors that modify or influence the response of the injured cell. Factors external to the cell, such as blood flow (or lack thereof) to the affected tissue, the impact of injury to other organ systems, the nature of the toxicant itself, absorption and distribution of the toxicant, the rate of metabolism and excretion of the toxicant, the innate inflammatory and immune response of the organism as a whole, and a large number of other factors, all have an impact on the reaction of the cell to a specific injury and, conversely, the reaction of the rest of the organism to the injured cell. Factors within the cell itself are also key in determining the exact morphologic pattern that will become manifest when the cell is injured or killed. Factors such as the degree of specialization, the function of the cell in the body, the dependence of the cell on oxidative phosphorylation, the degree of membrane turnover, and many, many others discussed here and elsewhere also contribute to the morphologic pattern of injury that is ultimately viewed and interpreted by the pathologist. The succeeding chapters in this book deal with many of these factors and situations from the standpoint of pecularities unique to each organ system and from the aspect of specific groups of toxicants and their mechanisms of causing injury.

SUGGESTED READING

Bosman, F. T., Visser, B. C., and van Oeveren, J. (1996). Apoptosis: Pathophysiology of programmed cell death. *Path. Res. Pract.* **192**, 676–683.

Cheville, N. F. (1994). Interpretation of acute cell injury: Degeneration. *In* "Ultrastructural Pathology: An Introduction to Interpretation" (N. Cheville, ed.), Chapter 2, pp. 51–79. Iowa State Univ. Press, Ames, IA.

Cheville, N. F. (1994). Consequences of acute cell injury: Necrosis, recovery and hypertrophy. *In* "Ultrastructural Pathology: An Introduction to Interpretation" (N. Cheville, ed.), Chapter 3, pp. 80–123. Iowa State Univ. Press, Ames, IA.

Cocoran, G., Fix, L., Jones, D. P., Moslen, M. T., Nicotera, P., Oberhammer, F. A., and Buttyan, R. (1994). Apoptosis: Molecular control point in toxicity. *Toxicol. Appl. Pharmacol.* **128**, 169–181.

Columbano, A. (1995). Cell death: Current difficulties in discriminating apoptosis from necrosis in the context of pathological processes *in vivo. J. Cell. Biochem.* **58**, 181–190.

Cotran, R. S., Kumar, V., and Collins, T. (1999) Cellular pathology. I: Cell injury and cell death. *In* "Robbins Pathologic Basis of Disease" (R. S. Cotran, V. Kumar, and T. Collins, eds.), 6th Ed., Chapter 1, pp. 1–29. Saunders, Philadelphia.

Cotran, R. S., Kumar, V., and Collins, T. (1999). Cellular pathology. II: Adaptations, intracellular accumulations and cell aging. *In* "Robbins Pathologic Basis of Disease" (R. S. Cotran, V. Kumar, and T. Collins, eds.), 6th Ed., Chapter 1, pp. 1–29, Saunders, Philadelphia.

Davis, M. A., and Ryan, D. H. (1998). Apoptosis in the kidney. *Toxicol. Pathol.* **26**, 810–825.

Duke, R. C., Witter, R. Z., Nash, P. B., Ding-E Young, J., and Ojcius, D. M. (1994). Cytolysis mediated by ionophores and pore-forming agents: Role of intracellular calcium in apoptosis. *FASEB J.* **8**, 237–246.

Farber, E. (1994). Programmed cell death: Necrosis versus apoptosis. *Mod. Pathol.* **7**, 605–609.

Farber, J. L. (1994). Mechanisms of cell injury by activated oxygen species. *Environ. Health Perspect.* **102** (Suppl. 10), 17–29.

Farber, J. L. (1982). Biology of disease: Membrane injury and calcium homeostasis in the pathogenesis of coagulative necrosis. *Lab. Invest.* **47**, 114–123.

Jones, T. C., Hunt, R. J., and King, N. W. (1996). Cells: Death of cells and tissues. *In* "Veterinary Pathology" (T. C. Jones, R. J. Hunt, and N. W. King, eds.), 6th Ed., Chapter 1, pp. 1–23. Williams & Wilkins, Baltimore, MD.

Kerr, J. F. R. (1971). Shrinkage necrosis: A distinct mode of cellular death. *J. Pathol.* **105**, 13–20.

Kerr, J. F. R., Wyllie, A. H., and Currie, A. R. (1972). Apoptosis: A basic biological phenomenon with wide-ranging implications in tissue kinetics. *Br. J. Cancer* **26**, 239–257.

King, N. W., and Alroy, J. (1996). Intracellular and extracellular depositions; degenerations. *In* "Veterinary Pathology" (T. C. Jones, R. J. Hunt, and

N. W. King, eds.), 6th Ed., Chapter 2, pp. 25–56, Williams & Wilkins, Baltimore, MD.

Lemasters, J. J., Nieminen, A. L., Qian, T., Trost, L. C., and Herman, B. (1997). The mitochondrial permeability transition in toxic, hypoxic and reperfusion injury. *Mol. Cell Biochem.* **174**, 159–165.

Levin, S. (1995). Commentary: A toxicologic pathologist's view of apoptosis or I used to call it necrobiosis, but now I'm singing the apoptosis blues. *Toxicol. Pathol.* **23**, 533–539.

Levin, S., Bucci, T. J., Cohen, S. M., Fix, A. S., Hardisty, J. F., LeGrand, E. K., Maronpot, R. R., and Trump, B. F. (1999). The nomenclature of cell death: Recommendations of an ad hoc committee of the Society of Toxicologic Pathologists. *Toxicol. Pathol.* **27**, 484–490.

Majno, G., and Joris, I. (1995). Apoptosis, oncosis and necrosis: An overview of cell death. *Am. J. Pathol.* **146**, 3–15.

Searle, J., Kerr, J. F. R., and Bishop, C. J. (1987). Necrosis and apoptosis: Distinct modes of cell death with fundamentally different significance. *Pathol. Ann.* **17**, 229–259.

Trump, B. F., and Berezesky, I. (1998). The reactions of cells to lethal injury: Oncosis and necrosis—The role of calcium. *In* "When Cells Die" (R. A. Lockshin, Z. Zkeri, and J. Tilly, eds.), pp. 57–96. Wiley-Liss, New York.

Weinberg, J. M. (1991). The cell biology of ischemic renal injury. *Kidney Int.* **39**, 476–500.

Wyllie, A. H., Kerr, J. F. R., and Currie, A. R. (1980). Cell death: The significance of apoptosis. *Int. Rev. Cytol.* **68**, 251–306.

Zakeri, Z., Bursch, W., Tenniswood, M., and Lockshin R. A. (1995). Cell death: Programmed, apoptosis, necrosis, or other? *Death Differ.* **2**, 87–96.

4

Organelle Biochemistry and Regulation of Cell Death

Myrtle A. Davis
Department of Pathology
University of Maryland School of Medicine
Baltimore, Maryland

Elizabeth H. Jeffery
Department of Food Science and Human Nutrition
Department of Veterinary Biosciences and College of Medicine
University of Illinois at Urbana-Champaign
Urbana, Illinois

I. Overview and Nomenclature

The terms apoptosis and oncosis are partly defined by morphological criteria, as outlined in a position paper written by the "Cell Death Nomenclature Committee" of the Society of Toxicologic Pathologists in 1998. The process of "oncosis" describes prelethal changes characterized by cytoplasmic swelling and karyolysis that are followed by cell death, whereas the term "apoptosis" describes a series of highly organized changes characterized by cell shrinkage and nuclear condensation prior to cell death. The term "necrosis" has always been used to describe all dead cells observed via fixed histopathology tissue section, regardless of the cause of death. Thus both oncotic necrosis and apoptotic necrosis can be used to describe the histophathologic features of dead cells in a tissue section. The term "programmed cell death" is sometimes used interchangeably with apoptosis, but more correctly denotes the clock-like timing of cell death that occurs during organ development and remodeling, rather than a pathological induction of death. This chapter reviews the cell biology and biochemical events that occur in key subcellular organelles involved in regulation of apoptosis, oncosis, or, in some cases, programmed cell death. This chapter is not an exhaustive description of all apoptotic pathways identified to date, or even all organelles that may play a role in apoptosis. Rather, it seeks, through reviewing the normal biochemistry of key organelles, to identify the underlying biochemical mechanisms responsible for the morphological changes described in the following chapter.

Cell death may be initiated by external signaling molecules binding to receptors on the surface of the plasma membrane that couple to the intracellular apoptotic machinery. Alternatively, cell death may be initiated from an internal signal such as DNA damage, disruption of normal mitochondrial function, or disturbances in the functioning of the endoplasmic reticulum (ER) resulting in ER stress, each of which, in its own way, triggers cellular signal transduction pathways that may lead to expression of gene products that regulate cellular response. The cell manages a complex array of pro-death pathways, balanced by an equally complex array of pro-survival pathways. Cell survival and death are constantly in balance, and as more is learned about these pathways, more checks and balances are found, pointing to a very finely controlled system. It will come as no surprise to the toxicologic pathologist that one of the controls is the dose of a toxicant and therefore the concentration of the activated signal transduction molecules: a low level may signal cell survival, whereas an exaggerated signal may swing the balance toward apoptosis. A massive dose may produce such extensive damage, for example, total loss of ATP, that the apoptotic pathway is overcome and oncosis results. Toxic substances may interfere with the normal function of the cell to initiate cell death in any of several ways, including acting as a mimic of a death ligand, or inhibiting an antiapoptotic or cell survival pathway. This chapter seeks to identify the roles that each organelle plays in this balance between life and death and the biochemical mechanisms that converge at key organelles.

II. Cell Membrane

A. INTRODUCTION

The cell membrane is a selective filter, protecting the cell from adverse aspects of the external environment and, through receptors, connecting the cell to the exterior via specific cell signaling molecules. A number of specific receptors act as the initial portal through which specific extracellular signals can trigger cell death. The membrane is attached to both the extracellular matrix and the intracellular cytoskeleton. During apoptosis, plasma membrane attachments to the extracellular matrix and the cytoskeleton are altered in an organized fashion, leading to the formation of membrane-bound apoptotic fragments. It is because membrane integrity is maintained during the early stages of apop-

totic change and during phagocytosis that the apoptotic cell, unlike the oncotic cell, is not associated with an inflammatory response. The cell membrane also plays an important role in directing the phagocytosis of membrane-bound apoptotic fragments.

B. MEMBRANE INTEGRITY AND SIGNALS FOR ENGULFMENT DURING APOPTOSIS

The cell membrane is an asymmetric bilayer consisting of a heterogeneous mixture of phospholipids, with phosphatidyl choline and sphingomyelin mainly on the exterior surface and phosphatidyl ethanolamine, phosphatidyl inositide, and phosphatidyl serine present on the inner surface. This asymmetry provides a difference in charge across the membrane. During the process of apoptosis, negatively charged phosphatidyl serine appears on the exterior surface. Annexin V or antibodies to phosphatidyl serine cannot enter the cell, but bind to these phosphatidyl moieties on the cell surface, confirming their location on the external surface in apoptotic cells. As the cytoskeleton disintegrates and the cell shrinks, blebs appear that bud off in the form of membrane-covered apoptotic fragments. N-Acetyl sugar moieties and the externalized phosphatidyl serine on the surface of these fragments are recognized by macrophages or neighboring cells, which then remove them by phagocytosis. The great speed with which these fragments are engulfed is reflected in the low number of apoptotic fragments present in a tissue at any given time.

C. RECEPTORS ASSOCIATED WITH THE CELL MEMBRANE

Receptors on the plasma membrane, many of which are transmembrane proteins, are involved in passing signals from the exterior to the interior of the cell. Binding of a ligand to a receptor can produce a conformational change in the receptor that leads to the production of signals within the cell. A common means to link receptors and the interior of the cell is through G proteins. Ligand-activated G proteins trigger a large number of enzyme-mediated pathways, such as adenylate cyclase and phospholipase C.

The latter catalyzes the metabolism of phospholipids on the inner surface of the membrane to produce cellular signal transduction molecules, such as inositol triphosphate (IP3) and diacylglycerol (DAG) from phosphatidyl sinositide. Other receptors act as catalytic receptors in that rather than participating in a G-protein link, the intracellular portion of the receptor has enzyme activity. Growth factors, such as epidermal growth factor (EGF), bind to transmembrane receptors that exhibit protein kinase activity on the cytoplasmic surface of the membrane and undergo autophosphorylation. This in turn triggers Ras and the mitogen-activated protein (MAP) kinases involved in cell growth and division.

When protein ligands that signal apoptosis arrive at the cell surface, these signals are interpreted by membrane receptors (death receptors), which then couple the external signal to the apoptotic pathway. This is a common mechanism for regulating initiation of apoptosis within the immune system. However, initiation of apoptosis by toxicants may be triggered from the cell surface or within the cell, bypassing the plasma membrane altogether.

A number of death receptors are associated with the cell membrane. A prototype example, the Fas receptor, is a major pathway for initiation of apoptosis. As with other members of the tumor necrosis factor receptor (TNFR) family, the Fas receptor is a transmembrane protein, having an external portion able to bind to a ligand and an internal portion that is activated when ligand binds externally, to transfer the death message to the cell. The Fas ligand may be present on the exterior of cells, such natural killer cells and macrophages, or it may be free in the extracellular space, secreted by other cells or by the cell to which it then binds. When the Fas ligand binds, it is thought to do so as a trimer, causing the Fas receptor protein to trimerize. It is the trimerization that is thought to produce the activation of the intracellular portion of the receptor, termed the death domain. Fas binding initiates a number of pathways for apoptosis, most particularly the caspase cascade, which leads to the destruction of proteins required for the maintenance of cytoskeleton and nuclear function.

The lipid ceramide is a metabolite of the cell membrane component sphingomyelin and acts as a second messenger mediating apoptosis. Ceramide is formed when ligand-activated plasma membrane receptors activate sphingomyelinase to cleave the bond between caramide and phosphoric acid of sphingomyelinase. It plays a key role in apoptosis following ligand binding to hormone and nerve growth factor receptors and TNFR family members, including Fas. Ceramide causes cell cycle arrest at G_0/G_1, as well as cell senescence, inhibition of DNA synthesis and inhibition of AP-1. Ceramide also causes a decrease in c-myc mRNA and triggers the activation of nuclear factor (NF)κB (see Section VI). The foregoing describes how receptor-mediated apoptosis is coupled to sphingomyelinase-dependent release of the proapoptotic molecule ceramide. Interestingly, apoptosis induced by DNA damage also triggers a ceramide pathway, but this ceramide is synthesized within the cell *de novo* rather than as a product of sphingomyelin hydrolysis.

III. Cytoskeleton

The cytoskeleton of the mammalian cell consists of a complex array of actin stress fibers (microfilaments), microtubules, and intermediate filaments. Actin has six isoforms, and each isoform is encoded by a separate gene that has tissue-specific expression. Microtubules are dynamic structures that serve as an intracellular scaffold and are composed of various microtubule subunit proteins. The intermediate filaments form a connection between the cell periphery and the nucleus, which facilitates linkages among the nuclear matrix, actin microfilaments, and extracellular matrix. Each of these components depends on a cellular equilibrium controlled by polymerization/depolymerization for proper function and each can play a critical role in mediating cellular processes such as cell polarity, cell division, cell adhesion, cell signaling, and cell death. We will specifically discuss the roles of each of these dynamic parts of the cytoskeleton in mediating cell death.

A. ACTIN MICROFILAMENTS

Intracellular actin exists as either a monomer (G-actin) or a polymer (filamentous or F-actin). The functions of the actin cytoskeleton are controlled by actin effector proteins that by binding actin, regulate a variety of cellular functions. The primary functions of actin effector proteins are polymerization, structural maintenance, and movement. The end result of the regulation of actin by effector proteins is a dynamic remodeling and quick response of the cytoskeletal network to stimuli. Many morphologic changes observed during cell death have been attributed to alterations in actin microfilament or actin-binding proteins. It has become apparent that during cell death, actin microfilament reorganization occurs early and is clearly detectable after an apoptotic stimulus. Second, the structure of various actin isoforms contains sites for caspase cleavage, and because caspases are activated during apoptosis, caspase-mediated actin cleavage has been hypothesized to occur during apoptosis. Surprisingly, actin cleavage has not been observed in several cell types induced to undergo apoptosis; however, in some cell types, β-catenin, a protein that connects cadherins (cell surface) to actin microfilaments (facilitating cell–cell adhesion), is cleaved proteolytically during apoptosis. Cleavage of β-catenin dissociates it from α-catatenin, which links to actin and α-actinin. Breaking this important link causes the cells to lose contact with each other and induces disorganization of the actin cytoskeleton.

The formation of cytoplasmic blebs during the apoptotic process also suggests a role for F-actin in cell death. In most cell types, apoptotic cell death is associated with a characteristic cytoplasmic membrane blebbing. When observing cells in culture, the blebbing process is highly active, showing both retraction and outward movement; the cell appears as though it were boiling. In contrast, blebs formed during oncotic forms of cell death do not retract but continue to expand unopposed until finally bleb rupture occurs. In oncosis, the disruption of plasma membrane cytoskeletal attachments also leads, at least in part, to bleb formation, but depletion of cellular ATP during oncosis may explain the difference in the type of blebs formed and early bleb rupture in oncosis. It is likely that several cellular events converge, resulting in actin cytoskeletal disruption in both apoptosis and swelling types of cell death.

B. MICROTUBULES

The vast majority of the evidence supporting a role for microtubules in cell death comes from observing the cellular effects of microtubule-interferring agents (MIA). In addition to antimitotic effects, the effects of MIAs on cells include activation of apoptosis. This response is thought to account for the cytotoxic actions of several MIAs. The popular chemotherapeutic taxol (a complex diterpone isolated from the western yew, *Taxus brevifolia*) binds specifically to microtubules. The binding of taxol to microtubules stabilizes the microtubules and induces microtubule bundling. Similarly, vinblastine, vincristine, nocodazol, and colchicines, by binding to efferent tubulin-binding sites, inhibit mitosis at G_2/M and induce apoptosis. Induction of G_2/M arrest by MIA may directly initiate apoptosis, or microtubule disruption may mediate apoptosis independent of G_2/M arrest via effects on apoptotic signaling pathways. Microtubule disruption has also been associated with the downregulation of antiapoptotic proteins bcl-2 or bcl-x_L. In addition, microtubule disruption can activate stress-activated protein kinases (JNK/SAPKs) and apoptosis signal regulation kinase (ASKI). It is an attractive possibility that the activation of apoptotic signaling may be mediated by microtubule disruption. However, it may be difficult to disassociate G_2/M arrest from the apoptotic response when using MIAs to induce apoptosis. This presents a unique challenge when attempting to confirm independent regulation of G_2/M arrest and apoptosis if microtubules are the primary targets.

C. INTERMEDIATE FILAMENTS

Intermediate filaments (IF) are referred to as intermediate because of their relative intermediate diameter of 10 nm compared to actin at 5–7 nm and microtubules at 20–25 nm. There are almost 50 IF proteins identified to date. These are classified by filament type. The filaments types are expressed in a manner specific for the tissue or organelle, e.g., neurofilaments occur in neurons, cytokeratin types are found in various epithelia, and nuclear lamins are found in the nuclear matrix of all cells. Proteolytic cleavage of IF proteins during the final phases of apoptosis has been hypothesized to facilitate final disposal of the dying cell. Just as the loss of actin cell membrane attachment will disrupt cellular attachment to ECM and cell–cell attachment, the breakdown of IF proteins during cell death will also disrupt cellular attachments. In addition, the cleavage of lamins (major structural proteins of the nuclear envelope) may mediate nuclear events such as DNA cleavage (see Section VI).

D. STRUCTURE MEETS GENE EXPRESSION AND CELL SIGNALING

The relationships among cell structure, cell signaling, and gene expression may provide important evidence connecting cytoskeletal structure to regulation of cell death. For example, Rho family proteins, members of the Ras superfamily of small GTPases, regulate a variety of cellular functions. Perhaps the most relevant of these to cell death are the effects of Rho proteins on organization of the actin cytoskeleton. In cell culture experiments that examined the cellular effects of Rho E and Rho 1 (from a subfamily of distinct Rho GTPases), it was demonstrated that microinjection of Rho E or Rho 1 into fibroblasts resulted in the breakdown of stress fibers, loss of cell adhesion, and cellular rounding. Similarly, stress-activated kinase p38 appears to regulate, at least in part, F-actin organization and early membrane blebbing in H_2O_2-induced apoptosis of endothelial cells. Taking these observations into account, it is interesting to further specu-late that Rho proteins may functionally regulate apoptotic morphology via cell signaling pathways. Furthermore, pharmaceuticals or environmental chemicals that specifically activate these signaling proteins may induce apoptotic morphology. These and other possible roles for Rho and other signaling proteins that regulate cytoskeletal function in the regulation of cell death are certain to emerge as studies progress in this rapidly expanding area.

IV. Mitochondrion

The origin, morphology, and biochemistry of the mitochondrion are somewhat complex compared to other organelles. The essential role that mitochondria play in the generation of cellular energy (ATP) and reactive oxygen species by oxidative phosphorylation make this unique cytoplasmic organelle a major regulator of various cell death response pathways. Several key biochemical steps that are essential to the induction and execution of cell death appear to converge on the mitochondrion and are tightly connected to the functional biochemistry of mitochondria. There are several basic features and functions of mitochondria that are important in regulating cell death. It is important to keep in mind that mitochondria among cell types are not biochemically identical; for example, enzyme composition and number of cristae differ between specialized cell types, but most of the functions and properties of mitochondria outlined here in relation to cell death are common to all mitochondria.

A. MITOCHONDRIAL COMPARTMENTS AND MEMBRANES: HISTORY AND FUNCTION

The origin of mitochondria is commonly traced back 1.5 billion years when it is proposed that an endosymbiotic association began between a glycolytic proeukaryotic cell and an oxidative bacterium. This essential hypothesis, explaining the origin of mitochondria, is key to understanding the biochemistry and the double membrane morphology of the mitochondrion. The inner membrane of the mitochondrion encloses the matrix space or lumen of the mitochondria and is phenotypically equivalent to the plasma membrane of an oxidative bacterium. The inner membrane is highly impermeable to ions and contains highly specialized translocators. Enzymes of the electron transport chain, essential for oxidative phosphorylation, are also embedded in the inner membrane. The matrix space resembles bacterial cytosol and remains isolated from cytosolic vesicular traffic. Several mitochondrial enzymes, DNA, ribosomes, and tRNAs are found in the mitochondrial matrix. The outer membrane is in contact with the cytosol and contains large pores constructed from porin and other ion channels, making it permeable to all cytosolic molecules and small proteins of 5000 Dal or less.

B. PERMEABILITY TRANSITION PORE (MITOCHONDRIAL MEGACHANNEL PORT)

Transport from the intermembrane space through the inner membrane is also regulated by specific pores and channels. One such pore, the permeability transition (PT) pore, (or mitochondrial megachannel port) is thought to be formed by a contact site between the inner and the outer mitochondrial membranes. An essential feature of apoptotic death signaling appears to be opening of the PT pore leading to a reduction in transmembrane potential. The protein composition and structural arrangement of the PT pore are only partly understood, but thus far it is thought to consist of the inner membrane protein, adenine nucleotide translocator (essential for ATP export to the cytosol), and the outer membrane protein, porin, which is a voltage-dependent anion channel. Regulation of the PT pore may involve several factors, including ions, glutathione, and sulfhydryl reduction. There also appear to be differences in the regulation of the PT pore between cell types and organs.

The open configuration of the PT pore may be key in the regulation of cell death by allowing proteins that are normally confined to *the mitochondrion* to gain access to the cytosol. In most cell types studied, the PT pore appears to be nonselective when opened. Opening of the PT pore results in dissipation of the H$^+$ gradi-

ent across the intermembrane space, uncoupling of the electron transport chain and expansion of the matrix space due to its hyperosmolality. Matrix expansion *due to the influx of water* can cause rupture of the outer membrane and release of matrix proteins into the cytosol.

The intermembrane space (between the outer membrane and the inner membrane) is biochemically similar to the cytosol; however, this space also contains several enzymes that utilize ATP and several cell death promoting factors including apoptosis-inducing factor (AIF), capsases, and cytochrome C. Movement of these proapoptotic factors from the intermembrane space to the cytosol is thought to be the key means by which mitochondria function to trigger a cell death cascade.

Because opening of the PT pore can result in a cascade of events that promote cell death, it is no surprise that antideath and pro-death signals converge at the PT pore. Anti-cell death bcl-2 family proteins are anchored to the outer MT membrane by a hydrophobic stretch of amino acids located within their carboxy terminus. It is not totally clear how the bcl-2 family proteins function at this membrane site. Experimental evidence suggests that bcl-2 may regulate opening of the PT pore, mitochondrial volume, release of proapoptotic factors, and/or release of mitochondrial cytochrome C. Although Bax and Bax-like proapoptotic proteins reside primarily in the cytosol, they too appear to act on the mitochondria by insertion into the mitochondrial membrane to form channels. These bax-induced pores can cause an increase in mitochondrial permeability or increase the permeability of the outer mitochondrial membrane, just as opening of the PT pore has been shown to do.

C. MITOCHONDRIAL SWELLING, PERMEABILITY, AND MECHANISM OF CELL DEATH

Mitochondrial swelling is a key morphologic feature of oncotic cell death. However, it appears *the cellular response (oncotic vs apoptotic cell death)* may be linked to that the extent of mitochondrial swelling. In oncotic cell death, the outer membrane ruptures, but in apoptotic cell death there appears to be an increase in mitochondrial permeability without rupture of the outer membrane. Thus, rupture of the outer membrane may be a major biochemical distinction between cells undergoing oncotic compared to apoptotic cell death. The extent and duration of pore opening and increased permeability *that results from this* may also be a determining factor in whether a cell dies by oncosis or apoptosis. Bcl-2 and $Bclx_L$ for example, have been shown to prevent toxicant-induced mitochondrial swelling associated with oncosis. Most toxicants that inhibit oxidative phosphorylation and decrease ATP cause severe mitochondrial swelling, and, in most cases, the cells show oncotic morphology.

The extent of mitochondrial swelling may also determine whether the cell recovers from an adverse event. It is possible for some degree of mitochondrial swelling to occur and this alteration can be a reversible, prelethal cellular change. Therefore, observations about mitochondrial swelling should not evitably lead to conclusions that the cell is dying or dead.

D. MITOCHONDRIAL PROTEIN TRANSLOCATION AND APOPTOSIS

Understanding the general means by which proteins are transported into the mitochondrial matrix is also helpful in understanding another potential role of mitochondria in apoptosis. Mitochondrial precursor proteins transported into mitochondria contain a signal peptide that has the potential to form an amphipathic helix. The mitochondria precursor protein is also unfolded during transport, and the unfolded precursor is protected in its unfolded state by cytosolic chaperone proteins known as chaperonins (i.e., Hsp 70 and Hsp 60 family proteins). Without these chaperones, mitochondrial proteins are not imported. Binding of the precursor protein to the chaperone requires an electrochemical gradient and release from the chaperone protein after translocation requires ATP hydrolysis. Once inside the matrix, the signal peptide is cleaved by a signal peroxidase, which gives rise to the mature protein.

The HSP chaperones may play a role in apoptotic cell death signaling by facilitating transport or retention proapoptotic proteins. An association between chaperone proteins Hsp 60 and Hsp 10 with procaspase 3 has been reported, and the activation of procaspase 3 is coupled to a dissociation of the procaspase 3 from the HSPS. Thus, mitochondrial chaperone proteins may function to retain proapoptotic proteins in the mitochondria and inhibit activation.

E. MITOCHONDRIAL ENERGY TRANSPORT AND CELL DEATH

Before discussion of the complex role of mitochondrial energy in cell death, a review of the pathway of energy production by the mitochondrion is helpful. Proteins involved in oxidative phosphorylation, i.e., electron transport chain components, ATP synthesis, and adenine nucleotide translocators, are located within the inner membrane. The transport of electrons from NAD^+ by the electron transport chain results in energy used to pump protons out of the inner membrane to create an electrochemical gradient (AU). The proton flux drives ADP phosphorylation to make ATP, which is exported to the cytosol by the adenine nucleotide translocator. The process of oxidative phosphorylation also produces reactive oxygen species (ROS; O_2^-, H_2O_2, and OH^-) as byproducts. Key enzymes such as glutathione peroxidase and mitochondrial superoxidase dismutase are essential for ROS detoxification.

Alteration in the production of ATP or ROS by the mitochondrial energy transport system can play an important role in cell death. Inactivation of iron centers of the electron transport chain proteins by oxidation inhibits mitochondrial ATP production. As stated earlier, it is not clear what the exact biochemical effects of antiapoptotic proteins $bclx_L$ or bcl-2 are on the mitochondria, but several key components of energy transport by mitochondria may be regulated by $bclx_L$ or bcl_2. $Bclx_L$ has been shown to promote the efficient exchange of ADP for ATP, permitting oxidative phosphorylation to be regulated by cellular ATP/ADP levels. Decreased ATP production will act in several ways to compromise the cell and ROS can cause similarly harmful effects. Increased production of ROS by the mitochondrial energy transport system or decreased detoxification of ROS can damage mitochondria directly (also indirectly by interfering with ATP production) and damage cellular protein lipids.

As with mitochondrial swelling, the results of several studies have suggested that the extent of ATP loss or ROS production is a crucial determinant as to whether a cell will undergo oncotic or apoptotic cell death. High levels of ROS production accompanied by extensive damage to mitochondria will induce oncosis in most cell types. The precise role of ROS in apoptosis is not clear, but ROS may promote an oncotic pathway by inhibiting the activities of proapoptotic caspases.

V. Endoplasmic Reticulum

The highly convoluted endoplasmic reticulum consists of a single lipid sheet or bilayer, enclosing a single space, the ER lumen. Morphologically, the ER exists in two forms: the rough ER, which resembles flattened membraneous sacs covered by ribosomes, and the smooth ER, devoid of ribosomes and appearing as an interconnected series of branching tubules. The rough and smooth ER carry out distinctly different roles in the cell. The smooth ER is involved in carbohydrates metabolism, lipid biosynthesis, fatty acid oxidation, and the detoxification of xenobiotics. The rough ER is involved in the synthesis of proteins and in their posttranslational modification.

A. THE "UNFOLDED PROTEIN RESPONSE" TO ER STRESS

Following synthesis, proteins pass into the ER lumen, where they undergo several types of post translational modifications. N-linked glycosylation (addition of an oligosaccharide chain to the terminal amino group of the protein) or attachment to membrane-bound glycolipids is a modification involved in directing the proteins to their final destination. Formation of tertiary

structure, or folding, also occurs within the ER lumen. Unfolded proteins are held in the correct conformation by chaperone proteins, while enzymatic modification stabilizes this conformation. For example, disulfide bond formation is catalyzed by protein disulfide isomerase within the uniquely oxidizing environment of the ER lumen. Several ER resident proteins are known as chaperone proteins because they are involved in directing the translocation of the folded proteins to their final destination within, or external to, the cell. Accumulation of unfolded proteins within the ER triggers an ER stress response in which a message, the "unfolded protein response" (UPR), is passed to the nucleus, resulting in the upregulation of ER-resident chaperone protein synthesis. It is the synthesis of chaperone proteins in response to heat stress that resulted in their common name: heat shock proteins. Further synthesis of unfolded proteins is downregulated and the N-linked glycosylation of proteins is halted during the UPR. If, following the increased synthesis of chaperone proteins, defective unfolded proteins cannot be folded and transported correctly, they may be "retrotranslocated" to the cytosol for ubiqitination and degradation. Disruption of posttranslational handling of proteins within the ER can also result in the initiation of apoptosis.

The major site of cellular phospholipid synthesis is at the cytoslic side of the ER membrane. The ER contains phospholipid-specific phospholipid translocators that can flip-flop lipids between cytosolic and lumenal sides of the membrane, permitting both faces of the membrane to grow by the insertion of newly synthesized phospholipids, while maintaining an asymmetry directed by the specificity and activity of the phospholipid-specific translocators. Vesicles can bud off the ER and fuse with membranes at other locations within the cell. Alternatively, phospholipid transfer proteins may catalyze the passage of phospholipids from the ER to other sites. The "UPR" signal produced during ER stress can also be triggered by changes in phospholipid metabolism in addition to changes in protein folding. In this

74

scenario, upregulation of the UPR occurs *as a result of* changes in inositol levels. Not only do unfolded protein and inositol levels trigger an UPR, but the UPR subsequently triggers the upregulation of both chaperone protein synthesis and some key enzymes in phospholipid biosynthesis.

B. ER STRESS AND CALCIUM

The ER is a major store of intracellular calcium (Ca), maintaining a gradient between cytosol ($10^{-7}\,M$) and lumen ($10^{-3}\,M$) similar to the gradient across the plasma membrane. Maintenance of the high ER lumenal Ca level is dependent on membrane-bound Ca ATPase that pumps Ca from the cytosol into the ER lumen. The high Ca ion concentration within the lumen of the ER facilitates posttranslational processing of proteins. The ER membrane also contains receptors, regulated by intracellular signals, for the release of Ca. Normally, inositol 1,4,5-triphosphate receptors are triggered by an IP3 signal to release the ER stores of Ca into the cytosol and trigger signaling by a variety of factors. In pathologic situations, Ca release from the ER can disrupt normal Ca homeostasis, decreasing ER lumenal Ca levels and raising cytosolic Ca. This shift in Ca homeostasis alters the activities of Ca-dependent enzymes in both the ER lumen and the cytosol. For example, the loss of Ca in the ER lumen can compromise protein processing. Within the cytosol, the increase in Ca can trigger a cascade of kinases resulting in transcription factor activation. Pro-apoptotic proteolytic enzymes (i.e., caspases, calpains) are also activated, indicating a link between the disruption in ER Ca homeostasis and apoptosis.

Toxicants such as thapsigargin, which inhibit the ER-dependent Ca ATPase that normally pumps Ca from the cytosol to the ER lumen, have been found to induce apoptosis and oncosis. Inhibition of the Ca-ATPase by thapsigargin is associated with release of both Ca and endogenous ROS from the ER into the cytosol. Normally, several enzymes at the smooth ER, including cytochrome P450, produce ROS as a by-product, which supplies the ER with an endogenous pool of ROS. Because ROS release into the cytosol following thapsigargin treatment can be inhibited by Ca chelators, ROS release is thought to be secondary to the alteration in Ca levels. Whether both ER depletion of Ca and cytosolic appearance of Ca are required for thapsigargin-induced release of ROS or cell death is not yet determined.

C. CASPASE 12 SPECIFICALLY RESPONDS TO ER STRESS

One of the caspase proteases associated with apoptosis has been specifically localized to the ER. Procaspase 12 is released from the ER in response to ER stress and is activated by the elevated Ca levels in the cytosol. Three toxins that have been associated with the disruption of ER biochemistry, initiation of ER stress and apoptosis—thapsigargin, brefeldin A, and tunicamycin—have been evaluated for their pro-apoptotic activity in embryonic fibroblast cells from caspase 12 null mutant mice and found to be compromised in their ability to trigger apoptosis. Whereas thapsigargin inhibits Ca release from the ER, brefeldin A inhibits transport from the ER to the Golgi and tunicamycin inhibits N-glycosylation of proteins in the ER lumen. This suggests that, irrespective of the mechanism of ER stress, there is a localized response in the ER that regulates cell death. Further experiments showing normal activities of pathways involved in plasma membrane and mitochondrial-induced apopotisis clearly implicate the specificity of caspase 12 to the ER-dependent proapoptotic pathways.

Because cells from caspase 12 knockout mice are not completely protected from the cytotoxic actions of ER proapoptotic toxins, alternative ER pathways for apoptosis that are not dependent on caspase 12 may be identified in the future.

VI. Nucleus

The nucleus is a major target for many cell death signals, presumably because of its essential role in long-term survival of the cell and maintenance of cellular function. In this way, the presence of a nuclear initiation site for a cell death pathway ensures that irreversible genetic damage is not perpetuated, by removing any chance of replication or continued cellular functions. Several lines of evidence show that the nucleus of the cell can functionally participate in the regulation of toxicant-induced cell death and cell survival pathways. Aside from the fact that a cell without a nucleus has a limited life span (i.e., mammalian red blood cells only live 120 days), the nucleus can play a critical role in activation, translation, and implementation of cell death signals. Essentially, the same molecular machinery that the nucleus uses to centrally control both heredity of cellular function and gene transcription can be used to regulate cell death.

A. A REVIEW OF NUCLEAR STRUCTURE DURING CELL DEATH

The nucleus of the cell is generally composed of 10–15% DNA, 80% protein, and 5% RNA. It is surrounded by a double membrane (nuclear envelope) that controls the exit of products from the nucleus and the entry of products from the cytoplasm. The nuclear envelope is composed of about 25% lipid (which is the majority of nuclear lipid), low levels of cholesterol, and sphingomyelin. Another characteristic feature of the nuclear envelope is the membrane-lined channels or pores (observed in 1876 by light microscopy) that fuse the outer and inner membranes. Enclosed in the nuclear envelope is the nuclear matrix (lamina) and the chromatin.

The nuclear matrix is mainly composed of a protein framework (nuclear lamina), which is key to the organization of chromatin and nuclear function. The lamins are type V intermediate filaments (similar to those found in the cytoplasm) that have been specifically targeted to the nucleus. The polymerized lamins (A, B, and C) make up the nuclear lamina, which is normally attached to the inner surface of the nuclear membrane and to the chromatin. During mitosis, the nuclear lamins are serine phosphorylated (by the maturation promoting factor p34Cdc2/28-cyclin B complex) and depolymer-

ized leading to disintegration of the nuclear lamina. The disintegration of the lamina meshwork is an essential step in mitosis because it facilitates breakdown of the nuclear envelope into small vesicles.

The chromatin is a highly organized and compact complex of DNA and protein. The most prevalent chromatin proteins are the histones, of which there are five major types (H1, H2A, H2B, H3, and H4). The chromatin is structurally organized within the nucleus by primary, secondary, and tertiary structures. The primary structure consists of the nucleosome (DNA and histone unit), the secondary structure consists of rosettes (six nucleosomes per rosette), and the tertiary structure of chromatin is the further folding of the rosettes into supercoiled loops. Chromatin condensation also occurs during mitosis, and the phosphorylation of histone proteins by p34 kinase is essential for this feature.

B. NUCLEAR STRUCTURE DURING CELL DEATH

Changes in nuclear structure and chromatin organization can be characteristic in both oncotic and apoptotic cell death pathways. Notable differences in the characteristic changes in nuclear structure exhibited during oncotic cell death versus apoptotic cell death are also mechanistically important. In oncotic pathways, the chromatin appears loosely packed or normal until very late in the process. In the late stages of oncotic cell death the nucleus swells and the nuclear membrane is degraded (see following Chapter 5). In many instances of oncotic pathway activation, it appears that the nuclear membrane is a major target damaged by direct or indirect mechanisms, such as covalent binding and lipid peroxidation, resulting in the decomposition of nuclear phospholipids.

Changes in chromatin structure during apoptosis appears to proceed via a well-organized series of biochemical events. In contrast to oncosis, during apoptotic death there is a characteristic aggregation, margination, and fragmentation of chromatin. The nuclear membrane remains intact around the chromatin fragments during apoptosis. Similar to mitosis, during apoptosis there is early degradation of lamina, leading to collapse of the nuclear lamina and aggregated heterochromatin (condensed uncoiled chromatin). The nuclear lamina however, is irreversibly degraded during apoptosis by proteolysis, in contrast to the reversible phosphorylation and depolymerization of the nuclear lamina during mitosis. Caspases mediate lamin degradation during apoptosis by cleaving lamins at a single site, causing collapse of the nuclear lamina and heterochromatin aggregation. The aggregated heterochromatin is then digested by proteases and nucleases to produce a characteristic DNA 200-bp "ladder" in most cell types and larger 50 and 300-kbp fragments in others. Interestingly, some studies have suggested that nuclear morphology (i.e., chromatin condensation) can occur independent of DNA fragmentation.

Several nucleases may be involved in DNA degradation during apoptosis. Interestingly, some of the nuclease activities that degrade DNA during apoptosis appear to be regulated by caspases. For example, caspase-activated DNAse (CAD) is a cytoplasmic DNAse complexed with an inhibitor subunit (ICAD). Caspase 3 cleaves the inhibitor subunit, which releases active CAD, which degrades nuclear DNA. Temporally, the nuclease-sensitive regions of the chromatin (i.e., the highly acetylated regions) are digested *directly* and early, whereas the more organized heterochromatin requires protease cleavage for further breakdown of the chromatin into DNA ladders. Similarly, there is a DNA fragmentation factor, a 40- to 45-kDa heterodimeric protein that may mediate DNA fragmentation and this factor is activated by caspase 3.

Several nuclear matrix proteins other than lamins are degraded during apoptosis, including topoisomerase II, poly(ADP-ribose) polymerase, and NuMa. Cleavage of these functionally diverse proteins, may work to ensure the irreversibility of the cell death process. It is interesting to note that changes in nuclear structure during mitosis and apoptosis in many ways appear to be morphologically similar and were once thought to be similarly regulated. As outlined

earlier, however, a major biochemical difference between the two is irreversible protein and DNA modifications such as proteolysis and DNA degradation that occur during apoptosis, but not during mitosis.

C. REGULATION OF CELL DEATH BY NUCLEAR TRANSCRIPTION FACTORS

A functional means by which the nucleus can regulate cell death is by the transcriptional activation of genes. Most evidence suggests that nuclear transcription factors and genes that have defined roles in other cellular responses (such as proliferation) are activated or induced during apoptosis and oncosis. The specific roles that these factors play in mechanisms of cell death may vary, but some transcription factors appear to have essential death regulatory functions. Two well-studied examples of death-regulating nuclear transcription factors, C-myc and NFkB, are described.

1. C-Myc

C-Myc protein is a member of a family of proteins that regulate cell proliferation and apoptosis. The ability of c-myc to regulate apoptotic cell death results from the coordinated activation of c-Myc and several protein partners (such as Max) that facilitate DNA binding and activate transcription. C-Myc can induce apoptosis in several cell types and appears to be a major regulator of apoptotic responses induced by a variety of insults, such as hypoxia, glucose deprivation, cancer chemotherapeutics, and DNA damage. The intrinsic function of c-Myc that is mechanistically linked to cell death is unclear; however, several cellular factors appear to be linked to c-Myc-induced apoptosis. For example, ornithine decarboxylase (ODC) is an enzyme involved in polyamine synthesis and is essential for cell proliferation. C-Myc induces ODC expression, which may cause excess polyamine synthesis and generation of reactive oxygen species, ultimately leading to cell death by oncosis or apoptosis. Several cell cycle regulatory genes that are induced by c-Myc have been suggested as regulators of apoptosis. For example, the phosphatase Cdc25A is a target of c-myc that dephosphorylates and activates Cdc2, which regulates the G_1 to S transition. It is unclear how cdc2 or cdc25A mediates cell death, but cdc25 appears to be required for some models of c-Myc-induced apoptosis. Alternatively, c-Myc may induce apoptosis and regulate the cell cycle by distinct and separate pathways. $P19^{ARF}$, a protein encoded by INK4, is regulated by the p53–mdm 2 complex and has been proposed to have a specific pro-apoptotic role; however, the mechanism of $P19^{ARF}$ pro-apoptotic function is not clear. The role of p53 in c-Myc-induced apoptosis is also unclear, but an interaction between c-myc and p53 is supported by several studies. It seems that p53 is required for c-myc-induced apoptosis in some cell types, but not in others. Some investigations have implicated p53 in the regulation of expression of bcl-2 family proteins. In any event, the regulatory role of c-Myc in apoptosis and oncosis are currently being actively explored.

2. NFκβ

The family of nuclear factor κβ nuclear transcription factors regulates cell survival by inhibiting or promoting apoptosis in several cell types. In resting cells, NFκβ is inactive in the cytoplasm and bound to IKβ. Upon stimulation (by environmental factors or extracellular signals), NFκβ is activated and it translocates to the nucleus. Degradation of IKβα is required for activation and nuclear translocation of NFκβ. Degradation of IKβα is initiated by serine phosphorylation and subsequent polyubiquitination of IKβα. Serine phosphorylation has been reported to be carried out by NFκβ-inducing kinase (NIK) and IKβα kinase (IKK). Following phosphorylation, the newly modified IKβα is then degraded rapidly by a ubiquitin-proteasome pathway. Once inside the nucleus, NFκβ binds to a K motif on DNA and regulates the transcription of several early response genes.

The anti-apoptotic role of $NF_κβ$ has been demonstrated in several models of apoptosis, including Ras-induced apoptosis of NIH3T3 cells, nitric oxide-induced apoptosis, and anti-IgM-induced apoptosis of -lymphoma cells. Although the regulation of $NF_κβ$ is the subject of intense study, the precise mechanism by which $NF_κβ$ regulates apoptosis is complex and to date remains somewhat elusive. Whether NFkB functions as a pro-apoptotic or anti-apoptotic factor is still the source of some discussion. Some investigations actually support an anti-apoptotic function for NFkB. Differences between studies in cell type and induction mechanisms of apoptosis may account for some of this apparent discordance.

D. DNA TUMOR VIRUSES AND REGULATION OF APOPTOSIS

Many DNA tumor viruses encode products that positively or negatively regulate apoptosis. Because viral replication is dependent on host cell DNA synthesis, the virus would benefit by inhibiting death of the host cell. However, viral induction of apoptosis may play a key role in mediating the exit of nonenveloped, nonlytic viruses from the host cell for the dissemination of progeny. The apoptotic cell may aid in viral dissemination because the membrane-bound apoptotic body does not incite an inflammatory response *in vivo*. Either way, the viral control of apoptotic machinery in the nucleus is key to this regulatory pathway. The mechanisms by which viral DNA proteins interact with the host cell to regulate apoptosis are diverse. For example, the human adenovirus encodes a bcl-2 homolog capable of inhibiting apoptosis (and possibly oncosis/necrosis) of the *infected* host cell. In another example, the hepatitis B virus p X protein inhibits cell death by interacting with caspase 3 and p53, although paradoxically the hepatitis B virus gene X appears to have proapoptotic activity. In some instances, viral proteins interact directly with apoptotic machinery. For example, Pox viruses encode the Crm A protein, which prevents or delays apoptosis by inhibiting proteases. The 35 protein, encoded by baculoviruses, appears to function like Crm A. In later stages of infection, viral proteins may function to induce apoptosis. For example, the human adenovirus also encodes an E3-11.6K product named the Ad death protein (ADP), which when expressed late in infection kills the host cell. Similarly, lentiviruses such as human immunodeficiency virus type 1 encode a viral transcription factor, Tat, that upregulates expression of the Fas ligand and induces apoptosis of $CD4^+$ T cells. Several examples of viral products that regulate apoptosis are reviewed by Young and colleagues (1997).

VII. Extracellular Matrix

The extracellular matrix consists of extracellular substrate adhesion proteins and receptors that mediate the attachment of epithelial or other cell types. Several cell types, especially epithelial cells and endothelial cells, require attachment to an extracellular matrix for proliferation, differentiation, and cell survival. When normal endothelial or epithelial cells are prevented from attaching to an extracellular substrate or basement membrane, they normally die. The type of death they undergo is a specific type of apoptosis termed "anoikis," which, specifically refers to death induced by detachment. In the body, this process may be important in preventing detached cells from surviving a move to a new and inappropriate location. Investigations have shown that increased cell contact with the ECM or cell spreading decreases cell susceptibility to anoikis/apoptosis.

A. INTEGRINS: CELL–MATRIX INTERACTION

Cell adhesion to an extracellular substrate is mainly mediated by the integrins. Integrins are a family of cell surface receptors that transmit signals to the cell upon binding to matrix proteins, such as laminin, collagen, or fibronectin. The signals transmitted by integrins result in a variety of intracellular signaling events, protein expression, and rearrangement of cytoskeletal architecture. Two of the integrin–matrix-regulated intracellular signal pathways that have been found to mediate cell death are the focal adhesion kinase (FAK) and phosphoinositide 3-kinase (PI3K) pathways.

The activation of FAK is associated with cell spreading and appears to play a role in the maintenance of cell–matrix interaction suppression of cell death. FAK is activated by tyrosine phosphorylation, which is induced by integrin attachment to the extracellular matrix. FAK translocation, dephosphorylation, and cleavage have been observed in renal epithelial cells undergoing apoptosis induced by several toxicants including the nephrotoxicant dichlorovinylcysteine (DCVC). In the DCVC model, FAK cleavage appears to be mediated by caspases, but FAK dephosphorylation is caspase independent. Other studies have suggested that FAK may prevent apoptosis by association with PI3K, phospholipase A_2, protein kinase C, or p53, but the nature of these interactions is presently unclear.

PI3K is a multisubunit enzyme that, when activated, generates 3'-phosphorylated inositol second messengers. Activation of PI3K requires binding of the enzyme, via a SH2 domain, to tyrosine-phosphorylated residues of a receptor such as insulin receptor substrate 1. Integrin engagement leads to PI3K activation in normal epithelial cells and in similar fashion to FAK, PI3K activities (and lipid products) decrease when cells are detached from the matrix. The serine/theonine kinase, AKT, appears to be one of the downstream target substrates of PI3K responsible for the anti-apoptotic effects of PI3K. Inhibition of PI3K or AKT usually leads to anoikis/apoptosis. The mechanism by which PI3K/AKT signaling regulates anoikis/apoptosis may involve the AKT-mediated phosphorylation of pro-apoptotic protein BAD, which may inhibit the pro-apoptotic activity of BAD in some cell types. There may be other cellular factors, however, that are involved in the AKT regulation of anoikis/apoptosis.

Integrins also link ECM to the intracellular cytoskeleton. The sites at which the extracellular matrix links to the actin cytoskeleton are called focal adhesions. Integrins have cytoplasmic tails that interact with the cytoskeleton through a series of cytoskeletal proteins such as talin and vinculin. Through these linkages, the extracellular matrix can control cell shape and cell survival.

B. MATRIX PROTEASES IN CELL DEATH

Alterations in extracellular matrix proteins may also contribute to the regulation of cell death. Enzymes that degrade ECM, mainly matrix metalloproteases (MMPS), as well as cell surface proteins, appear to be capable of regulating cell death during development. Transgenic knockout animals lacking MMPS show increased apoptosis of specific cell types. For example, lack of gelatinase B, a metalloprotease that cleaves collagen 5, results in delayed hypertrophic chondrocyte apoptosis and delayed vascularization, which results in aberrant ossification of the long bones. Similarly, loss of the MMP tissue plasminogen activator (TPA) renders neurons in the hippocampus resistant to cell death induced by excitotoxin. In TPA null mice, laminin (the matrix protein substrate for TPA) is not cleaved in the response to excitotoxin, implicating that the degradation of laminin may be important in the induction of hippocampal neuron cell death.

The control of cell death during development is tightly paired with MMP expression in both nonmammalian and mammalian systems. For example, the *xenopus* MMP gene, ST-3, is upregulated during tail resorption in cells where cell death takes place. In mammals, the upregulation of MMP genes has been observed in various tissues during remodeling (i.e., primary and connective tissue of the postlactational mammary gland). It is also important to note that the activities of MMPs can be inhibited by tissue inhibitors of MMPs (TIMPS). The expression and activities of TIMPS are usually the reciprocal of the expression and activities of MMPs during organ remodeling.

VIII. Summary

Research into the pathways involved in cell depth is one of the most rapidly moving fields today. A major reason for the intense interest in this field is the newly recognized relationship between apoptosis and cancer. When apoptosis is arrested, and therefore fails to remove genetically altered cells, proliferation goes unchecked

and carcinogenesis results. Only relatively recently have we started to realize that although many cancer chemotherapeutic agents induce oncosis, several also act through their ability to overcome the cancer cell's block in apoptosis and cause the natural demise of the genetically altered cell. Suppression of apoptosis has been proposed as a major mechanism for the action of nongenotoxic carcinogens and promoters such as clofibrate, phenobarbital, 2,3,7,8-tetradichlorbenzo-1,4-dioxin, and the tumor promoter used so commonly in experimental carcinogenesis, tetradecanoylphorbol ester. The latter is probably the best understood, activating protein kinase C to trigger the enhanced expression of Fos and Jun, resulting in increased AP-1 activation.

While the benefits of apoptosis relative to those of oncosis are commonly enumerated, there are circumstances where apoptosis has adverse effects on the organism. For example, apoptosis can aid in viral dispersal, as virally contaminated cells or cell fragments can be phagocytosed by neighboring cells. It remains to be seen whether there are circumstances where toxic metabolites, perhaps those causing oxidative damage, may also spread from cell to cell through phagocytosis of apoptotic fragments.

Until recently, receptor-driven pathways that initiated apoptosis at the plasma membrane or disruption of mitochondrial physiology leading to caspase 9 activation appeared to be the two major sites for the initiation of apoptosis. The unfolding of the role of caspase 12 in ER stress-induced apoptosis suggests (1) that caspases localized to organelles may also be independent sites for the initiation of apoptosis and (2) that new signaling pathways are bound to be uncovered in the future.

SUGGESTED READING

Filipski, J., Leblanc, J., Youdale, T., Sikorska, M., and Walker, P. R. (1990). Periodicity of DNA folding in higher order chromatin structures. *EMBO J* **9**, 1319–1327.

Gómez, J., García-Domingo, D., Martínez, A. C., and Rebollo, A. (1997). Role of NF-κB in the control of apoptotic and proliferative responses in IL-2-responsive T cells. *Front. Biosci.* **2**, d49–d60.

Kaufmann, S. H. (ed.) (1997). "Apoptosis: Pharmacological Implications and Therapeutic Opportunities". Academic Press, San Diego.

Kroemer, G., Dallaporta, B., and Resche-Rigon, M. (1998). The mitochondrial death/life regulator in apoptosis and necrosis. *Annu. Rev. Physiol.* **60**, 619–642.

Levin, S. (1998) Toxicological highlights. Apoptosis, necrosis, or oncosis: What is your diagnosis? A report from the Cell Death Nomenclature Committee of the Society of Toxicologic Pathologists. *Toxicol Sci.* **41**, 155–156.

Lockshin, R. A., Zakeri, Z., and Tilly, J. L. (eds.) (1998). "When Cells Die". Wiley-Liss, New York.

Margulis, L. (1975). Symbiotic theory of the origin of eukaryotic organelles; criteria for proof. *Symp. Soc. Exp. Biol.* **29**, 21–38.

Nagy, L., Thomazy, V. A., Heyman, R. A., and Davies, P. J. A. (1998). Retinoid-induced apoptosis in normal and neoplastic tissues *Cell Death Differ.* **5**:11–10.

Nakaagawa, T., Zhu, H., Morishima, N., Lu, E., Xu, J., Ynakers, B. A., and Yuan, J. (2000). Caspase-12 mediates endoplasmic-reticulum-specific apoptosis and cytotoxicity by amyloid-β. *Nature* **403**, 98–103.

Roberts, R. (ed.) (2000). "Apoptosis in Toxicology." Taylor & Francis

Thompson, E. B. (1998). The many roles of c-Myc in apoptosis. *Annu. Rev. Physiol.* **60**, 575–600.

Young, L. S., Dawson, C. W., and Eliopoulos, A. G. (1997). Viruses and apoptosis. *Br. Med. Bull.* **53**, 509–521.

Zamzami, N., Brenner, C., Marzo, I., Susin, S.A., and Kroemer, G. (1998). Subcellular and submitochondrial mode of action of Bcl-2-like oncoproteins. *Oncogene* **16**, 2265–2282.

81

———————————— *5* ————————————

Carcinogenesis

Stephen Mastorides
Department of Pathology
Memorial Sloan-Kettering Cancer Center
Division of Molecular Pathology
New York, New York

R. R. Maronpot
Laboratory of Experimental Pathology
National Institute of Environmental Health Sciences
National Institutes of Health
Research Triangle Park, North Carolina

"Cancer plays the part of a parasite of an organic species, whose object is to substitute itself for others."
Velpeau, 1854

I. Introduction

It is accepted today that cancer originates in single cells and develops through the clonal proliferation of their progeny. However, the search for a comprehensive theory of carcinogenesis has not been an easy road. Two predominant and antagonistic theories, humoralist and cellular, dominated most of the second half of the 19th century. The humoralist regarded cancer as originating from certain hereditary characteristics of the individual associated with susceptibility to contract the disease. Cellular pathologists such as Muller and Virchow, however, argued that cancer was related to a form of chronic irritation. This latter view was supported by experimental studies in mouse skin where wounding seemed to play a tumorigenic role. Experimental carcinogenesis has further defined our current view of neoplasia

ever since the experiments performed by Yamigawa, who induced skin cancer in rabbits by painting their ears continuously with benzene solutions of tar. Over the succeeding two centuries, hundreds of chemicals have been shown to transform cells *in vitro* and to be carcinogenic in animals. Some of the most potent have been extracted from fossil fuels or are synthetic products created by industry. However, a variety of occupational causes of cancer had been documented prior to the industrial revolution. In 1531, Paracelsus had described the "mala metallorum" among miners for silver and other metals, including uranium. This observation was later interpreted as radiation-induced lung cancer. In 1775, Pott attributed scrotal skin cancers to prolonged exposure to soot in chimney sweeps. A few years later, on the basis of this observation, the Danish Chimney Sweeps Guild ruled that its members must bathe daily. No public health measure since that time has so successfully controlled a form of cancer.

Cancers related to industrial activity were reported early in the industrial age in several locations with increasing frequency. Examples include the "analine" bladder cancer related to the systemic effects of napthylamines and the "paraffin cancer" caused by exposure to shale oil. The interest in industrial carcinogens coexisted with the realization that a definitive cause–effect relationship existed between tobacco and cancer. Early reports by Hill in 1761, which called attention to the association of "immoderate use of snuff" and the development of "polypusses," later received experimental confirmation by Roffo in 1931 when he induced skin cancer in rabbits by painting with tobacco-derived tar. However, tobacco tar was shown to be only a weak carcinogen in experimental models. Thus, a serious effort was undertaken to identify potential carcinogens using the mouse skin experimental model. Polycyclic aromatic hydrocarbons were the initial target of research. Benzopyrene, the most potent carcinogenic agent of tar, is present in the environment as a result of cigarette smoke and automobile exhaust fumes. It became the most intensely studied chemical carcinogen because of the belief that its chemical structure was related to that of steroid hormones. Steroidal hormones were at the time the only endogenous compounds reported to induce tumors in mice and humans. It was shown later that compounds with many different chemical structures could induce neoplasia. It also became clear that age and individual differences were contributing factors in the susceptibility to cancer, and these differences, presumably of genetic origin, could be inherited. Furthermore, it was observed that a long latent period could elapse from exposure to carcinogens to the development of cancer. In 1941, Rous and Kidd painted the skin of rabbits and found that if this painting was interrupted, tumors would disappear only to reappear if the application of tar was reestablished. It seemed, therefore, that a reversible process was taking place in those cells that did not attain the complete neoplastic state. These cells had undergone what Rous called "initiation." Further development of tumors would then require what was termed "promotion," the process by which the initiated cell expands clonally into a detectable cell mass that is either benign or preneoplastic.

Finally, cells must undergo additional changes in their "progression" to a malignant neoplasm. Today, it is known that for a normal cell to evolve into a malignant one, heritable changes involving multiple, independent genes are required. This multihit model is consistent with the incidence rates of cancer that increase exponentially with age.

It is estimated that 5% of human cancers are caused by viruses, 5% by radiation, and the remaining 90% by chemicals. Of these, an estimated 30% are caused by the use of tobacco products and the rest by diet, lifestyle, and environmental carcinogens. The importance of chemical products in the etiology of cancer is reflected in the fact that up to 8% of all human cancers are of occupational origin. All chemical carcinogens, or their derivatives, are highly reactive eletrophiles, which have electron-deficient atoms that can react with nucleophilic, electron-rich sites in the cell. Deoxyribonucleic acid (DNA), in particular, is made up of an array of nucleophilic centers at which these DNA-damaging agents can form adducts through one or more covalent bonds. To date, approximately 6 million chemicals have been identified and registered with the chemical abstracts services. Of these, more than 50,000 are estimated to be used regularly in commerce and industry. Less than 1000, however, have been scrutinized as to their carcinogenic potential.

II. The Spectrum of Proliferative Lesions

A. QUANTITATIVE CELL PROLIFERATION

1. Congenital Malformations

These proliferative growths consist of clusters of cells that are present at birth. They have limited growth potential, which is well coordinated with the rest of body growth. When body growth ceases in adulthood, these epithelial and/or mesenchymal cells also cease to grow. Examples of this type of cell proliferation include moles, hamartomas, and choristomas.

84

Teratomas can also be considered to fall into this category of cell proliferation but differ from those just described in that they represent true neoplasms. Teratomas result from faulty embryonic differentiation and organization brought about as a consequence of abnormal inductive influences. Teratomas are typically benign and are classically composed of cells from all three germ layers. They sometimes undergo malignant change.

2. Hyperplasia

Hyperplasia is characterized by an absolute increase in the number of cells per unit of tissue. It may be diffuse or nodular and is often accompanied by hypertrophy. Hyperplasia is typically nonprogressive in that it is limited in amount and terminates when the stimulus that evoked it has ceased. During hyperplasia, proliferating cells may appear less differentiated than their nonproliferating counterpart. This is believed to be a reflection of the fact that the cellular machinery is temporarily dedicated to cell division rather than to production of gene products for normal function of the fully differentiated cell. Different cells types have varying capacities to undergo hyperplasia (see Table I).

Hyperplasia is often classified to provide a basis for appreciating proximate underlying causes. It may be broadly thought of as either

TABLE I
Capacity of Tissues to Undergo Hyperplasia

High capacity: Surface epithelium
  Hepatocytes
  Renal tubules
  Fibroblasts
  Endothelium
  Mesothelium
  Hematopoietic stem cells
  Lymphoid cells
Moderate capacity: Glandular epithelium
  Bone
  Cartilage
  Smooth muscle of vessels
  Smooth muscle of uterus
Low capacity: Neurons
  Cardiac muscle
  Skeletal muscle
  Smooth muscle of gastrointestinal tract

physiological or pathological. Both categories of hyperplasia are characterized by an enhanced rate of cell proliferation.

a. Physiological Hyperplasia. Physiological hyperplasia is a normal process seen in development during maturation, e.g., bone growth, lymphoid tissue development, and liver growth. Hormonal hyperplasia is brought about by the influence of hormones on specific target tissues such as the mammary gland in response to prolactin or the thyroid gland in response to secretion of thyrotrophic hormone by the pituitary gland. Physiological adaptive hyperplasia, which may also be called compensatory, regenerative, or reparative hyperplasia, represents an attempt to repair an injury or disease that has resulted in loss of functional tissue. Frequently seen as a consequence of inflammation, it represents a response to an abnormal or pathological stimulus such as where lymphoid hyperplasia occurs secondary to local inflammation, in the healing of skin wounds, or in the union of bone fractures. The response here is normal or physiological even though the proximate cause may be pathological. Tissues undergoing adaptive hyperplasia do not exhibit excessive uncoordinated growth ("keloid" formation is an exception) and the proliferative response ceases when the stimulus is removed or the functional integrity of the damaged tissue has been restored.

Physiological adaptive hyperplasia may play an important role in the pathogenesis of neoplasia in that cells undergoing rapid cell division are at a greater risk to sustain a permanent genetic alteration that may result in the initiation or progression of the process of carcinogenesis. Clonal expansion of latent cancer cells may also occur as a result of regenerative or reparative proliferation.

Growth-promoting substances, such as cytokines, hormones, growth factors, and other mediators of growth control, play a critical role in the initiation, control, and arrest of adaptive or regenerative hyperplasia. These same substances and processes are probably involved in normal growth and differentiation and in neoplastic proliferation.

85

b. Pathological Hyperplasia. In pathological hyperplasia, proliferative cellular events are characterized by significant organization and cytological abnormalities. While the causes of pathological hyperplasia may be similar to those producing physiological hyperplasia, in pathological hyperplasia there is a change in intrinsic cell control that produces a subpopulation of cells that are less subject to normal tissue regulatory mechanisms. This cellular change leads to organizational and cytological abnormalities. Many forms of pathological hyperplasia represent instances of excessive hormonal stimulation of target cells, e.g., adenomatous hyperplasia of the endometrium.

In some instances, pathological hyperplasia may progress to neoplasia. Examples of this are found in human pathology where clinical observations and repeated biopsies provide a historic record supporting the association of pathologic hyperplasia and neoplasia. For example, endometrial carcinoma of the uterus is often preceded by or associated with pathological endometrial hyperplasia. Similarly, hepatocellular adenoma or carcinoma is closely related to compensatory hyperplasia of hepatic parenchymal cells seen in cirrhotic livers of chronic alcoholics and in hepatitis virus infection.

In humans and undoubtedly in animals, the majority of neoplasms develop without any previous reparative proliferation or hyperplasia of the tissues from which they arise. The coexistence of hyperplasia with neoplasia either in space or time is not proof of a cause–effect relationship between the two, although sustained elevated cell proliferation enhances the risk for cancer development

3. Hypertrophy

Hypertrophy is an increase in cell or organ size and results from an increase in the amount of cytoplasm and an increase in the number and size of cytoplasmic organelles. While not technically a proliferative change, hypertrophy deserves mention because it is sometimes diagnosed incorrectly as hyperplasia and because hypertrophy and hyperplasia may occur together. Hypertrophy is under various regula-

tory controls and, thus, is limited in amount and duration. Hypertrophy may be classified in a manner similar to how hyperplasia is classified. Compensatory or adaptive hypertrophy represents a physiological response to a stimulus such as is seen with muscle hypertrophy subsequent to prolonged exercise or in enzyme induction in the liver following exposure to chemical inducers such as phenobarbital. Hypertrophy can also be caused by hormones. For example, injection of growth hormone from the anterior pituitary induces hypertrophy of liver cells, which have an increase in their RNA content.

Whether the various types of hypertrophy are considered physiological or pathological depends on the philosophy of the person making the judgment. For example, because hypertension is a disease, then cardiac hypertrophy that occurs secondary to the hypertension can be considered pathologic. However, one could argue that cardiac hypertrophy is a normal physiological response to an increased demand for work, regardless of the proximate cause.

B. QUALITATIVE CELL PROLIFERATION

Qualitative changes such as metaplasia and anaplasia can occur in hyperplastic cells and represent one of the hallmarks of pathological hyperplasia. However, qualitative changes in the phenotype or in the association and organization of groups of cells can also occur in the absence of clear-cut evidence of increases in cell number.

1. Metaplasia

Metaplasia is the reversible substitution of one type of fully differentiated cell for another within a given tissue and is seen most commonly in epithelial tissues. The notion that metaplasia usually involves the substitution of a less specialized cell type should be avoided in that it involves a value judgment regarding whether a cell expressing a different set of genes is indeed less specialized. For example, squamous metaplasia occurring in an area normally populated by ciliated respiratory epithelium represents a situation where fully differentiated squamous cells have replaced the ciliated cells. The ability of the squamous cells to produce keratin is no less specialized than the ability of the ciliated cells to move the mucous blanket up the respiratory tree. Similarly, osseous metaplasia is the presence of cells capable of producing osteoid, a highly specialized function.

Metaplastic cells originate from cells capable of undergoing cell division. Each of these progenitor somatic cells carries the entire inherited genomic library of the individual. The phenotype of the metaplastic cell is merely a reflection of which genes from that library are expressed. Many highly specialized cells are terminally differentiated. Thus, they are not part of the mitotic pool in a given tissue and cannot serve as the origin of the metaplastic cell type. We generally consider that metaplastic cells originate from "reserve cells" (basal cells, stem cells) because these cell types are not specialized and appear to have their biochemical cellular machinery geared toward cell replication. However, even this notion has been challenged by the documentation that both respiratory basal cells and ciliated cells can originate from airway-lining serous cells, previously presumed to be terminally differentiated.

Metaplasia, especially in epithelial tissues, is frequently regarded as a protective response to insult such as irritation. It should be appreciated that this type of inference is teleological. The causes and regulatory mechanisms associated with metaplasia are unknown. Neoplastic transformation occasionally occurs at a site of metaplasia. This may be a consequence of a localized enhanced cell proliferation wherein genetic damage can be passed on to progeny cells before there is time to affect DNA repair. Alternatively, the insult may be sufficiently nonspecific in that it can alter genetic programming such that the cell may produce either metaplastic or neoplastic progeny.

2. Dysplasia

Abnormal formation or dysplasia of a tissue refers to alteration in its shape, size, and/or organization. Dysplasia usually affects but is not limited to epithelium and is generally reversible. In this form of qualitative cellular proliferation there is a lack of normal cell-to-cell relationships and orientations. In epithelial tissues, this is manifested as the disruption of normal cell layering. Dysplastic cells exhibit nuclear and cytological pleomorphism and increased mitotic activity. Dysplasia may be associated with chronic irritation, sometimes occurs along with metaplasia, and is occasionally associated with neoplastic transformation.

3. Anaplasia and Pleomorphism

Anaplasia is a qualitative alteration of differentiation. Anaplastic cells are typically poorly differentiated or undifferentiated and exhibit advanced cellular pleomorphism. In fact, anaplasia and pleomorphism are sometimes used incorrectly as synonyms. Pleomorphism refers to variation in the size and shape of cells. Several sizes and shapes of cells are usually present in anaplastic tissue, and true giant cells sometimes form. Anaplastic cells generally have hyperchromatic nuclei, prominent nucleoli, and a nucleus-to-cytoplasm size ratio that approaches 1:1. There is increased mitotic activity, sometimes with the formation of abnormal mitotic figures, loss of cell orientation, and lack of normal organization in the anaplastic tissue. Neoplasms, especially malignant neoplasms, are frequently composed of cells that are pleomorphic and anaplastic. In nonneoplastic tissue, anaplasia may represent the borderline between dysplasia and neoplasia.

C. PRENEOPLASIA

Patients or animals with preneoplastic lesions are at increased risk of developing neoplasia at the tissue site in which the preneoplasia is present. The preneoplastic lesions themselves are believed to progress to neoplasia, although unequivocal proof for this is difficult to document. Examples of preneoplasia from human medicine include leukoplakia of the oral cavity or vulva, senile keratosis, and xeroderma pigmentosum. Numerous putative preneoplastic lesions have been identified in laboratory animals, especially in animal models used to study the process of chemical carcinogenesis (Table II).

A well-studied example of preneoplasia is seen in experimental hepatocarcinogenesis studies. In experimental studies of liver neoplasia using rats exposed to potent hepatocarcinogens, the initial change detected in liver tissue consists of foci of cellular alteration. These foci consist of nests or islands of hyperplastic and/or hypertrophic hepatocytes that differe phenotypically from adjacent normal hepatocytes. Eventually, the rats develop hepatocellular neoplasms. There are several phenotypic types of foci of cellular alteration, and the ultimate neoplasms may resemble the foci phenotypically. Because of their consistent production by known hepatocarcinogens and their temporal relationship with ultimate neoplasia, these foci of cellular alteration are regarded operationally as preneoplastic lesions. Because the number of neoplasms eventually generated represents a very small proportion of the number of foci produced (estimates range from 1 neoplasm for every 1000 to 10,000 foci), conservative

pathologists regard the foci as "putatively preneoplastic."

The exact significance of hepatic foci of cellular alteration is unknown. Empirical observations speak both for and against their role in oncogenesis. On the one hand, hepatic foci of cellular alteration occur spontaneously in aging untreated rats that have a negligible background incidence of hepatic neoplasia. Also, in some experimental models, the stability or persistence of foci is dependent on continued exposure to a xenobiotic agent or feed ingredient. On the other hand, the consistent induction of foci by known hepatocarcinogens and the occasional observation of "foci within foci" suggest that these putatively preneoplastic lesions are related to hepatic neoplasia and may simply require an additional genetic perturbation to undergo neoplastic transformation. Despite the absence of definitive proof that hepatic foci of cellular alteration are precursor lesions for hepatic neoplasms, several investigators have identified chemicals as having hepatocarcinogenic activity based only on induction of foci by these chemicals. It has been proposed that regulatory decisions regarding the production, distribution, and use of chemicals can be based on the observation that they induce foci of cellular alteration in rat carcinogenicity studies.

D. NEOPLASTIC CELL PROLIFERATION

Benign comes from the Latin word "benignus" and means innocuous. A benign neoplasm is a localized growth. Its growth is by expansion and it may produce compression of adjacent normal tissues. Benign neoplasms ordinarily grow very slowly and are usually not life-threatening unless they interfere with normal function by blocking an organ, such as the intestine, or compressing vital areas, such as in the brain. Characteristic features of benign neoplasia are listed in Table III. Controversy regarding the significance of benign neoplasia with respect to the development of malignancy is similar to that associated with preneoplastic lesions. In chemical carcinogenicity tests using rodents, carcinogens frequently produce both

TABLE II
Examples of Presumptive Preneoplastic Lesions

Tissue	Presumptive preneoplastic lesion[a]
Mammary gland	Hyperplastic alveolar nodules Atypical epithelial proliferation Lobular hyperplasia Intraductal hyperplasia Hyperplastic terminal duct
Liver	Foci of cellular alteration Hepatocellular hyperplasia Oval cell proliferation Cholangiofibrosis
Kidney	Karyocytomegaly Atypical tubular dilation Atypical tubular hyperplasia
Skin	Increase in dark basal keratinocytes Focal hyperplasia/hyperkeratosis
Pancreas (exocrine)	Foci of acinar cell alteration Hyperplastic nodules Atypical acinar cell nodules

[a]Many of these presumptive preneoplasic lesions are seen in carcinogenicity studies utilizing specific animal model systems. Generalizations about these presumptive preneoplastic lesions are inappropriate outside the context of the specific animal model system being used.

TABLE III
Comparative Features of Benign and Malignant Neoplasms

	Benign	Malignant
General effect on the host	Little; usually does not cause death	Will almost always kill the host if untreated
Rate of growth	Slow; may stop or regress	More rapid (but slower than "repair" tissue); autonomous; never stops or regresses
Histologic features	Encapsulated; remains localized at primary site	Infiltrates or invades; metastasizes
Mode of growth	Usually grows by exansion, displacing surrounding normal tissue	Invades, destroys and replaces surrounding normal tissue
Metastasis	Do not metastasize	Most can metastasize
Architecture	Encapsulated; have complex stroma and adequate blood supply	Not encapsulated; usually have poorly developed stroma; may become necrotic at center
Danger to host	Most are without lethal significance	Always ultimately lethal unless removed or destroyed *in situ*
Injury to host	Usually negligible but may become very large and compress or obstruct vital tissue	Can kill host directly by destruction of vital tissue
Radiation sensitivity	Radiation sensitivity near that of normal parent cell; rarely treated with radiation	Radiation sensitivity increased in rough proportion to malignancy; often treated with radiation
Behavior in tissue	Cells are cohesive and inhibited by mutual contact	Cells do not cohere; frequently not inhibited by mutual contact
Resemblance to tissue	Cells and architecture resemble tissue of origin	Cells atypical and and plemorphic; disorganized bizarre architecture
Mitotic figures	Mitotic figures are rare and normal	Mitotic figures may be numerous and abnormal in polarity and configuration
Shape of nucleus	Normal and regular; show usual stain affinity	Irregular; nucleus frequently hyperchromatic
Size of nucleus	Normal; ratio of nucleus to cytoplasm near normal	Frequently large; nucleus-to-cytoplasm ratio increased
Nucleolus	Not conspicuous	Hyperchromatic and larger than normal

benign and malignant neoplasms of a given tissue, and morphologic evidence exists that the benign lesions progress to malignancy in some studies.

Malignant comes from the Latin word "malignus" and means malicious. Malignant neoplasms grow rapidly and are characterized by local invasiveness. Areas of necrosis seen in some malignant neoplasms presumably result when growth is so rapid that the neoplastic tissue outgrows the existing blood supply. Malignant growth is disorganized and such neoplasms may spread by extension into adjacent organs or by metastasis to distant sites via blood and lymphatic circulation. Characteristics of malignant neoplasms are listed in Table III. Although malignancy develops with greater frequency in chronic inflammation, hyperplasia, metaplasia, and even in benign neoplasia than in normal tissue, these lesions are not

necessarily precursors to malignancy. It is more probable that any malignancy that results is a consequence of the same stimulus that produced the other pathological proliferative lesions interacting with other critical intrinsic and/or extrinsic factors.

Some malignant neoplasms, particularly carcinomas, at some time in their evolution are at an intraepithelial or "*in situ*" stage. *In situ* carcinomas are microscopic lesions that have cytological criteria of malignancy, but are localized and have not gone beyond the basement membrane.

E. DIAGNOSTIC DISTINCTION AMONG PRENEOPLASIA, BENIGN NEOPLASIA, AND MALIGNANT NEOPLASIA

Given the presence of specific hallmarks of malignancy (e.g., anaplasia, local invasiveness, metastasis), there is usually little difficulty in obtaining consistent and concordant agreement among pathologists regarding the diagnosis of malignant neoplasms. More serious problems arise with benign proliferative lesions. Small lesions are especially difficult in that very little tissue mass is available to examine in a search for characteristic features that form the basis for diagnosis. A circular lesion consisting of 75 to 100 cells may be a preneoplastic change or, alternatively, a benign or a malignant neoplasm that has just started to grow. At this small size, even a true malignancy may not demonstrate features of local invasiveness. What the specific lesion is called becomes largely a matter of judgment by the pathologist. In the rat liver carcinogenesis model described earlier, such a small lesion would most probably be diagnosed as a focus of cellular alteration, even though it might in fact be a small hepatocellular carcinoma with minimal atypia. Alternatively, it might be a small hepatocellular adenoma but cannot be recognized definitively as such because it is too small to have caused significant compression of adjacent normal parenchyma.

Another problem associated with the evaluation of proliferative lesions, particularly in rodent chemical carcinogenicity studies, is the consistent categorization of lesions such as those that have some features of benign neoplasia and some features suggestive of malignant neoplasia. Even having well-defined diagnostic criteria, specific lesions will always be found that fall between two adjacent diagnostic categories. There is no easy resolution to this problem. Creating more diagnostic categories only creates more gray areas between the added categories of lesions. Pathologists must do their best to be consistent, particularly within a given study, and recognize the imprecision of the study results if diagnostic dilemmas were numerous. The hardest part will always be communicating to other scientists and administrators who use carcinogenicity data that even though some lesions carry the diagnosis of carcinoma, they could be equivocal and may be benign. The surgical pathologist can encounter a similar predicament. For example, the distinctions among a borderline ovarian tumor versus serous cystadenocarcinoma of the ovary, atypical ductal hyperplasia of the breast versus carcinoma *in situ*, the presence of stalk invasion in adenomatous polyps of the colon, and diagnosing dysplastic nevus versus early malignant melanoma are always difficult and diagnostically challenging.

One of the dogmas of diagnostic pathology is that size should not be a criterion for the diagnosis of neoplasia. Indeed, many slow-growing benign lesions, such as multinodular goiter, can grow to a very large size. All pathologists base a diagnosis of neoplasia versus preneoplasia or hyperplasia on definitive cytologic characteristics and patterns of growth. A size criterion would be helpful, for example, in categorizing focal pancreatic acinar proliferations or focal proliferative lesions in the pituitary gland when cytological characteristics of hyperplasia and neoplasia are identical and features such as compression are lacking. Furthermore, size has prognostic importance in soft tissue sarcomas and malignant melanoma. A size criterion would also be useful in consistently classifying rodent hepatocellular proliferative lesions when alterations in cytomorphology, growth pattern, compression, and other criteria are not found. Thus, in the absence of recognizable criteria for neoplasia, the pathologist could separate large foci of cellular alteration from small hepatocellular adenomas on the basis of size. In consideration of using a size criterion as described earlier, there are two caveats. First, size should not be used to categorize a proliferative lesion as malignant. Malignant neoplasms should have at least one feature of malignancy. Second, the size criterion should be used only in rare cases in categorizing specific proliferative lesions and not as a convenience.

III. Steps in the Neoplastic Process

A. OVERVIEW

The term "carcinogen" is generic. Under specific experimental conditions where dose and temporal sequence of dosing can be controlled, a given agent may behave as a complete carcinogen or as an incomplete carcinogen. The latter category includes tumor initiators, tumor promoters, and cocarcinogens. Even complete carcinogens may be without apparent effect when given at sufficiently low doses. In actuality, the practical limitations of our experimental studies may preclude obtaining absolute proof of whether there is a no effect level or threshold for a carcinogen. Whether there are actually chemical agents that are pure initiators or pure promoters is somewhat academic, as under sufficiently rigorous and specific experimental conditions, supposedly pure promoters and pure initiators have been shown to produce cancer. Thus, the terms complete carcinogen, initiator, promoter, and cocarcinogen are operational, being dependent on how the particular agent is employed in a given animal experiment.

Carcinogenesis may be considered as a form of toxicity in which cells achieve a different steady state from normal and do not respond normally to homeostatic mechanisms. The constitutive features of the cancer include an ability to invade, an ability to metastasize, and autonomous growth. The process of carcinogenesis is usually prolonged, requiring one-third to two-thirds of the life span to develop. While perturbations of cellular DNA are essential to the process, such interactions alone are not sufficient to bring about cancer in all cases. In some experimental situations, a few minutes of exposure to a carcinogen is enough to ultimately produce cancer, whereas in other experimental situations using the same carcinogen, usually at lower doses, cancer will not result unless the animal is subsequently exposed to additional types of chemical exposure. Simultaneous administration of a carcinogen and another agent may enhance, diminish, or block the carcinogenic process depending on the agents employed.

During the process of carcinogenesis, several phenomenological events have been documented. To be effective as an initiator of the process of carcinogenesis in the adult subject, a carcinogen must generally be mitogenic or cytotoxic, typically inducing cell death and restorative hyperplasia. This has been shown clearly in the rodent liver. Thus, cell death may play a key role as a rate-limiting step in the initiation of cancer in some tissues. Other evidence suggests that some carcinogens facilitate the growth of neoplasms by inducing immune suppression in the host. In addition, several environmental, hormonal, and dietary factors are known to affect the progression of transformed cells into malignant cancers. Loss of differentiation or possibly changes in patterns of differentiation and gene expression, such as altered cell morphology, alterations in nuclear-to-cytoplasmic ratio and chromatin composition, variations in DNA content, increased heterogeneity, loss of antigenicity, metaplasia, and dysplasia, are additional phenomenological changes that are documented in tissues undergoing neoplastic transformation. Finally, the chronological histopathologic study of chemically induced lesions shows repeatedly that many neoplasms appear to progress from hyperplastic proliferations to benign neoplasms and ultimately to malignant cancers. Thus, multiple stages in the evolution of proliferative lesions appear to accompany the carcinogenic process. These observations, taken together, provide strong empirical evidence that cancer is a multistep process and that a cascade of critical events is necessary for malignancy to develop.

B. MULTIPLE STEPS IN THE NEOPLASTIC PROCESS

Multistep models of carcinogenesis have proven useful for defining events in the neoplastic process and form the cornerstone of current hypotheses of the biological mechanisms of carcinogenesis. Multistage models of carcinogenic processes have been demonstrated in a variety of organ systems, e.g., skin, liver, urinary bladder, lung, kidney, intestine, mammary gland, and pancreas, by utilizing various experimental animal models. From use of these model systems, various agents have been categorized as initiators, promoters, and complete carcinogens. In the course of use of multistep models and development of hypotheses relative to carcinogenesis, the field of oncology research has been subjected to the generation of a lexicon that may cause confusion because of a discrepant use of terminology. Although there has been an attempt at standardizing terminology in cancer etiology internationally, there is still confusion. Practical and generally accepted definitions of commonly used terms are presented in Table IV. The operationally defined phases of carcinogenesis—initiation, promotion, and progression—are useful for discussion and understanding of carcinogenesis, but, in fact, each of these phases in the process may consist of multiple stages.

1. Initiation

The concepts of initiation and promotion were first described during experiments on mouse skin carcinogenesis but have since been applied to a variety of other tissues and species. During the initiation phase of chemical carcinogenesis, a normal cell undergoes an irreversible change characterized by an intrinsic capacity for autonomous growth. This capacity for autonomous growth remains latent for weeks, months, or years during which time the initiated cell may be phenotypically indistinguishable from other parenchymal cells in that tissue. Spontaneous

TABLE IV

Definition of Terminology Associated with Agents and Processes Related to Multistep Carcinogenesis[a]

Carcinogenesis: Process of generation of benign and malignant neoplasia in broadest possible sense.

Initiation: The first step in carcinogenesis whereby limited exposure to a carcinogenic agent produces a latent but heritable alteration in a cell permitting its subsequent proliferation and development into a neoplasm after exposure to a promoter.

Syncarcinogenesis: The synergistic enhancement of neoplasm formation by simultaneous or sequential administration of two different agents.

Cocarcinogenesis: The augmentation of neoplasm formation by simultaneous administration of a genotoxic carcinogen and an additional agent (cocarcinogen) that has no inherent carcinogenic activity by itself.

Promotion: The enhancement of neoplasm formation by the sequential administration of a carcinogen followed by an additional agent (promoter) that has no intrinsic carcinogenic activity by itself.

Anticarcinogenesis: The prevention or diminution of neoplasm formation by administration of an agent. Anticarcinogenic agents may be effective when given before, during, or after administration of the carcinogenic agent.

Progression: Processes associated with the development of an initiated cell to a biologically malignant neoplasm. Sometimes used in a more limited sense to describe the process whereby a neoplasm develops from a benign to a malignant proliferation or from a low-grade to a high-grade of malignancy. Progression is that stage of neoplastic development characterized by demonstrable changes associated with increased growth rate, increased invasiveness, metastases, and alterations in biochemical and morphologic characteristics of aneoplasm.

Carcinogen: An agent that causes neoplasia.

Genotoxic carcinogen: An agent that interacts with cellular DNA either directly in the parent form (direct carcinogen) or after metabolic biotransformation.

Direct carcinogen: Carcinogens that have the necessary structure to interact directly with cellular constituents and cause neoplasia. Direct acting carcinogens do not require metabolic conversion by the host to be active. They are considered genotoxic because they typically undergo covalent binding to DNA.

Procarcinogen: An agent that requires bioactivation in order to give rise to a direct acting carcinogen. Without metabolic activation these agents are not carcinogenic.

Proximate carcinogen: Metabolite of a carcinogen intermediate in the conversion to an ultimate carcinogen.

Ultimate carcinogen: That form of the carcinogen that actually interacts with cellular constituents to cause the neoplastic transformation, the final product of metabolism of the procarcinogen.

Epigenetic carcinogen: Carcinogen for which there is no evidence of direct interaction with cellular DNA. Synonymous with "nongenotoxic carcinogen."

Cocarcinogen: An agent not carcinogenic alone but that potentiates the effect of a known carcinogen.

Initiator: A chemical, physical, or biological agent that is capable of irreversibly altering the genetic component (DNA) of the cell. While initiators are generally considered to be carcinogens, they are typically used at low, noncarcinogenic doses in two-stage initiation – promotion animal model systems. Frequently referred to as a "tumor initiator."

Promoter: An agent that, when administered after an initiator or a low dose of acarcinogen, is capable of altering the expression of genetic information of the cell to cause clonal expansion of the initiated cell. Frequently referred to as a "tumor promoter."

Enhancer: Frequently referred to as a "tumor enhancer," an enhancer is an agent that increases the neoplastic response to a carcinogen or to a cryptogenic form of initiation. The term enhancer is used frequently in lieu of the term promoter in situations where there is no knowledge or implication regarding the agent's actual or temporal mechanism of action in increasing the neoplastic response.

[a] These definitions are considered operationally relevant and are in common usage. It should be appreciated that a given agent may function as a promoter in one circumstance and in a different temporal context may be a cocarcinogen. Depending on dosage, timing of administration, and/or frequency of administration, a given agent may function as an initiator, a promoter, or a complete carcinogen.

initiation refers to a situation in which the exact agent responsible for the initiating event is unknown. One possibility that can lead to spontaneous initiation would be a situation wherein there is infidelity in the action of DNA polymerase during normal cellular division or during DNA repair. Initiation operationally implies that there is alteration to cellular DNA at one or more sites in the genome. Such alteration represents a mutational event, which is hereditary.

Metabolic activation of a carcinogen to its chemically reactive products and their subsequent reaction with cellular targets (e.g., DNA bases) occurs within a few hours of exposure. Most tissues have the ability to repair this damage over a period of days or weeks. Currently accepted dogma suggests that the chemically damaged DNA, if not first repaired by normal cellular processes, is converted to a stable biological lesion (mutation, chromosomal rearrangement, etc.) during DNA replication. Thus, if a round of cell replication occurs before the DNA damage is repaired, the lesion in the DNA is said to be "fixed." This phenomenon may explain the high frequency of neoplasms in proliferating tissue where there is an intrinsically high rate of cell turnover coincident with exposure to a DNA-damaging agent. In contrast to the step of initiation, the conversion of an initiated cell to a fully malignant neoplasm is usually a prolonged process, lasting months in animals and years in humans.

Based on the hypothesis that most initiators are mutagenic or genotoxic, a battery of short-term *in vitro* and *in vivo* mutagenicity tests have been developed to permit the detection of chemicals with potential initiating activity. Identification of initiating agents is especially important because of the irreversible and hereditary nature of the alterations that occur during initiation. While useful when positive results are obtained, the predictiveness of short-term mutagenicity tests for the ultimate carcinogenic potential of xenobiotics is not absolute.

Exposure of experimental animals to chemicals with initiating activity may ultimately result in the induction of multiple neoplasms

in a given tissue. Each individual neoplasm is often found to be monoclonal in origin, having arisen from a single initiated cell. Application of techniques such as identification of cell surface immunoglobulin markers and glucose-6-phosphatase dehydrogenase variants, restriction fragment length polymorphisms, cytogenetic studies, single cell transplantation studies, and identification of chromosome inactivation mosaics has permitted identification of the monoclonal and polyclonal nature of individual neoplasms. The vast majority of human and animal neoplasms studied to date are monoclonal in origin.

There are several salient characteristics of initiation. It can occur following a single exposure to a known carcinogen. Changes produced by the initiator may be latent for weeks or months and are considered irreversible. The interval between initiation and promotion may be as long as 1 year in mouse skin painting studies and still yield skin neoplasms. Several lines of evidence indicate that initiation is additive and that the yield of neoplasms is dose dependent. Increasing the dose of initiator increases the incidence and multiplicity of resulting neoplasms and shortens the latency to manifestation of neoplasms. Because the initiating event must be "fixed" by a round of cell proliferation, it becomes obvious that initiation is dependent on the cell cycle. Finally, there is no readily measurable threshold dose for maximum and minimum responses to initiators. Unrealistically large numbers of animals would be required to demonstrate minimum responses, and confluence of multiple neoplasms following high doses precludes accurate quantitation of the neoplastic response. Properties of initiators are summarized in Table V.

Initiators interact with host cellular macromolecules and nucleic acids in specific patterns, typically involving the generation of reactive electrophiles, esters, or free radicals that bind covalently to nucleophilic sites in critical cellular macromolecules. The majority of known carcinogens have both initiating and promoting activity and can thus induce neoplasms rapidly and in high yield when given repeatedly. When

TABLE V
General Characteristics of Initiators and Promoters
of Neoplasia

Initiators/initiation

    Irreversible
    Additive
    Cannot identify initiated cells
    "Pure" initiation does not result in neoplasia unless promoter
      is subsequently applied
    Number of initiated cells dependent on dose
    No measurable threshold dose
    No measurable maximal response
    Agents are considered carcinogens
    Must be administered before the promoter
    Only one exposure may suffice
    Electrophile production and covalent binding to DNA
    Agents usually mutagenic

Promoters/promotion

    Reversible
    Nonadditive
    Agents not capable of initiation
    Modulated by diet, hormonal, environmental, and related
      factors
    Measurable threshold dose
    Measurable maximal response
    Agents not considered carcinogens but cocarcinogens
    Must be administered after the initiator
    Prolonged exposure is usually required
    No electrophile production and no covalent binding
      to DNA
    Agents usually not mutagenic

given at sufficiently low single doses, even a complete carcinogen may act as a "pure" initiator requiring subsequent promotion for the detection of any neoplasms. Under such circumstances, the agent can be regarded operationally as an "incomplete carcinogen."

A cell that has undergone the irreversible change that permits its ultimate neoplastic transformation may be phenotypically indistinguishable from adjacent normal parenchymal cells. However, when stimulated properly, it has an intrinsic capacity for autonomous growth. Most neoplasms are believed to be derived from the clonal proliferation of a single initiated cell. Usually at some point early in the clonal expansion, the differentially proliferating cells become phenotypically distinguishable from the surrounding normal parenchyma. Although such lesions may not as yet have sufficient characteristics to qualify as neo-

plasms, their recognition has led many to regard them as "preneoplastic."

2. Promotion

Promotion is classically considered that portion of the multistep carcinogenic process where specific agents, known as promoters, enhance the development of neoplasms from a background of initiated cells. The promoting agents themselves are so classified only in an operational sense. A promoter is typically given at some time after chemically induced or fortuitous initiation, and the doses of agent used are insufficient to produce cancer without prior initiation. It should be appreciated that when classical promoters are administered at sufficiently high doses and for prolonged intervals, neoplasia can occur without evidence of prior initiation. Under these conditions, a promoting agent must be considered a complete carcinogen unless fortuitous initiation from background radiation, dietary contaminants, environmental toxins, and so on is believed to have occurred. However, under typical experimental conditions commonly employed in short- and medium-term initiation–promotion experiments, neoplasia does not typically occur in animals that are not previously initiated.

The temporal sequence of promoter administration is critical to the operational definition of promotion. The agent must be administered after initiation and cause enhancement of the neoplastic process to be considered a promoter. If an agent is given simultaneously with an initiator and results in enhancement of the development of neoplasms, it is regarded as a cocarcinogen rather than a promoter. While some promoters such as phorbol esters are cocarcinogenic, not all promoters (e.g., phenobarbital, phenol) possess cocarcinogenicity and, conversely, not all cocarcinogens are promoters. Under these same conditions of simultaneous administration, a diminution in the neoplasm response is considered evidence of anticarcinogenic activity. Thus, several rodent liver tumor promoters (see Table VI), which are active when given after a variety of initiators, prevent or delay the development of liver

TABLE VI
Liver Neoplasm Promoters That Are Anticarcinogenic When
Added to Diets Containing an Active Carcinogen

α-Hexochlorocyclohexane
Cyproterone acetate
2,6-Di-*tert*-butyl-4-methylphenol
Orotic acid
Phenobarbital
Polychlorinated biphenyls
2-*tert*-Butyl-4-hydroxyanisole
3-*tert*-Butyl-4-methoxyphenol
1,1,1-Trichloro-2.2-bis (*p*-chlorophenyl)ethane

neoplasms when added to diets along with an active carcinogen. Finally, reversing the order of administration by giving a known promoter prior to an initiator may prevent the expression of carcinogenic activity on the part of the initiator.

While upper and lower thresholds have been demonstrated experimentally for promoters, some consider that, in an absolute sense, it is statistically impossible to unequivocally prove or disprove the existence of thresholds for promoters for much the same reasons that this cannot be done for initiators. One can never be certain that an apparent no effect level would, indeed, be without effect if a sufficiently large enough number of animals were used. Promoters include agents such as drugs, plant products, and hormones that do not interact directly with host cellular DNA (are not genotoxic) but somehow influence the expression of genetic information encoded in the cellular DNA. It has been suggested that promoting agents may cause gene repression and derepression in cells. Some experimental evidence suggests that the regulation of gene expression is unique to the nature of the promoting agent administered. Some promoters are believed to produce their effect by interaction with receptors in the cell membrane, cytoplasm, or nucleus (e.g., hormones, dioxin, phorbol ester, polychlorinated biphenyls). Alternatively, some hydrophilic–hydrophobic-promoting agents exert their effect through their molecular orientation at cellular inter-

faces. Other promoters are mitogenic, stimulating DNA synthesis and enhanced cell proliferation. This may occur directly or, alternatively, indirectly by selecting cells with a shortened G_1 phase, thereby giving them a selective proliferative advantage. At least in tissue culture, some promoters have been shown to inhibit intercellular communication (metabolic cooperation).

In some situations, metabolism appears to play little role in the action of promoters. Experimental evidence suggests that the molecule as a whole may exerts the promotional effect and that the molecular configuration determines the activity of the agent. When promoter metabolism does occur, it typically results in inactivation of the agent. Possible exceptions include D-limonene and trimethyl pentane (unleaded gasoline), which are promoters of renal tumors in rats.

Promoters appear to have a relatively high tissue specificity. Thus, phenobarbital functions as a promoter for rodent liver neoplasia but not in the urinary bladder. Saccharin, however, promotes urinary bladder neoplasia but not liver neoplasia in the rat. Similarly, 12-0-tetradecanoylphorbol-13-acetate is a potent skin and forestomach neoplasm promoter but has no appreciable activity in the liver. Antioxidants such as 3-*tert*-butyl-4-methoxyphenol and 2, 6-di-*tert*-butyl-4-methoxyphenol may act as promoters in one organ, antipromoters in another organ, and have no effect in a third organ. Thus, the practical definition of a promoter must include the designation of the susceptible tissue.

Tumor promotion may be modulated by several factors, such as age, sex, diet, and hormone balance. The correlation of increased rates of breast cancer in women following a "western" life style has implicated meat and fat consumption as playing an important role in breast cancer development. Experimental demonstration of the role of a high-fat diet in the promotion of mammary cancer in rats exposed to the mammary carcinogen dimethylbenzanthracene (DMBA) has been documented. Similarly, bile acids, as modulated by fat consumption, are known promoters of rat liver carcinogenesis. Age-and sex-associated modulations in hormonal levels of estrogens, progesterone, and androgens have been implicated as potential promoters of breast cancer on the basis of epidemiology studies in humans. Experimental studies have shown repeatedly that these hormones, in addition to pituitary prolactin, serve to promote mammary cancer in rats initiated with mammary carcinogens.

Some promoters cause hyperplasia and/or inflammation. This is particularly true in skin initiation–promotion studies using phorbol esters as promoters but is also seen in hyperplasia of hepatocytes following treatment with mitogenic agents such as phenobarbital. In the rodent liver, phenobarbital causes a transient hyperplasia of hepatocytes. It should be remembered that some materials can cause hyperplasia and inflammation but be without promoting effects. This has led some investigators to consider that the ability to stimulate DNA synthesis and cell division and the ability to induce inflammation are essential but not sufficient properties of promoters. Properties of promoters are summarized in Table V.

It has been suggested and confirmed experimentally that the process of promotion can be divided into at least two stages in the mouse skin painting initiation–promotion model. The two-stage promotion model is based on the stimulation of basal cell hyperplasia (dark basal keratinocytes) in stage 1 of promotion followed by enhancement of cell proliferation in stage 2. In the classical mouse skin carcinogenesis model, a phorbol ester binds to a membrane receptor, induces protein kinase C, and is effective with only one application, the process being at least partially irreversible, in the first stage of promotion. Weak or nonpromoting agents such as mezerein are effective as second-stage promoters but require multiple applications and do not always have receptor-binding properties. Similar multistage promotion has not yet been demonstrated in other experimental carcinogenesis model systems.

3. Progression

Progression is that part of the multistep neoplastic process associated with the development of an initiated cell into a biologically malignant cell population. In common usage, progression is used frequently to signify the stages whereby a benign proliferation becomes malignant or where a neoplasm develops from a low grade to a high grade of malignancy. During progression, neoplasms show progressively increased invasiveness, develop the ability to metastasize, and have alterations in biochemical, metabolic, and morphologic characteristics.

Tumor cell heterogeneity is an important characteristic of tumor progression. Expression of this heterogeneity includes antigenic and protein product variants, ability to elaborate angiogenesis factors, emergence of chromosomal variants, development of metastatic capability, altered metabolism, and decreased sensitivity to radiation. The development of intraneoplastic diversity may come about as a consequence of genetic change such as loss of polymorphic restriction fragments in DNA of malignant tumors or similar random processes such as additional genomic "hits" by genotoxic agents. Alternatively, the heterogeneity observed in tumor progression may be generated by epigenetic, regulatory mechanisms operative as a continuation of the process of promotion. More than likely, genetic and nongenetic events subsequent to initiation operate in a nonmutually exclusive manner during progression, possibly in an ordered cascade of latter events superimposed on earlier events.

The most plausible mechanism of progression invokes the notion that during the process of tumor growth there is a selection that favors enhanced growth of a subpopulation of the neoplastic cells. In support of this mechanism is the observation of increased phenotypic heterogeneity that is observed in malignant versus benign neoplastic proliferations. Presumably a variety of subpopulations arise and it is only a matter of time before the emergence of a subpopulation with more malignant biological characteristics or at least a differential growth advantage. This can occasionally be observed during early stages of experimental hepatocarcinogenesis when phenotypically distinguishable foci can arise within existing foci of cellular alteration. In addition, serial transplantation of tumors frequently shows an enhancement of malignant properties associated with increased numbers of passages. Here there is a presumed selection for more rapidly growing subpopulations because the subsequent serial passage is typically dictated by the size of the transplant growth in the recipient. Associated with progression is the development of an increased degree of karyotypic instability and of aneuploidy. This latter phenomenon may be related to the not infrequent observation of abnormal mitoses in malignant neoplasms. Finally, chromosomal rearrangement is associated with several clinically malignant neoplasms, especially leukemias. It is probable that such rearrangements are a consequence of karyotypic instability and that apposition of critical portions of genes upstream or downstream from genomic enhancers or derepressors impart a proliferative advantage and a metastatic capability to affected cells within an evolving neoplastic proliferation.

Distinction between tumor promotion and tumor progression is not readily discernible in the routine histopathologic evaluation of neoplasms. In fact, the distinction may be somewhat academic in that promotion may be considered part of the process of progression. In both situations the critical event is accentuated growth. What is believed to distinguish progression from promotion is the presence of structural genomic alterations in the former and the absence of definable structural changes in the genome of the latter. Both structural genomic changes and biochemical changes associated with tumor progression cannot be defined by conventional histopathology. Emerging technologies centered around histochemistry, immunocytochemistry, and *in situ* hybridization to identify products of protooncogenes and activated oncogenes offer promise to help distinguish various stages of progression in the evolution from benign to malignant neoplasms.

IV. Hypotheses of Mode of Action of Chemical Carcinogens

A. OVERVIEW

Four principal, but not necessarily mutually exclusive, hypotheses have been proposed to explain the development of cancer: the mutational genetic hypothesis, the nonmutational genetic hypothesis, the epigenetic hypothesis, and the viral hypothesis. According to the mutational genetic hypothesis, malignant transformation results from small structural molecular perturbations of cellular genetic material. An example of such a perturbations is a point mutation. Based on the nonmutational genetic hypothesis, large structural genomic changes that are not true mutations may cause neoplastic transformation. These are generally chromosomal alterations large enough to be seen microscopically, such as chromosomal rearrangements and recombinations, and gene amplifications.

According to the epigenetic hypotheses of carcinogenesis, structural alterations in genomic material are not required for the induction of neoplasia. Rather, changes in the intracellular regulatory processes controlling cell proliferation and differentiation result in or contribute substantially to neoplasia. Proposed mechanisms for nongenotoxic or epigenetic development of cancer include blocked differentiation, blockage of intercellular communication, irreversible changes in DNA transcription, altered methylation, chronic toxicity with attendant enhanced cell proliferation, and hormonal effects. There is no unequivocal proof for the proposed mechanisms of epigenetic induction of cancer. Some of the proposed mechanisms, such as hypomethylation and enhanced cell turnover, may be relevant for both the genetic and the epigenetic hypotheses of carcinogenesis.

The viral hypothesis of cancer induction postulates that infection by exogenous DNA or RNA viruses may play a role in malignant transformation. Vertically transmitted endogenous proviruses that are ubiquitous in the cellular genome may also be involved in the neoplastic process but their potential role is as yet undefined.

B. MUTATIONAL GENETIC HYPOTHESIS OF CHEMICAL CARCINOGENESIS

1. Mutational Events

There is strong evidence that a critical step in carcinogenesis is a structural alteration occurring in the genetic machinery of a somatic cell. This appears to be true whether the active agent is a chemical, ionizing radiation, or if the cancer has a viral etiology. According to the mutational hypothesis, one or more point mutations are responsible for initial and/or critical steps in the neoplastic process.

The origin of somatic mutation theory for cancer is generally credited to Boveri in 1914. According to the somatic mutation theory, cancer originates when an otherwise ordinary cell undergoes a mutation. An extension of this theory was proposed by Nordling in 1953 who postulated that if a large enough population of somatic cells lives for a sufficient length of time, gene mutations will occur in some of them. As the mutated cells proliferate, Nordling argued, there is a finite probability that some of them will sustain a second mutation. As the process of successive mutation and proliferation continues, cells will eventually sustain enough genetic alteration to become autonomous and result in cancer. The accumulation of successive mutations would be expected to increase as a function of age and of the degree of cell proliferation. Early occurrence of cancer might be expected to result from exposure to mutagens as well as to agents that increase the rate of cell proliferation.

The relevance of the somatic mutation theory to multistep carcinogenesis has been shown repeatedly to be the most probable explanation for the initiation of carcinogenesis. In more recent times, the possibility that malignant cancer can result from multiple genetic insults has been championed by several investigators and is supported experimentally. There seems little doubt that genetic mutation plays a causative role in the genesis of some cancers. However, it

has not been demonstrated unequivocally that mutation is a universal, sufficient, or necessary prerequisite for all cancers.

Supportive of the arguments for the mutational hypotheses of cancer causation is the correlation between mutagenicity and carcinogenicity, the correlation between faulty DNA repair mechanisms and some cancers, and the heritable nature of neoplastic transformation. While the correlation between mutagenicity and carcinogenicity is not perfect, many chemical carcinogens are mutagenic either alone or after metabolic activation. Because it is well known that some mutagens are not carcinogens and some carcinogens are not mutagens, invocation of the association between mutagenicity and carcinogenicity must necessarily be qualified. Practical considerations logically compel us to admit that no single mutagenicity test or even a battery of mutagenicity tests would be expected to reflect the complexity and diverse mechanisms of carcinogenesis. Nonetheless, the association between mutagenicity and carcinogenicity, where it occurs, is intuitively appealing as a potential mechanism for the genesis of some cancers.

Endogenous hereditary defects in mutational repair in the face of exposure to environmental mutagenic factors are known to lead to some cancers. Most notable is the occurrence of carcinomas and melanomas of the skin in xeroderma pigmentosum patients who sustain mutations caused by ultraviolet radiation. Because a constellation of biochemical abnormalities may be present in the same cells that have a defective excision repair of pyrimidine dimers, it cannot be adamantly stated that the observed skin cancers result exclusively from the accumulation of mutations resulting from deficient DNA repair. However, the association between defective DNA repair and carcinogenesis in xeroderma pigmentosum patients lends support to the somatic mutation hypothesis of cancer formation.

Finally, a large body of experimental data supports the contention that malignant cancer is generally not reversible. Even in initiation–promotion studies, the initial mutational changes constituting initiation may remain latent for weeks or months before being expressed by administration of a promoting agent. This "memory effect" is compatible with a stable somatic mutation.

Since the mid-1980s, oncogenes (mutated protooncogenes) have been identified in the tumor DNA of many human neoplasms as well as in spontaneous and chemically induced neoplasms in animals. These oncogenes are frequently in the *ras* oncogene family, and the activated *ras* oncogenes frequently differ from their homologous protooncogene by virtue of a single point mutation. In some experimental situations, carcinogen-induced activation of some oncogenes appears to be an early event in the carcinogenic process. While it can be argued that activation of protooncogenes may be a necessary event in the genesis of some cancers, it is unlikely that a single point mutation associated with an activated oncogene is sufficient in and of itself for the development of all cancers.

2. Interaction of Genotoxic Chemical Carcinogens with Their Cellular Targets

a. Nonalkylating Agents. This class of carcinogen directly substitutes for exocyclic amino groups of nucleosides. The substitution occurs either through oxidative mechanisms or by direct electrophilic attack and results in a change of base pairing because of deamination or a shift in tautomeric (structural isomer) equilibrium. Examples include nitrous oxide, which causes oxidative deamination, and formaldehyde, which forms cross-links within DNA. Formaldehyde also causes hydroxymethyl adducts and, thus, may also act as an alkylating agent.

b. Alkylating Agents. Alkylating chemical carcinogens either interact directly with cellular genomic material (direct acting carcinogens) or must first be metabolized by the host to a reactive species (indirect acting carcinogens). Examples of direct alkylating agents include methylnitrosurea, ethylnitrosourea, methylmethane sulfonate, and ethylmethane sulfonate. Indirectly acting alkylating agents require metabolic activation to an electrophilic intermediate and include chemicals such as dimethyl-

nitrosoamine, benzyo [*a*] pyrene, nitrofurans, nitroquinoline oxide, ethylene dibromide, ethylene dichloride, *N*-2-acetyl-2-aminofluorene, and dimethylhydrazine. Pathways for activation involve cytochrome P450, reduction with NADPH diaphorase, reaction with glutathione, or oxidation mediated by peroxidases or via prostaglandin synthetase. For specifics regarding metabolic activation of different types of chemical carcinogens, the reader is encouraged to consult cited reference material. For both direct and indirect acting agents, the reactive form of the carcinogen is an electron-deficient species (electrophilic form) that interacts nonenzymatically with electron-rich or nucleophilic molecular sites in the cell. These nucleophilic sites are not limited to DNA but also include RNA and cellular protein. Thus, the reaction is not specific for genomic material or for nucleic acids. The interaction of electrophilic forms of the carcinogen with host cellular material results in the formation of covalent adducts (addition products). These interactions take place primarily between the electrophilic form of the carcinogen and the nitrogen, oxygen, and sulfur atoms in the cellular macromolecules. The adducts that are formed may be small as is seen with simple alkylating agents or large, so-called "bulky adducts," as occurs with polycyclic aromatic hydrocarbons. In either case, configurational or conformational changes occur in the DNA, which can lead to steric hindrance and result in infidelity of DNA replication.

The electrophilic forms of carcinogens react at numerous macromolecular cellular sites and produce adducts and mutations throughout the genome. Some of these mutations may be lethal. Nonlethal reactions with cellular targets are the most relevant for carcinogenesis in that initiation occurs when one of these is in a critical genomic site. Nonlethal alteration in the somatic cell genotype is consistent with the heritable change that is observed in cancer cells. Evidence of alteration of the cellular genome is supported by the observation of chromosomal abnormalities and altered gene expression in cancer cells. Furthermore, adduct formation at DNA nucleophilic sites such as phosphate residues and hydrogen-bonding sites between base pairs can also result in miscoding or in sufficient distortion of DNA structure to result in infidelity of DNA replication. Because DNA damage (adduct formation) can be repaired efficiently by cellular enzymes, it is necessary for cell proliferation to occur prior to repair of the DNA damage in order for a heritable change to occur. Once a round of cell proliferation takes place, the genomic alteration is said to be "fixed" and the affected cell(s) is initiated. The round or rounds of cell replication that serve to fix the molecular lesions may occur *de novo*, may be induced by the inherent toxicity of the chemical carcinogen, or may be induced by the promoting activity of the chemical carcinogen.

C. NONMUTATIONAL GENETIC HYPOTHESIS OF CHEMICAL CARCINOGENESIS

1. Chromosomal Aberrations and Neoplasia

Numerical and/or structural chromosomal abnormalities and alterations are virtually universally present in neoplasms, particularly malignant neoplasms. Chromosomal aberrations are found in apparently spontaneous neoplasms as well as in those induced by chemical carcinogens or by oncogenic viruses. Against a backdrop of apparently random chromosomal aberrations observed in neoplasms, it is also apparent that there are a few constant karyotypic changes associated with specific neoplasms. Most notable is the association of the Philadelphia chromosome with the lymphoma/leukemia group of human diseases. However, in light of the relatively few constant karyotypic changes associated with specific histogenetic types of neoplasms and the random nature of the preponderance of chromosomal aberrations observed in neoplasms, it is difficult to establish a cause–effect relationship between specific chromosomal aberrations and cancer. Nonrandom chromosomal aberrations in animal neoplasms include trisomy 15 in T-cell lymphoma of the mouse, trisomy 13 in mouse mammary adenocarcinoma, and trisomy 4 in ethylnitrosurea-induced neurogenic neoplasms in the rat.

a. Gene Rearrangement, Transposition.

i. Reciprocal translocation Reciprocal translocation is a form of gene rearrangement where portions of two chromosomes are simply exchanged with no net loss of genetic information. This can result in an alteration of the structure of the genes by virtue of their new location and/or in abnormal expression of the translocated gene(s). A prototypical example of this phenomenon is represented by the Philadelphia chromosome associated with human lymphoma/leukemia. This specific chromosomal abnormality consists of a translocation between the long arms of chromosomes 9 and 22 and is seen in 85% of patients with chronic myelogenous leukemia. Translocations between other chromosomes are associated with different forms of leukemia.

ii. Nonreciprocal exchanges Nonreciprocal exchanges consist of deletions or additions of regions of chromosomes. While these types of changes are observed frequently in neoplasias, their specific functional or prognostic significance is generally unknown. The loss of genes involved in controlling carcinogenesis (i.e., tumor suppressor genes) may be important in many cancers.

In nonmammalian cells, transposons (modules of DNA material that are transposed to abnormal sites in the genome) are important for genetic variability and in the regulation of gene expression. The recent demonstration of transposon-like elements in the mammalian genome suggests that transposable elements, possibly promoted by repetitive endogenous sequences in the genome, may play a role in normal developmental processes as well as in neoplasia.

2. Gene Amplification

Gene amplification represents a situation where there is an increase in the amount of DNA present in a specific region of a chromosome. Chromosomal abnormalities observed in karyotype preparations such as homogeneously stained regions, abnormal banding patterns, and double minutes are the result of gene amplification. Assuming that the amplified

100

genes are transcriptionally active, an excess of the product encoded by the amplified genes would be anticipated. Drug-induced gene amplification, possibly with an associated specific karyotypic change, is known to result in drug resistance due to an increase in the amount of gene product. A number of observations have been made with respect to gene amplification and oncogenesis. The classical skin tumor promoter, phorbol ester, causes amplification of specific genes in cultured cells. DNA amplification has been shown to occur at the site of insertion of oncogenic retroviruses. It has been suggested that increased production of normal protein products of protooncogenes (e.g., c-*ras*) that have been amplified may contribute to the malignant phenotype. Amplification of c-*myc* is seen in small cell cancer of the lung in humans, and the degree of amplification is correlated with clinical aggressiveness of this cancer.

The causative role of DNA transposition, other types of DNA rearrangement, and even amplification of endogenous genes in either the origin or the development of neoplasia is difficult to ascertain at present. Even the mechanisms causing such somatic chromosomal abnormalities remain obscure. However, the sites for chromosomal rearrangement seem to correspond to specific fragile locations in the genome that may be uniquely susceptible to breakage. Further documentation of chromosomal abnormalities in various neoplasms may provide important clues about basic genetic mechanisms associated with carcinogenesis. In some cases, specific chromosomal abnormalities have been shown to have prognostic significance. Also, modulation of gene products may foster malignant behavior by causing uncontrolled cell proliferation and metastasis.

D. EPIGENETIC HYPOTHESIS OF CHEMICAL CARCINOGENESIS

1. Altered Methylation of Genes

The nonmutational genetic hypothesis postulates that a genomic perturbation other than a mutation may lead to cancer. One of the mechanistic explanations for this hypothesis relates to changes in the pattern of DNA methylation. Altered patterns of DNA methylation are associated with exposure to chemicals and are tissue specific. Consistent with a role of altered methylation in carcinogenesis are the observations that DNAs from specific tumors have evidence of hypomethylation, carcinogens are known to interfere with DNA methylation, and the drug 5-azacytidine, which causes undermethylation of genes, has been shown to enhance cell transformation. In general, genes from cancer cells are hypomethylated as compared to their normal counterparts, although important qualifications that relate to the test system used should be noted. Hypomethylation is believed to influence the regulation of transcription and gene expression and may be associated with cellular differentiation. Unfortunately, as with many abnormalities that are associated with cancer cells, we are faced with a dilemma in deciding if hypomethylation of genes is a cause of malignancy or a consequence of the altered metabolism of malignant cells.

2. Blocked Differentiation

An apparent characteristic of transformed cells is a partial or total block in terminal cell differentiation. A block of normal differentiation implies an alteration in normal gene expression. While it has been postulated that neoplasia may represent blocked or abnormal cellular differentiation, the paucity of knowledge relative to normal mechanisms that regulate differentiation makes it difficult to elucidate the potential role of abnormal cell differentiation in the genesis or development of cancer. In fact, experiments exploring the possibility that neoplasia is a disease of blocked differentiation have shown that, under specific environmental conditions, malignant cells have an intrinsic ability to revert to a normal phenotype. This suggests that if blocked differentiation plays a role in the development of neoplasia, the endogenous and/or exogenous factors regulating differentiation must be present continually to maintain the neoplastic phenotype. It has been argued, however, that cancer is not blocked differentiation but rather represents a new state of differentiation conferring a selective growth advantage to the altered phenotype.

3. Intercellular Communication

Among the potential regulatory factors associated with the phenotypic expression of transformed cells are those associated with intercellular communication. Intercellular communication, sometimes referred to as metabolic cooperation based on a popular assay for its measurement, is known to play an important role in the phenotypic expression of some transformed cells *in vitro*. In cocultivation studies, the presence of normal cells is sufficient to prevent the phenotypic expression of transformed cells. Apparently there is sufficient communication between cells, most probably occurring via gap junctions, such that biochemical substances elaborated by the normal cells block the expression of an abnormal phenotype by the transformed cells. Although not a ubiquitous characteristic of nongenotoxic carcinogens, it has been suggested that the inhibition of cellular communication may be the mode of action of many, but not all, chemicals that induce neoplasia but do not affect the genome directly. Current studies have shown that many tumor-promoting agents inhibit gap junction intercellular communication associated with the aberrant expression of connexin and the loss of function of cell adhesion molecules. It has also been suggested that the inhibition of intercellular communication may be one unifying mechanism for all forms of neoplasm promotion. Noncytotoxic levels of chemicals known to be promoters in lung, liver, skin, colon, breast, or esophagus have been shown to inhibit intercellular communication in cell culture systems.

An *in vivo* phenomenon that might be considered a different form of intercellular communication relates to the postulation that epidermal chalones are instrumental in the promotion of skin cancer. Chalones are tissue-specific substances that inhibit the proliferation of immature cells and probably operate through a cell membrane receptor mechanism rather than via gap junctions. Chalones are believed to be produced by neighboring cells and may operate as a type of paracrine control mechanism. Skin tumor promoters, such as phorbol esters, possibly inactivate the chalone receptor site, thereby switching off the mechanism of growth control in the affected cell(s). The existence of chalones has been debated. Some regard them as hormone-like substances with inhibitory activity. A number of growth inhibitory substances have been described (e.g., TGF-β). Many of these do not meet the tissue-specific definition of a chalone but nonetheless appear to regulate normal but not tumor cell growth.

4. Hormones

Hormones are chemical messengers that bind to specific cellular receptors and form a hormone–receptor complex that triggers a cellular response. The cellular response is specific for both the hormone and the target cell. The target cell response to hormone stimulation is typically an increase or decrease in cell division or an acceleration or deceleration in differentiation. There is an almost continual discovery of endogenous messenger substances and growth factors that fit the broad definition of "hormone." Like hormones, hormone-related peptides, commonly referred to as growth factors, play an important role in the control of growth and differentiation of cells, tissues, and organs. A major difference between hormones and growth factors is that hormones are produced in an endocrine tissue and act on cells at a distant site, whereas growth factors are secreted by a variety of normal and abnormal tissues and act on nearby responsive cells.

Endogenous hormone have long been known to be associated with the development of specific neoplasias and in some cases with the inhibition of carcinogenesis. Hormones or hormone imbalances undoubtedly play a major causative role in cancers of certain hormone-sensitive tissues (ovary, uterus, prostate, testes, endocrine organs). However, it is unlikely that they play a major causative role in the development of neoplasia in nonhormone-sensitive tissues. Through the use of two-stage animal models for mammary and thyroid cancer, hormones have been demonstrated to function as tumor promoters of neoplasia.

There is little evidence that there is direct interaction of endogenous hormones with DNA, although minimal DNA binding has been shown with some synthetic estrogens and some hormones do bind to protein. Most endogenous hormones are believed to act through a specific cellular receptor mechanism. Once there is binding to a specific membrane, cytosolic, or nuclear receptor, the receptor becomes activated and intracellular activity occurs that affects transcriptional or translational processes, resulting in the synthesis of specific proteins.

Just how hormonal interaction with a cell receptor leads to cancer is unknown, but one potential mechanism relates to an increase in cell turnover among cells that already possess latent genetic change. Thus, endogenous hormones may serve to promote spontaneously or otherwise initiated cells. Alternatively, hormonal imbalance could lead to increased proliferation in a sensitive cell population with secondary genotoxic damage from any one of several environmentally prevalent genotoxic agents. This certainly is consistent with the frequent observation of endocrine tumors developing against a previously existing background of hyperplasia. Furthermore, the two possibilities are not mutually exclusive. The precise signals and mechanisms by which hormones and related growth factors regulate cell proliferation and differentiation remain to be identified and are areas of active research. Evidence suggests that the mechanism of action of hormones and growth factors may be closely associated with and related to the action of oncogene protein products.

5. Cell Proliferation and Apoptosis

Increased cell proliferation can make an important contribution to the process of carcinogenesis. This can come about in either or both of two ways. First, the enhanced cell turnover could lead to "fixation" of spurious or spontaneous genotoxic damage. DNA damage is believed to occur continually from cellular exposure to endogenous or exogenous geno-

toxic insults or simply from endogenous errors in DNA replication. Fortunately, the vast majority of such DNA damage is repaired prior to cell division by efficient cellular enzymatic systems. The faster the cells are dividing, the greater the chance that genotoxic damage would not be repaired prior to cell division. Once cell division has taken place, the genomic alteration is "fixed" and is hereditary. If such a genomic alteration confers a selective growth advantage to the cell and its progeny, there will be clonal expansion and progressive development of neoplasia. A second way in which enhanced mitogenesis could contribute to neoplasia is to stimulate cell division in an already initiated cell, thereby providing the growth stimulus whereby it can expand clonally. In situations of continued exposure to a nongenotoxic mitogen, it is likely that both potential mechanisms could act in a complementary fashion. In either case, the mechanism of cancer "induction" would be considered secondary.

A variety of situations exist in animal carcinogenicity models where nongenotoxic chemicals given at sufficiently high doses may play a causative role in the development of neoplasia simply by enhancing cell proliferation. Examples of agents that may operate through this potential mechanism are given in Table VII. Confirmation of whether enhanced cell turnover is a realistic explanation for the observed carcinogenicity of nongenotoxic carcinogens will require carefully conducted studies that demonstrate enhanced cell turnover at doses that result in cancer and no increase in cell turnover at noncarcinogenic doses. If enhanced neoplasia in an animal test system is a consequence of increased cell proliferation and if the increased cell proliferation is related to exposure to excessive amounts of certain chemicals, then it becomes important to place the animal test results into the context of expected environmental exposure in assessing potential risk to human health.

Current data strongly suggest that cell death may be as essential as cell proliferation in carcinogenesis. The ratio between cell birth and counterbalancing cell death determines

TABLE VII
Nongenotoxic Carcinogens That May Act Indirectly through Enhanced Cell Proliferation

Agent	Target	Potential mode of action
Carbon tetrachloride	Liver	Necrosis and cytotoxicity
α-Hexachlorocyclohexane	Liver	"Additive" hyperplasia
Phenobarbital	Liver	"Additive" hyperplasia
Polybrominated biphenyls	Liver	"Additive" hyperplasia
Di (2-ethylhexyl)phthalate	Liver	"Additive" hyperplasia and peroxisome proliferation
Methyl clofenapate	Liver	"Additive" hyperplasia and peroxisome proliferation
Unleaded gasoline	Kidney	Toxicity from α_{2u}-globulin and resulting regenerative hyperplasia in male rats
Pentachloroethane	Kidney	α_{2u}-globulin induction in male rats
D-Limonene	Kidney	α_{2u}-globulin induction in male rats
Sodium saccharin	Urinary bladder	Hyperplasia
Biphenyl	Urinary bladder	Hyperplasia secondary to bladder calculi
Butylated hydroxytoluene	Urinary bladder	?

tumor growth. Two forms of cell death may be seen in cancer development: necrosis and apoptosis. Necrosis typically occurs when a developing cancer outgrows its blood supply. Apoptosis, however, is an energy-dependent process that involves active gene transcription and translation. In preneoplastic lesions, apoptosis is the predominant form of cell death that is observed. An increase in apoptosis often parallels the increase in cell proliferation observed in preneoplastic lesions and tumors. Enhanced apoptosis may be triggered by chemicals, food deprivation, certain cytokines, growth factors, tumor suppressor genes, and withdrawal of mitogenic agents in experimental *in vivo* carcinogenesis. It has been reported that the growth of dioxin-promoted preneoplastic liver foci in rat hepatocarcinogenesis is due to inhibition of apoptosis rather than to enhanced cell proliferation. An underlying principle of cancer chemotherapy is the selective induction of apoptosis in neoplastic cells. There is currently a large research effort to dissect out and understand the molecular controls of apoptosis.

E. VIRAL HYPOTHESIS OF CARCINOGENESIS

1. Exogenous DNA and RNA Viruses

The issue of whether a chemical carcinogen can activate a latent oncogenic virus as its primary mode of inducing neoplasia has been debated but never resolved. A variety of exogenous DNA viruses are known to cause cellular transformation and cancer in animals and humans. Of seven families of DNA viruses, six contain oncogenic members, such as hepatitis B virus, papilloma virus, herpes viruses, polyoma virus, and adenoviruses. The mechanisms whereby DNA viruses exert oncogenic activity are complex and not well understood. Complete or partial integration of virus into host genomic material appears to be critical for oncogenic transformation by some DNA viruses, but whether this is necessary for all oncogenic DNA viruses is not clear. While it is generally believed that exogenous DNA viruses require cooperation of unspecified endogenous and/or exogenous factors to produce neoplasia, a specific role for chemical carcinogens in this process has not been demonstrated.

Only 1 of 10 different groups of exogenous RNA viruses is associated with oncogenesis. This group contains the B-, C-, and D-type retroviruses, the best known being the C-type retroviruses. C-type retroviruses include acute and chronic transforming retroviruses.

While acute transforming retroviruses may be regarded as laboratory artifacts that do not cause malignant disease under natural conditions, they have been instrumental in contributing to the recent rapid advances in elucidating the role of molecular factors and oncogenes in the process of carcinogenesis. These actue transforming retroviruses contain homologues of mammalian protooncogenes. In fact, the retrovirus contains transforming sequences of cellular origin that were captured or transduced from a host cell following infection of that cell. Viruses in this category are generally defective in replication due to the loss of some viral genomic sequences necessary for replication. However, they can become replication competent when a "helper" virus containing the lost sequences is also present in the cell. Because retroviruses contain a viral oncogene (actually a transduced cellular protooncogene) that comes under the influence of efficient retroviral transcriptional promoters, the viral oncogene is expressed at high levels when cells are infected in the laboratory. Thus, cells in culture can be transformed and sarcomas or leukemias can be induced in a few days after laboratory infection of rodents or birds.

Another group of C-type retroviruses that do not have specific transforming sequences of cellular origin but can cause neoplasia under natural conditions are referred to as chronic transforming retroviruses. They are believed to induce neoplasia by insertion into the host DNA in locations where the strong transcriptional promoters of the viral genome will "activate" nearby structural cellular genes, known as protooncogenes, that are believed to control cell growth and differentiation. In this situation, cellular transformation is believed to occur as a consequence of increased transcription of the cellular protooncogene.

The viral hypothesis of carcinogenesis has gained steady support because of the frequency with which DNA and RNA viruses are isolated from animal neoplasms and human leukemias. However, these "tumor viruses" have subsequently been found to be widespread in healthy animals and humans. Because the probability that retroviruses without transforming genes will transform cells is low, on the order of 10^{-11}, and because relatively few cancers are caused by DNA viruses, it has been argued that viruses may not be a significant natural source of exogenous cancer genes. In fact, it

has been proposed that cellular transformation is typically a virus-independent event and that viral integration occurs during the process of clonal expansion of transformed cells.

2. Endogenous Proviral Sequences

Endogenous proviruses are found in a highly repetitive frequency in the mammalian genome. These provirus sequences are transmitted vertically through the germ line in the same fashion as cellular genes. It is estimated that approximately 0.4% of the total genome of the mouse consists of endogenous provirus sequences. This includes up to 50 type-C murine leukemia virus-related sequences and more than 600 intracisternal A particle sequences in addition to other defective and nondefective viral genomic sequences. The structure of these proviruses is highly conserved in evolution and some proviral sequences are transcribed in normal cells. These observations suggest that there is probably an important biological role for their polypeptide products, possibly in cellular differentiation.

The exact role of endogenous proviruses and the mechanisms involved in their regulation are poorly understood. The long terminal repeats of these endogenous proviruses may be transposed to new positions in the genome where they could act as enhancers or promoters of transcription of upstream or downstream cellular genes that control cellular growth and differentiation. In such a hypothetical situation these portions of the endogenous provirus sequences may play a role in neoplastic transformation. The observation that there is increased expression of endogenous retrovirus in some chemically induced neoplasms is suggestive evidence for their potential role in the development of some neoplasms. Mouse mammary tumor virus (MMTV) endogenous proviral sequences are activated during mammary carcinogenesis and this activation is associated with hypomethylation of the endogenous MMTV genome. Thus, interaction of chemical carcinogens with the host genome might produce a neoplastic response by virtue of inducing the transposition of endogenous proviruses to a new site in the cellular genome or by causing hypomethylation and subsequent activation of endogenous proviral sequences. Whether these or similar mechanisms are relevant or critical molecular events in chemical carcinogenesis is presently unknown.

V. Oncogenes and Tumor Suppressor Genes in Chemical Carcinogenesis

A. GENES AND ONCOGENES

Up to 10,000 genes are estimated to be present in the mammalian genome. These genes can be thought of as belonging to either of two general categories: structural genes or regulatory genes. Structural genes are nucleotide sequences that encode for the various protein products produced by the cell. Some structural genes function to maintain general housekeeping within the cell by encoding for proteins that are necessary for normal physiological functions, such as cell respiration, cell metabolism, detoxification, cell replication, growth, and differentiation. Other structural genes encode for specific protein products that are unique to the cell, such as immunoglobulin in B-lymphoid cells, hemoglobin in erythroblasts, collagen in fibroblasts, and albumin in hepatocytes. Regulatory genes, however, control the activity of structural genes as well as other regulatory genes and can be thought of as the switches that initiate, maintain, enhance, block, or stop the functioning or transcription of structural genes. The activity of specific regulatory genes is responsible for the fact that the erythroblast produces hemoglobin rather than collagen and for the fact that the fibroblast produces collagen rather than albumin. Considering that all nucleated somatic cells contain the entire genetic code for the species but that only specific genes are transcriptionally active in a given cell type, the proper functioning of regulatory genes is not a trivial matter.

Oncogenes are dominant-acting structural genes that encode for protein products capable of transforming the phenotype of a cell. Onco-

genes were first identified as the transforming genes of retroviruses. These oncogenes were not necessary for the life cycle of the virus but were responsible for transforming virally infected cells and producing cancer in the host. It was later learned that the transforming oncogenes were not intrinsic viral genes but rather were normal cellular structural genes captured from eukaryotic organisms previously infected by the retrovirus. The virus assimilated these normal cellular genes by a process called transduction. The transduced oncogene in the viral genome is referred to as a viral oncogene (v-onc). The homologous gene in the host genome is called a cellular oncogene (c-onc) or a protooncogene. In capturing the cellular protooncogene, the virus lost some of its own structural genes and, consequently, often became incapable of replicating in the absence of helper viruses.

As the genomes of various mammalian and submammalian species were examined, it was found that homologues to the retroviral oncogenes were present in species as diverse as yeast, fruit flies, amphibians, birds, and mammals. The high degree of evolutionary conservation of these protooncogenes suggested that they served important normal functions in the cell. It is now known that protooncogenes encode for proteins that are important in cell growth, development, and differentiation. Because cancer is a perturbation of normal cell growth and differentiation, the potential significance of alterations in protooncogenes becomes apparent. It is thus not surprising that examination of DNA from human and animal tumors has demonstrated the existence of dominant transforming oncogenes, some of which correspond to those responsible for the carcinogenicity of acute transforming retroviruses.

B. PROTOONCOGENE FUNCTION

Protooncogenes have derived their names from the respective retroviral diseases in which their homologues were discovered. Examples of different protooncogenes, their retroviral counterparts, species of origin, and their encoded protein products are presented in Table VIII.

TABLE VIII
Examples of Protooncogenes with Viral Counterparts

Oncogene product and oncogene	Source of name (species of origin)
Tyrosine protein kinase	
src	Rous sarcoma virus (chicken)
abl	Abelson leukemia virus (mouse)
fes	Feline sarcoma virus (cat)
Kinase related	
raf	3611 murine sarcoma virus (mouse)
mos	Murine sarcoma virus (mouse)
GTP-binding proteins	
H-ras	Harvey sarcoma virus (rat)
K-ras	Kirsten sarcoma virus (rat)
N-ras	Neuroblastoma (human)
Growth factor	
sis (platelet-derived growth factor)	Simian sarcoma virus (monkey)
Growth factor receptor	
erbB (epidermal growth factor receptor)	Avian erythroblastosis virus (chicken)
fms (colony-stimulating factor receptor)	McDonough sarcoma virus (cat)
Nuclear proteins	
c-myc	MC29 myelocytomatosis virus (chicken)
N-myc	Neuroblastoma (human)
myb	Myeloblastosis virus (chicken)
fos	FBJ osteosarcoma virus (mouse)

More than 30 protooncogenes have been identified by virtue of structural homology to retroviral oncogenes. In addition, at least 20 cellular transforming genes (putative oncogenes) and growth factors that do not have a viral oncogene counterpart have been identified by transfection studies and other methods. Protooncogenes encode for intracellular regulatory proteins, growth factors, and growth factor receptors that occupy specific intracellular and cellular membrane sites. Intracellular functions are important in cell growth and differentiation. Increased transcription of protooncogenes has been observed during embryogenesis, during stimulation of cell mitosis by growth factors, and during regeneration of lost tissue (e.g., following partial hepatectomy). As is obvious from Table VIII, protooncogenes encode for growth factors, growth factor receptors, regulatory proteins in signal transduction, nuclear regulatory proteins, and protein kinases. Protein kinase C, for example, controls such diverse functions as cell growth and specialization, metabolism, hormone action, nerve signal transmission, fertilization, and gene activity. Thus, proteins encoded by protooncogenes appear to play a role in multiple critical processes essential to normal cellular function. Perturbations in these encoded proteins brought about by protooncogene activation or enhanced expression could lead to alterations of growth and differentiation and, thus, contribute to neoplasia.

C. PROTOONCOGENE ACTIVATION

There is increasing evidence that cellular protooncogene (cellular oncogene) activation contributes to the neoplastic process. An activated protooncogene has come to be called an oncogene and is a protooncogene that has been altered quantitatively or qualitatively, resulting in inappropriate or overexpression. Activation can occur in several ways (see Table IX). Retroviral transduction had been shown to result in the acquisition of point mutations, deletions, or gene fusions within the coding sequence of the transduced protooncogene. This would lead to abnormal functioning and changes in levels and schedules of expression of encoded protein products. Retroviruses can also affect the expression of protooncogenes by a process called insertional mutagenesis. In this situation, the retroviral DNA integrates into the host cell DNA adjacent to or within the coding sequence of a protooncogene. The powerful retroviral promoters (regulatory genes) then drive transcription of the normal or truncated gene product of the protooncogene. Activation of protooncogenes can also occur by mechanisms independent of retroviral involvement. Point mutations and DNA rearrangements, such as translocations or gene amplifications, can result in protooncogene activation by leading to altered levels or schedules of expression of the normal protein product or in normal or altered levels of expression of abnormal protein.

TABLE IX
Mechanisms of Oncogene Activation

Protooncogene	Mechanism of activation	Oncogene
c-onc	Retroviral transduction	v-onc
c-myc	Chromosomal translocation	Ig/myc
c-abl	Chromosomal translocation	bcr/abl
N-myc	Gene amplification	DM/HSR
c-myc	Gene amplification	
K-ras	Gene amplification	
c-H-ras	Point mutation	12th, 13th, or 61st codon mutation
c-K-ras	Point mutation	12th, 13th, or 61st codon mutation
c-N-ras	Point mutation	12th, 13th, or 61st codon mutation
myc	Promoter/enhancer insertion	LTR/c-onc
myb	Promoter/enhancer insertion	LTR/common domain
erb B	Promoter/enhancer insertion	
mos	Promoter/enhancer insertion	
int-1	Promoter/enhancer insertion	
int-2	Promoter/enhancer insertion	

D. PROTOONCOGENE ACTIVATION IN CHEMICAL CARCINOGENESIS

The activation of protooncogenes in spontaneous and chemically induced neoplasia has received considerable attention in recent years. A variety of activated oncogenes have been documented in rodent neoplasms (see "Suggested Reading"). From some experimental studies it appears that certain types of oncogenes are activated by carcinogen treatment and that this activation is sometimes an early event in tumor induction. Other studies with human and rodent neoplasms suggest that oncogene activation is involved later in the carcinogenic process, specifically during tumor progression. While high levels of expression of a single *ras* oncogene are sufficient to transform cultured rodent cells in some systems, the concerted expression of at least two oncogenes is necessary for transformation in other *in vitro* culture systems. Furthermore, loss of specific regulatory functions such as tumor suppressor genes (discussed later) also appears to be a distinct step in neoplastic transformation. Thus, oncogenes may play an important role in chemical carcinogenesis. They may, in fact, be necessary for carcinogenesis but are not sufficient in and of themselves to cause cancer, consistent with a multistep process of carcinogenesis.

Study of the patterns of oncogene activation in spontaneous versus chemically induced rodent neoplasms has provided data that suggest that the molecular lesions associated with chemically induced cancer are sometimes different from those documented in spontaneous cancer. Furthermore, the patterns of oncogene activation in several rodent model systems appear to be carcinogen specific, are consistent with known or expected DNA adduct formation, and, in some cases, are similar to patterns of oncogene activation documented in human neoplasms.

The most frequently identified activated oncogenes detected in chemically induced neoplasms belong to the *ras* gene family. *Ras* oncogenes were originally detected and isolated by transfection of NIH3T3 cells (immortalized mouse fibroblasts) using DNA from tumors; this method of detection has been replaced by newer molecular techniques. Cloning of these genes from the tumor DNA revealed that many were H-*ras*, K-*ras*, or N-*ras* genes that differed from their protooncogene homologues by a single point mutation located in a specific codon. Thus, when adolescent rats are given a single exposure to nitrosomethylurea (NMU), mammary tumors result that have an activated H-*ras* oncogene with a G-A transition (mutation) in the 12th codon. G-A transitions are consistent with the O^6-methyl guanine adduct that is formed by methylating agents such as MNU, and such mutations would be expected to lead to nucleotide mispairing during DNA replication. The altered DNA would be expected to give rise to an abnormal protein product that could theoretically alter cell growth or differentiation. MNU is very labile with an estimated biological half-life of a few minutes. Thus, it is likely that the effect produced by this chemical carcinogen occurred as an early event in the carcinogenic process. Because hormone-stimulated cell division in the mammary tissue is also necessary for the development of mammary neoplasia in this model, it is unlikely that activation of the H-*ras* gene is sufficient in and of itself for the production of mammary neoplasia.

Another example of association of an activated H-*ras* gene with neoplasia is seen in the carcinomas produced in mouse skin by initiation with dimethylbenzanthracene (DMBA) followed by promotion with phorbol ester. In this instance there is an A-T transversion (mutation) in the 61st codon of the H-*ras* gene. Once again, the oncogene activation produced by the DMBA treatment was not sufficient to cause carcinoma development but required promotion by phorbol ester to obtain cancer.

Rodent test systems used for the *in vivo* detection of chemical carcinogens often depend on demonstration of an increased incidence of common neoplasms or on the induction of novel neoplasms in chronically treated animals. Using tumor DNA from the National Toxicology Program (NTP) carcinogenesis testing program to detect dominant transforming genes, patterns of oncogene activation have been documented for spontaneous and chemically induced neoplasms in Fischer 344 rats and in B6C3F1 mice. Results to date show a low frequency (about 3%) of activated oncogenes in spontaneous neoplasms of the Fischer 344 rats. In contrast, a variety of epithelial neoplasms induced by benzidine congeners as well as lung tumors induced by tetranitromethane inhalation have shown a high frequency of oncogene activation. In the B6C3F1 mouse there is a high frequency (55%) of oncogene activation in spontaneous liver tumors and a lower frequency (8%) in spontaneous nonliver tumors. The oncogenes in spontaneous liver tumors in the B6C3F1 mouse most frequently involve activation of the H-*ras* protooncogene by point mutations in the 61st codon. In chemically induced hepatic neoplasia in this mouse hybrid, there is also a high frequency of oncogene activation, but the pattern of oncogene activation differs from that observed in spontaneous liver tumors. In addition to a "background" level of mutations in the 61st codon identical to those observed in spontaneous hepatocellular neoplasms, additional point mutations were documented in codons 12 or 117 of the H-*ras* protooncogene in addition to the activation of K-*ras* and N-*ras* oncogenes in chemically treated mice that had an unequivocal increase in hepatocellular tumors. The induction of novel point mutations in chemically induced neoplasms suggests that it may be possible to distinguish between spontaneous and chemically induced neoplasms on the basis of patterns of oncogene activation. Further support for this contention has been obtained in an experimental model system using the strain A mouse. The strain A mouse has a high spontaneous incidence of lung tumors that can be exacerbated by treatment with known carcinogens. It was found that the pattern of oncogene activation differs between spontaneous and chemically induced lung tumors in the strain A mouse and that oncogene activation in some cases is chemical specific and is consistent with expected DNA adduct formation.

As was implied earlier with regard to methylnitrosourea (MNU)-induced mammary tumors and DMBA-induced skin tumors, activation of a *ras* oncogene appears to be a necessary but not sufficient step for the development of neoplasia. Further support for this hypothesis is afforded by *in vitro* transformation studies using primary rat fibroblasts. Malignant transformation required the successive introduction of two oncogenes into this cell line. Initial introduction of genes such as *myc* or p53 caused the cell line to become immortalized but not capable of causing tumors. Subsequent introduction of a *ras* oncogene resulted in malignant transformation. In this instance, the *ras* oncogene functioned as a late transforming gene in contrast to the situation with the MNU-induced mammary tumors in rats. In a similar study, Syrian hamster dermal cells were immortalized by treatment with the carcinogen MNU or with benzo [*a*] pyrene. The immortalized dermal cells underwent malignant transformation following subsequent treatment with activated *ras* oncogenes.

E. TUMOR SUPPRESSOR GENES AND CARCINOGENESIS

In vitro neoplastic transformation and somatic cell fusion studies provide evidence that malignant transformation represents a balance between genes for expression and for suppression of malignancy. There is also convincing evidence that growth suppressor genes, generally referred to as tumor suppressor genes or as antioncogenes, play a critical role in *in vivo* carcinogenesis. Growth suppressor genes are regulatory genes that normally function to limit or suppress normal growth by inhibiting the activity of structural genes responsible for growth. As such, when intact, they have a function opposite to that of oncogenes and might effectively oppose the action of an oncogene. While protooncogenes have to be activated to influence carcinogenesis, suppressor genes have to be inactivated for the transformed phenotype to be expressed. Inactivation can be achieved by chromosome loss, gene deletion, recombination, gene conversion, or point mutation. Protooncogene activation is generally the result of a somatic mutation. Mutant forms of tumor suppressor genes might be present in germ cells and may thus be hereditary. It is generally necessary for both alleles of a tumor suppressor gene to be inactivated to ultimately result in cancer. Exceptions include inactivation of a normal allele by genomic imprinting or by a dominant-negative mechanisms as is proposed for the p53 tumor suppressor gene. In common

human cancers, multiple tumor suppressor genes may be affected, supporting the notion that cancer development involves perturbation of several levels of growth control. Inactivation of the tumor suppressor gene p53 is a frequent occurrence in a variety of human cancers. Thus, inactivation or loss of tumor suppressor genes, working in concert with the activation of oncogenes and with a variety of endogenous and exogenous stimuli, plays an important part in the complex process of carcinogenesis.

VI. Cell Cycle Control and Carcinogenesis

The pivotal role of cell proliferation in all phases (e.g., initiation, promotion, progression) of the multistep process of carcinogenesis is inextricably linked to positive and negative cell cycle contol mechanisms as influenced by oncogenes, tumor suppressor genes, growth factors and their cognate receptors, hormones and their receptors, and the action of exogenous agents (e.g., chemicals and viruses) on cell cycle control. Uncontrolled cellular proliferation is the hallmark of neoplasia, and many cancer cells demonstrate damage to genes that regulate their cell cycles directly. The prevailing model of the cell cycle is that of a series of transitions at which certain criteria must be met before the cell proceeds to the next phase. The cell cycle is composed of an S (DNA synthesis) and an M (mitotic) phase, separated by two gap phases (G1 and G2). Progression through the cell cycle is tightly controlled by a group of heterodimeric protein kinases comprising a cyclin as a regulatory element and a catalytic subunit known as a cyclin-dependent kinase (Cdk). There are many combinations of cyclin/Cdk complexes, and each phase of the cycle is characterized by a specific pattern of expression and activity. Five major classes of mammalian cyclins (termed A–E) have been described. Cyclins C, D1–3, and E reach their peak of synthesis and activity during the G1 phase and regulate the transition from G1 to S phase. However, cyclins A and B1–2 achieve their maximal levels later in the cycle, during the S and G2 phases, and are regarded as regulators of the transition to mitosis. Association with cyclins not only activates cyclin–dependent kinases but also determines their substrate specificity. Depending on the cyclin partner and therefore the cell cycle stage, different key target molecules are phosphorylated. These events occur in a highly regulated temporal sequence that is maintained through a series of checkpoints. The presence of these checkpoints allows DNA repair before further progression into the cycle. The components of checkpoint control may not necessarily be essential to the workings of the cycle. Instead, their role is to "brake" the cycle in the face of stress or damage. Abrogation of cell cycle checkpoints with agents such as methylxanthine analogs or pentoxifylline increases the cytotoxicity of DNA-damaging agents. The importance of DNA damage in triggering a cell cycle shutdown is obvious. Replication of a damaged template would certainly result in irreversible chromosomal aberrations and a high mutation rate.

Two major checkpoints are thought to be particularly important following DNA damage and have been established at the middle to end of G1 (preceding DNA replication) and G2 (preceding chromosome segregation). Loss of the G1 checkpoint triggers genomic instability at the time of interaction of unrepaired DNA with the DNA replication machinery, leading to deletion type mutations and aberrant gene amplification. Inactivation of the G1 checkpoint serves as an initiation step that makes the cell susceptible to unregulated growth (initiation), increasing the probability of subsequent genetic alterations and establishing the fully developed neoplastic phenotype. Control at the G1 checkpoint is dependent on cyclin D1 (degraded at the G1/S transition) and cyclin E (degraded in mid-S phase). Overexpression of either cyclin D1 or cyclin E and subsequent activation of the cyclin D1 and cyclin E/Cdk complexes result in entry into S phase and decreased G1 time. Cyclin D1 is overexpressed in many human cancers, including breast and non-small cell lung carcinomas, sarcomas, mel-

anomas, B-cell lymphomas, and squamous cell carcinomas of the head and neck. Cyclin D1/cdk4 complexes act to phosphorylate pRB, the product of the retinoblastoma susceptibility gene. pRB does not seem to possess sequence–specific binding activity, but instead exerts a negative regulatory effect on gene expression through complex formation with DNA-binding proteins, including members of the E2F family. In nondividing or G0 (arrested) cells, underphosphorylated pRB is bound to E2F family members, leading to repression of E2F-mediated transcription. Upon phosphorylation by cyclin/cdk complexes, pRB dissociates from E2F proteins, leading to transcription of genes promoting S phase entry. Thus, underphosphorylated pRB maintains cells in G1, whereas phosphorylation inactivates pRB and allows exit from G1. In humans, inactivation of pRB is observed most commonly in retinoblastomas, osteosarcomas, carcinoid tumors, and non-small cell lung cancers. Another tumor suppressor gene, p53, is necessary for G1 phase arrest after DNA damage.

Mutations at the p53 locus are the most frequent genetic alterations associated with cancer in humans. The p53 protein can be divided into three main regions: the amino-terminal transactivation domain, the sequence-specific DNA-binding central core, and the multifunctional carboxy-terminal domain, which includes tetramerization and nuclear localization domains. The majority of p53 mutations involve several highly conserved regions within the DNA-binding core. Lack of p53 permits synthesis of damaged DNA and increases the incidence of selected types of mutations. This has been shown after a variety of DNA damage mechanisms, such as ionizing radiation (strand breaks), alkylation by methyl-methane sulfonate (MMS), ultraviolet irradiation (photo-dimers), and a variety of environmental carcinogens. Thus, one of the major roles of p53 is to ensure that, in response to genotoxic damage, cells arrest in G1 and attempt to repair their DNA before it is replicated. The wild-type p53 protein is normally kept at very low steady-state cellular levels by its relatively short half-life. However, it is stabilized and accumulates in cells undergoing DNA damage or in those responding to certain forms of stress. After DNA damage, p53 binds a consensus-binding site and activates the transcription of several "downstream" genes. One of these genes codes for the p21 protein. The p21 gene belongs to a family of negative cell cycle regulators, which function as cyclin-dependent kinase inhibitory molecules. Genes that encode these proteins are designated CKI genes. These negative regulators form stable complexes with cyclin/cdk units and inactivate them. p21 inactivates cyclin E-cdk2, cyclin A-cdk2, and cyclins D1, D2, and D3-cdk4 complexes, thereby inhibiting pRB phosphorylation and preventing progression of the cell cycle beyond G1. The p53 protein also activates the BAX gene, involved in the regulation of apoptosis. Apoptosis is a cell suicide mechanism that leads to "programmed cell death." Apoptotic cells undergo cell shrinkage and chromosomal condensation in response to DNA damage. These changes prevent the replication of cells that have sustained a degree of genetic damage beyond repair. The p53 protein regulates its own function through the activation of the MDM2 gene. The product encoded by MDM2 is a 90-kDa zinc finger protein (mdm2), which also contains a p53-binding site. The mdm2 protein binds to p53 and acts as a negative regulator, inhibiting wild-type p53 transcriptional activity and creating an autoregulatory feedback loop. A pRB-binding site has also been identified at the carboxy-terminal domain of mdm2 that interacts with pRB and restrains its functions. Thus, overexpression of mdm2 inactivates both p53 and pRB in a fashion similar to some viral oncoprotein products, demonstrating a potential link between p53 and pRB in cell cycle regulation, apoptosis, and tumor progression.

The cell cycle and its regulatory proteins are altered to the benefit of many viral agents. Progression of the cell cycle is advantageous for many viruses, as they require activation of host replication machinery to replicate their own genome. Several viral proteins have been shown to interact with and alter p53 and pRB.

The SV 40 large T antigen, the adenovirus E1B 55-kDa protein, and the human papillomavirus E6 protein each bind to p53 and inactivate it. Similarly, complex formation of underphosphorylated pRB with the SV 40 large T antigen, the adenovirus E1A protein, and the papillomavirus E7 protein leads to pRB inactivation and cellular immortalization. High transformation strains of tumor viruses encode proteins that bind and inactivate both p53 and pRB. In the normal cell, the growth deregulation caused by pRB inhibition can be counteracted by apoptotic cell death produced by normal p53. With the loss of both p53 and pRB, E2F activation stimulates unchecked cellular proliferation, leading to the emergence of neoplastic cell growth.

The high rate and mutation pattern of p53 and pRB in primary tumors have rendered them prototype tumor suppressor genes. Furthermore, detection of p53 and pRB mutations and altered expression of their encoded products appear to be of clinical prognostic significance when identified in specific cancers. Additional gene products known to be activated in response to DNA damage include transcription factors, growth factors, growth factor receptors, protective enzymes, and proteins associated with inflammation and tissue injury and repair. These findings are consistent with the current understanding of the molecular basis of carcinogenesis as a multistep process. Therefore, it is essential to further advance our understanding of the intricate molecular mechanisms that govern chemical carcinogenesis. This will allow us to improve strategies for assessing human cancer risk and to design effective treatment regimens.

VII. Tests for Carcinogenic Potential of Chemicals

Widespread and routine evaluation of chemicals for their carcinogenic potential began in earnest in the mid-1960s with the use of a standardized protocol for the "bioassay" program of the National Cancer Institute (NCI). The original NCI "bioassay" has evolved to the present-day National Toxicology Program (NTP) 2-year carcinogenicity study. Throughout this period a variety of alternative *in vivo* and *in vitro* assay schemes have been introduced in the hopes of identifying potential carcinogens in less time and for less money. Some of these alternative testing models have been highly beneficial tools to help explore the processes of carcinogenesis and the types of carcinogens, to identify and quantitative the genotoxicity of chemicals, and to identify the specific mechanisms whereby given agents produce a carcinogenic response in rodents. Testing batteries, tier approaches, and decision-point analyses have been proposed to provide a basis for prioritizing chemicals in the testing queue and to provide a larger database for risk assessment. These efforts serve to emphasize that, in the last analysis, there is no ideal test for identifying potential human carcinogens. In general, efforts to supplant the long-term carcinogen "bioassay" with less costly short-term tests have been frustrated by poor concordance of the latter with the traditional long-term test results. In the meantime, increasing costs for conducting long-term carcinogenicity studies have resulted in fewer chemicals being tested annually for potential carcinogenicity. Currently, much thought is being given to developing medium-term tests for carcinogenicity concomitantly with analyses of reasonable ways to reduce the cost of the standard long-term rodent carcinogenicity test.

A. *IN VIVO* CHRONIC RODENT CARCINOGENICITY STUDIES (RODENT BIOASSAYS)

The current strategy for identifying the potential carcinogenicity of chemicals involves systemic (including dermal) exposure of male and female rats and mice to high doses and fractions thereof of chemicals over a 2-year period. At the end of 2 years, the carcinogenicity of the chemical being studied is assessed by measuring the excess in neoplasm production above background levels, documenting the occurrence of rare neoplasms with negligible background levels, or demonstrating a reduced latency in neoplasm development in exposed animals versus controls. The original NCI "bioassay" was intended as a screen for carcinogenicity in the rodent. It was generally not intended to be used for risk assessment, determining carcinogenic potency, identifying subtleties of chronic toxicity, determining the mechanism of observed carcinogenic responses, or for establishing pathogenesis of lesions. The implication behind the original NCI "bioassay" was that if a chemical was found to cause neoplasms in treated animals, further studies would need to be designed and conducted to specifically determine parameters such as the mechanism of cancer induction, the nature of the dose–response, chemical metabolism, and target organ dosimetry. The more definitive testing of positive chemicals has generally not occurred. However, in the absence of such additional relevant data, "bioassay" results have been used as a basis for human risk assessment and regulation.

In an effort to consciously expand the original NCI "bioassay" and to make the test results more relevant for the interpretations being applied, considerable evolution has occurred in the design, conduct, and interpretation of long-term rodent carcinogenesis tests conducted under the auspices of the NTP. While the estimated maximum tolerated dose (EMTD) concept has been retained in principle, it is applied more conservatively in setting the high dose. However, a fundamental difference still exists in how the NTP selects the high dose in a chronic rodent carcinogenicity study and how industrial organizations determine the high dose in their otherwise similar chronic rodent carcinogenicity studies. High-dose selection relates to philosophic approaches to testing for toxicity and carcinogenicity. Governmental and similar organizations have traditionally conducted their studies to determine if exposure to a chemical can be harmful under any circumstances, whereas industry most frequently conducts their tests to determine if the chemical is reasonably safe. The first philosophic approach would tend to lead to situations where the animals might be overdosed, whereas the second approach would tend toward underdosing.

There is no right or wrong to either philosophy so long as the study results are interpreted appropriately.

In addition to the high dose or EMTD, at least two additional lower doses are employed in NTP rodent carcinogenicity studies with a conscious effort to utilize human and environmental exposure information to set the low doses. This permits better definition of dose–response and allows better utilization of data for risk assessment.

To more fully characterize the toxicity of chemicals, modifications to the chronic rodent carcinogenicity study protocol have been selectively introduced by the NTP. Interim sacrifices and "stop studies" are incorporated into the design of many carcinogenicity studies to better define the pathogenesis and biological relevance of the anticipated response. The route of administration of chemicals is chosen to mimic natural routes of human exposure whenever possible. Consequently, corn oil gavage of chemicals is rarely used in contemporary study design. Ancillary studies such as chemical disposition and metabolism, toxicokinetics, reproductive toxicity, teratology, behavioral testing, and immunotoxicity frequently complement contemporary 2-year carcinogenicity studies. In addition, *in vitro* and *in vivo* genotoxicity tests are conducted for each chemical. The quality of the pathology evaluation for both neoplastic and nonneoplastic lesions is rigorously peer reviewed. The final interpretation of study results is likewise subjected to intensive peer review, and any carcinogenic response is categorized according to levels of evidence (Table X) for the presence or absence of carcinogenicity in the study. All of this has resulted in a markedly imporved product, but has also resulted in expenditure of more time and money to evaluate each chemical.

There are positive and negative attributes of the contemporary NTP 2-year rodent carcinogenicity study. On the positive side, the test as performed currently is a thoroughly conducted and peer-reviewed assessment of carcinogenicity and chronic toxicity for the chemical under study. The study results are reasonably

TABLE X

National Toxicology Program's Levels of Evidence of Carcinogeniciy Used for Interpretative Conclusions Regarding Chronic Rodent Carcinogenicity Study Results

Clear evidence of carcinogenic activity

Demonstrated by studies that are interpreted as showing a dose-related (i) increase of malignant neoplasms, (ii) increase of a combination of malignant and benign neoplasms, or (iii) marked increase of benign neoplasms if there is an indication from this or other studies of the ability of such tumors to progress to malignancy

Some evidence of carcinogenic activity

Demonstrated by studies that are interpreted as showing a chemically related increased incidence of neoplasms (malignant, benign, or combined) in which the strength of the response is less that required for clear evidence

Equivocal evidence of carcinogenic activity

Demonstrated by studies that are interpreted as showing a marginal increase of neoplasms that may be chemically related

No evidence of carcinogenic activity

Demonstrated by studies that are interpreted as showing no chemically related increases in malignant or benign neoplasms

Inadequate study of carcinogenic activity

Demonstrated by studies that because of major qualitative or quantitative limitations cannot be interpreted as valid for showing either the presence or the absence of carcinogenic activity

interpreted and provide a better basis for risk assessment than previously designed rodent "bioassays" permitted. All data are published to allow for close scrutiny of the scientific basis for each interpretation. To date, the 2-year rodent carcinogenicity study appears to be the single best system for identifying carcinogenic potential. Not only has the 2-year rodent carcinogenicity test been sufficiently sensitive in identifying known human carcinogens, it has also identified carcinogens such as aflatoxin, 4-aminobiphenyl, bis(chloromethyl)ether, diethylstibesterol, melphalan, mustard gas, and vinyl chloride prior to discovery of their carcinogenicity in humans. Disadvantages of the chronic rodent carcinogenicity test relate primarily to the high cost of each study and to the long time interval required to obtain results. The high costs make the studies too expensive to repeat, thereby obviating the principle of reproducibility demanded by good science. However, in 70 "near-replicate" comparisons, good overall reproducibility of positivity, target site, and carcinogenic potency was found by comparing published studies done in rats, mice, or hamsters. The identification of rodent carcinogens on the basis of repeated exposure to high doses of chemical has been criticized as not realistic with respect to human exposure situations in all cases, although clear exceptions exist. Another criticism of the current 2-year rodent carcinogenicity study is that it does not define the mechanisms of any observed carcinogenesis. However, this criticism seems unfounded in that the "standard" chronic rodent carcinogenicity test is not designed to define mechanisms of carcinogenesis. While cost and lack of evidence of reproducibility remain valid criticisms of the chronic rodent carcinogenicity test, it still remains the best test system for definitively identifying potential human carcinogens.

An important issue relative to the chronic rodent carcinogenicity test is how the results are interpreted and used. Considering the results in black and white terms, namely carcinogenic or not carcinogenic, is clearly inappropriate. The studies determine only if a particular chemical under specific conditions could cause cancer in laboratory animals. Even this end point should be qualified by using judgment and scaling in assessing the significance of the carcinogenicity findings. For example, a chemical that causes an unequivocal increase in malignant neoplasia in multiple sites and in both sexes of rats and mice should be given different consideration than a chemical that causes a marginal increase of a benign neoplasm, whose background incidence is normally quite variable in one sex of one species. This approach is referred to as the "weight-of-evidence" method of interpretation and it goes further than just evaluating neoplasm incidence data. Also included in the "weight-of-evidence" method for assessing potential carcinogenic risk to humans is consideration of the nature of the dose–response curve, the pharmacokinetics of the chemical, whether the maximum tolerated dose (MTD) was exceeded in the carcinogenicity study, comparative species metabolism, route of administration, genotoxicity, cytotoxicity, and many other factors. The judgment that a chemical poses carcinogenic hazard should be made in light of the total evidence provided by all sources of available relevant information.

The MTD concept continues to be one of the most debated and controversial issues in toxicology. Studies that are negative for carcinogenicity and were conducted with doses below the MTD leave doubt about the adequacy of the chronic rodent carcinogenicity test. One never knows if the animals were sufficiently challenged with the chemical. Studies conducted at or above the MTD may compromise host homeostasis to such a degree that a positive result has little relevance to human exposure situations. Because it is not always possible to determine what the MTD will be prior to exposure of the animals over much of their life span, the real problem comes with how the study results are used in risk assessment. Thus, conclusions regarding carcinogenicity or lack thereof as determined in chronic rodent tests must be qualified as occurring under conditions of the specific study in question. The limitations of the particular study should be pointed out as they relate to MTD, the original design and purpose of the study, study conduct, confounding toxicity, and other study conditions. In addition, some standardized approach for describing the reasoning used to arrive at a conclusion about the carcinogenicity of a chemical is desirable conceptually and for consistent interpretation. For this purpose, categorization of the observed response using levels of evidence (see Table X) is helpful.

B. ADDITIONAL *IN VIVO* TESTS FOR CARCINOGENICITY

Definition of the following carcinogenicity models as "short term" is a probably a misnomer. When used with potent carcinogens, a preneoplastic or neoplastic response is often observed in a few weeks, hence the designation "short term." However, for less potent carcinogens and for noncarcinogens, tests are typically conducted for several months. In the case of the mouse skin-painting model, lifetime studies

115

may sometimes be conducted to assess carcinogenicity. Because of the sharp contrast in the study duration for these so-called "short-term" *in vivo* test models relative to truly "short-term" (days or weeks) *in vivo* test systems, they have more recently been referred to as "medium-term" bioassays for carcinogens, indicating a study shorter than the conventional 2-year rodent carcinogenicity study. "Short-term" or "medium-term" *in vivo* carcinogenesis animal models consist of an intact animal capable of chemical metabolism (activation and detoxification), complex tissue and hormonal interactions, and possessing repair mechanisms, all of which could influence the ultimate expression of carcinogenic responses to chemical exposure.

Various investigators have proposed specific "short-term" or "medium-term" *in vivo* rodent models to supplant the more costly chronic rodent carcinogenicity studies. In those instances where appropriate validation studies have been conducted, these models have shown unacceptable concordance with results obtained using the "gold-standard" chronic rodent carcinogenicity test. Few individuals seem to have considered simple questions such as "Why would a short-duration lung tumor assay system be expected to identify chemicals that produce renal cancer in a chronic rodent study?" Despite this unfortunate shortcoming, these alternative *in vivo* carcinogenicity models can play an important role in defining chemical carcinogenesis. First, *in vivo* "short-term" tests are useful in defining the nature of the carcinogenic response observed in a chronic rodent carcinogenicity study. For specific target tissues, they can identify whether a chemical is an initiator or promoter and they can help define the relative potency of the carcinogen. Second, they can help elucidate the mechanistic basis of carcinogenesis. Third, when used as part of a battery or tier approach to carcinogen testing, they help set priorities for more extensive carcinogenicity testing of chemicals.

A brief description of selected *in vivo* "short-term" and "medium-term" models is provided. These have been selected based on general popularity and recommendations for their use in decision point judgments and tier approaches to carcinogen identification.

1. Strain A Mouse Pulmonary Tumor Test

The strain A mouse lung tumor model has been in use since the 1940s and representatives from many classes of chemicals have been tested in this model. It has been found to be sensitive for some classes of chemicals and an insensitive assay for other classes. Typically, agents are administered to groups of 30 weaning male and female strain A mice by intraperitoneal injection three times a week for 8 weeks. Gavage and inhalation routes of chemical administration have also been used successfully. Mice are killed 24 weeks after the start of treatment when lungs are removed and fixed. Results (incidence and multiplicity) based on gross enumeration of lung nodules are compared to untreated and vehicle controls. Sensitivity of a given cohort of mice is assessed by running a positive urethan control. Although a typical pulmonary tumor test is based on gross observations, histologic examination reveals that both adenomas and adenocarcinomas are produced. A positive response should be confirmed in other animal studies, as the lung tumor response has shown poor agreement with chronic rodent carcinogenicity studies for some classes of compounds. An equivocal response indicates a need for retesting. The strain A pulmonary tumor test system is particularly useful for assessing the potency of pulmonary carcinogens and for mechanistic studies on carcinogenesis. It has been used to follow lung tumor progression as a function of chemical treatment and oncogene activation. Because there is a normal background incidence of pulmonary neoplasms in untreated strain A mice, this strain is considered especially sensitive to lung tumor induction.

2. Rat Mammary Neoplasm Test

The rat mammary neoplasm test is based on a carcinogenesis model first reported by Huggins and co-workers in 1959. Single or sometimes multiple doses of agent are given to virgin female Sprague–Dawley rats at around day 55 of age, which corresponds to maximum developmental activity of the mammary tissue. Animals are examined periodically by palpation for detectable masses over the next 6 to 9 months to determine mammary neoplasm incidence and multiplicity. DMBA is included as a positive control and typically results in the first detectable neoplasms in about 2 months and a 100% incidence of malignant mammary cancer after 9 months. Histopathologically, induced neoplasms are fibroadenomas, adenomas, adenocarcinomas, and sarcomas. A positive response is usually indicative that other carcinogenicity studies should be conducted for confirmation. This *in vivo* carcinogenesis model has been particularly useful in assessing the influence of hormonal enhancement of mammary carcinogenesis and in demonstrating the role of dietary fat in promoting mammary carcinogenesis.

3. Subcutaneous Injection Test

This relatively simple test consists of administering single or repeated subcutaneously injected doses of chemical to rats or mice (rats are generally considered more sensitive). Depending on solubility, the administered substance may remain in contact with subcutaneous tissues for prolonged periods of time. Developing sarcomas are detected clinically at the injection site by palpation and such data are used to determine time to tumor formation. In addition, primary neoplasms can occur at distant sites. Because some solid substances and persistent foreign body reactions can cause localized sarcomas in rodents, production of neoplasms at the injection site is indicative that further studies are needed. However, production of neoplasms at distant sites is generally regarded as evidence of carcinogenicity.

4. Mouse Skin-Painting Test

The mouse skin-painting model is used to determine potential carcinogenicity by repeated application of a chemical to the shaved skin of the back throughout all or most of the life span of the mouse. Clinical observation of papillomas and carcinomas in the treated area, with histopathologic confirmation, constitutes the most common end point. This test allows for the determination of time to neoplasm formation, neoplasm incidence, and neoplasm multiplicity (a measure of potency). In situations where there is systemic absorption of carcinogens, neoplasms in visceral organs can also be induced. A negative and/or vehicle control group and a positive control group (e.g., benzo [*a*] pyrene) are included in the experimental design. The chemical is usually given at the maximum dose (concentration) that does not produce shortening of the life span or excessive skin irritation. The mouse strain used should be sufficiently sensitive to chemically induced skin carcinogenesis but have a low incidence of spontaneous skin neoplasms. The relatively sensitive Sencar mouse will develop papillomas within 6 weeks when treated with a skin carcinogen. More resistant strains, such as the C57BL/6 mouse, develop skin neoplasms in the painted area after several months of treatment with potent carcinogens. The experimental protocol may be modified to permit assessment of the initiating and promoting potential of the chemical under test.

Practically all of our current concepts of cancer formation, i.e., initiation, cocarcinogenesis, promotion, progression, and, more recently, stages of promotion, have been derived from mouse skin-painting studies. Experimental mouse skin carcinogenesis dates back to 1915 when coal tar condensates were applied repeatedly to mouse skin to produce cancer. Highlights of the subsequent evolution history of the model include recognition of the role of epidermal irritation in the process of mouse skin tumor formation, discovery of cocarcinogens in the 1940s, recognition of the effects of interrupted chemical exposure and factors such as caloric restriction, discovery that phorbol ester promotion is mediated through a specific cell receptor, and demonstration that initiation is irreversible. With the establishment of the mouse skin-painting model as an indicator of multistage carcinogenesis, the door was opened for exploration of the biochemical and molecular mechanisms associated with successive steps in carcinogenesis.

Among the advantages of the skin-painting model are its long history of usage with many chemicals, the fact that testing conditions in the model have been optimized, the ability to measure initiating and promoting potential of carcinogens, and the fact that the model allows assessment of an actual carcinogenic effect in the whole animal. This test is particularly relevant for testing chemicals where human exposure is by the dermal route. Disadvantages of skin-painting studies are that they are relatively labor-intensive and may not be relevant for testing chemicals that are not activated metabolically in the skin.

5. In Vivo Rat Liver Neoplasm (Altered Focus) Model

A variety of treatment protocols have been proposed for *in vivo* rat liver carcinogenesis models. This test system is particularly useful for examining multistage hepatocarcinogenesis and for identifying liver tumor promoters. Examples of treatment protocols include sequential feeding of carcinogen and promoter, single treatment with a necrogenic dose of carcinogen followed by a proliferative stimulation in the presence of growth suppression (selection model), single treatment with a carcinogen during liver regeneration followed by repeated or continuous administration of a promoter (partial hepatectomy model), production of lipotrope deficiency following exposure to carcinogen, and initiation at birth with subsequent natural proliferation stimulation followed by promotion after weaning (neonatal rat model). A recently proposed test system for the detection of hepatocarcinogens involves quantitation of the number and size of diethylnitrosamine (DEN)-initiated placental glutathione S-transferase (PGST) positive foci of cellular alteration in the rat liver. In this latter test system, rats are initiated with a necrogenic dose (200 mg/kg) of DEN at 6 weeks of age, given the test substance 2 weeks later, given a partial hepatectomy 1 week later, and administered the test substance for an additional 5 weeks. At that time liver tissue is harvested and quantitative measurements (morphometrics and stereology) are made on histologically examined PGST-positive liver foci. While this assay permits screening of a large number of chemicals in a short time period, it does not work for all hepatocarcinogens (e.g., peroxisome proliferators) and is based on a nonneoplastic end point.

While known hepatocarcinogens produce PGST-positive and other histochemically identifiable foci, the occurrence of foci of cellular alteration is known to be modulated by a variety of factors (e.g., strain, sex, diet), many foci regress or remodel upon cessation of treatment, and only a few foci (estimated at between 1 out of 1000 to 1 out of 10,000) progress to actual liver neoplasms. Hence, an observed positive focus response should be qualified and is indicative of further confirmatory testing.

Rat liver neoplasm models have been extremely useful in confirming and extending the observations on the mechanisms of carcinogenesis made in mouse skin-painting models, and liver focus models may be useful in assessing carcinogen potency based on a quantitative end point.

6. Genetically Altered Mouse Models for Carcinogenicity

Several models that are currently being validated utilize genetically altered transgenic and gene-targeted knockout mice (see "Suggested Reading"). To produce transgenic mice, oncogenic genes or fusion genes are introduced at the pronucleus stage of embryogenesis, resulting in the early development of neoplasia at one or more target tissue sites. As more transgenic mice are developed, a potentially wide array of animal models with different types of neoplasms in different target tissues will be available. Production of gene–targeted knockout mice entails targeting specific genes such that their function is silenced. In a broad-based international effort, three popular contemporary models are being studied to assess their potential as models for assessing the carcinogenic potential of various chemical agents. These are the p53 +/− mouse, in which one allele of the p53 tumor suppressor gene has been silenced; the Tg.Ac skin-painting model, which contains a viral *ras* transgene; and the rasH2 mouse, which carries the normal human H-*ras* gene with its endogenous promoter sequence. Initial studies with these three genetically altered mouse models show promise as adjunct models that yield results in approximately 6 months. In addition to their potential use in hazard identification, genetically altered mice offer a test system to potentially assess how chemical agents may modulate the process and progression of neoplasia.

7. Other in Vivo Models for Assessing Carcinogenicity

Additional carcinogenicity models have been developed, including a rat urinary bladder model, a rat pancreatic cancer model, a gastric cancer model, a rat thyroid cancer model, a fish liver neoplasm model, and rat and mouse colon cancer models. A short-term multiorgan test system for carcinogens has been proposed in which rats are treated by multiple carcinogens to cause initiation in several target tissues followed by administration of the test chemical for 12 weeks. End points that lend themselves to quantitation include preneoplastic lesions in the liver, thyroid, lung, forestomach, urinary bladder, and esophagus.

Over the years it has become apparent that there is no philosopher's stone for identifying potential human carcinogens, there is no absolute reference for carcinogenicity, and virtually no human surrogate is ideal or immune to criticism. Equivocal results can occur in any animal model no matter how well a carcinogenicity study is designed. In the last analysis, carcinogenicity data are most relevant to the test model employed. The greatest potential of the various "short-term" organ-specific animal carcinogenesis models is in understanding the underpinnings of the carcinogenic process.

C. *IN VITRO* SHORT-TERM TESTS

It is beyond the scope of this chapter to extensively discuss short-term *in vitro* or *in vivo* models or combined *in vivo–in vitro* models for assessing genotoxicity of chemicals. Such models are more than adequately discussed in the cited references. End points include evidence of a chemical's mutagenic, clastogenic, and cell transformation activity. The utility of these tests as predictors of carcinogenesis has had mixed reviews. Data derived from *in vitro* and *in vitro* tests for genotoxicity are used in tier testing, in decision point analysis, and in using the "weight-of-evidence" method for risk assessment.

SUGGESTED READING

General Books of Reference

Barrett, J. C. (ed.) (1987). "Mechanisms of Environmental Carcinogenesis," Vols. I and II. CRC Press, Boca Raton, FL.

Tannock, I. F., and Hill, R. P. (eds.) (1987). "The Basic Science of Oncology." Pergamon Press, New York.

Pitot, H. C. (1986). "Fundamentals of Oncology," 3rd Ed. Dekker, New York.

Waalkes, M. P., and Ward, J. M. (eds.) (1994). "Carcinogenesis: Target Organ Toxicology Series." Raven Press, New York.

Introduction

Barrett, J. C., (1991). Relationship between mutagenesis and carcinogenesis. *In* "Origins of Human Cancer" (J. Brugge *et al.*, eds.). Cold Spring Harbor Press, Cold Spring Harbor, NY.

Barrett, J. C., and Weisman, R. W. (1987). Cellular and molecular mechanisms of multistep carcinogenesis: Relevance to carcinogen risk assessment. *Environ. Health Perspect.* **76**, 65–70.

Boyland, E. (1969). The correlation of experimental carcinogenesis and cancer in man (review). *Prog. Exp. Tumor Res.* **11**, 222–234.

Carrell, C. J. (1997). Benzo-a-pyrene and its analogues: Structural studies of molecular strain. *Carcinogenesis* **18**, 415–422.

Contran, R. R., Jumar, V., and Robbins, S. L. (1989). Neoplasia. "Robbins Pathologic Basis of Disease," (R. Cotran, ed), 4th Ed., pp. 239–305. Saunders, Philadelphia.

Couch, D. B. (1996). Carcinogenesis: Basic principles. *Drug Chem. Toxicol.* **19**, 133–148.

Doll, R., and Peto, R. (1981). The causes of cancer and quantitation estimates of avoidable risks of cancer in the United States today. *J. Natl. Cancer Inst.* **66**, 1193–1308.

Elesperu, R. K. (1996). Future approaches to genetic toxicology risk assessment. *Mutat. Res.* **365**, 161–173.

Mastorides, S., and Muro-Cacho, C. (1998). Carcinogenesis. "Hamilton and Hardy's Industrial Toxicology" (R. Harbison, ed.) 5th Ed., pp. 597–610. Mosby-Yearbook, St. Louis, MO.

Tennant, R. W. (1994). Evaluation of transgenic mouse bioassays for identifying carcinogens and noncarcinogens. *Mutat. Res.* **365**, 119–127.

Spectrum of Proliferative Lesions

Bannasch, P. (1986). Preneoplastic lesions as end points in carcinogenicity testing. I. Hepatic preneoplasia. *Carcinogenesis* **7**, 689–695.

Bannasch, P. (1986). Preneoplastic lesions as end points in carcinogenicity testing. II. Preneoplasia in various nonhepatic tissues. *Carcinogenesis* **7**, 849–852.

Nowell, P. C. (1986). Mechanisms of tumor progression. *Cancer Res.* **46**, 2203–2207.

Rotstein, J. B., and Slaga, T. J. (1988). Effect of exogenous glutathione on tumor progression in the murine skin multistage carcinogenesis model. *Carcinogenesis* **9**, 1547–1551.

Steps in the Neoplastic Process

Argyris, T. S. (1985). Promotion of epidermal carcinogenesis by repeated damage to mouse skin. *Am. J. Indust. Med.* **8**, 329–337.

Borzsonyi, M., Day, N. E., Lapis, K., and Yamasaki, H. (eds.) (1984). "Models, Mechanisms, and Etiology of Tumour Promotion." IARC, Lyon, France.

Fialkow, P. J. (1979). Clonal origin of human tumors. *Annu. Rev. Med.* **30**, 135–143.

Farber, E. (1984). Cellular biochemistry of the stepwise development of cancer with chemicals. *Cancer Res.* **44**, 5463–5474.

Foulds, L. (1969). "Neoplastic Development," Vol. 1. Academic Press, New York.

Foulds, L. (1975). "Neoplastic Development," Vol. 2. Academic Press, New York.

Gartler, S. M. (1977). Patterns of cellular proliferation in normal and tumor cell populations. *Am. J. Pathol.* **86**, 685–692.

Hecker, E. (1976). Definitions and terminology in cancer (tumor) etiology. *Z. Krebsforsch.* **86**, 219–230.

Hennings, H., and Yuspa, S. H. (1985). Two-stage tumor promotion in mouse skin: An alternative interpretation. *J. Natl. Cancer Inst.* **74**, 735–740.

Heppner, G. H., and Miller, B. E. (1983). Tumor heterogeneity:Biological implications and therapeutic consequences. *Cancer Metast. Rev.* **2**, 5–23.

Iversen, O. H., and Astrup, E. G. (1984). The paradigm of two-stage carcinogenesis: A critical attitude. *Cancer Invest.* **2**, 51–60.

Medina, D. (1988). The preneoplastic state in mouse mammary tumorigenesis. *Carcinogenesis* **9**, 1113–1119.

Nowell, P. (1978). Tumors as clonal proliferations. *Arch Cell Pathol.* **29**, 145–150.

Sisskin, E. E., Gray, T., and Barrett, J. C. (1982). Correlation between sensitivity to tumor promotion and sustained epidermal hyperplasia of mice and rat treated with 12-O-tetradecanoylphorbol-13-acetate. *Carcinogenesis* **3**, 403–407.

Tennant, R. W., Margolin, B. H., Shelby, M. D., Zeiger, E., Haseman, J. K., Spalding, J., Caspary, W., Resnick, M., Stasiewwicz, S., Anderson, B., and Minor, R. (1987). Prediction of chemical carcinogenicity in rodents from in vitro genetic toxicity assays. *Science* **236**, 933–941.

VanDuuren, B. L. (1982). Cocarcinogens and tumor promoters and their environmental importance. *J. Am. College Toxicol.* **1**, 17–27.

Vogelstein, B., Fearon, E. R., Hamilton, S. R., and Feinberg, A. P. (1985). Use of restriction fragment length polymorphisms to determine the clonal origin of human tumors. *Science* **227**, 642–645.

Hypotheses of Mode of Action of Chemical Carcinogens

Duesberg, P. H. (1987). Retroviruses as carcinogens and pathogens: Expectations and reality. *Cancer Res.* **47**, 1199–1220.

Frost, P., and Kerbel, R. S. (1983). On a possible epigenetic mechanism(s) of tumor cell heterogeneity: The role of DNA methylation. *Cancer Metast. Rev.* **2**, 375–378.

Iversen, O. H. (ed) (1988). "Theories of Carcinogenesis." Hemisphere, New York.

Nordling, C. O. (1953). A new theory on the cancer-inducing mechanism. *Br. J. Cancer* **7**, 68–72.

Saffhill, R., Margison, G. P., and O'Connor, P. J. (1985). Mechanisms of carcinogenesis induced by alkylating agents. *Biochim. Biophys. Acta* **823**, 111–145.

Singer, B., and Grunberger, D. (1983). "Molecular Biology of Mutagens and Carcinogens." Plenum Press, New York.

Weinstein, I. B., Gattoni-Celli, S., Kirschmeier, P., Lambert, M., Hsiao, W., Backer, J., and Jeffrey, A. (1984). Initial cellular targets and eventual genomic changes in multistage carcinogenesis. *In* "IARC Scientific Publication #56" M. Borzsonyi, N. E. Day, K. Lapis, and H. Yamasaki, eds.). IARC, Lyon, France.

Weisburger, J. H., and Williams, G. M. (1975). Metabolism of chemical carcinogens. *In* "Cancer: A Comprehensive Treatise" (F. F. Becker, ed.), Vol. 1. Plenum Press, New York.

5. Carcinogenesis

Weisburger, J. H., and Williams, G. M. (1975). Chemical carcinogens. *In* "Toxicology: The Basic Science of Poisons" (L. J. Casarett and J. Doull, eds.). Macmillan, New York.

Oncogenes and Tumor Suppressor Genes

Anderson, M. W., Maronpot, R. R., and Reynolds, S. H. (1988). The role of oncogenes in chemical carcinogenesis: Extrapolation from rodents to humans. *In* "Detection Methods for DNA-Damaging Agents in Men: Applications in Cancer Epidemiology and Prevention" (H. Bartsch, ed.). Oxford Univ. Press, Oxford, England.

Anderson, M. W., and Reynolds, S. H. (1988). Activation of oncogenes by chemical carcinogens. *In* "Pathology of Neoplasia" (A. E. Sirica, ed.). Plenum Press, New York.

Barrett, J. C., and Wiseman, R. W. (1987). Cellular and molecular mechanisms of multistep carcinogenesis: Relevance to carcinogen risk assessment. *Environ. Health Perspect.* **76**, 65–70.

Barbacid, M. (1986). Oncogenes and human cancer: Cause or consequence? *Carcinogenesis* **7**, 1037–1042.

Brodeur, G. M. (1987). The involvement of oncogenes and suppressor genes in human neoplasia. *Adv. Pediatr.* **34**, 1–44.

Burck, K. B., Liu, E. T., and Larrick, J. W. (1988). "Oncogenes: An Introduction to the Concept of Cancer Genes." Springer-Verlag, New York.

Franks, L. M., and Teich, N. (eds.) (1986). "Introduction to the Cellular and Molecular Biology of Cancer." Oxford Univ. Oxford, England.

Freifelder, D. (1983). "Molecular Biology." Jones and Bartlett, Boston.

Hong, H. L., Devereux, T. R., Boorman, G. A., and Sills, R. C. (1998). Predominant codon 61 K-ras CTA mutation in lung and Harderian gland neoplasms of B6C3F1 mice exposed to chloroprene or isoprene. *FASEB J.* **12** (S), A813, 2711.

Hong, H. L., devereux, T. R., Melnick, R. L., Eldridge, S. R., Greenwell, A., Haseman, J., Boorman, G. A., and Sills, R. C. (1997). Both K-ras and H-ras protooncogene mutations are associated with Harderian gland tumorigenesis in B6C3F1 mice exposed to isoprene for 26 weeks. *Carcinogenesis* **18**, 783–789.

Hong, H. L., Devereux, T. R., Roycroft, J. H., Boorman, G. A., and Sills, R. C. (1998). Low frequency of ras mutations in liver neoplasms from B6C3F1 mice exposed to tetrafluoroethylene. *Toxicol. Pathol.* **26**, 646–650.

Kahn, P., and Graf, T. (eds.) (1986). "Oncogenes and Growth Control." Springer-Verlag, New York.

Klein, G. (1987). The approaching era of the tumor suppressor genes. *Science* **238**, 1539–1545.

Maronpot, R. R. (1998). The potential of genetically altered mice as animal models for carcinogen identification. *Toxicol. Pathol.* **26**, 579–581.

Maronpot, R. R., Fox, T., Malarkey, D. E., and Goldsworthy, T. L. (1995). Mutations in the ras protooncogene: Clues to etiology and molecular pathogenesis of mouse liver tumors. *Toxicology* **101**, 125–156.

Massey, T. E., Devereux, T. R., Maronpot, R. R., Foley, J. F., and Anderson, M. W. (1995). High frequency of K-ras mutations in spontaneous and vinyl carbamate-induced lung tumors of relatively resistant B6CF1 (C57BL/6J x BALB/cJ) mice. *Carcinogenesis* **16**, 1065–1069.

Pimentel, E. (1986). "Oncogenes." CRC Press, Boca Raton, FL.

Pimentel, E. (1987). "Hormones, Growth Factors, and Oncogenes." CRC Press, Boca Raton, FL.

Sills, R. C., Boorman, G. A., Neal, J. E., Hong, H. L., and Devereux, T. R. (1999). Mutations in ras genes in experimental tumors of rodents. IARC Scientific Publications No. 146, pp. 55–86. Lyon, France.

Sills, R. C., Hong, H. L., Greenwell, A, Herbert, R. A., Boorman, G. A., and Devereux, T. R. (1995). Increased frequency of K-ras mutations in lung neoplasms from female B6C3F1 mice exposed to ozone for 24 or 30 months. *Carcinogenesis* **16**, 1623–1628.

Sills, R. C., Hong, H. L., Melnick, R. L., Boorman, G. A., and Devereux, T. R. (1999). High frequency of codon 61 K-ras A to T transversions in lung and Harderian gland neoplasms of B6C3F1 mice exposed to chloroprene (2-chloro-1, 3-butadiene) for 2 years, and comparisons with structurally related chemicals isoprene and 1, 3-butadiene. *Carcinogenesis* **20**, 657–662.

Stowers, S. J., Maronpot, R. R., Reynolds, S. H., and Anderson, M. W. (1987). The role of oncogenes in chemical carcinogenesis. *Environ. Health Perspect.* **75**, 81–86.

Tam, A. S., Foley, J. F., Devereux, T. R., Maronpot, R. R., and Massey, T. E. (1999). High frequency and heteogeneous distribution of p53 mutations in aflatoxin B1-induced mouse lung tumors. *Cancer Res.* **59**, 3634–3640.

Trukhanova, L. S., Hong, H. L., Sills, R. C., Bowser, A. D., Gaul, B., Boorman, G. A., Turusov, V. S., Devereux, T. R., and Dixon, D. (1998). Predominant p53 G to A transition mutation and enchanced cell proliferation in uterine sarcomas of CBA mice treated with 1, 2-dimethylhydrazine. *Toxicol. Pathol.* **26**, 367–374.

Watson, J. D., Tooze, J., and Kurtz, D. T. (1983). "Recombinant DNA: A Short Course." Freeman, New York.

Watson, M. A., Devereux, T. R., Malarkey, D. E., Anderson, M. W., and Maronpot, R. R. (1995). H-ras oncogene mutation spectra in B6C3F1 and C57BL/6 mouse liver tumors provide evidence for TCDD promotion of spontaneous and vinyl carbamate-initiated liver cells. *Carcinogenesis* **16**, 1705–1710.

Weinberg, R. A. (1988). Finding the anti-oncogene. *Sci. Am.* **44–51**, September 1988.

Overview of Cell Cycle Control

Cordon-Cardo, C. (1995). Mutation of cell cycle regulators: Biological and clinical implications for human neoplasia. *Am. J. Pathol.* **147**, 545–560.

Levine, A. J., Momand, J., and Finlay, C. A. (1991). The p53 tumour suppressor gene. *Nature* **351**, 453–460.

Sherr, C. J. (1996). Cancer cell cycles. *Science* **264**, 1672–1677.

Tests for Carcinogenic Potential of Chemicals

Ashby, J., and Tennant, R. W. (1988). Chemical structure, *Salmonella* mutagenicity and extent of carcinogenicity as indicators of genotoxic carcinogenesis among 222 chemicals tested in rodents by the U.S. NCI/NTP. *Mutat. Res.* **204**, 17–115.

Bull, R. J., and Pereira, M. A. (1982). Development of a short-term matrix for estimating relative carcinogenic risk. *J. Am. College Toxicol.* **1**, 1–15.

Calkins, D. R., Dixon, R. L., Gerber, C. R., Zarin, D., and Omenn, G. S. (1980). Identification, characterization, and control of potential human carcinogens: A framework for federal decision-making. *J. Natl. Cancer Inst.* **64**, 169–176.

Gold, L. S., Wright, C., Berstein, L., and deVeciana, M. (1987). Reproducibility of results in "near-replicate" carcinogenesis bioassays. *J. Natl. Cancer Inst.* **78**, 1149–1158.

Haseman, J. K., and Huff, J. (1987). Species correlation in long-term carcinogenicity studies. *Cancer Lett.* **37**, 125–132.

Haseman, J. K., Huff, J. E., Zeiger, E., and McConnell, E. E. (1987). Comparative results of 327 chemical carcinogenicity studies. *Environ. Health Perspect.* **74**, 229–235.

Hecker, E. (1987). Three stage carcinogenesis in mouse skin: Recent results and present status of an advanced model system of chemical carcinogenesis. *Toxicol. Pathol.* **15**, 245–258.

Interagency Regulatory Liaison Group (1979). Scientific basis for identification of potential carcinogens and estimation of risks. *J. Natl. Cancer Inst.* **63**, 241–268.

Lave, L. B., Ennever, F. K., Rosenkranz, H. S., and Omenn, G. S. (1988). Information value of the rodent bioassay. *Nature* **336**, 631–633.

Maronpot, R. R. (1998). The potential of genetically altered mice as animal models for carcinogen identification. *Toxicol. Pathol.* **26**, 579–581.

Maronpot, R. R., Shimkin, M. B., Witschi, H. P., Smith, L. H., and Cline, J. M. (1986). Strain A mouse pulmonary tumor test results for chemicals previously tested in the National Cancer Institute carcinogenicity tests. *J. Natl. Cancer Inst.* **76**, 1101–1112.

Milman, H. A., and Weisburger, E. K. (eds.) (1985). "Handbook of Carcinogen Testing," Noyes Publications. Park Ridge, NJ.

Mitsumori, K., Wakana, S., Yamamoto, S., Jodama, Y., Yasuhara, K, Nomura, T., Hyashi, Y., and Maronpot, R. R. (1997). Susceptibility of transgenic mice carrying human prototype c-Ha-ras gene in a short-term carcinogenicity study of vinyl carbamate and ras gene analyses of the induced tumors. *Mol. Carcinog.* **20**, 298–307.

Montesano, R., Bartsch, H., Vainio, H., Wilbourn, J., and Yamasaki, H. (eds.) (1986). "Long-Term and Short-Term Assays for Carcinogens: A Critical Appraisal." IARC Scientific Publication No. 83. IARC, Lyon, France.

Page, N. P. (1977). Concepts of a bioassay program in environmental carcinogenesis. *In* "Environmental Cancer: Advances in Modern Toxicology" (Kraybill and Mehlman, eds.), Vol. 3. Wiley, New York.

Saffiotti, U. (1980). Identification and definition of chemical carcinogens: Review of criteria and research needs. *J. Toxicol. Environ. Health* **6**, 1029–1057.

Shelby, M. D. (1988). The genetic toxicity of human carcinogens and its implications. *Mutat. Res.* **204**, 3–15.

Shubik, P. (1984). Carcinogenicity evaluation and regulatory decisions. *Regul. Toxicol. Pharmacol.* **4**, 322–324.

Slaga, T. J., Fischer, S. M., Triplett, L. L., and Nesnow, S. (1982). Comparison of complete carcinogenesis and tumor initiation and promotion in mouse skin: The induction of papillomas by tumor initiation-promotion a reliable short term assay. *J. Am. College Toxicol.* **1**, 83–99.

Society of Toxicologic Pathologists (1998). Focus on genetic altered mouse cancer models. *Toxicol. Pathol.* **26**, 461–584.

Squire, R. A. (1981). Ranking animal carcinogens: A proposed regulatory approach. *Science* **214**, 877–880.

Tennant, R. W. (1996). Evaluation of transgenic mouse bikoassays for identifying carcinogens and noncarcinogens. *Mutat. Res.* **365**, 119–127.

Ward, J. M., and Ito, N. (1988). Meeting Report: Development of new medium-term bioassays for carcinogens. *Cancer Res.* **48**, 5051–5054.

Weisburger, J. H., and Williams, G. M. (1981) Carcinogen testing: Current problems and new approaches. *Science* **214**, 401–407.

Williams, G. M., and Weisburger, J. H. (1981). Systematic carcinogen testing through the decision point approach. *Annu. Rev. Pharmacol. Toxicol.* **21**, 393–416.

Zeiger, E. (1987). Carcinogenicity of mutagens: Predictive capability of the *Salmonella* mutagenesis assay for rodent carcinogenicity. *Cancer Res.* **47**, 1287–1296.

6

Applied Clinical Pathology in Preclinical Toxicology Testing

G. S. Smith
CanBioPharma Consulting Inc.
Rockwood, Ontario, Canada

R. L. Hall
Covance Laboratories
Madison, Wisconsin

R. M. Walker
Pfizer Global Research
and Development
Mississauga, Ontario, Canada

I. Introduction

Clinical pathology testing is an integral component of evaluation of the toxicologic potential of therapeutic agents, pesticides, and industrial chemicals in laboratory animal species. Results of hematology, clinical chemistry, and urinalysis tests provide information regarding the overall health status of animals, as well as target organs and general metabolic, adaptive, or toxic processes associated with exposure to test articles. Clinical pathology results assist in establishing dose–response relationships and mechanisms of toxicity and provide a link with clinical observations and anatomic pathology findings. Knowledge of test article interference with laboratory tests is important from the standpoint of the interpretation of results in preclinical studies as well as in human trials. Clinical pathology is an important tool for monitoring the onset, course, and severity of toxic insults in preclinical animal models and thereby helps identify critical end points for monitoring the effects of the test article and/or its metabolites in the intended patient population or the population at risk. Valuable information regarding target organ effects can be compared across laboratory animal species and the importance and relevance of the findings extrapolated to humans or animal species that will be exposed to the test article.

Preclinical clinical pathology testing recommendations or requirements to support the study of potential therapeutic agents and other chemicals are outlined in guidelines provided by several national regulatory agencies (e.g., U. S. Food and Drug Administration, U. S. Environmental Protection Agency, Japanese Ministry of Health and Welfare). Globally recognized clinical pathology preclinical testing regulatory guidelines do not exist, and the International Conference on Harmonization of Technical Requirements for Registration of Pharmaceuticals for Human Use has not specifically

Handbook of Toxicologic Pathology, Second Edition
Volume 1

addressed clinical pathology testing. However, a joint scientific committee for International Harmonization of Clinical Pathology Testing, formed in 1992, has published minimum recommendations for clinical pathology testing of laboratory animals used in regulated safety assessment/toxicity studies (Table I).

Notwithstanding these recommendations, the clinical pathology component of the toxicology study protocol should be designed to meet specific study objectives. The elements that will be required to effectively interpret and report clinical pathology test results should be fully considered at the time of protocol preparation. Inclusion of test parameters that have unproven sensitivity or specificity for anticipated toxicities may be worthy of evaluation in an exploratory investigative study where the objective is to search for a potential marker of a difficult to monitor effect (e.g., coronary vasculitis). However, inclusion of unproven tests in definitive preclinical studies is likely to provide uninterpretable or confounding data and therefore such inclusion is not usually recommended. Judicious study design to permit discriminating interpretation of test results requires a knowledge of the characteristics of test parameters in health and pathologic states, species

differences, and causes of spurious or spontaneous variations in test results for a particular parameter/species. Riley (1992) lists 35 potential sources of preanalytical variation in clinical pathology analyses that may affect the predictive value of sample measurements. Test compound characteristics such as formulation, pharmacology, pharmacokinetics, and anticipated toxicity based on previous experience with the compound or pharmacologic class should be considered in selecting the species for study as well as time points and parameters for clinical pathology evaluation.

The intent of this chapter is to provide guidance on principles of interpretive clinical pathology in toxicology studies. It is not intended to provide a comprehensive, detailed description of characteristics of all potential test parameters in each laboratory species nor is it intended to describe analytical methodologies and potential assay interference. Such information is covered in texts referred to at the end of this chapter. Rather, the intent is to highlight aspects of hematology and clinical chemistry in particular that will be an aid to prudent study design and result interpretation. Understanding general principles common to hematology and biochemistry with specific knowledge of the properties of analytes in the species of interest is key to the accurate interpretation of results. Knowledge of the following properties of each analyte is required: source of origin or synthesis; kinetics of production; storage and specifics of release to circulation; circulating life span or half-life; and disposition/tissue fate or elimination. It is important that patterns of changes involving a number of clinical pathology parameters (hematology, clinical chemistry, and urinalysis) and associations of clinical pathology with other study findings (e.g., clinical signs, morphologic pathology, liver microsomal enzyme activities, toxicokinetics) be investigated and recognized as these patterns may be indicative of the overall metabolic, adaptive, or toxic process.

In order to provide a framework for interpretation of clinical pathology test results, this chapter provides an overview of key features of

TABLE I
Harmonization of Animal Clinical Pathology Testing in Preclinical Toxicity Studies[a]

Hematology	Chemistry	Urinalysis
WBC	Glucose	Overnight collection
Absolute differential	BUN	Appearance, volume
RBC, Hb, Hct	Creatinine	SG or osmolality
RBC morphology	Total protein	Protein
MCV, MCH, MCHC	Albumin	Glucose
Reticulocytes	Ca, Na, K	
Platelets	Cholesterol	
Bone marrow smears for potential cytology	Two of ALT, AST, SDH, GDH, or bile acids	
PT, APTT	Two of ALP, GGT, 5'NT, bilirubin, or bile acids	

[a]From Weingand et al. (1992, 1996).

hematology, such as the production of blood cellular elements and evaluation of erythrocyte (RBC), white blood cell (WBC), and platelet responses, as well as a brief summary of coagulation tests used most commonly in toxicology studies (see also Chapters 39 and 40). Similarly, an overview of plasma/serum clinical chemistry tests performed in preclinical toxicology studies is provided and the relevance of changes in these parameters is related to organs/body systems. Microsomal enzyme determinations are briefly alluded to as results may have implications for clinical and anatomic pathology result interpretation. Application of urinalysis in toxicology studies is also summarized. Based on this understanding, the design of the clinical pathology component of preclinical toxicology studies and the interpretation and reporting of clinical pathology results are discussed. Finally, the importance of integrating the clinical pathology findings with other study findings in the assessment of overall safety or risk assessment is stressed.

II. Hematology

A. PARAMETERS GENERALLY INCLUDED IN STUDY PROTOCOLS

Potential hematologic effects of test compounds are identified primarily by the evaluation of RBCs, WBCs, platelets, and coagulation. Automated determination of red cell parameters (RBC count, hemoglobin, hematocrit) and red cell indices [mean cell volume (MCV), mean cell hemoglobin (MCH), mean cell hemoglobin concentration (MCHC)] are performed routinely. Some instruments also calculate red cell distribution width (RDW). RDW is a numerical value for the variance of the size distribution curve of RBCs and is an index of the degree of anisocytosis of RBCs.

Quantification of blood reticulocyte counts is included in some protocols. Reticulocytes are immature anuclear RBCs that contain residual RNA and mitochondria and correspond to polychromatophilic RBCs observed in Wright's-stained blood smears. Reticulocyte enumeration is an index of bone marrow erythropoietic

activity and responsiveness. Species and age differences occur in the number of circulating reticulocytes in health with up to approximately 1% in adult dogs and monkeys, and 5% or more in rats and mice. Many laboratories prepare vitally-stained (e.g., new methylene blue) blood smears for the potential subsequent manual determination of reticulocyte counts, depending on peripheral blood RBC findings. A limited number of laboratories use flow cytometry to perform reticulocyte counts as a protocol required test, irrespective of peripheral blood findings. Evaluation of the reticulocyte response should be made on the basis of absolute rather than relative reticulocyte counts. Reticulocyte count changes, especially decreases, may occur prior to changes in red cell parameters and thus may be a more sensitive indicator of effects on the erythron, especially in short-term studies.

Total WBC and differential (relative and absolute) counts and platelet counts are integral components of most toxicology protocols. Interpretation of leukocyte responses should be made on the basis of absolute rather than relative counts. Some laboratories report instrument-calculated values for mean platelet volume (MPV) and, less often, platelet distribution width (PDW). PDW is a measure of platelet anisocytosis.

Assessment of RBC morphology is important when red cell parameters or indices have been affected by administration of the test article, although treatment-related alterations in cell morphology are relatively rare findings in toxicology studies. Many automated hematology analyzers are capable of flagging abnormal populations of peripheral blood cells and aberrations in cell morphology. However, regardless of whether such flagging occurs, a representative number of blood smears from control and high-dose animals should be screened microscopically.

Prothrombin time (PT), which measures extrinsic and common coagulation pathways, and activated partial thromboplastin time (APTT), which measures intrinsic and common pathways, are the coagulation tests performed most commonly.

Histopathologic examination of bone marrow is performed routinely in most toxicology studies, whereas the cytologic evaluation of bone marrow or the manual determination of bone marrow differential counts is generally contingent on the results of peripheral blood hematology and bone marrow histopathology. A limited number of laboratories perform bone marrow differential counts routinely using flow cytometry, regardless of peripheral blood hematology findings.

Function tests of RBCs, WBCs, or platelets are not performed routinely in toxicology studies. Such special investigative studies (e.g., neutrophil adherence, bactericidal ability, or chemotaxis: lymphocyte blastogenesis; *in vitro* and *in vivo* assays of lymphocyte effector functions; bleeding time; platelet aggregation or adhesion; release of platelet adenine nucleotides) can be conducted as required.

B. INTERPRETATIVE HEMATOLOGY

Understanding the fundamentals and kinetics of production, time in circulation, and fate of cellular blood elements, as represented schematically in Fig. 1, is key to the interpretation of hematology results. The pluripotent stem cell [colony-forming unit-spleen (CFU-S)] in marrow or spleen can differentiate along lymphoid or hematopoietic lines. Numerous cytokines or glycoproteins comprise the hematopoietic growth factors that stimulate or inhibit hematopoiesis at some level. Some are promiscuous and may affect erythropoiesis, granulopoiesis, and megakaryocytopoiesis [e.g., interleukin-3 (IL-3), granulocyte–macrophage colony-stimulating factor (GM-CSF)] whereas the growth factors erythropoietin and thrombopoietin are more restricted in their targets. The balance of hematopoiesis means that stimuli increasing stem cell input into a particular cell line may decrease the number of early progenitors being directed into other cell lines.

Test article-related changes in RBC, WBC, or platelet counts generally reflect an altered balance between production and peripheral loss or destruction. Hematology result interpretation needs to reflect the dynamic processes

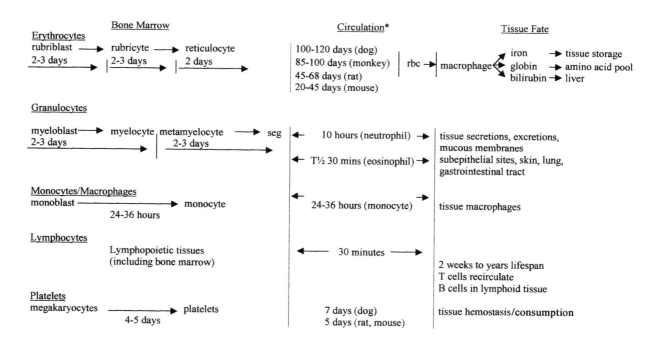

Figure 1. Kinetics of production, approximate time in circulation, and fate of blood cells.

involved. Ideally, results of samples collected at intervals should be evaluated to establish the temporal pattern of changes as an aid to understanding the processes involved. However, for practical reasons this is relatively seldom done in rodent studies.

1. Causes of Increases in Red Cells, Leukocytes, and Platelets

Increased numbers of blood cellular elements may occur for a number of reasons depending on the cell line involved. Increased production of marrow progenitors with concomitant increases in peripheral blood occurs following administration of biotechnology-derived growth or colony-stimulating factors in most common laboratory animal species, even though most of these manufactured products are human proteins. Increased tissue requirements for one or more of the blood cellular elements (e.g., following hemolysis, hemorrhage, or tissue inflammation) stimulate increased marrow production of specific cell lines (e.g., red blood cells, platelets, or neutrophils). Bone marrow is typically hypercellular. Increased bone marrow release of reticulocytes or segmented neutrophils from the neutrophil storage pool occurs relatively soon (i.e., within hours) following onset of the stimulus. If acute demand exceeds the rate of production in responsive situations, normal numbers of cells of a particular series can be maintained in peripheral blood for a short time due to the release of less mature, larger cells, such as nucleated RBCs, or neutrophil bands, metamyelocytes, or earlier forms (termed "left shift"). If the demand for cells is overwhelming, however, the number of circulating cells will be reduced regardless of enhanced marrow production. In the case of neutrophils and platelets, accelerated production and release of cells in excess of demand may result in moderate or marked increases in counts.

Proportionate increases in red cell numbers, hemoglobin, and hematocrit in toxicology studies generally reflect hemoconcentration/dehydration, which may also increase serum total protein and/or albumin concentrations.

Erythrocytosis is an anticipated finding when the test article is erythropoietin.

Increased peripheral blood leukocytes (generally neutrophils and/or lymphocytes) may reflect physiologic, pathologic, or xenobiotic-induced effects.

Physiologic neutrophilia occurs in response to fear, excitement, or exercise and is a mild (up to two-fold increase), short-lived (10–20 min) increase reflecting an epinephrine-mediated mobilization of neutrophils from the marginal pool to the circulating pool. Lymphocytosis may also occur, particularly in cats or non-human primates. Exogenous or endogenous (as in acute disease or stress) corticosteroids induce a mild to moderate neutrophilia (generally $< 25 \times 10^9$/liter in dogs) accompanied by lymphopenia, eosinopenia, and occasionally monocytosis. The neutrophilia is typically without a left shift and is due to increased bone marrow release of neutrophils and decreased migration of neutrophils from circulation to tissues, as well as a shift of cells from the marginal to circulating pool.

Inflammation occurs in response to mediators released in conjunction with tissue injury and/or infectious agents. Both marginal and circulating neutrophil pools are increased in inflammation, and a left shift may be present. Mild or long-standing inflammation may not produce a left shift. Severe inflammation may result in WBC counts in the range of 30–60 $\times 10^9$/liter or greater (e.g., 100×10^9/liter) in dogs. The neutrophilia of inflammation is frequently accompanied by lymphopenia and eosinopenia in the dog. Monocytosis is an inconsistent finding. WBC counts seldom extend beyond $30-40 \times 10^9$/liter in rodents or monkeys with inflammation. However, chronic lesions in older rats and mice (e.g., purulent heel sores) may be associated with WBC counts $> 50 \times 10^9$/liter. Lymphocytosis often contributes to the leukocytosis of inflammation in rodents. Neutrophilia may occur in association with hemorrhage or hemolysis.

Myeloproliferative and more common lymphoproliferative disorders are expected background findings in rats and mice on long-term toxicity studies. Myeloproliferative disorders are uncommon in nonrodents in toxicology studies.

Increased platelet counts are occasionally observed in toxicology studies. Primary thrombocytosis, an unusual finding, is an anticipated effect when the test article is a hematopoietic growth factor (e.g., thrombopoietin). Reactive or secondary thrombocytosis may occur secondary to catecholamine-induced splenic contraction or to generalized bone marrow stimulation as in hemolytic anemia, blood loss, or inflammation. Increased platelet production may be reflected in the presence of younger, larger platelets ("shift platelets"), which may cause increased MPV, although changes in MPV are inconsistently present. Rebound thrombocytosis may follow thrombocytopenia due to the reversible inhibition of platelet production by chemotherapeutic agents.

2. Causes of Decreases in Red Cells, Leukocytes, and Platelets

When peripheral demand for a cell type exceeds marrow and splenic (rodents) production, anemia, granulocytopenia, or thrombocytopenia occurs.

Anemia (defined as the condition characterized by a hemoglobin concentration below the lower reference limit) is broadly classified as regenerative or nonregenerative according to the presence or absence of reticulocytosis (or polychromasia and anisocytosis). Concomitant decreases in RBC count and hematocrit occur, which generally approximate the proportionate decrease in hemoglobin, depending on the cause of the anemia and effects on cell size. The evaluation of erythropoiesis, classification of anemia, and identification of mechanisms and agents associated with toxic effects on the erythroid system are described by Fried (1997), Dabrow and Gabuzda (1997), Salama (1997), and Means (1997). The term "anemia" connotes an adverse effect, and its judicious use depends on the extent of the decrease in hemoglobin. Decreases in red cell parameters may be due to hemorrhage, hemolysis, or decreased marrow production. An absolute increase in reticulocytes indicates a responsive marrow (regenera-

tive anemia) and that the cause of anemia is extra marrow (hemolysis or hemorrhage). In responsive situations, reticulocytosis is observable about 48–72 hr following the onset of anemia with maximum reticulocytosis occurring about 7 days postonset. Release of immature red cells from the bone marrow or spleen (extramedullary hematopoiesis is common for rodents) may be evidenced by reticulocytosis/polychromasia, an increase in MCV and RDW, decreased MCHC and hypochromasia, and, when the demand is extensive, nucleated red cells in circulation. The absence of reticulocytosis following the onset of anemia indicates an unresponsive marrow (nonregenerative anemia). Typical features of anemias of varying etiopathogenesis are summarized in Table II. Some of the features of anemia secondary to hemorrhage may resemble those of hemolytic anemia early in the process when the marrow may be responsive. However, with longstanding hemorrhage, iron loss may occur (external hemorrhage), marrow reserves become depleted, and marrow becomes hyporesponsive.

It can be readily appreciated from an awareness of red cell life span in different species that anemia due to decreased red cell production induced by a test article would take longer to occur in the dog or monkey as compared with the rat. As a corollary example, if the RBC count in a monkey is 3.1×10^{12}/liter after 2

TABLE II
General Causes and Characteristics of Anemia

Parameter	Anemia		
	Decreased Production	Chronic blood loss	Hemolysis
Reticulocytosis	−	+	+++
Polychromasia	−	+	+++
Nucleated RBC	−	+	+++
MCV	Normal or ↓	↓	↑
MCH	Normal or ↓	↓	Normal or ↑
Marrow cellularity	↓	Variable	↑
Serum protein	Normal	↓	Normal or ↑
Hyperbilirubinuria	−	−	±
Hemoglobinemia	−	−	±

weeks of test article treatment compared with 5.9×10^{12}/liter pretest (reference range 5.2–7.8 $\times 10^{12}$/liter), then decreased erythropoiesis can be ruled out as the primary mechanism underlying the effect. Therefore, the etiopathogenesis of the developing anemia is either hemorrhagic or hemolytic in nature. Also, based on circulating lifespan, it can be anticipated that agents causing direct injury to pluripotent hematopoietic stem cells or their stromal microenvironment (e.g., irradiation, chemicals, chemotherapeutics, antimetabolites, or cytotoxic agents) will manifest effects on peripheral blood granulocyte, platelet, and reticulocyte counts earlier than on RBC counts.

Granulocytes in peripheral blood have a short half-life of about 4–8 hr. In healthy animals, there is generally considered to be a large reserve of mature neutrophils present in the marrow storage pool. Thus it takes approximately 5–7 days for the suppression of granulopoiesis at the level of the proliferating pool (myeloblasts, promyelocytes, myelocytes) to be manifested by a drop in circulating neutrophil numbers. Removal of exposure to the inciting agent generally results in rapid recovery with return to approximately normal neutrophil numbers within 72 hr. The response of granulocytes to toxic injury, mechanisms underlying drug-induced hematotoxicity (e.g., immunogenicity, direct drug toxicity, accumulation of toxic metabolites, generation of toxic metabolites within neutrophils), and drugs associated with the development of agranulocytosis (e.g., phenothiazine derivatives, clozapine) are described by Pisciotta (1997).

Because the lifespan of platelets in peripheral blood is relatively short (e.g., about 7 days in dogs, 5 days in rats and mice), agents that impair thrombopoiesis result in the lowering of blood platelet counts within a relatively short time frame (e.g., 1–2 weeks). Recovery of blood platelet numbers is rapid following removal of the inciting agent, as platelet production time from megakaryocytes is short (about 4–5 days). In the example provided in Table III, dose-related decreases in group mean platelet counts occurred in treated rats following 4 weeks of

TABLE III
Hematology Data at Termination of 4-Week Rat Study (Mean ± SE)

Parameter	Treatment group			
	Control	Low dose	Mid dose	High dose
Platelets (10^9/liter)	1153±42	937±38[a]	829±17[a]	789±36[a]
Mean platelet volume (fL)	6.2±0.1	6.6±0.1	7.1±0.1[a]	7.1±0.2[a]

[a]Significantly different ($p < 0.01$) from control.

administration of a xenobiotic. While further investigations are necessary to establish the etiopathogenesis of the effect, increased MPV in treated groups indicates marrow responsiveness. The response of thrombocytes to toxic injury, and the toxicologic implications of modulation of platelet function by antiplatelet agents have been reviewed (Aster, 1997; Jakubowski, 1997). A large number of xenobiotics have been implicated in immune-mediated platelet destruction in humans.

Impairment of erythropoiesis takes longer to evidence as anemia in view of the comparatively longer red cell lifespan. Recovery following agent removal will start to be observed in peripheral blood within a few days (as the production time from committed stem cell to reticulocyte is about 4–5 days). However, recovery of circulating red cell numbers to pretest values may take weeks, depending on the degree of anemia caused by the inciting agent.

While follow-up investigative studies may be conducted to explore mechanisms of treatment-related anemia, neutropenia, or thrombocytopenia (e.g., [51]chromium RBC survival, erythropoietin quantification, [111]indium platelet mean lifespan determination), definitive identification of the underlying process is frequently not accomplished. In vivo rechallenge studies, with appropriately timed serial hematology sampling to monitor neutrophil or platelet counts, may be useful in identifying an immune basis for treatment-related cytopenias as well as indicating the stage of cell affected. Protein electrophoresis, immunoglobulin quantification, and antineutrophil or antimegakaryocye antibody tests may be instructive. A frequently asked question following the identification of treatment-related thrombocytopenia in animal studies is whether platelet function is altered. To address this question, a number of *ex vivo* evaluations can be performed, such as platelet aggregation, platelet adhesion, and clot retraction. Bleeding time, while a nonspecific and relatively crude test, can be used to investigate whether treatment-related effects on platelet numbers have *in vivo* functional relevance.

Decreases in blood lymphocyte counts in toxicity studies may reflect direct (e.g., chemotherapeutic or immunosuppressive agents) or indirect effects (e.g., inanition, stress). Distinction of direct from indirect causes of decreased counts is frequently difficult. Correlative histopathologic changes in lymphoid organs may be instructive. Total blood lymphocyte counts may remain within the reference range despite changes in subsets, and some immunosuppressive drugs may interfere with T-cell function without causing overt toxicity to lymphocytes (see also Chapter 39). Treatment-related changes in eosinophil counts rarely occur in toxicology studies, and basophils are seldom identified in peripheral blood of laboratory animal species other than the rabbit.

Changes in morphology of blood cells occur relatively infrequently in toxicology studies. Examples of treatment-related morphologic changes reported in animal studies are Heinz bodies (Heinz body hemolytic anemia), spherocytosis (immune-mediated hemolytic anemia), schistocytosis (associated with vasculitis or disseminated intravascular coagulation), and megaloblastoid red cell and neutrophil precursors (associated with folate inhibitors or agents that impair DNA synthesis). Intraerythrocytic plasmodium organisms are often observed in blood films from cynomolgus and rhesus monkeys, and while the infections are typically asymptomatic, they do have the potential to confound data interpretation.

3. Bone Marrow Evaluation

Bone marrow in sections of femur or sternum is generally included in the list of protocol-required tissues for histopathologic evaluation. Bone marrow smear cytologic examination should be performed in situations of unexplained reduction in RBC, WBC, or platelet counts or to investigate potential hematopoietic or nonhematopoietic neoplasia, marrow infiltrative disease, or osteomyelitis. There is limited scientific merit in performing manual differential counts on bone marrow samples from animals with a normal peripheral blood profile or where blood cellular elements are increased numerically. Cytologic marrow evaluations include cellularity of cell lines (erythroid, myeloid, lymphoid, megakaryocytes); maturation/progression of cells within cell lines; ratio of myeloid to nucleated erythroid cells (M/E ratio); and estimation of amount of iron present, although this is difficult to assess with confidence. Accurate interpretation of marrow smears depends on the quality of the preparation. For example, estimation of megakaryocyte numbers is very subjective and is affected by smear technique. In health about 80–90% of erythroid cells should be rubricytes and metarubricytes, and about 80% of the myeloid series should be in the maturation pool (segmented granulocytes, bands, metamyelocytes). Interpretation of the M/E ratio requires knowledge of peripheral blood cell counts. An increased or decreased M/E ratio is usually reflective of changes in the erythroid compartment when the WBC count is normal. When the M/E ratio is high and the WBC count is normal, anemia is likely due to erythroid hypoplasia. However, if both the M/E ratio and the WBC count are high, anemia cannot be attributed to decreased erythropoiesis with certainty, as granulocytic hyperplasia alone may be responsible for the high M/E ratio. Marrow iron can be anticipated to be absent or reduced in iron deficiency anemia and may be increased in anemia of chronic disease.

4. Coagulation Tests

The intrinsic and extrinsic coagulation pathways are evaluated routinely by the activated partial thromboplastin time (APTT) and one-stage prothrombin time (OSTP or PT), respect-

130

ively. These assays are relatively insensitive and nonspecific, as activity of a single clotting factor must be reduced to about 30% of normal before meaningful prolongation of APTT or PT occurs. Compounds that interfere with vitamin K absorption (e.g., high-dose levels of synthetic fat preparations) are examples of test articles that may cause prominent PT and APTT increases in laboratory animals. Small, statistically significant differences between the mean values for control and treated animals for these assays (e.g., < 2 sec) are observed occasionally in toxicology studies. Although usually not toxicologically meaningful, interpretation of these small differences requires consideration of many factors including, but not limited to, the pharmacologic activity of the test article, potential correlative clinical observations (e.g., retinal hemorrhage or melena), potential correlative histopathological findings (especially vascular or hepatic findings), the presence or absence of similar findings in earlier studies with the test article, and the possibility that the differences may be spurious because of difficulty with blood collection (e.g., it may be more difficult to acquire high-quality blood specimens from treated animals that are smaller, in poor health, or dehydrated). APTT and PT are insensitive measures of liver function. While almost all clotting factors are synthesized by the liver, the large liver functional reserve means that severe liver injury is generally required before coagulation times are affected. In the absence of obvious mechanisms for treatment-related, clinically relevant prolongation in APTT and/or PT (e.g., disseminated intravascular coagulation, decreased absorption of vitamin K, vitamin K antagonism, or liver failure), abnormal test results can be followed by determinations of specific clotting factor activities and plasma fibrinogen concentration.

III. Clinical Chemistry

Clinical chemistry tests are performed routinely in toxicology studies and generate information regarding the metabolism of carbohydrates, lipids, and proteins and the integrity of urinary, hepatobiliary, musculoskeletal, cardiovascular, and gastrointestinal systems. Routinely performed clinical chemistry tests are poor indicators of central nervous system (CNS) toxicity. Blood gas analyses are not generally a component of preclinical toxicology protocols. When included, blood gas results may provide some relatively nonspecific information regarding respiratory and gastrointestinal systems in particular. Other tests (e.g., gastrointestinal, pancreatic, or endocrine function) may be conducted as follow-up to determine the significance and relevance of initial clinical and clinicopathologic findings or to more accurately define test article effects on body systems or specific organs.

In assessing the significance of clinical chemistry and clinical pathology results in general, it is important that individual parameters are not evaluated in isolation but rather in concert with other study findings. Thus, inspection for associations between test parameters is necessary for accurate interpretation (Table IV).

Common causes of increases and decreases in clinical chemistry parameters measured in preclinical toxicology studies are indicated in Fig. 2.

A. CHOLESTEROL, TRIGLYCERIDES, AND GLUCOSE

Changes in cholesterol, triglycerides, or glucose are typically reflective of general metabolic events rather than serving as indicators of specific target organ toxicity, although cholesterol may be the pharmacologic target of hypolipidemic agents leading to extremely low serum cholesterol concentrations at dose levels used in toxicology studies. Cholesterol and triglycerides are components of chylomicrons and are derived from dietary intake and endogenous synthesis, particularly by the liver. Cholesterol is required for the synthesis of bile acids, corticosteroids, and sex steroids. Triglycerides are a source of energy. Changes (increases or decreases) in serum cholesterol or triglyceride concentrations are relatively frequent findings in toxicology studies, although the exact mechanisms involved are often unknown.

TABLE IV
Clinical Pathology Parameters in Preclinical Toxicology Study Protocols and Potential Associations with Body Systems

System	Clinical pathology parameters	System	Clinical pathology parameters
General metabolism	Total protein, albumin, cholesterol, triglycerides, glucose	Hepatobiliary Hepatic	ALT, AST, SDH, GDH, glucose, cholesterol, albumin, BUN, bilirubin, PT, APTT
Urinary	BUN, creatinine, electrolytes, calcium, phosphorus, protein, albumin, RBC parameters, urinalysis	Biliary	Bilirubin, ALP, GGT, 5'NT, bile acids
Gastrointestinal	Total protein, albumin, globulin, electrolytes, BUN		
Musculoskeletal	CK, AST, LDH	Cardiovascular	CK, AST, LDH
Immune	Total protein, globulin, serum protein electrophoresis, lymphocytes	Hematopoietic	Complete blood cell count, blood smear, bone marrow

Several factors may be involved, including food consumption and body weight changes, liver function, and hormone balance.

Serum glucose concentration depends on intestinal absorption, hepatic production, and tissue uptake of glucose. The balance is affected by several hormones. In particular, insulin reduces glucose concentrations by stimulating cellular uptake of glucose, and glucagon increases glucose concentrations by glycogenolysis and gluconeogenesis. Corticosteroids and catecholamines increase glucose concentrations via gluconeogenesis and gylcogenolysis, respectively. Also, corticosteroids, catecholamines, and growth hormone are insulin an-

tagonists and interfere with the action of insulin on cells. Common causes of increased glucose concentrations in toxicology studies include nonfasted samples, samples from moribund animals, and excitement/fear/pain (catecholamine release). *In vitro* glycolysis (primarily by erythrocytes), decreased food consumption, malabsorption, and hepatic disease may lead to decreased glucose.

B. SERUM PROTEINS

Total serum protein concentration reflects all of the different proteins in plasma with the exception of those that are consumed in clot formation, such as fibrinogen and the clotting factors.

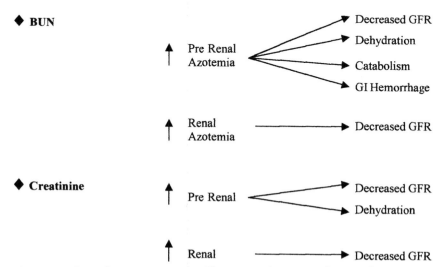

Figure 2. Some factors commonly affecting results in toxicology studies.

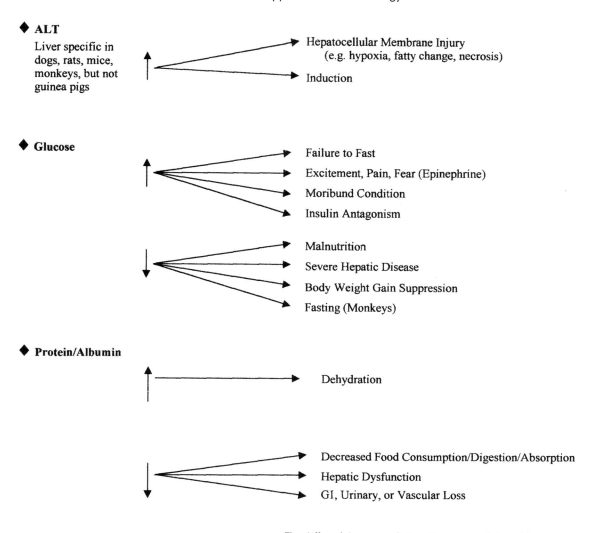

♦ **ALT**
Liver specific in dogs, rats, mice, monkeys, but not guinea pigs

→ Hepatocellular Membrane Injury (e.g. hypoxia, fatty change, necrosis)
→ Induction

♦ **Glucose**

→ Failure to Fast
→ Excitement, Pain, Fear (Epinephrine)
→ Moribund Condition
→ Insulin Antagonism

→ Malnutrition
→ Severe Hepatic Disease
→ Body Weight Gain Suppression
→ Fasting (Monkeys)

♦ **Protein/Albumin**

→ Dehydration

→ Decreased Food Consumption/Digestion/Absorption
→ Hepatic Dysfunction
→ GI, Urinary, or Vascular Loss

$T_{1/2}$ (albumin) approx. 2 days (mouse) or 8 days (dog)

Figure 2. (*Continued*)

Plasma protein is about 3–5 g/liter greater than serum protein. The hydration status of the animal should be considered when interpreting protein changes. Hypoproteinemia, like anemia, can be masked by dehydration. Albumin and globulins are increased proportionately in simple dehydration.

Albumin accounts for about 50% of total serum protein concentration in most species and for about 75% of plasma colloidal activity. Synthesis occurs in the liver. There is a direct correlation between albumin turnover and body size. For example, plasma albumin half-life is 2 and 8 days in the mouse and dog, respectively. Occurrence of hypoalbuminemia following 7 days of administration of a test compound could reflect decreased assimilation (e.g., decreased food consumption, digestion, or absorption or hepatic dysfunction) in the mouse. However, other underlying causes (e.g., gastrointestinal, urinary, or vascular loss of albumin) would be more likely causes of hypoalbuminemia in this time frame in the dog. Albumin is considered a negative acute-phase protein and decreased albumin can be an indicator of acute inflammatory conditions.

133

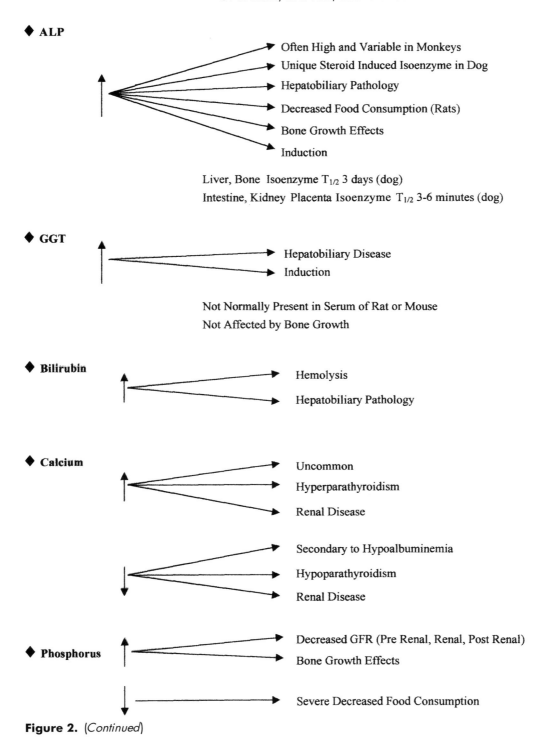

Figure 2. (*Continued*)

Globulins constitute a number of heterogeneous proteins, including coagulation factors, transport proteins, mediators of inflammation, and immunoglobulins. Electrophoretic separation identifies α, β, and γ fractions. Electrophoresis, while not generally included in most

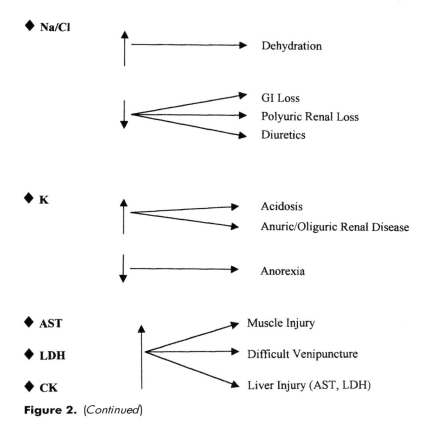

◆ **Na/Cl**

↑ ──────→ Dehydration

↓ ──────→ GI Loss
   ──────→ Polyuric Renal Loss
   ──────→ Diuretics

◆ **K**

↑ ──────→ Acidosis
   ──────→ Anuric/Oliguric Renal Disease

↓ ──────→ Anorexia

◆ **AST**

◆ **LDH**

◆ **CK**

──────→ Muscle Injury
──────→ Difficult Venipuncture
──────→ Liver Injury (AST, LDH)

Figure 2. (*Continued*)

preclinical toxicology protocols, may identify fractions affected in hyper- or hypoglobulinemia. Most globulins are synthesized by the liver. Immunoglobulins are synthesized by B lymphocytes and plasma cells and are generally found in the γ fraction of the electrophoretogram, although they may extend (particularly IgM) into the β region. The most frequent causes of hyperglobulinemia are dehydration and polyclonal gammopathy secondary to antigenic stimulation. Increased acute-phase proteins (e.g., α_2-macroglobulin, haptoglobulin, and ceruloplasmin) are frequently part of the increased globulins in the general response to inflammation.

Decreased Kupffer cell activity is rarely recognized in toxicology studies, but has been reported to occur with chronic fibrosing disorders and may also occur secondary to extensive Kupffer cell uptake of lipid/particulate intravenous formulations. The reduced Kupffer cell mass may allow delivery of enteric antigens

to the systemic circulation or to lymphoid tissues, resulting in excess antigen stimulation and hyperglobulinemia (polyclonal gammopathy).

Albumin/globulin (A/G) ratios reflect changes in the two major protein types. If albumin is selectively lost (e.g., glomerular disease) or not produced (e.g., hepatic disease), then the A/G ratio will be low. However, if there is a concomitant loss or failure to synthesize globulins (e.g., hemorrhage, enteropathy, exudation, malassimilation), then panhypoproteinemia and a normal A/G ratio may occur.

C. INDICATORS OF HEPATIC INTEGRITY AND FUNCTION

The most commonly affected target organs of xenobiotic administration in preclinical toxicology studies are the liver and kidneys, frequently reflecting test article tissue distribution, metabolism, and excretion patterns.

The metabolic, synthetic, and excretory roles of the liver, and the enzymes required to perform these functions, result in the potential for numerous biochemical alterations in response to perturbations caused by test article administration. Because the liver has large functional reserves, it is possible that a significant loss of functional tissue may occur with minimal or no detectable change in routine laboratory tests. Alterations in clinical chemistry parameters may be associated with hepatocellular injury, decreased functional mass, cholestasis, altered hepatic blood flow, metabolic adaptation (e.g., enzyme induction), or altered Kupffer cell activity. Clinical chemistry abnormalities may be due to one or a combination of these events. While no single test is superior in all situations, the pattern of findings in a selected battery of tests may indicate the location and severity of liver lesions.

Enzymes are not indicators of liver function *per se*, but rather several are indicators of cellular degeneration or necrosis and increased membrane permeability. The utility of an enzyme depends on a number of factors, including liver specificity, intrahepatic location, concentration gradient between the cell and serum, serum half-life, and *in vitro* stability, as well as ease, accuracy, and cost of measurement. Enzymes associated with hepatocellular integrity measured most commonly in preclinical toxicology studies are alanine aminotransferase (ALT) and aspartate aminotransferase (AST). ALT increases are generally regarded as indicative of effects on liver in dogs, nonhuman primates, rats, mice, and hamsters. Guinea pigs have low hepatocellular ALT activity, and therefore ALT is an insensitive indicator of liver injury in this species. Increased serum ALT activity has been reported in a dog with severe muscle but no liver pathology (Swenson and Graves, 1997). Notwithstanding this report, ALT is pragmatically regarded as a specific enzyme indicator of hepatocellular injury in most species used in preclinical toxicology studies. Hepatocellular ALT activity is up to about 10,000 times greater than in serum under normal circumstances. Serum activity increases within 12 hr and peaks in 1–2 days after toxic insult. The serum half-life of ALT is about 60 hr

in dogs. Activity may be misleadingly low several days after the occurrence of massive liver necrosis due to loss of liver tissue and/or exhausted coenzyme supply. Manual restraint methods in mice that involve grasping the abdomen may lead to increased ALT activities, presumably due to mechanical trauma to the liver. Routine handling of male C3H/HeJ mice has been reported to cause a five-fold increase in ALT activity (Swaim *et al.*, 1985).

Serum AST activity tends to parallel serum ALT activity in liver injury. However, AST is not a specific indicator of hepatocellular injury, as AST also has high activity in muscle. Cytosolic and mitochondrial AST isoenzymes exist. AST is present in red blood cells, and therefore increased serum activities may occur as an artifact associated with sample hemolysis. The serum half-life of AST is about 12 hr in dogs.

Serum ALT and AST activities can increase within hours of significant liver injury. In general, the magnitude of the increase in serum activity of ALT or AST correlates with the number of affected hepatocytes and is not necessarily an indicator of the severity or reversibility of the lesion on a pathologic basis. Altered hepatic blood flow can result in hypoxia with resultant increased hepatocellular membrane permeability and increased serum enzyme activities.

Other enzymes that may be elevated due to hepatocellular injury include lactate dehydrogenase (LDH), sorbitol dehydrogenase (SDH), glutamate dehydrogenase (GDH), isocitrate dehydrogenase, and arginase. LDH is not liver specific and is used more as an indicator of muscle injury. The other enzymes listed are considered liver specific; however, they are infrequently included in study protocols. GDH is located in mitochondria, and consequently determination of serum GDH activity had promise as an indicator of necrosis. Theoretically, determination of GDH activity should provide data complimentary to ALT (cytosolic) and AST (cytosolic and mitochondrial isoenzymes). However, GDH is not a sensitive predictor of hepatocellular injury in some models of hepatotoxicity.

Because urea synthesis depends on the hepatic uptake of ammonia absorbed from the gastrointestinal tract and subsequent liver urea cycle synthesis, liver dysfunction may lead to low blood urea nitrogen (BUN) concentrations. However, low BUN is seldom observed in toxicology studies. Clotting factors, bile acids, α and β globulins, albumin, cholesterol, glucose, and bilirubin may also be affected by decreased hepatic functional mass. However, measures of hepatic function may not be altered detectably until more than one-half of the hepatocellular mass is dysfunctional or nonfunctional.

Cholestasis may develop due to intra- (e.g., secondary to hepatocellular swelling) or extrahepatic obstruction of biliary flow. Cholestasis may also reflect abnormal secretory activity by hepatocytes (i.e., alterations in uptake, conjugation and secretion), although this is rarely identified in preclinical toxicology studies. Increased serum and urine bilirubin and increased serum bile acids, alkaline phosphatase (ALP), and γ-glutamyl transferase (GGT) activities are indicators of cholestasis. Leucine aminopeptidase and 5′ nucleotidase (5′NT) may be increased in cholestasis but are used less frequently in toxicology protocols. The mechanism underlying increased production of ALP and GGT in cholestasis is uncertain, but may involve bile acid-stimulated synthesis. Inclusion of conjugated and unconjugated bilirubin determinations in addition to total bilirubin is not warranted in most protocols. Unconjugated hyperbilirubinemia is uncommon in toxicity studies and its occurrence is usually due to marked hemolysis. Periportal and extrahepatic lesions generally cause greater conjugated hyperbilirubinemia than centrilobular lesions.

Alkaline phosphatase is a sensitive indicator of cholestasis in the dog but lacks specificity. Increased ALP activity may reflect the hepatic isoenzyme, but other isoenzymes, particularly bone and a steroid-induced enzyme in dogs, should also be considered as potential sources of increased serum ALP activity. The bone isoenzyme contributes significantly to serum activities in young growing animals, and thus ALP activities are high in young rats (typically about 6 weeks of age at study initiation) and in young dogs (typically about 6 months of age at study initiation). Serum half-life is about 3 days for liver and bone isoenzymes in dogs. The short half-life (about 3–6 min) for intestine, kidney, and placental isoenzymes makes it unlikely that any increase in serum ALP activity will be due to these isoenzymes in dogs. However, the intestinal isoenzyme contributes to serum activity in the rat to a greater extent than the liver isoenzyme. Serum GGT may be less sensitive than ALP to hepatobiliary disease in some species; however, serum activity is not affected by bone growth. Serum GGT activity in rats and mice is generally too low to be quantified in "normal" animals.

The time course of increases in hepatobiliary enzymes and serum bilirubin concentrations in a monkey with drug-induced multifocal hepatocellular necrosis and deposition of crystalline precipitates in bile canaliculi and within hepatocytes is demonstrated in Fig. 3. No concurrent control animals were used in the exploratory study from which this information was extracted. Serum ALT activity was increased moderately to markedly (compared with pretest and concurrent reference range values) as early as day 3 following initiation of daily administration of drug. Serum AST activity was also increased by day 3 compared with pretest; however, the magnitude of the increase was much less than for ALT. A toxicologically relevant increase in ALP was slow in developing, and the increase in the activity of this enzyme was not clearly treatment-related until day 10. Increased serum bilirubin concentration, outside the reference range, occurred by day 12. The increase was attributable to direct or conjugated bilirubin. Maximum values for all aforementioned parameters occurred at day 12 or 13. Interpretation of the results was that ALT was a sensitive indicator of drug-related hepatocellular injury that occurred early following initiation of treatment. Cholestasis, indicated by increased ALP and conjugated bilirubin, occurred relatively later in the study.

Increased serum activities of ALT, AST, ALP, and GGT may reflect enzyme induction

137

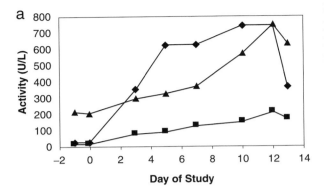

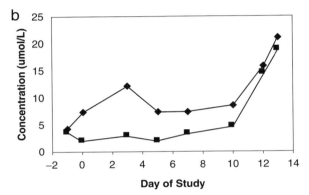

Figure 3. Time course of changes in serum clinical chemistry parameters in a monkey following daily xenobiotic administration. (a) Increased ALT(◆), AST(■), and ALP(▲) activities following daily xenobiotic administration. Moderate to marked increase in ALT by Day 3. Maximum values for each parameter occurred on Day 12. (b) Moderate increases in total (and direct) bilirubin on Days 12 and 13 following daily xenobiotic administration.

by administered xenobiotics (e.g., corticosteroids, anticonvulsants) rather than hepatobiliary injury. Most inducible enzymes are membrane associated. Increased serum enzyme activity may occur days following the inciting action, and several days to weeks may be required before peak activity is reached. Distinction between induction and leakage of enzymes may be difficult as some xenobiotics cause both.

D. INDICATORS OF RENAL FUNCTION

Serum urea nitrogen (generally referred to as blood urea nitrogen) and creatinine are used in conjunction with urine specific gravity or osmolality to evaluate renal function. BUN and creatinine are relatively insensitive to mild

renal injury. However, the commonly quoted paradigm that damage to 75% of nephrons is required prior to BUN elevation is not accurate in well-controlled toxicity studies, particularly in rat studies where the group size and narrow range of BUN values of untreated control rats facilitate the detection of relatively small but relevant increases in group mean BUN values secondary to renal insult. By the time 75% of nephrons are nonfunctional, the renal concentrating ability is usually impaired and urine is isothenuric (same specific gravity as glomerular fluid; about 1.008 to 1.012). "Normal" BUN values do not necessarily exclude renal pathology or test article-related renal effects. For example, in a subchronic study in monkeys, marked, multifocal deposition of drug metabolite crystalline precipitates throughout the cortex of the kidneys resulted in a multifocal giant cell response but did not cause changes in BUN or serum creatinine (unpublished data).

With renal toxicity, serum creatinine concentrations tend to parallel changes in BUN. Because creatinine diffuses throughout body water at a slower rate than urea (4 hr required for equilibration), serum creatinine concentration changes more slowly compared with BUN. Other potential clinicopathologic alterations in renal disease include nonregenerative anemia, hyperphosphatemia [reflecting decreased glomerular filtration rate (GFR)], hyperkalemia, metabolic acidosis (due to uremic acids), serum calcium alterations, hyponatremia and hypochloremia (urinary loss due to tubular failure), and hypoproteinemia/hypoalbuminemia (glomerular disease).

There are a number of nonrenal causes for elevations in serum concentrations of BUN and creatinine. Urea concentrations can vary with hydration status, diet, gastrointestinal hemorrhage, or protein catabolism. Serum creatinine concentration is influenced by muscle mass but is relatively independent of dietary influences and protein catabolism compared with BUN. The BUN/creatinine ratio, while not definitive, can be of value in the differential diagnosis of azotemia (accumulation of nitrogenous wastes, such as urea nitrogen and creatinine, in blood). Thus, in renal azotemia, BUN and creatinine can be anticipated to increase proportionately, whereas in prerenal azotemia, BUN may increase disproportionately.

E. ELECTROLYTES

While reference ranges for electrolytes (sodium, potassium, and chloride) are fairly wide, the range of results in a well-controlled study is generally quite narrow. Often the reasons for small, statistically significant differences in these parameters between treated groups and controls in toxicity studies are not apparent. Sodium (Na) is the major cation in serum and the major determinant of extracellular fluid volume. Hypernatremia is generally reflective of dehydration in which water losses exceed electrolyte losses. Hyponatremia may occur with gastrointestinal loss, renal tubular dysfunction with urinary loss or in hypoadrenocorticism (rare in toxicology studies). Potassium (K) is the major intracellular cation and is maintained within narrow limits because of its critical role in neuromuscular and cardiac excitability. Serum potassium is a relatively poor indicator of total body potassium because of shifts between intra- and extracellular compartments. Increased serum potassium may occur with acidosis due to the exchange of extracellular fluid (ECF) hydrogen ions for intracellular potassium ions. Chloride (Cl) is the major anion in serum. Hyperchloremia may occur secondary to dehydration (with a proportional increase in sodium) and is occasionally observed in conditions causing metabolic acidosis. Like sodium, serum chloride may decrease due to gastrointestinal or renal loss. However, vomiting may cause hypochloremia and normonatremia, as chloride (as HCl) may be lost in excess of sodium.

F. CALCIUM AND INORGANIC PHOSPHATE

Serum concentrations of calcium and inorganic phosphate are affected by parathyroid hormone, calcitonin, and vitamin D and represent a balance of intestinal absorption, bone formation/resorption, and urinary excretion. About 50% of serum calcium is in ionized form, which is biologically active in neuromuscular function, bone formation, coagulation, and other physiologic processes. About 40% of serum calcium is bound to albumin. The remaining serum calcium is complexed to anions such as citrate and phosphate. Mild hypocalcemia, secondary to hypoalbuminemia, is a common finding in toxicology studies. Because ionized calcium is unaffected, clinical signs of hypocalcemia do not occur. Hypercalcemia is uncommon in toxicology studies. Hypophosphatemia may be secondary to inanition. Serum inorganic phosphorus concentrations are high in young animals due to active bone growth. Hyperphosphatemia may occur in prerenal, renal, or postrenal azotemia, reflecting reduced GFR.

G. ENZYMES OF MUSCLE ORIGIN

Increased serum activities of creatine kinase (CK), LDH, and AST occur with degenerative or necrotizing muscle injury. CK is primarily cytosolic and three major isoenzymes exist. Most serum CK originates from muscle. Serum activity in healthy dogs varies with age, with pups having higher activity than adults. CK is generally the most sensitive indicator of skeletal or cardiac muscle injury with peak activity reached within about 6–12 hr. CK has a relatively short half-life (about 2–4 hr), and thus activity returns rapidly to normal following cessation of myodegeneration or necrosis. Persistent elevation indicates active muscle injury. All tissues contain various amounts of the five LDH isoenzymes; however, muscle, liver, and red blood cells (hemolysis) are the major sources of serum LDH activity. Species differences exist in the predominant tissue source of CK and LDH serum activities. AST is present in almost all tissues, and hence serum AST activity is nonspecific. Liver and muscle are considered the main sources of serum AST. Maximal AST activity is reached about 24–48 hr postinjury, whereas LDH activity peaks about 48–72 hr postinjury.

Interpretation of relatively small changes in CK, LDH, and AST in toxicology studies should be made with caution, as the variability of these parameters can be quite wide in healthy animals, particularly with regard to serum CK and LDH activities in nonhuman primates. Description of changes should also be made with the perspective that CK, for example, has the potential to increase manyfold (e.g., $\geq 100\times$) in generalized myopathies. Quantification of CK or LDH isoenzymes is of no interpretive benefit in treated animals with mild increases in total serum activities, particularly if values are within or approximate the reference range because the proportions of CK and LDH isoenzymes are variable in healthy animals. Also, there is little scientific merit in using CK or LDH isoenzyme determinations to assess myocardial toxicity at the end of a subchronic study because the amount of tissue damage necessary to produce a clear difference between control and treated animals would likely lead to early demise of the treated animals.

IV. Microsomal Enzyme Induction

The laboratory determination of microsomal enzyme induction in animals is frequently conducted as a component of the safety evaluation of new drug candidates and other chemicals. The primary purpose of conducting microsomal evaluations in preclinical safety evaluations is to determine whether hepatic P450 induction has occurred. The evaluation may also detect whether test compounds inhibit P450 enzymes. While evaluation of microsomal induction would not generally be considered a part of the scope of clinical pathology evaluation, P450 induction does have implications for clinical pathology result interpretation, as well as for metabolism and excretion of the test substance and other exogenous and endogenous substances. The advantage in conducting microsomal evaluations within toxicology studies lies in the potential wealth of other data, including clinical and anatomic pathology evaluations, for purposes of correlation and comparison.

Most drugs and other xenobiotics, as well as many endogenous compounds, must be bio-transformed or metabolized to more water-soluble forms before they can be eliminated from the body (see also Chapter 2). These biotransformations are divided into two groups called phase I and phase II reactions, which often occur sequentially. Phase I metabolism consists of hydrolysis, reduction, or oxidation and generally results in the introduction or loss of a functional group, such as $-OH$, $-NH_2$, $-SH$, or $-COOH$, producing a chemically reactive intermediate. Phase II reactions consist of conjugation of the substance with glucuronide, sulfate, glutathione, or an amino acid. Acylation and methylation are also phase II reactions. The metabolites of phase II reactions are readily excreted in urine or bile. The majority of the phase I biotransformations are catalyzed by the cytochrome P450 enzymes, a superfamily of heme-containing enzymes, which are located in the smooth endoplasmic reticulum of many different cell types. Quantitatively the highest cytochrome P450 concentrations, and hence the most biotransformations, occur in the liver. The subcellular component of homogenized tissue that corresponds to the smooth endoplasmic reticulum after ultracentrifugation at $100,000\,g$ or greater is called the microsomal fraction.

The capacity of the P450 system, as well as that of microsomal phase II reactions (e.g., glucuronidation), is augmented by the phenomenon of induction, which is the process whereby a drug or other xenobiotic increases the concentration and activity of one or usually multiple cytochrome P450 isoenzymes as well as phase II enzymes.

Total cytochrome P450 content and a variety of associated mixed function oxidase enzyme activities, as well as phase II enzyme activities, can be measured relatively easily by spectrophotometric or fluorometric methods. These assays have varying degrees of specificity for the major isoenzyme forms depending on the substrate used. Mixed function oxidase activities can also be determined by high-performance liquid chromatography for a variety of substrates, such as testosterone, which although technically more challenging, provide better sensitivity and specificity. Test article induction or inhibition of mixed function oxidase activities can be confirmed by the determination of specific isoenzyme concentrations by gel electrophoresis and immunoblotting (Western blotting) or ELISA, although these assays are labor intensive.

Microsomal induction data can be used to account for otherwise unexplained increases in liver weight and serum GGT, as well as alterations in other enzyme activities, such as ALT, AST, and ALP due to increased or decreased synthesis. Increased GGT activity has been used as an indirect index of hepatic enzyme induction with some compounds. The potent and prototypical inducer, phenobarbital, induces the levels and activities of multiple P450 isoenzymes and increases GGT activity in rat liver at the same time. Phenobarbital also causes an increase in liver weight attributable to hepatocellular hypertrophy due largely to the proliferation of smooth endoplasmic reticulum. It must be stated clearly, however, that many inducers do not cause an elevation in GGT, even in the presence of increased liver weight. Thus, an absence of increased GGT activity does not necessarily mean that induction has not occurred. Microsomal enzyme induction can also explain unexpected decreases in plasma or serum drug or metabolite levels with repeated dosing due to autoinduction by the test compound (the phenomenon whereby a chemical induces its own metabolism). Autoinduction needs to be distinguished from other causes of decreased drug levels with repeated dosing such as reduced absorption or increased excretion. In some cases, even a chemical that is not metabolized by P450 enzymes can induce microsomal enzymes.

Alterations in microsomal enzyme activities may impact the interpretation of thyroid hormone levels and thyroid morphologic changes (see also Chapter 41). Hepatic microsomal enzymes are important in thyroid hormone metabolism, as glucuronidation is the rate-limiting step in the biliary excretion of T_4 and sulfation is rate-limiting in T_3 excretion. Induction of these phase II pathways, and glucuronidation in particular, by a wide variety of chemicals can result in a shortened half-life of T_3 and T_4, which in turn causes thyroid-stimulating hormone (TSH) levels to increase as a consequence of removal of negative feedback inhibition. The resulting chronic stimulation of the thyroid gland can lead to changes in thyroid weight and thyroid pathology and ultimately lead to an increased incidence of follicular cell tumors. Rats are more susceptible to these hormone perturbations than nonhuman primates and humans because rat plasma T_4 has a short half-life and is not tightly bound to thyroxine-binding protein.

V. Urinalysis

Urinalysis is often included in preclinical toxicology study protocols and has the potential to provide specific evaluation of the urogenital tract as well as information concerning systemic changes. However, urinalysis is an imprecise tool in most toxicology studies. Urine samples are often taken at a single time point (e.g., at necropsy) rather than collected over a timed period. If determinations are made without reference to urine volume, tests are qualitative or semiquantitative at best. However, when samples are collected to permit expression of results according to a specific timed interval (e.g., overnight in rodents) and to urine volume, sample contamination may occur due to collection techniques.

Urinalysis usually consists of the evaluation of physicochemical properties and sediment examination. There is generally no justification for expending effort in evaluating microscopic sediment from animals in mid- and low-dose groups in toxicity studies if there are no treatment-related microscopic findings in a representative number of high-dose animals. Urine electrolyte excretion determinations, often a component of Japanese toxicity studies, and urinary enzyme activities for the identification of renal tubular toxicity are incorporated in some toxicity study protocols or in special investigations of potential nephrotoxins. Over-interpretation of results of urine electrolyte excretion (including fractional clearance) should be guarded against in view of the interanimal variability and the relative lack of experience of most laboratories in performing and interpreting these investigations. Numerous studies evaluating various urinary analytes (e.g., β_2-microglobulin, ALP, GGT, LDH, lysozyme, acid phosphatase, N-acetyl glucosaminidase) as specific indicators of segmental nephron injury have been published. Interlaboratory comparison of results is not possible due to a lack of standardization of methodologies. Urinary enzyme quantification may be useful in investigations designed to examine specific questions regarding nephrotoxcity; however, there is no convincing evidence to indicate that a particular enzyme or enzyme profile is superior over others as a screening tool for nephrotoxicity in general.

The scientific value of conducting urinalysis in terms of knowledge gained for labor invested is questioned frequently. It is recommended that the conduct of urinalysis in toxicity studies be performed under the same guiding principles as for other clinical laboratory parameters. That is, in general toxicity studies where the potential toxicity of the test article is unknown, the urinalysis component of the protocol should be designed efficiently to establish a minimum database of results that can be used as a platform for designing appropriate evaluations in subsequent studies as required. In initial repeat dose, subacute studies, urinalysis can be used effectively to screen for overt changes such as hematuria, pyuria, glucosuria, bilirubinuria, presence of casts, or abnormal crystalluria, as well as providing general information regarding hydration and concentrating ability (specific gravity or osmolality), acid–base balance (pH), and energy balance (ketones) of the animal at that point in time. In subsequent studies (e.g., subchronic or special investigative study), more targeted urine determinations, such as metabolite identification and quantification, characterization of abnormal crystalluria, electrolyte fractional excretion, or enzymuria determination may be added to the protocol as indicated.

VI. Clinical Pathology Study Design Considerations

General principles for consideration in designing the clinical pathology component of preclinical toxicology studies are highlighted in Table V.

Some laboratories include hematology and clinical biochemistry testing in acute rodent (i.e., single dose) study protocols. These evaluations are frequently unrewarding, particularly when samples are taken only to coincide with study termination at 14 days. It can be anticipated that animals surviving the toxic insult of a single high dose of a test article generally will have recovery of clinical pathology parameters to approximate concurrent control or reference range values by 14 days postdose. The potential to gain useful information regarding hematopoietic toxicity following a single dose of test article is limited unless sample timing is targeted to anticipate effects on a specific cell line and stage. Clinical pathology samples taken at 24 or 48 hr following a single dose at least have the potential to produce useful information.

Employing a battery of tests as outlined by the joint scientific committee for International Harmonization of Clinical Pathology Testing is recommended for single dose or rising dose studies in nonrodents, as well as for subacute studies in rodents and nonrodents, if the test article has unknown toxic potential. The clinical pathology protocol design for subsequent subchronic

TABLE V
Considerations in the Design of the Clinical Pathology Component of a Preclinical Toxicity Study

Study objectives
Scientific criteria
End points
Study type (acute, subacute, subchronic, chronic, carcinogenicity)
Species
Test article characteristics
Regulatory guidelines
Practical aspects
Appropriate controls

and chronic studies can be targeted more specifically based on clinicopathologic and morphologic pathology findings in subacute studies.

Consideration should be given to the optimal timing of clinical pathology samples according to anticipated targets rather than using only traditional study time points. For example, following the time course of development of a hematologic change early in a study may provide information regarding the type of process (e.g., direct toxicity or immune-based phenomenon). Development of tolerance to test article effects (e.g., hepatotoxicity) or of sequelae to initial effects (e.g., cholestasis subsequent to hepatocellular injury) may be demonstrated by serial sampling.

Selected toxicity studies, generally subchronic studies of 4 or 13 weeks duration, include a subgroup of animals that are maintained for a period of time following withdrawal of test article treatment in order to evaluate the potential reversibility of treatment effects. Customarily, the reversibility period is chosen to be 4 weeks. In general, 4 weeks does allow time for hematologic or clinical chemistry effects to show evidence of recovery in concert with recovery of morphology and function of the organs affected. However, it may be impractical to anticipate full recovery of all clinical pathology parameters within 4 weeks, depending on the parameter as well as the nature and severity of the injury. Closely following the time course to recovery of hematologic effects may be instructive in identifying the maturation stage of affected cells.

VII. Clinical Pathology Result Interpretation

The two fundamental questions to answer when evaluating an apparent difference in clinical pathology test results between control and treated animals or between pretest and post-treatment values are: "Is it real?" and "Is it bad?" The first question encompasses all the considerations that go toward deciding if the change truly reflects an effect of the treatment/test article or if the difference is a function of physiological or procedural effects. The answer to the second question is often more difficult to answer.

A large number of factors have the potential to influence the interpretation of clinical pathology results, and it is essential that these be taken into consideration in determining whether changes in parameters are artifacts or real, and incidental or treatment-related. Therefore, judgments need to be made based on a knowledge of test results in concurrent control animals and pretest values in nonrodent studies; expected variations due to artifacts and limitations of analytic methodologies; appropriateness of individual tests; effects of site of sample collection and anesthesia; effects of species, sex, and age; study design and procedure effects; statistical analysis; reference ranges for the species and the laboratory performing the analyses; and biological significance. Regarding this last point, interpretation of biological significance should not be made on the basis of change in a parameter in isolation, but rather with a broader knowledge of clinical observations, anatomical pathology findings, other clinicopathologic results (hematology, biochemistry, urinalysis), and other information as may be available (e.g., pharmacologic activity of test article; absorption, metabolism, distribution, excretion of test compound; toxicokinetics; liver microsomal enzyme studies; previous experience with compound or analogues; previous experience with pharmacologic class of compound). Classification of clinical pathology findings is summarized in Table VI.

A. POTENTIAL EFFECTS OF FACTORS UNRELATED TO TEST ARTICLE TREATMENT

1. Artifacts

Result artifacts may arise from a variety of causes, including improper collection technique (e.g., clumping of platelets with false reduction in platelet counts following tail bleeding in rodents; orbital sinus collection using a pipette causing glass activation of coagulation

TABLE VI
Classification of Findings in Preclinical Toxicology Studies

Artifact/spurious
Incidental (sporadic, spontaneous)
Test article-related
Dose-related
Gender-related
Statistically significant
Direct (primary) or indirect (secondary)
Pharmacologic
Metabolic
Toxic
Uninterpretable

cascade); improper specimen handling and storage (e.g., inadequate filling of collection tube; holding EDTA samples for more than 4 hr leads to high MPV values in dogs; instability of parameters on reanalysis such as CK; delay in separation of serum or plasma from blood cells leads to hypoglycemia due to *in vitro* glycolysis); hemolysis (causing spurious increases in serum AST, LDH, inorganic phosphorus, and, in some species, potassium); dilutional or evaporation errors; anticoagulant effects on cell morphology; and assay interference (e.g., factitious increases in creatinine due to cephalosporins; tetracycline interference with glucose; lipemia interference).

2. Physiological Influences

Physiological differences in test parameters may relate to species (CK, LDH, and ALP tend to be higher and more variable in nonhuman primates; GGT is not normally detectable in serum of rats or mice but is detectable in guinea pigs, rabbits, dogs, and nonhuman primates); age (e.g., typical changes associated with the maturation of young animals of most species include decreased reticulocytes, MCV, ALP, and inorganic phosphorus, and increased RBC count, Hct, Hb, total serum protein, and serum globulin concentration); gender (e.g., ALP is higher in male rats; Hct and WBC values tend to be higher in male rats); strain; excitement (endogenous catecholamine release); stress (endogenous corticosteroid release); and exer-

cise (increased Hct and WBC in postexercise samples).

3. Procedural Influences

Examples of procedural or study design effects include diet (e.g., influence on glucose, cholesterol, BUN, protein); fasting versus feeding prior to sample collection (overnight fasting of rats may result in increased RBC, Hb, and Hct, and decreased WBC, serum glucose, BUN, ALT, and ALP); decreased food consumption (results of food restriction studies in rats included decreased WBC and platelet counts, decreased triglycerides, cholesterol, total protein, ALT and ALP, increased serum bilirubin, and electrolyte derangements); restraint/handling methodologies (influence on ALT and AST in nonhuman primates and mice); anesthetic effects (decreased hemoglobin and RBC and increased AST and CK associated with ketamine administration in nonhuman primates); site of sample collection (WBC and platelet counts, total protein, and albumin vary according to site); and repeat bleeding (increased CK, LDH, and AST activities due to local tissue injury; anemia secondary to iatrogenic blood loss). Other aspects of study design that may affect test results include time of day of sampling, order of sampling within study (failure to randomize order of sample collection or analysis can lead to differences among groups for several analytes such as glucose, AST, LDH, platelet count, Na, K, and Cl), and placement of cages on room racks.

4. Species Differences

Species differences in clinical pathology parameters may influence result interpretation. For example, absolute neutrophil counts are low in rats and mice (e.g., $\leq 3.0 \times 10^9$/liter and often $\leq 1.0 \times 10^9$/liter) compared to dogs (3–10.5×10^9/liter). Platelet counts are high in rats and mice (e.g., $\geq 700 \times 10^9$/liter and often $\geq 1000 \times 10^9$/liter) compared with nonrodents (e.g., about 180–450×10^9/liter in dogs and nonhuman primates). Immature granulocytes described as ring form or "donut" cells are present in the marrow and occasionally in the circulation of rats, mice, and hamsters. Rabbit neutrophils or heterophils contain many large primary granules; rabbit eosinophils have larger, more rounded granules. The rabbit is the only laboratory species that normally has circulating basophils (up to 10%). Kurloff bodies are present as cytoplasmic inclusions in mononuclear cells, believed to be T lymphocytes, in guinea pigs. These bodies occur in less than 5% of circulating white blood cells, are more common in females during the first 3 months of life, and increase during pregnancy. Subclinical malarial infection (*Plasmodium* sp.) occurs frequently in imported cynomolgus and rhesus monkeys. Occasionally, this infection results in acute hemolytic anemia. Lymphocytes are commonly higher in bone marrow of rats and mice (e.g., up to 25% of nucleated cell count) compared with nonrodents. Unlike the rat and mouse, the spleen of the hamster does not normally contribute to hematopoiesis. APTT is severalfold longer in mice (reported as up to 110 sec) than for most other laboratory species (ca. 12–20 sec). Factor VII deficiency present in some laboratory-bred beagles may result in prolongation of prothrombin times and a tendency to bruising. Factor VII concentration is low in guinea pigs, therefore prothrombin time is relatively prolonged (50–100 sec) in this species. Thrombin time may also be relatively prolonged in guinea pigs, although APTT is similar to other laboratory species. Estrus-induced bone marrow hypoplasia occurs in ferrets. Affected ferrets have initial increases in platelet and white blood cell counts that are followed by pancytopenia.

ALP is more sensitive to cholestasis in the dog than in the rat or monkey. In rats, changes in serum activity of ALP may be reflective of changes in the intestinal isoenzyme rather than the heptobiliary isoenzyme and may increase or decrease secondary to decreased food intake. The dog has a unique steroid-induced ALP isoenzyme that is synthesized in the liver. Because serum ALP is higher and more variable in monkeys than for other species, serum GGT may be of more value in the diagnosis of hepatobiliary disease in monkeys. Serum GGT activity is gen-

erally undetectable in rodents but may increase secondary to hepatobiliary toxins or following microsomal enzyme induction. Bilirubinuria is a common finding in dogs and ferrets, as the threshold for bilirubin excretion is low compared with other species. Thus, serum bilirubin may be relatively slow to increase in cholestatic disease in these species. ALT is insensitive and nonspecific as a marker for hepatocellular injury in guinea pigs, reflecting low concentrations in the liver and high concentrations in other tissues (e.g., muscle). Also, ALT has higher mitochondrial compared with cytosolic distribution in guinea pigs. Subclinical enzootic hepatitis A infection in cynomolgus and rhesus monkeys causes transient ALT increases that may confound interpretation of ALT changes during toxicology studies. Increased ALT activity correlates with seroconversion to hepatitis A positivity. Rats, mice, and nonhuman primates have high red blood cell potassium concentrations, and therefore hemolysis will give spuriously high serum potassium concentrations (as well as LDH, AST, and, to a lesser degree, inorganic phosphorus and bilirubin concentrations). Red blood cell potassium concentrations are relatively low in dogs and ferrets. Serum cholesterol may be high in the hamster. LDH and CK increase in hereditary myopathy in Syrian hamsters. Total serum calcium is higher in rabbits (up to 4 mmol/liter) than in other species. This high serum calcium may lead to technical difficulties when performing coagulation tests. Unmodified, routine methods yield falsely elevated concentrations for albumin in rabbits as compared with electrophoretic values. The reason for this is not known. Total serum protein, albumin, and globulin concentrations tend to be higher in nonhuman primates than for other laboratory species. Serum electrolyte values may be higher (e.g., Na concentration up to 170 mmol/liter, Cl up to 125 mmol/liter) and more variable in unanesthetized compared with anesthetized monkeys.

5. Spontaneously Occurring Syndromes

Awareness of spontaneously occurring syndromes in the species under study is necessary, as such occurrences can influence posttreatment values and confound the determination of treatment effects. For example, the clinicopathologic features of necrotizing polyarteritis or "beagle pain syndrome" can complicate interpretation of toxicity studies. Affected dogs typically demonstrate pain, fever, stiff gait, neutrophilia, decreased red cell parameters, decreased albumin, increased α_2-globulins, thrombocytosis (some dogs), and necrotizing arteritis/periarteritis. This idiopathic syndrome is considered to be a latent condition, the expression of which can be precipitated in predisposed dogs by experimental treatment. Occurrences of a spontaneous wasting syndrome in marmosets may also complicate result interpretation and study conduct. The characteristics of this syndrome are poor weight gain or weight loss, muscle atrophy, alopecia, diarrhea, and colitis. Clinicopathologic features are macrocytic normochromic anemia, hypoproteinemia, hypoalbuminemia, increased serum AST and ALP, and thrombocytosis. Proteinuria is a common finding in control rats and mice, especially males, and severity increases with age and development of chronic progressive nephropathy.

B. COMPARATORS: CONCURRENT CONTROLS REFERENCE RANGES

The most important and relevant comparators for interpreting clinical pathology results in toxicology studies are results from appropriately matched concurrent control animals. Reference ranges provide an ancillary comparator database for consideration in the overall interpretation of test results. Reference ranges are generally constructed statistically to include the range of values found in 95% of a population of healthy individuals. There are many points for consideration when using reference ranges, and overreliance on reference ranges may lead to potential misinterpretation of results. For example, it can be anticipated that 1 out of 20 results for a specific test from a group of "normal" animals will be outside the historical reference range. As most often the test database for an animal consists of more

than 20 test results, it can be anticipated that a "normal" animal will have at least 1 test result outside the reference range. Reference ranges set cutoff points that may result in high false-positive or false-negative rates. Results within the reference range for a parameter or group of parameters associated with an organ do not ensure that the organ and its functional or metabolic processes are normal. Animals with severe organ pathology may still have clinical pathology values within the reference range. For example, liver enzymes may be within the reference range in cirrhosis in dogs, white blood cells may be within the reference range in leukemia in rodents, and serum potassium concentrations may be within the reference range, despite body/intracellular depletion. The relevance of a reference range depends on the population and conditions from which the reference range was derived, as well as the temporal relationship of when data constituting the reference range were generated compared to test study data.

Development of in-house reference ranges is essential as many variables affect study test results. Published reference ranges do not reproduce the conditions or methods by which test values were obtained in-house.

C. STATISTICAL ANALYSES

No standard statistical procedures are at present being used to analyze clinical pathology parameters. The first stage in the analysis of continuous data (which constitutes most clinical pathology data) should be to check for homogeneity of variances. Equality of variances in a set of samples is an important precondition for several statistical tests, such as the ANOVA and t-test. Information from this preliminary test dictates whether parametric or nonparametric tests should be used. Most laboratories assume that the variances of their data are homogenous and use parametric statistical tests. Clinical pathology data sets frequently do not display a Gaussian distribution, and the skewed distribution may produce too many statistically significant results in the ANOVA and t-tests. There are so many differences in the variance patterns from one test to another that attempting to use one or two statistical approaches to determine accurately the toxicologic significance of the results of the 30 to 40 clinical pathology tests commonly used would be difficult. Trend tests are useful; however, the use of multiple doses in safety assessment studies results in many borderline differences that are difficult to interpret. Thus, statistical analysis should not be regarded as the ultimate decision-making tool in the determination of treatment-related effects, but rather should be used to aid pattern recognition. Final decisions on the toxicologic significance of clinical pathology results must be based on sound biomedical judgment.

D. TREATMENT-RELATED VERSUS INCIDENTAL FINDINGS

In many studies, test article treatment-related changes in clinical pathology test parameters are clearly evident as statistically significant, dose-related effects. However, interpretive challenges occur when test results in treated animals differ from concurrent controls in a nondose-related manner, particularly when the changes were unanticipated based on previous studies conducted with the test compound or analogues or with agents of the same pharmacologic class, and when changes are not accompanied by corroborative morphologic pathology findings. For example, nondose-related increases (outside reference range values) in ALT activities were present at week 6 or 13 in several male monkeys (1/3 at low dose, 3/3 at mid dose, 1/3 at high dose level) administered daily oral doses of a vasoactive compound evaluated in a subchronic toxicity study (Table VII). Findings in females (data not shown) were similar to those in males. The increases in ALT were present inconsistently in particular individual monkeys over time. Pretest ALT activities for all treated monkeys were within the reference range. Also, ALT activities for the three control monkeys/sex remained within the reference range at pretest and weeks 6 and 13. No corroborative clinical, clinicopathologic, or liver histopathologic findings were present in treated monkeys.

TABLE VII
Individual Animal Data (Males): Subchronic Oral Monkey Study

Dose (mg/kg)	Toxicokinetic parameters[a]		ALT (U/liter)[b]	
	C_{max}[c] (μg/ml)	AUC 0–24[d] (μg·hr/ml)	Week 6	Week 13
50	3.3	10.7	71	76
50	0.8	3.3	114	58
50	4.8	20.9	843	182
500	0.9	3.7	146	748
500	2.8	11.0	107	748
500	2.1	5.5	1061	72
1000	0.3	1.3	634	790
1000	0.1	1.0	46	31
1000	0.3	0.7	37	32

[a] Week 9 toxicokinetic parameters.
[b] ALT upper reference range value: 138 (U/liter).
[c] Maximum plasma concentration of test drug.
[d] Area under the curve concentration (0–24 hr) of test drug.

The magnitude of the changes in ALT was marked in several monkeys, representing up to a 10-fold or greater increase compared with concurrent control and pretest values, as well as exceeding the upper limit of the reference range. The increased ALT activities were considered treatment-related and related to hepatocellular membrane "leakage" without overt evidence of altered liver morphology. The lack of dose-proportionality and inconsistency of ALT increases were attributed to the erratic oral bioavailability of the compound, as evidenced by the results of the toxicokinetic determinations conducted prior to week 13.

In a subchronic toxicity study of a CNS active compound, group mean CK activity was increased for high-dose male monkeys compared with controls at study termination (week 13) but not at week 6 (Table VIII). The increase was not statistically significant and values in treated females were similar to female control values at all time intervals. The difference in group mean CK activity for high-dose-treated males compared with controls was considered unrelated to treatment on the following basis: the magnitude of the change was small, particularly for a highly variable parameter,

TABLE VIII

CK Activities (U/liter) in Male Monkeys at Week 13 in
a Subchronic Toxicity Study (Mean ± SE)[a]

| Parameter | Treatment group | |
	Control	High dose
CK (U/liter)	137 ± 16	663 ± 491

[a]Upper limit of CK reference range: 1004 U/liter.

there were no increases in CK activity in mid-
and low-dose monkeys; there was no evidence
of treatment-related muscle pathology; there
were no treatment-related changes in other
serum enzymes that are muscle in origin (AST,
LDH); and the increase compared to the reference range occurred for only one monkey (this
could be anticipated based on the large standard error). Also, based on the number of monkeys evaluated at week 13 (i.e., $n = 24$; 3/sex/
group; three treated and one control group), it
could be anticipated that at least one CK value
would fall outside the reference range. This
study example also highlights that individual
animal results, as well as group mean values,
should be scrutinized, especially in nonrodent
studies because of the relatively small number
of animals per group.

E. DIRECT VERSUS INDIRECT EFFECTS

Once it is established that a change relates to
treatment, the importance of the change and
relevance to exposure of the intended population or population at risk needs to be established. Thus, it needs to be determined whether
the change is due to primary effects of the test
article or relates to effects secondary to test
article administration.

The most common hematology findings in
preclinical toxicology studies are mildly decreased (within 10–15% of concurrent control
values) red cell parameters without a corresponding increase in absolute reticulocyte
count or an apparent mechanism for the
effect. These findings are often present in animals with mild reductions in food consumption,
body weight, or weight gain, sometimes accompanied by mildly decreased serum total protein

and albumin (Table IX). Most often these
findings are considered to represent indirect or
secondary general metabolic effects of test article administration. Reduced caloric intake
can result in decreased T_3 and decreased
responsiveness to T_3 that may lead to reduced
erythropoietin production. The reductions in
red cell parameters are not due to direct toxic
effects of the test article on bone marrow, and
bone marrow histopathologic and cytologic
appearances are generally unremarkable, except
when food consumption and body weight
changes are prominent. In such circumstances,
the effects might be described as "mild decreases
in red cell parameters ($\leq 15\%$ decrease compared with controls), which were secondary to
body weight/food consumption changes, and
not of toxicologic importance."

A number of other changes in clinical pathology parameters may occur secondary to
decreased food consumption and body weight
gain supression or body weight loss in rodent
studies. Such changes may include hemocon-
centration; decreased WBC count (principally
lymphopenia), platelet count, total protein,
albumin, globulin, cholesterol, triglyceride,
inorganic phosphorus, ALT and ALP; increased
bilirubin; and electrolyte derangements. Also, a
fatal fasting syndrome can occur in monkeys
secondary to anorexia for any reason. Uremia
and other clinicopathologic findings (e.g., fatty
change of liver and proximal convoluted renal
tubules, renal tubular atrophy, and pancreatic
necrosis) characterize this syndrome. Results of
samples collected from animals *in extremis*
must be interpreted with caution, as the

TABLE IX

Selected Parameters at Termination of a 4-Week Rat Study
(Group Mean Values)

Group	Sex	Hematocrit (%)	Reticulocytes ($\times 10^9$/liter)	Total protein (g/liter)	Body weight (g)
Control	M	43	153	64	384
	F	42	117	66	242
Treated	M	40[a]	124	60[a]	347[a]
	F	37[a]	108	64	216[a]

[a]Significantly ($p < 0.05$) different from controls.

multiple and severe derangements in clinical pathology parameters may relate to the moribund state rather than directly to test article toxicity.

F. PHARMACOLOGIC VERSUS TOXIC EFFECTS

Treatment-related effects may reflect pharmacologic activity rather than toxic effects of test article administration. For example, decreased serum globulin concentrations occur in rodents administered antibiotics, likely reflecting effects of altered microbial populations on antigenic stimulation and immune response (Table X).

Mild reductions in red cell parameters are anticipated effects following the administration of angiotensin-converting enzyme (ACE) inhibitors in rats. These findings are likely due to pharmacologic effects, as ACE has been implicated in hematopoietic stem cell regulation by degrading a natural inhibitor of cell entry into S phase (Azizl, 1996).

Oral administration of high dose levels of a phosphodiesterase (PDE) III inhibitor to rats for 13 weeks resulted in treatment- and dose-related salivary gland hypertrophy and consequent increases in serum amylase activities (Table XI). The effects were considered secondary to the pharmacologic activity of the PDE III inhibitor with presumed increased intracellular cyclic AMP concentrations. Thus, the changes in rats were due to exaggerated pharmacologic effects rather than a toxicological phenomenon and were not important to the projected safety of administration of the compound in humans.

It is also possible, however, for an exaggerated pharmacologic effect (e.g., severe hypogylcemia due to insulin administration) to have

TABLE X
Serum Globulin Concentrations (g/liter) in Male Mice following 13 Weeks Oral Antibiotic Administration (Mean ± SE)

Parameter	Treatment group			
	Control	Low dose	Mid dose	High dose
Serum globulin (g/liter)	25 ± 1	23 ± 1	22 ± 0[a]	20 ± 1[a]

[a]Significantly ($p < 0.05$) different from controls.

TABLE XI
Serum Amylase Activities (U/liter) in Rats following 13 Weeks Oral Administration of a PDE III Inhibitor (Mean ± SE)

Parameter	Treatment group			
	Control	Low dose	Mid dose	High dose
Amylase (U/liter)	3741 ± 187	3861 ± 208	4359 ± 70[a]	4530 ± 137[a]

[a] Significantly ($p < 0.05$) different from controls.

more serious implications than a direct toxic effect.

G. BIOLOGIC IMPORTANCE OF TREATMENT-RELATED EFFECTS

Judgment is required in determining the toxicologic importance of a treatment-related change. For example, changes in analytes such as MCV, cholesterol, and triglycerides caused by high doses of test articles may reflect altered metabolic or adaptive changes, but may not be of toxicologic importance compared to changes such as compound-related neutropenia, thrombocytopenia, or increased ALT. Factors to consider include (1) does the test result indicate that the animal's health is compromised clinically or biologically, (2) are there clinical, clinicopathologic or pathologic correlates, (3) and what is the magnitude of the change?

An essential component of the interpretation of test results is to communicate the severity of treatment-related changes. This is generally done in comparison to concurrent control, pretest, or reference range values. To simply use qualifiers such as "minimal, mild, moderate, or marked" may be inadequate, as these terms are subjective according to individual experience. More instructive is to add a tangible perspective wherever appropriate, such as stating the numerical percentage or fold increase (or decrease) from concurrent controls or pretest values, or by provision of the actual value for the treated animal or group mean and the appropriate comparator.

Several factors should be considered when interpreting the potential toxicological importance of clinical pathologic findings. Knowledge of the characteristics of the test parameter is essential in arriving at an accurate perspective. The inherent analytical error must be taken into account. For example, inherent error is approximately 5% in automated WBC counts; therefore, attempting to interpret very small changes in WBC counts is of no merit. Understanding the extent of biological variation in the parameter in health is important. Because BUN concentrations and reference ranges in young, fasted, untreated control rats fall into a narrow range, relatively small differences in group mean values between treated and control values may be of biological significance. The most appropriate parameter needs to be evaluated. Thus, interpretation of leukocyte numerical changes should focus primarily on absolute counts and less so on relative differential counts. Knowledge of the characteristics of the parameter in the species tested is important. Moderate changes in ALP may be of no toxicological relevance in monkeys due to the inherent variability of this parameter in this species.

Temporal/kinetic characteristics of the parameter must be considered in result interpretation. For example, due to the relatively long RBC survival time in most species, significant decreases in RBC counts in short-term studies (e.g., 2-week studies in dogs or monkeys) should not be attributed to impaired bone marrow production, but rather to potential blood loss or hemolytic processes. However, in the same duration study, neutropenia could be a reflection of impaired neutrophil production in view of the short half-life of circulating neutrophils. Following similar logistics, as the half-life of albumin is about 8 days in the dog, significant hypoalbuminemia in a short-term study (e.g., 1-week study) in this species is not likely due to decreased food intake or decreased liver synthesis, but is more likely indicative of albumin loss from the body (e.g., acute external hemorrhage, gastrointestinal or urinary loss, or, less commonly, vascular loss) with or without inflammation (acute-phase reaction). The interpretation of hypoalbuminemia could be different in a study of similar duration in the mouse (albumin half-life of 2 days). Information regarding a subpopulation of cells may be

important. Absolute lymphocyte counts may be within the reference range, even though a subpopulation (e.g., CD4 lymphocytes) is absent. Interpretation of changes in a particular parameter should be made with knowledge of values of other analytes that may be linked pathophysiologically. For example, the attribution of increased serum ALP in young dogs to either bone growth or treatment-related hepatobiliary effects is influenced by the evaluation of serum GGT, bilirubin, and ALT and urine bilirubin values. Values for RBC count, serum creatinine, total protein, albumin, globulin, and urinalysis influence the attribution of increased BUN to prerenal, renal, or postrenal causes. Investigation of the etiopathogenesis of hyperbilirubinemia includes critical evaluation of RBC count, hemoglobin, ALP, GGT, ALT, and urine bilirubin determination.

Knowledge of the pharmacokinetic or toxicokinetic characteristics of the test material in the test species may help place clinical pathology findings in perspective. If administration of a xenobiotic leads to induction of its own metabolism, this could explain why some abnormalities noted early in a study may return to approximate concurrent control or pretest values later in the study. There may also be associated increases in serum activities of inducible enzymes (e.g., ALP, GGT). Nondose-related increases in clinical pathology test parameters may reflect erratic, nondose-related absorption of the test compound or saturation of absorption beyond a threshold-administered dose.

VIII. Reporting of Clinical Pathology Findings

The clinical pathology section of a toxicology study report should clearly identify test article treatment-related changes, their severity, their relationship to dose and gender, and their potential reversibility (where applicable). There needs to be distinction of biologically relevant from statistically significant findings, and identification of background changes with justification as to why these are not considered treatment-related. The appropriate use of terminology is important in accurate conveyance of the nature of findings. For example, terms such as pancytopenia, leukopenia, neutropenia, lymphopenia, and anemia must be used accurately, as these terms imply severity of effects. Such terminology should not be used to describe relatively mild decreases compared with concurrent controls or pretest values that may be statistically significant but remain within or very near the reference range for the species. These changes are best described factually as decreases compared with concurrent controls and appropriate quantifiers used. It is recommended that use of the term "significant" be restricted to the description of statistically significant results.

IX. Overall Result Reporting

To be effective, the safety or risk assessment of a drug, biologic, pesticide, or other agent must be based on accurately analyzed, interpreted, and presented data. The clinical pathology component of the report, as well as all other components, should clearly state an opinion as to what changes are test article-related and the relevance and importance of these changes. If, after rigorous scientific scrutiny, it cannot be established whether a change is treatment-related or incidental, then this should be clearly stated along with an opinion as to whether the finding merits clarification in a subsequent study. Reports should not be a simple listing of statistically significant changes, the importance of which is left up to the reader/reviewer to determine. Thus, the clinical pathology component of the report should support the overall reporting of the potential toxicity or effects of the test article in addressing the following.

1. Identification of test article treatment-related findings
2. Relationship of findings to administered dose and systemic exposure
3. Incidence of occurrence
4. Gender relationship

5. Correlations with clinical observations and anatomic pathology findings
6. Relationship to pharmacokinetic characteristics of test article
7. Potential reversibility of effects
8. Potential development of tolerance to effects
9. Perspective and importance of findings to the health of the test animals
10. Indication of whether changes are indicative of pharmacologic or toxic effects
11. Indication of whether changes were anticipated based on chemical structure or pharmacologic class of agent
12. Identification of no effect or no adverse effect dose

Ultimately, clinical pathology and other findings (e.g., clinical observations, microsomal enzyme assays, anatomic pathology, toxicokinetics) need to be integrated across toxicology studies in the compilation of an overall safety assessment of the test article, which includes the following: (1) perspective on relevance of findings to use of test article in intended species or exposure of individuals to test article and (2) statement of safety margin (dose/exposure at which toxic effects occur as a function of dose/exposure in population of interest).

X. Summary

Key features of hematology, clinical chemistry, and urinalysis in laboratory animal species have been described with respect to supporting judicious study design and interpretation of results from the clinical pathology component of preclinical toxicology studies. Numerous factors (e.g., artifacts, physiologic and procedural effects, spontaneously occurring syndromes, and species differences) have the potential to influence the interpretation of results, and it is essential that these be considered prior to determining what changes reflect test article/treatment effects. The most important and relevant comparators for interpreting findings are results in matched, concurrent control animals. Statistical analysis should be used to aid pattern recognition, but interpretation of the toxicologic importance and relevance of findings must be based on sound biomedical judgment. In result evaluation, associations among clinical pathology parameters and correlations of clinical pathology results with other study findings (e.g., clinical signs, microsomal enzyme analyses, anatomic pathology, and toxicokinetics) are essential for accurate interpretation. Test article treatment-related effects should be distinguished as direct (primary) or indirect (secondary) and toxic or pharmacologic. The severity of the effects, gender and dose relationships, and relevance to overall animal health should be addressed in the reporting of results. Clinical pathology results integrated with other study findings often provide important information regarding mechanisms of toxicity and dose–response relationships of target organ effects across different laboratory animal species, as well as the importance and relevance of study findings to humans or animal species potentially exposed to the test article.

SUGGESTED READING

Hematology

Anderson, T. D. (1993). Cytokine-induced changes in the leukon. *Toxicol. Pathol.* **21**, 147–157.

Aster, R. H. (1997). Response of thrombocytes to toxic injury. *In* "Comprehensive Toxicology" (G. Sipes, C. A. McQueen, and A. J. Gandolfi, eds.), Vol. 4, pp. 263–284. Elsevier Science, Oxford.

Badenhorst, P. N., and Kotze, H. F. (1997). Evaluation of platelets and thrombopoiesis. *In* "Comprehensive Toxicology" (G. Sipes, C. A. McQueen, and A. J. Gandolfi, eds.), Vol. 4, pp. 231–245. Elsevier Science, Oxford.

Beutler, E., *et al.* (1995). "Williams Hematology." 5th Ed. McGraw-Hill, New York.

Bloom, J. C. (1997). Introduction to hematotoxicology. *In* "Comprehensive Toxicology" (G. Sipes, C. A. McQueen, and A. J. Gandolfi, eds.), Vol. 4, pp. 1–10. Elsevier Science, Oxford.

Boon, G. D. (1993). An overview of hemostasis. *Toxicol. Pathol.* **21**, 170–179.

Dabrow, M. B., and Gabuzda, T. G. (1997). Nonimmune hemolysis and toxic methemoglobinemia. *In* "Compre-

hensive Toxicology" (G. Sipes, C. A. McQueen, and A. J. Gandolfi, eds.), Vol. 4, pp. 55–72. Elsevier Science, Oxford.

Deldar, D., and Parchment, R. E. (1997). Preclinical risk assessment for hematotoxicity: Animal models and *in vitro* systems. *In* "Comprehensive Toxicology" (G. Sipes, C. A. McQueen, and A. J. Gandolfi, eds.), Vol. 4, pp. 303–320. Elsevier Science, Oxford.

Duncan, J. R., Prasse, K. W., and Mahaffey, E. A. (1994). "Veterinary Laboratory Medicine." 3rd Ed. Iowa State Univ. Press, Ames, IA.

Fried, W. (1997). Evaluation of red cells and erythropoiesis. *In* "Comprehensive Toxicology" (G. Sipes, C. A. McQueen, and A. J. Gandolfi, eds.), Vol. 4, pp. 35–54. Elsevier Science, Oxford.

Frith, C. H., *et al.* (1993). The morphology, immunohistochemistry, and incidence of hematopoietic neoplasms in mice and rats. *Toxicol. Pathol.* **21**, 206–218.

Glomski, C. A., *et al.* (1982). Haemolytic anaemia in rhesus monkeys induced by methylcellulose. *Lab. Anim.* **16**, 310–313.

Green, R. A. (1999). Spurious platelet effects on erythrocyte indices using the CELL-DYN 3500 automated hematology system. *Vet. Clin. Pathol.* **28**, 47–49.

Hall, R. L. (1997). Evaluation and interpretation of hematologic data in Preclinical toxicology. *In* "Comprehensive Toxicology" (G. Sipes, C. A. McQueen, and A. J. Gandolfi, eds.), Vol.4, pp. 321–333. Elsevier Science, Oxford.

Hall, R. L. (2001). Principles of Clinical Pathology for Toxicology Studies. *In* "Principles and Methods of Toxicology" (A. W. Hayes, ed.). Taylor & Francis, Philadelphia.

Irons, R. D. (1997). Leukemogenesis as a toxic response. *In* "Comprehensive Toxicology" (G. Sipes, C. A. McQueen, and A. J. Gandolfi, eds.), Vol. 4, pp. 175–199. Elsevier Science, Oxford.

Jain, N. C. (1986). "Schalm's Veterinary Hematology." 4th Ed. Lea & Febiger, Philadelphia.

Jakubowski, J. A. (1997). Modulation of platelet function by xenobiotics: Toxicologic implications. *In* "Comprehensive Toxicology" (G. Sipes, C. A. McQueen, and A. J. Gandolfi, eds.), Vol. 4, pp. 247–261. Elsevier Science, Oxford.

Lawrence, J. B. (1997). Overview of hemostatic mechanisms. *In* "Comprehensive Toxicology" (G. Sipes, C. A. McQueen, and A. J. Gandolfi, eds.), Vol. 4, pp. 217–229. Elsevier Science, Oxford.

Liesveld, J. L., and Lichtman, M. A. (1997). Evaluation of granulocytes and mononuclear phagocytes. *In* "Comprehensive Toxicology" (G. Sipes, C. A. McQueen, and A. J. Gandolfi, eds.), Vol. 4, pp. 123–144. Elsevier Science, Oxford.

Manning, K. L., *et al.* (1996). Successful determination of platelet lifespan in C3H mice by *in vivo* biotinylation. *Lab. Anim. Sci.* **46**, 545–548.

Margolick, J. B., and Donnenberg, A. D. (1997). Evaluation of lymphoid cells and response to toxic injury. *In* "Comprehensive Toxicology" (G. Sipes, C. A. McQueen, and A. J. Gandolfi, eds.), Vol. 4, pp. 159–173. Elsevier Science, Oxford.

McGrath, J. P. (1993). Assessment of hemolytic and hemorrhagic anemias in preclinical safety assessment studies. *Toxicol. Pathol.* **21**, 158–163.

Means, R. T. (1997). Toxic effects on erythropoiesis. *In* "Comprehensive Toxicology" (G. Sipes, C. A. McQueen, and A. J. Gandolfi, eds.), Vol. 4, pp. 87–106. Elsevier Science, Oxford.

Novotny, W. R., and Love, T. W. (1997). Modulation of coagulation and fibrinolytic systems by therapeutic and nontherapeutic agents. *In* "Comprehensive Toxicology" (G. Sipes, C. A. McQueen, and A. J. Gandolfi, eds.), Vol. 4, pp. 285–302. Elsevier Science, Oxford.

Parchment, R. E., and Murphy, M. J., Jr. (1997). Human hematopoietic stem cells: Laboratory assessment and response to toxic injury. *In* "Comprehensive Toxicology" (G. Sipes, C. A. McQueen, and A. J. Gandolfi, eds.), Vol. 4, pp. 335–361. Elsevier Science, Oxford.

Pisciotta, A. V. (1997). Response of granulocytes to toxic injury. *In* "Comprehensive Toxicology" (G. Sipes, C. A. McQueen, and A. J. Gandolfi, eds.), Vol. 4, pp. 145–158. Elsevier Science, Oxford.

Reagan, W. J. (1993). A review of myelofibrosis in dogs. *Toxicol. Pathol.* **21**, 164–169.

Rebar, A. H. (1993). General responses of the bone marrow to injury. *Toxicol. Pathol.* **21**, 118–129.

Roth, J. A. (1993). Evaluation of the influence of potential toxins on neutrophil function. *Toxicol. Pathol.* **21**, 141–146.

Salama, A. (1997). Drug-induced immune hemolytic anemia. *In* "Comprehensive Toxicology" (G. Sipes, C. A. McQueen, and A. J. Gandolfi, eds.), Vol. 9, pp. 73–85. Elsevier Science, Oxford.

Shebuski, R. J. (1993). Interruption of thrombosis and hemostasis by anti-platelet agents. *Toxicol. Pathol.* **21**, 180–189.

Smith, J. E. (1997). Comparative biology and toxicology of the erythron. *In* "Comprehensive Toxicology" (G. Sipes, C. A. McQueen, and A. J. Gandolfi, eds.), Vol. 4, pp. 107–121. Elsevier Science, Oxford.

Valli, V. E., *et al.* (1990). Evaluation of blood and bone marrow, rat. *In* "Hemopoietic System" (T. C. Jones, J. M. Ward, U. Mohr, and R. D. Hunt, eds.), pp. 9–26. Springer-Verlag, Berlin.

Valli, V. E. O., and McGrath, J. P. (1997). Comparative leukocyte biology and toxicology. *In* "Comprehensive Toxicology" (G. Sipes, C. A. McQueen, and A. J. Gandolfi, eds.), Vol. 4, pp. 201–215. Elsevier Science, Oxford.

Weiss, D. J. (1993). Leukocyte response to toxic injury. *Toxicol. Pathol.* **21**, 135–140.

Weiss, D. J., Mirsky, M. L., Evanson, O. A., Fagliari, J., McClenahan, D., and McCullough, B. (2000). Platelet kinetics in dogs treated with a glycoprotein IIb/IIIa peptide antagonist. *Toxicol. Pathol.* **28**, 310–316.

Young, K. M., and Weiss, L. (1997). Hematopoietic structure-function relationships in bone marrow and spleen. *In* "Comprehensive Toxicology" (G. Sipes, C. A. McQueen, and A. J. Gandolfi, eds.), Vol. 4, pp. 11–34. Elsevier Science, Inc., Oxford.

Clinical Chemistry

Bauer, J. E. (1996). Comparative lipid and lipoprotein metabolism. *Vet. Clin. Pathol.* **25**, 49–56.

Boyd, J. W. (1983). The mechanisms relating to increases in plasma enzymes and isoenzymes in diseases of animals. *Vet. Clin. Pathol.* **12**, 9–24.

Boyd, J. W. (1988). Serum enzymes in the diagnosis of diseases in man and animals. *J. Comp. Pathol.* **98**, 381–404.

Burtis, C. A., and Ashwood, E. R. (1998). "Tietz Textbook of Clinical Chemistry," 3rd Ed. Saunders, Philadelphia.

Duncan, J. R., Prasse, K. W., and Mahaffey, E. A. (1994). "Veterinary Laboratory Medicine," 3rd Ed. Iowa State Univ. Press, Ames, IA.

Evans, G. O. (1991). Biochemical assessment of cardiac function and damage in animal species: A review of the current approach of the academic, government, and industrial institutions represented by the Animal Clinical Chemistry Associations. *J. Appl. Toxicol.* **11**, 16–21.

Ford, S. M. (1997). *In vitro* toxicity systems. *In* "Comprehensive Toxicology" (G. Sipes, C. A. McQueen, and A. J. Gandolfi, eds.), Vol. 7, pp. 121–141. Elsevier Science, Oxford.

Hall, R. L. (1992). Clinical pathology of laboratory animals. *In* "Animal Models of Toxicology" (E. Gad and C. Chengelis, eds.), pp. 765–811. Dekker, New York.

Hall, R. L. (2001). Principles of clinical pathology for toxicology studies. *In* "Principles and Methods of Toxicology" (A. W. Hayes, ed.). Taylor & Francis, Philadelphia.

Irausquin, H. (1992). The value of clinical chemistry data in animal screening studies for safety evaluation. *Toxicol. Pathol.* **20**, 515–518.

Kaneko, J. J., *et al.* (1997). "Clinical Biochemistry of Domestic Animals," 5th Ed. Academic Press, San Diego.

Kaplan, L. A., and A. J. Pesce. (1996). "Clinical Chemistry: Theory, Analysis, Correlation," 3rd Ed. Mosby, St. Louis.

Leard, B. L., *et al.* (1990). The effect of haemolysis on certain canine serum chemistry parameters. *Lab. Anim. Sci.* **24**, 32–35.

153

Loeb, W. F., and Quimby, F. W. (1989). "The Clinical Chemistry of Laboratory Animals." Pergamon Press, Oxford.

Plaa, G. L., and Zimmerman, H. J. (1997). Evaluation of hepatotoxicity: Physiological and biochemical measures of hepatic function. *In* "Comprehensive Toxicology" (G. Sipes, C. A. McQueen, and A. J. Gandolfi, eds.), Vol. 9, pp. 97–109. Elsevier Science, Oxford.

Sanecki, R. K., *et al.* (1993). Quantification of bone alkaline phosphatase in canine serum. *Vet. Clin. Pathol.* **22**, 17–23.

Stokol, T., and Erb, H. (1998). The apo-enzyme content of aminotransferases in healthy and diseased domestic animals. *Vet. Clin. Pathol.* **27**, 71–78.

Swenson, C. L., and Graves, T. K. (1997). Absence of liver specificity for canine alanine aminotransferase (ALT). *Vet. Clin. Pathol.* **26**, 26–28.

Tarloff, J. B., and Kinter, L. W. (1997). *In vitro* methodologies used to assess renal function. *In* "Comprehensive Toxicology" (G. Sipes, C. A. McQueen, and A. J. Gandolfi, eds.), Vol. 7, pp. 99–119. Elsevier Science, Oxford.

Thoreson, S. I., *et al.* (1992). Effects of storage time on chemistry: Results from canine whole blood, heparinised whole blood, serum, and heparinised plasma. *Vet. Clin. Pathol.* **21**, 88–94.

Wiedmeyer, C. E., *et al.* (1999). Semiautomated analysis of alkaline phosphatase isoenzymes in serum of normal cynomolgus monkeys (*Macaca fascicularis*). *Vet. Clin. Pathol.* **28**, 2–7.

Microsomal Enzyme Induction

Antoine, B., *et al.* (1987). Differential time course of induction of rat liver gamma-glutamyltransferase and drug-metabolizing enzymes in the endoplasmic reticulum, golgi and plasma membranes after a single phenobarbital injection: Evaluation of protein variations by two-dimensional electrophoresis. *Cell Biochem. Funct.* **5**, 217–231.

Carthew, P., Edwards, R. E., and Nolan, B. M. (1998). The quantitative distinction of hyperplasia from hypertrophy in hepatomegaly induced in the rat liver by phenobarbital. *Toxicol. Sci.* **44**, 46–51.

Goldberg, D. M. (1980). The expanding role of microsomal enzyme induction, and its implications for clinical chemistry. *Clin. Chem.* **26**, 691–699.

Guengerich, F. P. (1997). Cytochrome P450 enzymes. *In* "Comprehensive Toxicology" (G. Sipes, C. A. McQueen, and A. J. Gandolfi, eds.), Vol. 3, pp. 37–68. Elsevier Science, Oxford.

Johnson, S., *et al.* (1993). The effects on rat thyroid function of an hepatic microsomal enzyme inducer. *Hum. Exp. Toxicol.* **12**, 153–158.

Kauffman, F. C. (1997). Xenobiotic metabolism by the liver. *In* "Comprehensive Toxicology" (G. Sipes, C. A. McQueen, and A. J. Gandolfi, eds.), Vol. 9, pp. 73–95. Elsevier Science, Oxford.

Kitchen, K. T. (1999). Predicting chemical carcinogenicity by *in vivo* biochemical parameters. *In* "Carcinogenicity Testing, Predicting, and Interpreting Chemical Effects" (K. T. Kitchen, ed.), pp. 289–318. Dekker, New York.

Leeder, J. S., and Okey, A. B. (1996). Cytochromes P450 and liver injury. *In* "Drug-Induced Hepatotoxicity" (R. G. Cameron, G. Feuer, and F. A. de la Iglesia, eds.), pp. 119–153. Springer, Berlin.

Parkinson, A. (1996). An overview of current cytochrome P450 technology for assessing the safety and efficacy of new materials. *Toxicol. Pathol.* **24**, 45–57.

Urinalysis

Clemo, F. A. S. (1998). Urinary enzyme evaluation of nephrotoxicity in the dog. *Toxicol. Pathol.* **26**, 29–32.

Duncan, J. R., Prasse, K. W., and Mahaffey, E. A. (1994). "Veterinary Laboratory Medicine," 3rd. Ed. Iowa State Univ. Press, Ames, IA.

Hall, R. L. (1992). Clinical pathology of laboratory animals. *In* "Animal Models of Toxicology" (E. Gad and C. Chengelis, eds.), pp.765–811. Dekker, New York.

Hall, R. L. (2001). Principles of clinical pathology for toxicology studies. *In* "Principles and Methods of Toxicology" (A. W. Hayes, ed.). Taylor & Francis, Philadelphia.

Schardijn, G. H. C., and van Eps, L. W. S. (1987). β₂-microglobulin; its significance in the evaluation of renal function. *Kidney Int.* **32**, 635–641.

Stonard, M. D., *et al.* (1987). Urinary enzymes and protein patterns as indicators of injury to different regions of the kidney. *Fundam. Appl. Toxicol.* **9**, 339–351.

Zbinden, G., *et al.* (1988). Nephrotoxicity screening in rats; general approach and establishment of test criteria. *Arch. Toxicol.* **61**, 344–348.

Clinical Pathology Study Design, Result Interpretation, and Reporting

Azizl, M., *et al.* (1996). Acute angiotensin-converting enzyme inhibition increases the plasma level of the natural stem cell regulator N-acetyl-seryl-aspartyl-lysyl-proline. *J. Clin. Invest.* **97**, 839–844.

Baker, K. W., *et al.* (1996). A simple correlative technique for morphologic and energy dispersive analysis of glass-mounted paraffin sections. *In* "Proceedings:

Microscopy and Microanalysis" (G. W. Bailey, J. M. Corbett, R. V. W. Dimlich, J. R. Michael, and N. J. Zaluzec, eds.), pp.308–309. San Francisco Press Inc.

Bronson, R. T., *et al.* (1982). Fatal fasting syndrome of obese macaques. *Lab. Anim. Sc.* **32**, 187–192.

Capen, C. C. (1997). Mechanistic data and risk assessment of selected toxic end points of the thyroid gland. *Toxicol. Pathol.* **25**, 39–48.

Carakostas, M. C., and Banerjee, A. K. (1990). Interpreting rodent clinical laboratory data in safety assessment studies: Biological and analytical components of variation. *Fundam. Appl. Toxicol.* **15**, 744–753.

Carakostas, M. C. (1992). Interpreting clinical laboratory data in safety assessment studies. *Toxicol. Pathol.* **20**, 480–483.

Cavagnaro, J. A. (1992). Regulatory concerns in the current practices of clinical pathology. *Toxicol. Pathol.* **20**, 519–522.

Davies, D. T. (1992). Enzymology in preclinical safety evaluation. *Toxicol. Pathol.* **20**, 501–505.

Duncan, J. R., Prasse, K. W., and Mahaffey, E. A. (1994). "Veterinary Laboratory Medicine." 3rd. Ed. Iowa State Univ. Press, Ames, IA.

Dufour, D. R. (1996). Sources and control of analytical variation. *In* "Clinical Chemistry. Theory, Analysis, Correlation" (L. A. Kaplan and A. J. Pesce, eds.), pp.65–82. Mosby, St. Louis.

Fenner-Crisp, P. (1992). Regulatory concerns of the United States Environmental Protection Agency. *Toxicol. Pathol.* **20**, 523–525.

Friedman, R. B. and Young, D. S. (1989). "Effects of Disease on Clinical Laboratory Tests," 2nd Ed. AACC Press, Washington, DC.

Hall, R. L. (1997). Evaluation and interpretation of hematologic data in preclinical toxicology. *In* "Comprehensive Toxicology" (G. Sipes, C. A. McQueen, and A. J. Gandolfi, eds.), Vol.4, pp.321–333. Elsevier Science, Oxford.

Hall, R. L. (1997). Lies, damn lies, and reference intervals (or hysterical control values for clinical pathology data). *Toxicol. Pathol.* **25**, 647–649.

Hall, R. L. (2001). Principles of clinical pathology for toxicology studies. *In* "Principles and Methods of Toxicology" (A. W. Hayes, ed.). Taylor & Francis, Philadelphia.

Hayes, T. J., *et al.* (1989). An idiopathic febrile necrotizing arteritis syndrome in the dog: Beagle pain syndrome. *Toxicol. Pathol.* **17**, 129–137.

Khan, K. N. M., *et al.* (1996). Effect of bleeding site on clinical pathologic parameters in Sprague-Dawley rats: Retro orbital venous plexus versus abdominal aorta. *Contemp. Top.* **35**, 63–66.

Landi, M. S. (1990). The effects of four types of restraint on serum alanine aminotransferase and aspartate aminotransferase in the *Macaca fascicularis. J. Am. Coll. Toxicol.* **9**, 517–523.

Levin, S., *et al.* (1993). Effects of two weeks of feed restriction on some common toxicologic parameters in Sprague-Dawley rats. *Toxicol. Pathol.* **21**, 1–14.

Logan, A. C., and Khan, K. N. M. (1996). Clinical pathologic changes in two marmosets with wasting syndrome. *Toxicol. Pathol.* **24**, 707–709.

Lumsden, J. H. (1998). "Normal" or reference values: Questions and comments. *Vet. Clin. Pathol.* **27**, 102–106.

Mandell, C. P. (1991). Effect of repeated phlebotomy on iron status of rhesus monkeys *(Macaca mulatta). Am. J. Vet. Res.* **52**, 728–733.

Matsuzawa, T. (1992). Present status of animal clinical pathology examinations in the Japanese Pharmaceuticals Manufacturers Association. *Toxicol. Pathol.* **20**, 528–533.

Matsuzawa, T., *et al.* (1994). A comparison of the effect of bleeding site on haematological and plasma chemistry values of F344 rats: The inferior vena cava, abdominal aorta, and orbital venous plexus. *Comp. Haematol. Int.* **4**, 207–211.

Neptun, D. A., *et al.* (1985). Effect of sampling site and collection method on variation in baseline clinical pathology parameters in Fischer-344 rats. *Fundam. Appl. Toxicol.* **5**, 1180–1185.

Oishi, S. (1979). The effect of food restriction for 4 weeks on common toxicity parameters in male rats. *Toxicol. Appl. Pharmacol.* **47**, 15–22.

Riley, J. H. (1992). Clinical pathology: Preanalytical variations in preclinical safety assessment studies—effect on predictive value of analyte tests. *Toxicol. Pathol.* **20**, 490–500.

Scipioni, R. L., *et al.* (1997). Clinical and clinicopathological assessment of serial phlebotomy in the Sprague Dawley rat. *Lab. Anim. Sci.* **47**, 293–299.

Slighter, R. G., *et al.* (1988). Enzootic hepatitis A infection in cynomolgus monkeys *(Macaca fascicularis). Am. J. Primatol.* **14**, 73–81.

Stringer, S. K., and Seligmann, B. E. (1996). Effects of two injectable anesthetic agents on coagulation assays in the rat. *Lab. Anim. Sci.* **46**, 430–433.

Swaim, L. D., *et al.* (1985). The effect of handling techniques on serum ALT activity in mice. *J. Appl. Toxicol.* **5**, 160–162.

Szarfman, A., *et al.* (1997). Analysis and risk assessment of hematological data from clinical trials. *In* "Comprehensive Toxicology" (G. Sipes, C. A. McQueen, and A. J. Gandolfi, eds.), Vol. 4, pp.363–379. Elsevier Science, Oxford.

Waner, T. (1992). Current statistical approaches to clinical pathological data from toxicological studies. *Toxicol. Pathol.* **20**, 477–479.

Waner, T., and Nyska, A. (1994). The influence of fasting on blood glucose, trigylcerides, cholesterol, and alkaline phosphatase in rats. *Vet. Clin. Pathol.* **23**, 78–81.

155

Weingand, K., *et al.* (1992). Clinical pathology testing recommendations for nonclinical toxicity and safety studies. *Toxicol. Pathol.* **20**, 539–543.

Weingand, K., *et al.* (1996). Harmonization of animal clinical pathology testing in toxicity and safety studies. *Fundam. Appl. Toxicol.* **29**, 198–201.

Weissenger, J. (1992). Clinical pathology testing in preclinical safety assessment: Regulatory concerns. *Toxicol. Pathol.* **20**, 509–514.

Young, D. S. (1997). "Effects of Preanalytical Variables on Clinical Laboratory Tests," 2nd. Ed. AACC Press, Washington, DC.

Nomenclature

Ronald A. Herbert
National Institute of Environmental Health Sciences
Research Triangle Park, North Carolina

James R. Hailey
National Institute of Environmental Health Sciences
Research Triangle Park, North Carolina

John C. Seely
PATHCO Inc.
Research Triangle Park,
North Carolina

Cynthia C. Shackelford
Experimental Pathology Laboratories
Durham, North Carolina

Micheal P. Jokinen
Pathology Associates International
Durham, North Carolina

Jeffrey C. Wolf
Experimental Pathology Laboratories
Durham, North Carolina

Gregory S. Travlos
National Institute of Environmental Health Sciences
Research Triangle Park, North Carolina

I. Introduction
II. Terminology Issues
III. Suggested Practices
IV. Summary
Suggested Reading

I. Introduction

In rodent studies, histopathological evaluations are conducted to detect nonneoplastic and neoplastic structural changes in treatment groups versus controls that may be related directly or indirectly to administration of a test substance. The microscopic observations frequently form the basis of regulatory decisions concerning the hazards associated with exposure to many socially and economically important drugs and chemicals. Regulatory agencies often base their decisions regarding the potential carcinogenicity of a test compound primarily on increases in site-specific effects in animal studies. Thus, reliable pathology data are essential for interpretation of the chemical effects and for understanding the biological mechanisms by which chemically induced lesions develop.

The primary means of communicating histopathological findings is embodied within the terminology of diagnoses. Because histopatho-

logical diagnoses are based on subjective observations, the terminology used to classify lesions is crucial for analysis and interpretation of data derived from animal toxicological studies. Errors or inconsistencies in the diagnostic terminology used for specific structural changes could affect hazard identification and risk assessment significantly. Diagnostic terminology should therefore be precise and unambiguous and convey a clear picture of the important morphological changes.

Several factors can affect the application of specific diagnostic terms to individual lesions by pathologists contributing to the inconsistencies observed within and among toxicological studies. This chapter reviews the factors that commonly affect terminology usage in toxicologic pathology and proposes some basic methods or practices that may help minimize common problems.

II. Terminology Issues

Rodent toxicity and carcinogenicity studies have complex designs and incorporate large

Handbook of Toxicologic Pathology, Second Edition
Volume 1

numbers of animals. Microscopic examination of the tissues is often the most time-consuming phase of such studies. During this lengthy process, several factors can directly influence the diagnostic terminology and, consequently, the quality of pathology data.

A. TRAINING

Diagnostic terminology can be influenced by the type of training that the pathologist has received. Most veterinary anatomic pathologists are trained in a clinical setting where each animal case is considered unique. The primary objective of clinically trained pathologists is to identify the cause of disease or death for an individual animal and communicate the findings in a detailed fashion, i.e., each disease process identified and recorded as a separate entity. Consistency in terminology among cases is not a major concern if the pathologist can communicate the disease process(es) to the clinician. The situation is different in toxicological pathology where the emphasis is on identifying changes in relation to a treatment group rather than in an individual animal. Specifically, the goal of the toxicologic study pathologist is to determine whether there are differences in the incidences and/or severities of lesions in treated groups compared to control animals. Study pathologists must still identify the various tissue lesions, but generally have less freedom in the type and number of diagnoses that they may record; consistency and brevity aid in the statistical evaluation and interpretation of their findings.

A histopathological diagnosis is a qualitative judgement on the nature of a specific lesion and its apparent or expected biological behavior. Each diagnosis is a subjective observation, the accuracy of which depends on the totality of the pathologists' training and experience, the state of knowledge of the specific disease process, and the generally accepted diagnostic criteria and nomenclature within the profession. The proficiency of the pathologist can influence how lesions are interpreted and hence the selection of diagnostic terminology. Because most training occurs in domestic and companion ani-

mals, trainees are not exposed to the common background lesions of laboratory animals. This may lead to selection of inappropriate terminology by the novice pathologist evaluating rodent studies. Other common errors committed by novice pathologists include the use of multiple morphological descriptive terms or synonyms of a lesion or disease process; inconsistencies in the designation of topography, sites, and subsites; and duplication of diagnoses, all of which may result in misinterpretation of toxicologic data.

B. MULTIPLE PATHOLOGISTS

The practice of using multiple pathologists to evaluate a single study or a series of related studies is not uncommon and may cause variation in the diagnostic terminology used within and between studies. Due to the volume and breadth of toxicity/carcinogenicity bioassays, this practice often becomes unavoidable. Because training, experience, and abilities of pathologists differ, different criteria may be used by individual pathologists to distinguish lesions and designate thresholds for lesion diagnosis or severity grading. In addition, philosophical differences between pathologists or individual biases can influence the diagnostic terminology selected and, consequently, the consistency in pathology data. For example, different approaches for diagnosing treatment-related nonneoplastic lesions in the lungs of rats from an inhalation study may lead to different data. One pathologist may elect to combine the spectrum of lesions observed under a single diagnostic term, e.g., chronic active inflammation. Another pathologist, however, may choose to diagnose each lesion of the spectrum individually using the diagnostic terms inflammation, fibrosis, squamous metaplasia, regenerative hyperplasia, histiocyte infiltrate, and alveolar proteinosis. Arguments could be made for both approaches. Problems are encountered when comparing results between studies, particularly when comparing different studies on the same chemical or if similar lesions in the rat and mouse studies were diagnosed differently. This may be particularly problematic when the lesions are subtle or controversial or there is disagreement as to the nature of the lesion(s) observed. For example, reactive or regenerative epithelial hyperplasia adjacent to treatment-induced ulceration or an area of inflammation may be recorded by one pathologist and ignored by another who considers it a component of the spectrum of lesions associated with and secondary to ulceration.

C. DIAGNOSTIC DRIFT

Diagnostic drift is the phenomenon whereby variations in the application of diagnostic terminology or criteria occur during the histopathologic evaluation of a study. The microscopic examination of tissues in a toxicological study is performed over an extended period. Diagnostic drift is a result of such extended evaluations. Criteria used for diagnosing lesions are influenced by many qualitative and quantitative factors, and maintaining consistency over the long course of the histopathological evaluation is sometimes a challenge. The selection of multiple terms or a variety of modifiers for the same or morphologically or pathogenically similar lesions may be the most common form of diagnostic drift. Terminology may also change as the pathologist realizes the full spectrum of treatment-related effects. This may result in the application of slightly different diagnostic and grading criteria to distinguish between closely related lesions, e.g., hyperplasia vs early adenoma, over the course of a microscopic evaluation. Substantial delays between evaluation of dose groups can exacerbate this tendency. The amount of time between the original examination of the control and high-dose tissues and subsequent examination of tissues from lower dose groups may be enough to allow minor differences to occur within diagnostic criteria for a specific lesion. Severity grading of lesions is especially susceptible to diagnostic drift, particularly if the lesions are subtle and the treatment groups are known. In other cases, updated information obtained from the literature or from scientific meetings may change the way in which certain lesions are diagnosed during the course of the

evaluation. The result of diagnostic drift is an inconsistent use of diagnostic terminology, which may falsely create or mask treatment-related effects.

D. LESION COMPLEXITY

Some lesions consist of a variety of morphological features, the complexity or composition of which may affect diagnostic terminology used for classification. In these situations, some pathologists may elect to diagnose each component of the lesion. Others may elect to use a single general term to embrace the spectrum of changes present. This decision is influenced by training, experience, or the objectives of a specific study. In addition, synonymous terms exist for many lesions, and individual pathologists may have preferences or biases for alternative terms based on their training and experience. In general, lesions with similar characteristics and pathogenesis at a particular site should be consolidated in as few diagnoses as possible, preferably as a single diagnosis that reflects the biological significance of the pathologic process. Excessive splitting of diagnosis may lead to inconsistency in diagnosis and the masking of a treatment-related effect. A complex lesion that serves as an illustration is the spontaneous age-related renal disease that occurs in F344 rats. Microscopic features include alterations of the renal tubule such as degeneration, regeneration, dilatation, and the presence of protein casts, plus other components such as glomerulonephritis, glomerulosclerosis, interstitial fibrosis, chronic inflammation, and mineralization. Various labels for this syndrome include chronic nephrosis, progressive glomerulonephrosis, glomerular hyalinosis, and spontaneous glomerulosclerosis. The histomorphological appearance of the syndrome may vary among individual animals depending on the age of the animal and/or the degree of severity of disease. However, the vast majority of affected rats exhibit similar changes and disease progression. Thus, it has been suggested that the characteristic changes are classified under the single diagnosis of ''nephropathy.'' To diagnose each element of nephropathy separately clutters data, provides no additional useful information, and causes difficulty in analysis and interpretation. In addition, the danger inherent in such a practice is an inconsistent diagnosis. As a caveat, when using a single term such as nephropathy to cover a spectrum of changes, it is important to clearly define and characterize the term in the pathology narrative.

Conversely, situations exist in which diagnosing each component of a complex lesion is more appropriate. In general, multiple diagnoses should be used when important information about the pathogenesis or biology of a lesion must be conveyed. For example, squamous cell papillomas in the forestomach of rodents may occur secondary to focal ulceration that is often also accompanied by chronic submucosal inflammation and squamous epithelial hyperplasia. Frequently, some component of the lesion is absent in some tissue sections; primary ulceration and inflammation along with papillomas may be the only lesions observed. In other sections, prominent squamous epithelial hyperplasia may be observed with or without ulceration or papillomas, whereas, in other sections, all lesions may be observed. In this situation, it would be improper to combine the nonneoplastic changes under a single diagnosis of ulceration because information critical to understanding the pathogenesis of the forestomach papillomas would be lost.

E. THE NEED FOR STANDARDIZED NOMENCLATURE

Toxicologic pathologists have long recognized the need for a harmonization and standardization of nomenclature and diagnostic criteria among rodent studies conducted at different laboratories throughout the world. The lack of a universally accepted, standardized system of nomenclature has resulted in confusion, controversy, and additional costs and delays in the product review and approval by regulatory agencies.

Recent advances in computer technology have now made possible the usage of computer-based systems to capture pathology data. Well-designed systems can facilitate data recording, generate summary and statistical tables, and improve consistency among in-house pathologists. While computerized systems are inherently efficient, they may also exacerbate the lack of standardization that exists for diagnostic terminology. Many institutions and laboratories have developed in-house computerized pathology data acquisition systems or use commercially available systems with unique lexicons of diagnostic terminology. However, these lexicons are not standardized and may not be in harmony with established standardized nomenclature systems such as those used by the Society of Toxicologic Pathologists (STP) or the National Toxicology Program (NTP). Another problem is that some systems are somewhat restrictive in the available diagnostic terms, whereas others are overly flexible in that they do not limit pathologists to the terms already in the lexicon. Other software may even allow pathologists to build his or her personal diagnostic vocabulary. The availability of an excessively wide range of possible diagnostic terms can be a source of confusion and inconsistency for the experienced and inexperienced pathologist alike.

F. DATA COLLECTION

In toxicologic pathology, the pathologic diagnosis is the foundation of data collection. The approach to making a diagnosis is hierarchical and permits much flexibility and complexity in the range of diagnostic terminology used. A diagnosis is made by sequentially designating the topography (organ/tissue affected or site of occurrence), the disease process or morphology (predominant pathological change or type of lesion), and qualifiers. Topographic designations may include as many as three hierarchical terms: (1) organ, (2) site within an organ, and, if necessary, (3) a subsite of increasing specificity within sites. An example would be stomach, forestomach, epithelium. Morphological terms are used to describe the major pathological processes or abnormalities occurring in an organ or tissue. Qualifiers specify distribution, duration, character, and severity and are applied in conjunction with morphologies to define or characterize further the abnormalities. Each category of qualifiers has a large selection of terms from which to choose, thus permitting a variety of possible combinations and permutations in the final diagnosis. In many data collection systems, with the exception of the severity grade, any variation in topographical, morphological, or qualifier designations may define separate and distinct diagnosis categories when tabulated. It is therefore possible for pathologists to record more than one diagnosis for each type of lesion identified.

Qualifiers are often an important component of any diagnosis and can be used effectively to convey additional information about a lesion. Site qualifiers should be used to delineate lesions based on different regional anatomical differences, tissue-specific responses, or biological significance. For example, at different "levels" along its length, the nasal cavity is lined by squamous, respiratory, transitional, or olfactory surface epithelia. The response of these epithelia to inhaled toxicants frequently differs by location, and the use of a site qualifier helps characterize such site-specific effects. Likewise, chemically induced lesions in the larynx often have site specificity at the base of the epiglottis; thus, the designation "larynx, epiglottis" is appropriate. Examples of additional organs that require site-specific qualifiers include stomach, forestomach; stomach, glandular; adrenal gland, cortex; adrenal gland, medulla; pituitary gland, pars distalis; pituitary gland, pars intermedia; pituitary gland, pars nervosa; small intestine, duodenum; small intestine, jejunum; small intestine, ileum; eye, cornea; eye, retina; nose, squamous epithelium; nose, transitional epithelium; nose, respiratory epithelium; and nose, olfactory epithelium.

Alternatively, in some situations it may be best to refrain from using site qualifiers. As an example, for generalized inflammation in hollow organs or tissues that have surface epithelia, e.g., the nose, stomach, gastrointestinal tract, or urinary bladder, the use of qualifiers that indicate specific sites (lumen, epithelium,

mucosa, submucosa) may not be appropriate. In such instances, differences in lesion distribution may simply reflect the overall severity of the inflammation.

Distribution qualifiers are used to indicate an inherent feature of a lesion that has a particular biological significance or is a reflection of a specific pathogenesis. For example, centrilobular hepatic necrosis rarely has the same pathogenesis as hepatic necrosis, that is, multifocal and distributed randomly, so it is therefore important to include these types of modifiers. Likewise, it may be toxicologically relevant to the interpretation of a study to know whether hyperplasia of the forestomach is focal versus diffuse. Conversely, the use of distribution qualifiers is usually not warranted for common background or age-related lesions. The extent of such lesions is best conveyed by the use of severity grades.

Severity grading is the application of a subjective semiquantitative score to a lesion or process to denote the extent of tissue involvement, the degree of tissue damage, or a combination of these parameters. Severity grades are not absolute; rather, they represent degrees of changes relative to similar lesions in other animals in a study. Systems of severity grading and the subjective score vary in usage among pathologists. The following four-term system of severity grading is used frequently: "1, minimal; 2, mild; 3, moderate; or 4, marked." A fifth category, "5, severe," is sometimes incorporated to denote histopathological alterations that are especially profound, or perhaps related to the death of the animal. It is important that pathologists define the grading criteria adequately so that results are reproducible by the same or other pathologists. Severity grades are useful when making dose-related comparisons of qualitative changes, e.g., increases in average severity with increasing dose, or when comparing the relative toxicity of structurally related compounds. Severity grades are generally reserved for nonneoplastic lesions, whereas neoplasms are considered either present or not present. For some nonneoplastic lesions, however, severity grading adds little valuable information. Examples include ocular cataract or cysts of the pituitary pars distalis.

A few separate rules exist for the terminology applied to neoplasms. For neoplasms, each diagnosis should indicate whether the lesion is primary, that is, occurring within the tissue of origin, or metastatic. By convention, for neoplasms arising at sites distant from the primary, the qualifier "metastatic" is added to the diagnosis, and the site of the primary lesion is indicated parenthetically. An example would be lung, neuroblastoma, metastatic (nose). Also by convention, it is assumed that neoplasms not designated as metastatic are primary. For most neoplasms, the diagnosis should indicate whether the lesion is benign or malignant. Examples include stomach, glandular—neuro-endocrine cell tumor, benign; stomach, glandular—neuroendocrine cell tumor, malignant; adrenal gland, medulla—pheochromocytoma, benign; and adrenal gland, medulla—pheochromocytoma, malignant.

Diagnoses for neoplasms should not contain site qualifiers that signify a gross or subgross location of the lesion unless such qualifiers serve to distinguish the histogenesis of one neoplasm from another. For example, the site qualifiers "C cell" or "follicular cell" should be used to distinguished carcinomas of the thyroid gland. The occurrence of multiple and bilateral neoplasms should be indicated, especially when this occurrence appears to be a treatment-related phenomenon. Examples include "liver—hepatocellular adenoma, multiple" and "kidney, tubule—adenoma bilateral." Finally, inflammation and other types of paraneoplastic changes may result from the presence of neoplasms in any given tissue. These secondary lesions are usually not meaningful to the study and therefore should not be recorded as diagnoses.

III. Suggested Practices

Terminology problems originating from training may be addressed by adjusting the manner in which pathologists are trained. Training programs for potential toxicological pathologists must include a solid foundation in the pathology of common laboratory animals, which should include knowledge of the nature and distribution of common background and toxicant-induced lesions, common tissue-specific responses to toxicants, and the terminology used in diagnostic toxicological pathology. Coursework in basic principles of toxicology and toxicology testing should also be a component of a training program. The ability to deal effectively with many of the issues discussed in Section II are in part related to the training and extent of the experience of individual pathologists evaluating toxicological studies. For the inexperienced pathologist, histopathological evaluation should initially be performed in consultation with more experienced pathologists. Laboratories performing and evaluating toxicological studies should have procedures for comprehensive review and mentoring of trainee pathologists. Whenever practical, a pathology peer review should be incorporated into the histopathologic evaluation process.

Subchronic or chronic toxicity/carcinogenicity studies are usually conducted in male and female rats and mice. In the ideal situation, one pathologist should evaluate the control and treated groups of both sexes of the test species, as some chemicals are likely to cause similar effects, and comparisons of effects between the species are inevitable. In situations where this practice is not feasible, good communication among pathologists can maintain consistency. Comparison of lesions among pathologists conducting evaluations is essential, as they must be aware of the exact nature of the lesions observed in all sexes and species. Internal pathology peer reviews conducted before data are finalized are also highly desirable. By working together, pathologists can lessen the potential for inconsistencies in diagnostic terminology.

Diagnostic drift can be minimized by several methods. Initially, it is often helpful to examine a few animals from the control group and each dose group to determine the salient treatment effect(s). For example, the various treatment groups can be evaluated in replicates of 5 or 10 starting with the controls and high-dose groups and subsequently the mid and low doses. From the onset of the histopathological evaluation, pathologists should establish and use a limited set of diagnostic terms and clearly define the morphologic criteria used for classifying lesions under the terms utilized. In addition to establishing this diagnostic "dictionary" that is specific to a study, this preliminary evaluation allows the pathologist to set thresholds for severity grading. The overall goal of this exercise is to facilitate the consistent application of diagnostic terminology and criteria and acquaint the pathologist with the range of lesion severity, further facilitating consistency in diagnostic criteria used for the grading of lesions. At the end of the initial evaluation and the completion of the histopathologic evaluation, the diagnostic dictionary can be reviewed for duplications in terminology; the use of inappropriate terminology for topography, sites, and morphology; and terminology that is inconsistent with previous studies performed on the same or related compounds. If computerized systems are used to diagnose and record lesions, pathologists should be completely familiar with the system with particular respect to the manner by which it compiles, sorts, and analyzes microscopic diagnoses.

To address issues associated with lack of standardized terminology, initiatives have been started to harmonize diagnostic terminology by developing an internationally recognized standardized system of nomenclature and diagnostic criteria (SSNDC) for lesions of laboratory animals. These initiatives are encouraged and should be continual. The specific goals of these initiatives have been to reduce the confusion created by the plethora of diagnostic terms currently in use, improve the accuracy and consistency of pathology data generated, and facilitate the evaluation and interpretation of results from rodent toxicological studies. The program is a cooperative effort between the STP and domestic and international pathologists. A series of organ subcommittees were established that were in turn directed by a coordinating

committee composed of experienced toxicologic pathologists. Organ subcommittees were structured to include individuals with organ-specific expertise. The objective of the SSNDC was to develop and publish a series of guides for standardized diagnostic terms and criteria for each organ or system. During the compilation of these guides, input was solicited from many sources, including the general membership of the STP; regional discussion and working groups; professional societies, such as the American College of Veterinary Pathologists; the Society of Toxicology; the International Academy of Pathology; the Armed Forces Institute of Pathology; the American Registry of Pathology; the International Life Sciences Institute; the International Federation of Toxicologic Pathology; representatives of chemical and pharmaceutical industries; consultants; and government agencies. Internationally recognized publications produced by these initiatives include "Standardized System of Nomenclature and Diagnostic Criteria (SSNDC): Guides for Toxicologic Pathology)" generated by the STP and the "WHO/IARC: International Classification of Rodent Tumors" created by the International Agency for Research on Cancer (IARC). These publications provide recommended formats for the harmonization of diagnostic terminology and standardized diagnostic criteria that can be linked to specific lesions to achieve accuracy and consistency. Both the STP and the IARC have independently published monographs and fascicles on rat lesions; conversely, publication of mouse fascicles will be a joint STP–IARC effort. The STP guides contain complete morphological descriptions of lesions with color photomicrographs, nomenclature and diagnostic criteria, discussions, and reference lists. The SSNDC is now a widely accepted standardized system of nomenclature.

The IARC fascicles are the result of collaboration between chemical and pharmaceutical companies. The goal of this collaboration was to standardize the diagnostic terminology for the development of an animal historical control database for tumors and preneoplastic lesions in rats and mice so that such information could be used worldwide for regulatory purposes. Pathologists at participating companies determined the terminology used in the IARC fascicles, with some input from STP pathologists. The format of the fascicles is similar to that of the STP guides. Each fascicle is divided into data sheets, each of which presents the essential information on a specific lesion. Incorporated into the fascicles are the histogenesis and histology of selected lesions, including complete lesion descriptions plus black and white photomicrographs of salient morphologic features; nomenclatural criteria; lists of differential diagnosis(es); comments; and references. To be included in the fascicles, a lesion must have been documented photomicrographically in the literature. Information contained in the IARC fascicles has been combined with historical control data from carcinogenicity studies into an electronic database, the Registry Nomenclature Information System (RENI). The RENI system also includes NTP historical control data for neoplastic lesions in Fischer 344 rats and B6C3F1 mice.

Additional sources of standardized nomenclature can be found in other databases. The NTP uses a multifunctional computerized system, the Toxicology Data Management System (TDMS), to manage and collect in-life and toxicological data. Within the TDMS, the Post Experimental Information System (PEIS) includes a pathology module for the capture and retrieval of gross and microscopic pathology data. The PEIS uses a standardized system of nomenclature, the Pathology Code Table (PCT), to describe lesions. The PCT consists of a database that classifies gross and microscopic lesions by organ systems. It also partitions microscopic lesions into proliferative and nonproliferative categories. The system is hierarchical, and data are entered sequentially from a menu beginning with the topography, followed by sites and subsites within organs, the disease process, and qualifiers. Because the selected terms are stored in the TDMS system, a study-specific dictionary is compiled that facilitates review and correction of diagnoses,

data retrieval, and statistical analysis. The TDMS differs from other nomenclature systems in that diagnostic criteria for the terminology used are not included in the PCT, and it does not guide the user to those terms considered most appropriate for a given situation. It is necessary for pathologists using TDMS to provide additionally a narrative report that defines diagnostic terms and criteria.

Several published texts are excellent sources of standardized nomenclature. "Pathology of the Fischer Rat" (1990) and "Pathology of the Mouse" (1999) are authoritative and comprehensive pathology reference texts of both spontaneous and induced lesions observed in the Fischer 344 rat and the B6C3F1 mouse. The terminology in these texts is based on the NTP database of millions of extensively peer-reviewed histopathological slides from more than 500 short- and long-term toxicity/carcinogenicity studies conducted under the auspices of the NTP. Diagnostic categories included in these texts are based on standardized diagnostic criteria for the pathology terminology utilized by the NTP. The mouse text also contains references to lesions of transgenic mouse strains and mechanistic considerations. In both texts, the chapters follow the same basic format that includes normal anatomy and histology followed by discussions of congenital, degenerative, inflammatory, vascular, hyperplastic, proliferative, and miscellaneous lesions. The final section of each chapter addresses organ system toxicology and specific toxicological lesions observed within a particular organ system. Chapters include diagrams and photomicrographs to illustrate the salient morphological features of the lesions described. Additional reference texts include "Pathobiology of the Aging Rat" (1992), "Pathobiology of the Aging Mouse" (1996), "Rat Histopathology" (1984), and "Mouse Histopathology" (1990).

As mentioned previously, pathology peer review (PR) should be incorporated into the histopathologic evaluation process whenever practical. The PR process has been used by many institutions as a means to assess the reliability of and to increase confidence in histopathological data. Specifically, the purposes of PR are to verify the accuracy of the toxicologically significant microscopic findings, to ensure that the treatment-related effects are identified properly, to confirm that lesions are diagnosed similarly, and to check that the terminology used is contemporary. Pathology PR may be prospective or retrospective. In prospective PR, the general design for the review is included in the study protocol, and pathology data are not final until the review has been completed. In contrast, retrospective PR is conducted after pathology data are finalized. Basic protocols have been established in which the reviews of chronic and subchronic studies are flexible and based appropriately on study results and the size, duration, complexity, and purpose of each particular experiment. Many institutions routinely conduct an informal PR of the pathology data. This usually entails a review of the original diagnoses by a second pathologist who is a member of the same institution. Such reviews typically do not have standard operating procedures or study-specific protocols; they are often poorly documented, and it is the responsibility of the study pathologist to finalize data. Other institutions perform a more formal and rigorous PR, which involves separate quality assessment and Pathology Working Group reviews by pathologists outside the institution. This form of PR promotes a higher level of confidence in pathology data and result interpretations. It follows standard operating procedures and requires a study-specific protocol that states the extent of the review and the tissues to be examined.

While pathologists may disagree on the utility, format, and extent of PR procedures, regulatory agencies generally regard peer-reviewed data as more accurate and reliable; consequently, these agencies recommend the usage of independent peer review (EPA Pesticide Registration Notice 87–10, 1987). The submission of rigorously peer-reviewed data may reduce the extent to which pathology data are audited by a regulatory agency and may serve to expedite the review process of the agency. Peer review can also serve as an important source of continuing education for pathologists. For specific details on PR procedures, the reader is referred to several comprehensive reviews in *Toxicologic Pathology*.

Of particular importance in any histopathological evaluation is the pathology narrative section of the study report. The narrative is a discussion of the significant pathological findings, provides morphologic descriptions of the lesions observed, and places the major treatment-related lesions into a context that is supported by data and sound scientific arguments. In the pathology narrative, it is appropriate to describe the diagnostic terminology and criteria used for classifying lesions and treatment-related effects. Two of the most commonly encountered problems are inadequate morphological descriptions of lesions and the lack of information regarding any pertinent baseline diagnostic thresholds for lesion diagnosis and severity grading.

IV. Summary

Discerning differences between control and treatment groups and properly communicating these differences to the scientific community are the essence of toxicologic pathology. Communication is difficult under the best of circumstances. To communicate effectively, pathologists must consider the intended usage of data and that the larger audience of non-pathologists (regulatory toxicologist, risk assessor, risk manager) may be less familiar with pathology terminology and may approach study results with a different perspective. The goal for pathologists is to report findings in a manner that facilitates comparison of data among related studies. A systematic approach to the diagnosis and documentation of lesions and the consistent application of a standardized system of nomenclature are essential elements for assessing comparative toxicologic effects of different or structurally related chemicals. This task is not always easy.

SUGGESTED READING

Black, H. E. (1991). Peer review in toxicologic pathology: Some recommendations. *Toxicol. Pathol.* **19**, 290–292.

Black, H. E. (1997). Pebble in the pond. *Toxicol. Pathol.* **25**, 80–81.

Boorman, G. A., and Eustis, S. L. (1986). The pathology working group as a means for assuring pathology quality in toxicologic studies. *In* "Managing Conduct and Data Quality of Toxicologic Studies" (K. B. Hoover, J. K. Baldwin, A. F. Velner, C. E. Whitmire, C. L. Davies, and D. W. Bristol, eds.), pp. 271–275. Princeton Sci. Pub., Princeton, NJ.

Boorman, G. A., Eustis, S. L., Elwell, M. R., Montogomery C. A., Jr., and MacKenzie, W. F. (eds.) (1990). "Pathology of the Fischer Rat, Reference and Atlas". Academic Press, San Diego.

Copley, M. P. (1997). Environmental Protection Agency risk assessment – Process and toxicologic pathology. *Toxicol. Pathol.* **25**, 68–71.

Dua, P. N., and Jackson, B. A. (1988). Review of pathology data for regulatory purposes. *Toxicol. Pathol.* **16**, 443–450.

Eighmy, J. J. (1996). Study pathologist perspective of pathology peer review. *Toxicol. Pathol.* **24**, 647–649.

Environmental Protection Agency (1994). Pesticide Regulation (PR) Notice 94–5.

Faccini, J. M., Abbott, D. P., and Paulus, G. J. J. (1990). "Mouse Histopathology: A Glossary for Use in Toxicity and Carcinogenicity Studies." Elsevier, Amsterdam.

Faccini, J. M., Butler, W. R., Friedman, J. C., Hess, R., Reznik, G. K., Ito, N., Hayashi, Y., and Williams, G. M. (1992). IFSTP guidelines for the design and interpretation of the chronic rodent carcinogenicity bioassay. *Exp. Toxicol. Pathol.* **44**, 443–456.

Frantz, J. D. (1997). Pathology peer review. *Toxicol. Pathol.* **25**, 335–338.

Goodman, D. G. (1988). Factors affecting histopathologic interpretation of toxicity/carcinogenicity studies. *In* "Carcinogenicity: The Design, Analysis and Interpretation of Long-term Animal Studies: ILSI Monographs" (H. C. Grice, and J. J. Ciminera, eds.), pp. 109–118.

Greaves, P., and Faccini, J. M. (1984). "Rat Histopathology: A Glossary for Use in Toxicity and Carcinogenicity Studies" (J. M. Fanccini, D. P. Abbott, and G. J. J. Paulus, eds.). Elsevier, Amsterdam.

Hailey, J. R. (1994). Points of consideration relative to peer review of histological diagnoses. Society of Toxicologic Pathologists Newsletter, pp. 8–9.

Hardisty, J. F., and Boorman, G. A. (1986). National Toxicology Program pathology quality assurance procedures. *In* "Managing Conduct and Data Quality of Toxicology Studies" (K. B. Hoover, J. K. Baldwin, A. F. Velner, C. E. Whitmire, C. L. Davis, and D. W. Bristol, eds.), pp.263–269. Princeton Scientific Publishing, Princeton, NJ.

Hardisty, J. F., and Eustis, S. L. (1990). Toxicological pathology: A critical stage in study interpretation. *In* "Progress in Predictive Toxicology" (D. B. Clayson, I. C. Munro, P. Shubik, and J. A. Swenberg, eds.), pp. 41–62. Elsevier, Amsterdam New York.

Haseman, J. R., Huff, J., Rao, G. N., and Eustis, S. L. (1989). Sources of variability in rodent carcinogenicity studies. *Fundam. Appl. Toxicol.* **12**, 793–804.

Haseman, J. K., Thorrington, E. C., Huff, J. E., and McConnell, E. E. (1986). Comparison of site specific and overall tumor incidence analyses for 81 recent National Toxicology Program carcinogenicity studies. *Regul. Toxicol. Pharmacol.* **6**, 155–170.

Herbert, R. A., and Leininger, J. R. (1999). Nose, larynx and trachea. *In* "Pathology of the Mouse" (R. R. Maronpot, G. A. Boorman, and B. Gaul, eds.), pp. 259–292. Cache River Press, Vienna, IL.

International Agency for Research on Cancer (1992). International Classification of Rodent Tumors Part 1: The Rat. 2. Soft Tissue Tumors and Musculoskeletal System (U. Mohr editor-in-chief). IARC Scientific Publications, No. 122.

Mann, P. C. (1996). Pathology peer review from the perspective of an external review pathologist. *Toxicol. Pathol.* **24**, 650–653.

Maronpot, R. R., Boorman, G. A., and Gaul, B., (eds.) (1999). "Pathology of the Mouse". Cache River Press, Vienna, IL.

McConnell, E. E., and Eustis, S. L. (1994). Peer review in carcinogenicity bioassays: Uses and abuses. *Toxicol. Pathol.* **22**, 141–144.

McConnell, E. E., Solleveld H. A., Swenberg, J. A., and Boorman, G. A. (1986). Guidelines for combining neoplasms for evaluation of rodent carcinogenesis studies. *J. Natl. Cancer Inst.* **76**, 283–289.

Mohr, U., Dungworth, D., and Capen, C. C. (eds.) (1994). "Pathobiology of the Aging Rat", Vols 1 and 2. ILSI Press, Washington, DC.

Mohr, U., Dungworth, D. L., Capen, C. C., Carlton, W. W., Sundberg, J. P., and Ward, J. M. (eds.) (1996). "Pathobiology of the Aging Mouse", Vols. 1 and 2. ILSI Press, Washington, DC.

Montgomery, C. A., Jr. (1986). Good laboratory practices and the toxicology data management system. *In* "Managing, Conduct, and Data Quality of Toxicology Studies: Sharing Perspectives and Expanding Horizons," pp. 277–281. Princeton Publishing Co., Inc., Princeton, NJ.

Morgan, K. T., and Eustis, S. L. (1988). Criteria for classification of neoplasms for pathologists and statisticians. *In* "Carcinogenicity: The Design, Analysis and Interpretation of Long-Term Animal Studies" (H. C.

Grice and J. L. Ciminera, eds.), ILSI Monographs, Springer-Verlag, New York.

Peters, T. S. (1996). Pathology peer review: A concept for consideration. *Toxicol. Pathol.* **24**, 654–656.

Society of Toxicologic Pathologists (1997). Commentary: Documentation of pathology peer review. Position of the Society of Toxicologic Pathologists. *Toxicol. Pathol.* **25**, 655.

Street, C. S. (1988). Standardized systems of nomenclature and diagnostic criteria in toxicologic pathology. *Toxicol. Pathol.* **16**, 305–306.

Toxicology Data Management System Pathology Code Table Reference Manual. Document Number: TS-1006-5.1 Version 5.1 (1995). TDMS ADP Support Services for the National Toxicology Program prepared by Information Systems & Network Corporation.

Ward, J. M., Hardisty, J. F., Hailey, J. R., and Streett, C. S. (1995). Peer review in toxicologic pathology. *Toxicol. Pathol.* **23**, 226–234.

PART B
The Practice of Toxicologic Pathology

8

Basic Techniques

Thomas J. Bucci
Pathology Associates International
National Center for Toxicological Research
Jefferson, Arkansas

I. Introduction

Toxicologic pathology concerns the effect of potentially noxious products on the body. The question being asked about the product (test substance) usually involves its safety for humans or its efficacy as a medicament. The typical context is intentional controlled exposure of laboratory animals as surrogates for humans. The animal phase of toxicologic studies is comprehensive. Characterizing the morphologic response of exposed animals is an early step among many to establish the risk to humans who may be exposed to the same test substance. As an example, a description of the current U.S. National Toxicology Program (NTP) follows. Like other toxicologic investigations, this program evaluates chemicals for toxic and carcinogenic effects in laboratory animals. The description (Huff *et al.*, 1988), although succinct, indicates clearly the scope of the endeavor:

Ordinarily, a toxicology and carcinogenesis study of a chemical comprises an integrated approach of toxicological characterization: chemical disposition (absorption, distribution, metabolism, excretion); genetic toxicology (including assays of gene mutations in bacteria and in mammalian cells, chromo-some effects and transformation in mammalian cells, and DNA damage and repair); fertility and reproductive assessment (sperm morphology and vaginal cytology); systemic toxicology (14-day and 90–120 day exposures); specific studies as appropriate (immunological, biochemical, neurological, inhalation toxicology, and activated oncogenes); clinical pathology where applicable (hematology, urinalysis, endocrine function, and clinical chemistry); and long-term (two-year) toxicology and carcinogenesis studies. Each study on a chemical usually involves four individual, separate yet concurrent experiments: male rats, female rats, male mice, and female mice.

More recently, international and U.S. regulatory agencies have agreed to review carcinogenicity studies in only one rodent species when supplemented by an appropriate alternate test, e.g., a chronic study in rats plus a shorter-term validated carcinogenicity test in transgenic mice (USFDA (1997)).

In the broadest sense of the term, toxicologic pathology embraces all the elements alluded to in the quotation. Many short-term studies are conducted to elucidate the mechanism of action of the test compound, to give some idea of its toxicity, and to identify possible target organs. These studies incorporate standard histopathologic and clinical pathologic techniques. Sometimes specialized techniques, including electron microscopy, immunohistochemistry, autoradiography, and quantitative morphometry, are warranted.

Handbook of Toxicologic Pathology, Second Edition
Volume 1

Specific pathology protocols for testing of a compound may vary depending on the test substance or the sponsoring organization. Needless to say, the undertaking is important as judgements concerning risk to humans ultimately are based largely on these animal data. Whereas the rationale and procedures involved in risk assessment are beyond the scope of this chapter, some elements of concern to the toxicologic pathologist are germane, namely interspecies extrapolation and dose extrapolation.

Interspecies extrapolation encompasses all the genetic, physiologic, pharmacokinetic, and behavioral differences between humans and the species tested. Humans are genetically heterogeneous and are exposed to complex and variable mixtures of compounds, in contrast to the controlled conditions of the animal test. To provide the best data for subsequent extrapolations, it is the responsibility of the pathologist to make the most of the controllable aspects of the animal tests.

Dose extrapolation involves estimates of the effect of low doses (usually) on humans as inferred from the larger doses used in animal studies. The large doses are used to assure a measurable effect in the small populations tested. Unfortunately, the extrapolation is associated with many degrees of uncertainty and many assumptions must be made.

The first goal of toxicologic pathology is to establish the precise degree of risk posed to the test animals under the controlled exposure conditions. The process is similar to diagnostic pathology in lesion evaluation, but differs in the manner in which data are compiled. The focus is on representative response of a treatment cohort, versus individual patients, the objective being to quantify the average response of treated groups compared with untreated ones. There are standardized protocols, peer review procedures, and auspicious review by regulatory agencies.

These distinctive characteristics of toxicologic pathology, especially in such tests as the long-term rodent bioassays, often require different record keeping than the usual diagnostic description. Differences in records stem from

the need to establish quantitative risk to groups of animals exposed to graded doses of the test substance. The volume of morphologic data generated by a 2-year study in both sexes of two species of animals is huge. It must be collected in a standardized way and compiled in a condensed or manageable form.

The most undesirable characteristic of data in toxicologic pathology, short of inaccuracy, is inconsistency. Most of the factors that influence evaluation of morphologic change (e.g., poor fixation of tissue) have the undesirable effect of increasing the variability within groups and subsequently the range of data that the pathologist is forced to accept. This decreases the sensitivity of the methods used. When tissue fixation is poor, the pathologist cannot be sufficiently discerning to distinguish early toxic injury from early postmortem autolysis; thus the ability to detect a subtle effect of treatment is compromised. Similarly, spontaneous or nonspecific lesions that are similar to lesions associated with a test substance compromise evaluation. Vigilance is required to minimize the effect of these complicating factors. Toxicologic pathology requires the art of pathology to be used in conjunction with sound experimental design, methods, and analysis.

II. Factors Influencing the Evaluation of Altered Morphology

Many factors influence the interpretation of the significance of altered morphology, but this chapter emphasizes factors with special significance in toxicologic pathology. All pathologists, including toxicologic pathologists, rely heavily on clinical observation, analyses of blood and body fluids, and necropsy findings. Altered morphology is evaluated in the light of everything known about the animal, as the functional significance of the morphologic change can be quite different depending on the etiology involved. For example, proteinuria associated solely with nephrosis could plausibly be caused by toxicity of a test substance. In contrast, if an animal has a neoplasm of the urinary bladder with hydroureter and hydrone-phrosis, the proteinuria should be interpreted as secondary to urinary obstruction caused by the neoplasm.

The season of the year and the "occupation" of the animal are examples of factors that are particularly important in other aspects of pathology but have less influence in toxicologic pathology. Cognizance of such variables is essential for comparative purposes in diagnostic pathology. In other words, diagnostic pathology uses history and variation from the normal population to attain a diagnosis, whereas experimental toxicologic pathology uses comparison of differences among treatment groups of a normal population.

To exaggerate how individual variation can complicate the interpretation of bioassay results, we can imagine a hypothetical bioassay in which all animals in a toxicologic study would be histologically perfect. Their tissues would respond only to test substances and each animal's response would be identical qualitatively and quantitatively. Any morphologic change could, therefore, be attributed directly to exposure to the test substance. In reality, the task is performed with animals that are not identical. Their responses in the study are various and multifactorial, and may or may not be caused by the test material.

The routine bioassay is undertaken using two sexes, a minimum of three treatment levels, and one control group; usually two species are used. Each treatment group defined by species, sex, and dose is distinct The pathologist's task is to characterize the background changes, as reflected in the untreated animals, and to compare these changes with those found in each of the treated groups of the same species and sex. In effect, each bioassay is an exercise in population statistics. Rather than be concerned with each individual animal for its own sake, the pathologist must regard each animal as a statistical subunit of a set, the treatment group.

The focus on the representative response of each group necessitates the standardization of necropsy and histology procedures to minimize variation in histologic appearance among ani-

mals within or among treatment groups due to processing or artifact. It necessitates standardized classification of lesions so the diagnoses can be compared.

Subtle lesions are always difficult to interpret. Obviously, as lesions produced by the test substance become subtler with decreasing dose, they become more difficult to differentiate from background. The dose level at which they can no longer be distinguished is the "no observable adverse effect level" (NOAEL). Unfortunately, this level is not clearly defined, as background "noise" may interfere with the cutoff point. Identification of this dose has importance for subsequent extrapolation to humans and it forces the pathologist to wrestle with the threshold between "normal" and "least detectable change." The distinction is made more efficiently when the pathologist reads the slides with knowledge of the animals' treatment (i.e., not "blind") and then later rereads the slides without knowledge of treatment group ("blind") to confirm the interpretation. Table I includes some common factors (other than treatment) that affect the histologic

TABLE I
Factors That Influence Evaluation of Altered Morphology

Factors in collection and processing of tissue
    Standard operating procedures
    Quality of necropsy
    Accuracy of organ weights
    Fresh versus autolyzed tissue
    Type of fixative, adequacy of fixation
    Histologic preparation

Factors intrinsic to the animal
    Species, strain, sex, age
    Spontaneous disease
    Physiologic phenomena
    Normal histologic variation

Factors related to the environment
    Nutrition
    Temperature
    Illumination
    Sound

Factors related to nomenclature
    Standardization and consistency
    Pathologic process versus component stages
    Grading of lesions versus qualifiers
    "Blind" reading
    Combining of lesions

appearance of tissues in toxicologic pathology or that affect how histologic data are evaluated.

A. COLLECTION AND PROCESSING OF TISSUE

1. Standard Operating Procedures

This section does not contain specific "recipes" for handling tissue, as ample texts and periodical reports exist. Examples are included in the "Suggested Reading" section. The important message from this section is the reiteration that the procedures selected be codified into institutional standard operating procedures (SOPs). Unfailing adherence to well-selected SOPs is the most successful strategy to reduce variability in data, to ensure competently conducted studies, and to preclude the catastrophe of a failed experiment. There is no substitute, and regulatory agencies require them and audit their application.

2. Quality of the Necropsy

While the necrospy procedure is not an independent factor in the interpretation of morphologic change, it is the most critical single procedure in the entire toxicologic study. Many authors have emphasized this, but it bears repeating that the animal at the end of the study contains all of the previous effort that went into the study, as well as the results of the study. With respect to microscopic morphologic evaluation, a dependable standard procedure for necropsy is required to identify all gross lesions so none will be overlooked in subsequent correlations of gross and microscopic lesions; the same SOP should assure that technicians carefully collect all required tissues in a standard manner and that all lesions be described accurately. The trimming of tissues for subsequent processing and embedment is an opportunity to improve the quality of morphologic evaluation in at least three ways. The trimmer can confirm the prosector's observations and verify tissue accountability, can detect and describe additional lesions revealed upon trimming, and can effect a highly standardized protocol to provide identically trimmed sets of tissue from each animal. Tight standardization of trimming of tissue blocks is the first step in assuring uniform anatomical and histological sampling of each tissue, thereby reducing between-animal variation.

3. Accuracy of Organ Weights

Each of the factors relating to tissue processing is self-evident, but most are so pervasive in their impact on subsequent data that repetition is justified. Changes in organ weights, either absolute or relative to body weight, brain weight, or other reference, are sensitive indicators of early toxicity. In acute studies there may be no other indicator detected and weight change reveals the organ as a target (discussed further in Section II,B,4). In the case of testes and brain, where early morphologic lesions may not be demonstrable without expensive cytometry, weight change alone may serve as a valid biomarker of toxicity.

Knowledge of the weight of organs of treated animals versus controls can be a factor to cause the pathologist to reevaluate morphologic change. What previously may have been interpreted to be a spectrum of normal variation may now be seen (upon reexamination without knowledge of the treatment group) as two separable morphologic manifestations. The value of organ weight data is lost, however, if there is not a very rigorous SOP to prepare the organs for weighing. It is essential that fat and adventitia be removed in some highly uniform manner, that blood clots be removed consistently (e.g., from heart chambers), and that fluid be blotted uniformly. Small organs lose moisture rapidly under laboratory conditions. It was confirmed that a mouse thyroid gland would lose 25% of fresh weight if left uncovered in the laboratory for 15 min. Unless these variables are controlled carefully, much time and effort to obtain and use organ weight will be futile, as any real changes present may be obscured. When small tissues such as mouse thyroid or adrenal must also be examined histologically, serious consideration should be given to fixing the organ before trimming and weighing to reduce morphologic artifacts introduced by the handling and delay incident to obtaining their weight.

4. Fresh versus Autolyzed Tissue

No current techniques in pathology can restore autolyzed tissues, and to the extent that autolysis compromises the interpretation of tissue changes, all previous investment in that animal is wasted. Standard procedure should mandate two or more inspections of the animal colony each day for moribund or dead animals; they should be removed for immediate necropsy when feasible. Bodies should be refrigerated if prompt necropsy is not possible; 8 hr of refrigeration has been accepted arbitrarily as an upper limit for small rodents. Histologic postmortem changes in the rat have been described. Cells of lymph nodes, renal tubules, and intestinal villus tip were most vulnerable to autolytic change. Autolysis proceeds by degrees, and whereas the pathologist can "read through" mild degrees and detect well-developed lesions, the sensitivity of the study is compromised; advanced autolysis seriously compromises the pathologist's ability to detect the presence of toxic effects.

5. Type of Fixative and Adequacy of Fixation

Failure to achieve adequate fixation of fresh tissues causes the same loss of both data and investment as does loss through autolysis. The pathology laboratory may not be able to prevent the receipt of autolyzed tissues, but when tissues are fresh upon delivery, exercise of good SOPs for fixation should ensure well-preserved tissue. The author suspects there is more literature about fixatives and fixation than about most other techniques in pathology. Each organization has an abundant choice of chemical or physical fixation methods to best suit the objective of each study. Fixation by microwave and by vascular perfusion is used increasingly to prepare tissues for specialized examinations. Solutions of formaldehyde in various buffers are used universally because of their efficiency, versatility, and economy, although the carcinogenicity of this compound in rats has caused it increasing disrepute. Like other procedures in

the preparation of tissue sections, the specific reagents and techniques used are less important than the uniformity and consistency with which they are employed.

6. Histologic Preparation

To derive the greatest amount of information from the animal, the pathologist should examine a full set of tissues from each animal, with every organ sectioned in exactly the prescribed plane across the full face of the embedded tissue block. There should be no artifactual tearing or folding of the section and no extraneous debris or tissue. The sections should be of protocol-prescribed thickness and be stained uniformly in accordance with the SOP. Any deviation from the highest standard of quality risks compromise of the pathologists' ability to detect or quantify effects of toxicity. Missing tissues not only reflect doubt on the organization's ability to control a study, they also reduce the power of statistical analysis. Sections taken in the wrong plane can be tantamount to missing; worse, if unsuspected, they can lead to faulty interpretation. Artifacts can deprive the study of a full set of tissue by obscuring some features. Variations in stain quality and in tissue thickness interject additional variables that reduce the sensitivity of the examination to detect subtle change. Once again, there are many standard procedures that successfully produce high-quality sections for various purposes. No single one is advocated; however, slavish adherence to the SOPs should be practiced. For bioassay pathology, the volume of work virtually dictates the maximum use of automated methods. Automated methods have the added advantage of consistency and, increasingly, of computerized documentation of the steps in the procedure. As the equipment becomes more complex, there is an associated requirement that its calibration be performed, monitored, and documented carefully.

The final step in preparing the sections is to assure that every tissue of every animal is accounted for and that the animals' identification is correct. An accurate evaluation by the pathologist, attributed to an animal in the incorrect treatment group, is no better than an incorrect evaluation. It is worse still when mistaken identify is the result of exchanging animals between treatment groups, as then there are two incorrect sets of diagnoses. Quality control procedures, beginning with receipt of the animals, should be devised to detect and resolve errors at the earliest step and thus limit their effect on the study.

B. FACTORS INTRINSIC TO THE ANIMAL

1. Species, Strain, Sex, and Age

Some overriding considerations may dictate the choice of animal for the study. The relevance of the model to human should be a primary consideration (comparative physiology, pharmacodynamics if known, etc.). There may be regulatory requirements, and logistic and economic feasibility are factors. If the choice of animal is not proscribed by factors such as the foregoing, the animals selected should be the ones that have the most extensive database together with the lowest incidence of spontaneous disease in the organs of greatest interest. For chronic studies, special consideration should be given to age-dependent diseases, especially neoplasms. The species, strain, sex, and age of the animal influence the evaluation of morphologic change primarily as a function of the prevalence of spontaneous disease, in most applications. The animal's age influences the appearance of virtually every tissue. When a change is detected that is dissonant with the animal's chronologic age, that change requires special attention. Atrophy of the thymus is expected in aged animals. The same change in a young animal must be evaluated differently. Long-term (24-month) bioassays in rodents involve aged animals. By definition, aged populations of all species, including the human, are diverse pathologically. One characteristic of aging populations is marked individual variation in the expression of multiple aging changes; the individuals differ in the age when these changes first appear, their rate of progression, and their ultimate severity. Thus when rodents are used in long-term studies, thorough

documentation of age-dependent disease is essential to distinguish those processes from treatment-related changes.

2. Spontaneous Disease

a. Infectious Disease. Among spontaneous diseases, infectious diseases are serious considerations in all work with animals. In toxicologic pathology, infectious disease is more a problem for managers of the animal colony than for the pathologist, as epizootic infection in animals under test is a cause to terminate the study. However, most "clean" studies will harbor individual animals that have focal infections, as in rat preputial glands or middle ear, for example. These become factors in the evaluation of potential toxic effects, as interaction between infection and the metabolism of the test compound cannot be known with confidence. For the pathologist, the margin of uncertainty is increased with such animals. Some morphologic changes, such as stimulation (or depletion) in the immune system or the adrenal gland, may be caused by the infection, the test substance, both, or neither. Because random infections like these tend to vary in severity among individuals, the severity of the condition in the control animals may not resolve the uncertainty.

b. Neoplasms and Age-Related Nonneoplastic Disease. Except for epizootic infections, the problems posed by spontaneous disease are difficult to separate from considerations of species, strain, age, and sex of the animals, as each genotype has its own distinctive and sometimes dramatically different disease pattern. Complications of genotype-specific spontaneous neoplastic and nonneoplastic diseases of laboratory animals, particularly rodents, have been published; some examples are listed under "Suggested Reading." All animals in 24-month bioassays will have some age-dependent changes. Commonly a test substance will interact with these processes and affect their prevalence, severity, or progression. For example, Fischer rats, with a high prevalence of mononuclear cell leukemia, have various degrees of change in the liver and spleen associated with that malignancy, rendering those organs difficult to evaluate for potential treatment-related changes; depositions of amyloid are serious complications in many organs of older hamsters and mice; and age-related nephropathy has a variety of morphologic expressions in all species. These lesions obviously complicate the pathologists' effort to detect subtle patterns of treatment-related microscopic change.

A primary purpose of the 2-year study is to determine the carcinogenicity of the test substance. Cataloging the number of neoplasms in each treatment group is straightforward. Determining whether there is a treatment-related, biologically meaningful change in the prevalence of neoplasms can be elusive, however. There is often a high frequency of the same neoplasms in untreated animals, making the determination of an increase in treated groups proportionately less sensitive. In other situations, the prevalence of a spontaneous lesion at study termination may be reduced in the higher dosed groups relative to control groups when the disease is one that occurs late in life but is present and not fatal earlier (e.g., mononuclear cell leukemia in the Fisher 344 rat). In these instances there is the potential for interaction between the treatment's toxicity and the early stages of the disease. Because this combination may be debilitating or fatal, a significant number of these affected animals are removed from the study prematurely. One result is that the treated animals that survive to the study's end tend to be those without the spontaneous disease. The superficial appearance is that the treatment protected them, as the prevalence of that disease in the high-dose survivors is lower than in controls at the study's end. In such instances, analysis of each diagnosis as a function of time on study should reveal the "censoring" effect of the early fatal interaction. A detailed review of principles in the statistical evaluation of neoplasms in bioassays is available (Gart, 1986). Occasionally the untreated animals in a study will have a higher prevalence of a particular neoplasm than other recent controls in the same laboratory, further complicating evaluation of the number of neoplasms in their treated cohorts. Historical values for untreated animals in the same laboratory must then be considered to gain perspective, although only "recent" history may be relevant.

The magnitude of the problem presented by spontaneous neoplasia can be inferred from frequency data on Fischer 344 rats and B6C3F1 mice in recent 2-year dosed-feed bioassays reported by the NTP. Of approximately 900 untreated control rats of each sex, 28% of males and 51% of females had pituitary tumors, 89% of male rats had adenoma of testicular interstitial cells, and 29% (females) and 51% (males) had mononuclear cell leukemia. Overall, 93% of females and 93% of males were tumor bearing, with malignant tumors in 43 and 67% of them, respectively. Of 850 control mice of each sex, 70% of females and 76% of males were tumor bearing at 2 years; about 40% of these tumors were malignant. Hepatocellular neoplasms were particularly prevalent (32% in females and 51% in males), and lung tumors occurred in 24% of males.

Clearly, important consideration must be given to the frequency of spontaneous disease in the specific organ systems of interest. A mouse strain with high prevalence of pulmonary tumors early in life would be a poor choice for a carcinogenicity bioassay using inhalation exposure. [Having stated this principle, there is a seemingly large contradiction in the NTP's choice of the B6C3F1 hybrid mouse for its carcinogenicity bioassays, with its high average frequency of hepatocellular carcinoma in males, but the selection was a carefully considered compromise (Goodman, 1985).]

The chief strategies to reduce the spontaneous disease background are selection of the most appropriate species and strain to match the purpose of the study and maintaining the animals under conditions that minimize infectious and degenerative disease. Avoiding overnutrition is a particularly effective strategy (see Section II,C,1).

3. Physiologic Phenomena

Most physiologic phenomena have morphologic correlates, e.g., hyperplasia of reproductive structures is related to pregnancy and an increase in rough endoplastic reticulum in hepatocytes follows induction of mixed function oxidases. For a bioassay, the physiologic state of the animals in all groups should be similar throughout the period of the study. In particular, cyclic physiologic phenomena, when they have morphologic expression, must be defined carefully by appropriate control measures. One example is the storage of salivary secretion in secretory granules and their depletion with feeding activity. The size of the salivary acinar cells and the weight of the salivary glands can vary as much as fourfold between fasted and recently fed animals. The changes occur in a few hours in rats and mice. If both the high-dose group and the control group were moved to the pathology laboratory for necropsy at 8:00 AM after a night of feeding, the first set of animals killed would have secretion-depleted salivary glands. If the high-dose animals were killed first and the controls were to be killed beginning 3 hr later, the latter would have at least partially repleted secretory stores. Even if food remained in their cages, they would eat relatively little in full room light. In this example, awareness of feeding and killing schedules would influence the interpretation of size disparity in salivary acinar cells among the animals. If the disparity were a real treatment effect, it would be uniformly dose dependent and absent from controls as a first approximation.

4. Normal Histologic Variation

Differentiating treatment-related morphologic change from nontreatment related abnormal morphology is an important task for the toxicologic pathologist. Simply deciding whether a change from normal exists at all is sometimes difficult. The ability of pathologists using routine qualitative light microscopy to detect changes in the number or size of structures is undoubtedly a function of experience of the pathologist. At best, estimates credit pathologists with the ability to detect only those changes in number or size that deviate 20–30% from normal. The inherent variation in normal structures becomes a complicating factor in the evaluation of subtle morphologic change.

An experience in the author's laboratory illustrates that ancillary data can assist indetecting subtle morphologic change. Healthy young mice of most strains have moderate variation in hepatocyte size across each lobule, with the centrilobular cells larger, particularly in males. If the test substance causes mild centrilobular cytomegaly, it will be difficult to detect. If the pathologist is reading the liver slides only and has them segregated by sex and by treatment group, the change may be more apparent. If, at the opposite extreme, slides of all organs of each animal are read before moving to the next animal and the slides are read either randomly or "blindly" with respect to treatment group, especially if sexes are mingled, this mild change can be overlooked easily. In the author's episode, the pathologist did not detect centrilobular cytomegaly of hepatocytes until review of organ weight data revealed that livers of the high-dose males were on average 15% heavier than those from the control group. The pathologist then mingled sections of liver from control and high-dose groups and reread them without knowledge of their identity. He was then able to detect the difference in cell size and to separate them accurately on the basis of the mild cytomegaly in the treated group. The slightly enlarged cells had been overlooked, among the variety that were present, until the pathologist was "sensitized" to the possibility of their presence and was able to confirm this by direct comparison while "blinded" to their group of origin.

The underlying corollary is often overlooked—if cells are regarded as spheres, a change in cell area in the histologic section is evident as a function of the cell's radius squared, whereas its volume (and weight) is altered as a function of the cube of the new radius, thus rendering weight a more sensitive indicator of the change.

C. FACTORS RELATED TO THE ENVIRONMENT

1. Nutrition

Many husbandry-related conditions other than infectious disease can influence the outcome of toxicity and safety tests. Their effects must be distinguished from specific toxicity. These conditions normally would influence treated and control groups similarly so they would have the same epizootic manifestation as a spontaneous disease might. A bigger problem occurs when treated groups are handled differently from the controls during life, and are affected because of that difference, or when treated groups behave differently from controls, and their tissues reflect the difference. For example, an unpalatable test substance in the diet may reduce food consumption. This can cause variation in growth, body weight, longevity, and morbidity as a primary effect of nutrition but as only a nonspecific effect of the compound being tested. However, the high-dose animals will often be most affected and the changes could mistakenly be attributed to the test substance. Particularly confusing are situations in which animals at the upper level of dose consume less food, either because of unpalatability caused by the test substance or as an effect of toxicity. When otherwise untreated animals are deprived of food to the extent of 30–50% of what they would freely choose, they are healthier when judged by expected longevity (increased) and by morbidity and mortality rates and severity for most diseases at any age (decreased). In conformance with this effect of caloric restriction, treated animals that reduce their food intake by 30–50% may also outlive the control group and have a lower prevalence of most spontaneous diseases and neoplasms at any time point. This interaction of food consumption, dose, and prevalence of specific lesions can give the test substance the appearance of having protected the highest dosed group. By definition, aged populations of all species, including the human, are diverse pathologically. Their percentage survival could be higher and their disease prevalence lower than those of the controls when the study terminates. Such a group may actually have ingested less of the test compound than the next-lower dose group if the latter group consumes all of its feed. A corollary to the enhancement of health by caloric restriction is the emerging acknowl-edgment that the current rates of "spontaneous disease," especially tumors, are becoming epizootic in frequency in rodents and that the high rates of degenerative disease and of neoplasia are the result of overfeeding (see "Suggested Reading" and Chapter 11).

2. Temperature

Relatively small and transient changes in ambient temperature cause biologically significant change in the body temperature of rodents. Disturbances such as stormy weather or unaccustomed handling that last only minutes can cause 1- to 4-hr body temperature elevations of 1.0–1.5°C in mice. These effects would probably be proportionately less profound in larger species. In turn, body temperature is a reliable indicator of metabolic rate and therefore a sensitive determinant of metabolism of any test substance administered to the animals. A relatively small difference in ambient temperature has a dramatic impact on at least one morphologic characteristic of rodents: tail length. Rats raised in a 20°C environment have tails that are 3 cm shorter than littermates raised at 30°C. One can infer that proper timing and sufficiently sensitive methods would reveal a burst of increased cell proliferation in tails stimulated to grow at 30°C compared with the standard 22–24°C. Similar observations have been reported in mice. Thus ambient temperature, by stimulating heat exchange responses, is clearly another factor that can influence morphologic expression directly.

3. Illumination

Excess ambient illumination (light intensity) causes extensive retinal degeneration in rats and mice. If high-dose animals are housed routinely on upper shelves of cage racks, the degree of degeneration will appear to be dose related. Interacting with a carcinogen, light reportedly increased the leukemias and decreased skin carcinoma in DBA mice (cited by Clough, 1982). Long photoperiods caused regression of ovaries, Harderian glands and adrenal glands, and anestrus (Reiter, 1971), any of which could be attributed erroneously to a test substance.

4. Sound

Extraneous noise causes a biologically significant change in body temperature of rats and mice. Investigators who conduct toxicologic studies tend to be very much aware of the importance to provide controlled husbandry conditions for their animals, including control of extraneous noise. Nevertheless, most of us should probably be reminded that the auditory spectrum of rats and mice, unlike most other laboratory animals, is quite different from that of humans. The most sensitive hearing for most species is in the range of 0.5 to 10 kHz. Although mice cannot hear sounds below 1 kHz, they are exquisitely sensitive to sound in the 10- to 20-kHz range, the upper limit of which is beyond human perception. Therefore we can easily be unaware of sound frequencies, especially ultrasonic ones, that provoke stressful changes in mice via neuroendocrine stimulation. Many reports exist of adverse effects of sound on diverse species: behavioral and reproductive dysfunctions, changes in tumor susceptibility and immune response, hypertension, electrolyte metabolism, and body temperature. Extraneous sound clearly can be one source of variable outcome in toxicity tests.

There may be many yet-undetermined influences related to the animal colony environment that affect the incidence of neoplasia, other diseases, and physiologic conditions. These influences may contribute to some of the unexplained variations in prevalence data within and among laboratories.

D. FACTORS RELATED TO NOMENCLATURE

1. Standardization and Consistency

The rate of occurrence of any defined disorder cannot be determined accurately unless every case can be assigned to one of two classes: those with or those without the disorder. Classification of some kind is essential for any statistical comparison. Unfortunately, in pathology the gray zone between classes can be large, i.e., the classes are not mutually exclusive or exhaustive, making comparisons difficult. In addition, the nomenclature of pathology permits many variations in terminology for the same entity so even if the classification scheme were exclusive and exhaustive, inconsistent nomenclature can result in lost data. Possibly even worse than lost data is the confusion that is showered upon the uninitiated, who believe that any diagnosis is a positive finding. How is an administrator, or the computer, to know there is little difference among fibrosis, scar, and fibrous tissue?

The pathology lexicon uses topographic designations for systems, organs, sites within organs, and several subsites within sites. Morphologically we identify one or more of several major pathologic processes (e.g., inflammation, degeneration, proliferation) and apply qualifiers that specify distribution (focal, diffuse), duration (acute, chronic), severity (mild, moderate), and character (hemorrhagic, suppurative). Each class of qualifiers has a large selection of adjectives, supporting a vast number of permutations and combinations in the final written diagnosis. The essence of a diagnosis consists of a topographic designation, a process, and any essential qualifiers. If a record contains "liver, degeneration, fatty," and another one "median lobe, fatty change, focal," and a third, "hepatocyte, fatty change, multifocal," should they be considered as biological equals? Yes, they should. These results should be entered into the computer as three cases of a single entity, described identically, rather than as three different diagnoses. How should other records be compared to these if they contain the term "vacuolization" instead of "fatty change?"

Each pathologist must adopt, by convention or consensus, a limited set of diagnostic terms from among synonyms, sacrificing the rich diagnostic vocabulary in favour of terms that are more collective and amenable to statistical combination. By using fewer categories, treatment effects are not diluted by splitting classes into smaller categories that do not differ biologically.

Standard nomenclature must be adopted for neoplasia. Until the day of more sophisticated, truly "expert" computer programs that will untangle our synonym classes and hierarchical levels, it remains the pathologist's responsibility to reduce the data to permit meaningful statistical analysis.

Anticipating that there will be multiple animals in each of several treatment groups and further anticipating in chronic studies that most animals will have multiple lesions due solely to their age, the pathologist should maintain a list of diagnoses, and one pathologist should read the entire study to reduce operator bias. A typical two-species chronic study will contain 400–600 animals per species and could require up to 6 months for a pathologist to complete. Without a list of diagnoses, the pathologist may upgrade or downgrade diagnoses as time goes on ("diagnostic drift"). This is a significant factor in evaluation of morphologic change, as there are actually two components to the evaluation: "What is this change?" and "What should I call it?"

References included for "Suggested Reading" provide guidance for diagnostic criteria and nomenclature. The primary biologic significance of the pathologic process, not some secondary detail, should determine whether two lesions should have the same diagnosis. To disregard minor nuances in structure is a difficult assignment for pathologists, as it is contrary to much of their training. However, it is essential for comparative purposes and to limit operator bias and diagnostic drift.

2. Pathologic Process versus Component Stages

In the preceding section, a rigidly standardized and truncated set of diagnostic terms was recommended to facilitate both consistency over time and tabulation of results. The number of diagnoses can also be reduced by identifying and recording only the underlying pathologic process. This reduces markedly the number of diagnostic terms used, particularly in chronic studies. For example, all nonspecific kidney disease could be termed "nephropathy," rather than to provide a description of every recognizable component of the process. Once again this is counter to the training of most pathologists and is an "unlearning" step that is necessary in this specialized application.

With neoplastic diseases, consensus permits tissue changes secondary to the neoplasm to be disregarded in chronic studies, e.g., atrophy of seminiferous tubules associated with testicular interstitial cell tumor need not be recorded.

3. Grading of Lesions versus Qualifiers

Pathologic data are categorical in nature and are measured on a nominal scale, having no arithmetic relationship among the categories (acute versus chronic, mild versus moderate, focal versus diffuse). By attributing a subjective measure of degree (1+, 2+, 3+, etc.) to a process, such nominal characteristics can be converted to ordinal data that permit more powerful statistical analyses than those available for nominal data. For example, mild, moderate, and severe may translate into 1, 2, and 3. The grade of severity assigned to each such diagnosis is chosen to reflect a combination of the extent of the process (how many of its subordinate components are present), the distribution (focal to diffuse), and the actual degree of severity. This approach will eliminate dozens to hundreds of terms from the tables of diagnoses while enhancing the discriminating power of the examination and the statistical analyses.

4. "Blind" Reading

Most pathologists prefer to know the treatment history of the animals when they examine the tissues histologically. This knowledge enables the surest and fastest detection of treatment-related changes, as the pathologist's sensitivity and specificity increase when the baseline of altered morphology is known. Having seen the control animals, the pathologist then knows which spontaneous processes are present and how severe they are. These lesions can be graded in severity and recorded for comparison to treated groups. When ambiguous treatment changes are encountered, most pathologists examine a selection of tissues from all groups in a blind manner (without knowledge of treatment) to confirm whether the observed effects are, in fact, related to treatment. This method provides the best of both processes: speed and sensitivity to subtle change and complete objectivity through "blind" reading.

5. *Combining of Lesions*

It is often difficult to determine whether the prevalence of a particular neoplasm is truly increased in a treated group, exceeding that in the concurrent untreated control group. For example, should the number of benign and malignant neoplasms of a specific tissue, e.g., thyroid follicular cells, be combined to determine whether a greater number of neoplasms is present in treated versus untreated animals? Consider a control group of 50 animals containing 10 with an adenoma and 1 with a carcinoma of a particular cell type, while the treated group of 50 animals had 9 carcinomas and no adenoma of that cell type. The judgement of whether the treatment was carcinogenic would depend on whether the benign and malignant tumors in the control group are combined. If they are, the baseline rate is 11 neoplasms in 50 control animals, to compare with 9 of 50 in the treated group. This approach suggests no effect of treatment. Not combining the benign with the malignant tumors yields 1 malignancy in the controls versus 9 in the treated, a significant difference.

A further complication can occur when neoplasms in the same organ are histogenically different. Combining adenomas with carcinomas of follicular cells is one issue; combining the number of follicular cell tumors with C-cell tumors or with tumors of blood vessel origin in the same thyroid gland is another. If a control group of mice had a 10% prevalence of thyroid follicular cell adenoma and a treated group had 5% of each of C-cell adenoma, hemangioma, and follicular cell adenoma, can anyone be confident that the treatment caused neoplasia or that it did not? How should a test substance be classified when neoplasia in treated groups is not increased statistically in any single organ of the high-dose group but is significantly elevated statistically when tumors from all sites are combined?

How much weight should be placed on hyperplasia as an indication of preneoplastic stimulation of proliferation when it is increased in the treated animals? One factor that affects evaluation of this change is whether there is apparent progression from hyperplasia to neoplasia. If this is the case, hyperplasia is weighted more heavily.

There is no simple formula to resolve the questions concerning the combining of neoplasms. In practice, most studies are analyzed both combined and uncombined when there is uncertainty, and the outcome of both analyses is factored into the final assessment of carcinogenicity. The factors of food consumption, weight gain, and early death all affect tumor prevalence, as discussed in Section II,C,1, and these considerations must be part of the final assessment as well.

III. Summary

Toxicologic pathology differs in approach and methodology from diagnostic pathology. Usually, large numbers of rodents are used and pathologic interpretation of the effect of graded doses of some test substance is undertaken. The frequency of abnormalities in the untreated animals must be sufficiently low for detection of small increases in altered morphology over background in the treated animals. In carcinogenicity studies, most species have background neoplastic and nonneoplastic disease. These factors need to be separated from treatment-induced lesions. In addition, the amount of food consumed by the animals or the manner in which the tissues are handled during collection and processing may influence the experiment in a systematic manner. Variation in the morphologic expression of disease among animals has led to the adoption of precise simplified diagnoses; statistical separation of groups is facilitated by the use of less complex terminology.

Four major strategies contribute to reduction of the inherent variation in large bioassays: selection of animals for the study with consideration of their characteristic genetic and age-dependent lesions; husbandry to provide a rigidly controlled favorable environment for the animals; strictly standardized tissue-processing procedures selected carefully and followed faithfully to meet the needs of the study; and the disciplined use of nomenclature.

SUGGESTED READING

Introduction

Brown, S. L., *et al.* (1988). Review of interspecies risk comparisons. *Regul. Toxicol. Pharm.* **8**, 191–206.

Calabrese, E. (1988). Comparative biology of test species. *Environ. Health Perspect.* **77**, 55–62.

Contrera, J. F., and DiGeorge, J. A. (1998). *In vivo* transgenic bioassay and assessment of the carcinogenetic potential of pharmaceuticals. *Environ. Health Perspect.* **106** (Suppl.), 71–80.

Garattini, S. (1985). Toxic effects of chemicals: Difficulties in extrapolating data from animals to man. *CRC Crit. Rev. Toxicol.* **16**, 1–29.

Goodman, D. G. (1987). Animal testing of carcinogens. *Occup. Med.* **2**, 47–59.

Hacman, G. (1988). Prevention of cancer: Restriction of nutritional intake (joules): Mini-review. *Comp. Biochem. Physiol.* **91A**, 209–220.

Huff, J. E., *et al.* (1988). Carcinogenesis studies: Result of 398 experiments on 104 chemicals from the U. S. National Toxicology Program. *Ann. N. Y. Acad. Sci.* **534**, 1–30.

Maronpot, R. R. (1985). Considerations in evaluation and interpretation of long-term animal bioassays for carcinogenicity. *In* "Handbook of Carcinogen Testing," (H. A. Milman and E. K. Weisberger, eds.), pp. 372–383. Noyes, Park Ridge, NJ.

Rogers, A. E., and Longnecker, M. P. (1988). Dietary and nutritional influences on cancer: A review of epidemiologic and experimental data. *Lab. Invest.* **59**, 727–759.

United States Food and Drug Administration (1998). Guidance for Industry: S1B. Testing for Carcinogenicity of Pharmaceuticals. Federal Register (63 FR 8983) or http://www.fda.gov/cder/guidance/index.htm.

Factors That Influence Evaluation of Morphologic Changes

Collection and Processing of Tissue

Boorman, G. A., *et al.* (1985). Quality assurance in pathology for rodent carcinogenicity studies. *In* "Handbook of Carcinogen Testing," (H. A. Milman and E. K. Weisberger, eds.), pp. 345–357. Noyes Park, Ridge, NJ.

Carson, F. L. (1997). "Histotechnology: A Self-Instructional Text," 2nd Ed. American Society of Clinical Pathologists, Chicago, IL.

Farrow, M. G. (1987). Unique aspects of GLP pathology. *J. Am. Coll. Toxicol.* **6**, 207–211.

Fenwick, B. W., and Kruckenberg, S. (1987). Comparison of methods used to collect canine intestinal tissues for histologic examination. *Am. J. Vet. Res.* **48**. 1276–1281.

Fieldname, D. B., and Seely, J. C. (eds.) (1988). "Necropsy Guide: Rodents and the Rabbit." CRC, Boca Raton, FL.

Hayat, M. A. (1981) "Fixation for Electron Microscopy." Academic Press, New York.

Hopwood, O. (1985). Cell and tissue fixation 1972–1982. *Histochem J.*, **17**, 389–442.

Hopwood, O., *et al.* (1984). Microwave fixation: Its potential for routine techniques, histochemistry, immunocytochemistry and electron microscopy. *Histochem J*, **16**, 1171–1191.

Human, G. L. (1942). "Animal Tissue Techniques." Freeman, San Francisco.

Kanerva, R. L., Lefever, F. R., and Alden, C. L. (1983). Comparison of fresh and fixed organ weights of rats. *Toxicol. Pathol.* **11**, 129–131.

Luna, L. G. (ed.) (1968). "Manual of Histologic Staining Methods of the Armed Forces Institute of Pathology," 3rd Ed. McGraw Hill, New York.

McConnell, E. E. (1983). Pathology requirements for rodent two-year studies. I. A review of current procedures. II. Alternative approaches. *Toxicol. Pathol.* **11**, 60–76.

Moorlag, H. E., Boon, M. E., and Kok, L. P. (1986). Microwave methods for reducing staining time to seconds. *Stain Technol* **62**, 357–360.

National Toxicology Program General Statement of Work for the Conduct of Toxicity and Carcinogenicity Studies in Laboratory Animals (1987). USNIEHS, Research Triangle Park, NC.

National Society for Histotechnology. Educational Resources, 5900 Princess Garden Parkway, Suite 805, Lanham, Maryland 20706.

Preece, A. (1972). "A Manual for Histologic Technicians," 3rd Ed. Little Brown, La Jolla, CA.

Seaman, W. J. (1987). "Postmortem Change in the Rat: A Histologic Characterization." Iowa State Univ. Press, Ames, IA.

Sheehan, D., and Hrapchak, B. B. (1980). "Theory and Practice of Histotechnology," 2nd Ed. C. V. Mosby, St. Louis.

Thompson, S. W., and Hunt, R. D. (1966). "Selected Histochemical and Histopathological Methods." CC Thomas, Springfield, IL.

Thompson, S. W., and Luna, L. G. (1978). "An Atlas of Artifacts Encountered in the Preparation of Microscopic Tissue Sections." CC Thomas, Springfield, IL.

Factors Intrinsic to the Animal

Anver, M. R., and Cohen, B. J. (1979). Lesions associated with aging. *In* "The Laboratory Rat," (H. J. Baker, J. R. Lindsay, and S. H. Weisbroth, (eds.), Vol. I. Academic Press, New York.

Blumenthal, H. T., and Rogers, J. B. (1967). Spontaneous and induced tumors in the guinea pig, with special reference to the factor of age. *Prog. Exp. Tumor. Res.* **9**, 261–285.

Cline, J. M., and Maronpot, R. R. (1985). Variations in the histologic distribution of rat bone marrow cells with respect to age and anatomic site. *Toxicol. Pathol.* **13**, 349–355.

Davis, R. T., and Leathers, C. W. (eds.) (1985). "Behavior and Pathology of Aging in Rhesus Monkeys," Monographs in Primatology, Vol 8. A. R. Liss, New York.

Gart, J. J., *et al.* (1986) "Statistical Methods in Cancer Research," Vol. III. IARC Lyon.

Goodman, D. G., *et al.* (1979). Neoplastic and non-neoplastic lesions in aging F344 rats. *Toxicol. Appl. Pharmacol.* **48**, 237–248.

Goodman, D. G., Boorman, G. A., and Strandberg, J. D. (1985). Selection and use of the B6C3F1 mouse and F344 rat in long-term bioassays for carcinogenicity. *In* "Handbook of Carcinogen Testing," (H. A. Milman and E. K. Weisberger, eds.). Noyes, Park Ridge, NJ.

Greenman, D. L., Boothe, A., and Kodell, R. (1987). Age-dependent responses to 2-acetylaminoflorine in BALB/c female mice. *J. Toxicol. Environ. Health* **22**, 113–129.

Haseman, J. K., *et al.* (1984). Use of historical control data in carcinogenicity studies in rodents. *Toxicol. Pathol.* **12**, 126–135.

Haseman, J. K., *et al.* (1986). Comparison of site-specific and overall tumor incidence analyses for 81 recent National Toxicology Program carcinogenicity studies. *Regul. Toxicol. Pharmacol.* **6**, 155–170.

Portier, C. J., Heges, J. C., and Hoel, D. G. (1986). Age-specific models of mortality and tumor of mortality and tumor onset for historical control animals in the National Toxicology Program's carcinogenicity experiments. *Cancer Res.* **46**, 4372–4378.

Roe, F. J. C. (1988). Toxicity testing: Some principles and some pitfalls in histopathological evaluation. *Hum. Toxicol.* **7**, 405–410.

Sher, S. (1982). Tumors in control hamsters, rats and mice: Literature tabulation. *CRC Crit. Rev. Toxicol.* **11**, 49–79.

Solleveld, H. A., Haseman, J. K., and McConnell, E. E. (1984). Natural history of body weight gain, survival and neoplasia in the F344 rat. *JNCI* **72**, 929–940.

Tarone, R. E., Chu, K. C., and Ward, J. M. (1981). Variability in the rates of some naturally occurring tumors in F344 rats and B6C3F1 mice. *JNCI* **66**, 1175–1181.

Factors Related to the Environment

Al-Hilli, F., and Wright, E. A. (1983). The short term effects of a supra-lethal dose of irradiation and changes in the environmental temperature on the growth of tailbones in the mouse. *B. J. Exp. Pathol.* **64**, 684–692.

Clough, G. (1982). Environmental effects on animals used in biomedical research. *Biol. Rev.* **57**, 487–523.

Everett, R. (1984). Factors affecting spontaneous tumor incidence rates in mice: A literature review. *CRC Crit. Rev. Toxicol.* **3**, 235–251.

Maeda, H., *et al.* (1985). Nutritional influences on aging Fischer 344 rats. II. Pathology. *J. Gerontol.* **40**, 671–688.

Newberne, P. M. (1988). Importance of diet and nutrition in evaluating the safety of drugs. *Hum. Pathol.* **19**, 4–6.

Reiter, R. J., and Klein, D. C. (1971). Observations on the pineal gland, the Harderian glands, the retina, and the reproductive organs of adult female rats exposed to continuous light. *J. Endocrinol.* **51**, 117–125.

Roe, F. J. C. (1988). Toxicity testing: Some principles and some pitfalls in histopathological evaluation. *Hum. Toxicol.* **7**, 405–410.

Sales, G. D., *et al.* (1988). Environmental ultrasound in laboratories and animal houses: A possible cause for concern in the welfare and use of laboratory animals. *Lab Am.* **22**(4), 369–373.

Factors Related to Nomenclature

Anonymous (1998). Tumor incidence in control animals by route and vehicle of administration in $B_6C_3F_1$ mice. National Institute of Environmental Health Sciences, Research Triangle Park, NC.

Anonymous (1998). Tumor incidence in control animals by route and vehicle of administration in F344/N rats. National Institute of Environmental Health Sciences, Research Triangle Park, NC.

Anonymous Editorial (1986). Society of Toxicologic Pathologists' position paper on blinded slide reading. *Toxicol. Pathol.* **14**, 493–494.

Boorman, G. A., *et al.* (1985). Quality assurance in pathology for rodent carcinogenicity studies. *In* "Handbook of Carcinogen Testing," (H. Milman and E. Weisberger, eds.), pp. 345–357. Noyes, Park Ridge, NJ.

Boorman, G. A., Eustis, S. L., Elwell, M. R., Montgomery, C. A., Jr., and MacKenzie, W. F. (eds) (1990). "Pathology of the Fischer Rat." Academic Press, New York.

Gart, J. J., *et al.* (1986). "Statistical Methods in Cancer Research." Vol. III. IARC Lyon.

Maronpot, R. R., et al. (1986). National toxicology program nomenclature for hepatoproliferative lesions of rats. *Toxicol. Pathol.* **14**, 263–273.

Maronpot, R. R., Boorman, G. A. and Gaul, B. W. (1999). "Pathology of the Mouse." Cache River, IL.

McConnell, E. E., et al. (1986). Guidelines for combining neoplasms for evaluation of rodent carcinogenesis studies. *JNCI* **76**, 283–289.

Prasse, K., Hildebrandt, P., and Dodd, D. (1986). Letter to the editor from the Council of the American College of Veterinary Pathologists on their position regarding "blind" reading of slides. *Toxicol. Appl. Pharmacol.* **83**, 184–185.

Society of Toxicologic Pathologists. Standardized System of Nomenclature and Diagnostic Criteria. "Guides for Toxicologic Pathology." STP/ARP/AFIP Series.

9

Managing Pitfalls in Toxicologic Pathology

Peter C. Mann, Jerry F. Hardisty, and Mary D. Parker

Experimental Pathology Laboratories, Inc.
Research Triangle Park, North Carolina

I. Introduction

The practice of toxicologic pathology includes a number of areas that require the utmost diligence to avoid time-consuming, costly, or simply embarrassing errors in study design, data collection, or data reporting. The majority of these "errors" can be avoided by appropriate planning and attention to detail at certain crucial points in the conduct of toxicology studies. Some of the major areas of concern are discussed in this chapter, and potential solutions will be provided, so that these "pitfalls of toxicologic pathology" may be recognized and avoided.

II. Study Design

During the initial stages of study design, there are a number of issues that need to be resolved so that the ensuing stream of materials and data will not be hampered by needless delays or inappropriate omissions.

When designing a study, one must always ask what question is the particular study expected to answer. Different study types are designed to answer different questions: is the compound

acutely toxic, does it cause neoplasia, is the effect seen in a laboratory species relevant to that seen in humans, what are the mechanisms of a particular effect in a single organ, and so on. No single study can answer all questions, so it is important to design a study with specific questions in mind (see Chapter 14). This is becoming increasingly important as study directors try to learn as much from a single study as possible to avoid the extra costs and animal use of additional studies to elucidate mechanisms or to measure special parameters. As toxicology studies become increasingly complex, the possibility of errors occurring during the study increases exponentially. Errors that occur during the in-life portion of study, such as errors in dosing or measurement of clinical chemistry or hematology parameters, cannot be corrected at a later time point.

One should also be confident of the technical expertise of the laboratory performing the study. Some laboratories have expertise in routine toxicology studies, whereas others may have expertise in a specialized area. It would be naïve to assume that any particular laboratory has high levels of expertise in all areas of toxicology or to assume that because a particular laboratory provided excellent results for an acute inhalation study that they would be able to perform as well on a chronic infusion study.

Most contract laboratories desire to provide high-quality service, as their reputation depends on this. However, there is a tendency to perform studies according to the laboratory's usual "standards" unless the sponsor indicates strongly that a procedure or a complete study should be completed in a specific manner. For this reason, it is essential that a representative of the sponsor monitor the study closely during all phases of the study, from protocol development to final report, to assure that the study is conducted as expected. The monitor should go to the laboratory where the study is being conducted on a regular basis to review data, discuss problems, and generally maintain "ownership" of the study. These monitoring visits should be scheduled to coincide with key events or major milestones in a study, such as first day of dosing, interim sacrifices, or terminal sacrifices.

The majority of toxicology studies are designed as part of a submission to a regulatory agency and as such must be conducted under the auspices of the good laboratory practices (GLPs) act. Although the GLPs do ensure that a study is conducted in a manner that will fulfill regulatory requirements and help to ensure that data submitted are complete and accurate and that no fraudulent data are submitted, GLPs were not designed to dictate the most appropriate type of study. In today's increasingly complex world, the most appropriate test to elucidate a particular effect of a compound often changes more quickly than GLP regulations.

The expertise to conduct specific tests may exist only in an academic setting; these laboratories are often inadequate in terms of compliance with GLP regulations. Studies conducted in this situation can certainly be included as part of a submission package, but should not be the core studies. Similarly, studies in which one portion, for example, the in-life portion, was conducted at a non-GLP laboratory do not transform themselves into fully GLP compliant studies because another portion, for example, the pathology, was completed in a GLP facility.

Another commonly encountered problem concerns the differences between "good science" and regulated studies. Scientists may be conducting world class research in their laboratories, but if data appear corrupted or incomplete, the study will be treated with suspicion by the regulatory agencies. GLP regulations are basically good record keeping, validation of equipment and methods, and definition of personnel functions. They outline a set of practices that must be followed to submit studies to the regulatory agencies. The fact that a laboratory may conduct superior scientific research does not excuse it from complying with these regulations for submitted studies. The results of this type of scientific "arrogance" can be at best embarrassing and costly to the submitting sponsor, and at worst dangerous to the public's health.

When designing a protocol for a specific study, a number of issues should be considered. The correct number of animals per group and the number of treatment groups are determined by custom as well as by statistical considerations. Related to this is the question of whether one or two control groups are better for a chronic study. Although paired control groups may provide a more accurate picture of the normal variations in a population, the larger size may actually increase the significance of a treatment-related finding if the control groups are combined for analysis.

The age of animals should be considered when designing a study. Very young animals normally have high rates of growth and metabolism; this should be considered if one is contemplating studies of cell proliferation in a young population. Older animals, such as those in the later part of a 2-year study, will often have irregular estrous cycles and may react to treatments that affect the endocrine organs differently than younger animals of the same strain.

When designing a study, one should determine beforehand what clinical pathology parameters will be monitored so the collection process can be as noninvasive and nondisruptive as possible. Especially in shorter studies, hematology, clinical chemistry, and urinalysis results are often a much more accurate indicator of toxicity than histopathologic findings.

Another important decision concerns the number of tissues to be saved and processed when animals are examined postmortem. The tissue list is specified for studies to be submitted to either the Food and Drug Administration (FDA) or the Environmental Protection Agency (EPA) as part of a registration package. For smaller studies, which are often not GLP compliant, requests from study directors and sponsors range from all tissues to "just the major organs." Although examining all tissues might reveal the most information, this approach may have too high a cost/benefit ratio. One should choose a tissue list based on the knowledge of effects seen in other studies with the same compound or related compounds. In any case, it is wise to conduct a complete necropsy and save all the tissues, even if they are not initially examined, because once tissues are discarded they cannot be retrieved.

Much has been written about animal welfare issues in toxicologic pathology. Increased awareness of animal welfare has generally resulted in an improvement of treatment of laboratory animals. No study should be initiated without the approval of an institutional animal care and use committee (IACUC). In addition, continued research into ways to use fewer animals, such as using transgenic mice in short-term bioassays, as well as alternative methods of testing, should lessen our dependence on the use of large numbers of laboratory animals in the future.

III. Necropsy

The necropsy, or postmortem examination, is a pivotal procedure in any toxicology study. The necropsy is one of the few events in a study that cannot be repeated or recreated. Tissues that are not collected or samples that are missed are lost forever. Careful planning and a coordinated team approach are essential to a successful necropsy.

It is essential that every animal that comes to necropsy have its own unique individual animal necropsy record (IANR) so that all findings for the animal are located in one place. The IANR

should be simple, concise, and unambiguous. It should include areas for recording all essential information, including time and date of death, method of euthanasia, body weight, organ weights, gross findings, a checklist for tissues saved, and signature lines for all personnel involved in the necropsy (prosector, technician weighing tissues, pathologist). Generally speaking, all gross abnormalities should be recorded. In some cases, even normal physiological changes should be recorded grossly. An example of such normal physiological change is the dilation of the uterine horns seen in mice and rats during proestrus and estrus. Although this is a normal change, it may be affected by compounds such as endocrine modulators and should be recorded to determine if there is a treatment-related effect.

It is important that gross lesions are described as to size, color, and consistency rather than diagnosed. Diagnosis is appropriate only after the tissue has been examined microscopically. The pathologist must depend on the prosectors to recognize gross abnormalities, but it is the responsibility of the pathologist to determine the actual description of these abnormalities. The terms used should be clear, concise, and consistent so that similar gross lesions are always described in identical terms.

Although it is not required by regulation that the pathologist be present at necropsy, it is of utmost importance that, as the professional leader of the necropsy team, the pathologist be present. Although trained necropsy prosectors can generally recognize a tissue as abnormal, they are not trained to assess the biological significance of a particular lesion or set of lesions. It is the pathologist's responsibility to assure that all lesions from all animals are recorded accurately, as well as to maintain internal scheduling so that animals are euthanized on time, that tissues are weighed and trimmed properly, and that the necropsy proceeds in an orderly and efficient manner. It is crucial that the number of prosectors does not exceed the ability of the pathologist to maintain this orderly flow. The number of prosecting teams a pathologist can manage depends on the experience of the pathologist and the teams, as well as the type of study.

Each member of the prosecting team also has a specific set of duties. The prosector will usually be the most senior member of a team. Depending on the complexity of the study, there may be a trimmer, who assists the prosector, either by prosecting a subset of all tissues or by trimming organs prior to weighing and collection. The person weighing the organs can usually handle the organs from several teams at once. However, if tissues require special handling or need to be frozen quickly, an individual for each team may be required.

Similarly, the recorder, whose task it is to record all weights, gross lesions, and other findings, may be the trimmer or a second individual depending on the study design. It is important to carefully plan the duties of each member of the necropsy team well before the day of necropsy. The time spent planning the details of a necropsy can save time and prevent the aggravation of inadequate supplies or incorrectly preserved samples. A simple but often overlooked method of ensuring a smooth necropsy is to make sure that each member of the team has read and thoroughly understands the necropsy portion of the study protocol.

There are a number of ways to ensure that all protocol-required tissues are saved during necropsy. There should be a tissue list on the animal's necropsy record and two people should be involved in putting the tissue in fixative. One technician (prosector or trimmer) should place the tissues in fixative one tissue at a time and should verify the tissue for the recorder who is checking the tissue off on the necropsy record. In this manner the number of lost or missing tissues should be minimized.

Use of a tissue collection template (a card with an area marked for all tissues) under a sheet of plastic or a clear plastic tray with dividers or an ice cube tray labeled for various tissues will help ensure that all required tissues are collected from each animal. It is also important that tissues are not allowed to dry before immersion in fixative, as this will adversely effect the quality of tissue preservation. Tissues can be sprayed with saline on the necropsy table or in the collection tray. Larger tissues may be gently covered with a piece of gauze, which can then be moistened with saline.

The type of fixative is also determined by the type of study and the end points to be examined. Unfortunately, there is no universal fixative that will provide optimum fixation for all tissues and for every procedure. For most routine studies, 10% neutral-buffered formalin still remains the fixative of choice, because it is economical and provides good general fixation. Certain organs, especially the eyes and testes, require harder fixation and may be initially fixed in Davidson's, Bouin's, or, less commonly, Zenker's fixative.

Tissues should be trimmed to no more than 0.5 cm in thickness and placed in a volume of at least 10 times as much formalin as tissue. It is a good practice to change the formalin after 24–48 hr especially if there is a large amount of tissue in the container. Tissues that are to be examined on the transmission electron microscope (EM) need to be minced (no more than $1 \, mm^3$) and fixed quickly in a solution that contains gluteraldehyde. There are a number of formulas for EM fixatives, some of which (such as Mellonig's formalin) also produce acceptable results for light microscopy. With the increasing need for immunohistochemistry, the length of time a tissue spends in formalin has become important, as prolonged exposure to formalin can result in cross-linking of S bonds, which may impede the access of antibodies to target epitopes. For this reason, it is recommended that tissues for immunohistochemistry be changed from formalin to 70% ethanol within 48 hr of necropsy and that the tissues be trimmed and embedded as quickly as possible.

IV. Histology

From the moment of fixation on, all is artifact. The goal of the histology laboratory is to control this process so that the degree of artifactual change is minimal and consistent from organ to organ and animal to animal. Control of techniques and processes in the histology laboratory is essential to produce tissue sections that are of high quality.

As mentioned previously, formalin is still the most widely used fixative because it is both reliable and economical. Neutral-buffered formalin can be purchased premixed or made in the laboratory from concentrated formaldehyde. If making your own formalin, care must be taken to ensure that the correct percentage of formaldehyde and buffers is used so that tissues are fixed properly. Some laboratories add a small amount of eosin to color the solution to ensure that the tissues are not placed inadvertently in water rather than formalin. The relatively low cost of and convenience of premixed formalin make it preferable to making your own formalin.

Although formalin is quite stable and has a very long shelf life, certain situations can cause degradation. One example is freezing. Freezing of formalin causes the formaldehyde to crystallize and precipitate, resulting in an aqueous solution. If formalin is shipped in unheated trucks or left for extended periods on loading docks during winter months, it can freeze, resulting in autolyzed tissues. Similarly, the weather forecast should be considered before shipping tissues to a distant location. Although overnight courier services have improved shipping options, Nature still occasionally stymies people's best efforts and tissues end up either frozen in the winter or baking in the sun in the summer.

Formalin and other fixatives are mixtures that chemically alter biological molecules, both living and dead. With increasing regulations for transporting hazardous materials, it may become more difficult to ship formalin-fixed tissues by air, which will result in longer transit times. Some shippers also have strict regulations about the type of container for formalin shipments, including bagging and adsorbents. Be sure to check with your shipper before sending samples to a distant laboratory. Some contract laboratories provide a courier service for tissue pickup. This method provides control over the time in transit and temperature for tissues and allows for a strict chain of custody for all materials.

Once the tissues have reached the histology laboratory, there are several potential problem areas. Many laboratories process tissues by treatment group because this may make the clerical documentation of the process easier. One problem with this method is that if a processing artifact occurs, it may affect only one group, and thus appear to be a treatment effect. To eliminate such group bias, tissues should be processed by replicates so that tissues from animals of each group are included in all batches processed.

Improper fixation may cause nuclear digestion, which leads to improper staining. Improper pH of formalin, or the use of unbuffered formalin, destroys nuclear basophilia if overexposed (more than approximately 3 weeks) and alters the staining of some cells.

Several artifacts may be introduced during processing. If there is improper dehydration, the tissues may be spongy and impossible to section. Improper infiltration of paraffin gives a "parched earth" appearance to the resulting sections. A "moth-eaten" appearance may be caused by overexposure of tissues during dehydration, clearing, or paraffin impregnation.

When tissues are embedded, it is important that tissues of similar firmness be placed in the same cassette. If this is not done, for example, if bone and a soft tissue are placed together, the microtome knife will "hesitate" and may produce artifacts such as chatter marks, resulting from differences in the thickness of the tissue section. Other problems during microtomy include improper chilling of blocks or dull knives, both of which can cause compression of tissue sections, and damaged knife edges, which may cause tissue streaks or knife lines. Poor embedding practices or a loose knife or other microtome parts can cause a "venetian blind" effect, consisting of alternating thin and thick areas.

Other problem areas in the histology laboratory may be traced to equipment or a lack of understanding by operators. As an example, if tissue blocks are not chilled properly before they are sectioned, the resulting tissue ribbons may stretch or tear, resulting in artifacts. Artifacts may also occur during the staining process. Alum crystals may precipitate from improperly mixed hematoxylin or other dyes. A lack of proper agitation during the staining process may result in uneven staining. Improper dehydration during the staining process causes a murky, granular appearance to slides.

Several artifacts may occur during coverslipping. If the sections are allowed to dry before applying the cover glass, there may be stippling present, which resembles pigment. In addition, nuclei may appear black and glossy. Excessive mounting media will give sections a foggy appearance.

The lesson to be learned from all of the just-described potential artifacts is to hire the best histotechnologists one can and to treat them well, for without their efforts, the pathologist will have nothing (or only artifact) to examine.

A. SPECIALIZED HISTOLOGIC TECHNIQUES

Several tissues require special knowledge and techniques in the histology laboratory to ensure that maximum information can be obtained when the tissues are examined microscopically. These include the larynx, the nose, the thyroids, and the urinary bladder.

1. Larynx

Although the larynx is not included as a protocol-required tissue for most studies, it may be a target for some types of inhalation studies. The ventral diverticulum, the epithelium of the ventral mucosal glands, and the tip of the arytenoid cartilage appear to be most sensitive to inhaled toxicants so it is important that the larynx be embedded to reveal these areas. The technique for proper trimming and embedding of the larynx has been described well elsewhere (see "Suggested Reading").

2. Nasal Cavity

Similarly, tissues of the nasal cavity require special trimming and embedding to produce consistent results. There are four different types of epithelium in the nasal cavity: squamous, respiratory, transitional, and olfactory. Each type has a specific distribution in the nose. Unless specimens are trimmed and embedded consistently, it may not be possible to accurately assess common changes such as epithelial metaplasia. Schemes for trimming nasal specimens from rodents have been described in detail (see "Suggested Reading").

The orientation of some sections may effect the interpretation and results for that tissue. Examples include the thyroid glands in mice and rats and the urinary bladder in mice.

3. Thyroid Glands

Depending on the standard operating procedures (SOPs) for a particular laboratory, thyroids may be embedded either longitudinally (so that the trachea appears as two parallel walls) or as a cross section (so that the trachea appears to be a circular tube). Because C cells in the thyroid normally are distributed unevenly with a greater prominence near the center of the thyroid gland, the incidence of proliferative changes involving C cells in a longitudinal section will appear greater than in a cross section that was not taken from the central portion of the thyroid gland. This variation in distribution can affect study results, especially if different embedding techniques are used for different groups of animals in the study, i.e., interim versus terminal sacrifices, or spontaneous deaths versus scheduled sacrifices.

4. Urinary Bladder

For many years, the routine section of murine urinary bladder was a cross section, taken in the middle portion of the bladder. Recently, a unique lesion—the submucosal mesenchymal proliferative lesion of the urinary bladder of aging mice—has been described in several strains of mice (see "Suggested Reading"). This lesion apparently almost always occurs in the trigone area of the bladder so small lesions will not be observed if a cross section is taken. For this reason, many laboratories have now modified their SOPs to take a longitudinal section of mouse urinary bladder to include the area of the trigone.

B. ARTIFACTS VERSUS LESIONS

A number of changes occur during tissue processing that may appear to be treatment-related morphologic changes, but which are actually tissue artifacts. Knowledge of these changes will help the pathologist separate lesions from artifact. Several types of these artifacts are discussed and fall into three major classes: fixation or handling artifacts, processing artifacts, and sectioning artifacts, all of which may appear to be treatment-related "lesions."

1. Fixation and Handling

Although it is generally known that animal tissue should only be refrigerated prior to necropsy, occasionally tissues are frozen mistakenly before processing. The effect of freezing is recognizable microscopically as large empty spaces where the ice crystals formed. Similarly, if the formalin used to preserve the tissue was either chilled or frozen, there may be evidence of formalin crystals in the resultant slides (Fig. 1).

Suboptimal fixation can also produce an artifact that stimulates centrilobular hepatocellular vacuolation. True centrilobular vacuolation is the result of lipid accumulation in the hepato-cytes and occurs with many types of treatment. Artifactual vacuolation, which appears very similar microscopically, results when the time between euthanasia and prosection is excessive. In this case, there may be leakage of serum from the central vein into adjacent hepatocytes, giving the appearance of centrilobular vacuolation. The liver weight will be increased in these rats (see "Suggested Reading").

Several potential artifacts in the lungs are associated with handling at necropsy. If the lungs are infused with formalin using a syringe inserted in the trachea, excessive force will result in a widening of space around the vessels in the pulmonary parenchyma, which may be diagnosed incorrectly as perivascular edema. True edema will generally have some amount of eosinophilic proteinaceous fluid surrounding the vessels (Fig. 2). This fluid will not be present in lungs with artifactual "edema" (Fig. 3).

At the other end of the spectrum are lungs that have not been infused properly. The atalectatic appearance of these lungs may give the appearance of pneumonitis or interstitial pneumonia and present interpretive problems if a true alveolar change is present (Fig. 4).

A handling artifact observed in the brain is the result of the stretching of the trigeminal

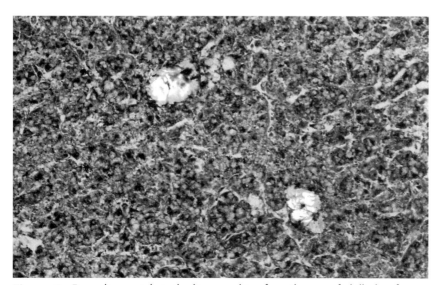

Figure 1. Formalin crystals in the liver resulting from the use of chilled or frozen formalin.

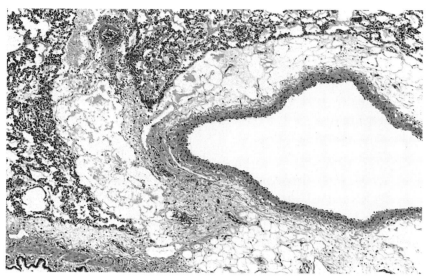

Figure 2. Pulmonary edema in the lung. Note the presence of eosiniophilic proteinaceous fluid in the space surrounding the vessels.

nerve tracts when the brain is removed from the skull. If the nerve roots are not cut, they stretch as the brain is lifted away, resulting in a vacuolated appearance to the trigeminal nerve tracts. Similar artifacts occur in the spinal cord, where the stretching of the myelinated nerve during removal may result in the appearance of swollen axons in the body of the spinal cord (Fig. 5).

2. Processing

Another type of artifact has been reported in the brain and spinal cord as a result of the method of processing. If the brain and spinal cord are placed on the tissue processor on Friday afternoon, actual processing generally does not begin until Sunday so that the tissue will be ready for embedding on Monday morning. This means

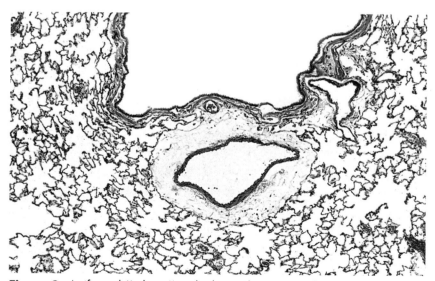

Figure 3. Artifactual "edema" in the lung. The perivascular space is widened by excess infusion pressure, but there is no proteinaceous fluid present.

194

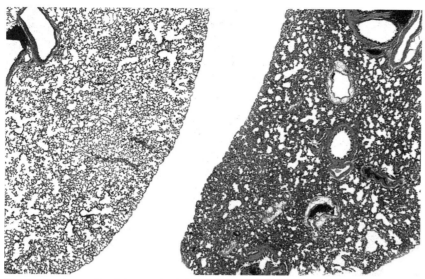

Figure 4. Lung. The lobe on the left has been infused correctly. The lobe on the right was not infused. Note the atelectatic appearance of the alveoli in the right lobe.

that the brain tissue sits in alcohol (the first stage on the processor) over the weekend, resulting in the appearance of vacuoles in the white matter of the brain and spinal cord (Fig. 6) (see "Suggested Reading").

There are three solutions to this problem. The simplest is not to process the brain and spinal cord over the weekend, as leaving these tissues in alcohol overnight (during the week) will not result in artifactual vacuoles. Another solution is to use formalin, rather than alcohol, as the first (or holding) solution in the tissue processor. A third solution is to process all tissues by replicate rather than by group (see

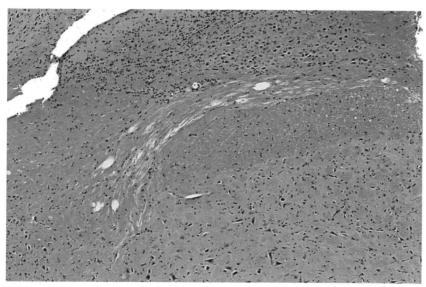

Figure 5. Brain. Note the vacuolated appearance of the trigeminal nerve tracts. This artifact is the result of stretching of the nerve roots as they are removed from the skull.

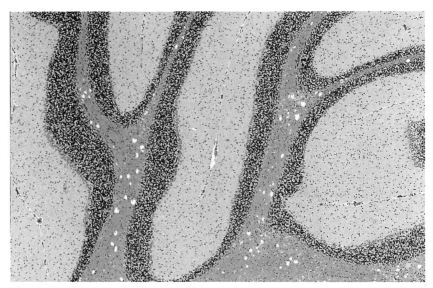

Figure 6. Brain. Vacuoles in the white matter are the result of prolonged immersion in alcohol.

earlier discussion) so that any artifactual changes will be spread across groups and will thus be less likely to be interpreted as an actual change.

3. Sectioning

Several changes are the result of mishandling during the sectioning of the tissue. If air is trapped between the tissue and the water bath, the tinctoral quality of the tissue will be affected and basophilic circles may appear in the tissue. Although these circles are quite regular in shape, they may be confused with basophilic foci in the liver of rats or mice (Fig. 7). Similarly, these air bubbles, which may be trapped under the tissue during embedding, will often pop and cause tears and holes in the tissue when it is mounted on the slide.

C. LESION INTERPRETATION

As has been seen in the previous section, there are many artifacts that could be interpreted incorrectly as lesions by the unwary pathologist. In addition, a number of true changes require knowledge of proper interpretation in order to produce consistent and meaningful data. Areas included in this section on lesion interpretation include rarely or poorly understood lesions, the differentiation of hyperplasia from neoplasia, sexual dimorphism in some organs in rodents, and changing terminology for necrosis.

1. Murine Pulmonary Eosinophilic Crystals

One type of poorly understood lesion is the presence of angular eosinophilic crystals in the lungs of mice. These crystals have been variously proposed to be hemoglobin or residue from the granules of eosinophils. Neither theory has been proved conclusively. These crystals occur both in macrophages, where they have been diagnosed as eosinophilic macrophage pneumonia, and free in the alveolar spaces. They were originally seen in "moth-eaten mice" that had lesions in the liver as well, but they have also been reported without lesions in other organs. The crystals in the lungs have been shown to be YM-1 or T lymphocyte-derived eosinophil chemotactic factor. The significance of and relationship to treatment of these crystals remain unknown (Fig. 8) (see "Suggested Reading").

2. Hepatic Lipomatous Cells

Another type of poorly understood lesion involves lipomatous cells in the liver (see

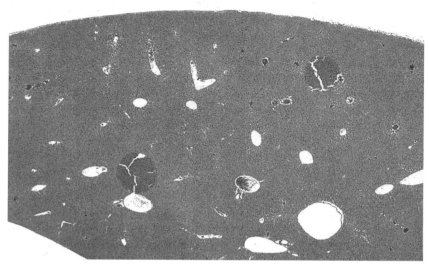

Figure 7. Liver. Round basophilic circles caused by trapped air may be confused with bosophilic foci.

"Suggested Reading"). The function of these cells is unclear, and the morphologic appearance often becomes clouded when there is a significant deposition of lipid in the liver. On rare occasions, these lipomatous cells may become neoplastic; in mice, these tumors have been diagnosed as Ito cell tumors based on morphologic features (Fig. 9) (see "Suggested Reading").

3. Hyperplasia vs Neoplasia

For some lesions encountered in the course of a study, the line between hyperplasia and benign neoplasia, or between a benign and a malignant tumor, is sometimes equivocal. For some lesions, criteria used to diagnose a particular lesion may have changed as we have learned more about the biologic behavior of a particular

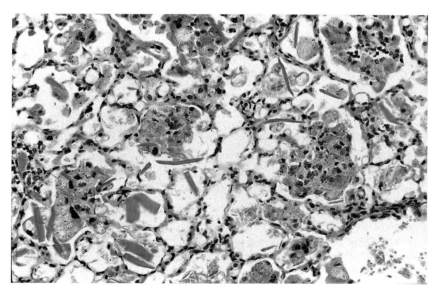

Figure 8. Lung. Murine pulmonary eosinophilic crystals. Note the presence of material both in macrophages and free in alveolar spaces.

197

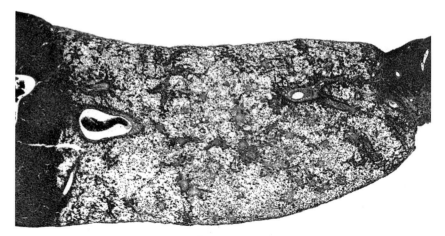

Figure 9. Liver. Lipomatous (Ito cell) tumor in a mouse.

process. For other changes, we are viewing a single point in time of a lesion that represents a long, continuous spectrum. The terminology we apply may therefore be considered somewhat ambiguous by an outside observer. Examples of this are discussed for the testes, lung, parathyroid, and thyroid.

For many proliferative lesions, including most endocrine tumors, the process of proliferation is a continuum so that there is not a distinct morphologic change that represents the difference between hyperplasia and neoplasia. For these types of lesions, arbitrary diagnostic criteria are sometimes necessary to distinguish between the two types of lesions.

a. Testes. Interstitial cell proliferation in the testes presents an interesting problem, as the proposed criteria for distinguishing between hyperplasia and neoplasia are different depending on the recommended nomenclature and diagnostic criteria that are followed. In the United States, the National Toxicology Program (NTP) has determined that any interstitial cell proliferation greater than one seminiferous tubule in diameter constitutes a benign neoplasm and should be diagnosed as such. On the other hand, several European authorities, as well as the Society of Toxicologic Pathologists (STP), feel that an interstitial cell proliferation must be at least three seminiferous tubules in diameter before it is called an adenoma (Fig. 10).

Adding to the confusion is the fact that a cross section of a proliferative lesion may not be cut across the greatest diameter of the lesion so that the lesion may appear smaller than it actually is and might be diagnosed incorrectly. Problems have occurred when interstitial cell proliferative lesions were originally diagnosed using one set of criteria and then peer reviewed using other criteria, resulting in a difference in the significance of the lesion in a particular study.

b. Lung. In the lung, the distinction between type II hyperplasia and an alveolar/bronchiolar adenoma may be difficult to make because the hyperplastic cells line the alveolar septae and, in more severe cases of hyperplasia, resemble small adenomas. One suggested criterion is that if more than three contiguous alveoli are filled with proliferating cells, it should be diagnosed as an adenoma (Fig. 11).

At the other end of the spectrum, some pathologists are comfortable diagnosing an alveolar/bronchiolar carcinoma only when the mass shows evidence of local invasion by penetrating through the pleura. Most pathologists would not require this much evidence of malignancy and would diagnose a carcinoma based on histomorphologic appearance and size, without the requirement for invasion.

Another controversial lesion in the lung is the spectrum of squamous-lined cystic lesions in the alveolar parenchyma (see "Suggested Reading"). Seen primarily in inhalation studies

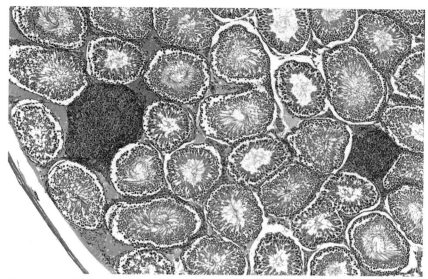

Figure 10. Testes. Both proliferative interstitial lesions would be diagnosed as adenomas using NTP criteria. Using other criteria (STP), both lesions would be diagnosed as hyperplasia.

involving metals and fibers, these lesions have been diagnosed by various pathologists and expert groups as epithelial cysts (pulmonary keratinizing cyst), benign squamous tumors (pulmonary cystic keratinizing epithelioma), and squamous cell carcinomas (Fig. 12).

Because the regulatory impact of a cyst is quite different from that of a carcinoma, it would seem appropriate to achieve agreement on the diagnostic criteria and nomenclature for the lesions and agreement on their biological significance.

c. Parathyroid. Proliferative lesions in the parathyroid result in a focal enlargement, usually in one of the two glands. Bilateral diffuse enlargement of both parathyroids in older rats is

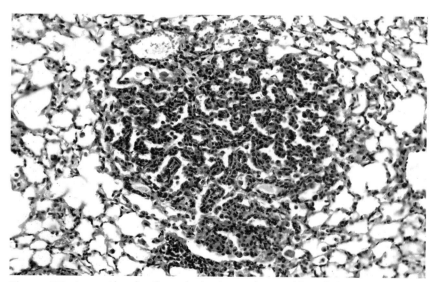

Figure 11. Lung. Alveolar/bronchiolar hyperplasia. Although this lesion is quite large, cells lining the alveolar walls do not fill the alveolar spaces.

199

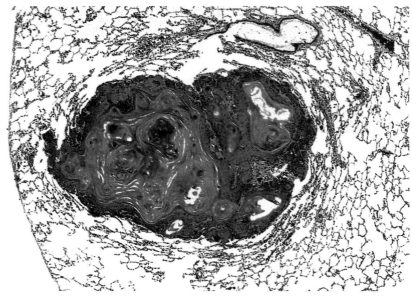

Figure 12. Lung. A pulmonary keratin cyst. Note the squamous epithelium lining the large keratin-filled spaces.

often the result of secondary renal hyperparathyroidism rather than neoplasia. For this reason, it is important that both parathyroids are examined grossly and microscopically; if only one is sectioned, differentiation between hyperplasia and neoplasia is more difficult.

d. Thyroid. In the thyroid, several lesions appear related. Cysts, cystic hyperplasia, and follicular hyperplasia all have been used to diagnose similar lesions in the follicular epithelium. The issue of whether a cyst should be considered a proliferative lesion is critical, as the impact of proliferative and nonproliferative lesions is different when they are reviewed by regulatory agencies.

4. Sexual Dimorphism

A number of organs exhibit normal sexual dimorphism. It is important to know these differences, both for the ability to recognize normal changes and to be able to diagnose changes caused by some compounds.

a. Kidney. One of the normal changes concerns the epithelium lining Bowman's capsule in the kidney of the mouse. In male mice this epithelium is cuboidal (Fig. 13),

whereas in females the epithelium is simple squamous (Fig. 14). The importance of knowing this normal variation was recently brought home when a group of researchers published an abstract describing the effect of a transgene on the renal epithelium of male mice—the "effect" was actually the normal male glomerulus.

b. Glands. There are sexual differences in several organs in rodents, including the submandibular salivary gland (Figs. 15 and 16) and preputial/clitoral glands. The normal appearance of these glands can be changed as a result of exposure to androgenic or estrogenic compounds, such as the synthetic androgen oxymethalone. (see "Suggested Reading").

The mammary gland in young rats undergoes age-related changes that might prove confusing. By 19 weeks of age, female rats have a tubuloalveolar pattern, whereas in males, the mammary gland is more florid, has an alveolar pattern, and lacks obvious tubular or ductal orientation. Exposure to certain compounds may cause male mammary glands to resemble those of females (Figs. 17 and 18) (see "Suggested Reading").

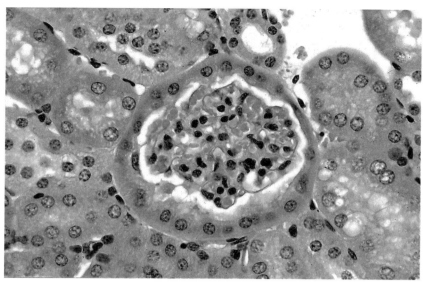

Figure 13. Mouse, kidney. Note the normal male glomerulus with cuboidal parietal epithelium lining Bowman's capsule. Reprinted from Maronpot (1999), with permission of the publisher.

5. Terminology of Cell Death

A final topic for confusion serves as an example of the continuing growth of knowledge in the filed of biomedical research. In the past few years, basic researchers have adopted the term "apotosis" to describe programmed cell death.

As pathologists, the morphologic changes seen with apoptosis are often difficult to separate from the classic diagnosis of necrosis. Some researchers have suggested the term "oncosis" to describe necrosis that involves cellular swelling. However, this term may be confused with a neoplastic process so most pathologists have

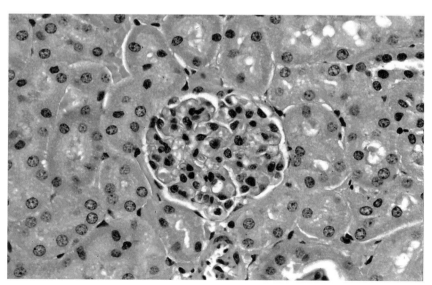

Figure 14. Mouse kidney. Note the normal female glomerulus with flattened parietal epithelium lining Bowman's capsule. Reprinted from Maronpot (1999), with permission of the publisher.

201

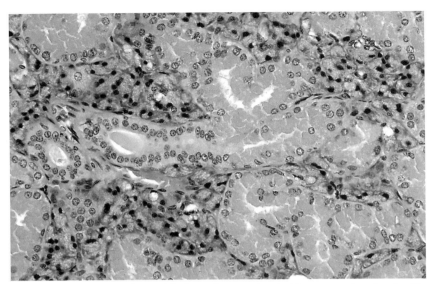

Figure 15. Mouse submandibular salivary gland. Normal male gland with prominent convoluted ducts lined by tall columnar cells with basally located nuclei, with numerous intracytoplasmic eosinophilic granules.

not generally accepted it. A special panel from the STP has issued recommendations for the nomenclature of necrosis. In this document, they recommend the use of the morphologic term necrosis, with modifiers such as apoptotic or oncotic if it will help with interpretation of a particular study or aid in the characterization of the necrotic process present in the specific tissue being examined (see "Suggested Reading").

V. Computer Systems

A number of problems may arise during data entry following morphologic interpretation and

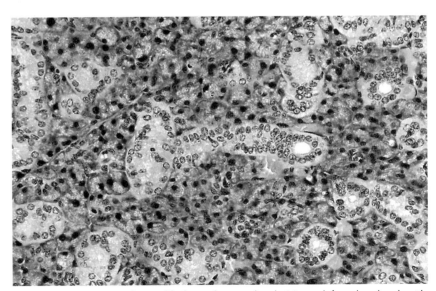

Figure 16. Mouse submandibular salivary gland. Normal female gland with smaller convoluted ducts lined by shorter columnar cells with centrally located nuclei, with fewer eosinophilic granules.

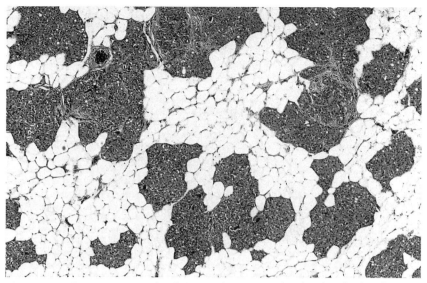

Figure 17. Rat mammary gland. Normal young male gland with alveolar pattern and no obvious tubular or ductal orientation.

severity grading of lesions. Many pathology software systems allow for direct entry by the pathologist as s/he examines the slides. The advantage to this system is that the pathologist has direct control of the entry. Another advantage is that the system administrators can tightly control the lexicon so that redundant diagnoses can be kept to a minimum. A disad-

vantage is that many systems require numerous keystrokes and/or shortcuts to reach a diagnosis. If the pathologist is not paying full attention to data entry, it is likely that keystroke errors may occur.

An alternative method involves dictation by the pathologist as s/he examines the slides. This method requires additional time for a pathology

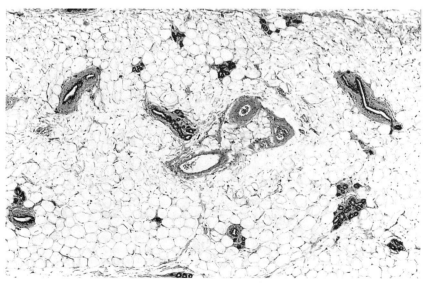

Figure 18. Rat mammary gland. Normal young female gland with tubuloalveolar pattern.

support technician to enter data into the software program. However, experience in our laboratory has shown that dictation is actually faster for the pathologist, especially if hands-free dictation devices are used, so that the pathologist does not have to look away from the slide to dictate a finding or enter a diagnosis directly into a computer. There is a much lower incidence of keystroke error because the data entry technician is paying full attention to the entry. In addition, a 100% quality control check of the data entry as compared to the dictation assures accuracy in study data. Using this method of data entry is by far more economical, as the time saved by the pathologist more than compensates for the time spent by the technicians in data entry.

A problem area has been encountered with several different direct entry software systems, which involves the use of a single keystroke for global entries. By using these single keystrokes, it is possible for a pathologist to record only positive findings and record all other tissues as "not remarkable" as the default diagnosis. Problems arise when tissues such as parathyroids or thymus, which are actually missing, are recorded as not remarkable rather than missing using the global entry key. In another case, a set of target tissues was marked as not remarkable, when in actuality they had never been trimmed in. Most software systems have the capability of turning this global capability either on or off; it is recommended that use of this type of global entry be avoided to prevent problems in tissue accountability and other diagnostic errors.

Problems in reporting and interpreting data can result from the use of duplicate or redundant terms. Regardless of whether one utilizes a direct input or dictation method of data entry, it is essential that attention be paid to the use of

diagnostic terminology. All members of a pathology group need to agree as to the terms used for common changes, such as chronic nephropathy in rats. It is also important that only one term be used for a particular lesion, as use of synonymous terminology may result in confusion or the dilution of an apparent effect.

Some pathology reporting systems truncate diagnoses on summary incidence tables. The full diagnosis with modifiers is reported only in the individual animal tables, whereas summary incidence tables only print the main morphologic diagnoses without modifiers. In these cases, the study pathologist does not have access to the full diagnoses when evaluating summary data and may misinterpret an effect.

An example of this problem is shown in Table I. The study pathologist diagnosed basophilic foci in the liver in several groups in a study. He used the modifiers of focal and multifocal to differentiate degrees of severity in individual animal data. However, the pathology reporting system that was in use at the laboratory only printed the total number of foci, without modifiers in the summary incidence tables.

When one examined the summary incidence tables, it appeared that there was no increase in the number of foci as a result of treatment. However, if one had access to individual animal data, as shown in Table II, it would be clear that the number of multifocal foci increased with treatment and that there was a clear relationship to treatment. With the particular reporting system in use at the laboratory, the only way to appreciate this trend would be to examine each individual animal report and to tabulate individual data manually.

Another reporting problem involves the use of merging or rationalization of diagnoses in

TABLE I

Incidence of Basophilic Foci Reported in Summary Incidence Tables (Original Study Data)

Tissue observation	0 mg/kg/day	1.5 mg/kg/day	5 mg/kg/day	15 mg/kg/day
Liver (no. examined)	50	50	50	50
Altered foci, basophilic	19	15	16	18

TABLE II
Incidence of Basophilic Foci as Reported in Individual Animal Reports

Tissue observation	0 mg/kg/day	1.5 mg/kg/day	5 mg/kg/day	15 mg/kg/day
Liver (no. examined)	50	50	50	50
Altered foci, basophilic, focal	16	7	8	8
Altered foci, basophilic, multifocal	3	8	8	10

summary incidence tables. This procedure allows for the combining of several terms used in individual animals into a single diagnosis that is recorded in the summary incidence tables. The final diagnosis may be one of the individual terms used or another diagnosis that attempts to reflect all the individual terms. In some systems, the rationalization process is tabulated, whereas in other systems it remains hidden. The rationalization process can result in different terminology on the summary incidence table than that recorded for the diagnosis in individual animal data, and the true incidence of a finding cannot be determined without teasing the information from the individual animal tables. In most cases, more attention should be paid to the development of an organized lexicon so that there is little need to combine terms in the summary incidence tables and so that the tables accurately reflect what has been recorded in individual animal data.

VI. Peer Review

Peer review of pathology data affords an opportunity to improve the quality and reliability of a toxicology report. Although peer review is not required by the regulatory agencies in most cases, it is clear that peer-reviewed studies are viewed with a greater degree of confidence than those studies that have not been reviewed. Because the process of peer review is covered elsewhere in this text, only a few points will be addressed.

A. STUDY REVIEW

Peer review is in many ways a quality assurance process in that the diagnoses are reviewed for correctness and consistency. At the same time, a thorough peer review also includes some quality-control aspects. An example is the review of slides for missing tissues. Occasionally, small tissues, such as parathyroids or lymph nodes, are recorded as normal by the pathologist, when they were actually missing. (The opposite situation also occurs.) The only way to determine whether a tissue is actually present or not is to reexamine the slide for the tissue in question. This type of error can only be recognized and corrected during a peer review.

Another type of quality-control function involves the audit of pathology specimens. Although not a part of most routine peer reviews, this step is included in all reviews conducted for the NTP. The audit includes the examination of wet tissue for animal identification and the identification of untrimmed gross lesions, as well as comparison of the microscopic slides with the corresponding paraffin blocks. This type of audit may reveal problems in animal or tissue accountability. This information can be especially helpful, as inspections by both the U.S. EPA and the U.S. FDA examine these types of accountability routinely.

B. PATHOLOGY WORKING GROUPS

Pathology working groups (PWGs) are generally convened to resolve a specific problem in a study. In most cases, the issues concern the criteria for neoplastic lesions, although there have been instances where PWGs focus on nonproliferative lesions. This latter type of PWG is often more complicated because there is less agreement, even among experienced pathologists, as to the diagnostic criteria for recording and grading the severity of nonproliferative lesions. There is one situation in which a PWG and a peer review are required by a regulatory agency. The U.S. EPA issued Pesticide (PR) Notice 94–5 in 1994, which requires both when a company is submitting a reevaluation of data from a previously submitted study. In this case, the agency requires the following action: (1) peer review of all neoplastic changes and all target tissues and (2) formation of a PWG that examines, as a minimum, all significant differences of opinion between the study pathologist and the reviewing pathologist, and (3) a PWG report that includes the diagnoses of the study pathologist, the reviewing pathologist, and the PWG. In the absence of these data, the EPA will ignore the new submission and base its evaluations on original data only when ruling on the resubmission.

VII. Conclusions

Although the practice of toxicologic pathology has matured considerably in the past several decades, there is still room for refinement. We have many new research tools to help with the practice of pathology, but there are still many pitfalls that may trap the unwary practitioner and result in data or reports that are incomplete, inconsistent, or even incorrect. This chapter has tried to outline some of the areas that can be eliminated by diligent attention to detail.

SUGGESTED READING

Boorman, G. A., Brockmann, M., Carlton, W. W., Davis, J. M. G., Dungworth, D. L., Hahn, F. F., Mohr, U., Richter Reichhelm, R., Turosov, V. S., and Wagner, B. M. (1996). Classification of cystic keratinizing squamous lesions of the rat lung: Report of a workshop. *Toxicol. Pathol.* **24**, 564–572.

Cardy, R. H. (1991). Sexual dimorphism of the normal rat mammary gland. *Vet. Pathol.* **28**, 139–145.

Dixon, D., Yoshitomi, K., Boorman, G. A., and Maronpot, R. R. (1994). "Lipomatous" lesions of unknown cellular origin in the liver of B6C3F1 mice. *Vet. Pathol.* **31**, 173–182.

Environmental Protection Agency (1994). Pesticide Regulation (PR) Notice 94–5. Requests for reconsiderations of carcinogenicity peer review decisions based on changes in pathology diagnoses.

Guo, L., Johnson, R. S., and Schuh, J. C. (2000). Biochemical characterization of endogenously formed eosinophilic crystals in the lungs of mice. *J. Biol. Chem.* **275**, 8032–8037.

Halliwell, W. H. (1998). Submucosal mesenchymal tumors of the mouse urinary bladder. *Toxicol. Pathol.* **26**, 128–136.

Harada, T., Enomoto, A., Boorman, G. A., and Maronpot, R. R. (1999). Liver and gallbladder. *In* "Pathology of the Mouse: Reference and Atlas," (R. R. Maronpot, G. A. Boorman, and B. W. Gaul, eds.), pp. 119–183. Cache River Press, Vienna, IL.

Lewis, D. J. (1992). Morphologic assessment of pathologic changes within the rat larynx. *Toxicol. Pathol.* **19**, 352–357.

Levin, S., Bucci, T. J., Cohen, S. M., Fix, A. S., Hardisty, J. F., LeGrand, E. K., Maronpot, R. R., and Trump, B. F. (1999). The nomenclature of cell death: Recommendations of an ad hoc Committee of the Society of Toxicologic Pathologists. *Toxicol. Pathol.* **27**, 484–490.

Maronpot, R. R., Boorman, G. A., and Gaul, B. W. (eds.) (1999). "Pathology of the Mouse: Reference and Atlas." Cache River Press, Vienna, IL.

McLarrin, G. M. (1982). Vacuoles in the fiber tracts of rat CNS tissues. *J. Histotechnol.* **5**, 171–173.

National Toxicology Program TR 485 (1999). Toxicology and Carcinogenesis Studies of Oxymetholone (CAS# 434071) in F344/N Rats and Toxicology Studies in B6C3F1 Mice (gavage studies). U.S. Dept. of Health and Human Services.

Renne, R. A., Gideon, K. M., Miller, R. A., Mellick, P. W., and Grumbein, S. L. (1992). Histologic methods and interspecies variations in the laryngeal histology of F344/N rats and B6C3F1 mice. *Toxicol. Pathol.* **20**, 44–51.

Sagartz, J. W., Madarasz, A. J., Forsell, M. A., Burger, G. T., Ayres, P. H., and Coggins, R. E. (1992). Histologic sectioning of the rodent larynx for inhalation toxicity testing. *Toxicol. Pathol.* **20**, 118–121.

Sykes, B. I., Penny, E., and Purchase, I. F. H. (1976). Heaptocyte vacuolation and increased liver weight occurring in anoxic rats. *Toxicol. Appl. Pharmacol.* **36**, 31–39.

Uriah, L. C., and Maronopot, R. R. (1990). Normal histology of the nasal cavity and application of special techniques. *Environ. Health Perspect.* **85**, 187–208.

Young, J. T. (1981). Histopathologic examination of the rat nasal cavity. *Fundam. Appl. Toxicol.* **1**, 309–312.

10

Special Techniques in Toxicologic Pathology

N. Gillett, C. Chan, C. Farman, and P. Lappin

Sierra Biomedical
A Division of Charles River Laboratories, Inc.
Sparks, Nevada

I. Introduction

Advances in cell and molecular biology have engendered a wide range of techniques that can be used to augment traditional morphologic tools to investigate mechanisms of disease or toxicity. In the team-oriented scientific world today, pathologists must be familiar with the technical basis and utility of a large variety of these techniques, some of which are slide based and some of which are solution based. In solution-based assays, the tissue is homogenized and DNA, RNA, or protein is extracted for analysis. In contrast, slide-based techniques, such as immunohistochemistry, *in situ* hybridization, *in situ* polymerase chain reaction (PCR), and laser capture microscopy, retain the tissue architecture and thus have the common ability to provide spatial localization of alterations in DNA, RNA, or protein at the cellular level in a heterogeneous cellular population, e.g., tissue. Slide-based techniques in particular reside more commonly in the pathology laboratory and require interpretation of the slide by a trained pathologist.

Pathologists within the pharmaceutical and chemical industries are increasingly using a variety of cellular and molecular biology techniques on a daily basis to answer different questions. This chapter focuses on some of the more common special techniques that a toxicologic pathologist utilizes, although it is by no means a comprehensive list of all methodologies. Although some technical aspects are discussed, the potential applications and limitations of each technique are the focus of the chapter review. This arena is a rapidly evolving field, and readers are encouraged to supplement their reading through the provided reference list and recent literature.

II. Immunohistochemistry in Toxicologic Pathology

A. INTRODUCTION

While microscopic examination of hematoxylin and eosin (H&E)-stained tissues remains the gold standard for the evaluation of toxicologic effects on animals following administration of pharmaceutical/biopharmaceutical compounds and potential toxins in general, immunohistochemistry (IHC) has great value in conjunction with H&E. IHC utilizes the precise antigen specificity of specialized proteins known as antibodies to localize target molecules in tissue sections. Antibodies can be produced to specifically recognize billions of different epitopes/antigens and can be created to recognize almost any molecule of interest. In IHC, an antibody that has specificity for a target molecule of interest is placed onto a tissue section and binds to its target molecule. This bound antibody can then be detected through a number of different techniques.

Antibodies can be labeled with fluorescent dyes for visualization (although direct labeling of the primary antibody often produces a signal that is insufficient for visualization). Alternatively, they can be tagged with molecules such as biotin or digoxigenin for further amplification or with reporter enzymes such as horseradish peroxidase or alkaline phosphatase to produce a visible colored precipitate at the site of antibody binding. In the more common IHC methods employed today, the primary antibody itself serves as the target for a secondary antibody, which has specificity for the Fc region of the primary antibody. Addition of the secondary antibody amplifies the signal and also allows the same reagents to be used for different primary antibodies. The development of IHC amplification procedures such as avidin–biotin complex (ABC) and catalyzed reporter deposition (CARD) has also increased the utility of IHC greatly as now even very rare antigens can theoretically be detected.

IHC can be used to visualize changes that are not apparent with routine H&E staining, which can greatly expand the amount of information obtained from a toxicologic study. For example, IHC can be used to detect the administered compound and/or its metabolites and may aid in determining the spatial and temporal distribution of the compound in the body. Additionally, various substances may be either increased or decreased in tissue in response to administration of a compound, and IHC may be useful in detecting such changes. Thus, the mechanisms of action and/or toxicity of the agent may be elucidated. These are just two examples of

the value of IHC in toxicologic pathology. This section focuses on various ways IHC can be utilized, using specific examples and including discussions of cell proliferation markers, markers of apoptosis, and cross-reactivity studies. The limitations of immunohistochemistry in toxicologic pathology are also covered, as well as suggestions for study planning and tissue collection and fixation.

B. TECHNICAL CONSIDERATIONS

1. Limitations of the Use of Immunohistochemistry in Toxicologic Pathology

a. Double-Labeling and Combination Techniques. It is possible to perform multiple labeling using two or more different antibodies, to label either the same cells or different ones. Labeling the same cells usually is most feasible using immunofluorescent techniques. It is also possible to use a combination of IHC and *in situ* hybridization. Double-labeling techniques may be useful in toxicologic pathology to determine the spatial location of an administered compound and a substance changed as a result of the compound or to look for activated inflammatory and/or immune cells infiltrating into tissue as a result of treatment with a certain compound.

b. Quantitative Data. A major limitation of IHC is that in most instances it cannot be used as a quantitative technique. An exception to this is in cell proliferation studies where the numbers of positively stained nuclei may be counted. There may be other instances in which the numbers of positively staining cells can be counted accurately and where such objective information is of vital importance to the study. In most instances, however, a qualitative evaluation of changes in staining patterns and intensity is sufficient to provide valuable information to the researcher.

2. Availability of Antibodies

A significant problem facing investigators wishing to use IHC to detect target molecules is the availability of antibodies specific for the

208

molecule (proprietary compounds will generally not have commercially available antibodies so the antibodies will have to be specially generated for this purpose). In addition, even if antibodies to the target compound are available, they may not work in IHC (commercial antibody vendors will generally have information of the applicability of their antibody to IHC; for specially generated antibodies, this information will have to be worked out experimentally).

For some molecules, a myriad of antibodies are available and the investigator must choose between a monoclonal (directed against a single epitope of the antigen) antibody made in one species and a polyclonal (directed against multiple epitopes of an antigen) antibody made in a different species. There is no general rule of thumb as to which type of antibody performs the best in immunohistochemistry, and the choice of antibody must often be made empirically.

Due to the widespread use of rodents in research, large numbers of antibodies specific for rodents have become available commercially. This is good news for those investigators using rodents in their studies. Some antihuman antibodies may cross-react with other species, but sometimes this information is not known and trial-and-error testing must be performed to determine the level of cross-reactivity. Many antihuman antibodies will cross-react with nonhuman primate tissue because of the close relationship among these species, but a surprising number do not. If long-term studies with an important compound are planned, a company may decide to synthesize (or have synthesized) a custom antibody for a specific purpose. Many antibodies available commercially, particularly those against CD markers will only work in frozen tissues. Therefore, it is important to plan ahead as far as tissue collection and fixation are concerned if it is at all possible that IHC will be performed. This is discussed in Section III.

3. Tissue Collection and Fixation

Sampling of desired tissues should be considered before a study is even designed in order to have adequate tissue samples for both standard histological examination and IHC. For larger species, a particular tissue usually can be split into two parts or, in the case of lymph nodes, two or more of a specific type of node may be collected. However, due to the small size of rodents and fetuses, it is not always possible to split tissues and therefore additional animals may need to be added to the study, with some dedicated to IHC and the others to histology.

It may be desirable in larger institutions that perform IHC on an extensive scale to establish banks of tissues from normal animals. In this way, control tissue is always available in the event that the cross-reactivity of a commercially available antibody needs to be tested or for small pilot experiments in which control animals may not have been included in the study.

Because of the possibility of diffusion, target molecules in tissue sections need to be immobilized prior to IHC. Target immobilization is usually accomplished through the fixation process (as in the case of formalin-fixed, paraffin-embedded tissue), but the choice of fixative may impact the ability of the antibody to bind to its target because not all antigens survive all fixation procedures.

Because only a subset of antibodies that work in immunohistochemistry also work with formalin-fixed, paraffin-embedded tissue, for novel antibodies, the desired method of tissue preparation for immunohistochemistry is freezing. Freezing the tissue allows investigators to have the most flexibility in optimizing conditions for a wide range of antibodies. Samples are usually frozen in isopentane or liquid nitrogen, using OCT embedding compound, and stored at $-70°C$ until used.

Alternatively, tissues may have been fixed in 10% formalin or 4% paraformaldehyde, particularly if IHC was not initially planned as part of the study. IHC may then be more problematic or even impossible, depending on the antibody and depending on the length of time the tissues have been in fixative. It is most desirable that tissues only be fixed for 1 to 2 hr and then transferred to 70% ethanol if IHC is to be performed. Lengthy fixation in formaldehyde-based fixatives may destroy any hopes of performing IHC using many antibodies. For many antibodies, retrieval of antigen in formalin-fixed, paraffin-embedded tissue may be necessary, using any of a variety of methods. Such methods have been published.

4. Controls

Anyone who has performed IHC is aware that there are many potential pitfalls to accurate performance of the assays and interpretation of the results. Proper controls are always essential to the correct interpretation of data. At a minimum, a serial section of tissue should be stained with an isotype-matched control antibody (for monoclonal antibodies) or pre- or nonimmune serum (for polyclonal antibodies) to demonstrate specificity of the primary antibody. In some cases, the IHC reagents may be the cause of nonspecific background staining. In this case, staining a series of sections where a different component of the IHC reaction is withheld would be useful in identifying the problematic reagent.

Many factors regarding the antibody and the technique need to be considered in order to perform IHC correctly and to get results that reflect the desired end point accurately. Johnson (1999) has summarized these factors in a review. A knowledge of the expected staining results based on prior studies is helpful. Otherwise, trial and error and thorough investigation of the reasons for unexpected staining are often necessary to ensure accuracy. As discussed earlier, in many cases IHC may reveal changes in patterns of cellular infiltration or expression of certain markers by cells, but functional changes may not be detectable and additional methods other than IHC may be necessary.

C. APPLICATIONS OF IMMUNOHISTOCHEMISTRY IN TOXICOLOGIC PATHOLOGY

1. Detection of Administered Compounds

The most direct application of immunohistochemistry in the evaluation of an administered compound is in the detection of the compound and/or its metabolites. This allows one to determine the spatial distribution of the test article and to specifically localize it to certain cell types. Distribution to unexpected organs may be detected. The ability to specifically localize the agent to certain cell types is an advantage over other methods to determine distribution, including the measurement of compound levels in plasma or digested tissue.

An example of the use of IHC to detect an administered compound was in a study of microcystin-LR-hepatotoxicity. In this study, IHC was used to localize microcystin-LR in mouse liver after intraperitoneal injection and was associated with the onset of hemorrhage and apoptosis. IHC may also allow evaluation of the temporal distribution of the compound, including the determination of shifts between organ compartments and the total time of duration of the agent in certain tissues. Oligonucleotide antisense compounds have been monitored in this manner using IHC.

When oligonucleotide antisense compounds are administered to an animal, basophilic granular material can be seen in the kidneys, liver, and lymph nodes on H & E-stained sections, particularly when higher doses are given. Using an antibody directed toward the antisense compound, it was determined that these granules represent either the compound itself or its metabolite. When new antisense compounds are developed, immunohistochemistry is commonly used to evaluate their distribution. This method is particularly useful when tissue levels are not high enough to cause the visible granule accumulation under standard H&E staining. A potential caveat to using IHC to detect administered compounds in tissues is that the method may not in some cases be sensitive enough to detect low levels of the test article. Combining IHC with other, more sensitive methods or using amplification techniques in the IHC protocol should resolve such problems.

2. Evaluation of Responses to Administration of a Compound

Immunohistochemistry is also valuable for evaluating alterations in host response to target organs following administration of a compound. In this respect it can generate much information about the mechanisms of action and/or toxicity of an agent. Several examples are discussed here.

a. Evaluation of CD Markers in Response to Immune-Modulating Agents. Immunohistochemistry can be used to evaluate changes in the cluster of differentiation (CD) antigens on immune/inflammatory cells in response to the administration of agents that modulate the immune system. The CD antigen convention is a system of naming cell surface markers on leukocytes that reflect either different stages of lineage-specific differentiation or different states of activation. Thus, it is possible to use antibodies directed against specific CD antigens to identify distinct lymphocyte subpopulations by staining immunohistochemically, for example, for CD2 (pan T cell), CD4 (helper T cell), CD8 (cytotoxic T cell), and CD20 (B cell) (Fig. 1, see color insert). The number of CD antigens and the availability of antibodies directed against them are constantly growing and investigators should thoroughly review if the CD antigen in which they are interested is appropriate for the question being asked.

If the administered compound targets a certain CD molecule, changes in the presence of that marker on cells may be evaluated by IHC. On numerous occasions in our experience, no apparent changes were present in lymphoid tissues based on H&E evaluation, whereas changes in numbers or distribution of lymphoid cell types were obvious using IHC evaluation of CD markers. However, because subtle differences in cell numbers may not be detectable by IHC, flow cytometry on peripheral blood cells and/or cells isolated from lymphoid tissues may be combined with IHC to provide more quantitative information on changes in certain cell types.

Evaluation of CD markers not only has value in adult animals but also can give information about the effects of a compound on the immune system of the developing fetus. Immunohistochemical evaluation of CD marker expression has illustrated on numerous occasions that there may be obvious effects on the numbers and distribution of various cell types without the presence of clinically detectable immunosuppression (including the lack of detectable opportunistic infections, a hallmark of clinical immunosuppression). This is often positive information for the developers of immunomodulatory compounds because it demonstrates that their drug has a desired, but not overwhelming, effect on the immune system.

One limitation of using IHC to evaluate changes in CD molecule expression is that it detects changes in numbers of cells and/or their distribution, but does not generally give any information about cellular function. The exception to this is the use of antibodies against CD markers found on activated cells of various types. A limitation of this method is that many activation markers are expressed on multiple cell types; therefore, double labeling with fluorescently labeled antibodies is often used to detect the subset of activated cells of interest. Commercial antibody suppliers are often very helpful in choosing appropriate activation markers via their catalogs and technical service representatives. Other methods that evaluate immune cell function more specifically can be combined with IHC to ensure that effects on the immune system are not missed.

b. Evaluation of Changes in Common Target Organs. Pharmaceutical/biologic agents can affect target organs in different ways and IHC can be used to study similar events in most organs. Thus, it is possible to compare changes in the kidney and liver in the distribution of organ-specific enzymes, cell-specific markers, and/or the composition of cellular infiltrates by using IHC.

The liver is commonly affected by a wide variety of pharmaceutical/biologic agents and toxins by virtue of its role in detoxification in the body. As a result, many substances in the liver may be altered. Many of these substances can be detected by IHC, making this a useful method for evaluation of effects on the liver. For example, various hepatocellular enzymes may be evaluated by IHC, and thus changes in these enzymes can be monitored.

211

Antibodies are available to mark various cell types within the liver, enabling evaluation of hypertrophy and/or hyperplasia of such cell types easier. Certain compounds may stimulate inflammation of the liver, causing influx of inflammatory cells and up regulation of cell adhesion molecules. These types of changes can often be detected using IHC. Finally, neoplastic and preneoplastic changes in the liver may be evaluated by detection of changes in growth factors, cell proliferation markers, and the protein products of oncogenes. An excellent review by Hall and Rojko (1996) on the use of immunohistochemistry in the evaluation of the liver is available. The liver has been used as an example because it is so commonly affected by pharmaceutical agents, but a similar approach using IHC may be useful in other target organs.

c. Immune Complex and Complement Deposition. Some pharmaceutical agents or toxic compounds, particularly biologic agents of a protein nature, may incite an immune response by the body. Such response may lead to deposition of immune complexes and complement in various organs, particularly in blood vessels and renal glomeruli. It is usually feasible to perform IHC for deposited complexes and complement when they are suspected based on histologic lesions. Methods are available to perform immunohistochemistry for these compounds on formalin-fixed, paraffin-embedded tissues.

d. Endocrine Disrupters. The evaluation of so-called endocrine disrupter compounds has become an active and controversial topic, concerning not only the administration of therapeutic compounds but also the effects of compounds found naturally and as contaminants in the environment (see Chapter 21). Recent U.S. legislation has mandated that a large number of potential endocrine disrupters be evaluated thoroughly. Many antibodies are already available against hormones and their receptors because of their importance in neoplasia of humans. Therefore, immunohistochemistry should prove to be feasible and valuable in the ongoing evaluation of agents acting on endocrine systems.

e. Biotransformation Enzymes. Drug-metabolizing enzymes, particularly the cytochrome P450 enzymes, are very important in the detoxification of many chemical compounds. Evaluation of changes in these enzymes by immunohistochemistry may help elucidate mechanisms of toxicity of certain compounds. Many antibodies are available that have been used by various investigators in numerous organs in both normal and chemically treated animals. As a specific example, a variety of cytochrome P450 enzymes have been localized to specific cell types in the nasal cavity, helping to explain the mechanisms of toxicity of numerous compounds that affect this region.

f. Mechanisms of Tumor Formation. Carcinogenicity of exogenous compounds may occur via either genotoxic or epigenetic mechanisms, and methods exist to use immunohistochemistry to investigate mechanisms of tumor formation by a wide variety of compounds. Genotoxic mechanisms of tumor formation by administered compounds may be evaluated by the use of immunohistochemistry to detect DNA adducts.

In recent years the tremendous importance of epigenetic mechanisms of tumor formation has been realized. Extensive research has determined that mutations in proteins and oncogenes such as p53 and k-ras, respectively, are very important in the formation of various types of neoplasms. Immunohistochemistry for the tumor suppressor protein p53 has proven to be very useful in the evaluation of neoplastic processes. When this protein is mutated, including after exposure to a carcinogenic compound, it becomes easier to detect with IHC because it becomes localized to the nucleus and is much more stable than normal p53. Examples of the use of IHC to detect mutated p53 abound. Belinsky *et al.* (1997) evaluated a large number of lung tumors induced in rats by a variety of agents and determined that mutation of p53 seemed to be important in certain tumor types but not in others.

Detection by immunohistochemistry of substances known to be produced by initiated or

must be administered exogenously to test animals by injection 1 to 2 hr prior to sacrifice, by means of subcutaneously implanted minipumps, or by administration in the drinking water. Antibodies against other compounds important in cell proliferation are becoming increasingly popular, including proliferating cell nuclear antigen (PCNA) and Ki67. The advantages of using such antibodies are that prior injections are not required and the antibodies can often be used on formalin-fixed, paraffin-embedded tissue, allowing retrospective studies to be performed in many cases.

One must recognize that while BrDU only detects cells in S phase, antibodies to PCNA and Ki67 detect cells in all stages of the replicative portion of the cell cycle (G1 + S + G2 + M). Some investigators believe that PCNA-positive cells can be separated out according to each of these stages based on characteristic differences in the pattern of nuclear staining. Studies using characteristic differences in nuclear staining of PCNA to compare S phase labeling of PCNA to that of BrDU have found that the labeling indices were similar for the two methods and thus concluded that the methods are equally useful for evaluating cell proliferation. One method may be preferred over the other depending on the specific situation.

Examples of the use of cell proliferation markers in toxicologic pathology abound in the literature, and it should not be difficult to find information appropriate for a desired situation. Experts in this field caution that with regard to evaluating cell proliferation in carcinogenesis studies, an increase in cell proliferation does not necessarily indicate that such proliferation will lead to neoplasia. Ghanayem et al. (1997) performed a specific study in which both proliferation and apoptosis were evaluated for two different compounds. They determined that the relative balance of the two different processes might be important in determining why carcinogenesis occurs with some nongenotoxic agents and not others.

Immunohistochemistry to evaluate changes in other compounds involved in cell cycle control, particularly cyclins and cyclin-dependent kinases, is becoming increasingly popular. Numerous antibodies are available commercially for this purpose. Various investigators have used IHC to evaluate changes in these cell cycle-related proteins in response to administration of various toxins.

5. Evaluation of Apoptosis

Apoptosis, or programmed cell death (PCD), is an active cell process that plays a critical role in a number of normal physiological events, including embryonic modeling, organization of the central nervous system, and metamorphosis. PCD has received widespread attention as a crucial component of a number of pathologic processes, including neoplasia and other disturbances in growth, inflammation, and immune responses. The best-defined biochemical alteration in cells undergoing PCD is generation of an endonuclease that cleaves nuclear DNA at the regions between the nucleosomes. This cleavage yields characteristic DNA fragments that are multiples of approximately 180–200 bp. Gel electrophoresis of DNA extracted from apoptotic cells shows a characteristic "DNA ladder" that is diagnostic for PCD. Morphologic criteria for PCD are also very specific at the ultrastructural level. Apoptotic cells are characterized by the shrinkage of the cytoplasm and nuclear chromatin condensation. The cellular shrinkage results in "apoptotic bodies," which are typically phagocytosed by macrophages or other surrounding cells.

Although the morphologic criteria of PCD are well defined, apoptotic cells can be very difficult to recognize in standard histologic sections. Two methods have been described that utilize the presence of DNA breaks in single cells to label cells undergoing PCD. One method uses DNA polymerase I and is called either in situ nick translation (ISNT) or in situ end labeling (ISEL) in the literature. The second method uses terminal deoxynucleotidyl transferase (TdT) and has been called either the tailing reaction or TdT-mediated bio-dUTP nick end-labeling (TUNEL). While these methods involve a combination of molecular biology and immunohistochemical techniques, they are covered here in order to include them in a discussion of immunohistochemical techniques used to evaluate various stages of the apoptotic pathway.

ISEL or ISNT, first described by Iseki in 1986 and later by Wijsman (1993), relies on the ability of DNA polymerase I (Pol 1) to add labeled nucleotides to 3'-hydroxyl ends of a DNA strand in the presence of a template, thereby extending the strand in a 5' to 3' direction. Thus, the term *"in situ* end labeling" has been used. It is hypothesized that ISEL probably detects the 3'-recessed DNA fragments formed in apoptosis. Because DNA Pol 1 is primer and template dependent, it cannot label the blunt-ended or 5'-recessed DNA fragments that may also occur in PCD. DNA Pol 1 also has an exonuclease activity that may start at single-stranded breaks and remove unlabeled nucleotides ahead of the enzyme, allowing their replacement by labeled nucleotides. Many vendors now offer the large subunit of DNA Pol 1, known as the Klenow fragment, for use in molecular biology and related applications. The Klenow fragment lacks any 3' to 5' exonuclease activity while retaining the primer extension and proofreading capabilities of DNA Pol 1 and has also been used with success in the ISEL procedure.

The TUNEL method is based on the specific binding of terminal deoxynucleotidyl transferase (TdT) to 3'-OH ends of DNA, with subsequent incorporation of biotinylated deoxyuridine at the sites of DNA breaks. Because TdT is template independent, it can label blunt-ended, 3'-recessed or 5'-recessed DNA fragments at hydroxylated 3' ends.

These methods have become very popular, and commercial kits (Oncor, Apoptag, CalBiochem) are available to specifically label apoptotic cells. However, controversy has arisen regarding the specificity of these enzymatic reactions. Both methods rely on the enzymatic detection of DNA fragments in tissue sections. Although DNA fragmentation is a key feature of PCD, DNA fragmentation also occurs in necrosis, albeit at a later stage in the death of the cell. Some groups feel that these methods do

not reliably detect apoptotic cells in tissue sections and are unable to differentiate them from necrotic cells or even from early postmortem autolysis. Other authors emphasize the value of these methods, but caution that they must be used in conjunction with the morphologic assessment of the labeled cell in order to distinguish necrosis from PCD.

Many antibodies and methods are now available for detecting earlier changes in the apoptotic pathway by immunohistochemistry. Arends and Wylie (1991) have written an excellent review describing these methods. Some of these are more specific than the TUNEL assay, although all have their limitations. Using multiple methods in combination may provide more valuable information than using the methods alone.

6. Evaluation of Infectious Disease Agents

Immunohistochemistry using antibodies against various infectious agents is commonly performed and can be useful in toxicologic pathology. If immunomodulatory compounds are administered, it is possible that increased susceptibility to infectious agents may occur in the test species due to immunosuppression, and such agents may be detected using IHC. Evaluation of background infectious diseases in a research animal colony is also possible. Animal models of infectious disease are used frequently to evaluate the efficacy of potential therapeutic compounds, and IHC for the particular infectious agent may help evaluate responses to therapy. Finally, viral vectors are often used to deliver gene therapy compounds, and IHC may be used to detect the presence of the viral vector to ensure delivery to the target organ (*in situ* hybridization is often used for this purpose as well).

D. CONCLUSION

In summary, it has been shown that immunohistochemistry has many important application in toxicologic pathology in answering the abundance of questions that arise in the development of pharmaceutical and biological agents for therapeutic purposes. Examples of its uses in this field are almost endless in the literature, and it is often applied very easily to novel questions that arise with new compounds.

III. *In Situ* Hybridization

A. INTRODUCTION

In situ hybridization (ISH) has emerged as an extremely sensitive method to evaluate gene expression at the cellular level in tissues. Much the way that immunohistochemistry evolved, utilizing the methods and reagents of immunology, ISH is the application of molecular biology methodologies and reagents to pathology. ISH was first described in 1969 and has primarily found applications in both basic and clinical research. In recent years, however, ISH has become an increasingly valuable technique in the arsenal of the toxicologic pathologist.

ISH is based on the principle that sequences of RNA or DNA that are complementary to the sequence of a target gene can be labeled and will specifically hybridize (bind) to cells in tissues, thereby localizing the site of the gene (DNA) or of gene expression (RNA). These complementary sequences, termed "probes," can be labeled with either radioisotopic or nonradioisotopic labels and, following hybridization to their target, can be visualized in tissue sections, cell preparations, and chromosome spreads. Prior to the development of ISH, molecular biology techniques such as Southern blots (for DNA) and Northern or dot blots (for RNA) were used to provide information on gene localization or expression at the tissue level. These techniques required the preparation of tissue homogenates from which DNA or RNA is extracted, run via electrophoresis through a gel, and then transferred to a support membrane that provides a matrix for subsequent hybridization. However, once the tissue has been homogenized and the nucleic acids extracted, any information regarding spatial localization will have been lost. ISH is valuable in that it preserves the tissue morphology and cellular origin of the target gene while also

providing information on the level of gene expression. ISH has also been used extensively in cytogenetics to identify genes on chromosomes, chromosomal rearrangements, etc. The focus of this review, however, is on the identification of gene expression in tissue sections.

B. TECHNICAL CONSIDERATIONS

A review of the literature reveals a plethora of ISH techniques using a variety of probe types, different labeling methods, etc. The truth that emerges from this survey is that similar to immunohistochemistry, there is probably not a single "best" method for ISH. Although some protocols work over a broad range of conditions, in general, experimental conditions must be customized for each target/tissue and, as always, appropriate controls must be run for the proper interpretation of data.

1. Selection of Probe Type

For many, the first technical consideration for ISH is the type of probe to use. Three main types of probes have been used in ISH: DNA (single or double stranded), RNA (riboprobes), or oligonucleotides. Of these types of probes, riboprobes and oligonucleotides are the most commonly used, and each has distinct advantages and disadvantages.

The advantages of riboprobes are that they probably offer the greatest sensitivity in detecting gene targets because of their length (typically 100–500 bp), their ability to be labeled to a high specific activity, and the greater stability of the DNA–RNA hybrids that are formed. In addition, sense riboprobes that are complementary to the antisense riboprobes and identical to the target gene can be used as negative controls on serial sections of tissues to identify areas of nonspecific tissue binding. Also, riboprobes have the advantage that RNase can be used in a posthybridization wash to degrade unbound RNA, thereby decreasing the background. One disadvantage of riboprobes is that RNA is quite labile, and, therefore, precautions must be used to ensure that the riboprobe is not degraded during the preparation of the probe or during the hybridization process. Another disadvantage of RNA probes is that they require some level of molecular biology skills to produce them. Riboprobes are generated by *in vitro* transcription from DNA templates containing RNA polymerase promoter sequences. Riboprobe templates can be created by subcloning the gene of interest into a plasmid ribovector or, alternatively, PCR techniques can be used to attach RNA polymerase recognition sites to the sequence of interest for subsequent *in vitro* transcription. Both methods of riboprobe template generation require at least a minimal level of molecular biology skills to be successful.

Oligonucleotides (oligo probes) are gaining popularity for use in ISH. Typically these are 20–50 nucleotide oligomers that are designed to hybridize specifically to target sequences. Many organizations already have in-house facilities that are able to synthesize oligonucleotides or, alternatively, oligonucleotides can be purchased from a number of commercial synthesis laboratories. Most synthesis laboratories can attach labels to the oligo probes at the time of synthesis or, alternatively, "kits" are available to label them prior to hybridization. Thus, oligo probes are often easier for the nonmolecular biologist to use. The main disadvantage of oligo probes is that they are much less sensitive than riboprobes due to their small size and require a relatively high copy number of mRNA in the tissue in order to detect a signal.

2. Selection of Probe Label

The other major technical consideration with ISH is the choice of probe label. There are two primary types: radioisotopic and nonisotopic. ISH was initially performed using radioisotopic lables, and is still the method of choice in many research laboratories. Types of radioisotopic labels are shown in Table I. The choice of label is a compromise between better cellular resolution, which requires relatively weak β emitters, and short exposure times, which are achieved by more energetic isotopes. At this time, medium energy β emitters such as ^{35}S and increasingly ^{33}P are the radioisotopes of choice in most laboratories using radioactivity. Most although not all, investigators feel that

TABLE I
β-Emitting Isotopes for *in Situ* Hybridization

Isotope	$T_{1/2}$	Max energy (MeV)	Resolution	Exposure time
^{3}H	12.35 years	0.018	High	Long
^{35}S	87.4 days	0.167	Moderate	Intermediate
^{33}P	28 days	0.250	Moderate	Intermediate
^{32}P	14.29 days	1.710	Poor	Short

ISH with radioisotopic-labeled probes is more sensitive in detecting low-level gene expression as compared to ISH with nonisotopic-labeled probes. Although isotopically labeled probes are generally more sensitive than nonisotopic probes, they require relatively long incubation times (some times weeks) and have poorer cellular resolution due to the pattern of radioactive emissions.

Protocols are available for ISH using isotopic-labeled probes that have been optimized and standardized for use on a variety of tissues and different probe sequences (Fig. 2, see color insert). This has not been possible for nonisotopic-labeled probes, where the protocol must be optimized for each new probe and tissue, similar to that required for antibodies in immunohistochemistry.

Nevertheless, ISH with nonisotopic-labeled probes will probes will probably be the method of choice for most laboratories in the future, as there are distinct advantages to working with nonisotopic labels, chief among them being not having to deal with the extra precautions associated with working with radioactivity. Nonisotopic labels for ISH probes are similar to those used in IHC (Table II). The most commonly used nonisotopic labels at this time are biotin- and digoxigenin-conjugated nucleotides, which can then be detected through a secondary detection system. Direct labeling, such as with a fluorescent tag, does not usually provide a strong enough signal for direct visualization. The choice of nonisotopic label is usually determined by the commercial availability of labeled nucleotides and the availability of sensitive detection systems to detect them. In addition to the benefit of not having to work with

TABLE II
Commonly Used Nonisotopic-Labeling Techniques

Direct
Fluorochromes (FITC, Texas Red, phycoerythrin)
Enzymes (horseradish peroxidase, alkaline phosphatase)
Indirect
Antibodies
DNA-RNA
RNA-RNA
Biotin
Digoxigenin
BrdU

radioactivity, the use of nonisotopic probes allows for markedly shorter detection times, lowers reagent costs, better cellular resolution, and increases the shelf life of reagents (nonisotopic labels do not decay like isotopic labels). In addition, new amplification strategies are being introduced that may increase the sensitivity of nonisotopic techniques markedly. Tyramide amplification, for example, uses the deposition of haptenized tyramide molecules in the vicinity of hybridized probes catalyzed by the enzyme horseradish peroxidase to greatly amplify the signal produced by digoxigenin- or biotin-labeled nucleotides.

C. APPLICATIONS OF ISH IN TOXICOLOGIC PATHOLOGY

To date, ISH has been used primarily as a research tool in molecular biology and pathology laboratories and is just starting to win acceptance in the clinical arena. Until recently, the use of *in situ* hybridization in toxicologic pathology has been limited to studies in very early discovery research and evaluation of efficacy in animal models. While useful in those environments, this technique also has broad applications in drug development, particularly for some biotechnology products such as gene therapeutics and antisense oligonucleotides.

1. ISH in Discovery Research

In early discovery research, ISH has been used to localize sites of gene expression for novel genes for which the function of the protein product may not be known. Determining the

cell type in which a gene is expressed can provide an insight into the potential function of the gene product. Northern and Southern blots allow investigators to localize gene expression at the tissue level, but ISH allows localization of gene expression to distinct cells in the probed tissues. For example, localization of a newly cloned guanylyl cyclase receptor to the photoreceptor layer of the eye provided an indication that this gene may function in phototransduction. Expression of guanylin mRNA was determined by ISH to be restricted to the intestine and helped confirm that guanylin was an endogenous activator of an intestine-specific receptor -guanylyl cyclase through which an *Escherichia coli*-derived enterotoxin worked. Leptin, the product of the *ob* gene, is secreted by fat cells and is involved in body weight regulation. ISH was used to demonstrate that expression of a form of the leptin receptor is expressed in the hypothalamus.

2. Study of Gene Expression in Animal Models

Although ISH has been traditionally thought of as a tool for early discovery research, today's toxicologic pathologists are increasingly using ISH as a tool for monitoring gene expression following drug administration. For example, in carcinogenicity testing, ISH for connexin 32 (Cx32) in liver samples of treated rats was used to determine if the compound might promote the formation of liver tumors. Although connexin genes are not oncogenes or tumor suppressor genes, they are integral to cell signaling and have been implicated in abnormal growth. ISH was used to demonstrate that renin mRNA expression was increased in the kidneys of rats treated with the angiotensin II antagonist ZENECA ZD8731. In the realm of environmental toxicology, ISH has been used to assess changes in the expression of genes associated with lung extracellular matrix (ECM) proteins such as collagen I and III, elastin, fibronectin, and interstitial collagenase. The deposition of some of these ECM proteins is increased in the lungs of animals following chronic ozone exposure.

219

3. ISH in the Study of Transgenic and Gene-Altered Animals

The study of transgenic and gene knockout animals in pharmaceutical research has provided a means to understand the function and interaction of specific genes *in vivo*. Animal models often provide the best means of studying disease because they can behave similarly to humans in many cases. ISH has been particularly valuable in the study of gene-altered animal models in characterizing tissue-specific transgene expression. In v-Ha-ras oncogene transgenic mice, ISH was used to verify expression of v-Ha-ras mRNA in both normal and neoplastic cells. The Laboratory of Environmental Carcinogenesis and Mutagenesis at the NIEHS has been evaluating the v-Ha-ras transgenic mouse model for its utility as a carcinogenic assay. Gene knockout animals provide an opportunity to study the effects of gene deletion *in vivo*. ISH was used to characterize the effects of estrogen receptor-α-dependent processes in estrogen receptor-α knockout (ERKO) mice. ISH of ovaries from ERKO mice showed a high level of LHR mRNA expression in the granulosa and thecal layers of antral follicles, indicating that ER-α action was not a prerequisite for LHR mRNA expression. Gene knockout animals can be used as models of human diseases. ISH was used to help determine the mechanism in the development of myasthenia gravis in interferon (IFN)-γ receptor-deficient mice. Lymphoid cells from these animals were examined by ISH for changes in the expression of various cytokine mRNAs, including IFN-γ. Upregulation of IFN-γ mRNA expression is believed to contribute to the susceptibility to myasthenia gravis in these mice.

4. Comparing Gene Expression across Species

ISH can also be used to explore mechanisms of disease in both animal models and humans. Because regions of gene sequences are often conserved across species, it is possible to design ISH reagents that can be used to examine gene expression in both animal models and the human disease. Because of the homology between mouse (flk-1) and human (KDR) growth factor receptors, it was possible to use the same probe to study expression in human colorectal liver metastases and a mouse model of colorectal liver metastases. Such evaluation of multiple species is often not possible using immunohistochemistry because of the lack of cross-reactivity of antibodies across species. Even when the sequence homology between species is not high enough to allow the use of the same reagents, ISH can still provide valuable information. ISH was useful in demonstrating the differential expression of two different cyclooxygenase isoforms in the kidneys of dogs, rats, monkeys, and humans.

5. ISH in the Evaluation of Gene Therapy and Antisense Therapeutics

The progression of gene therapy products and antisense oligonucleotides toward licensing increases the utility of ISH later in the drug development pathway. Because ISH allows cellular localization of gene expression, questions regarding the safety and efficacy of these products can be answered at a cellular level. For example, in the case of gene therapy, ISH has been used numerous times to localize the vector, indicate if the transferred DNA has entered the targeted host cell, and whether expression of the associated mRNA has occurred. In addition, ISH can determine if observed lesions are occurring at the site of cellular transduction or are spatially unrelated to the presence of the transferred DNA. ISH can also reveal whether transduction and/or gene expression is occurring in germ line cells in the testes or ovaries.

Following administration of antisense oligonucleotides, ISH can be used to evaluate the relative level of target mRNA in the cells of interest, both before and after oligonucleotide administration. Just as the advent of monoclonal antibodies as potential therapeutics has broadened the application of immunohistochemistry during the drug development process, it is likely that the development of sequences of DNA for use as drugs will increase the potential usefulness of ISH in drug development.

D. CONCLUSIONS

ISH can be a powerful tool for studying gene expression and distribution at the cellular level. While there are a number of parallels between IHC and ISH (indeed the two techniques complement each other as was discussed in Section II), there is some danger is overstating the similarities between the two techniques because the reagent requirements and technical expertise for each are quite different. An understanding of the principles underlying each method is essential to "trouble shooting" the procedures and interpreting the results.

Obviously, the most information regarding the gene and its protein product can be obtained if both IHC and ISH are performed. A variety of different patterns can be obtained if both IHC and ISH are performed on a given cell population (Table III). In recent years, dual detection methods have been developed where multiple genes or gene products can be detected in the same tissue section using a combination of IHC and ISH. Alternatively, these techniques can be used in serial sections from the

TABLE III
Interpretation of ISH and IHC Results

ISH	IHC	Interpretation
+	+	Detectable synthesis of mRNA Synthesis and storage of protein
+	−	Detectable synthesis of mRNA No detectable protein No storage of protein Rapid degradation of protein Below limit of detection
−	+	No detectable mRNA Rapid degradation of mRNA Protein synthesized in a different cell Below limit of detection Detectable protein Synthesis and storage of protein Uptake of protein
−	−	No detectable mRNA Rapid degradation of mRNA Protein synthesized in a different cell Below limit of detection No detectable protein No storage of protein Rapid degradation of protein Below limit of detection

same tissue block to determine the tissue distribution of the mRNA and protein. There are a number of instances where ISH and IHC will show differing patterns, depending on the storage or secretion of the protein product, the degree of posttranslational processing, and intracellular degradation of the protein. The decision to perform either IHC or ISH will often depend on the availability of the reagents and the nature of the scientific question. Often, antibodies will not be available for the gene product of interest to perform IHC. Usually the gene sequence is known prior to the availability of antibodies; thus, ISH may be the first procedure available to determine cellular localization for a given gene. In some cases, knowledge of the location of the protein product is more important than knowledge of the mRNA levels. Alternatively, in some cases, such as in endocrine tumors, the cells may be synthesizing a prohormone that is not detected by conventional antibodies, but can be detected by probes through ISH.

The obvious advantage of ISH as compared to PCR or Northern blots is that the mRNA can be localized to the cell. In some cases, ISH is more sensitive than Northern blots; for example, when a small proportion of the cell population is expressing mRNA at high levels, it is detected more easily by ISH than Northern blots. Conversely, when 100% of the cell population is expressing at low levels, it will be detected more easily by Northern blot than by ISH.

IV. Flow Cytometry

A. INTRODUCTION

Flow cytometry is an upcoming technology in toxicologic pathology that incorporates features of conventional microscopy and immunofluorescence in a high throughput system of cellular or particulate analysis. Flow cytometric evaluation of peripheral blood, bone marrow cells, dissociated tissue or tumor cells, or cultured cells provides a means to identify changes in the physical (cell phenotype, nucleic acid content) or biochemical (cell activity/function, cell proliferation/viability) attributes of cells, which may be induced by biopharmaceuticals. The utility of flow cytometry in preclinical evaluation comes from the capacity to examine large numbers of cells in a relatively short time interval. Using this high throughput capability coupled with a high degree of detector sensitivity, flow cytometry provides a means to identify subtle changes in cell attributes, some of which may represent indicators of altered immune function, delayed cellular/tissue repair, or neoplasia. Coupled with more traditional methods of preclinical testing, flow cytometry can be a powerful tool in the study of toxicologic pathology. In addition, many of the markers used to identify changes in cells from test animals have counterparts that react with similar constituents on human cells; as such, the results from some laboratory animal experiments can be correlated directly to effects that could be expected with similar manipulations in humans.

Flow cytometry is based on the examination of cells (or other particles) suspended in a hydrodynamically focused fluid stream that separates individual entities (cells or particles) for examination. Suspended particles pass individually through the flow cell where they are exposed to a focused laser light source. The light emission that results from the diffraction of laser light by the cells is filtered and directed to a series of photodetectors where the light signal is converted to electronic signals, which are digitized and displayed as cell attributes. Each cell type has a characteristic light scatter pattern that can be evaluated qualitatively and quantitatively. Many hematology analyzers currently in use incorporate this technology, converting light scatter properties of individualized blood cells (shape and granularity) to information used in blood cell differential analysis. Fluorescence-activated flow cytometry takes the technology a step further by adding signal detection from specific fluorochromes that can be attached to antibodies, specific proteins, and nucleic acids and, subsequently, to select cells or cell components. Flow cytometric

analysis of fluorochrome-conjugated probes can be used to detect and localize extracellular (membrane bound) and intracellular targets. The evaluation of cell components that may be altered by chemical or mechanical manipulation is enhanced by the examination of cellular structural and functional attributes using fluorescence flow cytometry.

In addition to standard light scatter/fluorescence evaluation, flow cytometers may also be equipped to sort cells or particles. With sorting, specific subpopulations of cells with one or more well-defined characteristics can be collected for additional analyses or experimentation. Viable cells can be collected in this manner for cell culture and manipulation or microscopy. More recently, laser-scanning cytometry (LSC; see Section IV,D) has been proposed as the next generation of fluorescence-activated cell analysis instruments, combining the fluorescence detection capabilities of a standard flow cytometer with the optics of a high-quality microscope. The analysis of a variety of cell preparations, including tissue sections with LSC, provides high-quality morphometry sufficient to map the location (cytoplasm, mitochondrial membrane, etc.) of specific labeled targets within individual cells.

B. APPLICATIONS OF FLOW CYTOMETRY IN TOXICOLOGIC PATHOLOGY

The use of biomarkers in preclinical drug evaluation has increased in recent years in an effort to provide the public with biopharmaceuticals and medical devices having a greater level of safety and efficacy. Much of the advancement in product quality has come about secondarily to the discovery and implementation of new analysis technology. Some of that technology has replaced or updated traditional analysis systems; more consistent data are generated at a faster rate. Some methodologies developed have shown increased detection sensitivity that can identify subtle changes much earlier after experimental manipulation than previously available. Speed, consistency, and sensitivity have helped take flow cytometry out of the research laboratory into toxicologic pathology, where the capabilities of this technology are only now being realized.

When first introduced in the late 1960s and early 1970s, flow cytometry was predominantly a research tool. Its value in clinical medicine quickly became apparent with subtyping of hematologic malignancies using cell-specific antibodies detected using fluorescence flow cytometry; valuable information about the cell type(s) involved in forms of leukemia provided the basis for treatment and prognosis. More recently, flow cytometry has been used to evaluate the progression of human immunodeficiency virus (HIV) and acquired immunodeficiency syndrome (AIDS) through the analysis of lymphocyte subsets. In both of these examples, flow cytometry has provided the ability to screen a large number of cells from a large number of individuals in a relatively short period of time using markers specific for known cell antigens. Given the abundance of labeled cell markers available, the speed at which a diverse cell population can be analyzed and the variety of sample types that can conceivably be evaluated, the merit of this technology in preclinical safety evaluation is evident. Some potential applications of flow cytometry in toxicologic pathology are described in the following sections with comments as to advantages and disadvantages of this technology over more traditional methods used in preclinical safety evaluation studies.

1. Cell Phenotyping

In addition to displaying certain structural attributes, all cells express one or more protein antigens on the cell membrane; these antigens define specific characters of the cell and may be expressed in patterns that can be used to differentiate morphologically similar cell subsets. As an example, cells of the immune system are characterized by the expression of clusters of differentiation antigens on the cell surface. One or more antibodies specific to a CD antigen can be used to identify subsets of immune cells within a mixture of cells (i.e., whole tissue, peripheral blood). With immunohistochemistry, tissue sections are treated with labeled anti-

bodies against different CD antigens to define the relative density and location of specific cell subpopulations within lymphoid and other tissue. Applying similar technology to peripheral blood, flow cytometry can be used to determine the presence of and relative frequency of subsets of immune cell in the blood (immunophenotyping of peripheral blood). Immunophenotyping can be used to track the redistribution of cell subsets in peripheral blood or tissue following cell or tissue stimulation (e.g., inflammation, transplantation). In addition to phenotyping of blood cells, flow cytometry can be used to characterize the attributes of normal and altered cells collected from bone marrow, tissue aspirates, and lavage fluid, as well as cells from solid tissues such as lymph nodes and malignant tumors (through mechanical or enzymatic dissociation). Isolated tissue cells can be analyzed for changes in phenotype that may be induced by culture conditions (i.e., purified islet cells destined for transplantation) or experimental manipulations (i.e., stimulated alveolar macrophages isolated from the lung after exposure to a pneumotoxicant).

While phenotyping can provide exquisite detail about individual cell types within a mixed cell population, care must be taken to avoid overinterpretation of these data. Phenotyping can expose subtle changes early in the pathogenesis of toxicity; subtle changes, however, may be indicative of minor variations of normal. Changes in the expression of markers on specific subsets of lymphocytes may suggest alterations in immune function; flow cytometry data must, however, be considered with other data generated during the evaluation (i.e., pharmacologic activity, clinical history, histology). Changes in discrete immune cell subsets in solid tissues can be discerned with flow cytometry, but data defining the spatial relationship of those subsets must be derived from other analysis methodologies (i.e., immunohistochemistry). Cellular or tissue effects of a biopharmaceutical agent may modulate multiple cellular antigens; the identification of changes in tissue morphology based on changes in antigen presentation (detected with IHC) may be

223

important to the discovery of functional changes in that tissue. The importance of extensive background/control data for flow cytometry cannot be overstated.

2. Quantitative Immunophenotyping

Standard cell phenotyping can be enhanced using additional techniques for flow cytometric quantitation. To date, these methods are still under development and not widely accepted for cytometric analysis in toxicologic pathology. With quantitative techniques, the number of antigens per cell is determined through the use of calibration beads labeled with a predefined amount of fluorescent dye. A fluorescence intensity value of the beads, measured as units of molecules of equivalent soluble fluorochrome (MESF), is determined for a set of labeled bead standards. The standard curve constructed is used to determine the MESF of the cells being labeled and evaluated. When this method is used with monoclonal antibodies conjugated 1:1 with the fluorescent dye phycoerythrin (PE), highly accurate values for the number of antibodies bound per cell can be determined. If the binding characteristics of antigen and antibody are also known, the number of antigens per cell can be calculated from fluorescent data. Knowledge of the binding characteristics of the antibody, as well as prevention of nonspecific antibody binding, is critical for accurate results using this method.

An alternative approach to quantitative immunophenotyping is the use of beads labeled with the antigen of interest (i.e., a specific CD antigen) combined with the appropriate antibody conjugated 1:1 with PE. As described earlier, a bead set containing three to four known antigen concentrations is necessary to generate the standard curve from which antigen/cell data can be derived. Although this method provides a higher level of precision than fluorochrome-tagged beads, sets are costly, as each is custom manufactured to user specifications.

Quantitative immunophenotyping can unmask subtle effects on target cells that may be defined incompletely by standard cell phenotyping. Reduced or enhanced antigen expression on target cells could represent an important toxicologic change induced by an experimental product; alterations of this type are potentially critical in cells of the immune system. Reduced or enhanced antigen availability may represent an effect of the pharmaceutical agent; saturation of antigen-binding sites secondary to the administration of a test agent may alter the cellular response to stimuli or increase the morbidity of some disease processes. It is apparent that changes of this nature would not be identified using traditional immunophenotyping unless that magnitude of the change was quite large. Quantitative immunophenotyping requires standardization of the methodology, a process that is ongoing at present. Careful accumulation and interpretation of normal range data, as well as standardization of reagents and instrumentation, will be necessary before this assay is widely used. As with standard phenotyping, overinterpretation of data must be avoided.

3. Cell Activation/Analysis of Cell Function

The effect of a toxicant on a target cell population may not be limited to morphologic alterations in those cells; cell function may be severely compromised with little immediate impact on cell morphology. In the immune system, immunosuppression with minimal to no effect on lymphocyte morphology may follow experimental manipulation. Traditionally, a series of lengthy assays have been done to measure changes in the proliferative ability or the functional capacity of immune cells. Standard lymphocyte proliferation assays can take 3–7 days, require large volumes of blood, and be costly in the amount of technical time required and reagents used. Cytokine production, an essential component of normal immune function, has also been measured by tedious, costly, and time-consuming traditional methods. Assays now available using flow cytometry have decreased turnaround time for the evaluation of cell activation by measuring activation-specific markers. Markers of cell activation include CD69, CD25, and HLA-DR that are expressed very early (minutes), early, and late (hours) after cell stimulation, respectively. Mitosis has been the cell activation marker of choice for many years, but may only be detectable for 12–24 hr or more after cell stimulation. The activation inducer molecule CD69 is expressed on most hematopoietic cells in response to proinflammatory stimuli; in T lymphocytes, CD69 may be involved in cell adhesion, cytokine production, and mitogenesis. The expression of CD69 occurs much earlier than cytokine production or cell proliferation (measured as tritiated thymidine incorporation) and can be identified and quantified by flow cytometry.

Cytokine production, typically measured by ELISA or fluorescence microscopy, can be detected with equal or greater precision at lower cost using highly specific antibodies and flow cytometry. ELISA and flow cytometry can provide similar information comparing cytokine production across multiple specimens; the addition of phenotyping can provide additional information about which cells in a mixed cell population are expressing the cytokine. The measurement of cytokine expression in conjunction with immunophenotyping has been used extensively to differentiate immune responses in CD4$^+$ T-helper cell (Th) subsets that are defined by the cytokines produced by each subset.

Although assays for cell activation markers can be done on fresh cell samples, functional assays may be impacted by the need for cell culture. Some assays may require several days of preparation, necessitating sterile incubation facilities. Changes in the phenotype or function of certain cells maintained in culture must be considered in the interpretation of results from these analyses. In addition, to avoid loss of cytokines into the culture milieu, cells being prepared for analysis must be treated with agents to prevent the egress of newly synthesized cytokine from the cells.

4. Cell Proliferation/Apoptosis

Traditional assays used to evaluate cell proliferation and apoptosis in tissues have centered on changes in whole organs or tissues, coupling organ weight with histologic alterations consisting of an increased mitotic index with proliferation and cell condensation/fragmentation with apoptosis. Histology provides good spatial orientation of altered cells within a tissue, but analysis requires a significant time input to evaluate sufficient cell numbers to attain significance. Flow cytometry is a useful adjunct to organ weight and histologic evaluation; a large number of different cells can be analyzed using specific markers to differentiate cell subtypes. In addition, attributes that define similar cells (i.e., hepatocytes) by age and/or cell cycle phase during exposure could be differentiated using DNA content and cell cycle protein markers. This combination could be used effectively to increase the detection of rare subpopulations of cells having specific characteristics. The precise information gained using individual cell analysis could aid in the defination of pathogenic mechanisms responsible for cellular proliferation and/or apoptosis in the whole tissues.

The drawback to analysis of whole tissue by flow cytometry is the issue surrounding tissue preparation. For tissues in which cells of interest are loosely attached to the connective tissue matrix (i.e., spleen, liver and lymph nodes), gentle mechanical or enzymatic dissociation can be used to individualize target cells without compromise of the structural components of the cells. Care must be taken using enzymatic methods that may digest protein antigens on the cell surface. Where cell attachment is well defined, dissociation may be associated with loss of cell membrane and cytoplasm, resulting in the loss of certain antigens; on cells isolated from tissues with an extensive connective tissue stroma, flow cytometric analysis may be limited to nucleic acid parameters.

5. Cell Sorting

Sorting a mixed population of cells using flow cytometry provides a means to acquire pure populations of cells defined by one or more light scatter or fluorescence emission characteristics. Sorting is accomplished by inducing a positive or negative charge into droplets

225

containing single cells with desired attributes defined in the interrogation region of the flow cytometer. Charged cells are subsequently deflected from the stream of analyzed cells and collected in sterile or nonsterile containers. Potential applications for cell sorting include the isolation of cells with identical attributes to be used for additional morphometric/functional analyses *in vitro*, collection of pure populations for cell culture, or the generation of isolated cells for experimental transplantation. The utility of cell sorting by flow cytometry for use in toxicologic pathology has yet to be recognized.

6. Other Applications

Efforts to employ flow cytometric technology in other aspects of preclinical evaluations have been investigated and, in some cases, utilized as an alternative way to measure changes induced by experimental manipulation. Most examples consist of converting particle (cell) analysis to an automated format using the flow cytometer from a manual method in which samples were evaluated and quantified by light microscopy. The first comparison of this type evaluated white blood cell differentials done manually compared to those done by a hematology analyzer (light scatter analysis). The prevalence of automated hematology analyzers in use confirms the acceptance of flow cytometry technology in clinical hematology, although manual differentials continue to be done for quality control. The analysis of other tissues (i.e., bone marrow) comparing traditional microscopy with flow cytometry remains to be done. Undoubtedly, flow cytometry will be used in a number of technologies where speed and numbers of cells analyzed are important, but will likely continue to be an adjunct to conventional microscopy.

C. LIMITATION OF FLOW CYTOMETRY

Some of the specific limitations of flow cytometric analysis have been described in the previous sections. Flow cytometers are high-tech and high-budget instruments that can rapidly perform sophisticated analyses precisely as

directed. It is critical that the operator has a solid understanding of the operation and capability of the instrument. Analyses to be done must be designed with specific end points in mind. Each machine must undergo rigorous setup and quality control checks at regular intervals to ensure that data gathered are reliable and consistent. Minor shifts in laser alignment and inadequate or incomplete compensation between fluorochromes can reduce the quality, quantity, and reliability of data derived by flow cytometry. In addition, a regimented and thorough cleaning program must be done after each analysis and regular maintenance of the hardware and software must be carried out at manufacturer-recommended intervals.

Sample preparation is as important to the success of flow cytometry as proper experimental design and instrument operation. Samples contaminated with particulate matter may yield erroneous data as particles of some sizes may be read as cells or may nonspecifically bind antibodies intended for specific cell surface proteins. Samples exposed to heat, light, or vigorous agitation may change and lose (or gain) properties that are "read" incorrectly in the interrogation region of the analyzer. Old samples submitted for labeling or labeled samples stored improperly may also give false results.

As stated previously, flow cytometry data must be interpreted in light of other information generated in the performance of a preclinical evaluation. The newness of this technology requires that baseline normal data be generated for each species evaluated as well as each marker tested. Intrinsic and extrinsic differences in animals, environment, and sample collection method must be considered in the interpretation of data generated by flow cytometry. For example, differences in antigen expression by certain cell types may occur due to differences in the strain, sex, or age of a test animal. The unexpected presence or absence of antibody cross-reactivity between species or organs within one species of test animal may result in false results. Sample preparation methods differ enough as to result in no signal by one method and abundant signal with another. It is likely that other considerations will arise as flow cytometry is implemented more fully in the standard toxicology assay.

D. LASER SCANNING CYTOMETRY

Laser-scanning cytometry combines cell imaging methods with flow cytometry with several distinct advantages over standard flow cytometry. Slides are used for cell preparation and analysis providing a semipermanent sample for archiving. Cells on the slide are mounted permanently to a specific location on the slide, making relocation and reanalysis convenient. Slides can accommodate touch preparations, tissue sections, smears, aspirates, or isolated/cultured cells. Centrifugation is not required in cell preparation, minimizing loss of sample and the use of smaller (rare) samples. Specimens can be restained with other fluorochromes or dyes for additional analyses; results of initial evaluations can be used to plan and institute additional labeling and analysis on the same samples. This methodology can be used not only to identify cell subtypes and characterize antigen expression or cell function, but also to map the expression of specific characteristics to locations on or within individual cells or relate expression to the cell cycle. The use of LSC in toxicologic pathology has not been fully realized, but will likely play a role in preclinical evaluation in the near future.

E. CONCLUSIONS

Flow cytometry and the associated fields of cell sorting and laser-scanning cytometry can be used for the identification of very specific changes in individual cells within a mixed cell population. While not able to replace traditional toxicologic testing, flow cytometry has the ability to detect subtle differences in a variety of cell types with high levels of speed and accuracy. For example, when used in conjunction with immunohistochemistry, flow cytometry can provide data about relative cell numbers to be incorporated with the spatial distribution of those cells within a tissue. As an adjunct to

traditional preclinical safety testing following experimental manipulation, flow cytometry has the potential to provide information about subtle events that occur early but may precede larger and more notable changes leading to significant effects. With the number of markers available, the addition of flow cytometry to a traditional preclinical analysis program will likely improve the quality of data generated and enhance the knowledge of positive and negative effects induced by novel biopharmaceuticals.

V. *In Situ* Polymerase Chain Reaction (PCR)/*in Situ* Reverse Transcriptase-PCR

A. INTRODUCTION

Although standard ISH permits localization of specific nucleic acid sequences at the cellular level, its relatively high threshold of detection sometimes limits its usefulness. Northern blots are capable of detecting mRNA levels approaching 10 copies per cell but do not localize the signal to specific cells. Most ISH protocols are incapable of detecting mRNA levels below 10–20 copies per cell and are not able to detect single copy DNA sequences.

The polymerase chain reaction is a powerful method, which is capable of specifically amplifying minute quantities of DNA. PCR has been shown to be able to amplify and identify a single copy of a gene in as little material as a single cell. However, before amplification, the target DNA must be extracted from the cellular material and, thus, the cellular localization is lost.

Among the newer morphological techniques that were particularly popular in the early 1990s are the *in situ* polymerase chain reaction (ISPCR) for the cellular detection of low-copy number DNA and the *in situ* reverse transcriptase polymerase chain reaction (IS RT-PCR) for the cellular detection of low-expression mRNAs. Both techniques combine the specificity and amplification of PCR with the cellular localization of standard ISH by targeting and amplifying specific signals within individual cells to detectable levels.

Most reports of ISPCR and IS RT-PCR have focused on the study of viral DNA sequences. Detection of endogenous DNA sequences by ISPCR and more recently mRNA sequences by IS RT-PCR have also been performed. However, the application of ISPCR to archival material has found limited success.

The principles of ISPCR and IS RT-PCR are straightforward in theory, but difficult to achieve in practice (Fig. 3). First, the cells or tissue samples are fixed and permeabilized in order to preserve tissue morphology, as well as to allow access of the PCR reagents (primers, nucleotides, and enzymes) for amplification. After fixation and permeabilization, the samples are placed into a thermal cycling unit to carry out the PCR amplification. Following amplification, the intracellular PCR products are visualized by standard ISH (indirect *in situ* PCR) or by the direct detection of labeled nucleotides, which have been incorporated during the PCR reaction (direct *in situ* PCR).

Several groups have reported the successful detection of specifically amplified DNA or RNA sequences. These groups have developed ISPCR protocols that share a number of key conceptual characteristics, yet all contain important experimental differences relating to sample preparation, amplification methodology, detection of amplified products, and the appropriate controls.

B. TECHNICAL CONSIDERATIONS

Early ISPCR studies were performed on single cells suspended in the PCR reaction mixture in tubes, which were thermal cycled in a block thermocycler. Following PCR, the cells were cytocentrifuged onto slides for ISH detection of amplified products. ISPCR has also been performed on cytocentrifuge preparations and tissue sections on glass slides placed directly on the heating block of a conventional thermal cycler or in a modified thermal cycling heating block. Manufacturers seeing the potential of these applications have manufactured thermal cycling units specifically for the amplification of material on slides (MJ Research, Perkin-Elmer, and Hybaid). IS RT-PCR has been performed successfully in suspended cells and tissue sections.

The choice of fixative and protease is crucial to the success of the ISPCR. If the fixation is not sufficient, then tissue morphology and target nucleic acids are not retained. Overfixation and/or insufficient permeabilization prevents the PCR reagents from entering the cells for amplification, and overpermeabilization destroys cellular morphology and allows diffusion of amplified PCR products into surrounding cells, thus compromising interpretation. This paradox is the essential difficulty of the technique. ISPCR has been performed successfully in samples fixed in paraformaldehyde, 10% buffered formalin, ethanol, and mixtures of alcohol and acetic acid. A number of different proteases of different concentrations or detergents have been tried with no clear consensus as to which is the best method. In most cases, a number of different fixation/permeabilization methodologies must be tried to find the optimal combination for each protocol.

Similar to the fixation/permeabilization steps, the choice of *in situ* amplification methodology is also crucial. Different strategies must be employed in an attempt to increase amplification efficiency, reduce false priming, and avoid the loss of PCR products. Many of the strategies employed are direct crossovers from

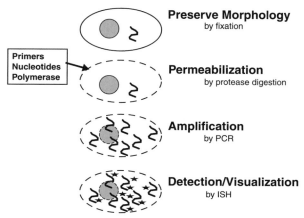

Figure 3. Theoretical basis for *in situ* PCR and *in situ* reverse transcriptase PCR.

solution PCR. To prevent false priming and increase target accessibility, some groups have employed Hot Start modifications, where a key component (typically the DNA polymerase) of the PCR reaction solution is withheld until the sample is heated beyond the temperature at which mispriming might occur. Heating the sample prior to the addition of a complete PCR solution also ensures complete target denaturation, or separation of the target DNA into single strands, which helps ensure the appropriate primer annealing when the sample is cooled. Variations in PCR reaction mixtures from those used in standard solution PCR have been used to increase amplification efficiency. Primer selection has ranged from single primer pairs to multiple primer pairs. With either strategy, it is important that the primers used for ISPCR work in solution PCR to assure specificity and amplification *in situ*. The number of PCR cycles for ISPCR has also been variable. As with the fixation/permeabilization steps, a number of different amplification strategies must be tested to find the optimum conditions for each study.

Two basic methodologies have been used to detect ISPCR products: indirect ISPCR (where standard ISH is used to detect the amplified products) and direct ISPCR (where labeled nucleotides are directly incorporated into the PCR products and detected directly through various means). Both direct and indirect ISPCR methods have been used with both radioactive and nonradioactive probes. In the case of nonradioactive direct ISPCR, a non-radioactive-labeled nucleotide such as digoxigenin dUTP is included in the PCR reaction mix and is incorporated directly into the PCR product. The labeled PCR product is then detected by immunohistochemical means via an antidigoxigenin antibody. Although direct ISPCR has been heralded as a rapid alternative to indirect ISPCR, the general consensus is that direct ISPCR is not as reliable as indirect ISPCR. This is due in part to the nonspecific incorporation of labeled nucleotides into fragmented endogenous DNA by the DNA polymerase.

C. CONTROLS

The use of appropriate controls for various steps in the ISPCR protocol is essential to rule out false-positive and false-negative results. On addition to the standard known negative and positive tissue samples, a number of other controls should be used. To identify nonspecific signals generated by the DNA repair component of the polymerase in direct ISPCR, a control reaction where primers have been omitted should be performed. Nonspecific probe hybridization in indirect ISPCR can be detected through the omission of either primers or polymerase in one set of controls because the target sequence will not have been amplified and thus would not be available for hybridization. When using immunological detection methods, a control slide substituting an irrelevant primary antibody should also be included. When performing IS RT-PCR, controls without reverse transcriptase and/or RNase pretreatment are required to detect false-positive signals resulting from the amplification of endogenous DNA sequences.

D. LIMITATIONS

Although potentially very powerful, ISPCR and IS RT-PCR have found only limited utility, primarily within the research area. Each type of starting material and protocol for ISPCR or IS RT-PCR requires its own set of conditions for successful amplification and detection. In addition, it has been shown that the degree of DNA or RNA amplification achieved with ISPCR or IS RT-PCR is much less than the exponential increase achieved with solution PCR.

The primary dilemma of ISPCR is that the very manipulations that are required to permit access of the PCR components into the cell increase the likelihood that the PCR product will diffuse out of the cell, losing the spatial localization of the product. In addition, PCR products that leak from the tissue become a target for solution phase PCR, thus increasing the amount of inappropriately localized PCR product. Although investigators have tried to control for diffusion artifacts by coamplifying positive and negative control tissue in the same reaction, the heterogeneity of the cell population in tissue makes this differentiation between positive and negative controls difficult at best. Frequently within a tissue, both negative and positive cell populations are present. To adequately adjust the conditions and controls to identify the negative and positive cells often means that one must know the results of the experiment prior to conducting it!

Many questions within toxicologic pathology do not require the spatial localization and identification of a single copy of RNA or DNA within a cell. In addition, other methodologies have become available that are capable of answering the same questions that have previously required the use of ISPCR. Amplification methods such as tyramide amplification have greatly increased the sensitivity of conventional ISH in some applications. Laser capture microscopy has even greater potential to answer similar questions as ISPCR. This method allows spatial localization through laser capture of an individual or small subset of cells, which can then be analyzed for gene expression through conventional solution molecular biology techniques. Although this technique requires availability of a laser capture microscope, the other technical aspects are much more straightforward than ISPCR.

VI. Laser Capture Microdissection

Until recently, cellular localization of molecular events in a heterogeneous cellular tissue has required molecular analysis on the slide itself, utilizing techniques such as *in situ* hybridization, *in situ* PCR, and *in situ* RT-PCR. While these techniques are useful, only a limited number of assays can be performed on the slide, and in some instances, e.g., *in situ* PCR, the technique is very difficult to perform. Further development of molecular genetics requires the molecular analysis of pure populations of cells extracted from their native tissues. The recent advent of laser capture microdissection (LCM) allows a similar degree of precision in localizing molecular changes at the individual cellular

level as *in situ* hybridization or *in situ* PCR and has the advantage that relatively large numbers of pure populations of cells can be collected for molecular analysis. Although only first described in 1996, this technique has already found wide application and is likely to continue to grow in popularity. Commercial LCM microscopes are available that will hasten the widespread utilization of this method.

LCM involves placing a thin transparent polymer film over a tissue section; visualizing the section with microscopy to identify the cells of interest; and then using a short-duration focused pulse from an infrared laser to selectively procure and attach the cells to the film. The technique can precisely target objects as small as individual cells with a resolution as small as 3–5 μm. The laser-heated polymer film expands focally and fills the voids in the tissue, resulting in a mechanically strong composite of polymer and cells. The film can then be lifted off from the tissue section, capturing the collected cells and leaving the noncollected cells and tissue still attached to the glass slide. The cells can then be placed directly into solution buffers for subsequent analysis of DNA, RNA, or protein levels by a variety of conventional molecular assays. LCM has the advantage of not requiring modification of standard techniques for molecular analysis, in contrast to the extensive method development that is necessary for *in situ* PCR.

LCM has already been used to study the pathogenesis of disease and to analyze protein or RNA expression in different populations of cells. Applications of this technique include analysis of gene expression in cells from various stages of tumor progression in different human malignancies; examination of RNA expression for leptin receptor isoforms in gastric epithelial cells; distribution of p53 mutations in aflatoxin B1-induced mouse lung tumors; and analysis of different cell populations. The combination of the ability to use standard molecular assays with the ability to selectively harvest distinct populations of cells indicate that LCM is likely to become the technique of choice for applications that require cellular localization of molecular analysis, possibly supplanting the use of *in situ* PCR and similar technically laborious methods.

VII. Confocal Microscopy

Advances in staining techniques such as immunofluorescence and in light microscopy technology continue to provide pathologists with new tools to analyze biologic systems. Traditional microscopy systems evaluate sections of tissue and provide information on what is essentially a two-dimensional snapshot of a three-dimensional system. Techniques such as stereology can provide a means to describe three-dimensional systems, but do not capture presentable images of these systems. Confocal microscopy integrates the power of computer technology with the optical precision of a scanning laser beam to capture and digitally compile high-resolution three-dimensional images from fluorescently labeled tissue specimens. The essential concept surrounding the confocal imaging system is that both illumination and detection are confined to the same spot in the specimen at any one time. In this way, only a highly resolved image is detected; out-of-focus regions are not captured.

Conventional epifluorescence microscopes illuminate and image all points of a specimen within the field of view at the same time. This is not usually a problem when observing a specimen visually, but capturing a representative image of specific fluorescently labeled structures can be problematic because the background fluorescence, whether occurring from sample autofluorescence or from the fluorescently labeled structures within the specimen themselves, overwhelms the signal from any particular focal plane of interest. These structures would be visible by eye, but representative images are difficult to capture.

Confocal microscopes have the advantage that they do not illuminate broad regions of a specimen. Instead, a tight beam of light (usually provided by a laser) illuminates a single point on the specimen. This beam of light is then scanned over the specimen, and information

from each point in a focal plane of interest is stored and integrated by computer to produce a high-contrast, two-dimensional image. Spatial filters are used to block unwanted fluorescence from both above and below the spatial point of interest so that images can be obtained from relatively thick sections, obviating the need for extensive fixation and sample preparation. A series of two-dimensional images can then be compiled to generate a high-resolution, three-dimensional image of fluorescently labeled structures within a specimen.

One of the largest advantages of confocal microscopy over other types of microscopy is that fluorescently labeled structures that are smaller than the limit of resolution can be observed in relatively thick specimens. This means that fluorescently labeled structures as small as cytoskeletal microtubules or small molecule drugs can be visualized in specimens that, because of the minimal fixation and processing of the tissue, more closely approximate an *in vivo* system. Thus it is possible to study the three-dimensional architecture of neurons in the brain without the need to dissect out the cell mechanically.

Researchers have also been able to use confocal microscopy to observe objects in living cells. This has been especially useful in looking at things such as gene expression and protein trafficking in cell lines. Because of the speed in which the laser is able to scan specimens and the ability to examine living cells, it is also possible to look at cellular events in real time. Using confocal microscopy, researchers were able to demonstrate internalization and transport pathways of insulin-like growth factor-I and insulin-like growth factor binding protein-3, the subcellular localization of metallothionein IIA, and trafficking differences in vascular endothelial growth factor isoforms. Confocal microscopy has also been used to evaluate slices of liver to examine liver viability and function after exposure to hepatotoxicants. Given the brevity of this review, only a small number of confocal microscopy applications used in toxicologic pathology could be presented. However, there are a number of good confocal microscopy review articles that describe other applications and provide more detail than what can be presented here.

VIII. Stereology

The traditional evaluation of morphologic end points on H&E slides, immunohistochemistry, or *in situ* hybridization yields a qualitative assessment of changes in cell numbers, morphology, and distribution based on the subjective evaluation of a trained observer. There is continual pressure to put more objectivity into this evaluation; one such effort involves the use of quantitation of morphologic parameters.

Quantitation potentially can yield increased information for the following reasons. First, differences that are subtle or difficult to detect qualitatively may be identified through quantitation. Second, the power of statistics can be used to analyze data and compare morphologic data to data from other end points. Finally, more reproducibly consistent data sets can be derived using similar quantitative techniques across different studies.

The direct two-dimensional measurement of cells or structures as they appear in histologic sections has been used extensively as a means of quantitating morphologic structures. However, these techniques are subject to artifacts that cannot be controlled. Thus, the numbers that are derived typically are biased numerically and can lead to false conclusions. A number of investigators believe that for quantitative purposes, two-dimensional section data must be related to three-dimensional spaces to derive meaningful quantitative data. Quantitation is only an improvement over qualitative evaluation if the numbers that are derived are accurate!

Sterology is the science that describes ways of quantitating objects in a three-dimensional space using two-dimensional sections. Initially, model-based methods were designed that relied on assumptions about particle shape, size, and orientation, and hence were also subject to numerical bias and erroneous conclusions. Because the assumptions could not be tested,

the degree of bias and hence the amount of error, could not be assessed. However, since the mid-1980s, the field of sterology has undergone a tremendous revolution with the development of new tools that are design based (assumption or model free) and essentially unbiased. Quantitation of morphologic parameters should be done using these stereologic principles in order to be assured of accurate results.

One advantage of the new tools is that they are highly efficient and require much less labor for measurements than previous morphometric techniques. However, sampling of tissues in a uniform nonbiased manner is still critical. It is extremely unusual that stereologic methods can be used on tissues that have been collected previously for other end points. In other words, stereology must be planned as part of the study to ensure a study design that considers non biased sampling and appropriate numbers of samples.

One of the most useful new stereologic tools is the dissector, which allows biological particles (e.g., cells or other discrete structures such as glomeruli) to be counted. With this technique, using defined counting rules, particles are counted using pairs of parallel planes that are separated by a known distance. Initially, physical dissector methods were used, e.g., two tissue sections a known distance apart could be evaluated. However, optical dissector techniques have essentially replaced the physical dissector. Focal planes within a thick tissue section can be used as the pairs for evaluation; confocal microscopy has particular advantages for this method.

In summary, new tools are available within the field of stereology that allow sophisticated and accurate quantitation of a variety of biological features. The danger is the inclination to attempt to "count" structures on sections taken from a standard toxicology study in an attempt to assign "real numbers" to the differences seen. There is a real danger of reaching the wrong conclusions unless the proper stereologic tools and appropriately collected samples are used for quantitation.

SUGGESTED READING

General

Ettlin, R. A., Oberholzer, M., Perentes, E., Ryffel, B., Kolopp, M., and Qureshi, S. R. (1991). A brief review of modern toxicologic pathology in regulatory and explanatory toxicity studies of chemicals. *Arch. Toxicol.* **65**(6), 445–453.

Gillett, N. A., and Chan, C. M. (1999). Molecular pathology in the preclinical development of biopharmaceuticals. *Toxicol. Pathol.* **27**(1), 48–52.

Malarkey, D. E., and Maronpot, R. R. (1996). Polymerase chain reaction and in situ hybridization: Applications in toxicological pathology. *Toxicol. Pathol.* **24**(1), 13–23.

Pilaro, A. M., and Serabian, M. A. (1999). Preclinical development trategies for novel gene therapeutic products. *Toxicol. Pathol.* **27**(1), 4–7.

Pilling, A. M. (1999). The role of the toxicologic pathologist in the preclinical safety evaluation of biotechnology-derived pharmaceuticals. *Toxicol. Pathol.* **27**(6), 678–88.

Schuh, J. C., and Harrington, K. A. (1999). Mechanisms of disease and injury: Utilization of mutants, monoclonals, and molecular methods. *Toxicol. Pathol.* **27**(1), 115–120.

Verdier, F., and Descotes, J. (1999). Preclinical safety evaluation of human gene therapy products. *Toxicol. Sci.* **47**(1), 9–15.

Immunohistochemistry

Anderson, L. M., Ward, J. M., Park, S. S., and Rice, J. M. (1989). Immunohistochemical localization of cytochromes P450 with polyclonal and monoclonal antibodies. *Pathol. Imunopathol. Res.* **8**, 61–94.

Arends, M. J., and Wyllie, A. H. (1991). Apoptosis: Mechanisms and roles in pathology. *Intl. Rev. Pathol.* **32**, 223.

Aschoff, A., Jantz, M., and Jirikowski, G. F. (1996). In-situ end labeling with bromodeoxyuridine: An advanced technique for the visualization of apoptotic cells in histological specimens. *Horm. Metab. Res.* **28**, 311–314.

Azimzadeh, A., Wolf, P., Dalmasso, A. P., Odeh, M., Beller, J.P., Fabre, M., Charreau, B., Thibaudeau, K., Cinqualbre, J., Soulillou, J. P., and Anegon, I. (1996). Assessment of hyperacute rejection in a rat-to-primate cardiac xenograft model. *Transplantation* **61**, 1305–1313.

Belinsky, S. A., Swafford, D. S., Finch, G. L., Mitchell, C. E., Kelly, G., Hahn, F. F., Anderson, M. W., and

Nikula, K. J. (1997). Alterations in the K-ras and p53 genes in rat lung tumors. *Environ. Health Perspect.* **105**, (Suppl. 4), 901–906.

Bogdanffy, M. S. (1990). Biotransformation enzymes in the rodent nasal mucosa: The value of a histochemical approach. *Environ. Health Perspect.* **85**, 177–186.

Bohle, R. M., Bonczkowitz, M., Altmannsberger, H. M., and Schulz, A. (1997). Immunohistochemical staining of microwave enhanced and nonenhanced nuclear and cytoplasmic antigens. *Biotech. Histochem.* **72**, 10–15.

Bursch, W., Oberhammer, F., and Schulte-Herman, R. (1992). Cell death by apoptosis and its protective role against disease. *TiPS* **13**, 245.

Cattoretti, G., Pileri, S., Parraviccini, C., Becker, M. H. B., Poggi, S., Bifulco, C., Key, G., D'amato, L., Sabattini, E., Feudale, E., Reynolds, F., Gerdes, J., and Rilke, F. (1993). Antigen unmasking on formalin-fixed, paraffin embedded tissue sections. *J. Pathol.* **171**, 83.

Center for Biologics Evaluation and Research. Points to Consider in the Manufacture and Testing of Monoclonal Antibody Products for Human Use (1997). USA Food and Drug Administration.

Charriaut-Marlangue, C., and Ben-Ari, Y. (1995). A cautionary note on the use of the TUNEL stain to determine apoptosis. *Neuroreport* **29**, 61–64.

Corcoran, G. B., Fix, L., Jones, D. P., Moslen, M. T., Nicotera, P., Oberhammer, F. A., and Buttyan, R. (1994). Apoptosis: Molecular control point in toxicity. *Toxicol. Appl. Pharmacol.* **128**, 169–181.

Cui, L., Takahashi, S., Tada, M., Kato, K., Yamada, Y., Kohri, K., and Shirai, T. (2000). Immunohistochemical detection of carcinogen-DNA adducts in normal human prostate tissues transplanted into the subcutis of athymic nude mice: Results with 2-amino-1-methyl-6-phenylimidazo[4,5-b]pyridine (phIP) and 3,2'-dimethyl-4-aminobiphenyl (DMAB) and relation to cytochrome P450s and N-acetyltransferase activity. *Jpn. J. Cancer Res.* **91**(1), 52–58.

D'Andrea, M. R., Rogahn, C. J., Damiano, B. P., and Adrade-Gordon, P. (1999). A combined histochemical and double immunohistochemical labeling protocol for simultaneous evaluation of four cellular markers in restenotic arteries. *Biotech. Histochem.* **74**, 172–180.

DeLisser, H. M., Newman, P. J., and Albelda, S. M. (1993). Platelet endothelial cell adhesion molecule (CD31). *Curr. Top. Microbiol. Immunol.* **184**, 37–45.

D'Herde, K., De Pestel, G., and Roels, F. (1994). In situ end labeling of fragmented DNA in induced ovarian atresia. *Biochem. Cell Biol.* **72**, 573.

Eichmuller, S., Stevenson, P. A., and Paus, R. (1996). A new method for double immunolabelling with primary antibodies from identical species. *Immuno. Meth.* **190**, 255–265.

Eldridge, S. R., and Goldsworthy, S. M. (1996). Cell proliferation rates in common cancer target tissues of

B6C3F1 mice and F344 rats: Effects of age, gender, and choice of marker. *Fundam. App. Toxico.* **32**, 159–167.

Fehrenback, H., Kasper, M., Haase, M., Schuh, D., and Muller, M. (1999). Differential immunolocalization of VEGF in rat and human adult lung, and in experimental rat lung fibrosis: light, fluorescence, and electron microscopy. *Anat. Rec.* **254**, 61–73.

Foley, J. F., Dietrich, D. R., Swenberg, J. A., and Maronpot, R. R. (1991). Detection and evaluation of proliferating cell nuclear antigen (PCNA) in rat tissue by an improved immunohistochemical procedure. *J. Histotechnol.* **14**, 237–241.

Fung, K. M., Messing, A., Lee, V.M.-Y, and Trojanowski, J. Q. (1992). A novel modification of the avidin-biotin-complex method for immunohistochemical studies of transgenic mice with murine monoclonal antibodies. *J. Histochem. Cytochem.* **40**, 1319–1328.

Garner, M. H., and Kong, Y. (1999). Lens epithelium and fiber Na, K-ATPases: Distribution and localization by immunocytochemistry. *Invest. Ophthalmol. Vis. Sci.* **40**, 2291–2298.

Gavrieli, Y., Sherman, Y., and Ben-Sasson, S. A. (1992). Identification of programmed cell death *in situ* with specific labeling of nuclear DNA fragmentation. *J. Cell Biol.* **119**, 493.

Ghanayem, B. I., Elwell, M. R., and Eldridge, S. R. (1997). Effects of the carcinogen, acrylonitrile, on forestomach cell proliferation and apoptosis in the rat: Comparison with methacrylonitrile. *Carcinogenesis* **18**, 675–680.

Gold, R., Schmied, M., Rothe, G., Zischler, H., Breitschope, H., Wekerle, H., and Lassmann, H. (1993). Detection of DNA fragmentation in apoptosis: application of *in situ* nick translation to cell culture systems and tissue sections. *J. Histochem. Cytochem.* **41**, 1023.

Grasl-Kraupp, B., Ruttkay-Nedecky, B., Koudelka, H., Bukowska, K., Bursch, W., and Schulte-Hermann, R. (1995). *In situ* detection of fragmented DNA (TUNEL Assay) fails to discriminate among apoptosis, necrosis, and autolytic cell death: A cautionary note. *Hepatology* **21**, 1465.

Hall, P. A., and Woods, A. L. (1990). Immunohistochemical markers of cellular proliferation: achievements, problems and prospects. *Cell Tissue Kinet.* **23**, 505–522.

Hall, W. C., and Rojko, J. L. (1996). The use of immunohistochemistry for evaluating the liver. *Toxicol. Pathol.* **24**, 4–12.

Harada, Y., and Yahara, I. (1993). Pathogenesis of toxicity with human-derived interleukin-2 in experimental animals. *Int. Rev. Exp. Pathol.* **34** (Pt. A), 37–55

Hierck, B. P., Iperen, L. V., Gittenberger-de Groot, C., and Poelmann, R. E. (1994). Modified indirect immunodetection allows study of murine tissue with mouse monoclonal antibodies. *J. Histochem. Cytochem.* **42**, 1499–1502.

Huppertz, B., Frank, H.-G, and Kaufmann, P. (1999). The apoptosis cascade: morphological and immunohistochemical methods for its visualization. *Anat. Embryol.* **200**, 1–18.

Iseki, S. (1986). DNA strand breaks in rat tissues as detected by *in situ* nick translation. *Exp. Cell Res.* **167**, 311.

Johnson, C. W. (1999). Issues in immunohistochemistry. *Toxicol. Pathol* **27**, 246–248.

Jones, H. B. (1988). The role of ultrastructural investigations in neurotoxicology. *Toxicology* **49**, 3–15.

Key, G., Becker, M. H., Baron, B., *et al.* (1992). Preparation and immunobiochemical characterization of new Ki-67 equivalent murine monoclonal antibodies (MIB 1–3) generated against recombinant parts of the Ki-67 antigen. *Anal. Cell. Pathol.* **4**, 181.

Knapp, W., Dorken, B., Reiber, E. P., *et al.* (eds.) (1989). "Leukocyte Typing IV: White Cell Differentiation Antigens." Oxford Univ. Press, New York.

Kressel, M., and Groscurth, P. (1994). Distinction of apoptotic and necrotic cell death by *in situ* labeling of fragmented DNA. *Cell Tissue Res.* **278**, 549.

Lee, C. C., Ichihara, T., Yamamoto, S., Wanibuchi, H., Sugimura, K., Wada, S., Kishimoto, T., and Fukushima, S. (1999). Reduced expression of the CDK inhibitor p27 (KIP1) in rat two-stage bladder carcinogenesis and its association with expression profiles of p21 (WAF1/Cip1) and p53. *Carcinogenesis* **20**, 1697–1708.

Li, S-L., Kaaya, E., Feichtinger, H., Biberfeld, G., and Biberfeld, P. (1993). Immunohistochemical distribution of leucocyte antigens in lymphoid tissues of cynomolgus monkeys (*Macaca fascicularis*). *J. Med. Primatol.* **22**, 285–293.

Li, Y., Chopp, M., Jiang, N., and Zaloga, C. (1995). *In situ* detection of DNA fragmentation after focal cerebral ischemia in mice. *Mol. Brain Res.* **28**, 164.

Mackay, F., and Browning, J. L. (1998). Turning off follicular dendritic cells. *Nature* **395** (6697), 26–27.

Mackay, F., Majeau, G. R., Lawton, P., Hochman, P. S., and Browning, J. L. (1997). Lymphotoxin but not tumor necrosis factor functions to maintain splenic architecture and humoral responsiveness in adult mice. *Eur. J. Immunol.* **27**, 2033–2042.

Migheli, A., Attanasio, A., and Schiffer, D. (1995). Ultrastructural detection of DNA strand breaks in apoptotic neural cells by *in situ* end-labeling techniques. *J. Pathol.* **176**, 27–35.

Monteith, D. K., Horner, M. J., Gillett, N. A., Butler, M., Geary, R., Burckin, T., Ushiro-Watanabe, T., and Levin, A. A. (1999). Evaluation of the renal effects of an antisense phosphorothioate oligodeoxynucleotide in monkeys. *Toxicol. Pathol.* **27**, 307–317.

Moore, M. M., Tsuda, H., Tamano, S., Hagiwara, A., Imaida, K., Shirai, T., and Ito. N. (1999). Marriage of a medium-term liver model to surrogate markers. A practical approach for risk and benefit assessment. *Toxicol. Pathol.* **27,** 237–242.

Mundle, S., Iftikhar, A., Shetty, V., Dameron, S., Wright-Quinones, V., Marcus, B., Loew, J., Gregory, S., and Raza, A. (1994). Novel *in situ* double labeling for simultaneous detection of proliferation and apoptosis. *J. Histochem. Cytochem.* **42,** 1533.

Nakamura, T., Sakai, T., and Hotchi, M. (1995). Histochemical demonstration of DNA double strand breaks by *in situ* 3′-tailing reaction in apoptotic endometrium. *Biotechnic. Histochem.* **70,** 33.

Nichol, K. A., Depczynski, B. B., and Cunningham, A. M. (1999). Characterization of hypothalamic neurons expressing a neuropeptide receptor, GALR2, using combined *in situ* hybridization: Immunohistochemistry. *Methods* **18,** 481–486.

Okudela, K., Ito, T., Mitsui, H., Hayashi, H., Udaka, N., Kanisawa, M., and Kitamura, H. (1999). The role of p53 in bleomycin-induced DNA damage in the lung. A comparative study with the small intestine. *Am. J. Pathol.* **155,** 1341–1351.

O'Reilly, M. A., Staversky, R. J, Watkins, R. H., and Maniscalco, W. M. (1998). Accumulation of p21 (Cip1/WAF1) during hyperoxic lung injury in mice. *Am. J. Respir. Cell. Mol. Biol.* **19,** 777–785.

Porter, H. J., Heryet, A., Quantrill, A. M., and Fleming, K. A. (1990). Combined non-isotopic *in situ* hybridisation and immunohistochemistry on routine paraffin was embedded tissue: Identification of cell type infected by human parvovirus and demonstration of cytomegalovirus DNA and antigen in renal infection. *J. Clin. Pathol.* **43,** 129–132.

Rimsza, L. M., Vela, E. E., Frutiger, Y. M., Richter, L. C., Grogan, T. M., and Bellamy, W. T. (1996). Combined *in situ* hybridization and immunohistochemistry for automated detection of cytomegalovirus and p53. *Mol. Diagn.* **4,** 291–296.

Roberts, R. A., Nebert, D. W., Hickman, J. A., Richburg, J. H., and Goldsworthy, T. L. (1997). Perturbation of the mitosis/apoptosis balance: A fundamental mechanism in toxicology. *Fundam. Appl. Toxicol.* **38,** 107–115.

Roslin, M. S., Tranbaugh, R. E., Panza, A., Coons, M. S., Kim, Y. D., Chang, T., Cunningham, J. N., and Norin, A. J. (1992). One-year monkey heart xenograft survival in cyclosporine-treated baboons. Suppression of the xenoantibody response with total-lymphoid irradiation. *Transplantation* **54,** 949–955.

Sabourin, C. L., Wang, Q. S., Ralston, S. L., Evans, J., Coate, J., Herzog, C. R., Jones, S. L., Weghorst, C. M., Kelloff, G. J., Lubet, R. A., You, M., and Stoner, G. D. (1998). Expression of cell cycle proteins in 4 - (methylnitrosamino)-1-(3-pyridyl)-1-butanone-induced mouse lung tumors. *Exp. Lung Res.* **24,** 499–521.

Sanders, E. J. (1997). Methods for detecting apoptotic cells in tissues. *Histol. Histopathol.* **12**(4), 1169–1177.

Sanders, E. J., and Wride, M. A. (1996). Ultrastructural identification of apoptotic nuclei using the TUNEL technique. *Histochem. J.* **28,** 275–281.

Sandusky, G. E., Horton, P. J., and Wightman, K. A. (1986). Use of monoclonal antibodies to human lymphocytes to identify lymphocyte subsets in lymph nodes of the rhesus monkey and the dog. *J. Med. Primatol.* **15,** 441–451.

Santella, R. M. (1999). Immunological methods for detection of carcinogen-DNA damage in humans. *Cancer Epidemiol. Biomark. Prev.* **8**(9), 733–739.

Schenk, D., Barbour, R., Dunn, W., Gordon, G., Grajeda, H., Guido, T., Hu, K., Huang, J., Johnson-Wood, K., Khan., K., Kholodenko, D., Lee, M., Liao, Z., Lieberburg, I., Motter, R., Mutter, L., Soriano, F., Shopp, G., Vasquez, N., Vandevert, C., Walker, S., Wogulis, M., Yednock, T., Games, D., and Seubert, P. (1999). Immunization with amyloid-β attenuates Alzheimer-disease-like pathology in the PDAPP mouse. *Nature* **400,** 173–177.

Schlossman, S., Bloumsell, S. L., Gilks, W., *et al.* (eds.) (1995). "Leukocyte Typing V: White Cell Differentiation Antigens." Oxford Univ. Press, New York.

Shapiro, F., Cahill, C., Malatantis, G., and Nayak, R. C. (1995). Transmission electron microscopic demonstration of vimentin in rat osteoblast and osteocyte cell bodies and processes using the immunogold technique. *Anat. Rec.* **241,** 39–48.

Shi, S-R., Gu, J., Kalra, K. L., Chen, T., Cote, R. J., and Taylor, C. R. (1995). Antigen retrieval technique: A novel approach to immunohistochemistry on routinely processed tissue sections. *Cell Vision* **2,** 6.

Speel, E. J. (1999). Robert Feulgen Prize Lecture 1999. Detection and amplification systems for sensitive, multiple-target DNA and RNA *in situ* hybridization: Looking inside cells with a spectrum of colors. *Histochem. Cell. Biol.* **112,** 89–113.

Stevens, H. P. J. D., van der Kwast, T. H., Timmermans, A., Stouten, N., and Jonker, M. (1991). Monoclonal antibodies for immunohistochemical labeling of immunocompetent cells in frozen sections of rhesus monkey tissues. *J. Med. Primatol.* **20,** 386–393.

Strater, J., Walczak, H., Krammer, P. H., and Moller, P. (1996). Simultaneous *in situ* detection of mRNA and apoptotic cells by combined hybridization and TUNEL. *J. Histochem. Cytochem.* **44,** 1497–1499.

Tuson, J. R., Pascoe, E. W., and Jacob, D. (1990). A novel immunohistochemical technique for demonstration of specific binding of human monoclonal antibodies to human cryostat tissue sections. *J. Histochem. Cytochem.* **38,** 923.

Wang, Q. S., Papanikolaou, A., Sabourin, C. L., and Rosenberg, D. W. (1998). Altered expression of cyclin D1 and cyclin-dependent kinase 4 in azoxymethane-induced mouse colon tumorigenesis. *Carcinogenesis* **19,** 2001–2006.

Wijsman, J. H., Jonker, R. R., Keijzer, R., Van de Velde, C. J. H., Cornelisse, C. J., and Van Dierendonck, J. H. (1993). A new method to detect apoptosis in paraffin sections: *In situ* end-labeling of fragmented DNA. *J. Histochem. Cytochem.* **41**, 7.

Willingham, M. C. (1999). Cytochemical methods for the detection of apoptosis. *J. Histochem. Cytochem.* **9**, 1101–1110.

Yang, Y., Nair, J., Barbin, A., and Bartsch, H. (2000). Immunohistochemical detection of 1,N(6)-ethenodeoxyadenosine, a promutagenic DNA adduct, in liver of rats exposed to vinyl chloride or an iron overload. *Carcinogenesis* **21**(4), 777–781.

Yawalkar, N., Egli, F., Hari, Y., Nievergelt, H., Braathen, L. R., and Pichler, W. J. (2000). Infiltration of cytotoxic T cells in drug-induced cutaneous eruptions. *Clin. Exp. Allergy.* **30**(6), 847–855.

Yoshida, T., Makita, Y., Tsutsumi, T., Nagata, S., Tashiro, F., Yoshida, F., Sekijima, M., Tamura, S., Harada, T., Maita, K., and Ueno, Y. (1998). Immunohistochemical localization of microcystin-LR in the liver of mice: a study on the pathogenesis of microcystin-LR-induced hepatotoxicity. *Toxicol. Pathol.* **26**(3), 411–418.

In Situ Hybridization

Abe, K., Ko., M., and MacGregor, G. (1998). A systematic molecular genetic approach to study mammalian germline development. *Int. J. Dev. Biol. G.* (7 Spec. No.), 1051–1065.

DeLellis, R. A. (1994). *In situ* hybridization techniques for the analysis of gene expression: Applications in tumor pathology. *Hum. Pathol.* **25**, 580.

Delker, D. A., Yano, B. L., and Gollapudi, B. B. (1999). V-Ha-ras gene expression in liver and kidney of transfenic Tg-AC mice following chemically induced tissue injury. *Toxicol. Sci.* **50**(1), 90–97.

de Sauvage, F. J., Keshav, S., Kuang, W. J., Gillett, N., Henzel, W., and Goeddel, D. V. (1992). Precursor structure, expression, and tissue distribution of human guanylin. *Proc. Natl. Acad. Sci. USA* **89**(19), 9089–9093.

Doughty, S., Ferrier, R., Hillan, K., and Jackson, D. (1995). The effects of ZENECA ZD8731, an angiotensin II antagonist, on renin expression by juxtaglomerular cells in the rat: Comparison of protein and mRNA expression as detected by immunohistochemistry and *in situ* hybridization. *Toxicol. Pathol.* **23**(3), 256–261.

Ettlin, R., Oberholzer, M., Perentes, E., Ryffel, B., Kolopp, M., and Qureshi, S. (1991). A brief review of modern toxicologic pathology in regulatory and explanatory toxicity studies of chemicals. *Arch. Toxicol.* **65**(6), 445–453.

Fetissov, S., and Marsais, F., (1999). Combination of immunohistochemical and *in situ* hybridization methods to reveal tyrosine hydroxylase and oxytocin and vasopressin mRNAs in magnocellular neurons of obese Zucker rats. *Brain Res. Brain Res. Protoc.* **4**(1), 36–43.

Fletcher, J. (1999). DNA *in situ* hybridization as an adjunct in tumor diagnosis. *Am. J. Clin. Pathol.* **112** (1 Suppl. 1), S11–S18.

Gall, J. G., and Pardue, M. (1969). Formation and detection of RNA-DNA hybrid molecules in cytological preparations. *Proc. Natl. Acad. Sci. USA* **63**, 378.

Gillett, N., and Chan, C. (1999). Molecular pathology in the preclinical development of biopharmaceuticals. *Toxicol. Pathol.* **27**(1), 48–52.

Holm, R., Karlsen, F., and Nesland, J. M. (1992). *In situ* hybridization with non-isotopic probes using different detection systems. *Mod. Pathol.* **5**, 315.

Hwang, P., Montone, K., Gannon, F., Senior, B., Lanza, D., and Kennedy, D. (1999). Application of *in situ* hybridization techniques in the diagnosis of chronic sinusitis. *Am. J. Rhinol.* **13**(5), 335–338.

Kadkol, S., Gage, W., and Pasternack, G. (1999). *In situ* hybridization: Theory and practice. *Mol. Diagn.* **4**(3), 169–183.

Khan, K., Venturini, C., Bunch, R., Brassard, J., Koki, A., Morris, D., Trump, B., Maziasz, T., and Alden, C. (1998). Interspecies differences in renal localization of cyclooxygenase isoforms: Implications in nonsteroidal anti-inflammatory drug-related nephrotoxicity. *Toxicol. Pathol.* **26**(5), 612–620.

Knowles, M., Noone, P., Hohneker, K., Johnson, L., Boucher, R., Efthimiou, J., Crawford, C., Brown, R., Schwartzbach, C., and Pearlman, R. (1998). A double-blind, placebo controlled, dose ranging study to evaluate the safety and biological efficacy of the lipid-DNA complex GR213487B in the nasal epithelium of adult patients with cystic fibrosis. *Hum. Gene Ther.* **9**(2), 249–269.

Lewis, M. E., Sherman, T. G., and Watson, S. J. (1985). *In situ* hybridization histochemistry with synthetic oligonucleotides: Strategies and methods. *Peptides* **6**, 75.

Lu, L. H., and Gillett, N. A. (1994). An optimized protocol for *in situ* hybridization using PCR-Generated 33-P-labeled riboprobes. *Cell Vision* **1**, 169.

Luoh, S., Di Marco, F., Levin, N., Armanini, M., Xie, M., Nelson, C., Bennett, G., Williams, M., Spencer, S., Gurney, A., and de Sauvage, F. (1997). Cloning and characterization of a human leptin receptor using a biologically active leptin immunoadhesin. *J. Mol. Endocrinol. F.* **1**, 77–85.

Malarkey, D., and Maronpot, R. (1996). Polymerase chain reaction and *in situ* hybridization: Applications in toxicological pathology. *Pathology* **24**(1), 13–23.

Moorman, F., De Boer, P. A., Vermeulen, J. L., and Lamers, W. H. (1993). Practical aspects of radio-isotopic *in situ* hybridization on RNA. *Histochem. J.* **25**, 251.

Oguro, K., Oguro, N., Kojima, T., Grooms, S., Calderone, A., Zheng, X., Bennett, M., and Zukin, R. (1999). Knockdown of AMPA receptor GluR2 expression causes delayed neurodegeneration and increases damage by sublethal ischemia in hippocampal CA1 and CA3 neurons. *J. Neurosci.* **19**(21), 9218–27.

Pacchioni, Papotti, M., Bonino, F., Bussolati, G., and Negro, F. (1992). Detection of cytomegalovirus by *in situ* hybridization using a digoxigenin-tailed oligonucleotide. *Liver* **12**, 257.

Parks, W., and Roby, J. (1994). Consequences of prolonged inhalation of ozone on F344/N rats: Collaborative studies. IV. Effects on expression of extracellular matrix genes. *Res. Rep. Health. Eff. Inst.* **65**, Pt 4, 3–29.

Phan, T., Gray, A., Nyce, J., and Mcginty, J. (1999). Autoradiographic evidence that intrastriatal administration of adenosine A(1) receptor antisense oligodeoxynucleotide decreases adenosine A(1) receptors in the rate striatum and cortex. *Brain Res. Mol. Brain Res.* **72**(2), 226–230.

Pilaro, A. M., and Serabian, M. (1999). Preclinical development strategies for novel gene therapeutic products. *Toxicol. Pathol.* **27**(1), 4–7.

Pilling, A. M. (1999). The role of the toxicologic pathologist in the preclinical safety evaluation of biotechnology-derived pharmaceuticals. *Toxicol. Pathol.* **27**(6), 678–688.

Poljak, M., Seme, K., and Gale, N. (1998). Detection of human papillomaviruses in tissue specimens. *Adv. Anat. Pathol.* **5**(4), 216–234.

Rihn, B., Bottin, M., Coulais, C., Zissu, D., and Edorh, A. (1995). Use of non-radioactive methods for the determination of the expression, the sequence and the copy-number of transgene in mice. *Cell. Mol. Biol.* **41**(7), 907–915.

Rudmann, D., and Durham, S. (1999). Utilization of genetically altered animals in the pharmaceutical industry. *Toxicol. Pathol.* **27**(1), 111–114.

Sasaki, M., Wizigmann-Voos, S., Risau, W., and Plate, K. (1999). Retrovirus producer cells encoding antisense VEGF prolong survival of rats with intracranial GS9L gliomas. *Int. J. Dev. Neurosci.* **17**(5–6), 579–591.

Schomberg, D. W., Couse, J., Mukherjee, A., Lubahn, D., Sar, M., Mayo, K., and Korach, K. S. (1999). Targeted distribution of the estrogen receptor-alpha gene in female mice: Characterization of ovarian responses and phenotype in the adult. *Endocrinology* **140**(6), 2733–2744.

Schuh, J., and Harrington, K. (1999). Mechanisms of disease and injury: Utilization of mutants, monoclonals, and molecular methods. *Toxicol. Pathol.* **27**(1), 115–120.

Shoda, T., Onodera, H., Takeda, M., Uneyama, C., Imazawa, T., Takegawa, K., Yasuhara, K., Watanabe, T., Hirose, M., and Mitsumori, K. (1999). Liver tumor promoting effects of fenbendazole in rats. *Toxicol. Pathol.* **27**(5), 553–62.

Shyjan, W., de Sauvage, F. J., Gillett, N. A., Goeddel, D. V., and Lowe, D. G. (1992). Retinal guanylyl cyclase: A photoreceptor specific membrane guanylyl cyclase. *Neuron* **9**, 727.

Singer, R. H., Lawrence, J. B., and Villnave, C. (1986). Optimization of *in situ* hybridization using isotopic and non-isotopic detection methods. *Biotechniques* **4**, 230.

Speel, E. J., Hopman, A., and Komminoth, P. (1999). Amplification methods to increase the sensitivity of in situ hybridization: Play card(s). *J. Histochem. Cytochem.* **47**(3), 281–288.

Speel, E. J., Saremaslani, P., Roth, J., Hopma, A., and Komminoth, P. (1998). Improved mRNA in situ hybridization on formaldehyde-fixed and paraffin-embedded tissue using signal amplification with different haptenized tyramides. *Histochem. Cell Biol.* **110**(6), 571–577.

Sterman, D. H., Treat, J., Litzky, L., Amin, K., Coonrod, L., Molnar-Kimber, K., Recio, A., Knox, L., Wilson, J., Albelda, S., and Kaiser, L. (1998). Adenovirus-mediated herpes simplex virus thymidine kinase/ganciclovir gene therapy in patients with localized malignancy: Results of a phase I clinical trial in malignant mesothelioma. *Hum. Gene Ther.* **9**(7), 1083–1092.

Stoler, M. H. (1993). In situ hybridization a research technique or routine diagnostic test? *Arch. Pathol. Lab. Med.* **117**, 478.

Suzuki, T., Ogata, A., Tashiro, K., Nagashima, K., Tamura, M., Yasui, K., and Nishihira, J. (1999). A method for detection of a cytokine and its mRNA in the central nervous system of the developing rat. *Brain Res. Brain Res. Protoc.* **4**(3), 271–279.

Tennant, R. W., Tice, R. R., and Spalding, J. W. (1998). The transgenic Tg.AC mouse model for identification of chemical carcinogens. *Toxicol. Lett.* **Dec. 28**, 102–103, 465–471.

Trabandt, A., Gay, R. E., Sukhatme, V. P., and Gay, S. (1995). Enzymatic detection systems for non-isotopic in situ hybridization using biotinylated cDNA probes. *Histochem. J.* **27**, 280.

Verdier, F., and Descotes, J. (1999). Preclinical safety evaluation of human gene therapy products. *Toxicol. Sci.* **47**(1), 9–15.

Viale, G., and Dell'Orto, P., (1992). Non-radioactive nucleic acid probes: Labeling and detection procedures. *Liver* **12**, 243.

Warren, R. S., Yuan, H., Matli, M. R., Gillett, N. A., and Ferrara, N. (1995). Regulation by vascular endothelial growth factor of human colon cancer tumorigenesis in a mouse model of experimental liver metastasis. *J. Clin. Invest.* **95**, 1789.

Wilmott, R., Amin, R., Perez, C., Wert, S., Keller, G., Boivin, G., Hirsch, R., De Inocencio, J., Lu, P., Reising, S., Yei, S., Whitsett, J., and Trapnell, B. (1996). Safety of adenovirus-mediated transfer of the human cystic fibrosis transmembrane conductance regulator cDNA to the lungs of nonhuman primates. *Hum. Gene Ther.* **7**(3), 301–318.

Xiao, W., Berta, S., Lu, M., Moscioni, A., Tazelaar, J., and Wilson, J. (1998). Adeno-associated virus as a vector for liver-directed gene therapy. *J. Virol.* **72**(12), 10222–10226.

Yang, H., Wanner, I., Roper, S., and Chaudhari, N. (1999). An optimized method for in situ hybridization with signal amplification that allows the detection of rare mRNAs. *J. Histochem. Cytochem.* **47**(4), 431–446.

Zhang, G. X., Xiao, B., Bai, X., van der Meide, P., Orn, A., and Link, H. (1999). Mice with IFN-gamma receptor deficiency are less susceptible to experimental autoimmune myasthenia gravis. *J. Immunol.* **162**(7), 3775–3781.

Flow Cytometry

Bigos, M., Baumgarth, N., Jager, G. C., Herman, O. C., Nozaki, T., Stovel, R. T., Parks, D. R., Herzenbert, L. A. (1999). Nine color eleven parameter immunophenotyping using three color flow cytometry. *Cytometry* **36**(1), 36–45.

Criswell, K. A., Bleavins, M. R., Zielinski, D., and Zandee, J. C. (1998). Comparison of flow cytometric and manual bone marrow differentials in Wistar rats. *Cytometry* **32**(1), 9–17.

Darzynkiewicz, Z., Bedner, E., Li, X., Gorczyca, W., and Melamed, M. R. (1999). Laser-scanning cytometry: A new instrumentation with many applications. *Exp. Cell Res.* **249**(1), 1–12.

Gossett, K. A., Narayanan, P. K., Williams, D. M., Gore, E. R., Herzyk, D. J., Hart, T. K., and Sellers, T. S. (1999). Flow cytometry in the preclinical development of biopharmaceuticals. *Toxicol. Pathol.* **27**(1), 32–37.

Gratama, J. W., D'hautcourt, J. L., Mandy, F., Rothe, G., Barnett, D., Janossy, G., Papa, S., Schmitz, G., and Lenkei, R. (1998). Flow cytometric quantitation of immunofluorescence intensity: Problems and perspectives. *Eur. Wor. Group Clin. Cell. Anal. Cytom.* **33**(2), 166–178.

Islam, D., Lindberg, A. A., and Christensson, B. (1995). Peripheral blood cell preparation influences the level of expression of leukocyte cell surface markers as assessed with quantitative multicolor flow cytometry. *Cytometry* **22**(2), 128–134.

Lappin, P. B., Ross, K. L., King, L. E., Fraker, P. J., and Roth, R. A. (1998). The response of pulmonary vascu-lar endothelial cells to monocrotaline pyrrole: Cell proliferation and DNA synthesis in vitro and in vivo. *Toxicol. Appl. Pharmacol.* **150**, 37–48.

Lee, T. K., Wiley, AL., Jr., Esinhart, J. D., Riley, R. S., and Blackburn, L. D. (1993). Variations associated with disaggregation methods in DNA flow cytometry. *Anal. Quant. Cytol. Histol.* **15**(3), 195–200.

Lenkei, R., Gratama, J. W., Rothe, G., Schmitz, G., D'hautcourt, J. L., Arekrans, A., Mandy, F., and Marti, G. (1998). Performance of calibration standards for antigen quantitation with flow cytometry. *Cytometry* **33**(2), 188–196.

Maino, V. C., and Picker, L. J. (1998). Identification of functional subsets by flow cytometry: Intracellular detection of cytokine expression. *Cytometry* **34**(5), 207–215.

Montenegro, V., Chiamolera, M., Launay, P., Goncalves, C. R., and Monteiro, R. C. (2000). Impaired expression of IgA Fc receptors (CD89) by blood phagocytic cells in ankylosing spondylitis. *J. Rheuatol.* **27**(2), 411–417.

Mossman, B. T. (1999). Environmental pathology:New directions and opportunities. *Toxicol. Pathol.* **27**(2), 180–186.

Omerod, M. G. (1998). The study of apoptotic cells by flow cytometry. *Leukemia* **12**(7), 1013–1025.

Ramanathan, M. (1997). Flow cytometry applications in pharmacodynamics and drug delivery. *Pharm. Res.* **14**(9), 1106–1114.

Rea, I. M., McNerlan, S. E., and Alexander, H. D. (1999). CD69, CD25, and HLA-DR activation antigen expression on CD3+ lymphocytes and relationship to serum TNF-alpha, IFN-gamma, and sIL-2R levels in aging. *Exp. Gerontol.* **34**(1), 79–93.

Rosen, J. L., Tran, H. T., Lackey, A., and Viselli, S. M. (1999). Sex-related immune changes in young mice. *Immunol. Invest.* **28**(4), 247–256.

Shapiro, H. M. (1995). "Practical Flow Cytometry" (H. M. Shapiro, ed.). Wiley-Liss, New York.

Steptoe, R. J., Li, W., Fu, F., O'Connel, P. J., and Thomson, A. W. (1999). Trafficking of APC for liver allografts of Flt3L-treated donors: Augmentation of potent allostimulatory cells in recipient lymphoid tissue is associated with a switch from tolerance to rejection. *Transpl. Immunol.* **7**(1), 51–57.

Yokoyama, W. M., Maxfield, S. R., and Shevach, E. M. (1989). Very early (VEA) and very late (VLA) activation antigens have distinct function in T lymphocyte activation. *Immunol. Rev.* **109**, 153–176.

In Situ PCR

Bagasra, O., Hauptman, S. P., Lischner, H. W., Sachs, M., and Pomerantz, R. J. (1992). Detection of human immunodeficiency virus type 1 provirus in mononuclear cells by *in situ* polymerase chain reaction. *N. Engl. J. Med.* **326**, 1385.

Bagasra, O., Seshamma, T., and Poomerantz, R. J. (1993). Polymerase chain reaction *in situ*: Intracellular amplification and detection of HIV-1 proviral DNA and other specific genes. *J. Immunol. Methods* **158**, 131–145.

Catzavelos, C., Ruedy, C., Stewart, A. K., and Dube, I. (1998). A novel method for the direct quantification of gene transfer into cells using PCR *in situ*. *Gene Ther.* **5**(6), 755–760.

Chiu, K.-P., Cohen, S. H., Morris, D. W., and Jordan, G. W. (1992). Intracellular amplification of proviral DNA in tissue sections using the polymerase chain reaction. *J. Histochem. Cytochem.* **40**, 333.

De Bault, L. E., and Gu, J. (1996). *In situ* hybridization, in situ transcription, and in situ polymerase chain reaction. *Scanning Microsc. Suppl.* **10**, 27–44.

Embleton, M. J., Gorochov, G., Jones, P. T., and Winter, G. (1992). In-cell PCR from mRNA: Amplifying and linking the rearranged immunoglobulin heavy and light chain V-genes within single cells. *Nucleic Acids Res.* **20**, 3831.

Embretson, J., Zupanic, M., Beneke, T., Till, M., Wolinsky, S., Ribas, J. L., Burke, A., and Haase, A. T. (1993). Analysis of human immunodeficiency virus-infected tissues by amplification and *in situ* hybridization reveals latent and permissive infections at single-cell resolution. *Proc. Natl. Acad. Sci. USA* **90**, 357.

Haase, A. T., Retzel, E. F., and Staskus, K. A. (1990). Amplification and determination of lentiviral DNA inside cells. *Proc. Natl. Acad. Sci.* **87**, 4971.

Heniford, B. W., Siu-Shum, A., Leonberger, M., and Hendler, F. J. (1993). Variation in cellular EGF receptor mRNA expression demonstrated by *in situ* reverse transcriptase polymerase chain reaction. *Nucleic Acids Res.* **21**, 3159.

Jilbert, A. R., Burrell, C. J., Gowans, E. J., and Rowland, R. (1986). Histological aspects of in situ hybridization. *Histochemistry* **85**, 505.

Jin, L., and Lloyd, R. V. (1997). In situ hybridization: Methods and applications. *J. Clin. Lab. Anal.* **11**, 2–9.

Komminoth, P., Heitz, P. U., and Long, A. A. (1994). In situ polymerase chain reaction: General methodology and recent advances. *Verh. Dtsch. Ges. Pathol.* **78**, 146–512.

Komminoth, P., and Long, A. A. (1993). *In-situ* polymerase chain reaction: An overview of methods, applications and limitations of a new molecular technique. *Virch. Arch. B Cell Pathol.* **64**, 67.

Komminoth, P., Long, A. A., Ray, R., and Wolfe, H. J. (1992). *In situ* polymerase chain reaction detection of viral DNA, single copy genes and gene rearrangements in cell suspensions and cytospins. *Diagn. Mol. Pathol.* **1**, 85.

Li, H. H., Gyllensten, U. B., Cui, X. F., Saiki, R. K., Erlich, H. A., and Arnheim, N. (1988). Amplification and analysis of DNA sequences in single human sperm and diploid cells. *Nature* **335**, 414.

Long, A. A. (1998). *In-situ* polymerase chain reaction: Foundation of the technology and today's options. *Eur. J. Histochem.* **42**, 101–109.

Long, A. A., Komminoth, P., Lee, E., and Wolfe, H. J. (1993). Comparison of indirect and direct *in-situ* polymerase chain reaction in cell preparations and tissue sections. Detection of viral DNA, gene rearrangements and chromosomal translocations. *Histochemistry* **99**, 151–162.

Malarkey, D. E., and Maronpot, R. R., (1996). Polymerase chain reaction and in situ hybridization: Applications in toxicological pathology. *Toxicol. Pathol.* **24**, 13–23.

Mee, A. P., Denton, J., Hoyland, J. A., Davies, M., and Mawer, E. B. (1997). Quantification of vitamin D receptor mRNA in tissue sections demonstrates the relative limitations of *in situ*-reverse transcriptase-polymerase chain reaction. *J. Pathol.* **182**, 22–28.

Nuovo, G. J. (1992). "PCR *in Situ* Hybridization." Raven Press, New York.

Nuovo, G. J., Gallery, F., Horn, R., MacConnell, P., and Bloch, W. (1993). Importance of different variables for enhancing *in situ* detection of PCR-amplified DNA. *PCR Meth. Appl.* **2**(4), 305–312.

Nuovo, G. J., Gallery, F., MacConnell, P., Becker, J., and Bloch, W. (1991). An improved technique for the in situ detection of DNA after polymerase chain reaction amplification. *Am. J. Pathol.* **139**, 1239–1244.

Nuovo, G. J., MacConnell, P., Forde, A., and Delvenne, P. (1991). Detection of human papillomavirus DNA in formalin fixed tissues by *in situ* hybridization after amplification by PCR. *Am. J. Pathol.* **189**, 847.

O'Leary, J. J., Chetty, R., Graham, A. K., and McGee, J. O. (1996). *In situ* PCR: Pathologist's dream or nightmare? *J. Pathol.* **178**(1), 11–20.

Patel, V. G., Siu-Shum, A., Heniford, B. W., Wieman, T. J., and Hendler, F. J. (1994). Detection of epidermal growth factor receptor mRNA in tissue sections from biopsy specimens using *in situ* polymerase chain reaction. *Am. J. Pathol.* **144**, 7.

Ray, R., Komminoth, P., Machado, M., and Wolfe, H. J. (1991). Combined polymerase chain reaction and *in-situ* hybridization for the detection of single copy genes and viral genomic sequences in intact cells. *Mod. Pathol.* **19**, 242.

Ray, R., Smith, M., Sim, R., Bruce, I., and Wakefield, A. (1995). *In situ* hybridization detection of short viral amplicon sequences within cultured cells and body fluids after the *in situ* polymerase chain reaction. *J. Virol. Methods* **52**, 247–263.

Saiki, R. K., Gelfand, D. M., Stoffel, S., Scharff, S. J., Higuchi, R. G., Horn, G. T., Mullis, K. B., and Erlich, H. A. (1988). Primer-directed enzymatic amplification of DNA with a thermostable DNA polymerase. *Science* **239**, 487.

Spann, W., Pachmann, K., Zabnieuska, H., Pielmeier, A., and Emmerich, B. (1991). *In situ* amplification of single copy gene segments in individual cells by the polymerase chain reaction. *Infection* **19**, 242.

Staskus, K. A., Couch, L., Bitterman, P., Retzel, E. F., Zupancic, M., List, J., and Haase, A. T. (1991). *In situ* amplification of visna virus DNA in tissue sections reveals a reservoir of latently infected cells. *Microb. Pathog.* **11**, 67.

Steel, J. H., and Poulsom, R. (1997). Making sense out of *in situ* PCR. *J. Pathol.* **182**(1), 11–12.

Teo, I. A., and Shaunak, S. (1995). Polymerase chain reaction in situ: An appraisal of an emerging technique. *Histochem. J.* **27**, 647–659.

Thaker, V. (1999). In situ RT-PCR and hybridization techniques. *Methods Mol. Biol.* **115**, 379–402.

Walboomers, J. M. M., Melchers, W. J. G., Mullink, H., Meijer, C. J. L. M., Struyk, A., Quint, W. G. J., van der Noordaa, J., and ter Schegget, J. (1998). Sensitivity of *in situ* detection with biotinylated probes of human papilomavirus type 16 DNA in frozen tissue sections of squamous cell carcinoma of the cervix. *Am. J. Pathol.* **139**, 587.

Laser Capture Microdissection

Banks, R. E., Dunn, M. J., Forbes, M. A., Stanley, A., Pappin, D., Naven, T., Gough, M., Harnden, P., and Selby, P. J. (1999). The potential use of laser capture microdissection to selectively obtain distinct populations of cells for proteomic analysis: Preliminary findings. *Electrophoresis* **20**(4–5), 689–700.

Bohm, M., Wieland, I., Schutze, K., and Rubben, H. (1997). Microbeam MOMeNT: Non-contact laser microdissection of membrane-mounted native tissue. *Am. J. Pathol.* **151**(1), 63–67.

Bonner, R. F., Emmert-Buck, M., Cole, K., Pohida, T., Chuaqui, R., Goldstein, S., and Liotta, L. A. (1997). Laser capture microdissection: Molecular analysis of tissue. *Science* **278**(5342), 1481–1483.

Breidert, M., Miehlke, S., Glasow, A., Orban, Z., Stolte, M., Ehninger, G., Bayerdorffer, E., Nettesheim, O., Halm, U., Haidan, A., and Bornstein, S. R. (1999). Leptin and its receptor in normal human gastric mucosa and in Helicobacter pylori-associated gastritis. *Scand. J. Gastroenterol.* **34**(10), 954–961.

Emmert-Buck, M. R., Bonner, R. F., Smith, P. D., Chuaqui, R. F., Zhuang, Z., Goldstein, S. R., Weiss, R. A., and Liotta, L. A. (1996). Laser capture microdissection. *Science* **274**(5289), 998–1001.

Fend, F., Emmert-Buck, M. R., Chuaqui, R., Cole, K., Lee, J., Liotta, L. A., and Raffeld, M. (1999). Immuno-LCM: Laser capture microdissection of immunos-

tained frozen sections for mRNA analysis. *Am. J. Pathol.* **154**(1), 61–66.

Goldsworth, S. M., Stockton, P. S., Trempus, C. S., Foley, J. F., and Maronpot, R. R. (1999). Effects of fixation on RNA extraction and amplification from laser capture microdissected tissue. *Mol. Carcinog.* **25**(2), 86–91.

Jin, L., Thompson, C. A., Qian, X., Kuecker, S. J., Kulig, E., and Lloyd, R. V. (1999). Analysis of anterior pituitary hormone mRNA expression in immunophenotypically characterized single cells after laser capture microdissection. *Lab. Invest.* **79**(4), 511–512.

Sgroi, D. C., Teng, S., Robinson, G., LeVangie, R., Hudson, J. R., Jr., and Elkahloun, A. G. (1999). In vivo gene expression profile analysis of human breast cancer progression. *Cancer Res.* **59**(22), 5656–5661.

Simone, N. L., Bonner, R. F., Gillespie, J. W., Emmert-Buck, M. R. and Liotta, L. A. (1998). Laser-capture microdissection: Opening the microscopic frontier to molecular analysis. *Trends Genet.* **14**(7), 272–276.

Sirivatanauksorn, Y., Sirivatanauksorn, V., Bhattacharya, S., Davidson, B. R., Dhillon, A. P., Kakkar, A. K., Williamson, R. C., and Lemoine, N. R. (1999). Evolution of genetic abnormalities in hepatocellular carcinomas demonstrated by DNA fingerprinting. *J. Pathol.* **189**(3), 344–350.

Tam, A. S., Foley, J. F., Devereux, T. R., Maronpot, R. R., and Massey, T. E. (1999). High frequency and heterogeneous distribution of p53 mutations in aflatoxin B1-induced mouse lung tumors. *Cancer Res.* **59**(15), 3634–3640.

Confocal Microscopy

Collan, Y. (1998). Alternatives for morphometric stereologic analysis in toxicopathology. *Toxicol. Lett.* **28**(102–103), 393–397.

Dailey, M., Marrs, G., Satz, J., and Waite, M. (1999). Concepts in imaging and microscopy: Exploring biological structure and function with confocal microscopy. *Biol. Bull.* **197**(2), 115–122.

Gandolfi, A. J., Wijeweera, J., and Brendel, K. (1996). Use of precision-cut liver slices as an in vitro tool for evaluating liver function. *Toxicol. Pathol.* **24**(1), 58–61.

Imbert, D., Hoogstraate, J., Marttin, E., and Cullander C. (1999). Imaging thick tissues with confocal microscopy. *Methods Mol. Biol.* **122**, 341–355.

Kuo, S. M., Kondo, Y., DeFilippo, J. M., Ernstoff, M. S., Bahnson, R. R., and Lazo, J. S. (1994). Subcellular localization of metalloghionein IIA in human bladder tumor cells using a novel epitope-specific antiserum. *Toxicol. Appl. Pharmacol.* **125**(1), 104–110.

Li, W., Fawcett, J., Widmer, H. R., Fielder, P. J., Rabkin, R., and Keller, G. A. (1997). Nuclear transport of insulin-like growth factor-I and insulin-like growth factor binding protein-3 in opossum kidney cells. *Endocrinology* **138**(4), 1763–1766.

Matsumoto, B., Hale, I. L., and Kramer, T. R. (1997). Theory and applications of confocal microscopy. *In* "Analytical Morphology" (J. Gu, ed.), pp. 231–244. Eaton Publishing Co., Natick, MA.

Maurer, J. K., and Jester, J. V. (1999). Use of *in vivo* confocal microscopy to understand the pathology of accidental ocular irritation. *Toxicol. Pathol.* **27**(1), 44–47.

Mongan, L. C., Gormally, J., Hubbard, A. R., d'Lacey, C., and Ockleford, C. D. (1999). Confocal microscopy: Theory and applications. *Methods Mol. Biol.* **114**, 51–74.

Paddock, S. W. (1999). Confocal laser-scanning microscopy. *Biotechniques* **27**(5), 992–1004.

Paddock, S. W. (1999). An introduction to confocal imaging. *Methods Mol. Biol.* **122**, 1–34.

Park, J. E., Keller, G. A., and Ferrara, N. (1993). The vascular endothelial growth factor (VEGF) isoforms: Differential deposition into the subepithelial extracellular matrix and bioactivity of extracellular matrix-bound VEGF. *Mol. Biol. Cell.* **4**(12), 1317–1326.

Peterson, D. A. (1999). Quantitative histology using confocal microscopy: Implementation of unbiased stereology procedures. *Methods* **18**(4), 493–507.

Petroll, W. M., Jester, J. V., and Cavanagh, H. D. (1994). In vivo confocal imaging: General principles and applications. *Scanning* **16**(3), 131–149.

Satoh, Y., Nishimura, T., Kimura, K., Mori, S., and Saino, T. (1998). Application of real-time confocal microscopy for observation of living cells in tissue specimens. *Hum. Cell* **11**(4), 191–198.

Takamatsu, T. (1998). Confocal microscopy: Applications in research and practice of pathology. *Anal. Quant. Cytol. Histol.* **20**(6), 529–532.

White, J. G., Amos, W. B., and Fordham, M. (1987). An evaluation of confocal versus conventional imaging of biological structures by fluorescence light microscopy. *J. Cell Biol.* **105**(1), 41–48.

Stereology

Bertram, J. F. (1995). Analyzing renal glomeruli with the new stereology. *Int. Rev. Cytol.* **161**, 111–172.

Bolender, R. P., and Charleston, J. S. (1993). Software for counting cells and estimating structural volumes with the optical disector and fractionator. *Micros. Res. Tech.* **25**, 314–324.

Bolender, R. P., Hyde, D. M., and Dehoff, R. T. (1993). Lung morphometry: A new generation of tools and experiments for organ, tissue, cell, and molecular biology. *Am. J. Physiol.* **265**, L521–548.

Cruz-Orive, L. M., and Weibel, E. R. (1990). Recent stereological methods for cell biology: A brief survey. *Am. J. Physiol.* **258**, L148–156.

Gunderson, H. J. (1992). Stereology: The fast lane between neuroanatomy and brain function—or still only a tightrope? *Acta. Neurol. Scand. Suppl.* **137**, 8–13.

Gunderson, H. J., Bagger, P., Bendtsen, T. F., Evans, S. M., Korbo, L., Marcussen, N., Moller, A., Nielsen, K., Nyengaard, J. R., Pakkenberg, B., et al. (1988). The new stereological tools: Disector, fractionator, nucleator, and point sampled intercepts and their use in pathological research and diagnosis. *APMIS* **96**, 857–881.

Gunderson, H. J., Bendtsen, T. F., Korbo, L. Marcussen, N., Moller, A., Nielsen, K., Nyengaard, J. R., Pakkenberg, B., Sorensen, F. B., Vesterby, A., et al. (1988). Some new, simple and efficient stereological methods and thier use in pathological research and diagnosis. *APMIS* **96**, 379–394.

Mayhew, T. M. (1992). A review of recent advances in stereology for quantifying neural structure. *J. Neurocytol.* **21**, 313–328.

Mayhew, T. M., and Gundersen, H. J. (1996). If you assume, you can make an ass out of u and me': A decade of the disector for stereological counting of particles in 3D space. *J. Anat.* **188**, 1–15.

Oorschot, D. E. (1994). Are you using neuronal densities, synaptic densities or neurochemical densities as your definitive data? There is a better way to go. *Prog. Neurobiol.* **44**, 233–247.

Peterson, D. A. (1999). Quantitative histology using confocal microscopy: implementation of unbiased stereology procedures. *Methods* **18**, 493–507.

Pitot, H. C., Dragan, Y. P., Teeguarden, J., Hsia, S., and Campbell, H. (1996). Quantitation of multistage carcinogenesis in rat liver. *Toxicol. Pathol.* **24**, 119–128.

West, M. J., and Gunderson, H. J. (1990). Unbiased stereological estimation of the number of neurons in the human hippocampus. *J. Comp. Neurol.* **296**, 1–22.

Application of New Technologies to Toxicologic Pathology

Bruce D. Car, Paul J. Ciaccio, and Nancy R. Contel

Department of Discovery Toxicology
DuPont Pharmaceuticals Company
Newark, Delaware

I. Introduction

Routine histology, immunohistochemistry, confocal microscopy, *in situ* hybridization, and electron microscopy collectively provide the descriptive cornerstone for evaluating the topographically specific effects of toxicants on tissues. The combination of descriptive technologies with novel technologies that permit large-scale evaluations of metabolic intermediates, proteins and mRNA, provide an enhanced insight into the biochemical lesions underlying morphologically detectable alterations. The precise lesion sampling afforded by laser capture microdissection allows the topographically discrete assessment of microscopic lesions by technologies such as the polymerase chain reaction (PCR).

The biochemical basis of histochemistry is the affinity of various dyes or immunoglobulin-conjugates for proteins, carbohydrates, and nucleic acids, allowing the visualization of microscopic structures. The trained pathologist registers subtle alterations in hue as meaningful indicators of function or injury in cells. Histologic staining of DNA relates to its degree of dispersion and thereby state of replication or transcription; RNA (e.g., the blueness of reticulocytes stained by a Romanowksy procedure) to its concentration in cells and protein to its concentration, distribution, and charge. Metabolic products of cells generally contribute little to their appearance. While descriptive histopathology provides an overall view of a cell's functional state, the novel technologies discussed in this chapter permit the examination of individual levels of cell function. Stages of metabolism and appropriate technologies to assay the quantitative and qualitative aspects of the products of those stages are shown in Table I.

The scope of this chapter is limited to a discussion of those novel technologies that permit large-scale assessments of tissues or organs in the evaluation of toxicity, as well as potential evaluation of xenobiotics for structural features associated with the genesis of toxicity. The scale of the analysis in this instance refers to the large number of measurable, distinguishable end

TABLE I
Selection of Assays for Metabolic Stages in the Evaluation of Toxicity[a]

Metabolic stage	Product	Traditional technology (scale)	Novel technology (scale)
Nucleus (cell division)	DNA	Microscopy (H)	Flow cytometry (L)
Transcription	mRNA	Northern blot (L)	Microarray (H) PCR (L)
Translation	Protein	Microscopy (H)	Proteomics (H)
Posttranslational modification	Decoration	Protein biochemistry (L)	Proteomics (H)
	Folding	X-ray crystallography (L)	
	Multimerization	Protein biochemistry (L)	Yeast two-hybrid (L)
	Processing	Protein biochemistry (L)	
Export from ER and/or cell	Functional	Immunomicroscopy (L)	Proteomics (H)
	Protein	Light microscopy (H)	
		Biochemistry (L)	
Assumption of activity	Metabolite	Biochemistry (L)	Metabonomics (H)
Catabolism of protein	Metabolite	Biochemistry (L)	Metabonomics (H)

[a]Metabolic stages appear chronologically from top (earliest) to bottom (latest). The throughput or number of products measurable in a single assay at a particular scale is indicated in parentheses (L, low; H, high).

points and not assay throughput. As is typical for new technologies, assay throughput was initially slow or poorly accessible but is improving for each of the following technologies.

II. Genomics: High-Density Nucleic Acid Microarrays

The ability to evaluate the expression of thousands of genes simultaneously with high-density nucleic acid microarrays (or DNA arrays) brings with it the promise that global, unbiased patterns of genetic regulation specific to toxicologic alterations may be identified early and be of predictive value.

DNA arrays consist of gridded membranes or glass slides covered with hundreds or thousands of ordered DNA targets, spotted by high-precision robotics. The position of a gene target on a grid is known as its address. Gene targets may be composed of short synthetic segments of DNA called oligonucleotides, full-length or partial-length cDNAs. The selection of genes provided on an array is often based on previously proven involvement in cellular processes potentially relevant to toxicology or pharmacology (Table II) and are termed "tox chips."

Following the dosing of animals with potentially toxic xenobiotics, mRNA is isolated from freshly collected tissues and reverse transcribed into cDNA. cDNA is labeled with a radioactive or fluorescent indicator and hybridized to the array. In Fig. 1 (see color insert), an example of a cDNA array is given, in which

TABLE II
Gene Categories Used in Evaluation of Toxic Mechanisms

Apoptosis	Xenobiotic metabolism
DNA replication and repair	Important CYP P450 polymorphisms
Oncogenes, tumor suppressor genes	Carbohydrate metabolism
Cell cycle genes	Lipid metabolism
Oxidative stress/redox homeostasis	Mesodermal differentiation
Heat shock proteins	Ecto/endodermal differentiation
Peroxisome proliferator response	Mitochondrial genes
Dioxin/PAH response	Housekeeping
Estrogen/testosterone responsive	Immune responses (T_H1, T_H2, T_H0)
Thyroid hormone responsive	Hypersensitivity reactions
Other endocrine—adrenal, pituitary, neuroendocrine	Inflammation
Structural genes	Hematopoiesis

of diverse technologies to resolve individual proteins or peptides. The direct measurement of proteins or peptides overcomes the main theoretical concern in the use of high-density DNA arrays; the accurate interpretation of biological events when processes are not regulated transcriptionally. Typically, proteomic approaches have utilized two-dimensional polyacrylamide gel electrophoresis with sophisticated image analysis of silver-stained gels, protein identification by peptide sequencing, mass spectrometry, Western immunoblotting, and protein quantitation by a variety of methodologies. More recently, protein "chip" arrays have allowed the large-scale, affinity capture of proteins via specific or general surface chemistries with highly sensitive detection by mass spectroscopic approaches. Computational analysis of data sets is, as with other large scale novel technologies, essential to the identification of patterns and key effects. Several proteomic databases exist on the internet, allowing results to be placed in the context of larger data sets.

Present shortcomings of proteomic technology include difficulty in the detection of low-abundance polypeptides, resolution of very basic and high molecular weight proteins, and the limited experience base in the field of toxicology.

IV. Metabonomics: Pattern Recognition Nuclear Magnetic Resonance Spectroscopy

The technology of nuclear magnetic resonance spectroscopy (NMR) has been developed in parallel with the DNA microarray revolution, albeit with considerable less fanfare. NMR spectrograms are high-resolution, ^{1}H NMR measurements of low molecular weight metabolites, generally obtained from low protein biofluids such as urine, bile, and cerebrospinal fluid following exposure to powerful magnetic fields. With newer instruments, as many as 6000 different metabolites in body fluids such as urine may be resolved. The science of analysis of NMR spectrograms has been dubbed "meta-

bonomics." In considerable part through the efforts of the group led by Dr. Jeremy Nicholson at the Imperial College of London, the utility of NMR pattern recognition approaches in toxicology has been well established.

Small molecular products of metabolism represent the end point of cellular events, as gene transcription frequently represents the point of initiation. Metabonomics is presently practically limited to the analysis of small molecules for which proton excitation spectra may readily be resolved. These metabolites must normally be in the range of 1–10 μM to be detected. A typical urine ^{1}H NMR spectrogram is depicted in Fig. 3, indicating clusters of peaks associated with certain aspects of metabolism or organ function.

The identification of meaningful patterns from thousands of genes or metabolites is beyond the scope of what can reasonably be achieved by the visual inspection of data. This overview is provided by powerful software that is able to deconvolute patterns and resolve the specificity of changes.

Pattern recognition approaches have been developed and applied to the classification of urinary ^{1}H NMR spectra from rats dosed with compounds that induce organ-specific damage in various tissues. ^{1}H NMR spectra are reduced to histograms with 256 intensity-related descriptors of the spectra. Toxin clustering behavior within spectra is detected by a principal components analysis (PCA) and using a soft independent modeling of class analogy (SIMCA) model. Regionally specific nephro-and hepatotoxicants are readily distinguished by this methodology and outliers or nonresponders readily detected. The SIMCA/PCA model can be used to predict and classify the toxicity of xenobiotics based on characteristic alterations in ^{1}H NMR spectra. The further analysis of toxicant-induced unique spectral peaks, or combinations thereof, can be exploited in the development of novel toxicity biomarkers. With increasingly more powerful and sophisticated instrumentation, the diversity of products detected by this technology and patterns deconvoluted within spectra will match or exceed the diagnostic

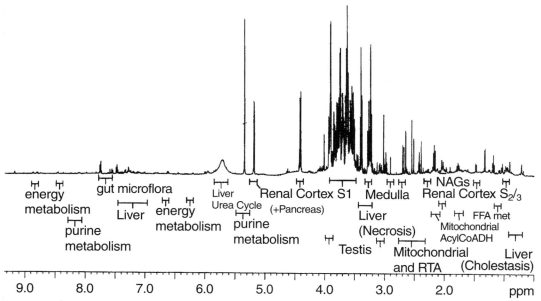

Figure 3. ^{1}H NMR Spectrum of abnormal not urine with biomacher regions. Reproduced with permission from Dr. Genemy Nicholson, Imperial College of Science, Technology, and Medicine, London.

information that may be obtained through genomic or proteomic technology.

Urinary biomarkers for hydrazine-induced hepatotoxicity and $HgCl_2$-induced renal toxicity are shown in Table IV. These biomarkers were shown to be robust in both Han–Wistar and Sprague–Dawley rats. Moreover, analysis of urine ^{1}H NMR spectra is also readily able to distinguish subtle metabolic differences between these rat strains.

As with genomic and proteomic technologies, the principal limitation of metabonomics is the lack of topographical specificity that can be inferred from data sets. The ability to discriminate patterns of change in ^{1}H NMR spectra specific for alterations in tissues or cells of defined locations is improving, as experience with this technology accumulates.

V. Laser Capture Microscopy

Laser capture microdissection (LCM) provides a topographical bridge to genomics and proteomics methodologies and can be utilized to overcome the problems arising from use of heterogeneous cell populations to study the effects of toxicants. LCM involves apposing a layer of transparent ethylene vinyl acetate to histologic sections. A low-power laser beam directed at the film causes it to extend its long chain polymers, capturing the cells or substructure of interest. The technique can be used on formalin-fixed, paraffin wax-embedded, frozen, and cytologic specimens. LCM has been utilized in combination with reverse transcription-PCR, immunohistochemistry, DNA microarray, and

TABLE IV
Hepatic and Renal Toxicants: Characteristic Urinary Changes
Detected by NMR

Hydrazine-induced hepatotoxicity		$HgCl_2$-induced nephrotoxicity	
Analyte	Concentration	Analyte	Concentration
Taurine	↑	Amino acids	↑
β-Alanine	↑	Organic acids	↑
Creatine	↑	Glucose	↑
2-Aminoadipate	↑	Citrate	↓
Citrate	↓	Succinate	↓
Succinate	↓	2-Oxoglutarate	↓
2-Oxoglutarate	↓	Hippurate	↓
Creatinine	↓		

proteomic analyses. In the cancer field, laser capture microdissection has been combined with DNA arrays to study gene expression in subpopulations of benign versus invasive, malignant breast epithelial cells in single biopsies of breast tissue.

VI. Computational Modeling

Currently most limited with respect to its extension to toxicologic pathology is the predictive use of quantitative structure–activity relationships (QSAR) based on computer algorithms. These algorithms combine aspects of physical molecular structure, solubility in biological membranes, chemical reactivity, ionization, pH characteristics, isomerization, binding affinity determinations for specific receptors, and extensive databases of structural alerts known to be associated with toxic events such as mutagenesis and metabolism to reactive molecular moieties. The prediction by a computer system of the complex outcomes of the interaction of chemicals with biological systems, given typical variables of absorption, distribution, metabolism, and excretion, is at best less than robust. The greatest utility of QSAR is in its application to structural series and with predication of effect on single outcomes, such as DNA damage, Ah receptor binding, or interaction with nuclear steroid receptors.

VII. Summary

Traditional and novel forms of microscopy provide topographic specificity and an initial level of understanding to the pathogenesis of xenobiotic-induced alterations in cells or tissues. Collectively, the generation and combined interpretation of data sets detailing the regulation of transcription (genomics), protein synthesis (proteomics), and end products of metabolism (metabonomics) with those providing topographic specificity will provide a greater understanding of mechanisms of xenobiotic-induced disease. The accurate determination of biochemical lesions allows the development of useful counterscreens for potential toxicants and

provides the necessary information to direct chemical synthesis toward reducing toxicity. Experience obtained with new technologies in the form of multiple "signatures" associated with established mechanisms of toxicology, pharmacology, and normal homeostatic events or responses will, in the future, facilitate the effective study of unknown potential toxicants for the mechanisms of their adverse activities.

SUGGESTED READING

Introduction

Car, B. D., and Robertson, R. T. (1999). Discovery toxicology: A nascent science. *Toxicol. Pathol.* **27**, 481–483.

Gillett, N. A., and Chan, C. M. (1999). Molecular pathology in the preclinical development of biopharmaceuticals. *Toxicol. Pathol.* **27**, 48–52.

Gossett, K. A., Narayanan, P. K., Williams, D. M., Gore, E. R., Herzyk, D. J., Hart, T. K., and Sellers T. (1999). Flow cytometry in the preclinical development of biopharmaceuticals. *Toxicol. Pathol.* **27**, 32–37.

Rodi, C. P., Bunch, R. T., Curtiss, S. W., Kier, L. D., Cabonce, M. A., Davila, J. C., Mitchell, M. D., Alden, C. L., and Morris, D. L. (1999). Revolution through genomics in investigative and discovery toxicology. *Toxicol. Pathol.* **27**, 107–110.

Rudmann, D. G., and Durham, S. K. (1999). Utilization of genetically altered animals in the pharmaceutical industry. *Toxicol. Pathol.* **27**, 111–114.

Ryan, A. M. (1999). Role of the pathologist in the identification and characterization of therapeutic molecules. *Toxicol. Pathol.* **27**, 474–476.

Genomics: High-Density Nucleic Acid Microarrays

Admundson, S. A., Bittner, M., Chen, Y., Trent, J., Meltzer, P., and Fornace, A. J., Jr. (1999). Fluorescent cDNA microarray hybridization reveals complexity and heterogeneity of cellular genotoxic stress responses. *Oncogene* **18**, 3666–3672.

Asfari, C. A., Nuwaysir, E. F., and Barrett, J. C. (1999). Applications of complementary DNA microarray technology to carcinogen identification, toxicology, and drug safety evaluation. *Cancer Res.* **59**, 4759–4760.

Burczynski, M. E., McMillian, M, Ciervo, J., Li, L., Parker J. B., Dunn, R. T., II, Hicken, S. A., Farr, S., and

Johnson, M. D. (2000). Toxicogenomics-based discrimination of toxic mechanism in HepG2 human hepatoma cells. *Toxicol. Sci.* **58**, 399–415.

Iyer, V., Eisen, M. B., Toss, D. T., Schuler, G., Moore, T., Lee, J. C. F., Trent, J. M., Staudt, L. M., Hudson, J. Jr., Moguski, M. S., Lashkari, D., Shalon, D., Botstein, D., and Brown, P. O. (1999). The transcriptional program in the response of human fibroblasts to serum. *Science* **283**, 83–87.

Lee, C.-K., Klopp, R. G., Weindruch, R., and Prolla, T. A. (1999). Gene expression profile of aging and its retardation by caloric restriction. *Science* **285**, 1390–1393.

Martin, M. J., DeRisi, J. L., Bennett, H. A., Iyer, V. R., Meyer, M. R., Roberts, C. J., Stoughton, R., Burchard, J., Slade, D., Dai, H., Bassett, D. E., Jr., Hartwell, L. H., Brown, P. O., and Friend, S. H. (1998). Drug target validation and identification of secondary drug target effects using DNA microarrays. *Nature Med.* **4**, 1293–1301.

Nuwaysir, E. F., Bittner, M., Trent, J., Barret, J. C., and Afshari, C. A. (1999). Microarrays and Toxicology: The advent of toxicogenomics. *Mol. Carc.* **24**, 153–159.

Rockett, J. C., Esdaile, D. J., and Gibson, G. G. (1999). Differential gene expression in drug metabolism and toxicology: Practicalities, problems and potential. *Xenobiotica* **29**, 655–691.

Sander, C. (2000). Genomic medicine and the future of health care. *Science* **287**, 1977–1978.

Sgroi, D. C., Teng, S., Robinson, G., LeVangie, R., Hudson, J. R., Jr., and Elkahloun, A. G. (1999). In vivo gene expression profile analysis of human breast cancer progression. *Cancer Res.* **59**, 5656–5661.

Waxman, D. J. (1999). P450 gene induction by structurally diverse xenochemicals: Central role of nuclear receptors CAR, PXR, and PPAR. *Arch. Biochem. Biophys.* **369**, 11–23.

Proteomics

Blackstock, W. P., and Weir, M. P. (1999). Proteomics: Quantitative and physical mapping of cellular proteins. *Trends Biotech.* **17**, 121–127.

Dove, A. (1999). Proteomics: Translating genomics into products? *Nature Biotech* **17**, 233–236.

Celis, J. E., Ostergaard, M., Jensen, N. A., Gromova, I., Rasmussen, H. H., and Gromov, P. (1998). Human and mouse proteomic databases: Novel resources in the protein universe. *FEBS Lett.* **430**, 64–72.

Metabonomics

Beckwith-Hall, B. M., Nicholson, J. K., Nicholls, A. W., Foxall, P. J., Lindon, J. C., Connor, S. C., Abdi, M.,

Connelly, J., and Holmes, E. (1998). Nuclear magnetic resonance spectroscopic and principal components analysis investigations into biochemical effects of three model hepatotoxins. *Chem. Res. Toxicol.* **11**, 260–272.

Holmes, E., Nicholls, A. W., Lindon, J. C., Ramos, S., Spraul, M., Neidig, P., Connor, S. C., Connelly, J., Damment, S. J., Haselden, J., and Nicholson, J. K. (1998). Development of a model for classification of toxin-induced lesions using ^{1}H NMR spectroscopy of urine combined with pattern recognition. *NMR Biomed.* **11**, 235–244.

Holmes, E. Nicholls, A. W, Lindon, J. C., Connor, S. C., Connelly, J. C., Haselden, J. N., Damment, S. J. P., Spraul M., Neidig, P., and Nicholson, J. K. (2000). Chemometric models for toxicity classification based on NMR spectra of biofluids. *Chem. Res. Toxicol.* **13**, 471–478.

Nicholson, J. K., and Wilson, I. D. (1989). High resolution proton magnetic resonance spectroscopy of biological fluids. *Prog. NMR Spect.* **21**, 449–501.

Timbrell, J. A. (1998). Biomarkers in toxicology. *Toxicology* **129**, 1–12.

Laser Capture Microscopy

Curran, S., McKay, J. A., McLeod, H. L., and Murray, G. I. (2000). Laser capture microscopy. *Mol. Pathol.* **53**, 64–68.

Computational Modeling

Barratt, M. D. (1998). Integration of QSAR and in vitro toxicology. *Environ. Health Perspect.* **106**, 459–465.

Benigni, R., Passerini, L., Gallo, G., Giorgi, F., and Cotta-Ramusino, M. (1998). QSAR models for discriminating between mutagenic and nonmutagenic aromatic and heteroaromatic amines. *Environ. Mol. Mutat.* **32**, 75–83.

Bradbury, S., Kamenska, V., Schmieder, P., Ankley, G., and Mekenyan, O. (2000). A computationally based identification algorithm for estrogen receptor ligands. 1. Predicting hERα binding affinity. *Toxicol. Sci.* **58**, 253–269.

Esdaile, D. J. (1998). Perpectives on the past, present and future of computer prediction in toxicology. *Toxicol. Lett.* **102–103**, 609–610.

Hall, A. H. (1998). Computer modeling and computational toxicology in new chemical and pharmaceutical product development. *Toxicol. Lett.* **102–103**, 623–626.

Mekenyan, O. G., Veith, G. D., Call, D. J., and Ankley, G. T. (1996). A QSAR evaluation of Ah receptor binding of halogenated aromatic xenobiotics. *Environ. Health Perspect.* **104**, 1302–1310.

Issues in Laboratory Animal Science for the Toxicologic Pathologist

Jeffrey I. Everitt and David C. Dorman
CIIT Centers for Health Research
Research Triangle Park, North Carolina

I. Introduction

As an integral member of the toxicology study team, the toxicologic pathologist needs to have a thorough understanding of the laboratory animal model that serves as a test system for studies with pathology requirements. Genetic, microbial, experimental, and environmental factors greatly effect lesion development in laboratory animals, and an understanding of the interplay of these factors with toxicant-induced effects is necessary for the pathologist to interpret study findings correctly. In addition to their role of assessing compound-induced effects, the toxicologic pathologist often identifies health-related issues in study animals and must be knowledgeable about the common disease states that all too often arise in long-term rodent studies. The pathologist must work closely with laboratory animal science professionals who are responsible for the oversight of rodent colony management.

Toxicologic research is becoming increasingly more complex with the advent of new and exciting advances in biotechnology. This is best ex-

emplified by the widespread use of genetically engineered mice and other rodents in toxicology testing facilities performing safety assessment bioassays as well as in basic research laboratories. In addition to the recent advances in the manipulation of the mammalian genome, there is an increasing sophistication in animal monitoring systems, such as telemetric assessment of physiological parameters, and imaging methods, such as magnetic resonance imaging (MRI). In the near future, these technologies will likely contribute to an improved understanding of the pathogenesis of many laboratory animal diseases and lesion states and will provide new and useful adjuncts to traditional pathology assessment.

Laboratory animal science is a diverse and complex discipline encompassing many different types of experimental animals. Remarks in this chapter will be limited to selected issues involving laboratory rodents, which are the most commonly utilized animals in toxicology studies. There are many questions in laboratory animal science that need to be considered during the planning and conduct of a toxicology study (Table I). Selected laboratory science issues that pertain to the work of pathologists and that influence lesion development will be

Handbook of Toxicologic Pathology, Second Edition
Volume 1

TABLE I
Laboratory Animal Science Issues to be Addressed by the Toxicology Study Team

IACUC

Review experiment from the standpoint of optimizing animal numbers and assuring proper statistical design

Review issues of animal pain and distress and consider methods to minimize pain or distress

Obtain IACUC review and approval of the experimental protocol

Review personnel training and training documentation issues

Define humane end points/criteria for euthanasia

Study issues

Assure compliance with regulatory test guidelines

Review staffing and associated concerns

Determine methods of allocation of animals to study without bias (randomization)

Determine animal identification and cage identification methods

Determine acclimation and quarantine periods (length, location, methods)

Review dosing methods and issues related to test compound (e.g., dose schedule, volume, vehicle, special monitoring needs)

Review all experimental manipulations of animals, including timing of events

Establish standard operating procedures for removing unscheduled animals from study and determine handling and disposition of animals

Animal model selection and use

Determine species and strain and review scientific rationale for model selection

Establish age, gender, weight, physiological status, and genetic needs

Choose source or supplier

Review genetic history and health history of source colony

Establish need for any prestudy health or genetic testing of supplied animals

Review strain-related causes of morbidity and mortality and institutional experience with chosen animal model

Animal environment

Review animal room issues (temperature, humidity, lighting, noise, air flow)

Establish methods and intervals for environmental monitoring

Review housing issues (group vs single housing, type of caging, type of bedding, frequency of cage change, room allocation, and methods to prevent bias in housing and handling such as rotation of cage or rack placement)

Review special housing needs (e.g., inhalation or metabolism caging) and methods for acclimation to equipment and special procedures

Determine whether other animals (e.g., sentinel animals) or studies (e.g., microbial infections in facility) pose danger to study animals and institute protective procedures if warranted

stressed in this chapter. For a more in-depth review of specific topics, the reader is directed to the "Suggested Reading" list.

II. Regulatory Issues

A. OVERVIEW OF RULES AND REGULATIONS

All scientists who utilize laboratory animals must be knowledgeable about government regulations and guidelines pertaining to the proper care and use of research animals. It is essential for every investigator to become familiar with the laws, regulations, and policies relating to the use of animals in research and to adopt a responsible attitude toward laboratory animal use. The following discussion will serve as an introduction to current government regulations and guidelines on the care and use of laboratory animal in the United States.

In the United States, oversight of animal care and use is primarily provided by two national laws: the Animal Welfare Act (7 USC 2131–2157) and the Health Research Extension Act (42 USC 289d). The latter was amended in 1985 by Public Law 99–158 to cover the care and use of animals in research. The regulations that implement the Animal Welfare Act are published in the Code of Federal Regulations (9 CFR 1–3) and are administered by the U.S. Department of Agriculture (USDA). For the purposes of this Act, animals are presently defined as "any live or dead dog, cat, nonhuman primate, guinea pig, hamster, rabbit, or any other warm-blooded animal which is being used, or is intended for use for research, teaching, testing, experimentation, or exhibition purposes, or as a pet" (9CFR 1.1). Rats and mice bred for use in research are currently exempted from these regulations, although this exemption may be eliminated in the next few years.

Among the provisions of the Animal Welfare Act are (1) standards to ensure the humane care of animals being transported; (2) standards for care of animals in research facilities, including minimum requirements for housing, feeding, watering, sanitation, handling, adequate veterinary care, and the appropriate use of anes-

thetic, analgesic, and tranquilizing drugs to ensure the minimization of pain and distress; (3)
the reporting of requirements to the USDA
showing that professionally acceptable standards for the humane care and use of animals
are in effect; (4) establishment of an institutional animal care and use committee (IA-
CUC); and (5) establishment of training for all
personnel involved in the care and use of animals.

The Health Research Extension Act is implemented by the Public Health Service Policy on
Humane Care and Use of Laboratory Animals
(PHS policy) and is administered by the National Institutes of Health, Office for Protection
of Research Risks (OPRR). The policy pertains
to all activities conducted and supported by the
public health service involving any live vertebrate animal used or intended for use in research, research training, experimentation,
biological testing, or related purposes. The
PHS policy requires compliance with the Animal Welfare Act and use of the "Guide for the
Care and Use of Laboratory Animals (Guide)"
(NRC, 1996) as a basis for developing and implementing an institutional program for activities involving animals. No activity supported
by the PHS involving animals may be conducted until the institution conducting the activity has provided a written assurance of
compliance with the PHS policy.

Many institutions that perform toxicology
research and testing are accredited by the
American Association for the Assessment and
Accreditation of Laboratory Animal Care, International (AAALAC). AAALAC is a nonre-
gulatory, not-for-profit organization whose
mission is to promote high standards of animal
care and use. Participation in the peer review
accreditation program is voluntary and at the
initiative of the individual institution. The
AAALAC council evaluates animal programs
by conducting site visits and reviewing reports.
It relies on the "Guide" as its primary standard
for the evaluation of laboratory animal care
and use programs. AAALAC accreditation demonstrates that a program has achieved a
standard of excellence beyond the minimum

required by law. It is presently the only accred-
iting body recognized by the PHS for activities
involving animals.

In addition to working under the auspices of
the Animal Welfare Act and in some cases PHS
policy, the work of many toxicologic pathologists is conducted under the guidelines of the
good laboratory practice (GLP) regulations of
the Food and Drug Administration (FDA) or
U.S. Environmental Protection Agency (U.S.
EPA). The GLP regulations contain additional
provisions for the care and use of laboratory
animals. Included among these are certain requirements for animal housing, separation of
species, quarantine of new and sick animals,
and separation of projects. There are also requirements for monitoring and documenting
the health of research animals, as well as documentation requirements for any treatments performed on research animals. There is a GLP
stipulation that all animals and animal enclo-
sures be properly identified. Identification requirements and documentation methods are of
particular importance to pathologists who must
also track tissues and biologic samples obtained
at necropsy.

B. INSTITUTIONAL ANIMAL CARE AND USE COMMITTEE

Both PHS policy and the Animal Welfare Act
require organizations using animals for research to designate the need to identify an institutional official responsible for the animal
care and use program and mandate the formation of the IACUC. The IACUC is responsible
for oversight of the animal care and use program. Specifically, the IACUC must assure that
consideration be given to the minimization of
pain and distress for all experimental animals.
This is particularly important in the toxicology
laboratory, where the administration of potentially deleterious xenobiotics can induce animal
suffering. A specific requirement of the IACUC
is to perform a semiannual review of the institution's animal care and use program, as well as
an inspection of the facilities where animals
are housed, using the "Guide" and the standards of the Animal Welfare Act as a basis for

evaluation. Reports of these reviews are sent to the designated institutional official with recommendations for programmatic improvements, if necessary, and corrective actions and time tables if deficiencies are noted. Among its duties, the primary task of the IACUC is the review of all animal use protocols prior to study initiation to assure compliance with applicable regulations such as the Animal Welfare Act and PHS policy.

The IACUC review of protocols requires an assurance that the animal model is appropriate and that the proposed experimental design uses the appropriate number of animals in a manner likely to achieve the scientific objectives of the study. There is a requirement that investigators consider alternatives to the use of animals where possible and that every effort be made to minimize pain and distress. IACUC review also includes review of the proposed method of euthanasia.

C. METHODS OF EUTHANASIA

The toxicologic pathologist should be involved in all facets of rodent bioassay study design and protocol development, and special attention should be directed to laboratory science issues that affect the necropsy. A very important part of the necropsy is performance of the euthanasia procedure. The pathologist needs to determine the proper method of euthanasia and assure proper oversight of the procedure. In general, the euthanasia method selected should be in accordance with the recommendations of the American Veterinary Medical Association (AVMA) panel on euthanasia. Euthanasia in the necropsy laboratory can present special challenges when it is associated with terminal surgical procedures, such as during the collection of certain samples and during the conduct of organ perfusion methods. These methods require a proper understanding of anesthetic management and monitoring procedures.

The method of euthanasia chosen should (1) have the ability to produce death without causing pain or distress to the animal; (2) be reliable; (3) be safe to personnel; (4) be nonreversible; (5) cause minimal emotional distress to necropsy personnel; and (6) be compatible with the scientific objectives of the experiment. There are many examples of untoward effects of the euthanasia method on research end points. Anesthetic overdose using injectable or inhalant anesthetic agents followed by exsanguination is a commonly utilized method favored by many toxicologic pathologists. This methodology is compatible with excellent tissue preservation and can be carried out efficiently. A variety of commonly used methods for rodent euthanasia are associated with tissue artifacts. These include pulmonary hemorrhage associated with carbon dioxide asphyxiation and tissue trauma associated with decapitation and cervical dislocation methods. Histopathologic assessment of tissues is often only one of several study end points, and thus the pathologist must understand the needs of the entire experiment (e.g., clinical biochemistry, hematology, body fluid analysis, immunologic assessments) so that the most appropriate euthanasia method can be chosen. Toxicology end points such as hormone levels, neurotransmitter activity, liver metabolism, and immune function parameters can be affected by certain anesthetic regimens and euthanasia methods.

III. Selection of Animal Models

A. OVERVIEW

The use of laboratory animal models will continue to play a critical role in toxicologic pathology. Laboratory rodents, primarily rats and mice, have proven to be useful in toxicology research and testing because they share many similarities with humans. There are metabolic, anatomic, and physiologic similarities that allow for comparisons in absorption, distribution, and excretion of xenobiotics. The small size, docile nature, short life spans and gestation periods, and large litter size make rodents very economical animal models to maintain, breed, and use in the conduct of lifelong studies. An extensive database on characteristics of mice and rats makes them invaluable animal models for toxicology studies.

For the proper interpretation of toxicology and pathology data, the age, gender, physiologic status, microbiologic status, nutrition, and genotype of the test animals must be considered. It is also necessary to consider the environment in which they are bred and maintained. Rodents are often classified according to microbiologic status (Table II). Most modern toxicology facilities use barrier-reared rodents with defined microbial flora. There is often a need to understand the environment of the source colony in which rodent models are bred and initially raised. The rodent supplier should provide information concerning diet and feeding methods, breeding procedures, genetic control, caging, and husbandry.

B. GENETIC ISSUES

There are many genetically determined responses of laboratory rodents to xenobiotics, and the effects of genotype often include interactions with the environment to create the phenotypic changes studied by the toxicologic pathologist. There are three main classes of laboratory rodents used in research and testing laboratories: isogenic strains, outbred stocks,

TABLE II
Classification of Rodents Based on Microbial Status

Classification	Criteria
Axenic animal	Derived by hysterectomy; reared and maintained in isolators with germ-free techniques
Gnotobiotic animal	As just described except that any acquired microbial forms are fully known and nonpathogenic
Defined microbially associated animal	An axenic animal that has been intentionally associated with one or more microorganisms
Barrier-maintained animal	A defined microbially associated animal that has been removed from the isolator and placed in a barrier. Such animals are tested to monitor for the presence of reconstituting flora and for the presence of accidentally acquired organisms
Conventional animal	An animal with an unknown and uncontrolled microbial burden. Generally reared under open animal room conditions

and mutants (spontaneous and genetically engineered). All three groups of rodents have been used extensively in toxicology research and testing, although critical evaluation of how rodent models were historically chosen has not been well elucidated in the literature. There has been a continuing debate concerning the choice of rodent strains most suitable for long-term toxicological studies. This debate has intensified recently because of apparent genetic drift in certain outbred stocks of rats, leading to significant declines in average life span and changes in certain reproductive parameters.

Isogenic rodents include inbred strains and F1 hybrid animals. Inbred strains are produced by at least 20 generations of sibling mating, with all individuals being derived from a single breeding pair in the 20th or subsequent generation. Members of an inbred strain are homozygous at all genetic loci without hidden recessive genes. As a result of this homozygosity, the inbred strain stays genetically constant for many generations. Each inbred strain of rodent has its own unique pattern of behavioral attributes, growth pattern, reproductive performance, neoplasm profile, lesion spectrum, and response to xenobiotics. When colonies of inbred animals are separated for a number of years, however, substrains occur as a result of new mutations, or residual genetic variation that was not eliminated at the time the colonies were separated. Currently, there are over 200 inbred strains of rats and many more inbred mouse strains.

F1 hybrids are the first-generation cross between two inbred strains. Like the parental inbred strains from which they are derived, they are also isogenic (i.e., all individuals are genetically identical). F1 hybrids have all the useful properties of inbred animals except that they are not homozygous at all genetic loci and they tend to be more vigorous than the parental strains. Many toxicologists feel that the level of heterozygosity in some F1 hybrids is a major advantage in that the animals may more closely resemble the noninbred animals of the species while still maintaining the advantages of a uniform genotype. Thus F1 hybrids have been favored for many biomedical studies, including toxicology research and testing experiments. Since 1972, the F1 hybrid (B6C3F1) of the cross between the C57BL/6N female and C3H/HeN male inbred mice has been the mouse model used by the National Cancer Institute and National Toxicology Program in the United States in the chemical carcinogenesis bioassay.

Many toxicology laboratories use outbred stocks of rodents. These animals are generally propagated in closed colonies using some form of random mating system that avoids the mating of close relatives. The result is a colony of rodents that is reasonably uniform in its characteristics, although each animal is genetically distinct. Outbred stocks of rodents are often known by generic names such as Sprague–Dawley rats or Swiss mice. As a result of genetic assortment, inbreeding, and selection, different colonies of outbred stocks will be genetically different from each other within a few years. It is important for scientists to understand that commercial rodent producers maintain multiple colonies of many of the important outbred stocks; therefore the relationship between the various colonies is dependent on the breeding practices utilized. Control of these breeding practices is critical to assure uniformity, even among single suppliers. Although genetic drift can be minimized using large colony sizes and specific breeding schemes, genetic quality control of outbred stocks is difficult and expensive and requires significant supplier effort.

Outbred stocks of rodents are occasionally considered to be analogous to the genetically variable human population, but this is misleading because the amount of genetic variation in rodent stocks is much less than in humans. Because there are profound strain differences in response to xenobiotics, some toxicologists have favored the use of genetically variable outbred stocks. Using more than a single genotype in rodent toxicology experiments is often desirable; however, there are a number of serious disadvantages to using outbred animals, including phenotypic variability and the need to use larger sample sizes to provide statistical

precision for end points that have substantial phenotypic variation within the population. Some toxicologists strongly advocate the use of multiple isogenic strains. This strategy has the advantage of long-term genetic stability and phenotypic uniformity of the test animal system but without the major disadvantage of using animals of only a single genotype. Rodent bioassays with multistrain designs can be somewhat more problematic for the toxicologic pathologist. Because fewer animals of each genotype are used, the databases of lesions are more limited, and familiarity with multiple strains is essential.

C. ISSUES INVOLVING THE USE OF HISTORICAL DATABASES

In general, toxicologic pathologists feel most comfortable using rodent models for which they have historical data on the incidence of spontaneous and xenobiotic-induced lesions. The lesion database for any rodent stock or strain is best when it is based on in-house studies with animals that have a similar genetic history and are maintained under identical environmental conditions to the study being conducted. Thus many institutions become reluctant to change the design of studies or to use new rodent models if they feel that the changes will negate their ability to utilize historical data. This is particularly true when studies need to be reported to regulatory agencies. Historical data can provide an extremely valuable tool for study interpretation, but sometimes the value of these databases is overstated. Genotypic qualities of rodent models change over time due to selection procedures, alterations in breeding schemes, and genetic drift. These genetic changes have led to changes in the historical incidences of many neoplasms and nonneoplastic findings in both isogenic strains and outbred stocks. In addition to alterations in genetic qualities of rodents, animal husbandry practices change over time, contributing to the need to view historical databases as living documents subject to change.

It is important to understand individual stock and strain characteristics when choosing rodent models for toxicology experiments. The longevity of the selected model is an important characteristic to consider for certain long-term studies. Regulatory requirements dictate certain survival criteria, and the decreasing longevity in certain stocks of *ad libitum*-fed rats in recent years has led to difficulty in some laboratories. Various approaches have been used in efforts to reverse the declining trends in survival. These efforts have included changes in breeding schemes and husbandry procedures (such as types of diets and the way in which rodents are fed).

A key point in properly selecting a rodent model is understanding the impact of strain-related spontaneous lesions on the proposed study end points. For instance, if the lung is a suspected target organ of toxicity, the Fischer 344 rat strain is probably not the animal model of choice for a long-term study. This strain has a very high incidence of leukemia, with pulmonary vascular infiltrates that would compromise the ability of the pathologist to diagnose interstitial lung disease. Similarly, if a nose-only method were the proposed route of exposure in a long-term inhalation study, one might not wish to choose a rat strain with a high incidence of spontaneous mammary tumors that would mechanically interfere with animal placement in the nose-only apparatus. In virtually all rodent stocks and strains, examples can be found of target organ compromise by a genetic predisposition to a high spontaneous background of lesions. There is no ideal rodent model for all types of toxicology studies, and one must critically evaluate model selection for each experiment.

D. CHALLENGES OF GENETICALLY ENGINEERED RODENTS

Although spontaneous mutant models have long been available in research laboratories, there has been an increasing reliance on the use of genetically engineered rodent models, particularly mice, in toxicology as in other areas of biological science. These new rodent models include animals created via insertional transgenesis experiments as well as animals cre-

ated with gene targeting approaches using homologous recombination in embryonic stem cells. The use of these valuable models has created special challenges for the toxicologic pathologist. The genetic background and lesion development of many of the genetically engineered mouse strains differs from those commonly used in rodent bioassays. Genetic background is extremely important to phenotype development, and thus the pathologist needs to have a working knowledge of the background incidence of lesions found in the parental genotypes. For instance, transgenic mice created on the commonly utilized FVB inbred background carry a genetic predisposition to retinal degeneration and thus are not useful for many types of ocular or neurobehavioral studies.

The usefulness of genetically engineered mouse models has created problems in toxicology testing in certain instances due to limited availability. Source colonies are sometimes relatively small, and animals may be difficult to breed, leading to difficulty in providing the age- and sex-matched group sizes needed for certain toxicology studies. Laboratories that have the need to purchase genetically engineered mouse models may not have the luxury of specifying the animal source because these models are often proprietary and breeding rights may be restricted. Limited source and supply create special challenges regarding isolation, quarantine, and health monitoring procedures. The experimental design of certain experiments may necessitate the cohousing of mice from multiple sources, with the resultant mixing of microbial flora. Significant animal health issues can also be associated with genetically engineered mice themselves, as many of the induced phenotypes vary depending on the immunomodulatory properties of the environment in which they are raised and maintained.

There are many examples of genetically engineered mice where phenotype varies with health status and husbandry practices. One such example is the so-called *Min* mouse (C57BL/6J-Apc$^{Min/+}$) used in carcinogenesis studies. The *Min* (multiple intestinal neoplasia) mouse bears a germline nonsense mutation in the mouse homologue of the human adenomatous polyposis gene (APC) and develops a high level of intestinal tumors by 4 months of age. On a C57BL/6 background, 100% of heterozygote animals develop a high incidence and high multiplicity of intestinal adenomas when fed a 10–15% fat diet. When fed a 3% fat diet, there are fewer tumors and smaller polypoid lesions. Fiber content is also known to be important in tumorigenesis in this model but less so than dietary fat intake. In addition to environmental modification of the phenotype, many of the genetically engineered mouse models are either more or less susceptible to murine pathogens than their parental strains, and the effect of these microbial infections on phenotype and lesion develop may be pronounced.

IV. Animal Health Considerations

A. ADVENTITIOUS AGENTS

The pathologist is often the toxicology study professional who is responsible for assessing the role and impact that pathogens have on the experimental results. Thus, the pathologist must be familiar with rodent pathogens and with the microbial factors that modify toxicity. Most modern toxicology research and testing facilities are relatively free of the adventitious murine pathogens that caused clinical disease in rodents and plagued bioassays in the past. This situation has come about because commercial rodent suppliers have instituted procedures of serologic screening of animals for antibodies to specific pathogens and employed subsequent elimination or cesarean rederivation of antibody positive colonies. There has been increasing awareness of the varied effects of natural pathogens in laboratory animals with ever-greater efforts to exclude these microbial agents from research subjects. Despite these efforts, microbial factors remain an important variable in toxicology research studies, and pathologists and laboratory animal science professionals must maintain a constant vigil against their untoward effects on experiments. Facilities

using genetically engineered mice are at particular risk for outbreaks of rodent pathogens.

Microbial infection indicates the presence of organisms that may be considered pathogenic, opportunistic, or commensals, of which the last two are most numerous. Few agents found in laboratory animals today cause overt clinical disease. Rodents that appear normal and healthy may be unsuitable as research subjects due to the unobservable but significant effects of the microbial infection. Over the past two decades, there has been a significant shift in the spectrum of murine pathogens, and there is a constant need to refine diagnostic testing methods, microbial containment, and disease prevention strategies. In addition to shifts in the spectrum of pathogens found in the toxicology laboratory, there have been significant changes over the years in rodent husbandry and caging methods that influence the spread of rodent infections. Many modern facilities now have very high animal stocking densities, and facilities that produce genetically altered mice can have multiple breeding colonies present in close proximity, factors that predispose to the spread of microbial diseases.

Microbial infections of laboratory rodents exert effects through a complex interplay of host and environmental factors. This is well illustrated by chronic respiratory disease of rats caused by *Mycoplasma pulmonis*. This mycoplasmal infection serves as a useful example of how an important murine pathogen can affect experimental results and, at the same time, be influenced by chemical toxicity factors and animal husbandry issues. *M. pulmonis* infection in the laboratory rat may cause overt clinical respiratory disease depending on a variety of host factors such as genotype and age. It can be exacerbated by high ammonia levels and thus influenced by husbandry conditions such as the type of bedding and caging and the schedule of cage changes. Similarly, there is a reported exacerbation of pulmonary lesions caused by the synergism of inhaled chemical compounds such as hexamethylphosphoramide with this respiratory pathogen.

B. SENTINEL MONITORING PROGRAMS

Many modern toxicology laboratories employ an ongoing microbial monitoring program during the course of subchronic and chronic studies. Rodent health status can change dramatically during the course of a study. Microbial infections can enter otherwise healthy colonies via newly supplied animals into the facility, feral rodents, insect pests, contaminated food, water, or bedding, contact with technical staff carrying organisms, entry of biological materials into the colony, or stress-induced spread of low-level, undetected infections that entered with the supplied animals. Specifically designated sentinel animals are often kept with study animals to facilitate the monitoring of the microbial status of rodent experiments. Important components of the sentinel monitoring program include a determination of the optimal number, age, strain, immune competence level, and exposure means of the sentinel animals. These sentinel animals are most commonly exposed to experimental animals through cohousing or exposure to contaminated bedding. There is no optimal design of a sentinel program. The design depends on study type, rodent model, microbial history, and equipment, staff, and physical layout of the laboratory.

Most rodent sentinel monitoring programs use serological assessment of animals against common murine viral and mycoplasmal agents. Molecular diagnostic techniques, such as polymerase chain reaction (PCR) examination of feces for viral pathogens and for the presence of bacterial infections such as those of the *Helicobacter* species, are extremely sensitive and specific diagnostic modalities that are becoming increasingly utilized. Less frequently employed, but an important component of some animal health monitoring programs, is the use of pathology screening of target tissues prior to and during the toxicity experiment.

Gross and microscopic evaluation of selected colony and sentinel animals provides study personnel with the ability to detect important infectious states for which the etiology is currently unknown. An important example of

this is the presence of inflammatory pulmonary lesions of idiopathic origin that have plagued studies in a number of toxicology facilities recently. This subclinical condition is believed to be a viral infection of unknown etiology that causes an age-dependent inflammatory lesion that can be quite severe. In addition to the detection of unknown infectious agents, target organ pathology screening allows the investigator to evaluate common environment-induced lesions. Certain targets of toxicity can be severely affected by environment-related background lesions. The rat nasal passages, a common target of xenobiotic-induced toxicity, provide one such example. Poor air quality from ammonia and cage contaminant buildup associated with insufficient cage changes can induce nasal epithelial alterations and obscure toxicant-induced change. Merely comparing dosed animals with controls is often not sufficient, but it may be necessary to determine if study animals are within normal limits for parameters being tested. The pathologist must always be cognizant of the fact that subclinical infection in chemically-exposed animals may be activated and manifested differently than in controls.

C. MICROBIAL EFFECTS ON TOXICITY

There are numerous ways in which murine pathogens can exert their effects as unwanted variables in toxicology studies. These effects can be exerted systemically on the whole animal (Table III) or can be exerted through specific local changes in the relevant target organs of toxicity (Table IV). Of great importance for the pathologist is the fact that subclinical infections with certain murine pathogens, particularly

TABLE III
Selected Systemic Effects of Microbial
Agents on Toxicology Studies

Alterations in longevity
Changes in food or water consumption
Alterations in fertility and fecundity
Alterations in metabolism
Immunomodulation
Changes in body weight

259

TABLE IV
Microbial Alteration of Respiratory Tract
That May Influence Toxicologic Responses

Alterations in airway epithelial cells
  Hypertrophy and hyperplasia
  Necrosis
  Syncytial cell formation
  Squamous metaplasia
  Mucous cell hyperplasia
Hyperplasia type II cells
Altered tumor response following
carcinogen
Decreased mucociliary function
Altered surfactant
Changes in airway cytokines
Alterations in pulmonary lymphocytes

those not found on the commonly utilized serologic screening profiles, are often first detected by noting lesions in target tissues. In recent years, chronic active hepatitis caused by *Helicobacter hepaticus* infection in mice has served as an excellent example of why the toxicologic pathologist is integral to an evaluation of colony health and provides needed input for the interpretation of study results. Depending on genotype, gender, and other host factors, such as immunocompetency, this infection can influence toxic and carcinogenic responses and can modify important metabolic processes.

In some instances, experimental procedures can interact with pathogens to induce adverse outcomes. For example, Syrian golden hamsters used in chronic inhalation bioassays have developed severe enteritis and mortality from latent clostridial infections triggered by the stress of immobilization in nose-only restraint tubes of the inhalation exposure apparatus. Rodent stress responses to experimental manipulations and chemical treatment must always be considered a possible trigger for the induction of pathogenicity and lesion development by opportunistic organisms. Immune modulation by chemical exposure must be considered a potential confounder in animals bearing potentially pathogenic organisms that do not induce lesions or systemic effects in the immunocompetent host. Microbial-induced lesions in the treated groups may not develop in control animals, potentially confusing the interpretation by the pathologist.

V. Housing and Husbandry Issues

A. ROLE OF ENVIRONMENT IN LESION PRODUCTION

Environmental factors in the animal room environment that affect rodents have been well studied and documented extensively. They include temperature, humidity, light, photoperiod, noise, housing methods, bedding, sanitation chemicals, airflow, diet, water, cage change methods, and handling. Although control of the environment is not the direct concern of the pathologist, environment-associated lesions are an extremely important aspect of rodent pathology.

A number of rodent lesion states that are associated in large part with environmental influences are listed in Table V. Many background rodent lesions that have an environmental component are strongly influenced by the interplay of environmental and genetic factors. For example, dystrophic cardiac calcinosis, a common

TABLE V
Selected Lesions Associated with Environmental Conditions

Lesion	Environmental condition
Phototoxic retinopathy	Light levels, photoperiodicity
Nephrocalcinosis	Diet
Cardiac calcinosis	Semipurified diet
Myocardial inflammation	Rancid dietary fat
Olfactory epithelial change	Bedding contaminants
Dental dysplasia	Powdered diet
Chronic progressive nephropathy	Dietary protein and caloric levels
Airway epithelial necrosis	High ammonia levels
Hepatic lipidosis	Semipurified diet
Obstructive genitourinary disease	Wire caging
Pododermatitis	Wire caging
Peripheral neuropathy	Wire caging
Ringtail	Temperature and humidity
Seizure-induced brain changes	Noise

cardiac lesion with a known genetic basis in certain mouse strains, is markedly influenced by type of diet. In addition to the marked interplay among environmental, microbial, and genetic factors, there can be significant interrelationships among various environmental conditions. For example, phototoxic retinal degeneration associated with high light levels and alterations in photoperiod can be markedly exacerbated by elevated ambient temperature.

The pathologist must carefully consider environmental conditions when comparing results from different rodent bioassays. For example, the type of housing conditions (groups vs single) and type of caging (direct contact bedding in polycarbonate shoeboxes vs suspended wire) can dramatically influence weight gain and tumor incidence in rodents. Therefore control of the environment and, more importantly, the documentation of environmental conditions are critical to the evaluation of rodent studies and to the establishment of rodent lesion databases. In the design of toxicology studies, the study team must consider the use of procedures to minimize sources of environmental variation. These procedures might include cage or rack rotation at various intervals throughout the study and variation in the order of certain husbandry and manipulative procedures.

In recent years, the laboratory animal science community has advocated a position that rodents should be housed in a manner that permits species-specific behaviors that contribute to their overall well-being. Most laboratory animal scientists believe that this is best accomplished by the use of direct contact bedding in solid floored caging under group housed conditions. Many toxicology studies are still conducted with individually housed animals in suspended wire caging to prevent variables that can be introduced by contact with metabolites in urine or feces or from the bedding itself. In the future, many rodent studies will probably be conducted with different husbandry conditions than in the past. Undoubtedly these changes will affect rodent lesion databases. There is ample evidence from the experience of the National Toxicology Program with

B6C3F1 mice to realize that group versus individual housing markedly influences tumor outcome data for certain sites where body weight gain is important. As has been mentioned previously, historical databases are subject to change and must be considered living documents.

B. STUDY DESIGN CONSIDERATIONS

It is critical that animals be allocated to study in a manner that minimizes bias. In most instances, this is accomplished by using randomization procedures based on body weight criteria. Many rodent suppliers ship animals based on body weight and estimate age from age/body weight growth charts. For certain types of studies (e.g., cell proliferation studies in young animals), age may be an extremely important factor, and relatively rigid criteria age as well as weight may be required for study subjects. There are correlations between body weight and certain site-specific tumors. Many long-term rodent toxicity studies result in body weight differences between dosed and control groups. When such differences are large, they could have an impact on the interpretation of study results for those tumor types showing a strong correlation with body weight.

Acclimation of animals to environment, personnel, and equipment is an often overlooked aspect of study design. Animals should be properly acclimated to all equipment used in a study. Rats that were not acclimated to metabolism caging prior to toxicant exposure were noted to have a 60-fold difference in LD_{50} to a nephrotoxic uranium compound due to differences in water intake caused by the housing change. In some instances, such as with nose-only inhalation exposure equipment, animal handling can have a dramatic influence on body weight gain.

At the outset of any toxicology experiment, the study director and pathologist should evaluate experimental procedures and consider whether any of the animal manipulations are likely to result in clinical or pathological effects. Numerous examples can be found in which study procedures led to lesion development.

For example, repeated prolonged immobilization of male rats in nose-only inhalation tubes is associated with testicular lesions, presumably from thermoregulatory and positional effects of blood flow on the testes. Extensive handling of mice has been associated with hepatic damage and changes in clinical chemistry parameters from thoracic compression. Similarly, bandage application in subchronic rat dermal toxicity bioassays has been associated with passive congestion of the liver leading to fibrosis. Administration of xenobiotics by gavage has been associated with pulmonary deposition and other causes of mortality. Gavage-associated mortality, noted to be more prevalent in female Fischer 344 rats than in other strains, has been reported to be due to irritant exacerbation of strain-related orpharyngeal degeneration. This serves as a reminder of the important interplay among experimental, chemical, genetic, and environmental factors in study interpretation.

In studies that measure cell proliferation using an exogenous label, the pathologist should be closely involved with in-life study design. The method, dosing regimen, and route of label administration to animals should be considered. These are challenging decisions. For instance, the condition of the animals at the time of manipulations, such as the implantation of osmotic pumps to deliver label, should be considered at the outset of the study. Anesthetizing an 8-week-old animal at an early interim sacrifice time point is often a simple procedure, but a very specialized anesthesia regimen may be required to perform the same procedure on an 18-month-old rodent with chronic renal dysfunction at time of terminal sacrifice. During protocol development, one must think through all of the stages of the experiment so that the proper treatment regimens can be employed with consistency throughout the entire study. Knowledge of the target organs of toxicity is often important to consider during study design, and thus the pathologist is often critical in decision making.

For the pathologist, one of the most important considerations in study design is the designation of how animals are to be removed from

the study at times other than scheduled sacrifice. Toxicology protocols have traditionally used the term moribund sacrifice to designate animals that are removed at nonscheduled times. Exactly what constitutes a moribund state may differ among individuals and may not reflect the strict definition of this term (dying or at the point of death). For many years, the primary objective of the moribund sacrifice was to provide the pathologist with tissues devoid of postmortem autolytic change. More recently, with renewed emphasis on animal welfare concerns, there has been an increasing pressure to replace the so-called moribund sacrifice with sacrifice for humane reasons. The primary objective of the change is a conscientious effort to reduce suffering associated with dying. Unfortunately, ascribing specific behavioral and physiological attributes that identify rodents in the process of dying is an exceedingly difficult task. Nonetheless, strict and consistent criteria and written procedures for the removal of animals from study for humane reasons should be in place. The study pathologist is well suited for interacting with the appropriate laboratory animal science personnel and the study director to develop the necessary criteria for determining removal for humane reasons.

VI. The Role of Diet in Toxicology Studies

A. INTRODUCTION

The diet represents the most complex mixture of chemicals to which animals are exposed and has been said to be the most important uncontrolled variable in chemical toxicity studies with rodents. Nonetheless, rodent diets draw relatively little attention as a research variable compared with microbial agents. The ingredients, essential nutrients, contaminant concentrations, and energy density of the diets influence the physiological processes and health of rodent models and their responses to administered chemicals. Over 40 nutrients are required in the diet of rodents. The diet must be adequate for the animal's gender, physiological condition (e.g., maintenance vs reproduction and lactation), and age.

An optimal rodent diet should have adequate concentrations of all the nutrients required for growth and maintenance without excessive fats, proteins, and other high-energy and growth-enhancing nutrients. Overnutrition linked to the common practice of *ad libitum* feeding of rodent chow has led to the increased growth and body weight of many important rodent strains used in toxicology experiments. This excessive caloric intake is associated with a number of important pathophysiologic processes that influence lesion development (Table V).

Feed consumption is a very commonly monitored clinical parameter in subchronic and long-term rodent toxicity and carcinogenicity studies. Decreased feed consumption may lead to malnutrition. Many subchronic rodent toxicity studies involve animal exposures sufficient to result in systemic toxicity, reduced feed consumption, and decreased terminal body weights. This observation may impair the toxicologist's ability to determine whether the observed adverse health effects are due to the chemical of interest, malnutrition, or an interaction of these two factors. For example, these interactions may influence the interpretation of neurotoxicity studies and studies in which growth and development are assessed. Anorexia and its accompanying weight loss are associated with a wide variety of behavioral changes in rats, including delayed pup development, increased motor activity, decreased hindlimb grip strength, increased escape behaviors, and cognitive learning deficits. These results indicate that reduced feed or water intake could mimic the behavioral effects of neurotoxic agents. Therefore, toxicologists reviewing study results cannot overlook the impact of reduced feed intake.

An animal's diet may also influence its response to a toxicant. There are numerous examples of the influence of diet on the development of both neoplastic and nonneoplastic lesions. Dietary modulation of lesion development can be through direct effects of dietary constituents or through secondary mechanisms such as the alteration of gut flora.

For example, 2,6-dinitrotoluene metabolism and hepatocarcinogenesis in rats fed diets with different pectin levels are influenced by diet-associated alterations in the flora of the lower intestinal tract.

B. TYPES OF DIETS

Three major types of diets are used in rodent toxicology studies: nonpurified diets, purified diets, and chemically defined diets. These diets can be fed in a variety of physical forms, although the use of pelleted chow is the most commonly employed. Nonpurified diets constitute the most widely used food in rodent toxicology studies. These diets are generally cereal-based diets composed primarily of unrefined plant and animal materials. They often contain added vitamins and minerals. These diets are characterized as open-formula or closed-formula diets. An open-formula diet is a diet in which the precise percentage composition of each ingredient is available to the investigator. A closed-formula diet is a diet that does not have the composition specified by type and amount of each ingredient by the manufacturer. Open-formula diets have been recommended for use in toxicology studies to reduce the variability in response that can arise because ingredients or their proportions are altered.

Purified diets are composed primarily of refined ingredients, including refined proteins, carbohydrates, and fat and added mineral and vitamin mixtures. These diets were called semi-synthetic or semipurified diets in the past. In general, purified diets are expensive, and standardized purified diet useful for long-term studies have not been established. A commonly utilized purified diet has been the AIN-76A formulation by the Council of the American Institute of Nutrition. This diet has been associated with periportal hepatic lipidosis, hemorrhagic changes, and soft-tissue calcifications in rodents. Purified diets are used selectively in studies in which the role of certain dietary constituents in tissue response is being examined. Chemically defined diets are characterized by nitrogen from pure amino acids, carbohydrates from refined monosaccharides or disaccharides, and fat from purified fatty acids or triglycerides. These diets are seldomly employed in toxicity studies.

C. CONTAMINANT ISSUES

Contaminants may be present in natural ingredient, nonpurified diets. For example, these diets may contain arsenic, lead, and other heavy metals, malathion and other pesticides, unintended antioxidants (e.g., BHA and BHT), phytoestrogens, mycotoxins, and other toxins. Whenever possible, the concentration of these contaminants should be kept as low as possible to prevent modification of the toxic response of the chemical under investigation. For example, a variety of natural ingredients such as estrogenic isoflavones in soybean meal have been shown to be chemoprotective and may prevent or decrease the development of spontaneous and experimental tumors. Estrogenic isoflavones such as genistein and daidzein may also affect the growth and development of rodents on natural ingredient diets that use soy as a source of protein. Standardized rodent diets with minimal estrogenic activity are desirable for some types of bioassays and are now available commercially.

Many toxicology facilities utilize the so-called certified diets. The pathologist should realize that the certification process deals with the issue of contaminant levels and has nothing to due with nutrient content. There are diet-associated lesions that can arise on study using certified diets. Several years ago, for example, multiple animal facilities had simultaneous outbreaks of scurvy in nonhuman primates fed certified chow in which the ascorbic acid was inadvertently left out. After lesions were noted, the diet was found to be lacking in vitamin C content. Lesions can also be associated with diets that deteriorate. Rancid fat in rodent diets that are stored and fed improperly have been associated with myocardial degeneration and inflammation.

D. DIETARY OPTIMIZATION

A decline in survival of rodents in 2-year chronic toxicity and oncogenicity bioassays

has been noted in many laboratories since the 1980s. This finding closely correlates with increases in food consumption and adult body weight over this same period of time. These changes have been observed in several commonly used toxicology models, including outbred Wistar and Sprague–Dawley rats, inbred Fischer 344 rats, and B6C3F1 hybrid mice. Since the early 1980s, rodent bioassays have had a steady increase in study-to-study variability, decreases in survival, and increases in the incidence, onset time, and severity of degenerative diseases, such as chronic progressive nephropathy and degenerative cardiomyopathy. In addition, spontaneous tumors have increased, primarily those that are endocrine related.

Changes in body weight of these multiple rodent stocks and strains have been influenced in large part by the breeding practices inherent in colony management. Commercial suppliers have understandably selected rodent breeding stock for more rapid growth and greater fecundity. Although genetic changes undoubtedly are partially responsible for changes in strain characteristics, these changes undoubtedly are partially responsible for changes in strain characteristics, these changes appear to be influenced greatly by the environmental conditions under which the animals are maintained. The practice of *ad libitum* feeding of rodent diets and the associated extremely high caloric intake are believed to be important factors in the alteration of these animal models (Table V). The decline in longevity and the high lesion content of study animals have led some scientists and policy makers to question the utility of the rodent bioassay for studies of safety assessment. The sensitivity of the rodent bioassay in distinguishing treatment effects from control requires adequate animal survival. Ironically, survival is often lower in *ad libitum*-fed control groups compared to high-dose groups given maximum tolerated doses of compounds that induce body weight loss from both toxicologic mechanisms and secondary effects.

Diet restriction is a well-established method of extending the life span of rodents. The restriction of fat, protein, minerals, and other nutritional components without caloric restriction does not increase the overall long-term survival of animals. A number of investigators have demonstrated that moderate diet restriction (70–80% of *ad libitum* levels) can significantly improve longevity in rodents and will support the maintenance of healthier animals with a lower incidence (or later onset) of certain degenerative and neoplastic diseases. Studies have shown that moderate diet restriction does not adversely affect metabolism, clinical chemistry, or toxicokinetic or toxicologic responses to pharmaceutical agents. Diet restriction has not yet received a clear endorsement as a standard of rodent husbandry, but it is being employed increasingly in long-term rodent studies in a number of laboratories. Studies conducted with these feeding practices have been accepted by regulatory agencies.

Not all laboratory animal scientists agree that diet restriction is the method of choice for optimizing how rodents are fed. Some have criticized that diet restriction imparts a significant disadvantage due to alteration in the pattern of how rodents consume feed, leading to potential changes in associated physiological processes. There has been an effort by the National Toxicology Program to formulate a new rodent open-formula diet (NTP 2000) that has a decreased protein content and slightly higher fat and fiber contents relative to older, commonly used open-formula diets such as NIH-07. Early indications are that this new diet is adequate for growth and maintenance in Fischer 344 rats and appears to prevent or decrease the severity of some diet-associated lesions such as chronic progressive nephropathy.

VII. Summary

Numerous genetic, microbial, environmental, and experimental factors work together to influence development of the lesions studied by the toxicologic pathologist. The pathologist needs to understand how factors associated with the laboratory animal and its experimental environment contribute to study findings so that the results of toxicity experiments can be evaluated properly. The changes that are occurring in laboratory animal husbandry practices are driven in part by recent advances in animal welfare concerns. Future standards for feeding and housing rodents will likely differ from those employed today. As advances are made in the use of genetically engineered animals, greater emphasis will be placed on understanding the mechanistic underpinnings of the interplay among host susceptibility factors, toxicant exposure, and environment.

SUGGESTED READING

Regulatory Issues

Regulations

Animal Welfare Act (1985). Pub. L. 99–198, 9 CFR (Parts 1, 2 and 3).
Health Research Extension Act of 1985. Pub. L 99–158, Animal in Research.
Hicks, J. M. (1997). Animal welfare and toxicology/safety studies: Making sense of the regulatory environment. *Contemp. Top. Lab. Anim. Sci.* **36**, 49–54.
Institute of Laboratory Animal Resources-Commission on Life Sciences-National Research Council (1996). "Guide for the Care and Use of Laboratory Animals," National Academy Press, Washington, DC.
Office for Protection of Research Risks. NIH (1996). Public Health Service Policy on Human Care and Use of Laboratory Animals.

Institutional Animal Care and Use Committees

Everitt, J., and Griffin, W. (1995). Proposed IACUC guidelines for the review of rodent toxicology studies. *Contemp. Top. Lab. Anim. Sci.* **34**, 72–74.
Hamm, T. E. (1995). Proposed Institutional Animal Care and Use Committee guidelines for death as an endpoint in rodent studies. *Contemp. Top. Lab. Anim. Sci.* **34**, 69–71.
Mann, M. D., *et al.* (1991). Appropriate animal numbers in biomedical research in light of animal welfare considerations. *Lab. Anim. Sci.* **41**(1), 6–14.
Stokes, W. S., and Jensen D. J. B. (1995). Guidelines for Institutional Animal Care and Use Committees:

Consideration of alternatives. *Contemp. Top. Lab. Anim. Sci.* **34**, 51–60.

Weigler, B.J. (1995). Justifying the number of animals in IACUC proposals. *Contemp. Top. Lab. Anim. Sci.* **34**, 47–50.

Euthanasia

American Veterinary Medical Association (1993). 1993 report of the AVMA Panel on Euthanasia. *J. Am. Vet. Med. Assoc.* **202**, 229–249.

Brooks, P. J., *et al.* (1999). The influence of euthanasia methods on rat liver metabolism. *Contemp. Top. Lab. Anim. Sci.* **38**, 19–24.

Butler, M. M., *et al.* (1990). The effect of euthanasia technique on vascular arachidonic acid metabolism and vascular and intestinal smooth muscle contractility. *Lab. Anim. Sci.* **40**(3), 277–283.

Howard, H. L., *et al.* (1990). The effect of mouse euthanasia technique on subsequent lymphocyte proliferation and cell mediated lympholysis assays. *Lab. Anim. Sci.* **40**(5), 510–514.

Toth, L.A. (1997). The moribund state as an experimental endpoint. *Contemp. Top. Lab. Anim. Sci.* **36**, 44–48.

Selection of Animal Models

Genetic Issues

Festing, M. F. (1979). Properties of inbred strains and outbred stocks, with special reference to toxicity testing. *J. Toxicol. Environ. Health* **5**(1), 53–68.

Festing, M. F. (1995). Use of a multistrain assay could improve the NTP carcinogenesis bioassay. *Environ. Health Perspect.* **103**(1), 44–52.

Kacew, S., *et al.* (1995). Strain as a determinant factor in the differential responsiveness of rats to chemicals. *Toxicol. Pathol.* **23**, 701–714.

Kacew, S., and Festing, M. F. (1996). Role of rat strain in the differential sensitivity to pharmaceutical agents and naturally occuring substances. *J. Toxicol. Environ. Health* **47**(1), 1–30.

Rao, G. N., *et al.* (1988). Mouse strains for chemical carcinogenicity studies: Overview of a workshop. *Fundam. Appl. Toxicol.* **10**(3), 385–394.

Wolff, G. L. (1996). Variability in gene expression and tumor formation within genetically homogeneous animal populations in bioassays. *Fundam. Appl. Toxicol.* **29**(2), 176–184

Historical Database Issues

Everett, R. (1984). Factors affecting spontaneous tumor incidence rates in mice: A literature review. *CRC Rev. Toxicol.* **13**(3), 235–250.

Germann, P. G., *et al.* (1998). Brief communication: Pathology of the oropharyngeal cavity in six strains of rats: Predisposition of Fischer 344 rats for inflammatory and degenerative changes. *Toxicol. Pathol.* **26**, 283–289.

Haseman, J. K., *et al.* (1984). Use of historical control data in carcinogenicity studies in rodents. *Toxicol. Pathol.* **12**, 126–135.

Haseman, J. K., *et al.* (1992). Value of historical controls in the interpretation of rodent tumor data. *Drug Inf. J.* **26**, 1–10.

Rao, G. N., *et al.* (1990). Growth, body weight, survival and tumor trends in F344/N rats during an eleven-year period. *Toxicol. Pathol.* **18**(1), 61–70.

Rao, G. N., *et al.* (1990). Growth, body weight, survival, and tumor trends in (C57BL/6 X C3H/HeN) F1 (B6C3F1) mice during a nine-year period. *Toxicol. Pathol.* **18**(1), 71–77.

Roe, F. J. (1994). Historical histopathological control data for laboratory rodents: Valuable treasure or worthless trash? *Lab. Anim.* **28**(2), 148–154.

Genetically Engineered Rodents

Harvey, M., *et al.* (1993). Spontaneous and carcinogen-induced tumorigenesis in p53-deficient mice. *Nat. Genet.* **5**, 225–229.

Tennant, R. W., *et al.* (1995). Identifying chemical carcinogens and assessing potential risk in short-term bioassays using transgenic mouse models. *Environ. Health Perspect.* **103**, 942–950.

Animal Health Issues

Adventitious Agents

Baker, D. G. (1998). Natural pathogens of laboratory mice, rats, and rabbits and their effects on research. *Clin. Microbiol. Rev.* **11**(2), 231–266.

Casebolt, D. B., *et al.* (1988). Prevalence rates of infectious agents among commercial breeding populations of rats and mice. *Lab. Anim. Sci.* **38**(3), 327–329.

Elwell, M. R., *et al.* (1997). "Have you seen this?" Inflammatory lesions in the lungs of rats. *Toxicol. Pathol.* **25**(5), 529–531.

Jacoby, R. O., *et al.* (1996). Rodent parvovirus infections. *Lab. Anim. Sci.* **46**(4), 370–380.

Sentinel Monitoring Program

Selwyn, M. R., and Shek, W. R. (1994). Sample sizes and frequency of testing for health monitoring in barrier rooms and isolators. *Contemp. Top. Lab. Anim. Sci.* **33**(3), 56–59.

Microbial Effects on Toxicity

Chomarat, P., *et al.* (1997). Distinct time courses of increase in cytochromes P450 1A2, 2A5 and glutathione S-transferases during the progressive hepatitis associated with Helicobacter hepaticus. *Carcinogenesis* **18**(11), 2179–2190.

Diwan, B. A., *et al.* (1997). Promotion by *Helicobacter hepaticus*-induced hepatitis of hepatic tumors initiated by N-nitrosodimethylamine in male A/JCr mice. *Toxicol. Pathol.* **25**, 597–605.

Everitt, J. I., and Richter, C. B. (1990). Infectious diseases of the upper respiratory tract: Implications for toxicology studies. *Environ. Health Persp.* **85**, 239–247.

Fox, J. G., (1983). Intercurrent disease and environmental variables in rodent toxicology studies. *Prog. Exp. Tumor Res.* **26**, 208–240.

Hiley, R. R., *et al.* (1998). Impact of *Helicobacter hepaticus* infection in B6C3F1 mice from twelve National Toxicology Program two-year carcinogenesis studies. *Toxicol. Pathol.* **26**, 602–612.

Nyska, A., *et al.* (1997). Alterations in cell kinetics in control B6C3F1 mice infected with *Helicobacter hepaticus*. *Toxicol. Pathol.* **25**, 591–596.

Overcash, R. G., *et al.* (1976). Enhancement of natural and experimental respiratory mycoplasmosis in rats by hexamethylphosphoramide. *Am. J. Pathol.* **82**(01), 171–189.

Peck, R. M., *et al.* (1983). Influence of Sendai virus on carcinogenesis in strain A mice. *Lab. Anim. Sci.* **33**(2), 154–156.

Rao, G. N., *et al.* (1989). Influence of viral infections on body weight, survival, and tumor prevalence of B6C3F1 (C57BL/6N × C3H/HeN) mice in carcinogenicity studies. *Fundam. Appl. Toxicol.* **13**(1), 156–164.

Schreiber, H., *et al.* (1972). Induction of lung cancer in germfree, specific-pathogen-free, and infected rats by N-nitrosoheptamethyleneimine: enhancement by respiratory infection. *J. Natl. Cancer Inst.* **49**(4), 1107–1114.

Housing and Husbandry

Role of Environment in Lesion Production

Bendele, A. M., and Carlton, W. W. (1986). Incidence of obstructive uropathy in male B6C3F1 mice on a 24-month carcinogenicity study and its apparent prevention by ochratoxin A. *Lab. Anim. Sci.* **36**(3), 282–285.

Bolon, B., *et al.* (1991). Toxic interactions in the rat nose: Pollutants from soiled bedding and methyl bromide. *Toxicol. Pathol.* **19**(4), 571–579.

Clough, G. (1982). Environmental effects on animals used in biomedical research. *Biol. Rev. Camb. Philos. Soc.* **57**, 487–523.

Everitt, J. I., *et al.* (1988). Urologic syndrome associated with wire caging in AKR mice. *Lab. Anim. Sci.* **38**, 609–611.

Haseman, J. K., *et al.* (1997). Body weight-tumor incidence correlations in long-term rodent carcinogenicity studies. *Toxicol. Pathol.* **25**, 256–263.

Losco, P. E. (1995). Dental dysplasias in rats and mice. *Toxicol. Pathol.* **23**, 677–688.

Steplewski, Z., *et al.* (1987). Effect of housing stress on the formation and development of tumors in rats. *Cancer Lett.* **34**(3), 257–261.

Young, S. S. (1987). Are there local room effects on hepatic tumors in male mice? An examination of the NTP eugenol study. *Fundam. Appl. Toxicol.* **8**(1), 1–4.

Study Design Considerations

Damon, E. G., *et al.* (1986). Effect of acclimation to caging on nephrotoxic response of rats to uranium. *Lab. Anim. Sci.* **36**(1), 24–27.

DePass, L. R., *et al.* (1986). Influence of housing conditions for mice on the results of a dermal oncogenicity bioassay. *Fundam. Appl. Toxicol.* **7**(4), 601–608.

Herzberg, A. M., and Lagakos, S. W. (1992). Cage allocation designs for rodent carcinogenicity experiments. *Environ. Health Perspect.* **97**, 277–280.

Martin, R. A., *et al.* (1986). Randomization of animals by computer program for toxicity studies. *J. Environ. Pathol. Toxicol. Oncol.* **6**(5–6), 143–152.

Role of Diet

General

Everitt, J. I., *et al.* (1988). Effect of a purified diet on cardiac calcinosis in mice. *Lab. Anim. Sci.* **38**, 426–429.

Goldstein, R. S., *et al.* (1984). Influence of dietary pectin on intestinal microfloral metabolism and toxicity of nitrobenzene. *Toxicol. Appl. Pharmacol.* **75**, 547–553.

Goldsworthy, T. L., *et al.* (1986). The effect of diet on 2,6-dinitrotoluene hepatocarcinogenesis. *Carcinogenesis* **7**, 1909–1915.

Hayashi, Y., *et al.* (1984). Nutritional factors influencing the results of toxicology experiments in animals. *J. Toxicol. Sci.* **9**, 219–234.

Newberne, P. M., and Sotnikov, A. V. (1996). Diet: The neglected variable in chemical safety evaluations. *Toxicol. Pathol.* **24**, 746–756.

Rao, G. N. (1988). Rodent diets for carcinogenesis studies. *J. Nutr.* **118**(8), 929–931.

Types of Diets

Mitchell, G. V., *et al.* (1989). Nutritional and pathological changes in male and female rats fed modifications of the AIN-76A diet. *Food Chem. Toxicol.* **27**(3), 185–191.

Rao, G. N., (1996). New diet (NTP-2000) for rats in the National Toxicology Program toxicity and carcinogenicity studies. *Fundam. Appl. Toxicol.* **32**, 102–108.

Contaminant Issues

Casanova, M., *et al.* (1999). Developmental effects of dietary phytoestrogens in Sprague-Dawley rats and interactions of genistein and daidzein with rat estrogen receptors alpha and beta *in vitro. Toxicol. Sci.* **51**, 236–244.

Kusewitt, D. F., *et al.* (1984). Fatal myocarditis in mice fed rancid purified diet. *Lab. Anim. Sci.* **34**, 70–74.

Rao, G. N., and Knapka, J. J. (1987). Contaminant and nutrient concentrations of natural ingredient rat and mouse diet used in chemical toxicology studies. *Fundam. Appl. Toxicol.* **9**(2), 329–338.

Thigpen, J. E., *et al.* (1987). The mouse bioassay for the detection of estrogenic activity in rodent diets: I. A standardized method for conducting the mouse bioassay. *Lab. Anim. Sci.* **37**, 596–609.

Diet Optimization

Albee, R. R., *et al.* (1997). Neurobehavioral effects of dietary restriction in rats. *Neurotoxicol. Teratol.* **9**, 203–211.

Blackwell, B. N., *et al.* (1995). Longevity, body weight, and neoplasia in *ad libitum*-fed and diet-restricted C57BL6 mice fed NIH-31 open formula diet. *Toxicol. Pathol.* **23**, 570–582.

Gumprecht, L. A., *et al.* (1993). The early effects of dietary restriction on the pathogenesis of chronic renal disease in Sprague-Dawley rats at 12 months. *Toxicol. Pathol.* **21**(6), 528–537.

Keenan, K. P., *et al.* (1994). The effects of overfeeding and dietary restriction on Sprague-Dawley rat survival and early pathology biomarkers of aging. *Toxicol. Pathol.* **22**(3), 300–315.

Keenan, K. P., *et al.* (1995). Diet, overfeeding, and moderate dietary restriction in control Sprague-Dawley rats: I. Effects on spontaneous neoplasms. *Toxicol. Pathol.* **23**(3), 269–286.

Keenan, K. P., *et al.* (1995). Diet, overfeeding, and moderate dietary restriction in control Sprague-Dawley rats: II. Effects on age-related proliferative and degenerative lesions. *Toxicol. Pathol.* **23**(3), 287–302.

Keenan, K. P., *et al.* (1996). The effects of overfeeding and moderate dietary restriction on Sprague-Dawley rat survival, pathology, carcinogenicity, and the toxicity of pharmaceutical agents. *Exp. Toxicol. Pathol.* **48**(2–3), 139–144.

Keenan, K. P., *et al.* (1999). Diet, caloric restriction, and the rodent bioassay. *Toxicol. Sci.* **52**(Suppl.), 24–34.

Levin, S., *et al.* (1993). Effects of two weeks of feed restriction on some common toxicologic parameters in Sprague-Dawley rats. *Toxicol. Pathol.* **21**, 1–14.

Rao, G. N. (1997). New nonpurified diet (NTP-2000) for rodents in the National Toxicology Program's toxicology and carcinogenesis studies. *J. Nutr.* **127**, 842S–846S.

Sheldon, W. G., *et al.* (1995). Age-related neoplasia in a lifetime study of *ad libitum*-fed and food-restricted B6C3F1 mice. *Toxicol. Pathol.* **23**, 458–476.

Thurman, J. D., *et al.* (1994). Survival, body weight, and neoplasms in *ad libitum*-fed and food-restricted Fischer 344 rats. *Toxicol. Pathol.* **22**, 1–9.

—————————————— *13* ——————————————

New Animal Models in Toxicology

Eugenia Floyd

Department of Drug Safety Evaluation
Pfizer Nagoya Laboratories
Taketoyo, Aichi, Japan

I. Many Strains of Genetically Engineered Rodents Are Available for Use in Toxicology

Since the first *in vivo* use of transgenic technology in 1976 and of targeted gene mutation by homologous recombination in 1989, many strains of genetically engineered rodents have been created and made available for use by researchers through commercial, collaborative academic and in-house sources. The advent of genomics has dramatically increased the production of new gene-altered mice for investigating the function of newly discovered genes (functional genomics) and for creating new animal models of disease. Some of these models are being used or evaluated for use as tools for toxicology research and toxicity testing. Transgenic and knockout or knockin mice

and rats will become increasingly important *in vivo* models for genetic toxicity testing, mechanistic toxicology research, specialized toxicity testing, and short-term carcinogenicity testing.

The toxicologic pathologist will need to develop and maintain a basic understanding of the continually evolving technologies used for genetic engineering (Fig. 1) because technology affects phenotype and its pathological manifestations in many ways, e.g., through the selection of background strain. Familiarity with the biology and spontaneous tissue changes of the gene-altered models will be required for accurate interpretation of findings from studies using these mice. Also, toxicologic pathologists who perform mechanistic and experimental studies will greatly broaden their research capabilities by understanding possible strategies for the use of genetically modified models. This chapter describes a selection of the many new rodent models available for use in toxicology and illustrates by example how these models have

Handbook of Toxicologic Pathology, Second Edition
Volume 1

Eugenia Floyd

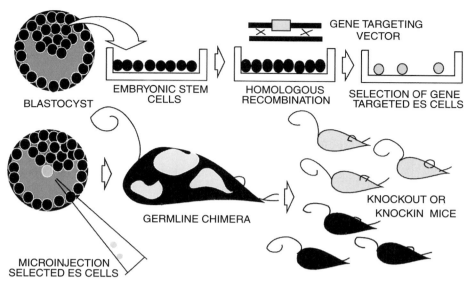

Figure 1. Targeted gene deletion for the creation of knockout mice is accomplished through homologous recombination in embryonic stem cells (ES). This process uses a DNA segment (targeting vector) that has flanking sequences identical to ES genomic segments flanking a targeted gene. The targeting vector hybridizes with the genomic DNA at the flanking sites and deactivates the targeted gene by replacing genomic DNA sequences critical for function of the targeted gene. The successfully targeted ES cells are retrieved and microinjected into developing blastocysts that are implanted into pseudopregnant dams. The resulting offspring will carry the genetic alteration in some tissues but not in others (chimeras). Chimeric offspring carrying the targeted deletion in the germline can be bred to produce lines of knockout mice.

been used to answer basic questions and solve specific problems in toxicological research and testing.

II. Genetically Engineered Mice Can Be Used for *in Vivo* Genetic Toxicity Testing

The primary purpose of genetic toxicology is to provide surrogate measures of the carcinogenic potential of a compound or chemical. The toxicologic pathologist, while maintaining ultimate interest in the endpoint of tumorigenicity, profits from an understanding of the relationship between genetic damage and the process of carcinogenesis. Building that understanding requires some knowledge of the methods, strengths, and limitations of the test systems used to measure genotoxicity, including genetically altered models.

A. MUTAMOUSE AND BIG BLUE TRANSGENIC MICE

The first mice genetically engineered for use in toxicology were the *lacZ* (MutaMouse) and *lacI* (Big Blue) transgenic mice created for *in vivo* mutagenicity testing. A *lacI* transgenic rat is also available. These two transgenes were derived from the bacterial *lac* operon that controls lactose metabolism through the regulated expression of β-galactosidase. The transgenes are in retrievable λ phage-shuttle vectors within the mouse genome where they act as untranscribed target genes for mutagenesis. An *ex vivo* bacterial plaque assay measures spontaneous and induced mutant frequencies in the *lacI* or Z genes retrieved from isolated genomic DNA (Fig. 2). Researchers have developed simpler and faster assays for mutational analysis using the *cI* or *cII* genetic segments of the λ shuttle vectors in these same transgenic mice. With either type of assay, *lac* transgenic mice can be

270

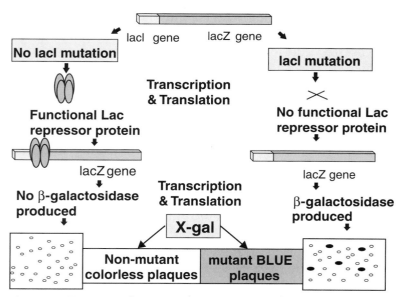

Figure 2. To measure *lacI* mutant frequency in Big Blue mice, genomic DNA is isolated from a tissue, and the transgenic λ shuttle vectors carrying the *lacI* genes are retrieved and packaged into viable phage particles. These λ phages can infect and lyse *Escherichia coli* to form plaques on a bacterial lawn. If the *lacI* gene carried by a phage is mutated, the bacterial *lacZ* gene will not be repressed, and the infected bacterium will produce β-galactosidase. In the presence of the substrate X- gal, this enzyme catalyzes a chromogenic reaction producing blue plaques so that *lacI* mutants can be counted readily. If the *lacI* gene carried by a phage is not mutated, *lacZ* will remain repressed so that the infected bacterial plaque will be clear. Big Blue is a registered trademark of Stratagene. Used with permission.

used to detect compound-induced point mutations and small genetic deletions in any tissue. Additional information about the mutation process can be obtained by sequencing the retrieved target gene (*lacI, lacZ* genes or *cI, cII* segments). Some mutagens produce mutational spectra that differ from the spontaneous mutation spectrum observed in the transgenic target DNA, which consists primarily (>50%) of G:C to A:T transitions at CpG sites. Spectral analysis by DNA sequencing may increase the sensitivity of the assay by allowing detection of mutagenesis produced by agents that can alter this spectrum even at low levels of mutation induction. Several laboratories—academic, governmental, and industrial—have evaluated these mice using a number of prototypical mutagens as well as nonmutagens, and the results of these studies are compiled in a historical database accessible through the internet (http://eden. ceh.uvic.ca/big-blue.htm). The site also contains background information on the various *lac* transgenic models and mutation assays used for *in vivo* genotoxicity testing.

B. *Aprt*-DEFICIENT MICE

A newer type of model for genetic toxicology testing has a site-directed inactivating point mutation in an endogenous gene that codes for an enzyme in the purine salvage pathway, adenosine phosphoribosyltransferase (APRT). The homozygous gene-altered mouse, which has two inactivated *Aprt* alleles, can be used to detect spontaneous or test agent-induced reverse mutations that restore functionality to at least one *Aprt* allele. Restored functionality is identified by an *ex vivo* assay that measures the uptake of adenosine by cells that contain the reverse mutation. The heterozygous (*Aprt*

+/−) mouse, however, will detect deletional loss of heterozygosity (LOH) that occurs most often as a mitotic recombinational event. The frequency of the LOH events is increased by exposure to some genotoxic carcinogens. Consequently, in contrast to the homozygote that detects point mutations, the *Aprt* +/− mouse may be useful for the *in vivo* identification of genotoxin-induced damage that occurs at the level of the chromosome.

C. *p^{un}* MUTANT MICE

A spontaneous mutant mouse can also be used for detecting agents that produce chromosomal deletions. The *p^{un}* mouse has white fur because it has a deactivating duplicated DNA segment in the *p* locus that controls coat color. Recombinational deletion of the duplicated segment is increased by treatment with some genotoxic carcinogens, producing mice with black-spotted coats. The disadvantage of this mouse, however, is its inability to detect genetic deletions in nonpigmented tissues.

D. OTHER NEW MODELS FOR MUTAGENICITY TESTING

Researchers continue to develop other new genetically engineered models for the *in vivo* assay of mutagenesis. Some models, like the *lac* transgenics, utilize bacterial target transgenes, e.g., mice with *gpt* transgenes in a pCGK shuttle vector. Others, such as thymidine kinase heterozygous (*TK*+/−) mice, utilize genetically altered endogenous genes, like the *Aprt* +/− mice. More research is needed to assess the utility of these newer models.

E. ADVANTAGES AND DISADVANTAGES OF GENE-ALTERED MICE FOR GENETIC TOXICOLOGY

Genetically engineered *in vivo* models have some advantages over standard *in vitro* tests of genetic toxicity, one of the most important being the subjection of the test compound or chemical to the normal physiological processes of absorption, distribution, metabolism, and elimination (ADME) that shape the activity of a compound *in vivo*. Another advantage is the ability to study organ-specific genetic toxicity and, of special interest to the toxicologic pathologist who studies carcinogenesis, to correlate tumor formation with mutagenesis or chromosomal alterations in the cells of a target organ. These models also may prove to be useful for assessing genetic toxicity in gonadal tissues, where genetic damage cannot be assayed readily by other techniques.

Among the disadvantages of these model systems are their high labor, time, and animal costs when compared to the standard battery of genetic toxicology tests (Ames, *in vitro* cytogenetics, *in vivo* micronucleus tests) now used by the chemical and pharmaceutical industries. Unlike the results from transgenic assays, results from standard battery tests are accepted routinely by governmental regulatory agencies around the world. Industry must rely most heavily on high-throughput systems capable of testing large numbers of compounds or chemicals quickly, inexpensively, accurately, and consistently. Additionally, some genetic toxicologists and regulatory scientists have judged the *lac* transgenic models to be inadequately sensitive because their target genes are not actively transcribed, as active expression of a gene increases its susceptibility to induced mutation. Bacterial target genes also have high spontaneous mutation rates because they have many CpG sites, which decrease their sensitivity for detecting induced mutations.

These criticisms have been addressed by some of the new *in vivo* models that utilize transcribed, endogenous genes as targets; however, none of these new *in vivo* models has been sufficiently validated for routine use in risk assessment. For these reasons, industry's current use of genetically engineered *in vivo* models for genetic toxicity testing will be limited to further evaluation of the models and to mechanistic or exploratory studies intended to solve particular problems that may arise during the routine testing of a compound or chemical. Gene-altered models will continue, nonetheless, to be very valuable tools for the toxicological research community.

272

III. Genetically Engineered Mice Can Be Used to Study Mechanisms of Toxicity *in Vivo*

A. ROLE OF XENOBIOTIC RECEPTORS IN TOXICITY

Some xenobiotics require receptor binding to initiate their pharmacological and/or toxic effects, and the role of some receptors important in the development of toxicities can now be explored *in vivo* using gene-altered mice. Two knockout models of particular interest were created by targeted deletion of the genes for the aryl hydrocarbon (AH) receptor and the peroxisome proliferator-activated receptor α (PPAR α).

1. Ahr-Null Mice

The AH receptor is a member of the basic helix–loop–helix superfamily of nuclear receptors. It binds halogenated and polycyclic aromatic hydrocarbons, many of which are highly toxic, carcinogenic, and teratogenic, e.g., dioxin and polychlorinated biphenyls. The AH receptor also mediates metabolism of some of its ligands through its transcriptional activation of the genes coding for cytochromes P450 1A1, 1A2, and 1B1, as well as several phase II metabolism enzymes, including glutathione-*S*-transferase (GST) and UDP-glucuronosyl-transferase 1A1. Experiments have shown that *Ahr*-null mice were resistant to the acute toxicity of dioxin, confirming that receptor binding was necessary to initiate the cascade of events that produced the toxicity of this chemical *in vivo*. Additionally, the teratogenic effects of dioxin were reduced, but not completely blocked, in these mice, indicating that some, but not all, of the developmental toxicity of dioxin is mediated through the AH receptor. These *Ahr*-null mice will be useful models for dissecting the receptor binding, cell signaling, and metabolic pathways responsible for the adverse effects of many other chemicals that are AHR ligands.

2. Ppar-Null Mice

PPAR α, and δ, and γ form a subfamily in the NR1 nuclear receptor gene family and share a common heterodimerization partner, the retinoid X receptor. PPARs, which are the natural receptors for free fatty acids and eicosenoids, regulate glucose and lipid homeostasis by controlling the expression of genes responsible for fatty acid synthesis, storage, and catabolism, including the P450 4A enzymes that catalyze the ω-hydroxylation of fatty acids.

PPAR α and γ also serve as receptors for xenobiotics that include the fibrate class of cholesterol-lowering drugs and the glitazones used for the treatment of type II diabetes, respectively. PPAR α ligands, which also include the phthalates used in the manufacture of plastics, cause the proliferation of peroxisomes in rodent hepatocytes after acute administration and hepatic tumors when administered chronically to rodents. Because of their widespread use as pharmaceuticals and in industry, peroxisome proliferators have been studied extensively to assess their toxicological risk to humans. Several early research findings suggested that the peroxisome proliferator activity and tumorigenicity of these compounds were rodent-specific responses related to the high-level expression of PPAR α in rodent hepatocytes. These findings included the inability to experimentally produce peroxisome proliferation in human hepatocytes *in vitro*, the lack of epidemiological evidence for fibrate-induced hepatocarcinogenesis in humans, and the relatively low-level expression of PPAR α in human tissues.

The *Ppar* α-knockout mouse has been useful for demonstrating *in vivo* that the hepatocellular peroxisome proliferation caused by di(2-ethylhexyl)phthalate and the hepatocarcinogenicity of WY-14,463 (a potent fibrate) were both entirely receptor mediated, strongly corroborating other evidence for the low carcinogenic risk of peroxisome proliferators to humans. Research has also shown that PPAR α functioning contributes to the maintenance of normal cellular redox balance, so the *Ppar* α-knockout mice will be useful for investigating oxidative stress as well as receptor-mediated toxicity.

B. ROLE OF CYTOCHROME P450 ENZYMES IN TOXICITY AND CARCINOGENESIS

1. P450 Knockout Mice

A number of the most exciting new models for use in toxicology are those having targeted deletions of some isoforms of the cytochrome P450 (CYP) mixed function oxidases. P450s, which form a superfamily of enzymes coded for by more than 12 gene families, catalyze the oxidative biotransformation of many endogenous substrates as well as xenobiotics. The CYP1, CYP2, and CYP3 enzyme subfamilies are responsible for the phase I metabolism of most drugs, and their enzymatic activity can detoxify toxic compounds or, in some cases, generate toxic metabolites.

Three P450 knockout mice, having targeted deletion of genes encoding CYP1A2, CYP2E1, and CYP1B1, have been reported in the literature. In the past, toxicological researchers had to rely on the coadministration of specific enzyme inhibitors, most of which had other pharmacological activities as well, to show that metabolism by a particular P450 enzyme was required for development of an agent's toxicity *in vivo*. Now, the use of gene-altered models can demonstrate more clearly how some toxicities are mediated *in vivo* by particular P450 isozymes, as illustrated in the following examples.

Acetaminophen is an analgesic that can produce toxicity in the liver and the kidney. *In vitro* and *in vivo* studies using enzyme inhibitors implicated both CYP1A2 and CYP2E1 in the production of a toxic electrophile judged to be responsible for causing both hepatic and renal tubular necrosis. Additionally, ethanol induction of CYP2E1 in rodents or its homologue in humans potentiated acetaminophen toxicity. The contribution of both of these enzymes to the development of this toxicity was confirmed elegantly in a series of *in vivo* studies using mice null for *Cyp1a2*, mice null for *Cyp2e1*, and cross-bred mice that were null for the genes of both isozymes. As anticipated, each of the single-gene knockout mice developed milder lesions than the wild-type

control mice when administered toxic doses of acetaminophen. Moreover, no hepatic or renal toxicity developed in the double knockout mice that were administered toxic doses equivalent to those given the single knockouts. These findings demonstrated that the metabolic activities of these two CYP isoforms were sufficient for producing all aspects of acetaminophen toxicity at the doses tested in mice in this study.

Other research using P450 knockout mice has generated results that were more unanticipated. Dimethylbenzanthracene (DMBA), a polycyclic aromatic hydrocarbon, is a highly potent carcinogen requiring metabolic activation. Like other aromatic hydrocarbons, DMBA binds the AH receptor, which then transcriptionally activates the gene for CYP1A1. DMBA is also metabolized extensively by CYP1A1, which is the P450 generally thought to mediate the carcinogenicity of polycyclic aromatic hydrocarbons. However, when *Cyp1b1* knockout mice were treated with carcinogenic doses of DMBA, they developed significantly fewer lymphomas than wild-type control mice, demonstrating that CYP1B1 was a primary mediator of DMBA carcinogenicity. CYP1B1, unlike 1A1, is expressed extrahepatically, and its expression in hematopoietic tissue, the site of tumor origin, indicates how local P450 activity can influence tissue susceptibility to carcinogenesis as well as other forms of toxicity.

2. P450 Transgenic Mice

The various models created by targeted deletion of P450 isoenzymes have been used to investigate the *in vivo* mechanisms of toxicity of many agents other than those presented earlier, including phenacetin, carbon tetrachloride, chloroform, benzene, and acetone. Only two P450 transgenic models have been reported in the literature, however, and few agents have been tested in them. These P450 transgenic mice were produced to better understand the role of human fetal metabolism in toxicity. Researchers created two lines of mice using the gene that codes for a human fetus-specific P450 enzyme, CYP3A7. In one line, the

CYP3A7 expression was directed to the liver, whereas in the other line, transgene expression was in the kidney. Studies with these mice demonstrated that this fetus-specific enzyme was capable of activating aflatoxin B1 (AFB1), a confirmed human carcinogen. The AFB1 activation produced significantly higher numbers of AFB1-N7-guanine DNA adducts, which are biomarkers of aflatoxin-induced genetic damage in humans, in the livers and kidneys expressing CYP3A7 than in the livers and kidneys of wild-type controls. These results suggest that, when exposed to AFB1, human fetuses may not be protected from the carcinogenic activity of this mycotoxin.

Additional P450 knockin or transgenic mice that will be developed in the future include models in which a human gene for a major P450 isoenzyme will replace its murine homologue in the mouse genome. These models should exhibit metabolic activity more comparable to that of humans and provide valuable tools for pharmacological and toxicological research.

C. ROLE OF PHASE II AND OTHER METABOLIC ENZYMES IN TOXICITY AND CARCINOGENESIS

Many enzymes other than the cytochrome P450s participate in the metabolism of xenobiotics. Among these are various oxidoreductases, dehydrogenases, monoamine oxidases, hydrolases, and esterases, as well as the different types of transferases that perform the conjugation reactions of phase II metabolism. Investigators have created several mouse strains with targeted deletions of some of these enzymes, and more strains are under development. These knockouts include mice with disruption of the genes encoding monoamine oxidases A and B, epoxide hydrolase, alcohol dehydrogenases (1, 3, and 4), NADPH:quinone oxidoreductase-1 (DT diaphorase), and GST P1/P2. Studies performed with mice having targeted deletions of the genes for microsomal epoxide hydrolase (mEH), GST, and three isozymes of alcohol dehydrogenase (ADH) illustrate the usefulness

of these knockouts in mechanistic toxicological research.

1. mEH-Null Mice

mEH has been implicated in the metabolic activation of carcinogenic polycyclic hydrocarbons such as DMBA through its ability to generate highly reactive aryl epoxide intermediates capable of alkylating DNA. The role of mEH in DMBA metabolic activation in vivo was tested using mice nullizygous for the mEH gene. When subjected to the classic two-step skin carcinogenesis bioassay using DMBA and when administered DMBA systemically in a standard carcinogenicity assay, these knockout mice were completely resistant to tumorigenesis. These results confirmed that mEH activity in vivo was required for the manifestation of DMBA-induced carcinogenicity.

2. Gst-Null Mice

Electrophilic intermediates produced by the P450 metabolism of compounds such as DMBA are conjugated to the tripeptide glutathione by GST. The catalytic activity of GST protects against the toxicity of these reactive intermediates as long as reduced glutathione is present in adequate supply. The protective activity of GST in vivo was examined by subjecting Gst-null mice to the two-step skin carcinogenesis bioassay using DMBA. When compared to wild-type controls, Gst-deficient mice developed significantly increased numbers of tumors, verifying the importance of glutathione conjugation in vivo for protection against the carcinogenicity of some metabolically activated polycyclic aromatic hydrocarbons.

3. Adh-Null Mice

Mice possess a number of ADH isoenzymes, and knockout mice have been created with targeted disruption of the genes encoding ADH1, ADH3, and ADH4. When administered toxic doses of ethanol, both Adh1-null and Adh4-null mice had significantly decreased blood ethanol clearance and increased incidences of embryonic resorption when compared to wild-type controls. However, only mice lacking ADH1 had longer ethanol-induced sleep times. *Adh1*-knockout and *Adh4*-knockout mice also showed reduced metabolism of retinol to retinoic acid. The *Adh3* knockouts, in contrast to the other two isozyme-null strains, had the same sensitivity as wild-type mice to ethanol intoxication, but they were significantly more sensitive to formaldehyde toxicity. Through the use of gene-altered mice in this series of studies, the *in vivo* activities of the various isozymes were clearly differentiated, showing that ADH1 and ADH4 redundantly regulated ethanol and retinol metabolism, whereas the preferred substrate for ADH3 was formaldehyde.

D. ROLE OF OXIDATIVE STRESS IN TOXICITY

Toxic damage inflicted by many xenobiotics and metals results from the metabolic generation of reactive oxygen species (e.g., hydroxyl radicals, hydrogen peroxide, superoxide radicals). Oxidative stress caused by these reactive molecules can be cytotoxic via direct damage to mitochondria, DNA, and cellular proteins and by the peroxidation of lipids, which damages cell membranes. These radicals are also generated by the biochemical reactions of normal physiologic processes such as respiration, and in response, the body has evolved a broad array of enzymatic and nonenzymatic defenses against oxidative stress (Fig. 3). Because pathways for protection against oxidative damage are redundant, studies in this field of research often require the simultaneous evaluation of multiple antioxidant parameters to determine whether perturbations in one pathway have been compensated for by augmented functioning of another pathway.

Targeted deletion of the genes encoding antioxidant enzymes and scavenger proteins has produced models that can be used to examine the role of these proteins in preventing oxidative stess. These models include mice with disrupted genes encoding glutathione peroxidase (GPX), copper-zinc superoxide dismutase

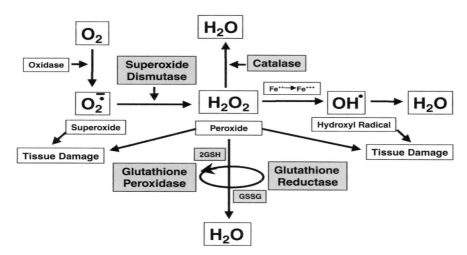

Figure 3. Enzymatic mechanisms of antioxidant defense include superoxide dismutase, which converts superoxide to peroxide; catalase, which accelerates conversion of hydrogen peroxide to water; and glutathione peroxidase, which catalyzes the reduction of hydroxyl radicals and peroxide by glutathione. Knockout and transgenic mouse models exist for each of these enzymes. Reprinted in modified form from Cotran, Kumar, and Robbins (eds.), "Robbins Pathologic Basis of Disease," 4th Ed., p. 10. Copyright 1996, with permission.

(CuZnSOD), heme oxygenase-2, and metallothionein I/II (MT-I/II). Some research has suggested that the protooncogene *Bcl-2*, which codes for a microsomal protein that inhibits apoptosis, may protect against oxidative stress, and a knockout model also exists for this gene. Although the manganese superoxide dismutase (*Mnsod*)-null mouse was not viable, the hemizygous mouse was. The *Mnsod+/−* mouse has been useful for investigating the gene dosage effects of this enzyme. Several strains of mice transgenic for antioxidant proteins or enzymes have also been created to investigate the potentially protective effects of overexpressing these genes. Mouse models now exist with transgenes for GPX, catalase, CuZnSOD, MnSOD, MT-I, MT-II, and Bcl-2. The body of research utilizing these models is extensive, but a few selected studies can illustrate the types of research questions that can be answered using these mice.

1. Mt-Null Mice

The *in vivo* roles of CYP2E1 and CYP1A2 in the bioactivation and toxicity of acetaminophen were discussed earlier. Other researchers have chosen to investigate *in vivo* mechanisms of oxidative stress that may contribute to the toxicity of this drug. Metallothionein is a protein that scavenges heavy metals such as cadmium, copper, lead, and zinc and protects against metal toxicities. A series of studies in *MtI/II*-null and transgenic mice verified, as expected, the *in vivo* role of MT in protection against cisplatin (platinum compound), cadmium, and mercury toxicities. However, some researchers have hypothesized, amidst some controversy, that these proteins are also scavengers for reactive metabolites and reactive oxygen species. In one test of this hypothesis, *MtI/II*-null mice were administered toxic doses of acetaminophen and were found to be more susceptible than wild-type mice to the development of hepatotoxicity and death. The degree of drug bioactivation and glutathione depletion was similar in both strains, demonstrating that their exposure to toxic metabolites was similar. These findings suggested that MT proteins

may play a protective role in removing either toxic intermediates generated during the metabolism of acetaminophen and/or reactive oxygen species produced by the toxic events following metabolic activation. *MtI/II*-null and transgenic mice will greatly aid further exploration of the possible role of these proteins in antioxidant defense.

2. Gpx1-Null Mice

Cellular glutathione peroxidase (GPX1), like other GPXs and GST, is an enzyme through which selenium is believed to provide its antioxidant activity. *Gpx1*-null mice were used in a series of studies to determine the importance of this particular isoenzyme for antioxidant protection *in vivo*. When exposed to highly toxic concentrations of the oxidant herbicides paraquat or diquat, wild-type mice survived, whereas *Gpx1*-null mice died. However, at lower exposures, both wild-type and null strains survived and developed toxicities of equal severity. These seemingly contradictory results probably reflected the redundancy of the antioxidant defense systems. The findings may have demonstrated that, over most ranges of oxidative stress, the degree of antioxidant protection was similar in wild-type mice and in mice lacking one element of the antioxidant defense system. The protective effect of GPX1 became evident only at the very highest levels of oxidative stress, a marginally additive effect consistent with redundancy. Alternatively, one could conclude that antioxidant defense is not a major function of GPX1. Better definition of the role of GPX1 and of the redundancy of antioxidant defenses could be explored in similar studies using mice genetically deficient for combinations of enzymes and proteins believed to be important for antioxidant defense.

E. *IN VIVO* STUDY OF REDUNDANCY IN ANTIOXIDANT PATHWAYS

The ability of one antioxidant pathway to compensate for another was supported by findings from studies using CuZnSOD (cellular SOD1) knockout mice and MnSOD (mitochondrial SOD2) hemizygous mice. *Sod1*-null mice had an apparently normal phenotype, unlike *Sod2*-null mice, which died postnatally. Tissue levels of MT-I and MT-II mRNA measured in *Sod1*-knockout mice were 10- to 12-fold higher than those of wild-type controls. This increase in MTs may have provided some compensation for the SOD1 loss by scavenging reactive superoxide radicals. Unfortunately, this investigation did not examine other antioxidant factors that may also have provided compensatory activity. Although tissue levels of MT in hemizygous *Sod2* mice have not been reported, the levels of mRNA for SOD1, catalase, and glutathione peroxidase were measured and showed no change from wild-type controls. *Sod2* hemizygous mice did, however, have 30 to 50% depletion of tissue glutathione levels when compared to wild-type mice, suggesting that increased scavenging by the tripeptide may have been able to compensate for the reduced SOD2 activity caused by the loss of one gene.

F. ROLE OF CYTOKINES AND OTHER MEDIATORS OF INFLAMMATION IN TOXICITY

There is increasing recognition that cytokines and other mediators of inflammation can be important determinants in the development and/or resolution of biological and chemical toxicities. The role of many of these mediators can now be dissected out using the numerous models that have induced alterations in genes of cytokines, cytokine receptors, and other factors and enzymes that participate in complex inflammatory processes (Table I).

1. Cytokine Receptor Knockout Mice

Some of the earliest work in this field involved the investigation of the role of cytokines in the development of endotoxic shock. Several experimental findings had identified tumor necrosis factor α (TNFα) as a potentially important player in the production of lipopolysaccharide (LPS)-induced endotoxic shock.

TABLE I
Cytokine Genes with Targeted Deletions in Mice

TNFR-1α/TNFR-1β	IL-4Rα
TNFR-1α/IL-1R1	IL-5
TNF	IL-6
IL-1R1	IL-7R
TNFRα	IL-10
TNFRβ	IL-12α
IFNγ	IL-12β
IFNγR	IL-12Rβ1
IL-2	IL-12Rβ2
IL-2Rα	LTα
IL-2Rβ	LTβ
IL-2Rγ	TGFβ1
IL-4	TGFβ3

These findings were corroborated *in vivo* by a study in which TNFα receptor knockout mice were found to be resistant to the lethal effects of low-dose LPS. In another series of studies on cytokines, recombinant interleukin-12 (IL-12) produced myelosuppression when administered to mice. IL-12 was also shown to secondarily induce increased release of interferon-γ (INFγ) through the activation of natural killer cells and T cells, suggesting that INFγ might mediate IL-12-induced myelosuppression. Administration of IL-12 to INFγ receptor knockout mice confirmed this suggestion by showing that the mice were resistant to myelosuppression, but it also demonstrated that the INFγ activity protected the mice against an IL-12-induced pulmonary toxicity.

Carbon tetrachloride (CCl₄) intoxication in mice is a popular experimental model for the study of hepatotoxicity. Several laboratories have investigated the role of cytokines, which are generally secreted by Kupffer cells in the liver, in the various processes that characterize the toxicity of this model. After the administration of toxic but nonlethal doses of CCl₄, hepatocellular necrosis is followed rapidly by hepatocellular proliferation that regenerates much of the damaged liver. Using two strains of mice, each of which was nullizygous for one of the two receptors of TNFα, researchers showed that signaling through TNFα-R1 was required for liver regeneration following CCl$_4$-induced injury. TNFα-R1 knockout mice exhibited a significantly weaker mitogenic response to CCl$_4$ than the wild-type controls and TNFα-R2 knockout mice. Lack of TNF receptors had little or no effect on sensitivity of the mice to CCl$_4$-induced necrosis.

In contrast, IL-6-deficient mice were significantly more susceptible than wild-type mice to acute CCl$_4$ necrosis. IL-6-null mice also exhibited less fibrosis in chronic CCl$_4$ toxicity, and this response was associated with secondarily decreased hepatic expression of transforming growth factor β (TGFβ), a factor known to promote fibrosis. Experiments using another gene-altered mouse deficient for IL-10 demonstrated that this cytokine limited neutrophil infiltration into the liver after CCl$_4$-induced acute necrosis and also decreased hepatic fibrosis in chronic toxicity.

2. TGFα Transgenic Mice

Creative use of transgenic mice to investigate the role of inflammatory mediators in toxicity was demonstrated in a study that employed several lines of mice expressing different levels of human transforming growth factor α (hTGFα). The transgenes were constructed using the surfactant protein C promoter, which directs gene expression to pulmonary epithelial cells. When exposed to Teflon fumes, mice showed dose-related increases in survival and decreases in the severity of pulmonary inflammation with an increase in hTGFα expression. Increased transgene expression correlated with secondary decreases in the expression of endogenous IL-6 and macrophage inflammatory protein-2 (MIP-2). Attenuation of the inflammatory response by TGFα through the downregulation of mediators such as IL-6 and MIP-2 may therefore have provided protection against acute toxic lung injury caused by Teflon fumes. In a cycle of similar studies, genetically altered mice have also been used to explore the roles of TGFα, TGFβ, and TNFα in bleomycin toxicity, another popular model for the study of pulmonary injury and oxidative stress.

3. Cox-2 Null Mice

Other proinflammatory factors include prostaglandins, leukotrienes, and bradykinins. Prostaglandins involved in inflammation are generated by the inducible enzyme cyclooxygenase-2 (COX-2). Knockout mice have been used to study the role of COX-2 in recovery from the hematopoietic toxicities of two compounds: the myelotoxic anticancer drug 5-fluorouracil (5-FU), and phenylhydrazine, which is hemolytic. Following treatment with 5-FU, myelosuppression was protracted in Cox2-null mice when compared to wild-type controls. Bone marrow in the knockout mice had significantly decreased numbers of erythroid and myeloid colony-forming cells even at day 12 after treatment. In contrast, the timing of erythropoietic recovery after phenylhydrazine administration was similar in Cox2-null and control mice. These studies did not explain the exact role of COX-2 induction in hematopoietic responses; however, they demonstrated that COX-2 was required for effective hematopoietic recovery following direct toxic damage to the marrow. COX-2 was not required for a simple erythroid regenerative response to hemolysis, which is a peripheral insult.

Toxicology studies using gene-altered mice can, as in this example, demonstrate and delimit new *in vivo* functions for a gene. These studies set the stage for additional research to further define the molecular and cellular mechanisms involved in the production of that functional phenotype. In this example, further studies might examine the role of COX-2 products (prostaglandins E$_2$, I$_2$, and thromboxane) in the survival, proliferation, and differentiation of bone marrow precursor cells.

IV. Genetically Modified Mice Can Be Used for Special or Customized Toxicity Testing

A. ALTERED PHENOTYPES REFLECTING TOXICITY

Genetically altered mice can themselves sometimes provide insight into the potential toxicities of certain chemical or biological agents.

Therapeutic compounds may be developed that are intended to increase or decrease the circulating levels, expression, or activity of biological targets (e.g., hormones, receptors, and enzymes) that are involved in disease processes. Some industrial chemicals may elicit similar increases or decreases in nontherapeutic biological targets. Transgenic or knockin mice that overexpress a target may exhibit exaggerated pharmacodynamic or toxic effects similar to those caused by a chemically induced increase in the activity of the same target. Mice that transgenically overexpress glucocorticoid receptors on pancreatic β cells illustrate this concept. The stable overexpression of these receptors increases sensitivity of the β cells to endogenous corticosterone in a manner that is analogous to their chronic exposure to exogenously administered corticosteroids. Chronic glucocorticoid therapy can be diabetogenic in addition to producing other serious side effects. Correspondingly, these transgenic mice exhibited decreased glucose tolerance and insulin secretion, indicating that one factor that can contribute to the production of diabetes is the direct chronic alteration by glucocorticoids of β cell function.

Similarly, knockout mice that lack the expression or activity of a particular target may exhibit some of the adverse effects that can result from downregulation or inactivation of that target by a chemical or biological agent. This concept is demonstrated by the skeletal growth abnormalities that developed in gelatinase-B-knockout mice. Gelatinase B, a matrix metalloproteinase (MMP-9), has been implicated in the pathogenesis of chronic arthritis and tumor metastasis, making it an attractive therapeutic target for these diseases. The toxic effects reported for some MMP inhibitor compounds include reversible skeletal growth abnormalities similar to those observed in gelatinase-B-null mice.

Interpretation of adverse findings in genetically altered mice as indicators of the activity-related toxicities of compounds or agents generally requires caution, however. A targeted gene has often been modulated throughout the ontogeny and life of a gene-altered mouse. This condition usually does not apply to therapeutic

interventions or chemical exposures, and compensatory expression of other genes can modify or mask the phenotypic expression of the altered gene function. Additionally, abnormalities in gene-altered mice may be developmental, thereby failing to accurately reflect adverse effects of the postdevelopmental modulation of a biological target. Among the numerous mouse models with misleading phenotypes for prediction of toxicity are cyclooxygenase-1 (COX-1) knockout mice. The most common toxicity caused by inhibitors of this enzyme, e.g., aspirin, is gastrointestinal (GI) ulceration; however, these genetically altered mice had no GI abnormalities.

B. IDENTIFYING ACTIVITY-RELATED TOXICITY

There are several new research applications for genetically altered mice in pharmaceutical toxicology that are poorly documented in the literature. The first involves use of knockout mice to differentiate activity-related (i.e., mechanism related) from structure-related toxicities of a therapeutic compound. Modern small molecule drugs are often designed by an iterative process that proceeds through the analysis of structure–activity relationships (SAR). In this process, medicinal chemists attempt to identify the active core of a compound and to optimize the chemical and biological properties of the compound by making small, sequential changes in its chemical structure. Toxic properties of a compound that are secondary to the same biological activity needed for effective disease treatment will manifest themselves regardless of the chemical structure of an active compound. Toxic properties that result from structural moieties not required for the activity of a compound can sometimes be identified and eliminated through SAR analysis. Whenever possible, it is therefore important to differentiate those toxicities that are activity related from those that are not.

Genetically altered mice that are null for a particular biological target can be useful for this purpose because they are capable of exhibiting only toxicities that are unrelated to a compound's activity upon that target. For example, consider two hypothetical compounds targeted against a particular enzyme. These compounds are from different chemical series, but both produce testicular degeneration, suggesting that the toxicity is activity related. If mice nullizygous for the enzyme fail to develop testicular degeneration when exposed to these compounds, whereas wild-type mice do, the results provide further evidence that the toxicity is activity related. The logic of this type of study is clear and elegant, but the biological complexity of *in vivo* systems, e.g., the existence of multiple receptor subtypes or isozymes with closely related structures and functions, can create the potential for generating ambiguous results in some studies.

C. CHARACTERIZING HUMAN–TARGET-SPECIFIC TOXICITY

Mice carrying human transgenes or knockin genes may also be useful in the specialized toxicity testing of some pharmaceutical compounds. Interspecies genetic homology of biological targets is generally high enough so that pharmaceutical compounds are active in several species. However, some compounds may exhibit pharmacological activity only against a human target. In these instances, activity-related toxicities cannot be characterized in the species used routinely for the toxicology testing of drugs (rodent, dog, nonhuman primate). For these species-specific compounds, transgenic or knockin mice that are genetically altered to express the human target may be useful for identifying activity-related toxicities. Certain preconditions, however, apply to this type of testing: the transgene or knockin gene should demonstrate tissue distribution patterns and levels of expression similar to those that occur in humans to avoid eliciting irrelevant toxicities.

V. Genetically Engineered Mice Can Be Useful for Short-Term Carcinogenicity Testing

In the 1980s and early 1990s, toxicology investigators and regulators began to recognize that the standard 2-year rodent bioassay used for carcinogenicity testing of drugs and chemicals had several intrinsic flaws and produced too many false-positive results. The debate on this subject spurred a search for better bioassay models that would allow faster, more accurate, and less expensive evaluation of a compound's carcinogenic risk to humans. At the same time, rational identification of potential models for use in carcinogenicity testing had been made possible by an increased understanding of the mechanisms responsible for tumor development.

A. MULTISTEP THEORY OF CANCER AS BASIS FOR NEW MODELS

The multistep theory of cancer development (Fig. 4), detailed during the last 30 years of cancer research, maintains that malignant tumors grow only after normal cells suffer multiple genetic changes in protooncogenes and tumor suppressor genes. These genetic changes often accumulate more rapidly when promoted by chronically recurring epigenetic events such as induced mitogenesis or cell proliferation secondary to chronic tissue damage or irritation. Working together, procarcinogenic genetic changes cause constitutive promotion of cell proliferation and survival while also inactivating intrinsic checks on cell growth. (A useful analogy for a cancer cell is a car with defective brakes *and* an accelerator frozen full-throttle.) According to this theory, a mouse model engineered to have a heritable predisposition to cancer development would need one fewer procarcinogenic event for its cells to become transformed, thereby allowing the model to respond more quickly to carcinogens than wild-type mice. Two of the most common genetic changes in human cancer cells are activating mutations of the *RAS* oncogenes and inactivating mutations of the *TRP53* tumor suppressor gene. To better model human cancer, the first genetically altered mice selected for evaluation in short-term carcinogenicity testing were therefore the *Trp53* hemizygous mouse and two *Ras* transgenic mice, the TG.AC and *Ras* H2 models. The *Xpa*-null mouse, which was also chosen

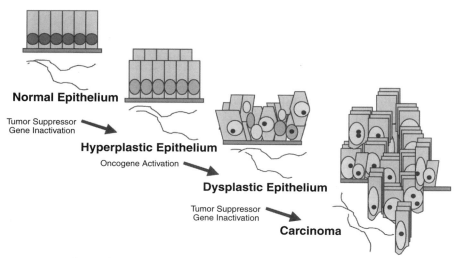

Figure 4. The multistep theory of carcinogenesis supports the use of genetically altered mice in accelerated carcinogenicity testing. It states that multiple, sequential alterations in protooncogenes and tumor suppressor genes compound over time to transform tissue from normal to hyperplastic, dysplastic, and, finally, cancerous tissue. Hereditary genetic alterations, such as Trp53 or XPA deficiency, that predispose to cancer shorten the number of steps, and therefore the time, required for tumor development.

for evaluation, is a model for xeroderma pigmentosa, a human disease characterized by defective DNA repair that predisposes to cancer.

B. GLOBAL COLLABORATION TO EVALUATE MODELS FOR SHORT-TERM CARCINOGENICITY TESTING

Interest in these new models grew quickly because of the immense resources spent yearly by industry and government for the carcinogenicity testing of chemicals and pharmaceuticals. Also, guidelines issued in 1997 by the International Conference on Harmonization (ICH) of requirements for the development of pharmaceuticals in Europe, Japan, and the United States provided further impetus for evaluation of these models through their acceptance of short-term carcinogenicity assays as alternatives for the 2-year mouse bioassay in regulatory submissions for drug approval. In a landmark collaboration, the International Life Sciences Institute (ILSI)/Health and Environmental Sciences Institue (HESI) brought to-

gether over 50 American, Japanese, and European laboratories from industry and government to participate in the conduct of an extensive battery of studies to evaluate selected new models for short-term carcinogenicity testing. ILSI-HESI data, together with other published data from the literature, form a baseline database that will allow better informed use of the models evaluated and aid in interpretation of data derived from accelerated bioassays conducted in the future.

C. THE Trp53 HEMIZYGOUS MODEL

Trp53 (P53, TP53) is a tumor suppressor protein that functions as a transcriptional regulator of genes that control the G1 cell cycle checkpoint, DNA repair, and apoptosis. Normal Trp53 responds to DNA damage, transactivates genes that delay the cell cycle prior to DNA synthesis, and facilitates functioning of the enzymatic complexes that repair damaged DNA before the entry of the cell into S phase. When the genetic damage is irreparable, Trp53 directs the defective cell into apoptosis. *Trp53* is the most commonly altered gene in human cancer, and loss of *Trp53* function permits DNA-damaged cells to remain in the cell cycle and proliferate, contributing to the genomic instability that underlies cancer development (Fig. 5).

Trp53 null mice are not used for carcinogenicity testing because more than half of them develop tumors and die by 6 months of age. In contrast, hemizygous mice are predisposed to tumor development while generally remaining tumor free for up to 6 or even 9 months. In a standard 2-year bioassay using outbred rodent strains, the background incidence of tumors in control animals is so high that large sample sizes ($n \geq 50$ per sex per dose) are required to obtain the sensitivity needed to detect statistically significant increases in tumor incidence caused by a test agent. Also, the inherent variability in background tumor incidences in 2-year studies can often produce false-positive test results. In contrast, smaller cohorts of *Trp53* hemizygous mice ($n=15$ to 25 per sex per dose) are needed for a 6-month bioassay because the low background tumor incidence does not obscure test results.

1. Results from Studies Using Trp53+/−Mice

The biology of *Trp53* function predicts that the hemizygous mouse should detect genotoxic carcinogens more rapidly than wild-type mice, and test results from completed short-term (6-month) bioassays generally bear this out (Table II). The *Trp53* hemizygous mouse developed tumors in response to treatment with almost all prototypical genotoxic carcinogens within 6 months; however, it failed to respond to a few, such as phenacetin, an analgesic and known human carcinogen. Importantly, the Trp53-deficient model has not responded to any non-carcinogens nor has it generated false-positive results for any nongenotoxic rodent-only carcinogens that are presumed to pose no carcinogenic risk for humans based on epidemi-

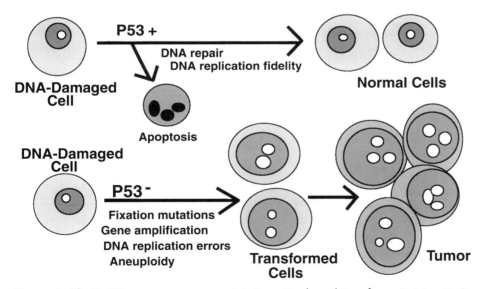

Figure 5. The Trp53 tumor suppressor protein is a critical regulator of genetic integrity. Its deactivation or loss allows many different types of genetic alterations to accumulate in proliferating cells, increasing the probability of tumor formation. The *Trp53* hemizygous mouse has one deactivated *Trp53* allele, and tumor formation in this model is often associated with loss of the other allele, leading to complete absence of Trp53 function.

TABLE II
Comparative Summary Results of Selected Short-term Carcinogenicity Assays[a]

Compound	Activity	Genotoxicity	2-year bioassay	Human carcinogen	Trp53+/-	TG.AC dermal	RasH2	Xpa-/-	Xpa-/- Trp53+/-
Benzene	Organic solvent	+	+	+	+	+	+	n.a.	n.a.
p-Cresidine	Industrial chemical	+	+	(+)	+	+	+	+	+
p-Anisidine	Industrial chemical	+	-	-	-	-	-	n.a.	n.a.
Cyclophosphamide	Antineoplastic	+	+	+	+	+/-	+	n.a.	n.a.
Methapyrilene HCl	Antihistamine	+/-	+	(-)	-	-	-	n.a.	n.a.
Cyclosporin A	Immunosuppressive	-	+	+	+	+	-	+	+
Phenobarbital	Sedative/hypnotic	-	+	-	-	+	-	-	-
Clofibrate	Hypolipidemic	-	+	-	-	+	+	n.a.	n.a.
17β-Estradiol	Estrogenic hormone	-	+	(+)	-	+	-	n.a.	n.a.
Diethylstilbestrol	Estrogenic hormone	-	+	+	+	+	+	+	+
Haloperidol	D₂R antagonist	-	+	(-)	-	n.a.	-	-	-
Sulfamethoxazole	Antibiotic	-	+	-	-	-	-	-	-
Ampicillin	Antibiotic	-	-	-	-	-	-	-	-

(-), presumed negative because of mechanism;
(+), sufficient evidence to assume positive;
n.a., not tested or results not available;
+, positive;
-, negative;
+/-, equivocal.

284

ological or mechanistic evidence, e.g., phenobarbital and clofibrate.

Interestingly, 6-month bioassays testing two human nongenotoxic carcinogens in *Trp53* +/− mice yielded positive results. These agents were the synthetic estrogen diethylstilbestrol (DES) and cyclosporin A, which cause tumor development through hormonal and immunosuppressive mechanisms, respectively. However, wild-type mice also developed tumors after 6 months of treatment with these drugs, suggesting that they are very potent carcinogens that can work effectively through Trp53-independent pathways.

2. Mechanisms of Tumor Induction in Trp53-Hemizygous Mice

Researchers have performed analyses to identify some of the secondary genetic changes responsible for the development of genotoxin-induced tumors in *Trp53* hemizygous mice. In studies using three different agents (benzene, phenolphthalein, and *p*-cresidine), most tumors of mesenchymal origin (lymphomas, sarcomas) exhibited loss of the remaining *Trp53* allele (LOH), indicating that complete absence of Trp53 tumor suppressor function contributed to the development of these tumors. However, in most transitional carcinomas that arose in the bladder of *p*-cresidine-treated mice, the remaining *Trp53* allele remained intact and unmodified, showing that tumor induction did not require mutation or LOH of the *Trp53* gene. These results suggested that mutational activation of an unidentified oncogene(s) and/or loss of the function of other tumor suppressor genes drove development of this epithelial tumor.

3. Spontaneous Tumors in Trp53+/− Mice

The most widely used strain of *Trp53* hemizygous mice (TSG-p53) has a predominantly C57BL/6 genetic background and may develop a few spontaneous tumors by 7 months of age, usually at a combined incidence below 6% (Table III). The two most common of these tumor types are malignant lymphomas and spindle cell sarcomas that arise in the connect-

ive tissues and skeletal muscle of the subcutis. Clearly differentiated osteosarcomas and bronchioloalveolar adenomas also occur spontaneously, but usually at very low incidences at 7 months. Administration of genotoxic carcinogens to *Trp53* hemizygous mice can often increase the incidence of background tumors rather than inducing the development of new tumor types.

Spindle cell tumors (Fig. 6) that develop in *Trp53* +/− mice are highly infiltrative and very poorly differentiated, but they may exhibit some areas of weak differentiation, often toward multiple sarcoma types within the same tumor: rhabdomyosarcoma, hemangiosarcoma, malignant fibrous histiocytoma, or fibrosarcoma. These sarcomas are also characterized by a highly variable cell size, high mitotic index, bizarre mitotic figures, large multinucleated cells, and marked nuclear pleomorphism. Spindle cell sarcomas have been induced by wounding and in response to the subcutaneous implantation of transponders used for the

TABLE III
Common[a] Spontaneous Tumors in Genetically Engineered Mice Used for Rapid Carcinogenicity Assays

Mouse strain	Tumor types
Trp53+/−	Malignant lymphoma Spindle cell sarcoma (subcutis) Osteosarcoma
TG.AC	Odontogenic tumors Squamous cell papilloma (forestomach, skin) Bronchioloalveolar adenoma Salivary duct carcinoma Erythroleukemia
RasH2	Hemangiosarcoma (spleen) Bronchioloalveolar adenoma, adenocarcinoma Squamous cell papilloma (skin, forestomach) Malignant lymphoma (female) Hardarian gland adenoma (female) Hepatocellular adenoma (male)
Xpa−/− and Xpa−/−; Trp53+/−	Malignant lymphoma Bronchioloalveolar adenoma Adrenal cortical adenoma (male) Sarcomas

[a]Incidence ≧ 1%.

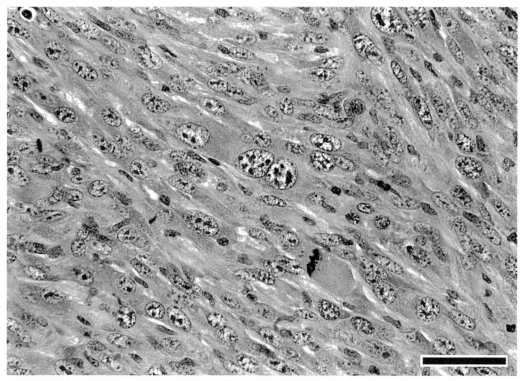

Figure 6. Soft tissue sarcoma from a *Trp53* hemizygous mouse. The sarcoma is composed of large, densely packed, poorly differentiated spindle cells with abundant cytoplasm and little stroma. Nuclei, which are large and vesicular, contain multiple large nucleoli. Atypical mitotic figures and multinucleated cells are common. Bar: 50 μm.

electronic identification of mice, factors that impact husbandry requirements for studies using this model.

Malignant lymphomas observed in *Trp53* hemizygous mice are generally highly proliferative, lymphoblastic (Fig. 7), and of thymic origin, although they often disseminate quickly to multiple organs. Another type of lymphoma, the splenic marginal zone lymphoma, also occurs rarely in the *Trp53* +/− mouse. Cells of these tumors, which express B220 and IgM at low levels, suggesting a B-cell origin, are more differentiated than thymic lymphomas in this strain of mouse.

D. THE TG.AC MOUSE

The TG.AC mouse carries a Harvey *ras* oncogene of retroviral origin. The transgene has transforming mutations (codons 12 and 59) and a ζ-globin promoter that was intended to direct gene expression selectively to erythrocytic precursor cells. The transgene is expressed constitutively at readily detectable levels only in the bone marrow and spleen of adult mice. However, this v-Ha-*ras* transgene also exhibits inducible expression in the skin when some test agents are administered topically and in internal organs other than the spleen and bone marrow when agents are administered systemically. The inducible expression of the transgene is not well understood, but it requires the unstable head-to-head arrangement of transgene promoter sequences, and it may be due, in part, to modulating effects of adjacent genomic sequences on transcription.

P21 Ras is a protein that transduces signals from activated membrane tyrosine kinase receptors to stimulate intracellular signaling cascades among seronine–threonine kinases that, in turn, initiate the transcription of

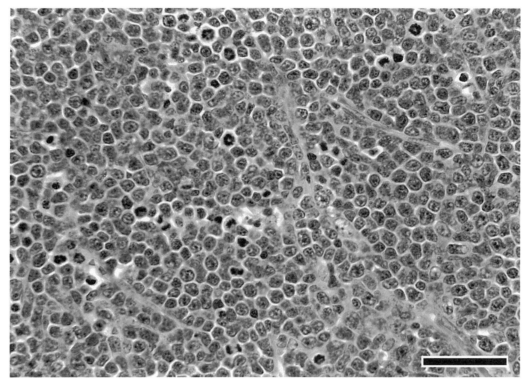

Figure 7. Thymic lymphoblastic lymphoma from a *Trp53* hemizygous mouse. The tumor is composed of a uniform population of large lymphoblasts having scant cytoplasm, large round nuclei, and multiple nucleoli. Mitotic figures are common. Xpa-deficient mice can develop similar tumors. Bar: 50 μm.

genes controlling cell proliferation (Fig. 8). Growth factor receptors, such as the epidermal growth factor receptors, signal through Ras. When altered by mutation at specific codons, Ras is constitutively membrane bound and activated, promoting the uncontrolled cell proliferation that contributes to tumor formation. In human cancer, *RAS* genes are the most commonly mutated oncogenes, occurring in approximately 30% of all tumors.

1. Results from Studies Using TG.AC Mice

The first agents shown to activate transcription of the v-H-*ras* transgene and produce tumors in the skin of TG.AC mice were chemical carcinogens previously characterized in the classic rodent two-step skin carcinogenesis assay. They included some prototypical genotoxic carcinogens, as well as nongenotoxic promoters of tumor development such as phorbol acetate

(TPA) and benzoyl peroxide. This transgenic mouse has been widely evaluated in 6-month bioassays, primarily because results can be scored by simple counting of squamous cell papillomas and carcinomas that develop at the dermal site where test agents are administered. Topical administration has its drawbacks, however, because appropriate doses can be difficult to determine and dermal and systemic metabolism of the same agent can be very different. Participants in the ILSI-HESI collaboration therefore chose to evaluate the performance of the TG.AC model using both oral and dermal routes of administration for many of the compounds.

In studies reported to date, the TG.AC mouse responded positively to most agents identified as two-species carcinogens in bioassays performed by the U.S. National Toxicology Program. Unlike the *Trp53* hemizygous

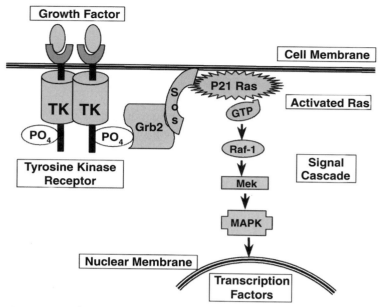

Figure 8. When growth factors bind their tyrosine kinase receptors, GDP is phosphorylated to GTP, which then activates the Ras protein. Ras in turn activates a complex intracellular signaling cascade through the MAPK pathway that leads ultimately to the transcriptional activation of genes that support cell proliferation. The growth stimulus is regulated by the ability of Ras to hydrolyze GTP and return to its inactive state. When mutated, the Ras protein remains membrane bound and incapable of hydrolyzing GTP so that it constitutively stimulates the cell to proliferate without any extracellular signal. TG.AC and *Ras*H2 mice have *Ras* transgenes. Reprinted in modified form from Ruddon, "Cancer Biology," 3rd Ed., Copyright 1995, with permission from Oxford University Press, and from *Trends Biochem. Sci.* **18**, 274, Copyright 1993, with permission from Elsevier Science.

mouse, the TG.AC model responded positively to a number of nongenotoxic as well as genotoxic agents when tested topically (Table II). Although the TG.AC mouse did not respond to a number of noncarcinogens (both genotoxic and nongenotoxic), this model produced a false-positive response to one noncarcinogen, resorcinol. The mouse also exhibited a robust dermal response to clofibrate, a nongenotoxic rodent carcinogen shown epidemiologically not to be carcinogenic in humans. Although nongenotoxic carcinogens such as DES and cyclosporin A produced positive dermal test results in the TG.AC, two potent human genotoxic carcinogens, cyclophosphamide and melphalan, yielded only equivocal results after dermal administra-

tion. These last two agents tested positively when administered orally to these mice, but, conversely, positive responses obtained dermally to several nongenotoxic chemicals were negative following oral administration. These studies demonstrated that results derived from testing by the favored dermal route were not always concordant with results obtained by oral dosing in TG.AC mice.

2. Mechanisms of Tumor Induction in TG.AC Mice

Studies to elucidate the mechanisms responsible for cutaneous papilloma and carcinoma formation in TG.AC mice have shown that tumors developed in response to test agents that induced expression of the Ha-*ras* transgene. Inflammatory cytokines and growth factors expressed during wounding were also able to induce transgene expression, a factor that impacts husbandry requirements for assays performed using this model. The challenge associated with true mechanistic understanding of this model, however, will be to clarify the function of the transgene's ζ-globin promoter, a genetic element not associated with known mechanisms of altered gene expression that induce tumor formation. More studies are needed to explain how palindromic sequences in adjacent ζ-globin promoters can produce an inducible Ha-*ras* transgene that responds to certain test agents, many of which are carcinogens.

3. Spontaneous Tumors in TG.AC Mice

The TG.AC mouse has an FVB/N genetic background and commonly develops several internal tumors that can arise spontaneously by 7 months of age (Table III). Because a carcinogenic response in genetically modified models can be manifested as an increase in the incidence of spontaneous tumors, the relatively high background incidence in TG.AC mice could complicate the interpretation of bioassays in which compounds are administered systemically. Odontogenic tumors (Fig. 9) occur spontaneously at highest incidence (up to 20%) in TG.AC mice, and forestomach squamous cell papillomas are the next most frequent (up to 10%). The odontogenic tumors may be one of three different morphologic subtypes (periodontally derived mesenchymal tumors, odontomas, and ameloblastomas), or they may be combinations of these subtypes. In contrast to the odontogenic and forestomach tumors, spontaneous dermal squamous cell papillomas have a lower incidence, generally less than 4%, making the model sensitive for detection of tumors induced by topical administration of test agents. Other internal tumors that can occur spontaneously by 6 to 7 months at incidences at or above 1% include bronchioloalveolar adenomas, salivary duct carcinomas, and erythroleukemia.

E. THE RasH2 MOUSE

Whereas the TG.AC mouse carries a mutated Ha-*ras* oncogene, the *RasH2* (or *H2ras*) model has a transgene composed of five to six contiguous copies of the normal human Ha-*RAS* protooncogene under the control of its own *RAS* promoter. The transgene is genomically stable and constitutively expressed in all tissues of the mouse, producing Ha-Ras levels up to three times the normal level. The genetic background of this model is an F1 cross of BALB/c and C57BL/6 strains (CB6F1).

1. Results from Studies Using RasH2 Mice

Like the TG.AC, this mouse has been evaluated extensively in short-term assays (6 months) using an array of model genotoxic carcinogens, nongenotoxic carcinogens, genotoxic noncarcinogens, and nongenotoxic noncarcinogens (Table II). Overall, the results suggest that when treated with transpecies genotoxic carcinogens, *RasH2* mice develop tumors with significantly higher incidences, shorter latencies, and sometimes increased malignancy when compared to control mice. An early study testing biweekly dosing of cyclophosphamide, an antineoplastic drug, reported that the *RasH2* mouse failed to respond to this potent human genotoxic carcinogen. However, in a subsequent study where the drug was administered daily, the response of the *RasH2* model was positive, illustrating the importance of study design when performing short-term carcinogenicity tests.

Some nongenotoxic rodent carcinogens, such as the peroxisome proliferators clofibrate and diethylhexylphthalate, produced equivocal or positive results in the *RasH2* mouse, indicating that the model could test positively for some compounds that pose no carcinogenic risk to humans. Additionally, this model failed to respond to the immunosuppressive human carcinogen cyclosporin A, although it did test positively for the hormone carcinogen DES. Unlike the other models evaluated, the *RasH2* mouse responded positively to phenacetin, a weak genotoxin that is carcinogenic in humans.

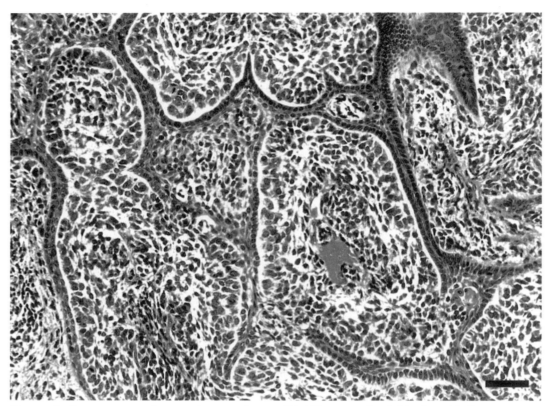

Figure 9. Spontaneous odontogenic tumor from a TG.AC mouse. Ameloblastic epithelium and stellate reticulum form patterns that resemble the enamel organ of a developing tooth. The section has one small focus of enamel or dentin. Photograph taken from a slide kindly provided by Paul Deslex, Pfizer Amboise Laboratories. Bar: 50 μm.

Finally, the *Ras*H2 mouse responded negatively to all noncarcinogens, as well as most rodent-only carcinogens, such as phenobarbital.

2. Mechanisms of Tumor Induction in the RasH2 Mouse

The mechanism(s) responsible for accelerated tumor formation in the *Ras*H2 mouse has been explored in several studies. The development of point mutations in codon 61 of the endogenous Ha-*Ras* gene has been implicated as a late event contributing to the progression of some spontaneous, but late-occurring hepatic hemangiosarcomas and hepatocellular carcinomas. Studies in the B6C1 wild-type strain have demonstrated that mutation of the Ki-*Ras* gene at codon 12 or 61 can be a common determinant of chemical-induced pulmonary tumor development. However, only a few chemicals tested in the *Ras*H2 mice induced tumors that exhibited high incidences of transforming point mutations in the Ha-*Ras* transgene or in the endogenous murine Ha-*Ras* or Ki-*Ras* genes, indicating that these particular genetic changes can contribute to, but are not required for, accelerated tumorigenesis. Additionally, chemically induced tumors did not have genetic alterations that affected *Trp53* function, e.g., mutation or loss of heterozygosity. Several carcinogens, however, uniformly increased expression of the *Ras*H2 transgene in tumor tissue twofold above background levels. This increase, while significant, is probably not adequate to completely account for accelerated tumor development in response to carcinogens, implicating the involvement of unidentified oncogenes or tumor suppressor genes in the induction of some tumors.

3. Spontaneous tumors of RasH2 Mice

At 8 months of age, the RasH2 mouse can exhibit a spectrum of spontaneous tumors, the most common of which are hemangiosarcomas in the spleen, bronchioloalveolar adenomas and adenocarcinomas, and squamous cell papillomas in the skin and forestomach (Table III). Females can also develop a significant incidence of malignant lymphomas and Harderian gland adenomas, whereas males can develop hepatocellular adenomas. The combined spontaneous tumor incidence in the RasH2 mouse can be 10% or more at 8 months of age, a factor to consider when determining sample sizes for studies with this model. In RasH2 mice, carcinogen treatment most commonly induced increased numbers of pulmonary and forestomach tumors similar to those that occur spontaneously.

F. Xpa-NULL AND Xpa-NULL/Trp53 HEMIZYOGOUS MICE

Humans lacking a functional XPA gene develop one form of xeroderma pigmentosa, a complex of diseases characterized, in part, by a greatly increased susceptibility to skin cancer. The Xpa-knockout mouse is one model of this human disease. XPA is a DNA-binding zinc-finger protein that functions in nucleotide excision repair (NER). It recognizes DNA adducts formed by some chemical mutagens or by ultraviolet light (UV-B) and sets off a cascade of events that culminate in DNA repair. Damage recognition by XPA is followed by DNA unwinding, strand incision, and excision of an oligomer that encompasses the site of damage. Synthesis and ligation of the corrected sequence complete the repair. Without functioning XPA, damaged nucleotides are not repaired, and they may induce the formation of persistent mutations during the DNA synthesis phase of the cell cycle.

Because Xpa-null mice were expected to respond only to carcinogens that produce DNA damage repaired by NER, researchers crossed this model with the hemizygous Trp53 mouse to create a new model having a broader reaction to genotoxic insults, decreased apoptotic response, and impaired cell cycle control. Laboratories using the Xpa-null mouse and participating in the ILSI-HESI collaboration on alternative models have included this double-targeted mutant mouse in their studies. Some investigators have suggested that, in addition to detecting most genotoxic carcinogens, this model might respond to nongenotoxic carcinogens that promote mutation accumulation indirectly through oxidative stress and increased cell proliferation. Unexpectedly, combination of the Trp53 mutation with Xpa deficiency increased the sensitivity of the mice to the toxicity of many of the compounds being tested, a factor to consider when setting doses for studies using this model.

1. Results from Studies Using Xpa-Null and Xpa-Null/Trp53 Hemizygous Mice

Xpa-null and double mutant models have been tested less extensively in short-term carcinogenicity assays than the TG.AC, RasH2, or Trp53 hemizygous models. UV-B light and topically applied DMBA, which were the first agents studied, induced a significantly increased formation of squamous cell carcinomas in Xpa-null mice by 3 to 4 months when compared to wild-type mice. Orally administered benzo[a]pyrene (B[a]P) treatment produced an increased incidence of lymphoma in Xpa-deficient mice that was significantly greater than that of the controls by 7 months. A classic murine hepatic carcinogen, 2-acetylaminofluorene (2-AAF), administered orally produced hepatocellular tumors in all female Xpa-knockout mice by 12 months. Male mice, in contrast, developed transitional cell tumors of the urinary bladder, with incidences that were increased significantly above those of controls by 12 months. Based on tumor latencies in these early studies with potent carcinogens, researchers using this model decided that the standard duration of studies with orally administered agents should be 9 months rather than 6 months as specified in most protocols for other genetically engineered models used in short-term bioassays.

As anticipated, genotoxic carcinogens produced positive test results in Xpa-null and

Xpa-null/*Trp53* hemizygous mice (Table II). Additionally, the two models responded negatively to noncarcinogens, such as ampicillin, and most nongenotoxic rodent-only carcinogens that have been tested, including phenobarbital. However, *Xpa*-null mice did respond positively when tested with WY-14,643, a potent peroxisome proliferator and putative rodent-only carcinogen. Like the *Trp53* hemizygous mouse, both XPA models and their wild-type counterpart produced positive results when tested with cyclosporin A.

2. Mechanisms of Tumor Induction in Xpa-Null and Xpa-Null/Trp Hemizygous Mice

Studies using mice that are nullizygous for *Xpa* and transgenic for *lacZ* have shown that with loss of XPA function, spontaneous accumulation of somatic mutations accelerated in tissues that maintain a capability for cell proliferation. Carcinogen treatment further accelerated the accumulation of mutations in the tumor target tissues of these mice. However, specific transforming mutations in oncogenes or tumor suppressor genes have not been identified. In the *Xpa*-null/*Trp53* hemizygous model, approximately half of all tumors exhibited loss of the remaining *Trp53* allele, indicating that complete loss of Trp53 function probably contributed to tumorigenesis in the dually targeted model.

3. Spontaneous Tumors of Xpa-Null and Xpa-Null/Trp53 Hemizygous Mice

Like the other genetically altered models being evaluated for short-term carcinogenicity testing, the *Xpa*-knockout mouse develops spontaneous tumors. These can occur at a total incidence of 5 to 7% by 11 months of age (Table III). The most common tumor types are malignant lymphomas, bronchioloalveolar adenomas, and adrenal cortical adenomas. Various types of sarcoma also occur at a low incidence. The double mutant mouse exhibits a similar spectrum of spontaneous tumors, but has higher background frequencies (total incidences 9 to 13%), a factor to consider when determining sample sizes for studies using this strain.

G. THE NEONATAL MOUSE ASSAY AND OTHER ALTERNATIVE CARCINOGENICITY ASSAYS

The neonatal mouse assay for tumorogenicity is not new, having been first used in 1959, nor does it employ genetically altered animals. However, after the issue of new ICH guidelines allowing the use of alternative models in carcinogenicity testing of pharmaceuticals, interest in this test system revived. The assay protocol uses neonatal mouse pups (CD1 and the B6C3F1 are the most commonly used strains) that are usually dosed two times with a test agent on days 8 and 15 after birth, unlike in standard bioassays where the compound is administered chronically. The route of administration used in the past for the neonatal mouse assay was usually intraperitoneal, a rare route for pharmaceutical dosing or chemical exposure. However, the ILSI-HESI studies evaluating the neonatal mouse model successfully adapted use of the oral gavage route, which allows for higher volumes and doses. The assay is terminated after 1 year when the mice are examined for gross and histopathological findings. Bronchioloalveolar and hepatocellular adenomas and adenocarcinomas have been the most common tumor types induced by carcinogens in the neonatal mouse model.

Because of its long-standing existence, the neonatal mouse assay has been used for many carcinogenicity studies, and most findings indicate that the model is sensitive to genotoxic carcinogens but insensitive to nongenotoxic carcinogens. Additionally, as with other models, background strain differences can profoundly affect results as exhibited by the relative insensitivity of C57BL/6 pups to dimethylnitrosamine (DMN)-induced hepatic tumors when compared to C3H pups.

Interest in a number of other older short-term assays for carcinogenicity has also resurfaced in some laboratories working outside of the ILSI-HESI collaboration. These tests include the standard two-step rodent skin carcinogenesis assay and the rat liver focus assay. Proponents of these test systems emphasize their ability to identify and distinguish between agents with tumor-initiating (genotoxic) and tumor-promoting (nongenotoxic) activities.

H. CURRENT AND FUTURE USE OF GENETICALLY MODIFIED MICE FOR SHORT-TERM CARCINOGENICITY TESTING

All of the genetically altered models evaluated through the ILSI-HESI collaboration (*Trp53* hemizygous, TG.AC, *Xpa* null, and *Ras*H2) have contributed greatly to our mechanistic understanding of carcinogenic processes through their use in basic tumor biology research. They will also continue to be useful models for mechanistic toxicological research designed to solve specific problems in carcinogenesis. The validity of their use in short-term carcinogenicity testing, however, is still under some debate, as are the relative merits of the various models and some protocol-related issues such as the appropriate study duration, sample size, and route of administration for each model. Most notably, support for use of the TG.AC mouse has been dampened somewhat because of the genomic instability of its transgene and the mechanistically problematic activity of the ζ-globin promoter. Proponents and opponents of the use of genetically engineered mice in carcinogenicity testing both agree that additional studies are needed to characterize the models further, e.g., more investigations of their xenobiotic-metabolizing capabilities compared with those of their wild-type counterparts. Currently, collective evidence indicates that these models are not overly sensitive, i.e., they have not responded positively to agents that were negative in the 2-year bioassay (which can detect rodent-only carcinogens in addition to human carcinogens). Additionally, some of the models, e.g., the *Trp* 53+/− mouse, may be more specific than the 2-year bioassay and therefore less likely to produce false-positive results for an agent's carcinogenic risk to humans.

Agencies that regulate chemical registration, such as the U.S. Environmental Protection Agency, are interested in but have not yet accepted the use of alternative models. However, pharmaceutical regulatory agencies participating in the ICH process have accepted data from short-term carcinogenicity studies, making use of these models a viable alternative to the standard 2-year mouse bioassay in drug development. At present, the drug regulatory agencies are continuing to review and approve protocols for short-term carcinogenicity studies submitted by sponsor companies as part of their regulatory filings for drug marketing approval. As the number of filings increases, the growing database of findings from these short-term bioassays will provide information for continued systematic evaluation of the performance of the models in predicting human risk.

In addition to the strains tested in the ILSI-HESI collaboration, a large number of other mutant and genetically engineered mice are predisposed to cancer development (e.g., the *min* mouse discussed in Chapter 30). Some of these strains will be useful for future evaluation as models for short-term carcinogenicity testing and for providing mechanistic information that may be useful for evaluating human carcinogenic risk. In particular, mice with genetic alterations in the p16^{ink4A}/cdk4/cyclin D/pRb pathway, which is estimated to be disrupted at one or more points in nearly all human tumors, are good candidates to assess. Genetically engineered rats and models with conditional mutations in oncogenes and tumor suppressor genes, in which expression of the altered gene can be controlled temporally, also hold promise for future use in carcinogenicity testing (Table IV).

VI. Caveats Apply to the Use of Genetically Engineered Mice in Research

Although gene-altered mice are powerful tools for research and testing, their use and the interpretation of results obtained through their use require thoughtful consideration. An understanding of the limitations of the technology used to create these models is useful for understanding some of the limitations of the models themselves.

Eugenia Floyd

TABLE IV
Genetically Engineered Mice Presented in Text with Selected Literature References

Mouse strain	Reference
Big Blue and MutaMouse	Schmezer, P., and Eckert, C. (1999). *IARC Sci. Publ.* (146), 367–394
Aprt deficient	Stambrook, P. J., *et al.* (1996). *Environ. Mol. Mutagen* **28**(4), 471–482
p^un	Schiestl, R. H., *et al.* (1997). *Proc. Natl. Acad. Sci. USA* **29**, 4576–4581
TK+/−	Dobrovolsky, V. N., *et al.* (1999). *Mutat. Res.* **25**, 125–136
Ahr null	Gonzalez, F. J., and Fernandez-Salguero, P. (1998). *Drug Metab. Dispos.*, **26**(12), 1194–1198
Pparα null	Lee, S. S., *et al.* (1995). *Mol. Cell. Biol.* **15**(6), 3012–3022
P450 null (2E1, 1B1, 1A2)	Buters, J. T., *et al* (1999). *Drug Metab. Rev.* **31**(2), 437–447
Gst null	Henderson, C. J., *et al.* (1998). *Proc. Natl. Acad. Sci. USA* **95**(9), 5275–5280
mEH null	Miyata, M., *et al.* (1999). *J. Biol. Chem.* **274**(34), 23963–23968
Gpx1 null	Cheng, W., *et al.* (1999). *FASEB J.* **13**(11), 1467–1475
Adh null	Deltour, L., *et al.* (1999). *J. Biol. Chem* **274**(24), 16796–16801
Mtl/II transgenic and Mtl/II null	Klaassen, C. D., and Liu, J. (1998). *J. Toxicol. Sci.* **23**(Suppl. 2), 97–102
Sod2 +/−	Van Remmen, H., *et al* (1999). *Arch. Biochem. Biophys.* **363**(1), 91–97
Sod1 null	Ghoshal, K., *et al.* (1999). *Biochem. Biophys. Res. Commun.* **264**(3), 735–742
INFγR null	Car, B. D., *et al.* (1999). *Toxicol. Pathol.* **27**(1), 58–63
IL6 null	Katz, A., *et al.* (1998). *Cytokines Cell Mol. Ther.* **4**(4), 221–227
IL10 null	Louis, H., *et al.* (1998). *Hepatology* **28**(6), 1607–1615
TNFα null	Yamada, Y., and Fausto, N. (1998). *Am. J. Pathol.* **152**(6), 1577–1589
TGFα transgenic	Hardie, W. D., *et al.* (1999). *Am. J. Physiol.* **277** (5 Pt 1), L1045–L1050
Cox2 null	Lorenz, M., *et al.* (1999). *Exp. Hematol.* **27**(10), 1494–1502
Trp53 +/− and TG.AC	Mahler, J. F, *et al.* (1998). *Toxicol. Pathol.* **26**(4), 501–511
RasH2	Mitsumori, K., *et al.* (1998). *Toxicol. Pathol.* **26**(4), 520–531
Xpa null	van Kreijl, C. F., and van Steeg, H. (1998). *Toxicol. Pathol.* **26**(6), 757–758
P16^INK4A null	Serrano, M. (2000). *Carcinogenesis* **21**, 865–869

A. EFFECTS OF GENETIC BACKGROUND ON PHENOTYPE

One factor that can significantly affect phenotype, as pointed out previously, is the genetic background of the mouse. Most transgenic mice are created using either FVB/N or C57BL/6 (B6) strains. Mouse models engineered using gene-targeting techniques, in contrast, are usually produced on a variably mixed background of the 129 strain, from which the embryonic stem cells are derived, and the B6 strain, which is the usual source of the blastocysts for microinjection. The targeted genetic alteration can eventually be bred onto a pure strain background by backcrossing, but 20 generations of breeding are required for this to be fully achieved. Cohorts of knockout or knockin mice with the same genetic alteration may ex-

press subtle phenotypic differences due to the effects of modifying genes from their variable genetic backgrounds. The effect of genetic background was illustrated by several examples presented earlier in the chapter, and many other examples can be cited, such as the different tumor spectra and latencies of *Trp53*-null B6 mice and *Trp53*-null 129 mice. When compared to the B6 background, the 129 background elicited a significantly higher incidence of teratomas (a common tumor type in the 129 strain), a lower incidence of lymphomas, and a generally shortened combined tumor latency.

B. EFFECTS OF GENETIC TECHNOLOGIES ON PHENOTYPE

Standard genetic engineering techniques are performed in embryos so that genetic alter-

294

ations are present, although not necessarily expressed, in all tissues throughout the ontogeny and lifetime of the mouse. This practice has resulted in embryonic or fetal lethality when targeted genes are critical for growth and development. It has also produced many mouse strains whose abnormal embryonic, fetal, or postnatal development has given rise to phenotypes not relevant for use in toxicology testing. An example of this would be the early lethality in mice with homozygous deletion of the SOD2 gene. Additionally, the lifelong existence of an induced genetic change can also bring about systemic adjustments in the regulation of other endogenous genes to create a misleading phenotype that does not accurately reflect the normal function of the gene of interest in adult animals. Systemic adjustments that develop slowly in some gene-altered mice will not interfere significantly with some toxicological studies. The potential may exist in longer studies, however, for chronic secondary physiological and histological alterations to influence the results of a study in ways that do not directly reflect the induced alteration in gene function. For example, after 9 months of age, AHR knockout mice exhibit early development of an array of age-related tissue changes, including cardiac and hepatic fibrosis, vascular hypertrophy, epidermal and gastric hyperplasia, and splenic T-cell depletion. The design and outcome of any chronic toxicology study using AHR-deficient mice will be impacted by these changes.

The existence of an endogenous murine homologue of a transgene or knockin gene can sometimes complicate the interpretation of study results. Monitoring of the continued or altered function of the homologue can provide useful data that can aid in the interpretation of studies in some circumstances. If the genetic homology of the endogenous gene and a non-murine transgene is high, one problem that can arise is the difficulty or even inability to obtain phenotyping reagents (antibodies, nucleotide probes) that can distinguish the transcription and protein products of the transgene from those of the endogenous homologue. In some reports, this problem was avoided through the creation of mice in which the endogenous gene was deleted before a homologous transgene was introduced, as in the human p-glycoprotein or multidrug-resistant (hMDR) transgenic mouse. P-glycoproteins transport drugs across cell membranes, and their name comes from the observation that their upregulation in a tumor cell can make that cell resistant to cytotoxic drugs.

C. IMPORTANCE OF GENETIC QUALITY CONTROL

Finally, there is the problem of animal quality control, most importantly for mice intended for use in regulatory testing. It is best practice to confirm both the genotype and the reported phenotype of a genetically engineered model before employing it in research or testing. Because environmental changes can alter the phenotype of genetically identical mice, confirmation is best carried out in the same laboratory and under the same laboratory conditions to be used for conduct of the research. Genotypes, like phenotypes, can also be unstable as illustrated by the following account of TG.AC "nonresponder" mice.

In a series of exploratory rapid carcinogenicity studies conducted by several laboratories, more than half of all heterozygous TG.AC mice failed to respond to the positive control agent (TPA) as they had in previously reported studies. Substitution of homozygous TG.AC mice increased the incidence of positive response, but did not solve the problem. Investigation by FDA scientists revealed that the source of the problem was a change in genotype not detected by the polymerase chain reaction or southern blotting assays routinely used to genotype this mouse.

Although the founder TG.AC mice had approximately 8 copies of the v-Ha-*ras* transgene, the TG.AC mice used in these studies had about 40 copies, indicating that there had been evolutionary reduplication of the transgene. Additionally, all nonresponder mice had lost a DNA fragment containing ζ-globin promoter sequences. Molecular genetic evidence suggested that with deletion of this DNA segment, there was loss of an inverted repeat (palindrome, e.g., GACCTTCCAG) that was required, for reasons that are not well understood, to induce transgene expression. Following microinjection of DNA into a mouse embryo, transgenes insert into the genome in tandem arrays with head-to-head or head-to-tail orientation. Palindromic DNA created by the head-to-head arrays can be unstable, causing gene duplication or deletion, and evidence suggests that both processes occurred in TG.AC mice.

A new screening protocol was developed that can identify TG.AC nonresponder genotypes, allowing them to be eliminated from the breeding colonies so that this problem can eventually be resolved. However, effective resolution requires implementation and maintenance of a rigorous quality control program that incorporates a standardized regimen for genotyping and phenotyping breeder mice and their offspring.

Quality control measures that can help avoid problems resulting from genetic instability include cryopreservation of embryos or sperm from founder animals so that colonies can be regenerated if necessary. Although in many cases engineered genotypes are evolutionarily stable, periodic reassessment of transgene copy number and integrity, of the fidelity of targeted gene alterations, and of phenotype will help ensure the validity of a model. It is worth noting that because models created for use in carcinogenesis research and testing often have gene alterations that promote genetic instability, some of these models may be more susceptible than others to spontaneous germline alterations and subsequent genetic drift over multiple generations.

VII. New Gene-Altering Technologies Will Produce More Sophisticated Mouse Models

Established genetic engineering techniques are constantly being improved, and new technolo-gies are being developed to help remove some of the limitations of the older technologies. New mouse models are introduced daily, many of which may become useful for research in toxicology. Maintaining a current knowledge of developments in the field of genetically engineered mice will be a growing challenge. However, new resources, such as an internet site containing databases that describe genetically altered models available for research (http://www.jax.org/resources/documents/imr/), will help scientists meet this challenge.

A. MODELS WITH MULTIPLE GENETIC ALTERATIONS

The simplest way to create a new model, as discussed in several examples cited previously, is to interbreed genetically modified models to produce mice carrying multiple genetic alterations. Additional examples of models already available for use in toxicology include the *Trp53* hemizygous/*lacI* transgenic mouse and the *Xpa* nullizygous/*Trp53* hemizygous/*lacZ* transgenic mouse. These mice are being used to investigate the relationship of tissue-specific mutagenicity and carcinogenicity *in vivo*. The popular *Trp53*-deficient mouse has also been crossed with many other targeted mutant and transgenic mice such as the telomerase-deficient TERC-null mouse and *Erbb2* transgenic mouse. Many models with multiple alterations in cytokines and cytokine receptors, such as the TNFR-1α/IL-1R1 double targeted mutant, are available for use by researchers. The possibilities for producing new models by this method are virtually limitless.

B. INDUCIBLE TRANSGENE SYSTEMS

The development of new tissue-specific gene promoters continues to advance, which permits increasingly precise tissue targeting of transgene or knockin gene expression. Inducible promoter systems (Fig. 10), such as the forward and reverse recombinant transactivator systems (TA, rTA) that use the tetracyline operator (tetO), allow temporal control of gene expression. Precise timing of the expression of modified genes will help avoid the creation of

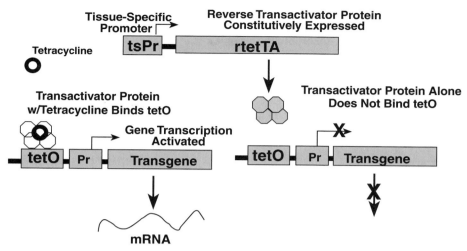

Figure 10. The reverse tetO inducible gene expression system is used to temporally activate transgene expression. This system requires two transgenes. The first codes for a transactivator protein that can bind the tet operon only when it is complexed with tetracycline. The other transgene is actively transcribed when the transactivator protein is bound to the tet operon. Transgene expression is therefore activated by the administration of tetracycline.

embryonic and fetal lethal phenotypes so genes critical for development can be studied in the adult mouse. Inducible expression systems will provide better models of cancer progression and late-onset chronic diseases. Additionally, they will permit the reversibility of phenotypic changes induced by transient or intermittent altered gene expression to be investigated.

One potential problem associated with these systems, and especially for their use in toxicological research, is their dependence on inducing agents such as tetracycline, doxycycline, dexamethasone, or other synthetic steroids. These compounds, especially the steroids, can have physiological and pharmacological effects of their own, and their use can complicate toxicology studies through pharmacokinetic and pharmacodynamic interactions. To avoid these interactions, inducible systems will need to be sensitive enough to respond consistently to subphysiologic doses of the inducers. Alternatively, the toxicology test protocols may need careful design to avoid concomitant administration of the test and inducing agents. A second problem with inducible systems is their "intrinsic leaki-

ness," i.e., low-level transcription in the absence of the inducing agent. However, continued engineering of the regulatory elements of these systems is already beginning to overcome these limitations. For example, the newly developed rtTA2^s-M2 variant of the rTA system is sensitive to 10-fold lower concentrations of doxycycline and causes no detectable background expression.

C. TISSUE-SPECIFIC GENETIC ALTERATIONS

Another new genetic engineering technology employs heterologous recombination systems such as the bacteria-derived *cre-loxP* and yeast-derived *flp-frt* systems to create tissue-specific genetic alterations (Fig. 11). Cre is a recombinase that deletes DNA segments positioned between *loxP* DNA sequences. *loxP* sites are placed in the genome of a mouse by targeted insertion around a gene of interest intended for inactivation or deletion. This mouse is bred to a mouse that carries a *cre* transgene under the control of a tissue-specific promoter, which will allow precise control of the tissue localization of the induced genetic change. When the tissue-specific promoter is also inducible,

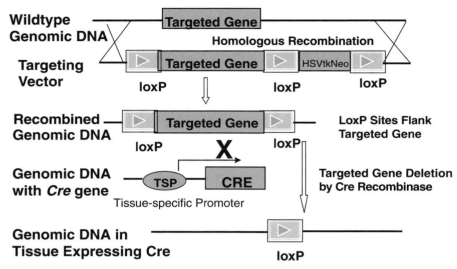

Figure 11. The Cre-loxP heterologous recombination system can be used for tissue-specific targeted gene deletion. In this process, a mouse is altered genetically by recombinational insertion of loxP sites into the flanking sequences of a targeted gene. This mouse is mated to another mouse that carries a Cre recombinase transgene under the control of a tissue-specific promoter. In the offspring, the targeted gene flanked by the loxP sites will be deleted in the tissue(s) where Cre is expressed.

the timing of the genetic alteration can be controlled as well. Activation of the Cre recombinase in a specific tissue will effect the targeted genetic deletion between *loxP* sites in that tissue. The *flp-frt* recombination system operates similarly. These systems have been used to create a number of genetically altered mice, but several limitations remain to be overcome before the technology will be as reliable as standard transgenic and gene targeting technologies.

D. FUTURE MODELS FOR USE IN TOXICOLOGY

The field of *in vivo* genetic engineering is evolving rapidly. Consequently, it is important to appreciate that some of the gene-altered models described in this chapter may soon be invalidated for their intended uses in toxicology or simply abandoned for a variety of technical reasons. However, genetic technologies will continue to improve to allow the creation of ever more sophisticated genetically altered models, which can replace those rejected for use in toxicology research and/or testing. Many of the new gene-altered mice, like the mouse models of the first genetically engineered generation, will be unique and valuable tools for the *in vivo* study of toxicological problems. Perhaps most significantly, they will continue to be useful for the *in vivo* confirmation of *in vitro* research findings. The new models will be designed to provide more accurate and relevant information for solving problems in toxicology and to significantly increase the predicitivity of animal testing for determining human toxicological risk. Success in that effort, if achieved, will be a major scientific accomplishment.

SUGGESTED READING

General Background

Frith, C. H., Highman, B., Burger, G., and Sheldon, W. D. (1983). Spontaneous lesions in virgin and retired breeder BALB/c and C57BL/6 mice. *Lab. Anim. Sci.* **33**(3), 273–286.

Frith, C. H., and Ward, J. M. (1988). "Color Atlas of Neoplastic and Non-neoplastic Lesions in Aging Mice." Elsevier, New York.

Li-Na, W. (1997). Transgenic animals as new approaches in pharmacological studies. *Annu. Rev. Pharmacol. Toxicol.* **37**, 119–141.

Mahler, J. F., Stokes, W., Mann, P. C., Takaoka, M., and Maronpot, R. R. (1996). Spontaneous lesions in aging FVB/N mice. *Toxicol. Pathol.* **24**(6), 710–716.

Maronpot, R. R., Boorman, G. A., and Gaul, B. W. (eds.) (1999). "Pathology of the Mouse: Reference and Atlas," Cache River Press, Vienna, IL.

Mohr, U., Dungworth, D. L., Capen, C. C., Carlton, W. W., Sundberg, J. P., and Ward, J. M. (eds.) (1996). "Pathobiology of the Aging Mouse," Vols. I and II. ILSI Press, Washington, DC.

Roths, J. B., Foxworth, W. B., McArthur, M. J., Montgomery, C. A., and Kier, A. B. (1999). Spontaneous and engineered mutant mice as models for experimental and comparative pathology: History, comparison, and developmental technology. *Lab. Anim. Sci.* **49**(1), 12–34.

Rudmann, D. G., and Durham, S. K. (1999). Utilization of genetically altered animals in the pharmaceutical industry. *Toxicol. Pathol.* **27**(1), 111–114.

Ward, J. M., Mahler, J. F., Maronpot, R. R., and Sundberg, J. P. (eds.) (2000). "Pathology of Genetically Engineered Mice." Iowa State Univ. Press, Ames, IA.

Genetic Toxicology Models

Ashby, J., Gorelick, N. J., and Shelby, M. D. (1997). Mutation assays in male germ cells from transgenic mice: Overview of study and conclusions. *Mutat. Res.* **14**, 111–122.

Cosentino, L., and Heddle, J. A. (1999). Effects of extended chronic exposures on endogenous and transgenic loci: Implications for low-dose extrapolations. *Environ. Mol. Mutagen.* **34**(2–3), 208–215.

Dobrovolsky, V. N., Casciano, D. A., and Heflich, R. H. (1999). *Tk+/−* mouse model for detecting in vivo mutation in an endogenous, autosomal gene. *Mutat. Res.* **25**, 125–136.

Dobrovolsky, V. N., Chen, T., and Heflich, R. H. (1999). Molecular analysis of *in vivo* mutations induced by N-ethyl-N-nitrosourea in the autosomal *Tk* and the X-linked *Hprt* genes of mouse lymphocytes. *Environ. Mol. Mutagen.* **34**(1), 30–38.

Gupta, P. K., Sahota, A., Boyadjiev, S. A., Bye, S., Shao, C., O'Neill, J. P., Hunter, T. C., Albertini, R. J., Stambrook, P. J., and Tischfield, J. A. (1997). High frequency *in vivo* loss of heterozygosity is primarily a consequence of mitotic recombination. *Cancer Res.* **57**(6), 1188–1193.

MacGregor, J. T. (1998). Transgenic animal models for mutagenesis studies: Role in mutagenesis research and regulatory testing. *Environ. Mol. Mutagen.* **32**(2), 106–109.

Monroe, J. J., Kort, K. L., Miller, J. E., Marino, D. R., and Skopek, T. R. (1998). A comparative study of in vivo mutation assays: Analysis of *hprt, lacI, cII/cI* as mutational targets for N-nitroso-N-methylurea and benzo[a]pyrene in Big Blue mice. *Mutat. Res.* **12**, 121–136.

Schiestl, R. H., Aubrecht, J., Khogali, F., and Carls, N. (1997). Carcinogens induce reversion of the mouse pink-eyed unstable mutation. *Proc. Natl. Acad. Sci. USA* **29**, 4576–4581.

Schmezer, P., and Eckert, C. (1999). Induction of mutations in transgenic animal models: BigBlue and Muta Mouse. *IARC Sci. Publ.* 1999;(146), 367–394.

Schmezer, P., Eckert, C., Liegibel, U. M., Klein, R. G., and Bartsch, H. (1998). Use of transgenic mutational test systems in risk assessment of carcinogens. *Arch. Toxicol. Suppl.* **20**, 321–330.

Skopek, T. R. (1998). Transgenic mutation models: Research, testing, and reality checks. *Environ. Mol. Mutagen.* **32**(2), 104–105.

Stambrook, P. J., Shao, C., Stockelman, M., Boivin, G., Engle, S. J., and Tischfield, J. A. (1996). APRT: A versatile *in vivo* resident reporter of local mutation and loss of heterozygosity. *Environ. Mol. Mutagen.* **28**(4), 471–482.

Swiger, R. R., Cosentino, L., Shima, N., Bielas, J. H., Cruz-Munoz, W., and Heddle, J.A. (1999). The *cII* locus in the MutaMouse system. *Environ. Mol. Mutagen.* **34**(2–3), 201–207.

Wijnhoven, S. W., Van Sloun, P. P., Kool, H. J., Weeda, G., Slater, R., Lohman, P. H., van Zeeland, A. A., and Vrieling, H. (1998). Carcinogen-induced loss of heterozygosity at the *Aprt* locus in somatic cells of the mouse. *Proc. Natl. Acad. Sci. USA* **10**, 13759–13764.

Zeiger, E. (1998). Identification of rodent carcinogens and noncarcinogens using genetic toxicity tests: Premises, promises, and performance. *Regul. Toxicol. Pharmacol.* **28**(2), 85–95.

PPAR and AHR

Aoyama, T., Peters, J. M., Iritani, N., Nakajima, T., Furihata, K., Hashimoto, T., and Gonzalez, F. J. (1998). Altered constitutive expression of fatty acid-metabolizing enzymes in mice lacking the peroxisome proliferator-activated receptor alpha (PPARalpha). *J. Biol. Chem.* **273**(10), 5678–5684.

Barclay, T. B., Peters, J. M., Sewer, M. B., Ferrari, L., Gonzalez, F. J., and Morgan, E. T. (1999). Modulation of cytochrome P-450 gene expression in endotoxemic mice is tissue specific and peroxisome proliferator-

299

activated receptor-alpha dependent. *J. Pharmacol. Exp. Ther.* **290**(3), 1250–1257.

Fernandez-Salguero, P. M., Ward, J. M., Sundberg, J. P., and Gonzalez, F. J. (1997). Lesions of aryl-hydrocarbon receptor-deficient mice. *Vet. Pathol.* **34**(6), 605–614.

Fernandez-Salguero, P. M., Hilbert, D. M., Rudikoff, S., Ward, J. M., and Gonzalez, F. J. (1996). Aryl-hydrocarbon receptor-deficient mice are resistant to 2,3,7,8-tetrachlorodibenzo-p-dioxin-induced toxicity. *Toxicol. Appl. Pharmacol.* **140**(1), 173–179.

Gonzalez, F. J. (1997). The role of peroxisome proliferator activated receptor alpha in peroxisome proliferation, physiological homeostasis, and chemical carcinogenesis. *Adv. Exp. Med. Biol.* **422**, 109–125.

Gonzalez, F. J., and Fernandez-Salguero, P. (1998). The aryl hydrocarbon receptor: Studies using the AHR-null mice. *Drug. Metab. Dispos.* **26**(12), 1194–1198.

Kersten, S., Seydoux, J., Peters, J. M., Gonzalez, F. J., Desvergne, B., and Wahli, W. (1999). Peroxisome proliferator-activated receptor alpha mediates the adaptive response to fasting. *J. Clin. Invest.* **103**(11), 1489–1498.

Lee, S. S., Pineau, T., Drago, J., Lee, E. J., Owens, J. W., Kroetz, D. L., Fernandez-Salguero, P. M., Westphal, H., and Gonzalez, F. J. (1995). Targeted disruption of the alpha isoform of the peroxisome proliferator-activated receptor gene in mice results in abolishment of the pleiotropic effects of peroxisome proliferators. *Mol. Cell. Biol.* **15**(6), 3012–3022.

Peters, J. M., Narotsky, M. G., Elizondo, G., Fernandez-Salguero, P. M., Gonzalez, F. J., and Abbott, B. D. (1999). Amelioration of TCDD-induced teratogenesis in aryl hydrocarbon receptor (AhR)-null mice. *Toxicol. Sci.* **47**(1), 86–92.

Ward, J. M., Peters, J. M., Perella, C. M., and Gonzalez, F. J. (1998). Receptor and nonreceptor-mediated organ-specific toxicity of di(2-ethylhexyl)phthalate (DEHP) in peroxisome proliferator-activated receptor alpha-null mice. *Toxicol. Pathol.* **26**(2), 240–246.

P450 Enzymes

Bondoc, F. Y., Bao, Z., Hu, W. Y., Gonzalez, F. J., Wang, Y., Yang, C. S., and Hong, J. Y. (1999). Acetone catabolism by cytochrome P450 2E1: Studies with CYP2E1-null mice. *Biochem. Pharmacol.* **58**(3), 461–463.

Buters, J. T., Doehmer, J., and Gonzalez, F. J. (1999). Cytochrome P450-null mice. *Drug. Metab. Rev.* **31**(2), 437–447.

Buters, J. T., Sakai, S., Richter, T., Pineau, T., Alexander, D. L., Savas, U., Doehmer, J., Ward, J. M., Jefcoate, C. R., and Gonzalez, F. J. (1999). Cytochrome

P450 CYP1B1 determines susceptibility to 7, 12-dimethylbenz[a]anthracene-induced lymphomas. *Proc. Natl. Acad. Sci. USA* **96**(5), 1977–1982.

Constan, A. A., Sprankle, C. S., Peters, J. M., Kedderis, G. L., Everitt, J. I., Wong, B. A., Gonzalez, F. L., and Butterworth, B. E. (1999). Metabolism of chloroform by cytochrome P450 2E1 is required for induction of toxicity in the liver, kidney, and nose of male mice. *Toxicol. Appl. Pharmacol.* **160**(2), 120–126.

Gonzalez, F. J., and Kimura, S. (1999). Role of gene knockout mice in understanding the mechanisms of chemical toxicity and carcinogenesis. *Cancer Lett.* **143**(2), 199–204.

Kimura, S., Kawabe, M., Ward, J. M., Morishima, H., Kadlubar, F. F., Hammons, G. J., Fernandez-Salguero, P., and Gonzalez, F. J. (1999). CYP1A2 is not the primary enzyme responsible for 4-aminobiphenyl-induced hepatocarcinogenesis in mice. *Carcinogenesis* **20**(9), 1825–1830.

Lee, S. S., Buters, J. T., Pineau, T., Fernandez-Salguero, P., and Gonzalez, F. J. (1996). Role of CYP2E1 in the hepatotoxicity of acetaminophen. *J. Biol. Chem.* **17**, 12063–12067.

Li, Y., Yokoi, T., Katsuki, M., Wang, J. S., Groopman, J. D., and Kamataki, T. (1997). *In vivo* activation of aflatoxin B1 in C57BL/6N mice carrying a human fetus-specific CYP3A7 gene. *Cancer Res.* **57**(4), 641–645.

Li, Y., Yokoi, T., Kitamura, R., Sasaki, M., Gunji, M., Katsuki, M., and Kamataki, T. (1996). Establishment of transgenic mice carrying human fetus-specific CYP3A7. *Arch. Biochem. Biophys.* **329**(2), 235–240.

Peters, J. M., Morishima, H., Ward, J. M., Coakley, C. J., Kimura, S., and Gonzalez, F. J. (1999). Role of CYP1A2 in the toxicity of long-term phenacetin feeding in mice. *Toxicol. Sci.* **50**(1), 82–89.

Pineau, T., Costet, P., Puel, O., Pfohl-Leszkowicz, A., Lesca, P., Alvinerie, M., and Galtier, P. (1998). Knockout animals in toxicology: Assessment of toxin bioactivation pathways using mice deficient in xenobiotic metabolizing enzymes. *Toxicol. Lett.* **102–103**, 459–464.

Sinclair, J., Jeffery, E., Wrighton, S., Kostrubsky, V., Szakacs, J., Wood, S., and Sinclair, P. (1998). Alcohol-mediated increases in acetaminophen hepatotoxicity: Role of CYP2E and CYP3A. *Biochem. Pharmacol.* **55**(10), 1557–1565.

Tonge, R. P., Kelly, E. J., Bruschi, S. A., Kalhorn, T., Eaton, D. L., Nebert, D. W., and Nelson, S. D. (1998). Role of CYP1A2 in the hepatotoxicity of acetaminophen: Investigations using Cyp1a2 null mice. *Toxicol. Appl. Pharmacol.* **153**(1), 102–108.

Valentine, J. L., Lee, S. S., Seaton, M. J., Asgharian, B., Farris, G., Corton, J. C., Gonzalez, F. J., and Medinsky, M. A. (1996). Reduction of benzene metabolism and toxicity in mice that lack CYP2E1 expression. *Toxicol. Appl. Pharmacol.* **141**(1), 205–213.

Wong, F. W., Chan, W. Y., and Lee, S. S. (1998). Resistance to carbon tetrachloride-induced hepatotoxicity in mice which lack CYP2E1 expression. *Toxicol. Appl. Pharmacol.* **153**(1), 109–118.

Zaher, H., Buters, J. T., Ward, J. M., Bruno, M. K., Lucas, A. M., Stern, S. T., Cohen, S. D., and Gonzalez, F. J. (1998). Protection against acetaminophen toxicity in CYP1A2 and CYP2E1 double-null mice. *Toxicol. Appl. Pharmacol.* **1**, 193–199.

Non-P450 Metabolic Enzymes and Antioxidant Defenses

Cheng, W., Fu, Y. X., Porres, J. M., Ross, D. A., and Lei, X. G. (1999). Selenium-dependent cellular glutathione peroxidase protects mice against a pro-oxidant-induced oxidation of NADPH, NADH, lipids, and protein. *FASEB J.* **13**(11), 1467–1475.

Deltour, L., Foglio, M. H., and Duester, G. (1999). Metabolic deficiencies in alcohol dehydrogenase Adh1, Adh3, and Adh4 null mutant mice: Overlapping roles of Adh1 and Adh4 in ethanol clearance and metabolism of retinol to retinoic acid. *J. Biol. Chem.* **274**(24), 16796–16801.

Fu, Y., Cheng, W. H., Porres, J. M., Ross, D. A., and Lei, X. G. (1999). Knockout of cellular glutathione peroxidase gene renders mice susceptible to diquat-induced oxidative stress. *Free Radic. Biol. Med.* **27**(5–6), 605–611.

Fu, Y., Cheng, W. H., Ross, D. A., and Lei, X. G. (1999). Cellular glutathione peroxidase protects mice against lethal oxidative stress induced by various doses of diquat. *Proc. Soc. Exp. Biol. Med.* **222**(2), 164–169.

Ghoshal, K., Majumder, S., Li, Z., Bray, T. M., and Jacob, S. T. (1999). Transcriptional induction of metallothionein-I and -II genes in the livers of Cu, Zn-superoxide dismutase knockout mice. *Biochem. Biophys. Res. Commun.* **264**(3), 735–742.

Henderson, C. J., Smith, A. G., Ure, J., Brown, K., Bacon, E. J., and Wolf, C. R. (1998). Increased skin tumorigenesis in mice lacking pi class glutathione-S-transferases. *Proc. Natl. Acad. Sci. USA* **95**(9), 5275–5280.

Ho, Y. S., Magnenat, J. L., Gargano, M., and Cao, J. (1998). The nature of antioxidant defense mechanisms: A lesson from transgenic studies. *Environ. Health Perspect.* **106** (Suppl. 5), 1219–1228.

Hochman, A., Sternin, H., Gorodin, S., Korsmeyer, S., Ziv, I., Melamed, E., and Offen, D. (1998). Enhanced oxidative stress and altered antioxidants in brains of Bcl-2-deficient mice. *J. Neurochem.* **71**(2), 741–748.

Jayanthi, S., Ladenheim, B., Andrews, A. M., and Cadet, J. L., (1999). Overexpression of human copper/zinc superoxide dismutase in transgenic mice attenuates oxidative stress caused by methylenedioxymethamphetamine (Ecstasy). *Neuroscience* **91**(4), 1379–1387.

Kang, Y. J., Chen, Y., Yu, A., Voss-McCowan, M., and Epstein, P. N. (1997). Overexpression of metallothionein in the heart of transgenic mice suppresses doxorubicin cardiotoxicity. *J. Clin. Invest.* **100**(6), 1501–1506.

Kang, Y. J., Chen, Y., and Epstein, P. N. (1996). Suppression of doxorubicin cardiotoxicity by overexpression of catalase in the heart of transgenic mice. *J. Biol. Chem.* **271**(21), 12610–12616.

Klaassen, C. D., and Liu, J. (1998). Metallothionein transgenic and knock-out mouse models in the study of cadmium toxicity. *J. Toxicol. Sci.* **23** (Suppl. 2), 97–102.

Klivenyi, P., St Clair, D., Wermer, M., Yen, H. C., Oberley, T., Yang, L., and Flint Beal, M. (1998). Manganese superoxide dismutase overexpression attenuates MPTP toxicity. *Neurobiol. Dis.* **5**(4), 253–258.

Liu, J., Liu, Y., Habeebu, S. S., and Klaassen, C. D. (1999). Metallothionein-null mice are highly susceptible to the hematotoxic and immunotoxic effects of chronic CdC12 exposure. *Toxicol. Appl. Pharmacol.* **159**(2), 98–108.

Liu, Y., Liu, J., Habeebu, S. S., and Klaassen, C. D. (1999). Metallothionein protects against the nephrotoxicity produced by chronic CdMT exposure. *Toxicol. Sci.* **50**(2), 221–227.

Liu, J., Liu, Y., Hartley, D., Klaassen, C. D., Shehin-Johnson, S. E., Lucas, A., and Cohen, S. D. (1999). Metallothionein-I/II knockout mice are sensitive to acetaminophen-induced hepatotoxicity. *J. Pharmacol. Exp. Ther.* **289**(1), 580–586.

Liu, J., Liu, Y., Habeebu, S. S., and Klaassen, C. D. (1998). Metallothionein (MT)-null mice are sensitive to cisplatin-induced hepatotoxicity. *Toxicol. Appl. Pharmacol.* **149**(1), 24–31.

Liu, Y., Liu, J., Iszard, M. B., Andrews, G. K., Palmiter, R. D., and Klaassen, C. D. (1995). Transgenic mice that overexpress metallothionein-I are protected from cadmium lethality and hepatotoxicity. *Toxicol. Appl. Pharmacol.* **135**(2), 222–228.

Lu, Y. P., Lou, Y. R., Yen, P., Newmark, H. L., Mirochnitchenko, O. I., Inouye, M., and Huang, M. T. (1997). Enhanced skin carcinogenesis in transgenic mice with high expression of glutathione peroxidase or both glutathione peroxidase and superoxide dismutase. *Cancer Res.* **57**(8), 1468–1474.

Merad-Saidoune, M., Boitier, E., Nicole, A., Marsac, C., Martinou, J. C., Sola, B., Sinet, P. M., Ceballos-Picot, I. (1999). Overproduction of Cu/Zn-superoxide dismutase or Bcl-2 prevents the brain mitochondrial respiratory dysfunction induced by glutathione depletion. *Exp. Neurol.* **158**(2), 428–436.

Mirochnitchenko, O., Weisbrot-Lefkowitz, M., Reuhl, K., Chen, L., Yang, C., and Inouye, M. (1999). Acetaminophen toxicity: Opposite effects of two forms of glutathione peroxidase. *J. Biol. Chem.* **274**(15), 10349–10355.

Miyata, M., Kudo, G., Lee, Y. H., Yang, T. J., Gelboin, H. V., Fernandez-Salguero, P., Kimura, S., and Gonzalez, F. J. (1999). Targeted disruption of the microsomal epoxide hydrolase gene: Microsomal epoxide hydrolase is required for the carcinogenic activity of 7,12-dimethylbenz[a]anthracene. *J. Biol. Chem.* **274**(34), 23963–23968

Przedborski, S., Jackson-Lewis, V., Kostic, V., Carlson, E., Epstein, C. J., and Cadet, J. L. (1992). Superoxide dismutase, catalase, and glutathione peroxidase activities in copper/zinc-superoxide dismutase transgenic mice. *J. Neurochem.* **58**(5), 1760–1767.

Radjendirane, V., Joseph, P., Lee, Y. H., Kimura, S., Klein-Szanto, A. J., Gonzalez, F. J., and Jaiswal, A. K. (1998). Disruption of the DT diaphorase (NQO1) gene in mice leads to increased menadione toxicity. *J. Biol. Chem.* **273**(13), 7382–7389.

van de Vrie, W., Marquet, R. L., Stoter, G., De Bruijn, E. A., and Eggermont, A. M. (1998). In vivo model systems in P-glycoprotein-mediated multidrug resistance. *Crit. Rev. Clin. Lab. Sci.* **35**(1), 1–57.

Van Remmen, H., Salvador, C., Yang, H., Huang, T. T., Epstein, C. J., and Richardson, A. (1999). Characterization of the antioxidant status of the heterozygous manganese superoxide dismutase knockout mouse. *Arch. Biochem. Biophys.* **363**(1), 91–97.

Yen, H. C., Oberley, T. D., Gairola, C. G., Szweda, L. I., and St Clair, D. K. (1999). Manganese superoxide dismutase protects mitochondrial complex I against adriamycin-induced cardiomyopathy in transgenic mice. *Arch. Biochem. Biophys.* **362**(1), 59–66.

Yoshida, M., Satoh, M., Shimada, A., Yasutake, A., Sumi, Y., and Tohyama, C. (1999). Pulmonary toxicity caused by acute exposure to mercury vapor is enhanced in metallothionein-null mice. *Life Sci.* **64**(20), 1861–1867.

Cytokines and Other Inflammatory Mediators

Car, B. D., Eng, V. M., Lipman, J. M., and Anderson, T. D. (1999). The toxicology of interleukin-12: A review. *Toxicol. Pathol.* **27**(1), 58–63.

Hardie, W. D., Prows, D. R., Leikauf, G. D., and Korfhagen, T. R. (1999). Attenuation of acute lung injury in transgenic mice expressing human transforming growth factor-alpha. *Am. J. Physiol.* **277**(5 Pt 1), L1045–L1050.

Katz, A., Chebath, J., Friedman, J., and Revel, M. (1998). Increased sensitivity of IL-6-deficient mice to carbon tetrachloride hepatotoxicity and protection with an IL-6 receptor-IL-6 chimera. *Cytokines Cell Mol. Ther.* **4**(4), 221–227.

Lorenz, M., Slaughter, H. S., Wescott, D. M., Carter, S. I., Schnyder, B., Dinchuk, J. E., and Car, B. D. (1999). Cyclooxygenase-2 is essential for normal recovery from 5-fluorouracil-induced myelotoxicity in mice. *Exp. Hematol.* **27**(10), 1494–1502.

Louis, H., Van Laethem, J. L., Wu, W., Quertinmont, E., Degraef, C., Van den Berg, K., Demols, A., Goldman, M., Le Moine, O., Geerts, A., and Deviere, J. (1998). Interleukin-10 controls neutrophilic infiltration, hepatocyte proliferation, and liver fibrosis induced by carbon tetrachloride in mice. *Hepatology* **28**(6), 1607–1615.

Madtes, D. K., Elston, A. L., Hackman, R. C., Dunn, A. R., and Clark, J. G. (1999). Transforming growth factor-alpha deficiency reduces pulmonary fibrosis in transgenic mice. *Am. J. Respir. Cell. Mol. Biol.* **20**(5), 924–934.

Natsume, M., Tsuji, H., Harada, A., Akiyama, M., Yano, T., Ishikura, H., Nakanishi, I., Matsushima, K., Kaneko, S., and Mukaida, N. (1999). Attenuated liver fibrosis and depressed serum albumin levels in carbon tetrachloride-treated IL-6-deficient mice. *J. Leukoc. Biol.* **66**(4), 601–608.

Ortiz, L. A., Lasky, J., Hamilton, R. F., Jr., Holian, A., Hoyle, G. W., Banks, W., Peschon, J. J., Brody, A. R., Lungarella, G., and Friedman, M. (1998). Expression of TNF and the necessity of TNF receptors in bleomycin-induced lung injury in mice. *Exp. Lung. Res.* **24**(6), 721–743.

Ortiz, L. A., Lasky, J., Lungarella, G., Cavarra, E., Martorana, P., Banks, W. A., Peschon, J. J., Schmidts, H. L., Brody, A. R., and Friedman, M. (1999). Upregulation of the p75 but not the p55 TNF-alpha receptor mRNA after silica and bleomycin exposure and protection from lung injury in double receptor knockout mice. *Am. J. Respir. Cell Mol. Biol.* **20**(4), 825–833.

Piguet, P. F., Kaufman, S., Barazzone, C., Muller, M., Ryffel, B., and Eugster, H. P. (1997). Resistance of TNF/LT alpha double deficient mice to bleomycin-induced fibrosis. *Int. J. Exp. Pathol.* **78**(1), 43–48.

Ryffel, B. (1997). Impact of knockout mice in toxicology. *Crit. Rev. Toxicol.* **27**(2), 135–154.

Yamada, Y., and Fausto, N. (1998). Deficient liver regeneration after carbon tetrachloride injury in mice lacking type 1 but not type 2 tumor necrosis factor receptor. *Am. J. Pathol.* **152**(6), 1577–1589.

Special Toxicity Testing

Delaunay, F., Khan, A., Cintra, A., Davani, B., Ling, Z. C., Andersson, A., Ostenson, C. G., Gustafsson,

J., Efendic, S., and Okret, S. (1997). Pancreatic beta cells are important targets for the diabetogenic effects of glucocorticoids. *J. Clin. Inves.* **100**(8), 2094–2098.

Langenbach, R., Loftin, C., Lee, C., and Tiano, H. (1999). Cyclooxygenase knockout mice: Models for elucidating isoform-specific functions. *Biochem. Pharmacol.* **58**(8), 1237–1246.

Markovits, J., and Gunson, D. (1999). Matrix metalloprotease inhibitor induced metaphseal and physeal changes in growing animals. *Vet. Pathol.* **36**, 491. [Abstr. No. 43].

Vu, T. H., Shipley, J. M., Bergers, G., Berger, J. E., Helms, J., Hanahan, D., Shapiro, S. D., Senior, R. M., and Werb, Z. (1998). Gelatinase B-null mice exhibit deficient growth plate angiogenesis and hypertrophic chrondrocyte apoptosis. *Cell* **93**, 411–422.

Short-time Carcinogenicity Testing

Ames, B. N., and Gold, L. S. (1990). Chemical carcinogenesis: Too many rodent carcinogens. *Proc. Natl. Acad. Sci. USA.* **87**(19), 7772–7776.

Contrera, J. F., and DeGeorge, J. J. (1998). In vivo transgenic bioassays and assessment of the carcinogenic potential of pharmaceuticals. *Environ. Health Perspect.* **106**(Suppl. 1), 71–80.

Eastin, W. C., Haseman, J. K., Mahler, J. F., and Bucher, J. R. (1998). The National Toxicology Program evaluation of genetically altered mice as predictive models for identifying carcinogens. *Toxicol. Pathol.* **26**(4), 461–473.

Gold, L. S., Slone, T. H., and Ames, B. N. (1998). What do animal cancer tests tell us about human cancer risk? Overview of analyses of the carcinogenic potency database. *Drug Metab. Rev.* **30**(2), 359–404.

International Conference on Harmonisation (1998). Guidance on testing for carcinogenicity of pharmaceuticals. *Fed. Regul.* **63**, 8983–8986.

ILSI Health and Environmental Sciences Institute. (2000). Poster abstracts from: Workshop on the evaluation of alternative methods for carcinogenicity testing. Leesburg, VA. USA.

Tennant, R. W. (1998). Evaluation and validation issues in the development of transgenic mouse carcinogenicity bioassays. *Environ. Health Perspect.* **106**(Suppl. 2), 473–476.

Tennant, R. W., Stasiewicz, S., Mennear, J., French, J. E., and Spalding, J. W. (1999). Genetically altered mouse models for identifying carcinogens. *IARC Sci. Publ.* **146**, 123–150.

U.S. Food and Drug Administration Center for Drug Evaluation and Research. (2000). Draft Guidance for Industry: Carcinogenicity Study Protocol Submissions. *Fed. Regul.* **65**, 66757.

Trp53 Hemizygous Mouse

Blanchard, K. T., Barthel, C., French, J. E., Holden, H. E., Moretz, R., Pack, F. D., Tennant, R. W., and Stoll, R. E. (1999). Transponder-induced sarcoma in the heterozygous p53 +/− mouse. *Toxicol. Pathol.* **27**(5), 519–527.

Dass, S. B., Bucci, T. J., Heflich, R. H., and Casciano, D. A. (1999). Evaluation of the transgenic p53 +/− mouse for detecting genotoxic liver carcinogens in a short-term bioassay. *Cancer Lett.* **143**(1), 81–85.

Donehower, L. A. (1996). The p53-deficient mouse: A model for basic and applied cancer studies. *Semin Cancer Biol.* **7**(5), 269–278.

Donehower, L. A., Harvey, M., Slagle, B. L., McArthur, M. J., Montgomery, C. A., Jr., Butel, J. S., and Bradley, A. (1992). Mice deficient for p53 are developmentally normal but susceptible to spontaneous tumours. *Nature* **356**(6366), 215–221.

Donehower, L. A., Harvey, M., Vogel, H., McArthur, M. J., Montgomery, C. A., Jr., Park, S. H., Thompson, T., Ford, R. J., and Bradley, A. (1995). Effects of genetic background on tumorigenesis in p53-deficient mice. *Mol. Carcinog.* **14**(1), 16–22.

Dunnick, J. K., Hardisty, J. F., Herbert, R. A., Seely, J. C., Furedi-Machacek, E. M., Foley, J. F., Lacks, G. D., Stasiewicz, S., and French, J. E. (1997). Phenolphthalein induces thymic lymphomas accompanied by loss of the p53 wild type allele in heterozygous p53-deficient (+/−) mice. *Toxicol. Pathol.* **25**(6), 533–540.

Finch, G. L., March, T. H., Hahn, F. F., Barr, E. B., Belinsky, S. A., Hoover, M. D., Lechner, J. F., Nikula, K. J., and Hobbs, C. H. (1998). Carcinogenic responses of transgenic heterozygous p53 knockout mice to inhaled 239PuO2 or metallic beryllium. *Toxicol. Pathol.* **26**(4), 484–491.

Harvey, M., McArthur, M. J., Montgomery, C. A., Jr., Butel, J. S., Bradley, A., and Donehower, L. A. (1993). Spontaneous and carcinogen-induced tumorigenesis in p53-deficient mice. *Nat. Genet.* **5**(3), 225–229.

Jacks, T., Remington, L., Williams, B. O., Schmitt, E. M., Halachmi, S., Bronson, R. T., and Weinberg, R. A. (1994). Tumor spectrum analysis in p53-mutant mice. *Curr. Biol.* **4**(1), 1–7.

Kemp, C. J. (1995). Hepatocarcinogenesis in p53-deficient mice. *Mol. Carcinog.* **12**(3), 132–136.

Kemp, C. J., Wheldon, T., and Balmain, A. (1994). p53-deficient mice are extremely susceptible to radiation-induced tumorigenesis. *Nat. Genet.* **8**(1), 66–69.

Kemp, C. J., Donehower, L. A., Bradley, A., and Balmain, A. (1993). Reduction of p53 gene dosage does not increase initiation or promotion but enhances malignant progression of chemically induced skin tumors. *Cell* **5**, 813–822.

Mahler, J. F., Flagler, N. D., Malarkey, D. E., Mann, P. C., Haseman, J. K., and Eastin, W. (1998). Spontaneous and chemically induced proliferative lesions in Tg.AC transgenic and p53-heterozygous mice. *Toxicol. Pathol.* **26**(4), 501–511.

Morimura, K., Salim, E. I., Yamamoto, S., Wanibuchi, H., and Fukushima, S. (1999). Dose-dependent induction of aberrant crypt foci in the colons but no neoplastic lesions in the livers of heterozygous p53-deficient mice treated with low dose 2-amino-3-methylimidazo[4,5-f]quinoline. *Cancer Lett.* **138**(1–2), 81–85.

Park, C. B., Kim, D. J., Uehara, N., Takasuka, N., Hiroyasu, B. T., and Tsuda, H. (1999). Heterozygous p53-deficient mice are not susceptible to 2-amino-3, 8-dimethylimidazo[4,5-f]quinoxaline (MeIQx) carcinogenicity. *Cancer Lett.* **24**, 177–182.

Sagartz, J. E., Curtiss, S. W., Bunch, R. T., Davila, J. C., Morris, D. L., and Alden, C. L. (1998). Phenobarbital does not promote hepatic tumorigenesis in a twenty-six-week bioassay in p53 heterozygous mice. *Toxicol. Pathol.* **26**(4), 492–500.

Stoll, R. E., Holden, H. E., Barthel, C. H., and Blanchard, K. T. (1999). Oxymetholone. III. Evaluation in the p53+/− transgenic mouse model. *Toxicol. Pathol.* **27**(5), 513–518.

Venkatachalam, S., Shi, Y. P., Jones, S. N., Voge, H., Bradley, A., Pinkel, D., and Donehower, L. A. (1998). Retention of wild-type p53 in tumors from p53 heterozygous mice: Reduction of p53 dosage can promote cancer formation. *EMBO J.* **17** (16), 4657–4667.

Ward, J. M., Tadesse-Health, L., Perkins, S. N., Chattopadhyay, S. K., Hursting, S. D., Morse, H. C., III (1999). Splenic marginal zone B-cell and thymic T-cell lymphomas in p53-deficient mice. *Lab. Invest.* **79**(1), 3–14.

TG.AC Transgenic Mouse

Asano, S., Trempus, C. S., Spalding, J. W., Tennant, R. W., and Battalora, M. S. (1998). Morphological characterization of spindle cell tumors induced in transgenic Tg.AC mouse skin. *Toxicol. Pathol.* **26**(4), 512–519.

Cannon, R. E., Spalding, J. W., Trempus, C. S., Szczesniak, C. J., Virgil, K. M., Humble, M. C., and Tennant, R. W. (1997). Kinetics of wound-induced v-Ha-ras transgene expression and papilloma development in transgenic Tg.AC mice. *Mol. Carcinog.* **20**(1), 108–114.

Cardiff, R. D., Leder, A., Kuo, A., Pattengale, P. K., and Leder, P. (1993). Multiple tumor types appear in a transgenic mouse with the ras oncogene. *Am. J. Pathol.* **142**(4), 1199–1207.

Delker, D. A., Yano, B. L., and Gollapudi, B. B. (1999). V-Ha-ras gene expression in liver and kidney of transgenic Tg.AC mice following chemically induced tissue injury. *Toxicol. Sci.* **50**(1), 90–97.

Hansen, L. A., Trempus, C. S., Mahler, J. F., and Tennant, R. W. (1996). Association of tumor development with increased cellular proliferation and transgene overexpression, but not c-Ha-ras mutations, in v-Ha-ras transgenic Tg.AC mice. *Carcinogenesis* **17**(9), 1825–1833.

Holden, H. E., Stoll, R. E., Spalding, J. W., and Tennant R. W. (1998). Hemizygous Tg.AC transgenic mouse as a potential alternative to the two-year mouse carcinogenicity bioassay: Evaluation of husbandry and housing factors. *J. Appl. Toxicol.* **18**(1), 19–24.

Humble, M. C., Szczesniak, C. J., Luetteke, N. C., Spalding, J. W., Cannon, R. E., Hansen, L. A., Lee, D. C., and Tennant R. W. (1998). TGF alpha is dispensable for skin tumorigenesis in Tg.AC mice. *Toxicol. Pathol.* **26**(4), 562–569.

Leder, A., Kuo, A., Cardiff, R. D., Sinn, E., and Leder, P. (1990). v-Ha-ras transgene abrogates the initiation step in mouse skin tumorigenesis: Effects of phorbol esters and retinoic acid. *Proc. Natl. Acad. Sci. USA* **87**(23), 9178–9182.

Spalding, J. W., French, J. E., Tice, R. R., Furedi-Machacek, M., Haseman, J. K., and Tennant, R. W. (1999). Development of a transgenic mouse model for carcinogenesis bioassays: Evaluation of chemically induced skin tumors in Tg.AC mice. *Toxicol. Sci.* **49**(2), 241–254.

Tober, K. L., Cannon, R. E., Spalding, J. W., Oberyszyn, T. M., Parrett, M. L., Rackoff, A. I., Oberyszyn, A. S., Tennant, R. W., and Robertson, F. M. (1998). Comparative expression of novel vascular endothelial growth factor/vascular permeability factor transcripts in skin, papillomas, and carcinomas of v-Ha-ras Tg.AC transgenic mice and FVB/N mice. *Biochem. Biophys. Res. Commun.* **247**(3), 644–653.

Trempus, C. S., Mahler, J. F., Ananthaswamy, H. N., Loughlin, S. M., French, J. E., and Tennant, R. W. (1998). Photocarcinogenesis and susceptibility to UV radiation in the v-Ha-ras transgenic Tg.AC mouse. *J. Invest. Dermatol.* **111**(3), 445–451.

Trempus, C. S., Haseman, J. K., and Tennant, R. W. (1997). Decreases in phorbol ester-induced papilloma development in v-Ha-ras transgenic TG.AC mice during reduced gene dosage of bcl-2. *Mol. Carcinog.* **20**(1), 68–77.

RasH2 Transgenic Mouse

Hayashi, S., Mori, I., Nonoyama, T., and Mitsumori, K. (1998). Point mutations of the c-H-ras gene in spontaneous liver tumors of transgenic mice carrying the human c-H-ras gene. *Toxicol. Pathol,* **26**(4), 556–561.

Mitsumori, K., Koizumi, H., Nomura, T., and Yamamoto, S. (1998). Pathological features of spontaneous and induced tumors in transgenic mice carrying a human prototype c-Ha-ras gene used for six-month carcinogenicity studies. *Toxicol. Pathol.* **26**(4), 520–531.

Mitsumori, K., Wakana, S., Yamamoto, S., Kodama, Y., Yasuhara, K., Nomura, T., Hayashi, Y., and Maronpot, R. R. (1997). Susceptibility of transgenic mice carrying human prototype c-Ha-ras gene in a short-term carcinogenicity study of vinyl carbamate and ras gene analyses of the induced tumors. *Mol. Carcinog.* **20**(3), 298–307.

Mitsumori, K., Yasuhara, K., Mori, I., Hayashi, S., Shimo, T., Onodera, H., Nomura, T., and Hayashi, Y. (1998). Pulmonary fibrosis caused by N-methyl-N-nitrosourethane inhibits lung tumorigenesis by urethane in transgenic mice carrying the human prototype c-Ha-ras gene. *Cancer Lett.* **129**(2), 181–190.

Umemura, T., Kodama, Y., Hioki, K., Inoue, T., Nomura, T., and Kurokawa, Y. (1999). Susceptibility to urethane carcinogenesis of transgenic mice carrying a human prototype c-Ha-ras gene (rasH2 mice) and its modification by butylhydroxytoluene. *Cancer Lett.* **145**(1–2), 101–106.

Yamamoto, S., Mitsumori, K., Kodama, Y., Matsunuma, N., Manabe, S., Okamiya, H., Suzuki, H., Fukuda, T., Sakamaki, Y., Sunaga, M., Nomura, G., Hioki, K., Wakana, S., Nomura, T., and Hayashi, Y. (1996). Rapid induction of more malignant tumors by various genotoxic carcinogens in transgenic mice harboring a human prototype c-Ha-ras gene than in control non-transgenic mice. *Carcinogenesis* **17**(11), 2455–2461.

Yamamoto, S., Urano, K., Koizumi, H., Wakana, S., Hioki, K., Mitsumori, K., Kurokawa, Y., Hayashi, Y., and Nomura, T. (1998). Validation of transgenic mice carrying the human prototype c-Ha-ras gene as a bioassay model for rapid carcinogenicity testing. *Environ. Health Perspect.* **106**(Suppl. 1), 57–69.

Yamamoto, S., Urano, K., and Nomura, T. (1998). Validation of transgenic mice harboring the human prototype c-Ha-ras gene as a bioassay model for rapid carcinogenicity testing. *Toxicol. Lett.* **102–103**, 473–478.

Xpa-Deficient Mouse

Berg, R. J., de Vries, A., van Steeg, H., and de Gruijl, F. R. (1997). Relative susceptibilities of XPA knockout mice and their heterozygous and wild-type littermates to UVB-induced skin cancer. *Cancer Res.* **57**(4), 581–584.

Bol, S. A., van Steeg, H., Jansen, J. G., Van Oostrom, C., de Vries, A., de Groot, A. J., Tates, A. D., Vrieling, H., van Zeeland, A. A., and Mullenders, L. H. (1998). Elevated frequencies of benzo(a)pyrene-induced Hprt mutations in internal tissue of XPA-deficient mice. *Cancer Res.* **58**(13), 2850–2856.

de Vries, A., Dolle, M. E., Broekhof, J. L., Muller, J. J., Kroese, E. D., van Kreijl, C. F., Capel, P. J., Vijg, J., and van Steeg, H. (1997). Induction of DNA adducts and mutations in spleen, liver and lung of XPA-deficient/lacZ transgenic mice after oral treatment with benzo[a]pyrene: Correlation with tumour development. *Carcinogenesis* **18**(12), 2327–2332.

de Vries, A., van Oostrom, C. T., Dortant, P. M., Beems, R. B., van Kreijl, C. F., Capel, P. J., and van Steeg, H. (1997). Spontaneous liver tumors and benzo[a]pyrene-induced lymphomas in XPA-deficient mice. *Mol. Carcinog* **19**(1), 46–53.

de Vries, A., van Oostrom, C. T., Hofhuis, F. M., Dortant, P. M., Berg, R. J., de Gruijl, F. R., Wester, P. W., van Kreijl, C. F., Capel, P. J., van Steeg, H., *et al.* (1995). Increased susceptibility to ultraviolet-B and carcinogens of mice lacking the DNA excision repair gene XPA. *Nature* **14**, 169–173.

Frijhoff, A. F., Krul, C. A., de Vries, A., Kelders, M. C., Weeda, G., van Steeg, H., and Baan, R. A. (1998). Influence of nucleotide excision repair on N-hydroxy-2-acetylaminofluorene-induced mutagenesis studied in lambda lacZ-transgenic mice. *Environ. Mol. Mutagen.* **31**(1), 41–47.

Giese, H., Dolle, M. E., Hezel, A., van Steeg, H., and Vijg, J. (1999). Accelerated accumulation of somatic mutations in mice deficient in the nucleotide excision repair gene XPA. *Oncogene* **18**(5), 1257–1260.

van Kreijl, C. F., and van Steeg, H. (1998). Transgenic mouse models for the identification of human carcinogens: A European perspective. *Toxicol. Pathol.* **26**(6), 757–758.

van Oostrom, C. T., Boeve, M., van Den Berg, J., de Vries, A., Dolle, M. E., Beems, R. B., van Kreijl, C. F., Vijg, J., and van Steeg, H. (1999). Effect of heterozygous loss of p53 on benzo[a]pyrene-induced mutations and tumors in DNA repair-deficient XPA mice. *Environ. Mol. Mutagen.* **34**(2–3), 124–130.

van Steeg, H., Klein, H., Beems, R. B., and van Kreijl, C. F. (1998). Use of DNA repair-deficient XPA transgenic mice in short-term carcinogenicity testing. *Toxicol. Pathol.* **26**(6), 742–749.

Neonatal Mouse, Other Short-Term Assays, and Models for Future Assessment

Arfandi, S. E., Chang, S., Lee, S., Alson, S., Gottlieb, G. J., Chin, L., and DePinho, R. A. (2000). Telomere dysfunction promotes non-reciprocal translocations and epithelial cancers in mice. *Nature* **406**, 641–645.

Enzmann, H., Bomhard, E., Iatropoulos, M., Ahr, H. J., Schlueter, G., and Williams, G. M. (1998). Short-and intermediate-term carcinogenicity testing: A review. 1. The prototypes mouse skin tumour assay and rat liver focus assay. 2. Available experimental models. *Food Chem. Toxicol.* **36**(11), 979–1013.

Flammang, T. J., Tungeln, L. S. V., Kadlubar, F. F., and Fu, P. P. (1997). Neonatal mouse assay for tumorigenicity: Alternative to the chronic rodent bioassay. *Regul. Toxicol. Pharmacol.* **26**(2), 230–240.

Miyauchi, M., Nishikawa, A., Furukawa, F., Kasahara, K., Nakamura, H., Takahashi, M., and Hirose, M. (1999). Carcinogenic risk assessment of MeIQx and PhIP in a newborn mouse two-stage tumorigenesis assay. *Cancer Lett.* **142**(1), 75–81.

Serrano, M. (2000). The *INK4a/ARF* locus in murine tumorigenesis. *Carcinogenesis* **21**, 865–869.

Von Tungeln, L. S., Xia, Q., Bucci, T., Heflich, R. H., and Fu, P. P. (1999). Tumorigenicity and liver tumor rasprotooncogene mutations in CD-1 mice treated neonatally with 1- and 3-nitrobenzo[a]pyrene and their trans-7, 8-dihydrodiol and aminobenzo[a]pyrene metabolities. *Cancer Lett.* **137**(2), 137–143.

Quality Control of Induced Genetic Alterations

Collick, A., Drew, J., Penberth, J., Bois, P., Luckett, J., Scaerou, F., Jeffreys, A., and Reik, W. (1996). Instability of long inverted repeats within mouse transgenes. *EMBO J.* **1**, 1163–1171.

Lewis, S., Akgun, E., and Jasin, M. (1999). Palindromic DNA and genome stability: Further studies. *Ann. N. Y. Acad. Sci.* **18**, 45–57.

Thompson, K. L., Rosenzweig, B. A., and Sistare, F. D. (1998). An evaluation of the hemizygous transgenic Tg.AC mouse for carcinogenicity testing of pharmaceuticals. II. A genotypic marker that predicts tumorigenic responsiveness. *Toxicol. Pathol.* **26**(4), 548–555.

New Technologies in Genetic Engineering

Chin, L., and DePinho, R. A. (2000). Flipping the oncogene switch: Illumination of tumor maintenance and regression. *Trends Genet.* **16**, 147–150.

Muller, U. (1999). Ten years of gene targeting: Targeted mouse mutants, from vector design to phenotype analysis. *Mech. Dev.* **82**, 3–21.

Rosenberg, M. P. (1997). Gene knockout and transgenic technologies in risk assessment: The next generation. *Mol. Carcinog.* **20**(3), 262–274.

Sauer, B. (1998). Inducible gene targeting in mice using the Cre/lox system. *Methods* **14**(4), 381–392.

Urlinger, S., *et al.* (2000). Exploring the sequence space for tetracycline-dependent transcriptional activators: Novel mutations yield expanded range and sensitivity. *Proc. Natl. Acad. Sci. USA* **97**(14), 7963–7968.

Pathology Issues in the Design of Toxicology Studies

Ricardo Ochoa
Drug Safety Evaluation
Pfizer Inc.
Groton, Connecticutt

I. Introduction

A. TOXICOLOGY STUDIES AND THEIR UTILITY

Any discussion of the design of safety studies to support the eventual registration of new compounds that will have human exposure will have to take into consideration the following points:

1. The type of compound.
2. The compound's intrinsic toxicity for the individual species.
3. Any transspecies toxic effects.
4. The route of exposure.
5. The length of administration.
6. The dose and exposure levels.
7. The effects of absorption, elimination, and distribution on exposure to the compound.
8. The reason for exposure with a risk-benefit ratio.
9. The numbers of individuals to be exposed.
10. The degree of knowledge of exposure and acceptance of risk by the exposed population.
11. Gender, age, concomitant therapies, and health status of exposed population.

Toxicologic studies are carried out for compounds being developed for human use in order to assure the safe exposure of humans to new chemical entities (NCE). These studies should define the toxicity or hazards associated with the NCE in order to adequately assure safety in humans. Additionally, the effects of compounds are also studied in target animal species for compounds developed for veterinary use. NCEs that have the potential to become part of the food chain or to be present in the environment of humans or animals are also studied in order to identify their toxic effects and their possible impact on humans or other at-risk species.

The number of studies that a toxicologic pathologist gets involved with is large and varied. Therefore this chapter will, by necessity, be limited. It highlights issues concerning studies leading to the registration of compounds for human use, either as a treatment or as a preventive for disease. It also attempts to cover some aspects of studies of compounds to be used in animals that may become part of the human food chain or that share the environment with humans.

II. Landmarks in Compound Development

Major landmarks in the development of a human pharmaceutical development are the discovery and patenting of a new chemical entity, application to the regulatory agency for approval to test the drug in human clinical trails, and an application for authorization to market the drug.

A. APPROVAL FOR HUMAN CLINICAL TRAILS

An application usually must be made to a regulatory authority in which the applicant proposes to conduct clinical trials in humans. This document (or series of documents) summarizes the initial preclinical information developed in studies carried out in at least two species (one nonrodent), with a multiple of the dose of the drug intended for humans. Animals should be exposed for at least the same time or a multiple of the time of human exposure during clinical trials. In addition, genotoxicity and some preliminary pharmacokinetic studies are given in support of this application.

1. United States and Canada

The investigational new drug submission (IND, USA; INDS Canada) is the documentation filed with the Food and Drug Administration (FDA) of the United States or the Therapeutic Products Programme of Health Canada to request permission to administer the new drug to humans for the first time. Approval must be obtained before clinical trials begin. The clinical trial plan still must meet with the ethics review boards' (ERB) approval at all institutions where human testing will be undertaken. Institutional review boards and research ethics boards can sometimes act as an ERB to ensure

that informed consent and other ethical issues have been addressed by the sponsor. In addition, comments concerning study design may be given to the sponsor.

2. Europe

First use in humans is unencumbered by the need to formally request permission from a regulatory agency in Europe or the general European Agency for the Evaluation of Medical Products before the compound is used in humans. This approach relies on the responsibility of the organization, or sponsor, that is attempting to study the new drug in question. Human candidates entering the trials are protected by the institutional review boards (IRB) of the research institutions, which review the information and authorize the use of the compound in human subjects. The lack of a formal IND process in Europe has produced a marked increase in the number of initial clinical studies performed by pharmaceutical companies in Europe in recent years.

3. Japan

A formal application to test a new drug in humans must be obtained from the Japanese Ministry of Health and Welfare. The equivalent document in Japan is called the clinical trial planning notification (CTPN).

B. APPLICATION FOR A LICENSE TO MARKET A DRUG

All countries with applicable law regarding therapeutic products require some form of application to permit selling of the drug. Often, based on risk assessment and risk management procedures, each drug may be classified or scheduled as a drug that is a controlled substance, prescription medicine, etc. Generally, documentation required for obtaining a license to sell a drug is substantial. However, it is the responsibility of the sponsor to demonstrate that the new drug is safe, efficacious, and of acceptable quality.

Both the United States and Canada require detailed documentation for all aspects of the development of the new drug application

(NDA, United States) and new drug submission (NDS, Canada). In Japan the Shinsei-sho application document is required, whereas in Europe a marketing authorization application (MAA) is necessary. These documents contain the clinical and preclinical studies necessary to document the safety, efficacy, and quality of the drug and drug substance. These materials are submitted to the regulatory agency for review and, if adequate, an authorization to market it in the specific country or region is obtained.

Similar documents exist in other countries. In addition to data demonstrating safety, efficacy and quality of the drug, most countries require a summary of the submission. In the United States, an integrated summary of safety (ISS) and an integrated summary of efficacy (ISE) are required. Similarly, Canada requires a comprehensive summary (CS). In other countries, experts in the field are asked to provide "expert reports." Europe requires a preclinical and clinical expert report to be signed by the author. The Japanese expert report, called the Gaiyo, incorporates a preclinical section. As in other expert reports, this section places into context all the nonclinical findings for the particular compound and as such should include the overall review by the pathologist involved in the development of the particular NCE. The involvement of the pathologist in this phase assures the correct interpretation of pathology data. It should correlate morphologic and clinical pathology findings among the different animal models used to obtain safety data and place them in context with human clinical adverse effects.

III. Role of the Pathologist in Compound Development

Because of their training in medicine (human or veterinary) and their understanding of basic pathophysiology, toxicologic pathologists are uniquely qualified to participate in all phases of the compound development process. In the past, pathologists in the pharmaceutical industry were utilized almost exclusively in a limited role to identify changes in tissues from animals in toxicology studies. Increasingly, however, pathologists are being recruited to participate in the broader aspects of pharmaceutical discovery and development. Their unique contributions in helping to clarify and understand the pathophysiology of effects of compounds in animals are being complemented by an often extensive training with animal models of toxicity and efficacy and in various aspects of biotechnology.

The increase in the use of transgenic animals in the pharmaceutical industry has created a demand for pathologists to phenotype and to help explain the mechanisms of unexpected findings in these strains. Equally important is the need to participate in the very early evaluation of the efficacy and toxic potential of NCEs. As combinatorial chemistry has increased the numbers of compounds synthesized, and high throughput screening has increased the numbers of compounds that are selected for potential development, early data become more critical to improve the chances of success. By exploiting their comprehensive understanding of comparative physiology, pathology, toxicology, and medicine, the toxicologic pathologist can advise development teams and can serve as a natural conduit between the discovery laboratories and the physicians utilizing these compounds in humans. By understanding the needs and constraints of both, the pathologist can have a great impact in the development process.

Toxicology studies are designed to create conditions that increase the possibility of observing toxic effects of compounds. Consequently, an important role for the pathologist is to place the effects observed in animals into proper perspective. Overinterpretation of the information presented is often one of the major challenges in the evaluation of pathology data by third parties.

We will explore specific issues regarding the role of the pathologist in discovery, exploratory toxicology, regulatory, mechanistic, and carcinogenicity studies.

A. DISCOVERY STUDIES

1. Objective

Studies performed during the process of compound discovery are designed to select quality compounds to enter development. They provide data that allow early decision on new compounds. As the number of compounds that are explored for possible development increases, it becomes more challenging to provide accurate data for decision making. Such decisions are necessary to select likely candidate compounds that enter the very expensive development process.

The early selection of high-quality candidates has several beneficial effects, such as increasing the chance for success in developing a safe and efficacious compound. In addition, it decreases the time it takes to develop these drugs and decreases the probability that unexpected complicating findings will surface later in the drug development process.

By giving early indication of the nature and biological significance of morphology and clinical pathology changes, the development team can address these issues and thereby determine a context for compound effects (and adverse effects). This also enables the team to suggest possible ways of monitoring these effects in humans before expensive clinical trials start. Additionally, participation in discovery teams places the toxicologist and toxicologic pathologist in a pivotal position within the organization as contributors to the process of both compound discovery and development. It also increases the quality of the information that teams receive, even when that information has the potential to stop the compound from further development.

2. Participation in Discovery Teams

One very important aspect of participation of the toxicologic pathologist in discovery studies is the need to have intimate knowledge of the objectives of the team, the ongoing activities,

and the individuals involved in the drug discovery process. One common mistake made by the team is to consider the pathologist as a consultant, i.e., the team considers that the contribution of the pathologist is independent of the objectives of the team. The consequences of this approach include the improper collection and preservation of samples to be examined, as well as missed opportunities for creative intervention by the pathologist to help solve factual or potential problems in efficacy or toxicity that develop during the early stages of lead searching. A thorough understanding of the compound class, the known effects of compounds in that class, and the efficacy model used for "proof of concept" will allow the pathologist to provide better advice to the team on the direction to follow to reach their objectives.

3. Types of Discovery Studies

Studies that are carried out in animals during the discovery process are of two major categories: screening and exploratory toxicology studies.

a. Screening Studies. These studies are intended to select from several compounds the ones with better characteristics to be presented for development. They generally involve the identification of one or several end points that are used as criteria to rank the different candidates.

i. Efficacy models These studies may address the efficacy of the compounds using animal models of the human condition for which the compound is being developed. They may also identify a single end point in a healthy animal (such as glucose or cholesterol lowering) and therefore may not require reproduction of the disease condition.

The contribution of the pathologist in the selection and validation of the best animal model of a human condition can be invaluable. Although other biologists involved in the team may be well versed in the specific models that are considered standard for a given disease, the pathologist can identify refinements to the end points or, alternatively, propose more optimal efficacy models.

310

ii. Eliminating undesirable side effects These studies are based on the knowledge that a particular class of compounds produces an undesirable effect that the team would like to eliminate or reduce. As many of these side effects have a morphologic or biochemical counterpart, the pathologist can assist in setting up and validating the model, and may simplify its implementation.

iii. Formulation screening The pathologist's association with colleagues in the formulation development group can produce improvements in the absorption and safety of formulations early in the development process. When the pathologist develops morphologic information regarding the effect of specific vehicles and whole formulations at local and systemic levels, formulators gain tremendous insight that allows them to select optimal formulations. This is particularly true with respect to parenteral formulations, but also for novel oral and topical preparations.

b. Exploratory Toxicology Studies. These studies intend to mimic, on a smaller scale, the studies that are going to be applied to compounds in development to satisfy regulatory requirements. They are intended to increase the chances of success of the particular compound by establishing end points of toxicity. These studies have both advantages and constraints to the development of the drug. An understanding of the advantages and disadvantages of these studies is necessary so that false assumptions concerning the suitability of the compound for further development are not made.

Involving the toxicologic pathologist in exploratory toxicology studies affords certain benefits, including a fast turnaround and a reduction in compound and animal use.

1. *Fast turnaround:* Because these studies are short in duration and use few animals, the investment of time is low and therefore the team can obtain information relatively promptly.

2. *Sparing the compound:* At this time in the discovery process, compound production is usually highly time- and resource-intensive and therefore supplies are at a premium. It is

important to use these studies to their maximum advantage in order to optimize the amount of information obtained with the few grams of compound available.

3. *Sparing of animals:* These studies utilize few animals and are designed to prevent the performance of unnecessary regulatory studies. Regulatory studies require multiple doses and many more animals than these earlier studies.

Several factors affect the design and execution of discovery studies that need to be taken into consideration.

1. *Compound availability:* As described earlier, these studies often suffer from lack of availability of compound. This can force the pathologist to utilize fewer animals than are needed or to utilize a delivery route that is not the intended one in order to maximize exposure. Care should be taken not to decrease the number of animals to an inadequate number, which would provide no useful data or, worse, information that misleads the team.

2. *Compound information:* As few studies have been performed with these compounds at this stage, there is a paucity of information regarding absorption, metabolism, elimination, half-life, length of occupancy of receptors, and other information that may be very important for interpretation of the obtained results. Whenever possible, these studies should also be used to advance the team's knowledge of these parameters.

3. *Formulation problems:* As there is very scant information about these compounds, its formulation is often suboptimal. Formulation may have a tremendous effect on exposure, and the lack of absorption due to inadequate formulation may lead to false assumptions of safety. It is therefore crucial to build some measure of exposure into these studies so as to address the adequacy of data obtained.

4. *Opportunity for false assumptions:* Because the number of animals is small and the information is inadequate, there is a higher risk of over-interpretation of information in these studies.

5. *Screening is tedious:* By its nature, screening constitutes the application of new variables

(compounds) to well-established and routine models. As morphological evaluation is a highly labor-intensive activity, systems may eventually be developed that streamline and eventually significantly reduce or replace morphology as an end point. Systems such as high throughput screening and gene chip technology are being developed to decrease the cost and increase the speed of making decisions. The pathologist's input in the development and validation of these methods is critical.

6. *Predictability of models:* This is probably the most important aspect of early evaluation of compounds. There is a natural tendency to over-interpret data obtained in these studies. It is important to keep in mind that studies in animals are approximations to what may happen in human subjects. Often there is not enough information about the mechanism or the cause of altered morphology, and without this information it is impossible to predict whether human responses to exposure will be similar to those of the animals tested at this early stage. It is all too easy to assume cross-species applicability and therefore eliminate promising new compounds from development. Correspondingly, accepting compounds into development without obtaining information regarding mode of action and predictability of response may result in selecting the wrong compound and using other less important criteria (such as early compound availability) as selection criteria. This lack of information may result in unnecessary exposure of human subjects. In addition, wasted time and resources will occur in developing a compound that will be later dropped from development, as toxicity in humans becomes apparent. The solution is to gather information about the mechanism of any inadequately understood effect that may be used to apply selection criteria to compounds chosen for development.

4. Study Design

Discovery and toxicology exploratory studies generally use rodents, and less often dogs. Small nonrodents such as small simian species like marmosets (*Sanguinus* sp.) are now being used more often.

Small animals help in sparing compound. However, they also limit the collection of samples for clinical pathology and pharmacokinetics. Monkeys such as cynomolgus (*Macaca fascicularis*) are perceived as being more predictive of the human response based on the phylogenetic proximity of simians to humans. The claims of higher predictability of simian studies to the human condition should be accepted only when there is documentation that supports such claims. Information regarding the similarity of receptors and pharmacokinetics is important to place these models in their proper context.

Generally, a dose is chosen that produces a drug concentration that is a multiple of the effective dose. This estimate is generally based on *in vitro* screens or early efficacy models. These doses are increased until some intolerance and/or toxicity is observed. From there, doses are decreased somewhat and given over several days, varying between 5 and 14 days, depending on compound availability.

It is important to collect pathology data in these early studies. Occasionally, some laboratories fail to do this in the belief that such information is either irrelevant or too expensive to obtain. Concurrent controls should be used in these studies, as is general practice for any proper scientific investigation. The lack of vehicle controls often results in data that are difficult or impossible to interpret.

Another common practice is the return of animals to the colony for reuse. The reuse of animals for toxicological studies (regulatory or not) complicates the interpretation of pathological changes. An essential part of the pathological evaluation is the ability to define the time of appearance of a lesion. The interpretation of histopathology changes is complicated by the inability to identify whether the change is recent and therefore due to the administration of the new compound or preexistent and related to a previous exposure in studies that reuse animals previously exposed to the same or different compounds. Additionally, there is the possibility of predisposing animals to biochemical or tissue damage thereby exaggerating the effects of the "new" compound. Alternatively, there is the possibility of decreasing the sensitivity of the animal to the injurious effects of a compound due to the induction of protective effects, such as enzyme induction, therefore also leading to false conclusions.

IV. Regulatory Studies

Regulatory animal studies used most frequently in pharmaceutical development may be divided into several categories.

A. STUDIES TO SUPPORT FIRST IN HUMAN EXPOSURE

1. Acute toxicity and short-term tests: mutagenicity tests and acute toxicity tests in two species.
2. Range-finding studies: 2-week study in rodents and nonrodents.

B. STUDIES TO SUPPORT LONGER EXPOSURES IN HUMANS

1. Subchronic studies: 2- to 13-week study in rodents and nonrodents.
2. Chronic toxicity: 6-month study in rodents and 6- to 12-month study in rodents and nonrodents.
3. Two-year carcinogenicity study in rats and mice.
4. Reproductive toxicology and teratology: fertility and early development, pre- and postnatal development, and embryo and fetal development.

C. LENGTH OF STUDIES

The International Committee on Harmonization (ICH) has been organized to create consensus among representatives of the pharmaceutical industry and regulatory agencies of the three major pharmaceutical markets (European community, Japan, and the United States). The object of this effort is to simplify the complex regulations that direct the process of filing for the approval of compounds in the international market. Although this committee has been working for several years, many drug safety recommendations of the ICH are not yet final. Nonetheless, great advances have been made in defining aspects of the toxicology studies to be performed. A significant achievement of this process is defining what kinds of studies need to be performed to carry out clinical trials in the different regions. Although differences still exist, there is consensus in some aspects. Table I attempts to summarize the length of the studies that are necessary to support clinical trials of different lengths.

There is wide consensus that preclinical toxicology studies generally support clinical studies of equal length. Some exceptions exist to these rules, particularly when the risk–benefit analysis reveals that exposure to the potential harmful effects of a compound is less detrimental to the patient than the withdrawal of a drug presenting obvious benefits.

These exceptions occur more often in compounds that are being developed for serious life-threatening diseases for which there is no alternative treatment. Examples of these conditions are chemotherapeutic agents used for terminal cancer or drugs for diseases such as AIDS.

TABLE I
Duration for Toxicology Studies (ICH)

Duration of clinical trial	Rodents	Nonrodents
Single dose		
USA	1–14 days	1–14 days
European community (EC)	2 weeks	2 weeks
Japan	4 weeks	2 weeks
Up to 2 weeks	2 weeks (4 weeks, Japan)	2 weeks
Multiple dose		
Up to 1 month	1 month	1 month
Up to 3 months	3 months	3 months
Up to 6 months	6 months	6 months
> 6 months	6 months	Chronic (EC, 6 months; USA and Japan, 6, 9, or 12 months)

The length of the animal toxicology studies increases as development proceeds in order to protect an increasing number of humans being exposed to the experimental compounds for a longer period of time. As the compound progresses in development, the number of individuals exposed may reach tens of thousands of people. This mass exposure places increased responsibility in the correct interpretation of the longer term toxicology studies and is the basis for some regulatory requirements.

The entity that sponsors the development of the particular compound has the responsibility to inform the U.S. regulatory agency when new, unexpected, and significant findings in toxicology studies may change the risk to human subjects participating in clinical studies. This information must be provided promptly within 2 weeks of the finding, and there may be additional requirements to disclose the new finding to clinical investigators and even patients.

This requirement places a responsibility on the pathologist to address these changes expeditiously and to reach a conclusion as to their biological significance in the shortest time possible. Because these findings occur during the latest stages of development of the compound, when the sponsor's investment is already considerable, frequently there is a need for thorough and urgent consultation to define whether the finding fits within this category.

V. General Considerations for the Use of Pathology in Regulatory Studies

A. WHAT IS IN A DIAGNOSIS?

There are some considerations in designing toxicology studies to support drug registration that will enhance the ability of the pathologist to provide useful information to the assessment of risk to humans.

First, pathological evaluation in these studies should not be limited to providing tables that divide the diagnoses into every component of their description to be treated as exact data. Rather, diagnoses should be the synthesis of those different components into a meaningful diagnosis, which is placed into perspective by a professional who is well versed in pathophysiology and medicine. Thus, pathological diagnoses are the interpretations of a well-trained pathologist as to what all the components of a morphologic response mean in biological terms.

Second, to achieve a useful interpretation, information regarding the treatment group, clinical signs, necropsy findings, clinical pathology, and any other relevant information should be taken into consideration when making diagnoses. Therefore, the initial evaluation of any changes should not be done blindly, as this ancillary information is critical to arriving at a good diagnosis.

Blind interpretation of histological findings is defined as that in which the treatment group and ancillary data are not identified to the pathologist. This method has been advocated by some regulators and is practiced by some laboratories. The most effective function of the pathologist follows the clinical model, where all the available information enters into the evaluation of the particular condition to assess its significance.

Performing a blinded assessment becomes useful at a later stage when a change is identified and one wants to decide whether the controls or the treated animals have a higher incidence or severity of the change. In such situations, blinding the slides for that organ allows the pathologist to remove the possible bias of knowing which animals were treated and which animals were given control substance such as vehicle.

Third, there is the issue of "background changes" seen in the tissues evaluated. Experienced pathologists who look at animal tissues on a regular basis know that ancillary information about an animal is critical to interpret all observed morphological changes. Researchers unfamiliar with the process of diagnosing lesions may assume that every tissue that deviates from control should be given a diagnosis and entered into the study tables. This action is of course an ideal concept that has little to do with reality.

Like all living things, laboratory animals have variations in their normal morphology as well as underlying conditions that reflect their exposure to pathogens and other environmental influences, the peculiarities of the species and strain, and marginal changes that are difficult to differentiate from pathological processes. There are also occasionally subtle artifacts that complicate interpretation. To make things more complicated, in every study between 75 and 80% of the animals are treated, and only 20–25% of the animals are used in the control group(s). Consequently, the probability that a spontaneous change will be observed in treated animals is $p=0.75-0.80$.

This bias is more likely to occur in larger species (dogs, monkeys), as fewer animals are used in these studies. This phenomenon is particularly challenging when working with simians that often have a large number of spontaneous conditions because they are seldom laboratory reared and free of all pathogens. The role of the pathologist is to discern compound-induced effects from the background changes and to provide clear interpretation.

In addressing spontaneous changes, two common methods are used to determine their importance. Some findings should be recorded into the database, as compounds may have effects on the expression of background changes and because of the need to have accurate historical data. Other changes should be ignored because they constitute variation in normality and would produce random noise in data, complicating interpretation and statistical evaluation of the data set. Selection of changes that need to be recorded and reported, and those that should be ignored, must be agreed upon with other pathologists, particularly the peer reviewer, and should follow a defensible argument for the decision.

Fourth, once a change is identified in a target organ, the pathologist has to decide what events are considered primary and which are secondary to the compound administration. For ex-

ample, when observing decreases in erythroid and white blood cell counts, one has to distinguish between bone marrow toxicity and the indirect effects of chronic illness, as in chronic stress or inflammatory processes. In the first case, the effect of the compound is direct, whereas in the second case one would have to monitor for the primary effect to prevent the secondary one from occurring.

B. PEER REVIEW AND QUALITY CONTROL

The subject of peer review has been debated throughout the pathology community since the early 1980s. Peer review has come to represent a standard in the industry, although the way it is applied varies among companies and laboratories. As there is no agreed upon standard that directs how, and in what studies, peer review should be conducted, this section represents the individual opinion of the author based on experience and does not claim to represent general practice.

Peer review is practiced universally in carcinogenicity studies, although many laboratories practice it on most other studies. There has been a range of proposals to consider peer review as a quality assurance issue. At one end of the spectrum, a designated authority, generally external to the pathology group performing the slide evaluation, would undertake slide review. At the other extreme, there are pathologists who consider peer review to be informal consultations among pathologists when there is doubt about the diagnosis.

The most accepted present position is that peer review should be a formalized consultation that helps the study pathologist arrive at the most accurate interpretation of the changes in a study or to feel comfortable with the lack of such changes. As understood by the author, the peer-review process works best when the responsibility for the decision on the significance of the changes is left in the control of the study pathologist. The peer-reviewer's role should be to assist in the interpretation of histological changes, discuss the changes observed as to treatment association, and to call the pathologist's attention to missed or inconsistent

315

diagnoses. The peer reviewer and the study pathologist should discuss their differences and reach consensus on the nomenclature and significance of the changes in question.

At the end of the process, a statement is placed in the study file as to the extent of the peer-review process and whether the diagnoses in the study reflect, or do not reflect, the consensus of the two pathologists. There is no regulatory need to document every single discrepancy, and this process should be performed outside good laboratory procedure audits.

There should not be a preconceived idea that the best individual to assist in peer review is the individual with the most experience. When there are well-trained pathologists working together, the less experienced pathologist may identify changes that the more experienced pathologist may have missed as a consequence of familiarity, bring new focus on old practices, or both. The peer-review process can thus become a mutual learning experience for both pathologists involved. It can also bring cohesiveness to a group and strengthen the position of the individual pathologist when the changes have to be discussed with management or regulatory agencies.

C. SHARING STUDIES

Drug safety studies with tight deadlines are often on the critical path to compound development. Examination of tissues is imperative, but is often viewed as time-consuming or rate-limiting. One solution is the sharing of studies, particularly carcinogenicity studies, among two or more pathologists in order to cut the time it takes to produce a report.

Although some people argue that this can be accomplished successfully, it is fraught with potential bias that can affect data. For example, group or sex differences may arise based on individual histopathological interpretation, which may not reflect actual effects of the compound. Alternatively, assigning random numbers of animals to different pathologists may eliminate any group or sex bias, but differences in interpretation by the individuals may lead to operator bias and inaccurate conclusions.

There is enough variability between individual pathologists in their approach to histopathological interpretation that the most common practice is still to have one pathologist responsible for the total interpretation of a study.

D. RECUTTING AND RESTAINING

Histotechnicians may feel the need to cut additional tissue sections from paraffin blocks for a variety of reasons. This effort is usually performed in search of the perfect section. However, multiple sectioning should be done judiciously.

Every slide of the tissue should be examined and all lesions recorded. Inconsistent sampling procedures may lead to inaccurate incidence data. Therefore, it is important to take into consideration the number of sections obtained from an animal when summarizing lesion incidences.

E. EVALUATING ONLY HIGH-DOSE AND CONTROL GROUPS

It is customary in the industry to perform histopathological evaluation of high-dose and control groups, and only target organs in intermediate- and low-dose groups. The reason for this convention is obvious savings in labor. The scientific rationale for this practice is based on the concept of linearity of response. Although most toxicological responses are linear, this may not always be the case. Notoriously, hormonal effects may have biphasic response curves. Therefore, the practice should be followed judiciously.

VI. Studies to Support First in Human Exposure

In general, the toxicology package to support first in human exposure includes acute and short-term repeated dose studies in two species, generally by two routes (when the intended route is other than oral). Two alternative types of studies are available to facilitate the rapid evaluation of compounds in the clinical setting (phase I). These alternatives are "single dose to single dose" studies and the "screening IND." Both are explored later.

A. ACUTE TOXICITY STUDIES

1. Objectives

Acute toxicity studies are designed to determine the dose that will produce mortality or serious toxicological effects when given once or over a few administrations. They also serve to provide information regarding doses that should be used in subsequent studies. These studies provide another opportunity to determine compound-induced effects as observed by morphology, clinical chemistry, or other evaluations. Acute studies can also give an early indication of the possible target organ(s).

2. Study Design

By definition, single-dose studies are limited to administration of a single dose, although this definition is often extended to include multiple administrations of the compound over a 24 h period. These studies can be designed to have a multistage exposure, with escalating doses to find intolerance. There is generally a "washout" period allowed between exposures based on the pharmacokinetics of the compound.

If the "washout" period is not sufficient to clear the compound and its effects, the study becomes a multiple-dose exposure. Animals may be sacrificed and necropsy performed in these studies. The number of animals in these studies is variable, but in general it includes 3 to 4 animals per sex per group for larger laboratory animal species and 5 to 10 rodents per sex per group.

End points for these studies vary. Most studies include clinical observations and clinical pathology determinations. Some studies are limited to determining the number of animals that die during the study, often necropsies are not performed, and tissues are not collected. This decision misses the opportunity of obtaining data that can be used for the design of later studies. However, these studies are generally not very informative because the changes that occur are often peracute without time to de-

velop clinicopathological or morphologic abnormalities.

In general, acute toxicity studies are carried out at doses that reach the limits of practicality of administration, and often doses cannot be given that directly produce intolerance because of the low acute toxicity of the compound. In such cases, it may not be necessary to exceed the dose of 2 g per kilogram of body weight for pharmaceuticals and 5 g per kilogram of body weight for pesticides.

a. LD_{50} Determinations. This is a subset of the acute toxicity studies. The median lethal dose (LD_{50}) is defined as the dosage that kills 50% of the animals exposed. This determination has been useful to compare the acute toxicity of substances and has served as a basis for classifying industrial and environmental toxicants.

Pharmaceutical development used to start with a formal determination of LD_{50}. Experience showed that the LD_{50} did not provide much useful information for the development of pharmaceutical products and used too many animals. The formal determination of a traditional LD_{50} is no longer necessary for the development of pharmaceutical products. Such a determination is still required for chemical products and represents a way to compare the relative toxicity of compounds to which humans, or the environment, are potentially exposed.

b. Acute Toxicity Categories. In order to compare the toxicity of different compounds under acute exposure, the EPA has created four "hazard categories" that apply to compounds with eventual environmental exposure. Regulatory agencies generally agree that once a compound reaches a dose of 5 g/kg by the oral route (category IV), it can be considered "generally regarded as safe (GRAS)."

Of course, these categories deal with acute toxic effects and do not take into consideration repeated exposure. The hazards of repeated exposure (such as chronic, cumulative damage, and carcinogenicity potential) may limit exposure to levels much lower than the acute toxicity studies. Table II presents the categories as published in the review manual of the U.S. of

TABLE II
Acute Toxicity Categories

Hazard indicators	I	II	III	IV
Oral LD_{50} (mg/kg)	≤ 50	50–500	500–5000	>5000
Inhalation LC_{50} (mg/liter)	≤ 0.05	0.05–0.5	0.5–2	> 2
Dermal LD_{50} (mg/kg)	≤ 200	200–2000	2000–5000	>5000

America Environmental Protection Agency in 1994.

B. ALTERNATIVE STUDIES TO SUPPORT "FIRST IN HUMAN" EXPOSURE

1. Single-Dose to Single-Dose Toxicity Studies

These studies are intended to support single-dose toxicity studies in humans when one or several compounds of the same class need to be chosen on the basis of pharmacokinetic profiles in humans. This plan has the advantage of sparing compound production for multidose animal and clinical trials and decreasing the time for early development, as several compounds can be screened at the same time.

a. Study Design. Although there is a single administration to the animals, the design of these studies requires full tissue histopathology at 24 hr after administration and after a 2-week recovery period. Two species and two routes, other than intravenous, are necessary for intended administrations. The ICH guidelines require two routes unless the intended use is intravenous and then only that route may be used. If an acceptable formulation is not available for the parenteral use of oral compounds, then the intravenous route may be avoided.

2. Screening IND

Screening IND studies are meant to require a minimum amount of information before single-dose studies can be performed in volunteers with several candidates. The premise is similar to the single-dose to single-dose studies, although there are some differences. The screening IND assumes the opening of a formal IND for several candidates and then the opening of a formal

IND for the chosen compound to continue into development. This is different from the opening of several concurrent IND files (one per compound tested) for the single-dose to single-dose protocols. When only one or two compounds are compared, it is often more convenient to present two initial IND documents than to restart the process in the screening IND paradigm. Nonetheless these two alternatives are available for FDA-regulated studies in humans. As indicated before, these paradigms are not required for European first in human studies, as there is no formal IND-like process in Europe.

C. SUBACUTE, SUBCHRONIC, AND CHRONIC TOXICITY STUDIES

The objective of these studies is to define the toxic effects over a period of repeated administration that is related to the length of use in humans. This objective is accomplished by administering the compound at multiples of the therapeutic dose that will produce intolerance in the animals. This method is known as defining the target organ toxicity. Additionally, these studies may also be designed to identify doses that are safe to animals. Finally, these studies may be designed to address whether the changes observed are progressive, stable, or reversible.

1. No Observed Effect Level (NOEL)

The NOEL is interpreted as the highest dose where there are no differences between the control and the treated group. The no observed adverse effect level (NOAEL) is defined as the highest dose where the effects observed in the treated group do not imply an adverse effect to the subject.

One common example of this difference is the observation of immunosuppression in animals treated with compounds being developed for use in transplantation or autoimmune diseases. These compounds are expected to produce immunosuppression at low levels, which is considered a pharmacologic effect. Therefore the NOEL is expected to be low in these individuals, but the NOAEL would be higher because one has to define the adverse effects beyond the issue of immunosuppression. Another common example is the presence of organ changes that are adaptive, such as hepatocellular hypertrophy. Many scientists consider this change as a normal response to increasing metabolism of a xenobiotic, and it is not considered "adverse" unless accompanied by liver damage, generally evidenced by an elevation of liver enzymes.

2. Lowest Observed Effect Level (LOEL)

The LOEL is interpreted as the lowest dose where there are differences between the control and the treated group. The lowest observed adverse effect level (LOAEL) is defined as the lowest dose where the effects observed in the treated group imply an adverse effect to the subject. The utility of the LOEAL and NOAEL is when used together a dose range is given. Usually the LOEL/LOEAL is the dose above the NOEL/NOAEL. By giving both values, the reader can see the gap between doses that the real NOEL/NOAEL and LOEL/LOAEL probably lie.

3. Study Design

Selection of the experimental animal species and strains is of the utmost importance when addressing the toxicity of a compound and cross-species relevancy should not be assumed. The choice should enhance the predictivity of the studies for humans. Several points should be taken into consideration when choosing species and strain of animals. The similarity of the therapeutic target in the experimental animals to that of the human is an important consideration.

Similarities in the pharmacokinetic and metabolic profiles between species are important, although frequently unknown. The similarity of the physiological mechanisms in the target organ should also be taken into consideration.

D. CARCINOGENICITY STUDIES

1. General Considerations

a. Objective(s). Carcinogenicity studies are designed to identify the risk of development of cancer in humans when exposed to xenobiotics. The general premise is that long-term exposure of animals will allow compounds to express any carcinogenic potential. The two most common models for carcinogenicity testing are the 2-year administration of the candidate compound to mice and rats.

Most compounds intended for chronic use will have to be tested in both species in the United States and Japan, although for the European community, only one species is required, generally the rat. In the European community, carcinogenicity studies are required for the registration of compounds intended for continuous use for more than 6 months; in the United States they are generally required if the intended continuous use is longer than 3 months. They may also be required for compounds intended for intermittent but frequent use for chronic or recurrent conditions.

Carcinogenicity studies may sometimes be completed postmarketing. They can also be averted altogether for certain compounds with life-saving indications or if intended for severely debilitating or terminal diseases.

The issue of carcinogenicity testing has probably received the most scrutiny of all subjects in toxicology since the 1950s. At the center of the controversy is whether these tests are good predictors of human risk. Regulatory agencies are faced with the need for assessment of the carcinogenicity hazard in models other than humans (or other target populations). Data collected since the 1960s indicate that the rodent model often overpredicts carcinogenic risk.

Fifty percent of all compounds tested in these models are considered positive. Some compounds, such as phenobarbital, are carcinogenic in animals, but show no evidence of carcinogenicity in humans, despite large amounts of epidemiological human data.

It is not difficult to agree on the effect of clear carcinogens, which produce marked and early effects in animals. On these occasions it is necessary to identify the conditions in which these effects would be seen in humans, if at all. The issue of a "safe dose" becomes important, although there is controversy.

The controversy of the "safe dose" is based on whether the compound is genotoxic or is not genotoxic, and the classification of compounds into so-called genotoxic and nongenotoxic carcinogens. More difficult to place into context is the case of an unexpected tumor that is statistically significantly increased, but in a marginal way, when compared to controls (and even historical tables). In many cases, these may be statistical aberrations, although their interpretation becomes extremely difficult. Unfortunately, some regulators may consider such tumors as evidence of carcinogenesis.

The scientific and clinical training of the pathologist and experience in the interpretation of lesions in older animals are valuable assets when interpreting the results of carcinogenicity studies. The ability of the pathologist to understand species differences is very helpful to place these effects into the proper context for human risk.

b. Alternative Methods. The FDA has expressed a willingness to accept alternative methods of carcinogenicity evaluation that may be more mechanism based. These studies may eventually complement or even replace traditional carcinogenicity testing. Currently the 2-year rat carcinogenicity test is required in order to attain compound registration, although the mouse carcinogenicity study may be replaced with other studies.

The rationale for replacing the mouse carcinogenicity study with alternative tests should be based on clear scientific arguments of their adequacy. Alternative methods include transgenic animals, such as the TgAc +/+, p53+/−, and XPA −/− strains, other alternative and mechanistic studies, such as the neonatal

mouse, and the liver proliferation model. At the time of this writing, there is considerable activity to define and characterize these models. The future utility of these alternatives will be assessed after more information is gathered on their predictivity of carcinogenic risk to humans. Acceptability of these methods in other countries that still require two animal models as well as other regulatory agencies in the United States, such as the EPA, is still to be decided.

c. The Delaney Clause. In 1952, the U.S. congress created a law in which the Delaney clause can be found. It states: "No additive shall be deemed to be safe if it is found to induce cancer when ingested by man or animal or if it is found, after tests which are appropriate for the evaluation of the safety of food additives, to induce cancer in man and animals" (United States Code, 1987). This regulation is based on the expectation that the results of the animal carcinogenicity tests can be extrapolated predictably to human risk. As there are many exceptions to this premise, it is now untenable, but the regulation is still enforced.

The Delaney clause is applied by U.S. regulatory agencies to compounds that fall in the category of "unwillfull exposure," such as compounds that may stay in the environment or become part of the food chain for humans and other species. Therefore the clause applies to compounds to be used in food animals, as well as to compounds that are categorized as foods or food additives. Regulations similar to the Delaney clause do not apply to registration in Europe, Japan, and other countries.

d. Nomenclature and Standardization Efforts. The most important end point in carcinogenicity studies is the histopathological evaluation of tissues. Pathologists bring their experience and training to the interpretation of the changes observed. These are often unique to the individual. Pathologists may have their own interpretation of certain changes, which may not reflect the majority position. The utilization of individual or outdated nomenclature for the changes observed creates confusion and an inability to compare the findings between studies.

Several organizations have attempted to create standardized classification criteria for diagnoses. The World Health Organization (WHO) has published the International Classification of Rodent Tumors through its International Agency for Research on Cancer (IARC). In recent years, the Society of Toxicologic Pathologists (STP) in conjunction with the Armed Forces Institute of Pathology (AFIP) of the United States has published a comprehensive list of diagnoses applicable to toxicology studies. This list has become the unofficial standard for diagnoses and is followed by most major groups.

It is important for pathologists to realize that use of the standard nomenclature is in the interest of a common understanding of the particular change observed. Following a standardized nomenclature should not be viewed as capitulating on the individual's knowledge and expertise to interpret changes. The use of standardized nomenclature creates a common language for understanding the changes observed. When a pathologist differs strongly from the nomenclature utilized, the diagnostic term should reflect the standard nomenclature, and the text of the document should address the interpretation of the pathologist.

e. Historical Databases. Interpretation of histopathology data can be best performed when the context of the diagnoses can be put into perspective with the help of historical data. The use of historical control data brings into consideration the incidence of changes observed in the particular species or strain. They should compare studies of similar length as the one in question.

Because 75–80% of the animals in the study are given the compound and only 20–25% of the animals are controls, it is quite likely that spontaneous, yet unusual, changes will appear in the treated animals. This is an inherent bias in test systems and is more often a problem in the interpretation of studies where there are a limited number of animals, as in the case of nonrodent species, as well as in carcinogenicity studies.

Historical controls then bring the variability inherent in the system, which may exceed the variability of concurrent controls, into the interpretation. Historical controls cannot replace the role of concurrent controls, which help in addressing environmental biases. An important issue of the utilization of historical controls is the use of a common nomenclature. Without a common understanding of the criteria for diagnoses, the historical controls become of limited utility.

In recent years, the Fraunhoffer Institute in Hanover has championed the use of databases for carcinogenicity studies, creating two databases: one in Europe (RITA) and another one in North America (NACAD). These efforts help in the sharing of databases between laboratories and increase understanding of spontaneous conditions in experimental animals.

Historical databases are also very important in the interpretation of shorter term studies, although there are no intercompany databases developed. The larger companies and contract research organizations (CRO) have developed their own databases to be applied to their studies. Also, some of the laboratory animal procurement companies provide actuarial tables that may help in the interpretation of study data. Nonetheless, actuarial tables are often subject to the vagaries of lack of common nomenclature and may not be up to date.

The subject of the contemporaneity of databases has been debated hotly among regulatory circles, academia, and industry. This debate arises in the observation that the background incidence of lesions will change with time as a consequence of multiple factors. There is "genetic drift" to consider as well as changes in husbandry and the health of the animals.

Although these influences are undeniable, in the past, databases have been more variable because of a lack of general agreement in a nomenclature than due to these causes. With the advent of computers and more standardized nomenclature, the databases can be used with more confidence. Changes in diet, husbandry, or strains should be taken into consideration before the databases can be used.

For carcinogenicity studies, the length of the study and the age of the animals at the time of death are important. Mortality begins after the first year in study and accelerates after 18 months. Therefore, comparisons should be made with animals that survive to a period close to the time of death of the animal expressing the changes in question. In general, databases do not include treated animals, as the changes observed may not be interpretable as spontaneous.

2. Study Design

Carcinogenicity studies are designed to optimize the expression of compound-related carcinogenesis and minimize the confounding effects of other toxicity, background, or indirect effects. A good carcinogenicity study design starts with a preliminary dose selection or feeding study. The objective of this study is to find the doses at which the compound can be given optimally for the period necessary for carcinogenesis evaluation.

The optimum dose is defined as the dose that will allow the expression of any carcinogenic potential, while minimizing increases in mortality produced by complications of either acute or chronic toxicity. Therefore, the dose selection studies should address the dose at which effects will interfere with the long-term survival of the animals.

For those studies in which the compound will be mixed with the diet, it is necessary to assess palatability of the diet and food consumption. Dose selection for a carcinogenicity study is generally determined from a 3-month feeding or gavage study. Other data, such as pharmacokinetic information, are important to assess the frequency of administration needed and the exposure of animals to the compound.

a. Dose Selection. An important aspect of the carcinogenicity studies is the selection of dose. As indicated earlier, too high a dose may confound the interpretation of the carcinogenicity study by producing multiple toxic changes that will interfere with the expression of a carcinogenic effect. Too high a dose may also, and frequently does, interfere with the long-term survival of particular groups.

The maximum tolerated dose (MTD) is the highest dose that will produce exposures at which the toxic effects of the compound will be maximized, but that will not likely compromise the long-term survival of the animals. Based on molecular technologies and high-throughput screening, compounds are more selective in their mode of action. There has also been a recent decrease in regulatory tolerance, with elimination of compounds from development with the most toxic side effects. These two factors and the near elimination of clearly genotoxic compounds based on *in vitro* genotoxic assays from most drug development have increased the difficulty in arriving at an MTD.

Some authorities accept that an alternative to the MTD is a dose that will produce up to but no more than a 20% decrement in body weight gain in a 3-month study, not due to palatalicity-related decreases in food consumption. A multiple of at least 25 times the maximum exposure in humans is now considered an acceptable alternative, when higher doses would be impractical or impossible and the drug candidate is not genotoxic.

This multiple of exposure does not apply unless there are reasons of practicality of administration or in situations when there is a flat dose–response curve when exposure does not increase with increasing doses. Before engaging in carcinogenicity studies, however, it is a good idea to consult with the regulatory agency (ies) for concordance with the intended doses. Many a carcinogenicity study has been invalidated, criticized severely, or had to be repeated on the basis of inadequate dose selection.

b. Strain (Stock) Selection. Most carcinogenicity studies are carried out in either mice or rats. These are not technically strains, but outbred stocks of these species. The term "strain" will be used due to the universality of its use, but the reader is cautioned to understand this frequent error. The most commonly used mouse is the CD-1. Regarding rats, there has been considerable controversy regarding the strains to be used.

Attempts to standardize the strains to be used in a carcinogenicity study have failed, as all strains have certain unwanted characteristics. The most commonly used strain in Europe is the Wistar. The most common ones in the

United States are the Sprague–Dawley and the Fisher. Fewer laboratories use the Long Evans strain.

During the 1980s and 1990s the length of survival of the Sprague–Dawley strain had been decreasing. In the past it was the practice of breeders to select the largest animals in the belief that they would have enhanced litter sizes and fecundity. These practices produced animals that overate, becoming very heavy, and had shortened life spans, particularly males.

Increased body weight is associated with increased mortality and appearance of neoplasia. Food restriction or optimization in these studies prevents overeating and controls body weight, increasing the longevity of these animals and decreasing background neoplasia. It has been proposed that when these strains are used, food consumption should be restricted in carcinogenicity studies in order to assure sufficient animals surviving to the intended length of the study.

Although some companies are now routinely optimizing food consumption between controls and treated animals, food restriction continues to be controversial. To address the problem of premature mortality, some suppliers of Sprague–Dawley rats have rederived their stock and have suspended the selection of larger animals, achieving an adequate survival to the end of the 2-year studies.

c. Length of Studies. There is very little agreement on the necessary length of carcinogenicity studies. Most designs expect the studies to last between 18 and 24 months in the mouse and 24 months in the rat. The rationale for the length of these studies is based more in tradition than in strict scientific validation. Some studies are carried out up to 36 months in the hope that they will pick up effects that would not be apparent in the 24-month period. Others argue that most compounds that are clearly carcinogenic express their effect quickly and unequivocally and that increasing the time of the test will lead to false positives.

It is generally agreed that genotoxic compounds will act early, although most of these compounds have not advanced to obtain market registration in recent times. Longer studies would increase the probability of recognizing effect in nongenotoxic compounds. These effects are frequently difficult to place in the context of risk assessment because they often are not applicable to human exposure and mechanisms of toxicity and create an opportunity for these compounds to produce statistical significance of uncertain biological significance.

The expectation of a carcinogenicity study is that enough animals would survive to the end of the 2-year period (rats) for an evaluation to be made. Traditionally, regulatory agencies have expressed an expectation for a 50% survival in the high dose and the controls at the end of 2 years, although there are no clear scientific data that support this figure. Because traditional studies are designed with 50 animals per sex per dose group, one can conclude that the logical reason is that carcinogenicity studies require the survival of 25 animals to the end of the study in order to reach a convincing conclusion. This thinking has led to some study designs that start with 65 or more animals per set per dose group, hoping that the minimum number of 25 animals per group will survive until the scheduled sacrifice. It is noteworthy that the expectation of the number of survivors has not been arrived at by a thorough validation of the carcinogenicity models, but rather by customary demands by some of the people involved in review of data generated.

d. Number of Groups. Most toxicology studies utilize three or four treatment groups and one vehicle control group. In some studies, where comparison with a standard may be desirable, a positive control group may also be included. Because the end point for carcinogenicity studies resides in a variable incidence of histological changes and because of the confounding effects of old age in these animals, the need to address variability of the test system is higher. This has led some laboratories to use two separate control groups, both of which receive vehicle.

The statistical analysis may be carried out first with both control groups combined or against one of the two control groups. In case of statistical significance in combined control data or against one control group, the treated groups are then compared statistically for significance against each of the control groups. If the statistical significance disappears with one of the control groups, it is obvious that the effect can be ascribed to spontaneous variability in the incidence of the particular change. Although this exercise requires the use of more animals, it can save a study from a spurious significance. There is not universal agreement on the utility of this practice, but it can be useful in some occasions.

e. Statistical Analysis. The most utilized statistical analysis for histopathological changes in carcinogenicity studies is the Peto trend analysis, which takes survival and cause of early mortality into consideration. For statistical analysis of other data, such as clinical pathology and organ weights, the pairwise method can be utilized, although a suitable trend test may be more appropriate. In case of statistical significance, which may be suspected of being due to variability in the system, the Bonferoni method may be applied. The *p* value for statistical significance may vary depending on the spontaneous incidence of the tumor type, with more common tumors requiring a 0.01 rather than 0.05. For further statistical information, please see Chapter 5.

VII. Clinical Pathology

Guidance for the conduct of clinical pathology testing in toxicological studies has been published. These recommendations emanated from a committee on harmonization of clinical pathology testing, sponsored jointly by the Society of Toxicologic Pathologists (STP), the American College of Clinical Chemistry (ACCC), and the American Society of Veterinary Clinical Pathology (ASCVP). The use of clinical pathology end points, particularly hematology, after the 12-month period is considered unadvisable due to the impact of chronic disease and age-related changes in clinical pathology parameters. In carcinogenicity stud-

ies, after 12 months, the only clinical pathology end point recommended is the use of blood smears at the end of the study to serve in identifying lymphomas and leukemias.

It is important to recognize that too-frequent bleeding of rats, if performed by the retrobulbar route, may induce ocular damage, which may complicate the histological evaluation of the eyes. In mice, the general practice is not to perform clinical pathology evaluation on the principal groups that may obviate the presentation of these data. In mice, one can perform clinical pathology at terminal sacrifice or by establishing satellite groups exclusively for this purpose. It is also customary, for mice and rat studies, to include a few satellite animals to obtain pharmacokinetic data to document actual exposure up to 12 months.

VIII. Reproductive Toxicology

The pathologist plays an important role in the evaluation of reproductive toxicity in animals. As the reproductive studies are performed generally after the first human studies have been initiated or even completed, interaction between the pathologist and the reproductive toxicologist is essential, as information from previous animal studies is relevant. This information often helps in establishing doses for the formal reproductive studies and in identifying possible mechanisms for any reproductive damage. The correlation of morphological data with the results of specialized tests, such as sperm analyses, is essential to place the results in perspective.

Knowledge of embryonic development by the pathologist is often useful in identifying the exact time of damage that produces malformations. This information is valuable in the identification of the mechanism of action of teratogenic xenobiotics.

Male fertility testing is not required for early clinical trials but may be encouraged in Japan. However, evaluation of the male reproductive tract is necessary. This is generally satisfied by the thorough routine histological evaluation of the tract in preclinical studies. Therefore the male reproductive tract is evaluated carefully in repeated dose toxicity studies, and there may not be a need to perform this examination in reproductive studies if the conditions of exposure remain comparable. The male fertility test is recommended prior to therapeutic confirmatory studies (clinical phase III).

More controversy surrounds how and when is the best time to address female reproductive effects. In the 1977 guidelines, a woman of childbearing potential was defined very rigidly and referred to all premenopausal women physiologically capable of becoming pregnant. This led to a very cautious approach to the use of women in clinical phase I and phase II studies.

The FDA has removed the restriction for the inclusion of women in early trials because patient behavior and laboratory testing can minimize the risk of fetal exposure. This change in policy was intended to develop more information about the use of compounds in women. Nonetheless, there is no regulatory basis for requiring women or women of childbearing potential in particular trials such as Phase I studies and there is a high level of concern for the unintentional exposure of the conceptus before the potential risks of such exposure are evaluated. Consequently, this change in definition is unlikely to, by itself, cause drug companies or Internal Review Boards (IRB's) to alter restrictions that they might impose on the participation of women of childbearing potential in early clinical trials.

IX. Pediatric Populations

The FDA has produced guidelines intended to increase the number of compounds developed for childhood diseases. In general, the support of pediatric trials has been based on information gathered from extensive experience with adult populations, and the performance of specific studies in very young animals is not generally considered necessary. Occasionally, when specific effects need to be clarified, the performance of studies in neonatal or very young animals is unavoidable before children are exposed.

X. Special Studies

A. ANIMAL HEALTH PRODUCTS

Most products for the treatment of animal diseases in the United States are registered with the FDA Center for Veterinary Medicines, although biologics such as vaccines are regulated by the U.S. Department of Agriculture. In general, there is little need for classical safety studies for vaccines, with the exception of injection site reactions. Studies performed in the process of registration of other veterinary products can be divided into two categories: compounds intended for use in food animals and compounds intended for use in companion animals.

Generally, compounds for use in companion animals require studies only in the target species. This may be preceded by preliminary dose-range finding studies in laboratory animals. Target animal species studies are carried out at a series of multiples of the therapeutic dose in the intended species (usually $1\times$, $3\times$, and $5\times$), and histopathologic evaluation is essential. Chronic toxicity studies are performed when the therapeutic regimen indicates prolonged exposure. Reproductive studies may be necessary in the targeted species.

Studies intended to register compounds for use in food animals (the definition of which varies with the culture and country) have two purposes. The first type of study is intended to define the toxicity in the target species using trials similar to those for companion animals. The second objective is to define the risk of exposure to humans that are expected to consume products from these animals (milk, eggs, meat). Not only should these studies define the limits of toxicity, but also the time of withdrawal, when concentration of the compounds will reach safe levels for human consumption after the animals receive the treatment with the product (residue studies).

SUGGESTED READING

Calabrese, E. J., and Baldwin, L. A. (1999). The marginalization of hormesis. *Toxicol. Pathol.* **27**(2), 187–194.

Calabrese, E. J., and Baldwin, L. A. (1999). Chemical hormesis: Its historical foundations as a biological hypothesis. *Toxicol. Pathol.* **27**, 195–216.

Choudary, J., *et al.* (1996). Response to Monro and Mehta proposal for use of single-dose toxicology studies to support single-dose studies of new drugs in humans. *Clin. Pharmacol. Ther.* **59**, 265–267.

Davies, T. S., and Monro, A. (1994). The rodent carcinogenicity bioassay produces a similar frequency of tumor increases and decreases: Implications for risk assessment. *Regul. Toxicol. Pharmacol.* **20**(3 pt 1), 281–301.

DeGeorge, J. J., *et al.* (1999). The duration of non-rodent toxicity studies for pharmaceuticals. *Toxicol. Sci.* **49**, 143–155.

Eastin, W. C., *et al.* (1998). The National Toxicology Program evaluation of genetically altered mice as predictive models for identifying carcinogens. *Toxicol. Pathol.* **26**(4), 461–473.

Gonzalez, F. J. (1996). Use of transgenic animals in carcinogenesis studies. *Mol. Carcinog.* **16**, 63–67.

Guideline for the study and evaluation of gender differences in the clinical evaluation of drugs. *CFR* **58**, 139, July 22, 1993.

Keenan, K. P., *et al.* (1998). Need for dietary control by caloric restriction in rodent toxicology and carcinogenicity studies. *J. Toxicol. Environ. Health B* Apr–Jun; **1**, 135–148.

"Label Review Manual Chapter 8: Precautionary Labeling." (Online) http://www.epa.gov/oppfead1/labeling/lrm/chap-08.htm. January 5, 2000.

Mahler, J. F., *et al.* (1998). Spontaneous and chemically induced proliferative lesions in Tg.AC transgenic and p53-heterozygous mice. *Toxicol. Pathol.* **26**(4), 501–511.

Memorandum of Understanding Between the Environmental Protection Agency and the Food and Drug Administration; Drug/Pesticide Products for Use on or in Animals (1983) *Fed. Regist.* 49 Friday May 20.

Merkatz, R. B., *et al.* (1993). Women in clinical trials of new drugs: A change in Food and Drug Administration policy. *N. Engl. J. Med.* **329**, 292–296.

Monro, A., and Mehta, D. (1996). Are single-dose toxicology studies in animals adequate to support single doses of a new drug in humans? *Clin. Pharmacol. Ther.* **59**, 258–64.

Peto, R., *et al.* (1980). Guidelines for simple, sensitive significance tests for carcinogenic effects in long-term animal experiments. *In* "Long-Term and Short-Term Screening assays for Carcinogenesis: A Critical Appraisal." AIARC Monographs Supplement 2, Lyon, International Agency for Research on Cancer, pp. 311–426.

Roe, F. J. (1998). A brief history of the use of laboratory animals for the prediction of carcinogenic risk for man with a note on needs for the future. *Exp. Toxicol. Pathol.* **50**, 271–276.

Standardized System of Nomenclature and Diagnostic Criteria in Guides for Toxicologic Pathology, STP/ARP/AFIP, Washington, DC, 1990–1999.

United States Food and Drug Administration (1999). International Conference on Harmonization: Guidance on the duration of chronic toxicity testing in animals (rodent and nonrodent testing); Availability. *Fed. Regist.* **64**, 34259–34260.

Weingand, K., *et al.* (1992). Clinical pathology testing recommendations for non-clinical toxicity and safety studies. *Toxicol. Pathol.* **20**, 539–543.

Weisburger, J. H. (1994). Does the Delaney clause of the U.S. Food and Drug laws prevent human cancers? *Fundam. Appl. Toxicol.* **22**, 483–493.

Use and Misuse of Statistics in the Design and Interpretation of Studies

Shayne C. Gad

Gad Consulting Services
Raleigh, North Carolina

Colin G. Rousseaux

Department of Cellular and Molecular Medicine
Faculty of Medicine
University of Ottawa
and Therapeutic Products Programme
Health Canada
Ottawa, Ontario, Canada

1. Introduction

This chapter has been written for both practicing and student toxicologic pathologists as a practical guide to common statistical problems encountered using differing research strategies in toxicologic pathology and the methodologies available to solve them. First we will give an overview of the areas of research that the toxicologic pathologist is presently, or may be in the future, involved in. Next, core issues in mathematical decision making are discussed. The chapter then details some of the principles used in making mathematical inferences and includes discussions of why a particular procedure or interpretation is recommended. Enumeration of assumptions that are necessary

Handbook of Toxicologic Pathology, Second Edition
Volume 1

for procedures to be valid are described, and problems often seen in the practice of toxicology and toxicologic pathology are discussed.

Since 1960, as the field of toxicologic pathology has evolved, it has also become increasingly complex and controversial in both its theory and practice. As in all other sciences, toxicologic pathology started as a descriptive science. Initially, pathologists described morphological changes seen following accidental exposure to xenobiotics. The need to understand the dose–response effects of specific xenobiotics on tissues and organisms so that prediction of adverse effects could be extrapolated to a target population could be made resulted in predictive toxicologic pathology. Prediction could only be made when animals were dosed with, or exposed to, chemical or physical agents and the resultant adverse effects were observed. With the accumulation of these results, it has become possible to infer and study underlying mechanisms of action for adverse effects observed. Toxicologic pathology has now developed to the mechanistic stage, where active contributions to the field encompass both descriptive and mechanistic studies. This stage mainly requires determination of dose–response relationships for adverse effects so that predictions of response can be made when the dose is known. In the future, toxicologic pathology may be key to resolving therapeutic product-related adverse health effects in addition to adverse health effects caused by environmental chemical exposures.

Studies continue to be designed and executed to generate results in the form of measurements or observations referred to as data. As questions asked by the researcher increase in complexity, the data analyses have become more complex. The field of statistical analysis has also grown since the mid-1960s, mostly to assist interpretation of data generated in the field of toxicology. These simultaneous changes have led to an increasing complexity of data generated and the introduction of confounding factors, which may severely limit the utility of the resulting data.

The toxicologic pathologist is well trained to assist in interpretation of the biological importance of analyzed data from inferential experiments. The biological meaning of results must be evaluated as to their importance, use, and extrapolation to either risk characterization or safety assessment. In addition, the peculiarities of toxicological data need to be understood before procedures are selected and employed for analysis.

A number of characteristics of toxicology experiments in animals impact their extrapolation to human populations. First, relatively small sample sets of data are collected from the members of an experimental animal population, which is not actually the human or target animal population of interest. Second, sample data are often censored on a basis other than by the investigator's design. Censoring occurs when the data points are not obtained as planned. This censoring usually results from

biological factors, such as death or morbidity of an animal, or from a logistic factor, e.g., equipment failure or a tissue not collected during necropsy. Third, the conditions under which experiments are conducted are extremely varied. In pharmacology, the possible conditions of interaction of a chemical or physical agent with a person are limited to a small range of doses given via a single route of exposure over a short course of treatment to a defined patient population. In toxicology, however, the investigator controls all test variables, such as dose, route, timespan, and subject population. Fourth, time frames available to identify, assess, and give opinions to issues are limited by practical and economic factors. This frequently means that there is no time to repeat a critical study so a true iterative trial-and-error approach to toxicologic pathology is not possible.

The training of most pathologists in statistics remains limited to a single introductory course, which concentrates on some theoretical basics. As a result, the armamentarium of statistical techniques of most toxicologic pathologists is limited and the tools that are usually present in the workplace, such as t tests, χ^2, analysis of variance, and linear regression, are neither optimized nor well understood. Before we elaborate on these tools, we need to go back to an overview of toxicologic pathological research, some basic issues surrounding "results," classification, type of numbers generated, and the meaning of statistical and biological significance. Once the stage is set we hope to illustrate the appropriate use of certain statistical procedures, what the statistical method does, and the assumptions required for validity of the output.

A. RESEARCH AND THE TOXICOLOGIC PATHOLOGIST

The introduction described the toxicologic pathologist as an individual who is central to the generation of adverse health effects data for the generation of safety assessment of a new compound or evaluating risk following an unintended exposure to a xenobiotic. As seen in other chapters, the toxicologic pathologist is becoming involved in fields other than safety assessment, such as novel compound discovery. In fact, if one takes a broader view of toxicologic pathologists in industry, academia, and government, it can be seen that they are involved in practically all types of research, ranging from the description of new chemically related disease states to highly controlled experiments from which inferences are made.

Although the core expertise of the toxicologic pathologist is centered on making diagnoses, the medical and veterinary training often required as a prerequisite for the discipline makes the toxicologic pathologist an excellent resource for observational and associative research. Most readers will remember their basic epidemiology training. This training, combined with other skills of the toxicologic pathologist, places them in prime position to assist in the identification and interpretation of adverse events following market authorization of pharmaceuticals, biologics, agrochemicals, and other xenobiotics. For this reason, we include this type of research in the overview of research types undertaken by the toxicologic pathologist in Table I.

From Table I, the reader will recognize how descriptive research is underpinned by clear and detailed description, quantification of findings, and morphological diagnoses. The process of creating standards for describing a specific diagnosis of clinical, clinical pathology, and morphological findings to create a diagnosis is essential in all aspects of toxicologic pathology. Anatomy and taxonomy use such description to *classify* normal tissues and species so that all tissues or individuals with the descriptive criteria are included, and all tissues or individuals without the criteria are excluded, from the group (class). These *classification* requirements mean that individuals in the class must be only in one class. Classes must be *mutually exclusive* (those cannot be both in the class and excluded from it) and *mutually exhaustive* (all of those meeting the criteria are included in the class). The easiest toxicologic pathological classification occurs when lesions are pathognomonic for a specific cause. Unfortunately, these occurrences are rare, hence the requirement for standardization. The importance of standard

classes of neoplastic and nonneoplastic lesions can be found in chapter 7.

The importance of classification is discussed in more detail later in this chapter. It is essential that the best effort be made to make sure that lesions fit only one class, as many of the statistical methods described later require that the variables (in this case lesion class) be independent for analysis; i.e., if there is a gray zone where a lesion could be in either class, the assumptions behind many analyses are violated. Violation of the assumptions of these statistical tests brings the validity of the analysis into question.

Descriptive research is not limited to defining classes. Observation is a powerful tool in establishing an understanding of disease processes and how diseases develop. In addition, associations can be made between risk factors and the lesions described. This type of research is commonly referred to as associative research and is the cornerstone of epidemiology. Postmarket surveillance of adverse heath effects typifies associative research.

Associative research can range from a simple cross-sectional survey, where at a specified time point a "crosssection" of those individuals with or without the lesions(s) are associated with specific risk factors, such as drug exposure, to complex prospective cohort studies. These studies usually evaluate lesion development of two or more groups (e.g., exposed vs unexposed) over time. For example, the development of mesothelioma in asbestos workers vs nonasbestos-exposed individuals may be studied prospectively over a number of years. The main difficulty seen in this type of research is the lack of control of other factors that may cause or may influence the development of mesotheliomas. This unknown source of systematic influence confounds the association, hence these factors are known as *confounding factors* or variables. The importance of control and sources of systematic influence is discussed later.

The final type of research, and the type that is presently central to the practice of most toxicologic pathologists, is inferential research. Here experiments are developed to control all

TABLE I

An Overview of Research Methods Available to the Toxicologic Pathologist

Type of Research	Descriptive		Associative				Inferential	
	Case report	Case series	Retrospective study	Cross-sectional survey	Cohort studies	Clinical trials	Animal experiments	In vitro assays
	Description of lesions seen in accidental poisoning in one case	Description of lesions seen in accidental poisoning in a number of similar cases	Evaluation of autoimmune hemolytic anemia cases with a history of a specific drug treatment	Survey of those taking a drug who have or have not the adverse effect under examination	Comparison of smokers with nonsmokers over time to evaluate the incidence of lung cancer	Comparison of a new drug with the present gold standard for comparative safety and efficacy in patients with a defined disease	Experiments designed to evaluate the carcinogenicity of a test substance, e.g., the bioassay	Cell or tissue models used in experiments to determine some property of a test article, e.g., Ames assay
Control	None	None	Poor	Fair	Average–good	Average–good	Good–excellent	Excellent
Confounding variables	—	—	Very high	High	Moderate	Moderate–low	Low	Low
Extrapolation to target species	—	—	Excellent	Excellent	Excellent	Excellent	Good	Fair
Role of toxicologic pathologist	Description and classification of the lesions	Description and classification of the cases	Definition of disease vs nondiseased; interpretation	Definition and classification of the adverse effect; interpretation	Definition and classification of tumors; interpretation of degree of severity	Definition and interpretation of drug-related lesions in those who die	Description and classification of lesions in exposed animals	Relating results to other preclinical findings

possible factors that may affect the outcome except for the factor under study. For example, a typical bioassay controls species, environment, manipulations, and so on, so that all animals are essentially the same except for the treatment they receive. The treatments are planed *before* the observations and measurements are made (*a priori*) and before mathematical inferences concerning the probability of the treatment causing the outcome are made. Inferences following, or during the experiment, are central to the current role of the toxicologic pathologist, and hence make the core of this chapter. Again, the biological importance of the effect needs to be interpreted by the toxicologic pathologist.

B. OBSERVATIONS AND MEASUREMENTS

Observations and measurements are essential to all aspects of toxicologic pathology. Even when describing a new case, observations are described as to distribution, color, size, and texture. These observations are then summarized as to severity and distribution disease process affecting a specific tissue as a morphological diagnosis. An example of a gross morphological diagnosis is ileitis, severe, fibrinopurulent, segmental; and an example of a histological morphological diagnosis is hepatic necrosis, periacinar, acute, generalized. Measurements may also be made regarding size, weight, and so on to define the disease further.

All measurements and observations produce scalar measurement, ordered severity, and categories, each of which have implications regarding the type of statistical analysis that should be undertaken and how inference can be made using that analysis. We describe three types of outputs, which an understanding of each is necessary to select the correct method to derive inference of treatment effect. Regardless of its type, each measurement and each individual piece of experimental information gathered are called a *datum*. However, as we gather and analyze multiple measurements at one time, the resulting outputs are called *data*.

Data are collected on the basis of their association with a treatment, intended or otherwise, as an effect (a property) that is measured in the experimental subjects of a study. These identifiers, i.e., treatment and effect, are termed *variables*. Treatment variables previously selected and controlled by the researcher are termed *independent variables*. Effect variables, measurements, and observations such as weight, life span, and number of neoplasms are termed *dependent variables*. The measures of these variables are believed to be *dependent* on the "treatment" being studied.

All possible measures of a given set of variables in all the possible subjects that exist are termed the *population* for those variables. Such a population of variables cannot be truly measured. For example, one would have to obtain, treat, and measure the weights of all the Fischer 344 rats that were, are, or ever will be. Instead, we deal with a representative group called a *sample*. If our sample of data is collected appropriately and of sufficient size, it serves to provide good estimates of the characteristics of the parent population from which it was drawn.

Regardless of the type of data, optimal design and appropriate interpretation of experiments require that the researcher understand both the biological and the technological underpinnings of the system being studied and of the data being generated. From the point of view of the statistician, it is vitally important that the experimenter both knows and is able to communicate the nature of the data and understand its limitations. A summary of data types is presented in Table II.

The nature of data collected is determined by three considerations: the biological source of the data (the system being studied), the instrumentation and techniques being used to make measurements, and the design of the experiment. The researcher has some degree of control over each of these, at least over the biological system (s/he normally has a choice of only one of several models to study) and most over the design of the experiment or study. Such choices, in fact, dictate the type of data generated by a study. The following discussion aims to clarify the differences seem

TABLE II
Types of Variables (Data) and Examples of Each Type

Classified by		Type	Example
Scale	Continuous	Scalar	Body weight
		Ranked (ordinal)	Severity of a lesion
	Discontinuous	Scalar	Weeks until the first observation of a tumor in a carcinogenicity study
		Ranked (ordinal)	Clinical observations in animals
		Attribute (nominal)	Eye colors in fruit flies
		Quantal (nominal)	Dead/alive or present/absent
Frequency distribution		Normal	Body weights
		Bimodal	Some clinical chemistry parameters
		Others	Measures of time to incapacitation

among data types commonly seen in toxicologic pathology.

1. Categories

Categories, also referred to as "classes," are quintessential to toxicologic pathology. The most common category the toxicologic pathologist is familiar with is the definitive diagnosis. Here there may be a number of categories (diagnoses) into which the toxicologic pathologist places his or her observations, e.g., hepatocellular carcinoma and chronic interstitial nephritis. The categories only allow accumulation of "whole" events. It is not possible to have a partial diagnosis or make an "average" diagnosis. Either the diagnosis is made or it is not. These data are grouped on the basis of name or category; hence they are usually termed *nominal* or *categorical* data.

A special type of category results in only one of two outcomes: yes or no. Typical examples include live or dead, pregnant or not, etc. These data are referred to as *dichotomous, quantal,* or *binary* and are often seen in safety studies. Again, there is only one choice, partial choices cannot be made, i.e., an animal cannot be both dead and alive.

2. Nonmeasured Scales

Toxicologic pathologists are also familiar with the use of scales to express degrees of severity. These arbitrary scales are not measured, but the scale shows an internal relationship; i.e., in the case of severity, mild (+) is less than moderate (++), which is less than severe (+++). Because the severity is ordered, the resulting data are often called *ordinal* in nature. This scale does not define a measured parameter to which a known measurement scale can be applied, and hence is call a "nonparameter." In fact, both nominal and ordinal data are called *nonparametric* data, often where nonparametric statistical analysis is required for inference as to cause and effect.

3. Measurements

All are familiar with measured parameters. These measured parameters are scalar, as in ordinal scales, but use a recognized scale of measurement such as grams. Measurements can be either *continuous*, such as length and weight, or *discontinuous*, where measurements are made in whole numbers. White blood cell numbers and other hematological parameters are examples of discontinuous measurements. The difference between the categorical events described earlier and this discontinuous measurement relates to numbers. Again, a partial white cell cannot be recorded, but because there are so many cells, data approximate a continuum. Situations where discontinuous data can be considered as a continuum for the purpose of analysis are discussed later.

4. Proportions and rates

Data can be recorded as proportions ratios and rates, e.g., percentage affected with a specific tumor, 1:2 male:female ratio, and incidence of occurrence. These data are continuous, as fractions are possible. They are, however, seldom measured parameters and are not usually distributed normally. These data require distribution-free (i.e., nonparametric) statistical analysis unless a specified mathematical distribution can be approximated for the data set. Analyses of these data are discussed later.

332

Proportions can be misleading without reference to the *absolute values* from which they were calculated. For example, a "50% affected" rate represents one of two animals affected, or one million affected in a population of two million. Unscrupulous allusions as to effectiveness can be attempted using proportions without reference to the number in the study population.

5. *Type of data and statistical methods*

Statistical methods are based on specific assumptions. *Parametric statistics*, those that are most familiar to the majority of scientists, have more stringent underlying assumptions than nonparametric statistics. Parametric statistical analyses reflect analysis of *measured parameters*, e.g., weight. Nonparametric techniques should be used whenever the requirements for parametric tests cannot be verified or are not reasonably expected to be true. For example, continuous data such as cadmium concentrations in kidney tissue from an exposed versus unexposed population could be studied using nonparametric statistics when the assumptions for parametric analysis cannot be met. *Nonparametric* data refer to data that were not measured, such as with a ruler, but were gathered as types or classes, such as numbers of classified observations and whether the experimental unit fits a defined state. An example of such data includes the number of fetuses with a specific defect and the number of pregnant females in a teratology study. There are data, however, not measured, but show a continuous scale such as subjective severity scores. These data are common in toxicologic pathology and may be analyzed using parametric analysis, provided that the assumptions of the tests can be met.

Among the underlying assumptions for many parametric statistical methods (such as the analysis of variance) is that data are continuous. The nature of data associated with a variable (as described earlier) imparts a "value" to that data, the value being the power of the statistical tests that can be employed. For this reason, except for situations where nonpara-metric data can be transformed to approximate normally distributed parametric data, parametric statistical analyses should not be used for nonparametric data.

Continuous variables are those that can at least theoretically assume any of an infinite number of values between any two fixed points (such as measurements of body weight between 2.0 and 3.0 kg). Discontinuous variables, meanwhile, are those that can have only certain fixed values, with no possible intermediate values (such as counts of five and six dead animals, respectively).

II. Prerequisites to Statistical Analysis

Statistical analyses are tools that aid us in inferring whether experimental manipulations caused an effect, or that associations between putative risk factors and outcomes are likely. As statistical analysis is a supportive tool to assist in decision making, it is not always necessary to analyze data. If all events occur in one group, but not in any other, it is obvious where the treatment effect lies (subject, of course, to reasonable sample sizes and appropriate conduct of experiments). Unfortunately, biology is rarely this simple. Usually, events of interest are seen in most, if not all, experimental groups. The question that statistical analysis attempts to answer is whether the difference in the frequency or severity observed in different groups is due to chance or a result of the experimental manipulation.

A. BIOLOGICAL VARIATION

Biological variation is central to all our lives. Diversity allows life to fill our planet with rich mixtures of life forms. Within each species, diversity is essential for survival and finding a niche in which to develop. Without exploring the theory of evolution, diversity in our own species is recognized in a number of visible characteristics, such as height, and functional characteristics, such as biotransforming abilities. The latter source of variability has led to the developing field of pharmacogenomics. Unfortunately, biological diversity interferes with efforts to test treatment effects, even when the experiment is designed and controlled *a priori*. No matter how inbred study animals are, there is always a range of response displayed in measurements made on these animals.

The normal variability in the test species is called normal biological variation. The distribution of measurements typically follows a *normal* or *Gaussian distribution*. This distribution is described as a "bell-shaped" curve (as shown in Fig. 1), an essential underpinning of many statistical analyses. In essence, this is the background of "noise" against which backdrop observations are made. Mathematics can help clarify whether the results seen in an experiment are a result of biological "noise" or a treatment-related "signal." Just as the experimenter cannot be sure that the treatment did have an effect, statistical analyses do not give a definite yes or no answer, rather a probability statement.

The mathematics used in the analysis results in a probability that the variability in results is caused by biological variation and not the treatment (Fig. 2). The experimenter

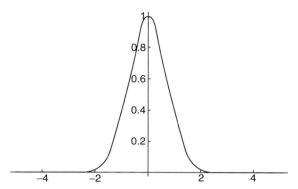

Figure 1. Normal biological variability. *X* axis reports the frequency of the observation; *Y* axis reports the measurements.

can then review the probability of the treatment groups being the same and then decide whether to reject that they are or not. This decision point is referred to as rejecting the null hypothesis; the null hypothesis being that the variability of effects is due to normal biological variation, and hence groups are the same. By convention, we reject this hypothesis when the probability of making a false rejection is 5% or less. Hypothesis testing is discussed in more detail later.

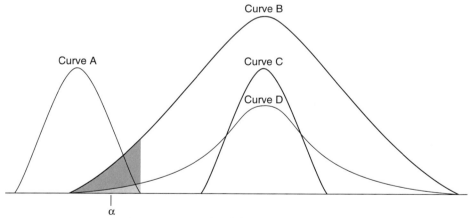

Figure 2. Experimental outcome mixed with biological variability. If comparison is made between curve A (e.g., the control group response) and curve C (e.g., treatment response), then the separation of the two groups is obvious. However, if curve A (e.g., response of controls) is compared with curve B or D it is not obvious as to whether the groups are different or represent subsets of biological variation within the experiment. The null hypothesis would state that all curves are part of the variability shown within the experiment rather than caused by the treatment. The probability, less than which the experimenter is willing to reject this hypothesis, is given by α.

B. DESCRIBING DATA

Limitations in our ability to measure restrict the extent to which the real-world situation approaches the theoretical, but many of the variables studied in toxicology are in fact continuous. Examples of these are lengths, weights, concentrations, temperatures, periods of time, and percentages. An experiment can result in the collection of thousands of data. These data usually have a distribution, which may be normal in nature. Regardless of the type of distribution, efforts are made to describe the data for visible inspection and comparison. The number that summarizes a number of data is termed a *descriptive statistic*. Descriptive statistics are used to summarize the *location* or *central tendency* of data and to provide a measure of the *dispersion* of data in and about this central location. The mean (the average), the median (the 50th percentile), and the mode (the most common result) give description of the location, whereas the standard deviation (or the standard error of the mean), the semiquartile range, coefficient of variation, and range give descriptions of dispersion. It should be noted that the choice of descriptive statistic implies a particular type of distribution for data.

1. Mean and Standard Deviation

Most commonly, *location* or *central tendency* is described by giving the (arithmetic) mean and *dispersion* by giving the *standard deviation* (SD) or the *standard error of the mean* (SEM). The statistics that we are most familiar with are the mean, denoted by the symbol $\bar{x}$ (also called the arithmetic average), and the SD, which is denoted by the symbol σ and the SEM. The SD can be calculated as in Eq. (1):

$$\sqrt{\frac{\sum X^2 - \dfrac{(\sum X)^2}{N}}{N-1}}, \qquad (1)$$

where X is the individual datum and N is the total number of data in the group.

Similarly, the SEM can be calculated using Eq. (2)

$$SEM = \frac{SD}{\sqrt{N}}. \qquad (2)$$

The SD and the SEM are related to each other, but yet are quite different. The SEM is quite a bit smaller than the SD, making it very attractive to use in reporting data. This size difference is because the SEM actually is an estimate of the error (or variability) involved in measuring the means of samples and not an estimate of the error (or variability) involved in measuring data from which means are calculated. This difference is implied by the *central limit theorem*.

The central limit theorem states that the distribution of sample means will be approximately normal regardless of the distribution of values in the original population from which the samples were drawn. Second, it defines the mean value of the collection. Finally, the theorem states that the SD of the collection of all possible means of samples of a given size, called the SEM, depends on both the standard deviation of the original population and the size of the sample.

The SEM should be used only when the uncertainty of the estimate of the mean is of concern, which is almost never the case in toxicology. Rather, researchers are usually concerned with an estimate of the variability of the population for which the SD is appropriate.

2. Median and Semiquartile Range

The use of the mean with either SD or SEM implies, however, that there is reason to believe that the samples of data for summary are from a population that is at least approximately normally distributed. If this is not the case, then it is preferable to use a set of statistical descriptions that do not require a normal distribution. These are the *median*, for location, and the *semiquartile* distance (or interquartile range), for a measure of dispersion. Another situation can arise: sometimes data are log normally distributed or distributed according to some other distribution that can be relatively easily transformed to give a normal distribution. For lognormal data, the geometric mean and geometric standard deviation are appropriate descriptors of central tendency and dispersion.

335

When all the numbers in a group are arranged in a ranked order (i.e., from smallest to largest), the median is the middle value, i.e., the 50th percentile. If there is an odd number of values in a group, then the middle value is obvious, e.g., for 13 values the seventh largest is the median. When the number of values in the sample is even, the median is calculated as the midpoint between the $(N/2)^{\text{th}}$ and the $([N/2]+1)^{\text{th}}$ number. For example, in the series of numbers 7, 12, 13, and 19, the median value would be the midpoint between 12 and 13, which is 12.5.

When all the data in a group are ranked, a quartile of the data contains one ordered quarter of the values. Typically, the borders of the middle two quartiles $Q1$ and $Q3$, which together represent the semiquartile distance and which contain the median as their center, describe dispersion. Given that there are N values in an ordered group of data, the upper limit of the jth quartile (Q_j) may be computed as being equal to the $[jN \div 1)/4^{\text{th}}]$ value. Then the semiquartile distance can be computed, which is also called the quartile deviation and interquartile range (QD) with the formula $QD = (Q_3 - Q_1)/2$. For example, for the 15 value data set 1, 2, 3, 4, 4, 5, 5, 5, 6, 6, 6, 7, 7, 8, and 9, the upper limits of Q_1 and Q_3 can be calculated as:

$$Q_1 = \frac{1(15+1)}{4} = \frac{16}{4} = 4$$
$$Q_3 = \frac{3(15=1)}{4} = \frac{48}{4} = 12 \qquad (3)$$

The 4th and 12th values in this data set are 4 and 7, respectively. The semiquartile distance can then be calculated as

$$QD = \frac{7-4}{2} = 1.5.$$

3. Mode and Range

Rarely is the mode and range used as descriptive statistics. Their use may be considered when data are very skewed or may have a different distribution from normal. The mode describes the most common event, whereas the range describes the distance between the lowest and the highest measurement.

4. Coefficient of Variation

There are times when description of the relative variability of one or more sets of data is desired. The most common way of doing this is to compute the *coefficient of variation* (CV), which is calculated as the ratio of the standard deviation to the mean.

$$CV = \frac{SD}{\bar{X}} \qquad (4)$$

A CV of 0.2 or 20% thus means that the standard deviation is 20% of the mean. Due to the inherent variability of biological response in toxicologic pathology studies, the CV is frequently between 20 and 50%, and may exceed 100%.

5. Statistical Graphics

The use of graphics in one form or another in statistics is the single most effective and robust statistical tool and, at the same time, one of the most poorly understood and improperly used. Graphs are used for one of four major purposes. Each of the four is a variation on the central theme of making complex data easier to understand and use. These four major functions are exploration, analysis, communication and display of data, and graphical aids.

Exploration, simply summarizing data or trying to expose relationships between variables, shows the characteristics ("behavior") of data sets, allowing a decision on one or more appropriate forms of further analysis, e.g., the scatter plot.

Analysis is the use of graphs to formally evaluate some aspect of the data, such as whether there are outliers present or if an underlying assumption of a population distribution is fulfilled. As long ago as 1960, some 18 graphical methods for analyzing multivariate data relationships were developed and proposed. Table III presents a summary of major graphical techniques that are available.

Communication and *display* of data are the most commonly used functions of statistically graphics in toxicologic pathology. These graphics are used for internal reports, presentations at meetings, or formal publications in the

336

TABLE III
Forms of Statistical Graphs by Function Used for Preliminary Assessment of Data

Exploration		
Data summary	Two variables	Three or more variables
Box and whisker plot	Autocorrelation plot	Biplot
Histogram	Cross-correlation plot	Cluster trees
Dot-array diagram	Scatter plot	Labeled scatter plot
Frequency polygon	Sequence plot	Glyphs and metroglyphs
Ogive		Face plots
Stem and leaf diagram		Fourier plots
		Similarity and preference maps
		Multidimensional scaling displays
		Weathervane plot

Analysis		
Distribution assessment	Model evaluation and assumption verification	Decision making
Probability plot	Average versus standard deviation	Control chart
Q-Q plot	Component plus residual plot	Cusum chart
P-P plot	Partial residual plot	Half-normal plot
Hanging histogram	Residual plots	Ridge trace
Rootagram		Youden plot
Poissonness plot		

Communication and display of data		
Quantitative graphics	Summary of statistical analyses	Graphic aids
Line chart	Means plot	Confidence limits
Pictogram	Sliding reference distribution	Graph paper
Pie chart	Notched box plot	Power curves
Contour plot	Factor space/response	Nomograms
Stereogram	Interaction plot	Sample-size curves
Color map	Contour plot	Trilinear coordinates
Histogram	Predicted response plot	
	Confidence region plot	

literature. In communicating data, graphs should not be used to duplicate data that are presented in tables, but rather to show important trends and/or relationships in the data. Although such communication is most commonly of a quantitative compilation of actual data, graphs can also be used to summarize and present the results of statistical analysis.

Graphical aids to calculation are graphs that are becoming outdated, as microcomputers become more widely available. This fourth and final function of graphics includes nomograms and extrapolating and interpolating data graphically based on plotted data. The classic example of a nomogram in toxicology is that presented by Litchfield and Wilcoxon for determining median effective doses.

There are many forms of statistical graphics (a partial list, classified by function, is presented in Table III), and a number of these, such as scatter plots and histograms, can be used for each of a number of possible functions. Most of these plots are based on a Cartesian system, i.e., they use a set of rectangular coordinates. Our review of construction and use focuses on these forms of graphs.

Construction of a rectangular graph of any form starts with the selection of the appropriate form of graph followed by the laying out of the coordinates, or axes. Even graphs that are going to encompass mulivariate data, i.e., more than two variables, generally have as their starting point two major coordinates. The horizontal axis, or ordinate, also called the X axis, is used to present an independent variable, e.g., dose. The vertical axis, or ordinate, also called the Y axis, is used to present an dependent variable, e.g., response. Each of these axes is scaled in the units of measure that will most clearly present the trends of interest in data. The range covered by the scale of each axis is selected to cover the entire region for which data are presented. The actual demarcating of the measurement scale along an axis should allow for easy and accurate assessment of the coordinates of any data point, yet should not be cluttered.

Some rules apply to diagrammatic representation of data. Data points should be presented by symbols that present the appropriate indicators of location. If symbols represent a summary of data from a normal data population, some indication of the variability, or uncertainty, associated with that population should be used. It should be noted that error and variability are not synonymous. Both represent uncertainty, but variability is inherently irreducible, whereas error can be reduced through design and analysis. "Error bars" represent the standard deviation, or standard error, of the mean. If data are not normal or continuous, location should be represented by the median with the range or semiquartile distance showing the variability estimates.

Symbols used to present data points can also be used to present a significant amount of additional information. Distinct symbols, such as circles, triangles, and squares, are used to provide a third dimension of data, most commonly the treatment group. Further complexity can be used to present even more information. Methods, such as Chernoff's faces, can be used to present a large number of different variables on a single graph. In Chernoff's method, faces are used as symbols of the data points. Aspects of the faces present additional quantal or nominal data, such as the presence or absence of a lesion, or class of lesion.

The three other forms of graphs that are commonly used are histograms, pie charts, and contour plots. *Histograms* are graphs of simple frequency distribution. The abscissa (x axis) contains the variable of interest, such as life span or litter size, and is generally shown as classes or intervals of measurements, e.g., age ranges of 0 to 10, 10 to 20 weeks. The ordinate (y axis) displays the incidence or frequency of observations. The result is a set of vertical bars, each of which represents the incidence of a particular set of observations. Measures of error or variability about each incidence are reflected by some form of error bar on top of, or in the frequency bars, as shown in Fig. 3. The size of class intervals may be unequal (in effect, one can combine, or pool, several small class intervals), but it is proper in such cases to vary the width of the bars to indicate differences in interval size. Bias can be introduced by not addressing interval size, as the appearance of a distorted volume of the bars gives the view an incorrect impression of data distribution.

Pie charts are the only common form of quantitative graphic representation that is not rectangular. The figure is presented as a circle, out of which several "slices" are delimited. The pie chart presents a breakdown of the components of a group. Typically the entire set of data under consideration, such as total body weight, constitutes the pie, whereas each slice represents a percentage of the whole, such as the organ weight as a percentage of total body weight. The total number of slices in a pie should be small for the presentation to be effective. Variability or error can be presented readily by creating a subslice of each sector shaded and labeled accordingly.

Finally, the *contour plot* is used to depict the relationships in a three-variable, continous data system. A contour plot visually portrays each contour as a locus of the values of two variables associated with a constant value of the third variable. An example would be a relief map that gives both latitude and longitude of constant altitude using contour lines.

The most common misuse of graphs is to either conceal or exaggerate the extent of

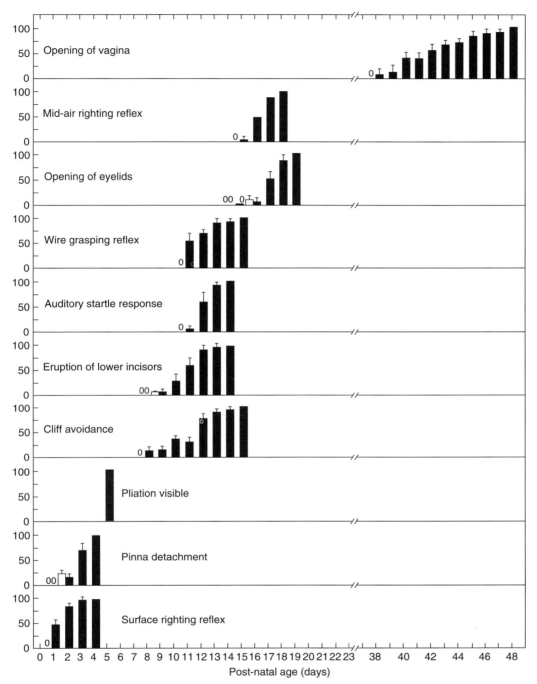

Figure 3. Acquisitions of postnatal development landmarks in rats.

differences by using inappropriately scaled or ranged axis. There is a statistic for evaluating the appropriateness of scale size called the lie factor. This statistic is calculated as the ratio of the shown effect size to the range of potential change or effect. An acceptable range for the lie factor is within 0.95 to 1.05. If the lie factor is less than 0.95, the size of an effect is being understated, whereas a lie factor greater than 1.05 suggests that the effect is being exaggerated. A number of excellent references are available for those who would like to pursue statistical graphics further.

C. BIOLOGICAL AND STATISTICAL SIGNIFICANCE

It is essential that a professional who firmly understands three concepts interprets any analysis of study results. These concepts include the *nature and value of different types of data*, the difference between *biological significance and statistical significance*, and *causality*. For the first concept, the reader is referred to Section B. The second item is essential for the toxicologic pathologist to have a sound concept when interpreting study data. The determination of causality is the subject of other chapters and is in its own section later in this chapter.

1. False Negatives and Positives

To illustrate the importance of biological vs statistical significance, we shall consider the four possible combinations of these two different types of significance, for which we find the relationship shown in Table IV.

Cases IV and I in Table IV give us no problems, for the answers are the same statistically and biologically. However, cases II and III present problems. In case II (the "false positive"), we have a circumstance where there is statistical significance in the measured difference between treated and control groups, but there is no true biological significance to the finding. This is not an uncommon happening, for example, in the case of clinical chemistry parameters. This is called *type I error* by statisticians, and the probability of this happening is called the α level. When this type of error occurs, the null hypothesis (i.e., no difference) is rejected when it is true.

In case III (the "false negative"), we have no statistical significance, but the differences between groups are significant biologically/toxicologically. Statisticians call this *type II error*, and the probability of such an error happening by random chance is called the β level. In this situation, the null hypothesis is accepted when it is false. An example of this second situation is when we see a few of a very rare tumor type in treated animals.

In both case II and case III, numerical analysis, no matter how well done, is no substitute for professional judgment. Along with this, however, one must have a feeling for the different types of data and for the value or relative merit of each. Note that the two error types interact, and in determining sample size we need to specify both α and β levels. Table V demonstrates this interaction in the case of tumor or specific lesion incidence.

2. True Biological Positive Effects

By now the reader may be puzzled as to how we agree that a result is "the truth." Even when it is established that an effect is of biological importance, the illustration shown earlier shows that there are always some false positive and negative outcomes based on the set false positive level, the sample size, and the resulting false negative probability. In addition to uncertainties of biological importance based on clinical judgment and statistical probability, there are other sources of uncertainty that should be recognized.

The generation of data through laboratory tests, particularly immunologic, hematologic, and enzymatic, all inherently show false negative and positive results. These results may occur because of the test itself or because of disease classification criteria used for defining the "normal" and "abnormal" ranges for the parameter of interest. For example, an immunocytochemical stain may not stain all tissues adequately that have the agent to be stained present. Conversely, some normal tissue may stain positive due to background staining. In this example we can see false negative and positives occurring not as a result of statistical error,

TABLE IV
Four Possible Combinations of Biological and Statistical Significance

Biological significance	Statistical Significance	No	Yes
	No	Case I	Case II
	Yes	Case III	Case IV

TABLE V
Sample Size Required to Obtain a Specified Sensitivity at $P < 0.05$ Treatment Group Incidence

Background tumor incidence	P^a	α level									
		0.95	0.90	0.80	0.70	0.60	0.50	0.40	0.30	0.20	0.10
0.30	0.90	10	12	18	31	46	102	389			
	0.50	6	6	9	12	22	32	123			
0.20	0.90	8	10	12	18	30	42	88	320		
	0.50	5	5	6	9	12	19	28	101		
0.10	0.90	6	8	10	12	17	25	33	65	214	
	0.50	3	3	5	6	9	11	17	31	68	
0.05	0.90	5	6	8	10	13	18	25	35	76	464
	0.50	3	3	5	6	7	9	12	19	24	147
0.01	0.90	5	5	7	8	10	13	19	27	46	114
	0.50	3	3	5	5	6	8	10	13	25	56

^{a}Power for each comparison of treatment group with background tumor incidence.

but as a result of error inherent to the test. The concept of false negatives and positives can be followed through reagents used in the test and so on.

The researcher requires knowledge of true positives, i.e., the probability of the test demonstrating positive findings in diseased subjects (*sensitivity*), and true negatives, i.e., the probability of a negative test in the absence of disease (*specificity*). The researcher also needs to know the ability of the test to give the same answer on a number of runs (*precision*) and the ability to give data that correspond to the true value of a measured parameter (*accuracy*).

If one examines Table VI for the combinations of biological and statistical significance, it can illustrate the relationship between test results and disease state.

Using Table VI, one can now define sensitivity, specificity, and other test predictions. Because precision and accuracy require data other than those described earlier, they will not be addressed further. However, we can now give values to other characteristics of the test in question, including sensitivity and specificity.

Equation (5): Determination of the test sensitivity from the 2 × 2 table

$$d/b + d$$

Equation (6): Determination of the test specificity from the 2 × 2 table

$$a/a + c$$

Equation (7): Determination of the test false positive rate (probability of a positive test when the disease is absent) from the 2 × 2 table

$$c/a + c$$

Equation (8): Determination of the test false negative rate (probability of a negative test when the disease is present if the test is positive) from the 2 × 2 table

$$b/b + d$$

Equation (9): Determination of the test positive predictive value (probability that the

TABLE VI
Four Possible Combinations of Biological and Statistical Significance

Disease?		No	Yes
Test result?	No $(a + b)$	Case I (a)	Case II (b)
	Yes $(c + d)$	Case III (c)	Case IV (d)
Total	$(a + b + c + d)$	$(a + c)$	$(b + d)$

a, the number of individuals that do not have the disease and test negative (true negative); b, the number of individuals that the have the disease and test negative (false negative); c, the number of individuals that do not have the disease and test positive (false positive); and d, the number of individuals that do not have the disease and test negative (true negative).

341

disease is present if the test is positive) from the 2 × 2 table

$$d/c + d$$

Equation (10): Determination of the test negative predictive value (probability that the disease is absent given a negative test) from the 2 × table

$$a/a + b$$

Equation (11): Determination of the test positive predictive value (probability that the disease is present given a positive test) from the 2 × 2 table

$$d/c + d$$

Although all these values have utility, it is the positive predictive value ($d/c + d$) that gives the experimenter the most information concerning the reliability of data.

3. Causality

The reasons that biological and statistical significance is not identical are multiple, but a central one is certainly *causality*. Through our consideration of statistics, we should keep in mind that just because a treatment and a change in an observed organism are seemingly or actually associated with each other does not "prove" that the former caused the latter. For example, the fact that the number of storks' nests found each year in England is correlated with the number of human births that year does not mean that storks bring babies. Although spurious correlation is widely recognized, similar errors hold true for statistical significance. In other words, sometimes two variables will appear to respond in step with one another, while the relationship is not to one another but to a third variable, which was not studied.

Proof that treatment causes an effect requires an understanding of the underlying mechanism and proof of its validity. At the same time, it is important that we realize that not finding a good correlation or suitable significance associated with a treatment and an effect likewise does not prove that the two are not associated. In other words, failure to show a correlation

does not mean that a treatment does not cause an effect. At best, it gives us a certain level of confidence that under the conditions of the current test, these items are not associated.

These points will be discussed in greater detail in the "assumptions" section for each method, along with other common pitfalls and shortcomings associated with the method. To help in better understanding the chapters to come, terms used frequently in discussion throughout this book should first be considered. These are presented in Table VI.

Causality is more difficult to address in observational research because of the difficulty associated with the inability to control the "experimental" environment. In this case, numerous factors may be associated with an observed outcome. To address the issue of causality, a number of questions can be asked of the association(s) that may help clarify these situations.

a. Time Sequence. It is obvious that for a factor to cause a lesion, exposure to it must precede the lesion. This criterion is automatically met in experiments and well-designed prospective cohort studies. The design of the study must ensure, to an extent that is practical, that candidates do not have the lesion before the study commences. For example, a small lesion could be present before exposure but not be found by palpation until after exposure. However, in many cross-sectional and retrospective types of investigation it may be difficult to establish the temporal relationship.

b. Strength of Association. In observational analytic studies, the strength of association is measured by relative risk or odds ratios [Eq. (12)]. The greater the departure of these statistics from unity (1.00), the more likely that the association is causal. For the calculation of relative risks and odds ratios, a 2 × 2 table can be used.

Lesion		Yes	No
Drug	Yes ($a+b$)	(a)	(b)
	No ($c+d$)	(c)	(d)
Total	($a+b+c+d$)	($a+c$)	($b+d$)

The **relative risk** can be calculated as:

TABLE VII
Some Frequently Used Terms and Their General Meanings[a]

Term	Meaning
95% confidence Interval	A range of values (above, below, or above and below) the sample (mean, median, mode, etc.) has a 95% chance of containing the true value of the population (mean, median, mode). Also called the fiducial limit equivalent to the $P < 0.05$.
Bias	Systemic error as opposed to a sampling error. For example, selection bias may occur when each member of the population does not have an equal chance of being selected for the sample.
Degrees of freedom	The number of independent deviations usually abbreviated df.
Independent variables	Also known as predictors or explanatory variables.
P-value	Another name for significance level, usually 0.05.
Power	The effect of the experimental conditions on the dependent variable relative to sampling fluctuation. When the effect is maximized, the experiment is more powerful. Power can also be defined as the probability that there will not be a type II error $(1 - \beta)$. Conventionally, power should be at least 0.07.
Random	Each individual member of the population has the same chance of being selected for the sample.
Robust	Having inferences or conclusions little affected by departure from assumptions.
Sensitivity	The number of subjects experiencing each experimental condition divided by the variance of scores in the sample.
Significance level	The probability that a difference has been erroneously declared to be significant, typically 0.005 and 0.001 corresponding to 5 and 1% chance of error.
Type 1 error (false positives)	Concluding that there is an effect when there really is not an effect. Its probability is the α level.
Type II error (false negatives)	Concluding there is an effect when there really is an effect. Its probability is the α level.

[a] From Maniott (1991).

$$\frac{a/(a+b)}{c/(c+d)}$$

The **population relative risk** can be calculated as:

$$\frac{(a+b)/n}{c/(c+d)}$$

The **odds ratio** can be calculated as:

$$\frac{ad}{bc}$$

The **population odds ratio** can be calculated as:

$$\frac{d(a/c)}{c(b/d)}$$

Although no explicit statistic is used when the dependent variable is measured, the relative difference in level of this variable with and without a particular factor may be used to assess the likelihood of producing the observed differences. For example, the relative difference in the incidence of massive hepatic necrosis could be related to treatment (or lack of treatment) with a specific drug suspected of causing an adverse drug reaction.

Strength of association is used as an indication of a causal association because for a confounding variable to produce or nullify an association between the lesion and the treatment, that confounding variable must have just as strong an association with the treatment. Although the fraction and/or the population is not used as a direct measure of strength of association, they must be kept in mind when interpreting the size of the relative risk or odds ratio. In fact, a given odds ratio could be given more credence if the population attributable fraction was large rather than small. The reasons for this credibility are the same as those given before under the discussion of proportions.

c. Dose–Response Relationship. An association is more likely to be causal if the frequency of lesions increases directly with exposure. Dose–response relationships, trends, and other evaluations of prospective experiments are discussed in detail later. However, the tenet that causality relates to increasing dose and response holds true for observational studies. For example, the incidence of liver-related adverse drug reactions that increase with the dose that the patient receives of the drug is indicative of causation. This criterion is not an absolute one, as in lesions that are threshold based there may not be a monotonic dose–response relationship.

d. Coherence. A biologically sensible explanation for the association gives support to causality. However, an association that is not biologically plausible, given the current state of knowledge, may still be correct. Lack of a biologically sensible explanation does not necessarily infer lack of association. Because almost any association is explainable after the fact (*post hoc*), it is necessary to predict the nature of the expected association and explain its biological meaning prior (*a priori*) to analyzing data. This is particularly important during the initial research when one is collecting information on a large number of unrefined factors to see if any are associated with the disease. For example, when investigating the severe liver pathology in the previous example, it is important to evaluate other possible causes of the lesions: the drug is innocent until proven guilty.

e. Consistency. An association gains credibility if it is supported by similar findings in different studies under different conditions. Therefore, consistent results in a number of studies are the observational equivalent of replication in experimental work. In the case of the example of drug-associated liver lesions, preclinical safety data and adverse reactions seen with other drugs of the same class all add consistency and hence support causality.

f. Specificity of Association. Initially, it was assumed that an association was more likely to be causal if the putative cause appeared to produce only one or a few effects. Today, this criterion is not widely used because it is known that a single causal agent may produce a number of effects. Specificity of the association may be of more value in studies where the risk factors and the lesions or disease are highly re-

fined. In initial studies where the variables are often composite in nature, the application of this criterion likely will be unrewarding.

g. Elaborating Causal Mechanisms. If an association is assumed to be causal, one can investigate the nature of the association using a number of methods. Initially, it is useful to sketch out the potential pathogeneses of lesion development. Next, consideration should be given to any direct or indirect cause of the lesions. For example, liver lesions may occur as a direct effect of the drug or metabolite or may result from ischemia secondary to anemia or poor tissue perfusion. Third, for each of the potential causes listed in the second step, the question of whether the cause is necessary and sufficient should be answered. From the adverse drug reaction example given earlier, closer evaluation of the preclinical and clinical pharmacokinetics of the compound may show that the metabolite demonstrated some hepatotoxicity, whereas the parent compound did not. Regardless of the method used to define the pathogenesis of the lesions, there is no fixed method to determine causal mechanisms. Good judgment is useful in generating such hypotheses as to the pathogenesis, but until *a priori* experimentation confirms or refutes the hypothesis, the pathogenesis can only be considered as hypothetical.

Observational studies have excellent applicability to the population on which they were undertaken. However, because of the lack of control and potential confounding variables, inference is limited. Well-controlled inferential experimentation enables the researcher to infer with some certainty that an effect was caused by the experimental manipulation or not.

III. Functions of Statistical Analyses

In addition to describing data, statistical methods may serve to do any combination of three possible tasks: (1) hypothesis testing, (2) models, and (3) reduction of dimensionality. The one most readers will be most familiar with is *hypothesis testing*, i.e., determining if two (or more) groups of data differ from each other at a predetermined level of confidence. A second function is the construction and use of *models* that may be used to predict future outcomes of chemical–biological interactions. The use of models is seen most commonly in linear regression or in the derivation of some form of correlation coefficient. Model fitting allows us to relate one variable (typically a treatment or "independent" variable) to another. The third function, *reduction of dimensionality*, is utilized less commonly than the first two. This final category includes methods for reducing the number of variables in a system while only minimally reducing the amount of information, therefore making a problem easier to visualize and to understand. Examples of such techniques are factor analysis and cluster analysis. A subset of this last function, discussed later under descriptive statistics, is the reduction of raw data to single expressions of central tendency and variability (such as the mean and standard deviation). There is also a special subset of statistical techniques, which is part of both the second and the third functions of statistics. This is *data transformation*, which includes such activities as the conversion of numbers to log or probit values.

A. HYPOTHESIS TESTING AND PROBABILITY (P) VALUES

A relationship of treatment to some toxicological end point is often stated to be "statistically significant ($p < 0.05$)." What does this really mean? A number of points have to be made. First, statistical significance need not necessarily imply biological importance if the end point under study is not relevant to the animal's well-being. Second, the statement will usually be based only on data from the study in question and will not take into account prior knowledge. In some situations, e.g., when one or two of a very rare tumor type are seen in treated animals, statistical significance may not be achieved but the finding may be biologically extremely important, especially if a similar treatment was previously found to elicit a similar response. Third, the p value does not describe the probability that a true effect

of treatment exists. Rather, it describes the probability of the observed response, or one more extremes, occurring by chance alone. When a "chance" event is sufficiently unlikely ($p < 0.05$), it is reasonable to conclude that the observed event was due to something other than chance, namely the treatment or other etiologic agent under study. A p value that is not significant is consistent with a treatment having a small effect, not detected with sufficient certainty in this study. Fourth, there are two types of p value. A "one-tailed (or one-sided) p value" is the probability of getting by chance a treatment effect in a specified direction as great as or greater than that observed. A "two-tailed p value" is the probability of getting, by chance alone, a treatment difference in either direction that is as great as or greater than that observed. By convention, p values are assumed to be two tailed unless the contrary is stated. Where, which is unusual, one can rule out in advance that the possibility of a treatment effect except in one direction, a one-tailed p value should be used. Often, however, two-tailed tests are preferred, and it is certainly not recommended to use one-tailed tests and *not* report large differences in the other direction. In any event, it is important to make it absolutely clear whether one- or two-tailed tests have been used.

When presenting results of statistical analyses, it is a great mistake to mark, as do some laboratories, results simply as significant or not significant at one defined probability level (usually $p < 0.05$) by an asterisk or some other symbol. This practice does not allow the reader any real chance to judge whether the effect is a true one. Some statisticians present the actual p value for every comparison made. While this gives precise information, it can make it difficult to assimilate results from many variables. One practice is to mark p values routinely using plus signs to indicate positive differences (and minus signs to indicate negative differences) as follows: $+ + + p < 0.001$, $+ + 0.001 \leq p < 0.01$, $+0.01 p < 0.05$, $(+0.05 \leq p \leq 0.1$. This description highlights significant results more clearly and also allows the reader to judge the whole range from "virtually certain treatment effect" to "some suspicion." Note that using two-tailed tests, bracketed plus signs indicate findings that would be significant at the conventional $p < 0.05$ level using one-tailed tests but are not significant at this level using two-tailed tests.

This "fiducial limit" ($p < 0.05$) implies a false positive incidence of 1 in 20 and, though now embedded in regulation, practice, and convention, was somewhat an arbitrary choice to begin with. In interpreting p values it is important to realize that they are only an aid in judgment to be used in conjunction with other available information. One might validly consider a $p < 0.01$ increase as chance when it was unexpected, occurred only at a low dose level with no such effect seen at higher doses, and was evident in only one subset of data. In contrast, a $p < 0.05$ increase might be convincing if it occurred in the top dose and was for an end point one might have expected to be increased from known properties of the chemical or closely related chemicals.

B. MULTIPLE COMPARISONS

When a p value is stated to be < 0.05, this implies that, for that particular test, the difference could have occurred by chance less than 1 time in 20. Toxicological studies frequently involve making treatment-control comparisons for large numbers of variables and, in some situations, also for various subsets of animals. Some statisticians worry that the larger the number of tests, the greater is the chance of picking up statistically significant findings that do not represent true treatment effects. For this reason, an alternative "multiple comparisons" procedure has been proposed in which if the treatment was totally without effect, then 19 times out of 20 *all* the tests should show nonsignificance when testing at the 95% confidence level. Automatic use of this approach cannot be recommended. Not only does it make it much more difficult to pick up any real effects, but there is also something inherently unsatisfactory about a situation where the relationship between a treatment and a particular response depends arbitrarily on which other responses

happened to be investigated at the same time. It is accepted that in any study involving multiple end points that there will inevitably be a gray area between those showing highly significant effects and those showing no significant effects, where there is a problem distinguishing chance and true effects. However, changing the methodology so that the gray areas all come up as nonsignificant is not the answer.

C. ESTIMATING THE SIZE OF THE EFFECT

It should be clearly understood that a p value does not give direct information about the size of any effect that has occurred. A compound may elicit an increase in response by a given amount, but whether a study finds this increase to be statistically significant will depend on the size of the study and the dispersion of data. In a small study, a large and important effect may be missed, especially if the end point is measured imprecisely. In a large study, however, a small and unimportant effect may emerge as statistically significant.

Hypothesis testing tells us whether an observed increase can or cannot be reasonably attributed to chance, but not how large it is. Although much a statistical theory relates to hypothesis testing, current trends in medical statistics are toward confidence interval estimation with differences between test and control groups expressed in the form of a best estimate, coupled with the 95% confidence interval (CI). Thus, if one states that treatment increases response by an estimated 10 units (95% CI 3–17 units), this would imply that there is a 95% chance that the indicated interval includes the true difference. If the lower 95% confidence limit exceeds zero, this implies the increase is statistically significant at $p < 0.05$ using a two-tailed test. One can also calculate, for example, 99 or 99.9% confidence limits, corresponding to testing for significance at $p < 0.01$ or $p < 0.001$.

In screening studies of standard design, the tendency has been to concentrate mainly on hypothesis testing. However, presentation of the results in the form of estimates with confidence intervals can be a useful adjunct for some analyses and is very important in studies aimed specifically at quantifying the size of an effect.

Two terms refer to the quality and reproducibility of our measurements of variables. The first, *accuracy*, is an expression of the closeness of a measured or computed value to its actual or "true" value in nature. The second, *precision*, reflects the closeness or reproducibility of a series of repeated measurements of the same quantity.

If we arrange all of our measurements of a particular variable in order as a point on an axis marked as to the values of that variable, and if our sample were large enough, the pattern of distribution of data in the sample would begin to become apparent. This pattern is a representation of the frequency distribution of a given population of data, i.e., the incidence of different measurements, their central tendency, and dispersion.

As mentioned in the introduction, the most common frequency distribution is the *normal (Gaussian) distribution*. The normal distribution is such that two-thirds of all values are within 1 SD of the mean (or average value for the entire population) and 95% are within 1.96 SD of the mean. Symbols used are μ for the mean and σ for the standard deviation. Other common frequency distributions can be used, such as the binomial, Poisson, and χ^2.

Contrasted with these continuous data, however, are discontinous (or discrete) data, which can only assume certain fixed numerical values. In these cases the choice of statistical tools or tests is, as described later, more limited. Before detailing with some of the statistical methods available for data evaluation from experiments, a brief discussion of aspects of experimental design and its impacts on analysis is warranted.

IV. An Overview of Experimental Design

Toxicological experiments generally are designed to answer two questions. The first question is whether an agent results in an *effect* on a biological system. The second question, never far behind, is *how much* of an effect is present. It has become increasingly desirable that the results and conclusions of studies aimed at assessing the effects of environmental agents be as clear and unequivocal as possible. It is essential that every experiment and study yield as much information as possible and that the results of each study have the greatest possible chance of answering the questions it was conducted to address. The statistical aspects of such efforts, so far as they are aimed at structuring experiments to maximize the possibilities of success of answering the questions, are called experimental design. Before addressing the issue of experimental design it should be remembered that removal or control of bias is necessary to make sure that the experimental work is not flawed and that results are usable.

A. CONTROL

Control in experimentation is central to determining treatment effect. *Control* is the term used to describe efforts made by the researcher to remove any known systematic influence on the experiment; i.e., all variables except for the independent variables under study are removed. Failure to control for other systematic influences on the dependent variables means that the researcher cannot determine whether the effect was due to the experimental independent variable(s) or some other source of systematic variation. It should be noted that there are numerous sources of systematic variation, ranging from the obvious, such as gender of the test species, to those that are easy to overlook, such as differences in handling by two different animal care attendants.

All inferential experiments have one or more control groups. These groups are assumed to be free of all systematic sources of variation, including the independent variable(s). It may be necessary to have both negative and positive controls, where in addition to the absence of independent variables another group is treated with a known positive outcome for the purposes of comparison. Multiple negative controls may be used where a systematic source of variation is expected. For example, a negative and pair-fed control may be used when treatment-related anorexia is known from previous studies. It is of interest that the French term for control is *temoin*, which, when translated, means "witness." Obviously, a witness should not be biased to the outcome of an investigation.

B. BIAS AND CHANCE

Any toxicological study aims to determine whether a treatment elicits a response. An observed difference in response between a treated and control group need not necessarily be a result of treatment. There are, in principle, two other possible explanations: *bias*, or systematic differences other than treatment between the groups, and *chance*, or random differences. A major objective of both experimental design and analysis is to try to avoid bias.

As mentioned previously, treated and control groups should be alike in respect of all factors other than the independent variable under test. Differences that cannot be controlled and remain must be corrected for in the statistical analysis. Chance cannot be wholly excluded because identically treated animals will not respond identically. This is due to inherent biological variability between individuals. While even the most extreme difference might in theory be due to chance, a proper statistical analysis will allow the experimenter to assess the likelihood, or probability, of this possibility. The smaller the probability of a "false positive," the more confident the experimenter can be that the effect is real. A good experimental design improves the chance of picking up a true effect with confidence by maximizing the ratio between "signal" and "noise."

Bias is any factor that makes results depart systematically from the values representative of the population. Bias can also be defined as: "*A process at any stage of inference tending to produce results that depart systematically from the true values.*" Bias must be distinguished from random error or chance as mentioned previously. The types of bias that may affect studies involving the toxicologic pathologist are described in more detail in Section VI,A. Bias

is particularly difficult to address in observational studies.

C. BASIC PRINCIPLES OF EXPERIMENTAL DESIGN

The four basic statistical principles of experimental design are replication, randomization, concurrent ("local") control, and balance. These may be summarized as follows.

1. Replication

Any treatment must be applied to more than one experimental unit (animal, plate of cells, litter of offspring, etc.). This provides more accuracy in the measurement of a response than can be obtained from a single observation, as underlying experimental errors and biological variability tend to be averaged over the replicates. It also supplies an estimate of the experimental error derived from the variability among each of the measurements taken (or "replicates"). In practice, this means that an experiment should have enough experimental units in each treatment group (i.e., a large enough "N") so that reasonably sensitive statistical analysis of data can be performed. The estimation of sample size is addressed in detail later. A distinction needs to be made between replication and duplication. Replication is the method of using different experimental units to increase the experimental number, e.g., giving a degree of severity rank to similar lesions from two mice. However, duplication is characterized by repeated measurements on the same experimental unit, e.g., blind rereading lesions and giving a second severity rank to the same lesion. The purpose of duplication is to gain an understanding of the precision of the measurements, in this case the severity rank. The distinction between replication and duplication is important to make when the toxicologic pathologist discusses the need, or not, to reread sections of a study blind.

2. Randomization

Randomization is practiced to ensure that every treatment shall have its fair share of results from among the spectrum of possible outcomes.

348

It also serves to allow the toxicologist to proceed as if the assumption of "independence" is valid; i.e., there is not avoidable (known) systematic bias in how one obtains data.

3. Concurrent Control

Comparisons between treatments should be made to the maximum extent possible between experimental units from the same closely defined population. Therefore, animals used in the "control" group should come from the *same* source, lot, age, and so on as test group animals. Except for the treatment being evaluated, test and control animals should be maintained and handled in exactly the same manner. Concurrent control should remove all sources of variation except for the treatment being evaluated. A number of controls are used in toxicologic pathology: negative, positive, and sham. A negative control is the control discussed earlier. There are, however, different types of negative controls. First, treatment controls are those that come from the *same* source, lot, age, and so on as test group animals and are given the treatment being evaluated without the test article and all animals are maintained and handled in exactly the same manner. Second, an experimental control group may be used where animals come from the *same* source, lot, age, and so on as other groups of experimental animals, but are maintained in exactly the same manner as the test and treatment control groups. Positive controls are animals from the *same* source, lot, age, and so on as test group animals, except they are given a treatment with a known response. This type of control ensures that under the experimental conditions, positive results can be obtained. The final type of control, the sham control, is used where an experimental manipulation of the animals under treatment occurs. Here the sham control is manipulated, but not treated.

4. Balance

If the effect of several different factors is being evaluated simultaneously, the experiment should be laid out in such a way that the contributions of the different factors could be separately distinguished and estimated. There are several ways of accomplishing this using different forms of design, as will be discussed later. It is important to recognize that mathematical comparisons are best when group sizes are similar. It may be tempting to place more animals in the treated group to "see" the effect, but such an action weakens statistical analysis of the experiment.

D. DETECTING TREATMENT EFFECTS

There are 10 facets of any study that may affect its ability to detect an effect of a treatment. The first six concern minimizing the role of chance and the last four relate to the avoidance of bias.

1. Choice of Species and Strain

Ideally, the responses of interest should be rare in untreated control animals but should be reasonably readily evoked by appropriate treatments. Some species or specific strains, perhaps because of inappropriate diets, have high background tumor incidences, which make increases both difficult to detect and difficult to interpret when detected.

2. Sampling

Sampling is an essential step upon which any meaningful experimental result depends. Sampling may involve the selection of which individual data points will be collected, which animals to collect tissue samples from, or taking a sample of a diet mix for chemical analysis. There are three assumptions about sampling which are common to most of the statistical analysis techniques that are used in toxicology. The assumptions are that the sample is collected without bias, each member of a sample is collected independently of the others, and members of a sample are collected with replacements.

Precluding bias, both intentional and unintentional, means that at the time of selection of a sample from a population, each portion of that population has an equal chance of being selected. Independence means that the selection of any portion of the sample is not affected by, and does not affect, the selection of any other portion. Finally, sampling with replacement means that, in theory, after each portion is selected and measured, it is returned to the total sample pool and thus has the opportunity to be selected again. This last assumption is a corollary of the assumption of independence. Violation of this assumption, which is almost always the case in toxicology and all the life sciences, does not have serious consequences if the total pool from which samples are selected is sufficiently large (30 or greater) that the chance of reselecting that portion is relatively small.

3. Sampling Methods

There are four major types of sampling methods: random, stratified, systematic, and cluster.

a. Random. Random sampling is by far the most commonly employed sampling method in toxicology. It stresses the fulfillment of the assumption of avoiding bias. When the entire pool of possibilities is mixed (or randomized), then the members of the group are selected in the order that they are drawn from the pool. Procedures for randomization are presented in a later chapter.

b. Stratified. First dividing the entire pool into subsets or strata, and then conducting randomized sampling from within each stratum, is how stratified sampling is performed. This method is employed when the total pool contains subsets that are distinctly different but within which each subset contains similar members. An example is a large batch of a powdered pesticide in which it is desired to determine the nature of the particle size distribution. Larger pieces or particles are on the top, whereas progressively smaller particles have settled lower in the container and are at the bottom, and the material has been packed and compressed into aggregates. To determine a representative answer to whether there is a particle size distribution as hypothesized, appropriately subsets from each subset should be selected, mixed, and sampled randomly. This method is used quite commonly in diet studies.

c. Systematic. In systematic sampling, a sample is taken at set intervals, e.g., every fifth container of reagent is sampled, or a sample is collected from a fixed sample point in a flowing stream at regular time intervals. This is employed most commonly in quality assurance and quality control procedures.

d. Cluster. In cluster sampling, the pool is already divided into numerous separate groups, such as bottles of tablets. Small sets of these groups, such as several bottles of tablets, are selected. Finally, a few members from each set are selected for analysis. The result is a cluster of measures. Like systematic sampling, this method is used commonly in quality control or in environmental studies when the effort and expense of physically collecting a small group of units are significant.

4. Sampling in Toxicologic Pathology Studies

In classical studies where toxicologic pathology is used, sampling arises in a practical sense in a limited number of situations. First, sampling occurs by selecting a subset of animals or test systems from a study to make some measurement, which either destroys or stresses the measured system or is expensive, at an interval during a study. This may include interim necropsies in a chronic study or collecting blood samples from some animals during a study. Second, samples may be taken to analyze inhalation chamber atmospheres to characterize aerosol distributions with a new generation system. Third, samples of diet to which test material has been added may be collected. Fourth, quality control samples may be performed on an analytical chemistry operation by having duplicate analyses performed on some materials. In addition, duplicates, replicates, and blanks are used to ensure that the results can be relied upon. By using duplicates, replicates, and blanks, the specificity, sensitivity, accuracy, precision, limit of quantitation, and ruggedness can be determined. Finally, samples of selected data may be required to audit for quality assurance purposes.

5. Dose Levels

The selection of dose levels and dosing methodology are very important and controversial aspects of study design. In screening studies aimed at hazard identification, it is normal to test at dose levels higher than those to which humans likely will be exposed, but not so high that overt toxicity occurs in order to avoid requiring unreasonably large numbers of animals. A range of doses is usually tested to guard against the possibility of a misjudgment of an appropriate high dose. It is important that the "appropriate high dose" induce some toxicity, however. Because the metabolic pathways at high doses may differ markedly from those at lower doses, it is important to ensure a range of doses be used. In studies aimed more at risk estimation, more and lower doses may be tested to obtain better information on the shape of the dose–response curve. Unfortunately, in practice, the shape of the curve in the very low dose range is not known. This is particularly important in assessing the risk to cancer where the incidence of cancer that could be detected in a typical rodent bioasseay is on the order of 2%. For the purposes of risk assessment, risk estimates are at least 1000-fold lower (i.e., 10^{-5}). For this reason, this type of study does not have much ability to give the shape of the curve for this assessment.

6. Number of Animals

This is obviously an important determinant of the precision of the findings. The calculation of the appropriate number depends on the critical difference, i.e., the size of the effect it is desired to detect. The number is also impacted by the false positive rate, i.e., probability of an effect being detected when none exists, equivalent to the "α level" or "type I error." Similarly, the false negative rate influences the number of experimental units required, i.e., probability of no effect being detected when one of exactly the critical size exists, equivalent to the "β level" or "type II error." Finally, the measure of the variability of response by the animals influences the number required.

Tables relating numbers of animals required to obtain values of critical size, α, and β are given in many references in the Suggested Reading following this chapter and software is

also available for this purpose. As a rule of thumb, to reduce the critical difference by a factor n for a given α and β, the number of animals required will have to increased by a factor n^2.

7. Duration of the Study

It is important not to terminate a study too early, especially where the incidence of effects of interest is strongly age related. The death datum is a powerful quantal point giving a definite yes or no answer. However, it also important not to allow a study run for too long, i.e., beyond the point where further time on the study would provide any useful incremental information. The last few weeks or months may produce relatively little valuable incremental information at a disproportionately high cost, and partly because diseases of extreme old age may obscure the detection of adverse effects of interest. In addition, deaths may become unacceptably high to ensure the continuing validity of the assumptions used in the analysis of data generated from the experiment. For nonfatal conditions, the ideal stop point is to sacrifice the animals when the average prevalence of death is around 50%. Greater mortality than this often invalidates the assumptions used in the statistical analysis.

8. Stratification

To detect a treatment difference with accuracy, it is important that the groups being compared are as homogeneous as possible with respect to all other (nontreatment) variables, whether or not such variables are known or suspected causes of the response. Unfortunately, there are a number of reasons why groups may not be homogeneous. Suppose that there is another known important cause of the response for which the animals vary; i.e., there are two, not one, systematic sources of variation (factors) in the experiment, even though the experiment was designed for one source (the treatment). An example of such a situation may be a mixture of hyper- and hyporesponders to the treatment. Because the randomization scheme did not account for the hyper- and hyporesponse seen in this experiment, it is possible that the treated group may have a higher proportion of hyperresponders. This bias will lead to a higher response in the treatment group regardless of whether the treatment has an effect of not. Even if the proportion of hyperresponders is the same as in the controls, it will be more difficult to detect an effect of treatment because of the increased between-animal variability.

If the second factor (sensitivity) is known before the experiment begins, it should be taken into account in both the design and the analysis of the study. In the design, it can be used as a "blocking factor" to correct for potential allocation bias. This "blocking factor" will ensure that animals with hyper- or hyposensitivity are allocated equally, or in the correct proportion, to control and treated groups. In the analysis, the factor should be treated as a stratifying variable, with separate treatment-control comparisons made at each level, and the comparisons combined for an overall test of difference. This is discussed later, where the factorial design is provided as an example of more complex experimental designs to investigate the separate effects of multiple treatments.

9. Randomization

Randomization is the arrangement of experimental units so as to simulate a chance distribution, reduce the interference by irrelevant variables, and yield unbiased statistical data. If randomization is not carried out, one can never be sure whether treatment-control differences are due to treatment or to "confounding" by other systematic sources of variation; i.e., unless randomization is used, one cannot determine whether the experimental treatments had an effect or whether an observed effect was due to allocation of the animals among experimental groups. The ability to randomize easily is a major advantage that animal experiments have over epidemiological studies.

While randomization is expected to eliminate allocation bias, simple randomization of all animals may not be the optimal technique for obtaining the most sensitive test. If there is another major source of variation, e.g., sex or

batch of animals, it will be better to carry out stratified randomization, i.e., carry out separate randomization within each level of the stratifying variable. This stratified randomization is similar to the example of hyper- and hypersensitivity given earlier.

The need for randomization applies not only to the allocation of the animals to the treatment, but also to any method, person, or practice that can materially affect the recorded response. The same random number that is used to apply animals to a treatment group can be used to determine cage position, order of weighing, order of bleeding for clinical chemistry, order of sacrifice at termination, technician attending, pathologist evaluating gross necropsy, and so on.

10. Adequacy of Control Group

While historical control data can, on occasion, be useful, a properly designed study demands that a relevant concurrent control group be included with which results for the test group can be compared. The principle that like should be compared with like, apart from treatment, demands that control animals should be randomized from the same source as treatment animals. Careful consideration should also be given to the appropriateness of the control group. Thus, in an experiment involving treatment of a compound in a solvent, it would often be inappropriate to include only an untreated control group, as any differences observed could only be attributed to the treatment–solvent combination. To determine the specific effects of the compound, a comparison group given the solvent only, by the same route of administration, would be required.

It is not always recognized that the location of the animal in the room in which it is kept may affect the animal's response. An example is the strong relationship between the incidence of retinal atrophy in albino rats and the closeness to the lighting source. Systematic differences in cage position should be avoided, preferably via randomization.

We have now become accustomed to developing exhaustively detailed protocols for an experiment or study prior to its conduct. *A priori* selection of statistical methodology, as opposed to the *post hoc* approach, is as significant a portion of the process of protocol development and experimental design as any other and can measurably enhance the value of the experiment or study. Prior selection of statistical methodologies is essential for the proper design of other portions of a protocol, such as the number of animals per group or the sampling intervals for body weight. Implied in such a selection is the notion that the toxicologic pathologist has an in-depth knowledge of the area of investigation and an understanding of the general principles of experimental design. The analysis of any set of data is dictated to a large extent by the manner in which data are obtained.

E. CENSORING

Censoring is a second concept essential to the design of experiments in toxicologic pathology. Censoring involves the exclusion of measurements from certain experimental units, or indeed of the experimental units themselves, from consideration in data analysis or inclusion in the experiment. Censoring may occur either prior to initiation of an experiment as a planned procedure, during the course of an experiment as an unplanned procedure, e.g., death of animals, or after the conclusion of an experiment, when usually data are excluded because of being identified as some form of outlier.

In practice, *a priori* censoring in toxicology studies occurs in the assignment of experimental units, usually animals, to test groups. The most familiar example is that in the practice of assignment of test animals to acute, subacute, subchronic, and chronic studies, where the results of otherwise random assignments are evaluated for body weights of the assigned members. If the mean weights are found not to be comparable by some preestablished criterion, such as a 90% probability of difference by analysis of variance, then members are reassigned, or censored, to achieve comparability in terms of starting body weights. Such a pro-

cedure of animal assignment to groups is known as a *censored randomization*.

F. IMPACTS OF SAMPLE SIZE

The first precise or calculable aspect of experimental design encountered is determining sufficient test and control group sizes to allow one to have an adequate level of confidence in the results of a study; i.e., the ability of the study design with the statistical tests used to detect a true difference, or effect, when it is present. The statistical test contributes a level of power to such detection. Remember that the power of a statistical test is the probability that a test results in rejection of a hypothesis, H_0 say, when some other hypothesis, H_1 say, is valid. This is termed the power of the test "with respect to the alternative hypothesis H_1."

If there is a set of possible alternative hypotheses, the power, regarded as a function of H_1, is termed the *power function* of the test. When the alternatives are indexed by a single parameter θ, simple graphical presentation is possible. If the parameter is a vector θ, one can visualize a *power surface*.

If the power function is denoted by $\beta(\theta)$ and H_0 specifies $\theta = \theta_0$, then the value of $\beta(II)$ is the probability of rejecting H_0 when it is in fact valid. This is the *significance level*. A test's power is greatest when the probability of a type II error, the probability of missing an effect, is the least. Specified powers can be calculated for tests in any specific or general situation. Some general rules to keep in mind are as follows.

1. The more stringent the significance level, the greater the necessary sample size. More subjects are needed for a 1% level test than for a 5% level test.
2. Two-tailed tests require larger sample sizes than one-tailed tests. Assessing two directions at the same time requires a greater investment.
3. The smaller the critical effect size, the larger the necessary sample size. Subtle effects require greater efforts.
4. Any difference can be significant if the sample size is large enough.

5. The larger the power required, the larger the necessary sample size. Greater protection from an incorrect conclusion requires greater effort. The smaller the sample size, the lower the power, i.e., the greater the chance of missing detection of a true difference.

6. The requirements and means of calculating a necessary sample size depend on the desired (or practical) comparative sizes of test and control groups.

This number (N) can be calculated, for example, for equal sized test and control groups using the following equation:

$$N = \frac{(t_1 + t_2)^2}{d^2} S, \qquad (13)$$

where t_1 is the one-tailed t value with N-1 degrees of freedom corresponding to the desired level of confidence, t_2 is the one-tailed t value with N-1 degrees of freedom corresponding to the probability that the sample size will be adequate to achieve the desired precision, and S is the sample standard deviation, derived typically from historical data.

G. CONSIDERATIONS MADE BEFORE DESIGNING THE EXPERIMENT

There are a number of aspects of experimental design, which are specific to the practice of toxicologic pathology. Before we look at a suggestion for a step-by-step development of experimental designs, the following aspects should first be considered.

1. *Differing group variability.* Frequently, data gathered from specific measurements of animal characteristics are such that there is wide variability in data. Often, such wide variability is not present in a control or low dose group, but in an intermediate dosage group, variance inflation may occur, i.e., there may be a large standard deviation associated with the measurements from this intermediate group. In the face of such a set of data, the conclusion that there is no biological effect based on a failure to show a statistically significance effect might well be erroneous.

2. *Involuntary censoring.* In designing experiments, one should keep in mind the potential effect of involuntary censoring on sample size. In other words, although a study might start with five dogs per group, this provides no margin should any die before the study is ended and blood samples are collected and analyzed. Just enough experimental units per group frequently leaves too few at the end to allow meaningful statistical analysis and allowances should be made accordingly in establishing group sizes.

3. *Meta-analysis.* It is certainly possible to pool data from several identical toxicological studies. One approach to this is meta-analysis, considered in detail later. For example, after first having performed an acute inhalation study where only three treatment group animals survived to the point at which a critical measure, such as analysis of blood samples, was performed, there would be insufficient data to perform a meaningful statistical analysis. The protocol would then have to be repeated with new control and treatment group animals from the same source. At the end, after assuring that the two sets of data are comparable, data could be combined, or pooled, from survivors of the second study with those from the first. However, the costs of this approach would be both a greater degree of effort expended than if we had performed a single study with larger groups and increased variability in the pooled samples, which would decrease the power of statistical methods used in the analysis.

4. *Unbalanced designs.* Another frequently overlooked design option in toxicology is the use of an unbalanced design, i.e., various group sizes for different levels of treatment. There is no requirement that each group in a study, be it control, low dose, intermediate dose, and high dose, have an equal number of experimental units assigned to it. Indeed, there are frequently good reasons to assign more experimental units to some group than to others. All the major statistical methodologies have provisions to adjust for such inequalities, within certain limits. The two most common uses of the unbalanced design include those that have larger groups assigned to either the highest or lower dose

groups. This change in number is done to either compensate for losses due to possible deaths during the study or to give more sensitivity in detecting effects at levels close to an effect threshold or more confidence to the assertion that no effect exists.

5. *Undesirable variables.* We are frequently confronted with the situation where an undesired variable influences our experimental results in a nonrandom fashion. Such a variable is called a *confounding variable.* Its presence, as discussed earlier, makes the clear attribution and analysis of effects at best difficult, and at worst impossible. Sometimes such confounding variables are the result of conscious design or management decisions, such as the use of different instruments, personnel, facilities, or procedures for different test groups within the same study. Occasionally, however, such a confounding variable is the result of unintentional factors or actions, in which case it is sometimes called a "lurking variable." Such variables are almost always the result of standard operating procedures being violated, e.g., water not connected to a rack of animals over a weekend, a set of racks not cleaned as frequently as others, or a contaminated batch of feed used.

6. *Experimental unit.* The experimental unit in toxicology encompasses a wide variety of possibilities. It may be cells, plates of microorganisms, individual animals, litters of animals, etc. The importance of clearly defining the experimental unit is that the number of such units per group is the "N", which is used in statistical calculations or analyses, and critically affects such calculations. The experimental unit is the unit that receives treatments and yields a response that is measured and becomes a datum.

7. *Concurrent control.* A true concurrent control is one that is identical in every manner with the treatment groups except for the treatment being evaluated. This means that all manipulations, including gavaging with equivalent volumes of vehicle or exposing to equivalent rates of air exchanges in an inhalation chamber, should be duplicated in control groups just as they occur in treatment groups.

The goal of the seven principles of experimental design is *statistical efficiency* and the *economizing of resources.* The single most important initial step in achieving such an outcome is to define clearly the objective of the study, i.e., get a clear statement of what questions are being asked.

For the reader who would like to further explore experimental design, a number of more detailed texts are available that include more extensive treatments of the statistical aspects of experimental design.

V. Designs Commonly Used in Toxicologic Studies

There are five basic experimental design types used in toxicology: *completely randomized, completely randomized block, Latin square, factorial design*, and *nested design.* Other designs that are used are really combinations of these basic designs and are employed very rarely in toxicologic pathology. Before examining these four basic types, however, we must first examine the basic concept of blocking.

Blocking is the arrangement or sorting of the members of a population, such as all of an available group of test animals, into groups based on certain characteristics, which may, but are not sure to, alter an experimental outcome. Characteristics, which are frequently blocked, may cause a treatment to give a differential effect. These include genetic background, age, sex, overall activity levels, and so on. The process of blocking attempts to distribute members of each blocked group evenly to each experimental group.

A. COMPLETELY RANDOMIZED DESIGN

A completely randomized design uses the arrangement of experimental units so as to simulate a chance distribution. There are no attempts made to evaluate the effects of any other source of variability except the treatment. This is the most common type of design particularly found in acute and subacute toxicologic pathological studies. Here animals are assigned randomly to any treatment group.

B. COMPLETELY RANDOMIZED BLOCK DESIGN

We should now recall that randomization is aimed at spreading out the effect of undetectable or unsuspected characteristics in a population of animals, or some portion of this population. The merging of the two concepts or randomization and blocking leads to the first experimental design that addresses sources of systematic variation other than the intended treatment; the *completely randomized block design*. This type of design requires that each treatment group have at least one member of each recognized group, e.g., age, the exact members of each block being assigned in an unbiased random fashion. In toxicologic pathology studies where the application of the treatment may take some time, the experiment may be blocked so that the first group of animals is assigned randomly in equal numbers to each and every treatment group. For example, the duration of surgery required to implant an experimental medical device may be such that blocking is necessary to account for the systematic variation caused by the time of implantation.

C. LATIN SQUARE DESIGN

The *Latin square design* is the second experimental design that addresses sources of systematic variation other than the intended treatment. It assumes that one can characterize treatments, whether intended or otherwise, as belonging clearly to separate sets. These categories are arranged into two sets of rows, e.g., source litter of test animal, with the first litter as row 1, the next as row 2, etc. The secondary set of categories is arranged as columns, e.g., ages of test animals, with 6 to 8 weeks as column 1, 8, to 10 weeks as column 2, and so on. Experimental units are then assigned so that each major treatment, such as control, low dose, and intermediate dose, appears once and only once in each row and each column. If one denotes test groups as A (control), B (low), C (intermediate), and D (high), such as assignment would appear as in Table VIII, where it can be seen that randomized

TABLE VIII
Diagrammatic Representation of Treatment Allocation in a Latin Square Design

Source litter	Age (weeks)			
	6–8	8–10	10–12	12–14
1	A	B	C	D
2	B	C	D	A
3	C	D	A	B
4	D	A	B	C

experimental units are assigned to a treatment group and then assigned randomly to a place in the Latin square.

In the study on the effect of a xenobiotic on development given in Table VIII, treatment, age grouping, and litter sources of variation have been addressed in the design.

D. FACTORIAL DESIGN

The third type of experimental design that addresses sources of systematic variation other than the intended treatment is *factorial design*. In a factorial design there are two or more clearly understood factors, such as exposure level to test chemical, animal age, or temperature. The classical approach to this situation, and to that described under the Latin square design, is to hold all but one of the treatments constant and, at any one time, to vary just that one factor. If it is suspected that two factors are independent and have an effect on the outcome, a factorial design may be used to either obtain greater information regarding the effect of each factor and/or determining whether there is an interaction of the factors altering the outcome. In the factorial design, all levels of a given factor are combined with all levels of every other factor in the experiment. When a change in one factor produces a different change in the response variable at one level of a factor than at other levels of this factor, there is an interaction between these two factors, which can then be analyzed as an interaction effect. The terminology used to describe a factorial design is (number of levels of factor 1) × (number of levels of factor 2). For example, one can make design and evaluate the dose–response on two different strains off mouse. If four dose levels are used in three strains of mouse, then a 4 × 3 factorial design could be used to show treatment effect, strain effect, and, if an effect is seen, whether there is an interaction between dose and strain.

E. NESTED DESIGN

The last of the major varieties of experimental design are the *nested designs*, where the levels of one factor are nested within, or are subsamples of, another factor, i.e., a subfactor. That is, each subfactor is evaluated only within the limits of its single larger factor at each level except the first, or highest. The subfactors are versions of subfactors in other groups except that they have a higher level factor that differs. Figure 4 shows the form of this design.

In Fig. 4, the generic terms could be replaced with an example of individual animal observations coming from animals of different batches and from different suppliers. In this case the supplier would represent the factor and the batch of animals the subfactor. Animals are selected from each batch for examination. In a nested design, there is never any uncertainty as to whether factors are crossed between batches, i.e., there can be no interaction between factors.

Nested designs can be balanced as in Fig. 4 or unbalanced. In an unbalanced nested design the number of subfactors and observations may not be the same for each factor. Also, there may be a number of stages, depending on the number of subsamples selected. Figure 4 is a two-stage nested design, whereas a one-stage nested design would not have a subfactor in its organization.

VI. Managing Data

Data must be generated and recorded in an unbiased manner. It is recognized that many options exist for analysis, which will be discussed later. However, biased data generation, with the knowledge of the operator, is fraudulent. Good laboratory practices (GLPs) have been implemented to ensure that data analyzed represent data generated from the experiment. GLPs have three main components: requirements for personnel, requirements for facilities, and requirements to create standard operating procedures (SOPs) and records of events undertaken in the study. Even with the implementation of GLPs and SOPs, systematic error, or bias, can enter the experiment.

A. BIAS

1. Bias of Design

Design bias is seen most commonly in inadequately controlled studies where a major source of variability confounds the experiment. However, *true bias* such as circadian rhythm may confound studies without being detected. When fundamental *changes in methods* occur during the experiment, another source of variation is introduced. Obviously, the systematic or *nonrandom allocation* of cases to treatment group may make comparison impossible, e.g., comparing medical vs surgical treatments of disease to treatment with a drug. *Sample bias* can occur in associative research through confounding factors (e.g., nutrition) and clinical "walk in" adverse drug reaction studies. In this case the worker has no way of randomizing the spontaneity of the disease; it either occurs or does not. *Nonsimultaneous comparisons* can

Factor	1				2				3			
Sub-factor	1	2	3	4	1	2	3	4	1	2	3	4
Observation	Y111	Y121	Y131	Y141	Y211	Y221	Y231	Y241	Y311	Y321	Y331	Y341
	Y112	Y122	Y132	Y142	Y212	Y222	Y232	Y242	Y312	Y322	Y332	Y342
	Y113	Y123	Y133	Y143	Y213	Y223	Y233	Y243	Y313	Y323	Y333	Y343

Figure 4. An illustration of a two-stage nested design.

be an overlooked source of bias in observational studies, e.g., when a comparison of experimental results with "results" prior to treatment is made.

2. Bias of Observation

Knowledge of the treatment group can influence the observer's actions and records through conscious or unconscious bias. The bias does not always result in a shift in data that is more likely to reject the null hypothesis. In fact, some operators may be so aware of bias that overcompensation can cause a reverse bias. *Blinding* is the term used to describe a method or coding where the researcher has no knowledge of the treatment group that an animal, or sample, comes from. Data can be biased if researcher judgment is used and no form of blinding has been taken. A paradox exists in toxicologic pathology: on the one hand, knowledge of the treatment group is necessary to permit the use professional judgment to distinguish unimportant morphological changes from treatment-related lesions, whereas on the other hand, knowledge of the treatment groups results in the potential for bias when subjective scales are used. Therefore, although it is necessary for the toxicologic pathologist to first determine the lesions showing a dose–response with knowledge of the treatment groups, blind rereading of the study, or parts of the study, may be necessary to remove observation bias. Data that are easily biased in this way include subjective scales or convention categories selected from data gathering, e.g., improved, unchanged, or worse.

Observer bias may also occur when multiple observers have different handling and judgment methods, which can add systematic error unless this error is distributed equally among treatment groups. *Work-up bias* occurs when heightened observation of a specific effect occurs once a particular "discovery" of such an effect has been noted ("before" and "after" effect). An example in toxicologic pathology is the recognition of a lesion part way through reading a study. Increased vigilance will result in a high number of this type of lesion recorded from this point on in the reading. Blind rereading of the study or lesions in question can remove this type of bias.

3. Bias of Estimation

As has been described earlier, statistical inference is of two types: estimation and hypothesis testing. Both methods of inference involve assumptions and systematic procedures, which may introduce bias. Bayesian methods may be involved that incorporate prior information or convictions into the analysis, which may give a "wished" effect rather than a real effect if not scrutinized carefully. *Bias of estimator* occurs when a systematic procedure is used to make the "best estimate" of a true value (which is not known). This usually occurs when the mean of the sample is assumed to approximate the mean of the population. We make this assumption with all our statistical methods and have no way of testing this effect unless we measure the whole population. Variance is the sum of squares of deviations of observed values from the sample mean divided by the number of observations. It does not represent the true variance of the population, but a representative sample. In addition, because the sample estimate of the mean is subject to sampling error, instead of n, n-1 is used for degrees of freedom in calculations as an attempt to remove the knowledge bias of the last event to be tested probabilistically. In other words, there is a probability associated with all units taken from a sample except the last: the last sample is known.

Bias in the *assumptions* underlying the statistical analysis, such as different estimates obtained from different models, may occur. One has to assume either that these biases do not exist in the analysis or that they have little effect to bias the end point. *Description bias* can occur when the wrong descriptor is used to describe a population or sample, e.g., mean vs median and standard deviation vs range for normal vs skewed data. *Prior conviction* bias may exist as to how to handle "outliers," or data that may "bias" the results because the value is so large or small in comparison to the other data points.

4. Bias in Hypothesis Testing

Violation of assumptions of a test introduces bias into probabilistic testing. *Postfactor hypothesis* bias occurs when in testing a hypothesis: when one is committed to accept/reject a conjecture on experimental evidence using an appropriately applied statistical procedure, failure to do so is an obvious bias, if not fraud. Goodness-of-fit tests by their nature are weak and can only show a good fit and cannot demonstrate a *lack of fit*.

5. Other Forms of Bias

Forms of bias can exist in interpretation, presentation, and reporting of results. The *a factori argument*: "It is certainly true that the treatment group was older than the control group, but this would clearly work against the efficacy of treatment, and, had animals been comparable, the treatment would have been more effective...." The statement may have a plausible ring to some readers, but complex biological problems are involved. For example, it is assumed that age is a monotonic trend, and it is not assumed that drugs may act in a biphasic or polyphasic manner. It behooves the toxicologic pathologist to recognize the impacts of nonevidence-based comments made in their reports. This topic is discussed in detail in Chapter 14. Acceptance of these conclusions cannot be compelled by evidence. There are many other types of biases that are more problematic in associative than inferential research. These are beyond the scope of this chapter.

B. BIAS AND THE TOXICOLOGIC PATHOLOGIST

Two distinct sources of systematic bias may occur in data recording by the toxicologic pathologist. Observer bias can occur when the observer is aware of treatment. This knowledge may consciously influence the observer through true bias of observation, or unconsciously as reading bias, referred to earlier as work-up bias. In reading and work-up bias, the observer increases his or her attention to a lesion, once noted in the sections. This effect on the observer has also been call "diagnostic drift." In some situations it may be necessary to reread all the slides blind and in random order to be sure that diagnostic drift is avoided. Elimination bias occurs when data are eliminated for various reasons. Usually, such protocol violations should be recorded; however, it should be noted that valid analysis could not be conducted unless one can distinguish animals that were examined and did not have the relevant response and animals that were not examined. Therefore, it is important clearly to identify which data are missing and for what reason. The following list is given as a guide to make sure that such situations do not occur.

1. Forms should be used when some form of repetitive data must be collected. They may be either paper or electronic.

2. If only a few (two or three) pieces of data are to be collected, they should be entered into a notebook and not onto a form. This assumes that the few pieces are not a daily event, with the aggregate total of weeks/months/years ending up as lots of data to be pooled for analysis.

3. Forms should be self-contained, but should not try to repeat the content of the SOPs or method descriptions.

4. Column headings on forms should always specify the units of measurement and other details of entries to be made. The form should be arranged so that sequential entries proceed down a page, not across. Each column should be clearly labeled with a heading that identifies what is to be entered in the column. Any fixed part of entries (such at °C) should be in the column header.

5. Columns should be arranged from left to right so that there is a logical sequential order to the contents of an entry as it is made. An example would be data/time/animal number/body weight/name of the recorder. The last item for each entry should be the name or unique initials of the individual who made the data entry.

6. Standard conditions that apply to all the data elements to be recorded on a form or the columns of the form should be listed as footnotes at the bottom of the form.

7. Entries of data on the form should not use more digits than are appropriate for the precision of data being recorded.

8. Each form should be clearly titled to indicate its purpose and use. If multiple types of forms are being used, each should have a unique title or number.

9. Before designing the form, carefully consider the purpose for which it is intended. What data will be collected, how often, with what instrument, and by whom? Each of these considerations should be reflected in some manner on the form.

10. Those items that are common/standard for all entries on the form should be stated as such once. These could include such things as instrument used, scale of measurement (°C, F, or K), or the location where the recording is made.

VII. Statistical Methods

One approach for the selection of appropriate techniques to employ in a particular situation is to use a decision tree method. Figure 5 is a decision tree that leads to the choice of one of three other trees to assist in technique selection, with each of the subsequent trees addressing one of the three functions of statistics that was defined earlier in this chapter. Figure 6 is a decision tree for the selection of hypothesis-testing procedures, Figure 7 represents a decision tree for modeling procedures, and Figure 8 shows a decision tree for the reduction of dimensionality procedures. For the vast majority of situations, these decision trees will guide the user's choice of the appropriate technique. The tests and terms in these trees will be explained subsequently.

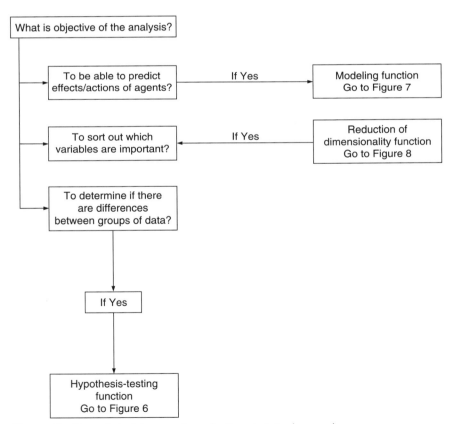

Figure 5. Overall decision tree for selecting statistical procedures.

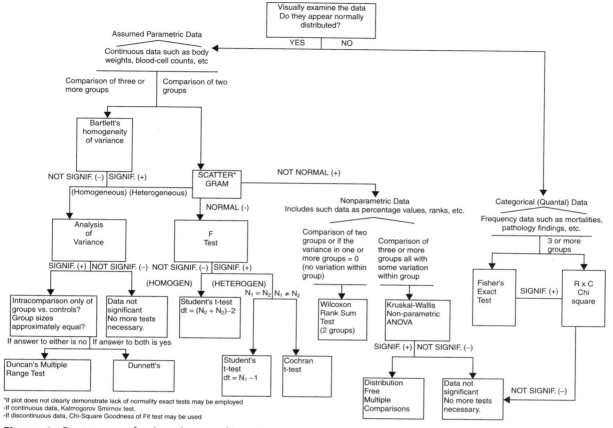

Figure 6. Decision tree for the selection of hypothesis-testing procedures.

A. STATISTICAL ANALYSIS: GENERAL CONSIDERATIONS

1. Variables to be Analyzed

Although some toxicologic pathologists still regard their discipline as providing qualitative rather than quantitative data, it is abundantly clear that pathology has to be quantitative to at least some degree. When applied to routine screening of animal toxicity and carcinogenicity studies, quantitative data generation is necessary so that statistical inferences and statements can be made about possible treatment effects. Inevitably, there will be some descriptive text that will not be appropriate for statistical analysis. However, the main objective of the toxicologic pathologist should be to provide information on the presence or absence, with severity grade or size where appropriate, of a list of conditions. These lesions should be con-

sistently recorded from animal to animal and classified by well-defined criteria, which can be validly used in a statistical assessment (see Chapter 7).

The toxicologic pathologist can generate a plethora of data. Should one then analyze all the end points recorded? Some arguments have been put forward against analyzing all the end points in studies; in the opinion of the authors, none of these arguments justifies the exclusion of end points. Nevertheless, these arguments are presented to make the reader familiar with them, and corresponding counter arguments.

One argument is that some end points are "not of interest." Perhaps the study is essentially a carcinogenicity study so that non neoplastic end points are not considered as important. They are considered to be "background pathology" and are almost *per se* unrelated to treatment. However, if the pathologist has been

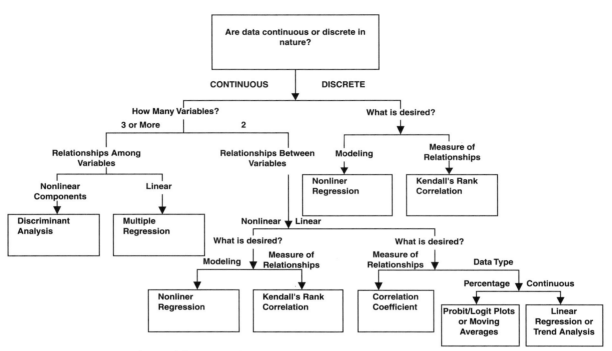

Figure 7. Decision tree for modeling procedures.

diligent in recording data correctly and completely, then, in general, these data should be analyzed. The incremental costs of the additional statistical analysis are much less than those of doing the study and the pathology. While one might justify failure to analyze non neoplastic data where tumor analysis has already shown that the compound is clearly carcinogenic and

no longer of market potential, the general rule should be to analyze everything that has been specifically investigated.

Another argument put forward against doing multiple analyses on data generated by the toxicologic pathologist is that it may yield many "chance" significant *p* values that have to be considered and evaluated for biological

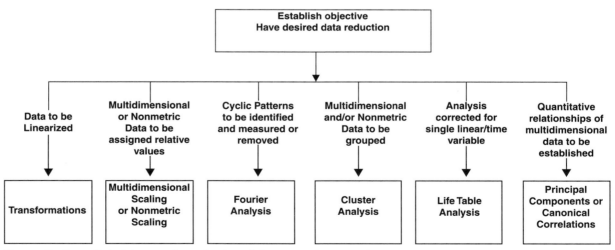

Figure 8. Overall decision tree for reduction of dimensionality procedures.

significance in the context of the entire set of available data. The global context of dose–response, as summarized in Table IX, must be kept in mind when deciding whether to exclude any data from analysis. A detailed look at the data can only aid interpretation, provided that one is not hide-bound by the false argument that statistical significance necessarily equates with biological importance and definitely indicates a true effect of treatment.

Finally, some end points occur only very rarely. One must then be clear what can be considered for classification as a "very rarely" occurring event. For a typical study with a control and three dose groups of equal size, one would compute a significant trend if all three cases of a "very rarely" observed morphological alteration occured in the top dose level or in the control group (two-tailed $p \approx 0.03$). In this case, a total of three cases will normally be enough for statistical analysis. End points occurring once or twice only are not worth analyzing formally, although, if only seen in the top dose group, they may be worth noting in the report. This is especially true if they are lesions that are rarely reported.

2. Combination of Pathological Conditions

There are four main situations where combining pathological morphological alterations in a statistical analysis can be considered. The first is when essentially the same lesion has been recorded under two or more different names, or even under the same name in different places. Here failure to combine these conditions in the

analysis may severely limit the chances of detecting a true treatment effect. It should be noted, however, that grouping together conditions that are actually different might also result in the masking of a true treatment effect, particularly if the treatment has a very specific effect.

The second situation is when separately recorded lesions form successive steps on the pathway of the same process. The most important example of this phenomenon is for the incidence of related types of malignant tumor, benign tumor, and focal hyperplasia. It will normally be appropriate to carry out analyses of (1) incidence of malignant tumor, (2) incidence of benign or malignant tumor, and, where appropriate, (3) incidence of focal hyperplasia, benign or malignant tumor. It will not normally be appropriate to carry out analyses of benign tumor incidence only or of the incidence of focal hyperplasia only.

The third situation for combining is when the same pathological condition appears in different organs as a result of the same underlying process. Examples of this are the multicentric tumors, such as myeloid leukemia, reticulum cell sarcoma, and lymphosarcoma, or certain nonneoplastic conditions, such as arteritis/periarteritis and amyloid degeneration. Here analysis will normally be carried out only of incidence at any site.

The final situation where an analysis of combined pathology findings is appropriate is for analysis of overall incidence of malignant tumor at any site, of benign or malignant tumor at any site, or of multiple tumor incidences. While analyses of tumor incidence at specific sites are normally more meaningful, as treatments often affect only a few specific sites, these additional analyses are usually required to guard against the possibility that treatment had some weak but general tumor-enhancing effect that would not be otherwise evident. In some situations, one might also envisage analyses of other combinations of specific tumors, such as tumors at related sites, e.g., endocrine organs if the compound demonstrates a hormonal effect, or of similar histopathologic type.

TABLE IX
The Three Dimensions of Dose–Response

Dose	Response
↓ Increasing dose	Incidence of responders in an exposed population increases
↓	Severity of response in affected individuals increases
	Time to occurrence of response or of progressive stage of response decreases

3. Taking Severity into Account

The argument that all data recorded by the toxicologic pathologist should be analyzed can be extended to grading of lesions. If the pathologist chooses to grade a condition for severity, the grade should be taken into account in the statistical analysis. There are two ways to analyze data when the grade is to be taken into account. In one, data are analyzed when the animal has a condition and the condition is at least grade 2, at least grade 3, etc. In the other approach, nonparametric methods utilizing ranked data are used. The latter approach is more powerful, as it uses all the information in one analysis. Unfortunately, those without some statistical training may not understand the output as easily.

Note that *consistent grading* is necessary for meaningful analyses based on grade. If a condition has been scored only as present/absent for some animals, but has been graded for others, it is not possible to use graded analyses unless the pathologist is willing to go back and grade the specific animals showing the condition.

4. Using Simple Methods Which Avoid Complex Assumptions

Different statistical analytical methods can vary considerably in their complexity and in the number of assumptions they make. Statistical analysis should be used for the clarification of effects rather than being performed only to obtain a "*p* value." Wherever possible, use statistical methods that are simple, robust, and make few assumptions. The use of statistical models has its place, however, more for effect estimation than for hypothesis testing and in studies of complex design rather than in those of simple design. There are three reasons for this. First, the toxicologic pathologist usually understands simpler methods, and hence s/he can justify the outputs. Second, seldom are there adequate data in practice to validate fully the assumptions of any formal statistical model. Third, even if particular models are shown to be appropriate for use, the loss of power in using

appropriate simpler methods is often very small.

Methods for the routine statistical analysis of tumor incidence do not use formal parametric statistical models. For example, when evaluating the relationship of treatment to incidence of a well-defined pathological finding, and adjusting for other factors, in particular age at death, which might bias the comparison, methods involving "stratification" are recommended. These should be used in preference to a multiple regression approach, or time-to-tumor models.

Analyses of variance (ANOVA) methods can be useful for estimating treatment effects when continuously distributed data are obtained. However, the appropriateness of ANOVA as a tool depends on the validity of the fundamental assumptions of normally distributed variables and equal variability in each group. If these assumptions are violated, or cannot be reasonably demonstrated or assumed, nonparametric methods are more appropriate for hypothesis testing. These may be based on the rank of observations, rather than their actual value, and do not depend on the assumptions common to the parametric methods.

5. Using all Data

In addition to evaluating treatment and effect relationships, there are situations where determination of the effect of other sources of systematic differences among individuals are warranted. Gender differences, differing times of sacrifice, and differing secondary treatments may be considered. A source of systematic difference can be considered a *factor*. It is often important to evaluate the effect of these factors so that a more powerful analysis of the treatment effects can be made. These factors can be evaluated for relationships within each level of the factor (e.g., factor–sex; level–male, female) and combined to see whether data can be pooled. Some scientists consider that conclusions for males and females should always be drawn separately, but there are strong statistical arguments for a joint analysis.

6. Combining, Pooling, and Stratification

Table X is a hypothetical study of a toxic agent that induces tumors without shortening the lives of tumor-bearing animals. Hypothetical data for the number of animals with tumor number examined are shown in Table X.

Table X shows that if the time of death is ignored, and *pooled* data are evaluated, the incidence of tumors is the same in each group. This leads to the *false* conclusion that treatment had no effect. However, by evaluating the *time to death* on treatment an increased incidence in the exposed group can be seen. An appropriate statistical method would *combine* a measure of difference between the groups based on the early deaths and a measure of difference based on the late deaths, and conclude *correctly* that incidence, after adjustment for time of death, is greater in the exposed groups.

In this example, time of death is the stratifying variable with two strata: early deaths and late deaths. The essence of the methodology is to make comparisons only within strata so that one is always comparing like with like except in respect of treatment. Then combine the differences over strata. Stratification can be used to adjust for any variable, or combinations of variables.

Some studies are of factorial design, in which combinations of treatments are evaluated. The simplest such design is one in which four equal-sized groups of animals receive no treatment, treatment A only, treatment B only, and treatments A and B. The basic assumption for analysis of this type of experiment is that the two treatment effects are *independent*. In this factorial experiment, one can use stratification to enable more powerful tests to be conducted of the possible individual treatment effects. Thus, to test for effects of treatment A, for example, one conducts comparisons in two strata, the first consisting of groups 1 and 2 (not given treatment B) and the second consisting of groups 3 and 4 (given treatment B). Combination of results from the two strata is based on twice as many animals and is therefore markedly more likely to detect possible effects of treatment A than is a simple comparison of groups 1 and 2. There is also the possibility of identifying *interactions*, such as synergism and antagonism, between the two treatments.

In some routine long-term screening studies, the study design involves five groups of usually 50 animals of each sex, three groups of which are treated with increasing doses of a compound, and two of which are untreated controls. Assuming that there is no systematic difference between the control groups, e.g., the second control group in a different room or from a different batch of animals, the main analyses will pool the control groups, resulting in a single groups of 100 animals. Pooling the control groups should only occur following a preliminary analysis to show no difference in the incidence of effects in these control groups. If there is a difference between control groups, the "cause" of the difference needs to be evaluated and determined how this "cause" may have affected, or not, the experimental groups. Once this has been determined, the most appropriate method of analysis for the situation is used.

7. Trend Analysis, Low-Dose Extrapolation and NOEL Estimation

While comparisons of individual treated groups with the control group are important, a more powerful test of a possible effect of treatment is a test for a dose-related trend. *Trend tests* use all data in a single analysis to evaluate the effects of treatment that result in a positive or negative dose–response relationship. In interpreting the results of trend tests, it should be noted that a significant trend does not necessarily imply a significant effect at lower doses. Conversely, a lack of a significant increase at lower doses does not necessarily indicate

TABLE X
Sample Data from a Hypothetical Bioassay

	Control	Exposed	Combined
Early deaths	1/20 (5%)	18/90 (20%)	19/110 (17%)
Late deaths	24/80 (30%)	7/10 (70%)	31/90 (34%)
Total	25/100 (25%)	25/100 (25%)	50/200 (25%)

evidence of a threshold, i.e., a dose below which no increase occurs.

Testing for trend is a more sensitive method than simple pair-wise comparisons of treated and control groups for showing a possible treatment effect. Attempting to estimate the magnitude of effects at low doses, typically below the lowest positive dose tested in the study, is a much more complex procedure and is heavily dependent on the assumed functional form of the dose–response relationship.

Low dose extrapolation is typically conducted for tumors believed to be caused by a genotoxic effect. Given severe limits in understanding the biology of low dose genotoxicity, and the inability to generate data in the very low response range of the dose–response curve, "no threshold" is ordinarily assumed. This assumption is based on a current understanding of initiation and a lack of evidence for a less conservative (i.e., protective) approach. However, some, but by no means all, scientists believe these tumors have no threshold. For other types of tumors, and for many nonneoplastic end points, a threshold cannot be estimated directly from data at a limited number of dose levels. A no observed effect level (NOEL) can be estimated by finding the highest dose level at which there is no significant increase in treatment-related effects. It should be noted that the NOEL addresses any treatment-related effect, whereas the no observable adverse effect level (NOAEL) defines the effect as detrimental. The other statistic of great importance to understanding where on the dose curve the response occurs is the lowest effect level (LOEL), or lowest adverse effect level (LOAEL). These levels are the lowest dose at which an effect, or adverse effect, occurred. The true threshold for the effect of *interest under the conditions of the study* is bracketed by the NOEL and LOEL (i.e., the threshold t is given by NOEL $< t \leq$ LOEL).

8. Need for Age Adjustment

Where there are marked differences in survival among treated groups there is a need for an age adjustment, i.e., an adjustment for age at death or onset. This is illustrated in Table X where,

because of the greater number of deaths occurring early in the treated group, the true effect of treatment disappears if no adjustment is made. Thus, a major purpose of age adjustment is to avoid temporal bias.

It is not always recognized that even where there are no survival differences, age adjustment can increase the power to detect group differences. This is illustrated by the example in Table XI.

In Table XI, treatment results in an earlier onset of a condition causing mortality, which eventually occurs in all animals. Failure to age adjust will result in a comparison of 29/50 with 21/50, which is not statistically significant. Age adjustment will essentially ignore early and late deaths, which contribute no comparative statistical information, and be based on the comparison of 9/10 with 1/10, which is statistically significant. By avoiding diluting data capable of detecting treatment effects with data that are of little or no value for this purpose, age adjustment sharpens the contrast rather than avoiding bias.

9. Need to Take Context of Observation into Account

Age adjustment cannot be used unless the context of the end point is clear. There are three relevant contexts, with the first two relating to the situation where the condition is only observed at death, e.g., an internal tumor, and the third where it can be observed during life, e.g., a skin tumor. In the first context the condition is assumed to have caused the death of the animal, i.e., to be *fatal*. Here the incidence rate for a time interval and a group is calculated as the number of animals dying because of the lesion during the interval divided by the

TABLE XI
The Effect of Age Adjustment on Mortality Data

	Control	Exposed
Early deaths	0/20	0/20
Middle deaths	1/10	9/10
Late deaths	20/20	20/20
Total	21/50	29/50

number of animals alive at the start of the interval. In the second context, the animal is assumed to have died of another cause; i.e., the internal tumor is *incidental*. In the case of incidental lesions the rate is calculated as the number of animals with the lesion dying during the interval divided by the total number of deaths during the interval. In the third context, where the lesion is *visible*, the rate is calculated as the number of animals with the condition during the interval divided by the number of animals without the condition at the start of the interval.

The method of Peto and colleague takes the context of observation into account. Sometimes, the nature of the lesion does not always allow the toxicologic pathologist to decide whether a condition is fatal or incidental. However, in experiments where marked survival differences are seen, the toxicologic pathologist should attempt to decide upon the context of the lesion. Failure to do so may result in the inability to conclude reliably whether a treatment is beneficial or harmful.

For those reading carcinogenicity studies, the definition of what constitutes a fatal tumor sometime conflicts with the needs of the statistician regarding hard measurable end points. Here we have a paradox: the statistician requires mutually inclusive and mutually exclusive groups of fatal vs nonfatal tumors for the analysis, whereas the pathologist rarely is able to judge without question as to whether the lesion was fatal. To demonstrate the problem, and pose a solution, we shall use examples to show the need for data for the statistician and the weakness of data generated by the toxicological pathologist.

The effect of lack of definition of context, and the need to have context for statistical purposes, is well illustrated by the evaluation of *N*-nitrosodimethylamine (NDMA) for carcinogenicity. Here it was assumed that all pituitary tumors were fatal. This resulted in the false conclusion that NDMA was carcinogenic. In contrast, if it were assumed that these lesions were incidental, the false conclusion that NDMA was protective would result. By using

the toxicologic pathologist's contextual opinion as to which tumors were, and which were not, likely to be fatal, the resulting analysis concluded correctly that NDMA had no carcinogenic effect in the pituitary. It is imperative that the toxicologic pathologist attempts to judge the context the lesions in question, as s/he is the most competent to make such a judgment. Failure to put the lesions in context may result in either an erroneous conclusion or no conclusion at all.

Many toxicologic pathologists have entered the Peto variable, a quantal categorization as to whether the tumor in question was incidental or fatal, whenever s/he felt that a particular tumor was why the animal came to necropsy that day. For example, an animal that has been slowly deteriorating in a bioassay was found to have a 10-cm pituitary mass at necropsy. The histological evaluation of the mass revealed that is was a *pars distalis* adenoma. The clinical history of no neurological signs with this space-occupying lesion indicated that the tumor was slow growing. It may seem that the Peto variable in this case should be marked as "fatal"; however, such an action would be a mistake, as described in the following paragraph.

The Peto variable is collected for the purpose of determining the *duration* of the tumor's presence. A fatal classification represents a tumor that has been interpreted as *"rapidly fatal."* Tumors are classified by the pathologist as incidental, fatal, or mortality independent (observable). Incidental tumors are those tumors deemed not directly or indirectly responsible for the animal's death, but observed at necropsy. Fatal tumors are tumors deemed to have killed the animal either directly or indirectly. Mortality-independent tumors are tumors that are detected at times other than at necropsy. The distinction between fatal and incidental tumors is important because it is essential to distinguish between a chemical that reduces survival by shortening the time to tumor onset, or the time to death following tumor onset (a real carcinogenic effect), and one that reduces survival, but for which tumors are observed earlier simply because they are dying of competing causes (noncarcinogenic effect). In the example given earlier, collection of a fatal rather than an incidental classification misrepresents the "real" findings for the Peto variable, as the tumor was present for a long time. In fact, the problem resides with the interpretation of what the Peto variable represents. Obviously, dichotomous data must result from a simple yes/no question, but often two questions are asked: was the tumor the cause for necropsy of the animal and/or was the tumor rapidly fatal?

The Peto variable represents the second question and not the first. For this reason it has been suggested that only tumors recognized as rapidly fatal receive the fatal Peto variable designation. To make sure that only rapidly fatal tumors are included as fatal, malignant lymphomas and leukemias would be marked as fatal, whereas all other tumors should be marked as incidental. It is our opinion that the conservative use of the fatal Peto variable is preferable to misclassification of an incidental datum to fatal to make sure that overly conservative assessments are not made in carcinogenesis studies that are quite conservative in their output without the introduction of this statistic. Regardless of violating the assumptions of the test, it is preferable to record tumor-related deaths for Peto's trend test evaluation than not to have any data regarding premature mortality in a bioassay.

Although it is normally good practice for the toxicologic pathologist to ascribe "factors contributing to unscheduled death" for each animal, it is not strictly necessary to determine the context of observation for all conditions at the outset. An alternative strategy is to analyze data under differing assumptions. Multiple analyses of data may be done using a different context for unscheduled deaths. Typically, analyses of decedents would assume that all cases are incidental and use the context of no cases fatal, all cases fatal, or all cases of the same defined severity occurring in decedents fatal.

If the conclusion for all scenarios is the same, or if the toxicologic pathologist states that one scenario is the most likely, it may not be necessary to know the context of observation for the condition in question for each individual animal. Using this alternative strategy might result in analysis cost reductions and time savings by allowing evaluations to focus on a limited number of lesions where the conclusion seems to hang on correct knowledge of the context of observation. Finally, it should be noted that although many nonneoplastic conditions observed at death are never causes of death, it is in principle as necessary to know the context of observation for nonneoplastic conditions as it is for tumors.

10. Experimental and Observational Units

Animals in a study are often both the "experimental unit" and the "observational unit," but this is not always so. For determining treatment effects by the methods of the next section, it is important that each experimental unit provides only one item of data for analysis, as the methods all assume that individual data items are statistically independent.

In many feeding studies, where the cage is assigned to a treatment, it is the cage rather than the animal that is the experimental unit. In contrast, histopathologic observations for a tissue may be based on multiple sections per animal. In this case the section is the observational unit, whereas the animal is the experimental unit. Similarly, in reproduction and teratology studies the dam is the experimental unit, whereas fetuses are the observational units. Multiple observations per experimental unit should be combined in some suitable way into an overall average for that unit before analysis. Often these multiple observations are not distributed normally, hence median and semiquartile ranges are used commonly for describing multiple observation data for an experimental unit (Table XII).

For these data, a series of calculations would be necessary before statistical analysis could be undertaken. As these observations are unlikely to be distributed normally, median and semiquartile ranges would be used. To obtain a datum for each bitch, first the median score per pup (in parentheses under pup number)

TABLE XII
An Example Addressing the Experimental Unit, Offspring, and Hepatic Pathology

Animal number	Treatment	Pup number	Hepatic pathology score
E-9991	B	1	0
(0)		(0)	0
		2	0
		(0)	0
		3	0
		(0)	0
		4	0
		(0)	
E-9992	A	1	3
(2.5)		(2.5)	2
E-9993	D	–	–
E-9994	A	1	3
1.5		(3)	3
		2	1
		(1.5)	2
		2	1
		(1.5)	2
E-9995	C	1	1
(0.5)		(1)	1
		2	0
		(0)	0
		3	1
		(0.5)	0
E-9996	D	–	–
E-9997	B	1	0
(0)		(0)	0
		2	0
		(0)	0
		3	0
		(0)	0
		4	0
		(0)	0
		5	0
		(0)	0
E-9998	C	1	1
(1)		(0.5)	0
		2	0
		(1)	2
		3	1
		(1)	1
		4	2
		(1.5)	1

is derived. Then the median score per pup per dam (in parentheses under animal number) would be used for describing the multiple observations for the experimental unit, the bitch.

11. Missing Data

Missing data is a common problem in toxicologic pathology. Missing tissues and inadequate blood samples for analysis are not uncommon, even under GLP conditions. How missing data are handled in statistical evaluation is critical to obtaining a valid interpretation of results.

Animals with missing data can simply be removed from the analysis. There are, however, some situations where removal of the experimental unit can be inappropriate. Particularly of note is when a lesion assumed to have caused the death of the animal is analyzed. For example, an animal dies at week 83 of a bioassay for which the section was unavailable for microscopic examination. This animal cannot contribute to the group comparison at week 83. However, as it was alive in previous weeks it should contribute to the denominator of the calculations in all previous weeks.

Missing observations also occur when histopathologic evaluation is only done when an abnormality is seen at postmortem. In such an experiment, hypothetical data may appear as in Table XIII.

The following statistics could be derived for the data. Ignoring animals with no microscopic sections, one would compare 2/2 = 100% with 14/15 = 93% and conclude that treatment nonsignificantly decreased incidence. This is likely to be a false conclusion, and it would be better

TABLE XIII
Data Generated from a Hypothetical Experiment Where Histopathologic Evaluation Is Only Done in Animals Where Gross Lesions Were Seen

	Control group	Treated group
Number in group	50	50
Number with gross lesions	2	15
Histopathologic evaluation	2	15
Classified neoplasm	2	14

here to compare the percentages of animals that had a postmortem abnormality that turned out to be a tumor, i.e., 2/50 = 4% with 14/50 = 28%. Unless some aspect of treatment made tumors much easier to detect at postmortem, one could then conclude that treatment did have an effect on tumor incidence.

Particular care has to be taken in studies where the procedures for histopathologic examination vary by group; otherwise observer bias will affect the data generated. The protocol often requires a full microscopic examination of a given tissue list in decedents in all groups and in terminally killed controls and high-dose animals. In other animals (terminally killed low- and mid-dose animals), microscopic examination of a tissue is only conducted if the tissue is found to be abnormal at postmortem. Such a protocol is designed to save money but can lead to invalid comparisons among treatment groups. Suppose, for example, responses in terminally killed animals are 8/20 in the controls, 3/3 (with 17 unexamined) in the low-dose, and 5/6 (with 14 unexamined) in the mid-dose animals. Is one supposed to conclude that treatment at the low- and mid-doses increased response, based on a comparison of the proportions examined microscopically (40, 100, and 83%)? Or should one conclude that it decreased response, based on the proportion of animals in the group (40, 15, and 25%)? It could well be that treatment had no effect but that some small tumors were missed at postmortem. In this situation, a valid comparison can only be achieved by ignoring the low- and mid-dose groups when carrying out the comparison for the age stratum "terminal kill." This may seem wasteful of data, but actually represents the *appropriate* use of *relevant* data.

12. Use of Historical Control Data

In some situations, particularly where incidences are low, the results from a single study may suggest an effect of treatment on tumor incidence. Statistical analysis may fail to demonstrate a treatment effect. The possibility of comparing treated group results with those of historical control groups from other studies in

the institution is then often raised. By doing this, a nonsignificant incidence of 2 out of 50 cases in a treated group may seem much more significant if no cases have been seen in, say, 1000 animals representing controls from 20 similar studies. Conversely, a significant incidence of 5 out of 50 cases in a treated group as compared with 0 out of 50 in the study controls may seem far less convincing if many other control groups had incidences around 5 out of 50.

While not understating the importance of looking at historical control data, it must be emphasized that there are a number of reasons why variation between study may be greater than variation within study. Hence the utility of data from historical controls may be of lesser value than would appear on the surface. Differences in diet, duration of the study, intercurrent mortality, and the study pathologist may all contribute to variation between studies. Statistical techniques that ignore this variation and test treatment incidence against a pooled control incidence may give results that are seriously in error, and are likely to overstate statistical significance.

B. METHODS FOR DATA EXAMINATION AND PREPARATION

Data from toxicology studies should always be examined before any formal statistical analysis commences. The preliminary review should determine whether data are suitable for analysis and, if so, what form the analysis should take (see Fig. 5). If the data as collected are not suitable for analysis or if they are only suitable for low-powered analytical techniques, one may wish to use one of the many forms of data transformation to change the data characteristics so that they are more amenable to analysis. A number of tools are available to aid in data examination and preparation. Following examination, exploratory data analysis (EDA) can be done. EDA is a broad collection of techniques and approaches to "probe" data so as to both examine and perform some initial, flexible analysis of the data. Two major points made throughout this section are the use of the appropriate statistical tests, and the effects of small sample sizes, as is often the case in toxicologic pathology, on our selection of statistical techniques. The reader should be careful not to "look" at the data prior to formal statistical analysis as a method of finding which test will give the most "desirable" result. In other words, the form and completeness of the data should suggest the right test. The desired conclusion must not direct the choice of test to evaluate the data.

1. Data Examination

Two major techniques are commonly used for data examination: the *scattergram* and *Bartlett's test*. Simple examination of the nature and distribution of data collected from a study frequently can suggest patterns and results that were unanticipated. These unanticipated patterns often require the use of additional or alternative statistical methodology. Scattergrams describe these patterns, whereas Bartlett's test may be used to determine whether groups of data are homogeneous. If data are homogeneous and are from a continuous distribution, parametric analytical methods are applicable. However, if group continuous data fail Bartlett's test (i.e., are heterogeneous), we cannot be secure in our belief that parametric methods are appropriate until we gain some confidence that the values are distributed normally.

a. Scattergram. Parameters of the population can be computed, in particular kurtosis and skewness, using large groups of data. From these parameters it is possible to determine if the population is normally distributed with respect to the parameter of interest with a certain level of confidence. If concern is

especially marked with respect to the normality of the data, a χ^2 goodness-of-fit test will determine normality. When each group of data consists of 25 or fewer values, kurtosis, skewness, and χ^2 goodness of fit are not accurate indicators of normality. For smaller groups of data, preparation and evaluation of a scattergram of the data will help give a visual estimate of the normality of the data.

The scattergram procedure is a simple histogram of the data followed by a visual appreciation of the location and distribution of the data. The abscissa (horizontal scale) should be in the same scale as the values and should be divided so that the scale of the abscissa covers the entire range of observed values. Across such a scale we then simply enter symbols for each of our values (see Table XIV and Fig. 9).

Figure 9 is a traditional and rather limited form of scattergram or scatterplot. It can be seen that such plots can reveal significant information about the amount and type of associations between the two variables, the existence and nature of outliers, the clustering of data, and a number of other two-dimensional factors.

Current technology allows us to add significantly more graphical information to scatterplots by means of graphic symbols for the plotted data points. An example of this approach is shown in Fig. 10. Here, dermal dose, dermal irritation, and white blood cell count are presented. Figure 10 quite clearly suggests that as dose (variable x) is increased, dermal irritation (variable y) also increases; and as irritation becomes more severe, the white blood cell count (variable z), an indicator of

TABLE XIV
Hypothetical Data

Time	1	2	3	4	5	6	7	8	9	10	11	12
C	4.5	5.4	5.9	6.0	6.4	6.5	6.9	7.0	7.1	7.0	7.4	7.5
Tx	4.0	4.5	5.0	5.1	5.4	5.5	5.6	6.5	6.5	7.0	7.4	7.5
Time	13	14	15	16	17	18	19	20	21	22	23	24
C	7.5	7.5	7.6	8.0	8.1	8.4	8.5	8.6	9.0	9.4	9.5	10.4
Tx	7.5	8.0	8.1	8.5	8.5	9.0	9.1	9.5	9.5	10.1	10.0	10.4

Group 1:

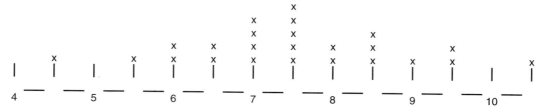

Group 2:

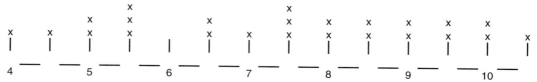

Figure 9. Scattergram derived from data in Table XIV. Group 1 approximates a normal distribution; therefore, the appropriate parametric tests can be performed on such data. In contrast, group 2 clearly dose not appear to be distributed normally. In this case, the appropriate nonparametric techniques must be used.

immune system involvement, suggesting infection or persistent inflammation, also increases. However, there is no direct association of variables x and z.

b. Bartlett's Test for Homogeneity of Variance. Bartlett's test is used to compare the variances among three or more groups of data, where data in the groups are continuous sets, such as body weights, organ weights, red blood cell counts, or diet consumption measurements. It is expected that such data will be suitable for parametric methods as normality of data is assumed. Bartlett's test is used frequently as a test for the assumption of equivalent variances. Bartlett's test is based on the calculation of the corrected χ^2 value by the formula:

$$\chi^2_{corr} = 2.3026 \frac{\sum df \left(\log_{10} \left[\frac{\sum [df(S^2)]}{\sum df} \right] \right) - \sum [df(\log_{10} S^2)]}{1 + \frac{1}{3(K-1)} \left[\sum \frac{1}{df} - \frac{1}{\sum df} \right]},$$

(14)

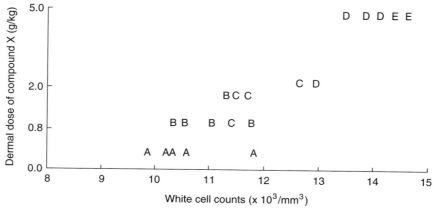

Figure 10. Descriptive scattergram for the dermal irritation study. Skin necrosis observation at termination: A, none; B, slight; C, moderate; D, marked; E, severe.

where

$$S^2 = \text{variance} = \frac{n\sum X^2 - (\sum X)^2}{\frac{n}{n-1}},$$

X is individual datum within each group,
n is number of data within each group,
K is number of groups being compared, and
df is degrees of freedom for each group $= (n-1)$.

Assumptions and Limitations

1. Bartlett's test does not test for normality, but rather homogeneity of variance (also called equality of variances or homoscedasticity).
2. Homoscedasticity is an important assumption for Student's t test, analysis of variance, and analysis of covariance.
3. The F test (covered in the next chapter) is actually a test for the two sample (i.e., control and one test group) case of homoscedasticity. Bartlett's test is designed for three or more samples.
4. Bartlett's test is very sensitive to departures from normality. As a result, a finding of a significant χ^2 value in Bartlett's test may indicate nonnormality rather than heteroscedasticity. Outliers can bring about such a finding, and the sensitivity to such erroneous findings is extreme with small sample sizes.

The corrected χ^2 value yielded by the calculations just shown is compared to the values listed in the χ^2 table according to the numbers of degrees of freedom. If the calculated value is smaller than the table value at the selected p level, traditionally 0.05, the groups are considered homogeneous and the use of ANOVA is assumed proper (subject, or course, to the verification of normality of the distributions to be compared). If the calculated χ^2 is greater than the table value, the groups are considered heterogeneous. In the case of heterogeneity, other tests are necessary. For a decision tree for the selection of the correct test, see Fig. 6.

c. *Statistical Goodness-of-Fit-Tests.* A goodness-of-fit test is a statistical procedure for comparing individual measurements to a specified type of statistical distribution. For example, a normal distribution is completely specified by its arithmetic mean and variance (the square of the standard deviation). The null hypothesis, which the data represent a sample from a single normal distribution, can be tested by a statistical goodness-of-fit test. Various goodness-of-fit tests have been devised to determine if data deviate significantly from a specified distribution.

Another goodness-of-fit method is maximum likelihood test. If a significant departure occurs, it indicates only that the specified distribution can be rejected with some assurance. This does not necessarily mean that the true distribution contains two or more sub-populations. The true distribution may be a single distribution based on a different mathematical relationship, e.g., lognormal. In the latter case, logarithms of the measurement would not be expected to exhibit by a goodness-of-fit test a statistically significant departure from a lognormal distribution. A sample size of 200 or more is required to conduct a valid analysis of mixtures of populations. When the means of subpopulations are less than 3SD apart and sample sizes are less than 300, the maximum likelihood method should be used with extreme caution, or not at all.

None of the available goodness-of-fit methods establish bimodality conclusively. Bimodality may occur when separation between the two means (modes) exceeds 2SD. Conversely, inflections in probits or separations in histograms *less than* 2SD apart may arise from genetic differences in test subjects.

i. Fisher's skewness statistic and Engelman and Hartigan test An example of the correct test under bimodal conditions is provided by Mendal, who compared eight tests of normality to detect a mixture of measurements that consisted of two normally distributed components with different means, but equal variances. *Fisher's skewness statistic* was preferable when one component comprised less than 15% of the total distribution. However, when the two components comprised more nearly equal proportions

(35–65%) of the total distribution, then the *Engelman and Hartigan test* was preferable. For other proportions, the maximum likelihood ratio test was best. Thus, the maximum likelihood ratio test appears to perform very well, with only a small loss from optimality, even when it is not the best procedure.

ii. Maximum likelihood ratio test The method of *maximum likelihood ratio test* provides estimators of a parameter that are usually quite satisfactory. These estimators have the desirable properties of being consistent, asymptotically normal, and asymptotically efficient for large samples under quite general conditions. The estimators are often biased, but the bias is frequently removable by a simple adjustment. Other methods of obtaining estimators are also available, but the maximum likelihood ratio test is the most frequently used.

These maximum likelihood methods can be used to obtain *point estimates* of a parameter, but we must remember that a point estimator is a random variable distributed in some way around the true value of the parameter. The true parameter value may be higher or lower than our estimate. It is often useful to obtain an interval within which we are reasonably confident the true value will lie, and the generally accepted method is to construct what are known as *confidence limits*. Maximum likelihood estimators also have another desirable property: *invariance*.

The mathematical description of the maximum likelihood estimator is as follows. Let us denote the maximum likelihood estimator of the parameter θ, where x is a random variable, by $f(x;\theta)$. Then, if $f(x;\theta)$ is a single-valued function of θ, the maximum likelihood estimator of $f(\theta)$ is $f(x_1;\theta)^*f(x_2;\theta)^*f(x_3;\theta)\ldots f(x_n;\theta)$. The principle of maximum likelihood tells us that we should use as our estimate that value that maximizes the likelihood of the observed event.

iii. Confidence intervals The following procedure will yield upper and lower 95% confidence limits. This procedure will with the property give limits that include the true value of the parameter 95% of the time, with a 5%

probability that the interval will not include the true value of the parameter. Calculating the upper and lower 95% confidence limits.

1. Choose a (test) statistic involving the unknown parameter and no other unknown parameter.
2. Place the appropriate sample values in the statistic.
3. Obtain an equation for the unknown parameter by equating the test statistic to the upper 2.5% point of the relevant distribution.
4. The solution of the equation gives one limit.
5. Repeat the process with the lower 2.5% point to obtain the other limit.

Usually it is best to have a confidence interval as narrow as possible. With a symmetric distribution such as the normal or t, this is achieved using equal tails. One can also construct 95% confidence intervals using unequal tails, e.g., using the upper 2% point and the lower 3% point. The same procedure very nearly minimizes the confidence interval with other nonsymmetric distributions, e.g., χ^2 and has the advantage of avoiding rather tedious computation.

When the appropriate statistic involves the square of the unknown parameter, both limits are obtained by equating the statistic to the upper 5% point of the relevant distribution. The use of two tails in this situation would result in a pair of nonintersecting intervals. When two or more parameters are involved, it is possible to construct a region within which the true parameter values will most likely lie. Such regions are referred to as *confidence regions*.

2. Preparing Data

Preparing data requires cleaning it for statistical evaluation. First, data should be checked for completeness, and numbers rounded to the correct number of significant figures for the procedure that generated the data. In addition, data points that appear to be outliers should be evaluated for inclusion or exclusion, using the methods described earlier. Once data are ready for use in analysis, two other techniques may be required before the analysis commences randomization, including a test for randomness in a sample of data and transformation of data.

a. Randomization. Randomization is the act of assigning a number of items, e.g., plates of bacteria or test animals, to groups in such a manner that there is an equal chance for any one item to end up in any one group. Randomization is a control against any possible bias in the assignment of subjects to test groups.

A variation on this is censored randomization, which ensures that the groups are equivalent in some aspect after the assignment process is complete. The most common example of a censored randomization is one in which it is ensured that the body weights of test animals in each group are not significantly different from those in the other groups. This is done by analyzing group weights both for homogeneity of variance and by analysis of variance after animal assignment and then again randomizing if there is a significant difference at some nominal level, such as $p \leq 0.10$. The process is repeated until there is no significant difference.

There are several methods for actually performing the randomization process. The three most commonly used are card assignment, use of a random number table, and use of a computerized algorithm.

i. Card assignment For the card-based method, individual identification numbers for items (e.g., plates or animals) are placed on separate index cards. These cards are then shuffled and placed one at a time in succession into piles corresponding to the required test groups. The results are a random group assignment.

ii. Random number table method The random number table method requires only that one have unique numbers assigned to test subjects and access to a random number table. One simply sets up a table with a column for each group to which subjects are to be assigned. Randomization starts from the head of any

one column of numbers in the random table. Each time the table is used, a new starting point should be utilized. If the test subjects number less than 100, only the last two digits in each random number in the table are used. If they number more than 99 but less than 1000, only the last three digits are used. To generate group assignments, read down a column, one number at a time. As digits are found that correspond to a subject number, the subject is assigned to a group (enter its identifying number in a column) proceeding to assign subjects to groups from left to right filling one row at a time. After a number is assigned to an animal, any duplication of its unique number is ignored. As many successive columns of random numbers are used as is required to complete the process.

iii. Computerized random number generation The third (and now most common) method is to use a random number generator that is built into a calculator or computer program. Procedures for generating these are generally documented in user manuals.

b. Transformations. If initial inspection of a data set reveals an unusual or undesired set of characteristics, or a lack a desired set of characteristics such as normality, there is a choice of three courses of action. First, a method or test appropriate to the present conditions that have assumptions not violated by the conditions may be selected. Second, analysis may not be attempted on the grounds that data cannot be analyzed using the planned techniques. Finally, attempts can be made to transform the variable(s) under consideration in such a manner that the resulting transformed variates (X' and Y', for example, as opposed to the original variates X and Y) meet the assumptions of the test to be employed or have the characteristics that are desired.

The key to transformation is recognizing that the scale of measurement of most (if not all) variables is arbitrary. That is to say that the relationship of each variable or variate to one another is important, whereas the unit of measurement is arbitrary. For example, a linear scale of measurement may have been used to record the data; however, this scale could have been changed to a logarithmic scale to represent the data. Often such scales are used because they are easier to read. Familiar logarithmic measurements are that of pH values or the Richter earthquake intensity. Transforming a set of data (converting X to X') is really as simple as changing a scale of measurement. Transformation does not alter the relationship of variables, just their representation.

Data transformation is commonly done to normalize data. As the assumptions for the common statistical analyses require normality of data, transformation is necessary to permit analysis by our most common parametric statistical techniques, such as analysis of variance (ANOVA). Transformation does not guarantee normally distributed data. A simple test of whether a selected transformation yields a distribution that satisfies the underlying assumptions for ANOVA is to plot the cumulative distribution of samples on probability paper. This paper is a commercially available paper that has the probability function scale as one axis. One can then alter the scale of the second axis, i.e., the axis other than the one that is on a probability scale, from linear to any other scale, e.g., logarithmic, reciprocal, square root. When the plot is complete, check to see if a previously curved line indicating a skewed distribution becomes linear to indicate normality. The slope of the transformed line gives an estimate of the standard deviation. If the slopes of the lines of several samples or groups of data are similar, the variance of the different groups is homogenous. These transformed data can be analyzed.

The second reason to transform data is to create a linear relationship between a paired set of data, such as dose and response. This transformation is used commonly in toxicologic pathology and is discussed in more detail in the section under probit/logit plots.

Third, transformation of data may be done to adjust for the influence of another variable. This procedure is an alternative in some situations to the more complicated process of analysis of covariance. An example of where this transformation is used is the calculation of organ weight to body weight ratios in *in vivo* toxicity studies. Here the resulting ratios serve as "raw data" for an analysis of variance performed to identify possible target organs, provided that the assumption of the ANOVA is met. If these ratios need to be normalized, data can be transformed again to achieve normality.

Finally, transformation of data may be undertaken to make the relationships between variables clearer. Removing, or adjusting for, interactions with other uncontrolled variables that may influence the pair of variables to be analyzed achieve this clarification. This case is discussed in detail in the section under time series analysis. Common transformations are presented in the Table XV.

C. EXPLORATORY DATA ANALYSIS

Since the early 1980, an entirely new approach has been developed to get the most information out of the increasingly larger and more complex data sets that scientists are faced with. This approach involves the use of a very diverse set of fairly simple techniques that comprise exploratory data analysis (EDA). There are four major ingredients to EDA.

1. Displays

Displays visually reveal the distribution; variance and trends are sometimes referred to as the behavior of data. They suggest a framework for analysis. The scatterplot demonstrated earlier is an example of this approach.

2. Residuals

Residuals are data remnants, or data filtered out, following a fitted model. The analysis has removed these residuals. Residuals are the remnants of error or variability that remain following the fitting of a model. These residuals are seen as deviation from a linear plot, as in a linear regression. Residuals provide an expression of lack of fit of the model to a specific region. If the regression model is adequate, they should be without structure; i.e., they should present no pattern. The evidence of a

TABLE XV
Common Data Transformations

Transformation	How calculated[a]	Example of use
Arithmetic	$x' = \dfrac{x}{y}$ or $x' = x + c$	Organ weight/body weight
Reciprocals	$x' = \dfrac{1}{x}$	Linearizing data, particularly rate phenomena
Arcsine (also called angular)	$x' = \text{arcsine } \sqrt{x}$	Normalizing dominant lethal and mutation rate data
Logarithmic probability (probit)	$x' = \log x$ $x' = \text{probability } X$	pH values Percentage responding
Square roots	$x' = \sqrt{x}$	Surface area of animal from body weights
Box Cox	$x' = (x^v - 1)v$: for $v \neq 0$ $x' = 1nx$: for $v = 0$	A family of transforms For use when one has no prior knowledge of the appropriate transformation to use
Rank transformations	Depends on nature of samples	As a bridge between parametric and nonparametric statistics (Conover and Iman, 1981)

[a] x and y are original variables; x' and y' are transformed values. "C" stands for a constant.
[b] Plotting a double reciprocal (i.e., $\frac{1}{x}$ vs $\frac{1}{y}$) will linearize almost any data set. So will plotting the log transforms of a set of variables.

pattern indicates an area on regression in which the function of the model is not optimal.

3. Reexpressions

Reexpression involves "redrawing" data to different scales so as to visualize which scale would serve best to simplify and improve the analysis of data. Simple transformations, such as those presented earlier in Section III,B, are used to simplify data behavior and clarify analysis, e.g., linearizing or normalizing data.

4. Resistance

Resistance requires decreasing the sensitivity of analysis. It also involves clarifying summary statistics so that the occurrence of a few outliers, for example, will not complicate or invalidate the methods used to analyze data. For example, the median, not the arithmetic mean, is a summary statistic that is highly resistant to the effect of outliers.

These four ingredients are utilized first in an exploratory phase and then a confirmatory phase. The exploratory phase isolates patterns in and features of data and reveals them, allowing an inspection of data before any firm choice of actual hypothesis testing or modeling methods has been made. Confirmatory analysis allows evaluation of the reproducibility of the patterns or effects. Its role is close to that of classical hypothesis testing, but also often includes steps such as incorporating information from an analysis of another, closely related set of data and validating a result by assembling and analyzing additional data. These techniques are in general beyond the scope of this text but can be in Velleman and Hoaglin (1981) and Hoaglin *et al.* (1983).

5. Robustness

A concept related to resistance and exploratory data analysis is that of robustness. Robustness generally implies insensitivity to departures from assumptions surrounding an underlying model, such as normality. In summarizing the location of data, the median, although highly resistant, is not extremely robust, but the mean is both nonresistant and nonrobust.

6. An Example

a. Data. Toxicology has long recognized that no population, whether it is animal or human, is completely uniform in its response to any particular toxicant. Rather, a population is composed of a (presumed normal) distribution of individual animals, some of which are resistant to intoxication (hyporesponders), the bulk that respond close to a central value (such as an LD_{50}), and some that are very sensitive to intoxication (hyperresponders). This distribution requires that data are examined and prepared as described in Section III,B.

b. Determination of Outliers. The sensitivity of techniques such as ANOVA is reduced markedly by the occurrence of outliers, either extreme high or low values, including hyper- and hyporesponders, which serve to markedly inflate the dispersion of data points, and hence variance, of the sample. Such variance inflation is particularly common in small groups of experimental units that are exposed or dosed around a threshold level. This exposure or dosing results in a small number of hypersensitive individuals in the sample responding markedly. Such a situation is displayed in Fig. 11 showing a plot of the mean and standard deviations of methemoglobin levels in a series of groups of animals exposed to successively higher levels of a hemolytic agent.

Although the mean level of methemoglobin in group C is more than double that of the control group (A), no hypothesis test will show a significant difference because of the large variance of the data. This "inflated" variance exists because a single individual has such a marked response. The occurrence of the variance inflation is certainly an indicator that data need to be examined closely for potential out-

lying events as described in Section III,B. Indeed, all tabular raw data in toxicologic pathology should be inspected visually for both trend and variance inflation. Summary statistics may hide important information concerning trend and variance inflation.

D. HYPOTHESIS TESTING OF CATEGORICAL DATA

Categorical data presented in a contingency table contain any single type of data. The contents of the contingency table are classified treatment and control groups, with the members of each group classified as to one of two or more response categories, such as tumor/no tumor or normal/hyperplastic/neoplastic. In these cases, two forms of analysis can be used: Fisher's exact test for the 2×2 contingency table and the RXC χ^2 test for large tables. It should be noted, however, that there are versions of both of these tests that permit the analysis of any size of contingency table.

Nonparametric statistical analysis of ranked data is an exact parallel of the more traditional parametric methods. There are methods for a single comparison, similar to Student's t test, and for the multiple comparisons, similar to ANOVA, with appropriate *post hoc* tests for exact identification of the significance with a set of groups. Four tests for these situations are described: the Wilcoxon rank sum test, distribution-free multiple comparisons, Mann–

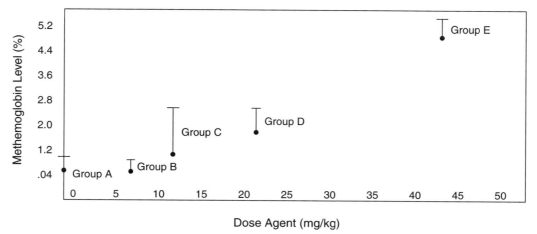

Figure 11. Variance inflation (mean + SD).

378

Whitney U test, and the Kruskall–Wallis non-parametric analysis of variance. For each of these tests, tables of distribution values for the evaluations of results can be found in any of a number of reference volumes. It should be noted that for data that do not fulfill the necessary assumptions for parametric analysis, these nonparametric methods are either as powerful as, or more powerful than, the equivalent parametric test.

1. Fisher's Exact Test

Fisher's exact test should be used to compare two sets of discontinuous, quantal data. Quantal data are categorical all-or-none type of data such as live or dead. Contingency data tables can check small sets of quantal data. Larger data sets, however, require computation. Examples of such data include incidences of mortality or certain histopathological findings. These data can also be expressed as ratios. These data do not fit a continuous scale of measurement but usually involve numbers of responses classified as either negative or positive. The analysis is started by setting up a 2×2 contingency table to summarize the numbers of "positive" and "negative" responses as well as the totals of these responses as shown in Fig. 12. Using the set of symbols shown in Fig. 12, the formula for P^1 appears as follows:

$$P = \frac{(A+B)!(C+D)!(A+C)!(B+D)!}{N!A!B!C!D!}. \qquad (15)$$

The exact test produces a probability (P) that is the sum of the calculation repeated for each possible arrangement of the numbers in the cells (i.e., A, B, C, and D) showing an association equal to or stronger than that between the two variables. The P resulting from these computations will be the exact one- or two-tailed probability depending on which of these two approaches is being employed. This value tells us if the groups differ significantly, e.g., probability less than 0.05, and the degree of significance.

---

[1]A! is A factorial. For 4! – as an example this would be (4) (3) (2) (1) = 24.

Assumptions and Limitations

1. Tables are available that provide individual exact probabilities for small sample size contingency tables.
2. Fisher's exact must be used in preference to the χ^2 test when there are small cell numbers, i.e., less than six.
3. The probability resulting from a two-tailed χ^2 test is exactly double that of a one-tailed from the same data.
4. Ghent has developed and proposed a good (though, if performed by hand, laborious) method extending the calculation of exact probabilities to 2×3, 3×3, and RXC contingency tables.
5. Fisher's probabilities are not necessary symmetric. Although some analysts will double the one-tailed p value to obtain the two-tailed result, this method is usually overly conservative.

2. $2 \times 2 \, \chi^2$

Although Fisher's exact test is preferable for analysis of most 2×2 contingency tables in toxicologic pathology, the χ^2 test is still used widely and is preferable in a few unusual situations. χ^2 is used when cell sizes are large yet only limited computational support is available [Eq. (16)]:

$$X^2 = \frac{(0_1 - E_1)^2}{E_1} + \frac{(0_2 - E_2)^2}{E_2}$$
$$= \sum \frac{(0_i - E_1)^2}{E_1} \qquad (16)$$

where 0 are observed numbers (or counts) and E is expected numbers.

The common practice in toxicologic pathology is for the observed figures to be test or treatment group counts. The expected statistic is calculated for each box or cell in the contingency table as

$$\sum = \frac{(column\ total)(row\ total)}{grand\ total}.$$

The degrees of freedom for this statistic are (R-1)(C-1) = (2-1)(2-1) = 1. Looking at a χ^2 table for one degree of freedom, we can see where our test statistic lies at the 0.05 and 0.01 probability levels.

Group	"Positive"	"Negative"	Total
Group I	A	B	A + B
Group II	C	D	C + D
Totals	A + C	B + D	A + B + C + D = N_{total}

Figure 12. An example of a 2 × 2 contingency table.

Assumptions and Limitations

Assumptions:
1. Data are univariate and categorical
2. Data are from a multinomial population
3. Data are collected by random, independent sampling
4. Groups are of approximately same size, particularly for small group sizes

When to use:
1. When data are of a categorical (or frequency) nature
2. When data fit the assumptions just given
3. To test goodness to fit to a known form of distribution
4. When cell sizes are large

When not to use:
1. When data are continuous rather than categorical
2. When sample sizes are small and very unequal
3. When sample sizes are too small (e.g., when total N is less than 50 of if any expected value is less than 5)
4. For any 2 × 2 comparison (use Fisher's exact test instead)

3. R × C χ^2

The R × C χ^2 test can be used to analyze discontinuous frequency type data as in the Fisher's exact or 2 × 2 χ^2 tests. However, in the R × C test (R, row; C, column), we wish to compare three or more sets of data. An example would be comparison of the incidence of tumors among mice on three or more oral dosage levels. We can consider data as "positive" (tumors) or "negative" (no tumors). The expected frequency for any box is (row total) (column total)/(N_{total}). As in the Fisher's exact test, the initial step is setting up an R × C contingency table as shown in Fig. 13.

Using the symbols shown in Fig. 3, the formula for χ^2 is

$$\chi^2 = \frac{N_{tot}^2}{N_A N_B N_K} \left(\frac{A_1^2}{N_1} + \frac{A_2^2}{N_2} + \cdots \frac{A_K^2}{N_K} - \frac{N_A^2}{N_{tot}} \right). \quad (17)$$

The resulting χ^2 value is compared to table values according to the number of degrees of freedom, which is equal to (R-1)(C-1). If χ^2 is smaller than the table value at the 0.05 probability level, the groups are not significantly different. If the calculated χ^2 is larger, there is a difference among the groups. A 2 × R χ^2 or Fisher's exact tests will have to be undertaken to determine which group(s) differs from which other group(s).

Assumptions and Limitations

1. Based on data being organized in a table so that there are *cells* (A, B, C, and D are "cells").

	"Positive"	"Negative"	Total
Group I	A_1	B_1	$A_1+B_1=N_1$
Group II	A_2 ↓	B_2 ↓	$A_2+B_2=N_2$
Group R	A_R	B_R	$A_R+B_R=N_R$
Totals	N_A	N_B	N_{total}

Figure 13. A typical R × C contingency table.

380

	Columns (C)		
	Control	Treated	Total
No effect	A	B	A + B
Rows (R)			
Effect	C	D	C + D
Total	A + C	B + D	A + B + C + D

2. None of the "expected" frequency values should be less than 5.0.
3. χ^2 test is always one tailed.
4. Without the use of some form of correction, the test becomes less accurate as the differences between group size increase.
5. The results from each additional column (group) is approximately additive. Due to this characteristic, χ^2 can be used readily for evaluating any R × C combination.
6. Results of the χ^2 calculation must be a positive number, which is an inevitable outcome given the other conditions.
7. Test is weak with either small sample sizes or when the expected frequency in any cell is less than 5 (this latter limitation can be overcome by "pooling" – combining cells).
8. Test results are independent of order of cells, unlike Kolmogorov–Smirnov.
9. Can be used to test the probability of validity of any distribution.

E. HYPOTHESIS TESTING OF ORDINAL DATA

1. Wilcoxon Rank-Sum Test

The Wilcoxon rank-sum test is used commonly for the comparison of two groups of nonparametric interval or not normally distributed data. Typically, these data are measured within certain limits on a continuum. For example, how many animals died during each hour of an acute study? The test is also used when there is no variability (variance = 0) within one or more of the groups we wish to compare.

Data in both groups are initially arranged and listed in order of increasing value. Then each number in the two groups must receive a rank value. Beginning with the smallest number in either group, which is given a rank of 1.0,

each number is assigned a rank. If there are multiples of the same numbers, called "ties," then each value of equal size will receive the median rank for the entire identically sized group. Thus if the lowest number appears twice, both figures receive a rank of 1.5. This, in turn, means that the ranks of 1.0 and 2.0 have been used and that the next highest number has a rank of 3.0. If the lowest number appears three times, then each is ranked as 2.0 and the next number has a rank of 4.0. Thus, each tied number gets a "median" rank. This process continues until all of the numbers are ranked. Each of the two columns of ranks (one for each group) is totaled, giving the "sum of ranks" for each group being compared. As a check, we can calculate the value:

$$\frac{(N)(N+1)}{2}, \tag{18}$$

where N is the total number of data in both groups.

The result should be equal to the sum of the sum of ranks for both groups. The sum of rank values is compared to table values to determine the degree of significant differences, if any.

These tables include an upper and a lower limit value that are dependent on the probability level. If the number of data is not the same in both groups ($N_1 \neq N_2$), then the lesser sum of ranks (smaller N) is compared to the table limits to find the degree of significance. Normally the comparison of the two groups ends here and the degree of significant difference can be reported.

Assumptions and Limitations

1. Too many tied ranks increase false positive results, i.e., rejection of the null hypothesis may occur at less than 5%, even though the α level is set at 0.05
2. The Wilcoxon rank-sum test can be highly biased in the presence of censored data.

2. Distribution-Free Multiple Comparison

The distribution-free multiple comparison test should be used to compare three or more groups of nonparametric data. These groups are then analyzed two at a time for any significant differences. The test can be used for data similar to those compared by the rank-sum test. We often employ this test for reproduction and mutagenicity studies where we wish to compare survival rates of offspring of rats fed various amounts of test materials in the diet.

Two values must be calculated for each pair of groups: the difference in mean ranks and the probability level value against which the difference will be compared. To determine the difference in mean ranks we must first arrange data within each of the groups in order of increasing values. Then we must assign rank values, beginning with the smallest overall figure. Note that this ranking is similar to that in the Wilcoxon test except that it applies to more than two groups. The ranks are then added for each of the groups. As a check, the sum of these should equal:

$$\frac{N_{tot}(N_{tot} + 1)}{2} \tag{19}$$

where N_{tot} is the total of all groups.

Next we can find the mean rank (R) for each group by dividing the sum of ranks by the numbers in the data (N) in the group. These mean ranks are then used in those pairs to be compared, usually each test group vs the control, and the differences are found $|R_1 - R_2|$. This value is expressed as an absolute figure; i.e., it is always a positive number. The second value for each pair of groups, the probability value, is then calculated:

$$z = \left[\frac{\alpha}{K}(K - 1)\right]\sqrt{\frac{N_{tot}(N_{tot} + 1)}{12}}\sqrt{\frac{1}{N_1}\frac{1}{N_2}}, \tag{20}$$

where a is the level of significance for the comparison (usually 0.05, 0.01, 0.001, etc.), K is the total number of groups, and z is a figure obtained from a normal probability table and determining the corresponding "Z score."

The result of the probability value calculation for each pair of groups is compared to the corresponding mean difference $|R_1 - R_2|$. If $|R_1 - R_2|$ is smaller, then there is no significant difference between the groups. If the difference is larger, the groups are different and $|R_1 - R_2|$

must be compared to the calculated probability values for $\alpha = 0.01$ and $\alpha = 0.001$ to find the degree of significance.

Assumptions and Limitations

1. As with the Wilcoxon rank-sum test, too many tied ranks inflate the false positive.
2. Generally, this test should be used as a *post hoc* comparison after Kruskall–Wallis.

3. Mann–Whitney U Test

This is a nonparametric test in which data in each group are first ordered from lowest to highest values. Then the entire data set, both control and treated values, is ranked, with the average rank being assigned to tied values. The ranks are then summed for each group and U is determined:

$$U_t = n_c n_t + \frac{n_t(n_t + 1)}{2} - R_t$$
$$U_c = n_c n_t + \frac{n_c(n_c + 1)}{2} - R_c, \tag{21}$$

where n_c and n_t are the sample sizes for control and treated groups and R_c and R_t are sums of ranks for the control and treated groups.

For the level of significance for a comparison of the two groups, the larger value of U_c or U_t is used. This is compared to critical values as found in tables. The Mann–Whitney U test is employed for discontinuous count data, but the choice of test to be employed for percentage variables should be decided on the same grounds as described later under reproduction studies.

Assumptions, Limitations, and Comments

1. It does not matter whether the observations are ranked from smallest to largest or vice versa.
2. This test should not be used for paired observations.
3. Test statistics from a Mann–Whitney are linearly related to those of Wilcoxon. The two tests will always yield the same result. The Mann–Whitney is presented here for historical completeness, as it has been much favored in reproductive and developmental toxicology studies. However, it

should be noted that the authors do not include it in the decision tree for method selection.

4. Kruskal–Wallis Nonparametric ANOVA

The Kruskal–Wallis nonparametric one-way analysis of variance should be the initial analysis performed when three or more groups of nonparametric data are to be evaluated. Typically, data are not distributed normally, are discontinuous, or all the groups to be analyzed are not from the same population, but the data are not of a categorical, or quantal, nature. Commonly, these data are either rank type evaluation data, such as behavioral toxicity observation scores, or reproduction study data.

The analysis is initiated by ranking all the observations from the combined groups. Ties are given the average rank of the tied values, i.e., if two values that would tie for 12th rank—and therefore would be ranked 12th and 13th—both would be assigned the average rank of 12.5. The sum of ranks of each group ($r_1, r_2, \ldots r_k$) is computed by adding all the rank values for each group. The test value H is then computed:

$$H = \frac{12}{n(n+1)}\sum(r_1^2/n_1 + r_2^2/n_2 + \ldots + r_k^2/n_k) - 3(n+1), \quad (22)$$

where $n_1, n_2, \ldots n_k$ are the number of observations in each group.

The test statistic is then compared with a table of H values, available in a number of statistical texts. If the calculated value of H is greater than the table value for the appropriate number of observations in each group (degrees of freedom), there is significant difference between the groups. However, further testing using the distribution-free multiple comparisons method is necessary to determine which groups are different from one another.

Assumptions and Limitations

1. The test statistic H is used for both small and large samples.
2. When we find a significant difference, we do not know which groups are different. It is incorrect to then perform a Mann–Whitney U test on all possible combinations. Rather, a multiple comparison method must be used, such as distribution-free multiple comparisons.
3. Data must be independent for the test to be valid.
4. Too many tied ranks will decrease the power of this test and also lead to false positive results.
5. When $k = 2$, the Kruskal–Wallis χ^2 value has 1 df. This test is identical to the normal approximation used for the Wilcoxon rank-sum test. A χ^2 with 1 df can be represented by the square of a standardized normal random variable. In the case of $k = 2$, the H statistic is the square of the Wilcoxon rank-sum (without the continuity correction).
6. The effect of adjusting for tied ranks is to slightly increase the value of the test statistic, H. Therefore, omission of this adjustment results in a more conservative test.

5. Log Rank Test

The log rank test is a statistical methodology for comparing the distribution of time until the occurrence of an event of interest in independent groups. In toxicologic pathology, the most common event of interest is death or occurrence of a tumor, but it could be any other event that occurs only once in an individual. The elapsed time from initial treatment or observation until the *event* is the *event time*, often referred to as "survival time," even when the *event* is not "death."

The log rank test provides a method for comparing "risk-adjusted" event rates, useful when test subjects in a study are subject to varying degrees of opportunity to experience the event. Such situations arise frequently in toxicology studies due to the finite duration of the study, early termination of the animal, or interruption of treatment before the event occurs.

The log rank test might be used to compare survival times in carcinogenicity bioassay animals given a new treatment with those in the control group. Another example is comparison

383

of time to liver failure for several dose levels of a new drug where the animals are treated for 10 weeks or until cured, whichever comes first. If every animal were followed until the event occurrence, the event times could be compared between two groups using the Wilcoxon rank-sum test.

However, some animals may die or otherwise complete the study before the event occurs. In such cases, the actual time to the event is unknown because the event does not occur while under study observation. The event times for these animals are based on the last known time of study observation and are called "censored" observations because they represent the lower bound of the true, unknown event times. The log-rank test is preferable in this case, as the Wilcoxon rank-sum test can be highly biased in the presence of censored data.

The null hypothesis tested by the log-rank test is that of equal event time distributions among groups. Equality of the distributions of event times implies similar event rates among groups not only for the clinical trial as a whole, but also for any arbitrary time point during the trial. Rejection of the null hypothesis indicates that the event rates differ among groups at one or more time points during the study.

The principle behind the log-rank test for comparison of two life tables is simple; if there were no difference between the groups, the total deaths occurring at any time should split between the two groups at that time. So if the numbers at risk in the first and second groups in (say) the sixth month were 70 and 30, respectively, and 10 deaths occurred in that month we would expect

$$10 \times \frac{70}{70 + 30} = 7$$

of these deaths to have occurred in the first group, and

$$10 \times \frac{30}{70 + 30} = 3$$

of the deaths to have occurred in the second group.

A similar calculation can be made at each time of death (in either group). By adding to-

gether for the first group the results of all such calculations, we obtain a single number, called the extent of exposure (E_1), which represents the "expected" number of deaths in that group if the two groups had the distribution of survival time. An extent of exposure (E_2) can be obtained for the second group in the same way. Let O_1 and O_2 denote the actual total numbers of deaths in the two groups. A useful arithmetic check is that the total number of deaths $O_1 + O_2$ must equal the sum $E_1 + E_2$ of the extents of exposure. The discrepancy between the O's and E's can then be measured:

$$\chi^2 = \frac{(|O_1 - E_1| - 1/2)^2}{E_1} + \frac{(|O_2 - E_2| - 1/2)^2}{E_2}. \quad (23)$$

For rather obscure reasons, χ^2 is known as the log-rank statistic. An approximate significance test of the null hypothesis of identical distributions of survival time in the two groups is obtained by comparing x^2 to a χ^2 distribution on 1 degree of freedom.

The log-rank test can use the product-limit life table calculations rather than the actuarial estimators shown earlier. The distinction is likely to be of little practical importance unless the grouping intervals are very coarse. It has been suggested that the approximation in treating the null distribution of χ^2 as a χ^2 is conservative, so that it will tend to understate the degree of statistical significance.

In the formula for χ^2, the continuity correction of substracting $1/2$ from $|O_1 - E_1|$ and $|O_2 - E_2|$ has been used before squaring. This is recommended when, as in nonrandomized studies, the permutations argument does not apply. Further details of the log-rank test and its extension to comparisons of more than two treatment groups and to tests that control for categorical confounding factors are available.

Assumptions, Limitations, and Comments

1. The end point of concern is or is defined so that it is "right censored"—once it happens, it does not reoccur. Examples are death or a minimum or maximum value of an enzyme or physiologic function (such as respiration rate).

2. The method makes no assumptions on distribution.

3. Many variations of the log-rank test for comparing survival distributions exist. The most common variant has the form:

$$X^2 = \frac{(O_1 - E_1)^2}{E_1} + \frac{(O_2 - E_2)^2}{E_2},$$

where O_i and E_i are computed for each group, as in the formulas given previously. This statistic also approximates a χ^2 distribution with 1 degree of freedom under H_0. A continuity correction can also be used to reducing the numerators by $\frac{1}{2}$ before squaring. Use of such a correction leads to further conservatism and may be omitted when sample sizes are moderate or large, i.e., greater than or equal to 15 per cell.

4. The Wilcoxon rank-sum test could be used to analyze the event times in the absence of censoring. A "generalized Wilcoxon" test, sometimes called the Gehan test, based on an approximate χ^2 distribution, has been developed for use in the presence of censored observations.

5. Both the log-rank and the Wilcoxon tests are nonparametric tests and require no assumptions regarding the distribution of event times. When the event rate is greater early in the trial than toward the end, the generalized Wilcoxon test is the more appropriate test because it gives greater weight to the earlier differences.

5. Survival and failure times often follow the exponential distribution. If such a model can be assumed, a more powerful alternative to the log-rank test is the likelihood ratio test. This parametric test assumes that event probabilities are constant over time. That is, the chance that a patient becomes event positive at time t given that he is event negative up to time t does not depend on t. A plot of the negative log of the event times distribution showing a linear trend through the origin is consistent with exponential event times.

6. Life tables can be constructed to provide estimates of the event time distributions. Estimates commonly used are known as the Kaplan–Meier estimates.

F. HYPOTHESIS TESTING ON UNIVARIATE PARAMETERS

Univariate case, i.e., where each datum is defined by one treatment and one effect variable, data from normally distributed populations generally have a higher information value associated with them than nonnormal and nonparametric data sets. However, the traditional hypothesis testing techniques are generally neither resistant nor robust. All data analyzed by these methods must be continuous, i.e., any number may represent the data and each such data number has a measurable relationship to other data numbers.

1. Student's "t" Test (Unpaired t Test)

Pairs of groups of continuous, randomly distributed data are compared via this test. This test can be used to compare three or more groups of data, but they must be compared by examination of two groups taken at a time and are preferentially compared by ANOVA. Usually this means comparison of a test group versus a control group, although two test groups may be compared as well.

To determine which of the three types of t tests described in this chapter should be employed, the F test is usually performed first. This test will reveal whether the variances of data are approximately equal, which is a requirement for the use of parametric methods. If the F test indicates homogeneous variances and the numbers of data within the groups (N) are equal, then the Student's t test is the appropriate procedure. However, if the F is significant (i.e., data are heterogeneous) and the two groups have equal numbers of data, the modified Student's t test is applicable. The value of t for Student's t test is calculated using the following formula:

$$t = \frac{\overline{X_1} - \overline{X_2}}{\sum D_1^2 + \sum D_2^2} \sqrt{\frac{N_1 N_2}{N_1 + N_2}(N_1 + N_2 - 2)}, \quad (24)$$

where the value of $\sum D^2 = \frac{N \sum X^2 - (\sum X)^2}{N}$.

The value of t obtained is compared to the values in a t distribution table according to the appropriate number of degrees of freedom (df) from standard statistical texts. If the F value is not significant, i.e., variances are homogeneous,

385

the $df = N_1 + N_2 - 2$. If the F was significant and $N_1 = N_2$, then the $df = N - 1$.

Even though a nonrandom distribution may exist, the modified t test is still valid. If the calculated value is larger than the table value at $p = 0.05$, it may then be compared to the appropriate other table values in order of decreasing probability to determine the degree of significance between the two groups.

Assumptions and Limitations

1. The test assumes that data are univariate, continuous, and normally distributed.

2. Data are collected by random sampling.

3. The test should be used when the assumptions in 1 and 2 are met and there are only two groups to be compared.

4. Do not use when data are ranked, when data are not approximately normally distributed, or when there are more than two groups to be compared. Do not use for paired observations.

5. This is the most commonly misused test method, except in those few cases where one is truly only comparing two groups of data and the group sizes are roughly equivalent. Not valid for multiple comparisons (because of resulting additive errors) or where group sizes are very unequal.

6. Test is robust for moderate departures from normality and, when N_1 and N_2 are approximately equal, robust for moderate departures from homogeneity of variances.

7. The main difference between the Z test and the t test is that the Z statistic is based on a known standard deviation, σ, while the t statistic uses the sample standard deviation, s, as an estimate of σ. With the assumption of normally distributed data, the variance σ^2 is more closely estimated by the sample variance s^2 as n gets large. It can be shown that the t test is equivalent to the Z test for infinite degrees of freedom. In practice, a "large" sample is usually considered $n \geq 30$.

2. Cochran t Test

The Cochran test should be used to compare two groups of continuous data when the vari-

ances, as indicated by the F test, are heterogeneous and the numbers of data within the groups are not equal ($N_1 \neq N_2$). This is the situation when data expected to be randomly distributed were not. Two t values are calculated for this test: the "observed" t (t_{obs}) and the "expected" t (t'). The observed t is obtained by using the following equation:

$$t_{obs} = \frac{\bar{X}_1 - \bar{X}_2}{\sqrt{W_1 + W_2}}$$

where $W = \text{SEM}^2$ (standard error of the mean squared)

$$= S^2/N$$

where S (variance) can be calculated from:

$$S = \frac{\dfrac{N \sum X^2 - \left(\sum X\right)^2}{N}}{N - 1} \qquad (25)$$

The value for t' is obtained from:

$$t' = \frac{t_1' W_1 + t_2' W_2}{W_1 + W_2},$$

where t_1' and t_2' are values for the two groups taken from the t distribution table corresponding to $N - 1$ degrees of freedom (for each group) at the 0.05 probability level (or such level as one may select).

The calculated t_{obs} is compared to the calculated t' value (or values, if t' values were prepared for more than one probability level). If t_{obs} is smaller than a t', the groups are not considered to be significantly different at that probability level.

Assumptions and Limitations

1. The test assumes that data are univariate, continuous, normally distributed, and that group sizes are unequal.

2. The test is robust for moderate departures from normality and very robust for departures from equality of variances.

3. F Test

This is a test of the homogeneity of variances between two groups of data. It is used in two separate cases. The first is when Bartlett's indicates heterogeneity of variances among three or more groups, i.e., it is used to determine which pairs of groups are heterogeneous. Second, the F test is the initial step in comparing two groups of continuous data that we would expect to be parametric (two groups not usually being compared using ANOVA), with results indicating whether data are from the same population and whether subsequent parametric comparisons would be valid. The F is calculated by dividing the larger variance (S_1^2) by the smaller one (S_2^2). S^2 is calculated as follows:

$$S^2 = \frac{N \sum X^2 - \left(\sum X\right)^2}{N-1} \quad (26)$$

where N is the number of data in the group and X represents the individual values within the group.

Frequently, S^2 values may be obtained from ANOVA calculations. The calculated F value is compared to the appropriate number in an F value table for the appropriate degrees of freedom ($N-1$) in the numerator (along the top of the table) and in the denominator (along the side of the table). If the calculated value is smaller, it is not significant and the variances are considered homogeneous (the Student's t test would be appropriate for further comparison). If the calculated F value is greater, F is significant and the variances are heterogeneous (the modified Student's t test would be appropriate if $N_1 = N_2$, or the Cochran t test should be used if $N_1 \neq N_2$). See Fig. 5 to review the decision tree.

Assumptions and Limitations

1. This test could be considered as a two-group equivalent of the Bartlett's test.
2. If the test statistic is close to 1.0, the results are not significant.
3. The test assumes normality and independence of data.

4. Analysis of Variance

ANOVA is used for comparison of three or more groups of continuous data when the variances are homogeneous and data are independent and normally distributed. A series of

calculations are required for ANOVA, starting with the values within each group being added ($\sum X$) and then these sums being added ($\sum \sum X$). Each datum within the groups is squared, these squares are then summed ($\sum X^2$), and these sums added ($\sum \sum X^2$). Next the "correction factor" (CF) can be calculated:

$$CF = \frac{\left(\sum_1^K \sum_1^N X\right)^2}{N_1 + N_2 + \cdots N_k} \quad (27)$$

where N is the number of values in each group and K is the number of groups. The total sum of squares (SS) is then determined as follows:

$$SS_{total} = \sum_1^K \sum_1^N X^2 - CF \quad (28)$$

In turn, the sum of squares between groups (bg) is found from:

$$SS_{bg} = \frac{\left(\sum X_1\right)^2}{N_1} + \frac{\left(\sum X_2\right)^2}{N_2} + \cdots \frac{\left(\sum X_k\right)^2}{N_k} - CF \quad (29)$$

The sum of squares within group (wg) is then the difference between the last two equations:

$$SS_{wg} = SS_{total} - SS_{bg} \quad (30)$$

There are three types of degrees of freedom (df) to determine. The first, *total df*, is the total number of data within all groups under analysis minus one ($N_1 + N_2 + \ldots N_k - 1$), where k is the last measurement. For the second equation, the *df between groups* is the number of groups minus one ($K - 1$). The last equation (the *df within groups* or "error df") is the difference between the first two figures ($df_{total} - df_{bg}$).

The next set of calculations requires determination of the two mean squares (MS_{bg} and MS_{wg}). These are the respective sum of square values divided by the corresponding df figures ($MS = SS/df$). The final calculation is that of the F ratio. For this, the MS between groups is divided by the MS within groups ($F = MS_{bg}/MS_{wg}$).

For interpretation, the F ratio value obtained in the ANOVA is compared to a table of F values. If $F \leq 1.0$, the results are not significant and comparison with the table values is not necessary. The degrees of freedom (*df*) for the greater mean square (MS_{bg}) are indicated along the top of the table. Then read down the side of the table to the line corresponding to the df for the lesser mean square (MS_{wg}). The figure shown at the desired significance level (traditionally 0.05) is compared to the calculated F value. If the calculated number is smaller, there are no significant differences among the groups being compared. If the calculated value is larger, there is some difference but further (*post hoc*) testing will be required to determine which groups differ significantly.

Assumptions, Limitations, and Comments

1. The one-way analysis of variance ANOVA is the workhorse of toxicology. Many other forms exist for more complicated experimental designs.
2. The test is robust for moderate departures from normality if the sample sizes are large enough. Unfortunately, this is rarely the case in toxicologic pathology.
3. If the sample sizes are approximately equal, ANOVA is robust for moderate inequality of variances (as determined by Bartlett's test).
4. It is not appropriate to use a t test (or a two groups at a time version of ANOVA) to identify where significant differences are within the design group. A multiple-comparison *post hoc* method must be used.

5. Post Hoc Tests

A wide variety of *post hoc* tests are available to analyze data after finding a significant result from an ANOVA. Each of these tests has advantages and disadvantages, proponents and critics. Four of the tests used commonly in toxicologic pathology will be presented here. These are Duncan's multiple range test, Scheffe's multiple comparisons, Dunnett's t test, and Williams' t test. If ANOVA reveals no significance, it is inappropriate to proceed to perform a *post hoc* test in hope of finding differences. To do so would result in multiple comparisons, which increase the type I error rate beyond the desired level.

a. Duncan's Multiple Range Test. Duncan's multiple range test is used to compare groups of continuous and randomly distributed data such as body weights and organ weights. The test is used to determine where significant differences exist in three or more groups taken by evaluating one pair at a time. This test, as with other *post hoc* tests, should only follow observation of a significant F value in the ANOVA. It serves to determine which group (or groups) differ(s) significantly from other group (or groups).

There are two alternative methods of calculation. The selection of the proper one is based on whether the number of data (N) is equal or unequal in the groups.

i. Groups with equal numbers of data Two sets of calculations must be carried out: (1) determination of the difference between the means of pairs of groups and (2) preparation of a probability rate against which each difference in means is compared.

The means are determined (or taken from the ANOVA calculation) and ranked in either decreasing or increasing order. If two means are the same, they take up two equal positions in the rank. Thus, for four means we could have ranks of 1, 2, 2, and 4 rather than 1, 2, 3, and 4. Unlike nonparametric tests where the average rank is assigned to ties, this case would be 1, 2, 5, 2, 5, and 4. The groups are then taken in pairs and the differences between the means ($\bar{X}_1 - \bar{X}_2$), expressed as positive numbers, are calculated. Usually, each pair consists of a test group and the control group, although multiple tests groups may be compared if so desired. The relative rank of the two groups being compared must be considered. If a test group is ranked "2" and the control group is ranked "1," then we say that there are two places between them, whereas if the test group were ranked "3," then there would be three places between it and the control. To establish the probability table, the standard error of the mean (SEM) must be calculated:

$$\sqrt{\frac{\text{error mean square}}{N}} = \sqrt{\frac{\text{mean square within group}}{N}} \quad (31)$$

where N is the number of animals or replications per dose level.

The mean square within groups (MS_{wg}) can be calculated from the information given in the ANOVA procedure (refer to the earlier section on ANOVA). The SEM is then multiplied by a series of table values to set up a probability table. The table values used for the calculations are chosen according to the probability levels (note that the tables have sections for 0.05, 0.01, and 0.001 levels) and the number of means apart for the groups being compared and the number of "error" degrees of freedom (df). The "error" df is the number of df within the groups. This last figure is determined from the ANOVA calculation and can be taken from ANOVA output. For some values of df, the table values are not given and should thus be interpolated.

ii. Groups with unequal numbers of data This procedure is very similar to that discussed earlier. As before, the means are ranked and the differences between the means are determined ($\bar{X}_1 - \bar{X}_2$). Next, weighting values ("a_{ij}" values) are calculated for the pairs of groups being compared:

$$a_u = \sqrt{\frac{2N_iN_j}{(N_i + N_j)}} = \sqrt{\frac{2N_1N_2}{(N_1 + N_2)}} \tag{32}$$

This weighting value for each pair of groups is multiplied by ($\bar{X}_1 - \bar{X}_2$) for each value to arrive at a "t" value. It is the "t" that will later be compared to a probability table. The probability table is set up as before except that instead of multiplying the appropriate table values by SEM, SEM^2 is used. This is equal to $\sqrt{MS_{wg}}$.

For the desired comparison of two groups at a time, either the ($\bar{X}_1 - \bar{X}_2$) value (if $N_1 = N_2$) is compared to the appropriate probability table. Each comparison must be made according to the number of places between the means. If the table value is larger at the 0.05 level, the two groups are not considered statistically different. If the table value is smaller, the groups are different and the comparison is repeated at lower levels of significance. Thus, the degree of

significance may be determined. We might have significant differences at 0.05 but not at 0.01, in which case the probability would be represented at $0.05 > p > 0.01$.

Assumptions and Limitations

1. Duncan's assures a set α level or type I error rate for all tests when means are separated by approximately regular intervals. Preserving this α level means that the test is less sensitive than others are, such as the Student–Newman–Keuls test. The test is inherently conservative and not resistant or robust.

b. Scheffe's Multiple Comparisons. Scheffe's multiple comparison test is another *post hoc* comparison method for groups of continuous and randomly distributed data. It compares three or more groups and is widely considered a more powerful significance test than Duncan's.

Each *post hoc* comparison is tested by comparing an obtained test value (F_{contr}) with the appropriate critical F value at the selected level of significance (the table F value multipled by $K - 1$ for an F with $K - 1$ and $N - K$ degrees of freedom[2]). F_{contr} is computed as follows:

(a) Compute the mean for each sample (group)
(b) Denote the residual mean square by MS_{wg}
(c) Compute the test statistic as

$$F_{contr} = \frac{(C_1\bar{X}_1 + C_2\bar{X}_2 + \cdots + C_k\bar{X}_k^{12})}{(K - 1)MS_{wg}(C_1^2/n_1 + \cdots + C_K^2/n_k)}, \tag{33}$$

where C_k is the comparison number such that the sum of $C_1, C_2 \cdots C_k = 0$.

Assumptions and Limitations

1. The Scheffe procedure is robust to moderate violations of the normality and homogeneity of variance assumptions.
2. It is not formulated on the basis of groups with equal numbers (as one of Duncan's procedures is), and if $N_1 \neq N_2$, there is no separate weighing procedure.
3. It tests all linear contrasts among the population means (the other three methods confine themselves to pair-wise

comparison, except they use a Bonferroni type correlation procedure).

4. The Scheffe procedure is powerful because of it robustness, yet it is very conservative. The type I error (the false positive rate) is held constant at the selected test level for each comparison.

c. Dunnett's t Test.

Dunnett's t test assumes that what is desired is a comparison of each of several means with one other mean and only one other mean. In other words, it assumes that one wishes to compared each and every treatment group with the control group, but not compare treatment groups with each other. This causes a problem if a comparison of a treatment group with another treatment group is required. However, if one wants only to compare treatment groups versus a control group, Dunnett's is a useful approach.

To illustrate the method, let us evaluate a study with K groups (one of them being the control) where we wish to make $K - 1$ comparisons. In such a situation, we want to have a P level for the entire set of $K - 1$ decisions (not for each individual decision). The Dunnett's distribution is predicated on this assumption. The parameters for utilizing a Dunnett's table, such as found in his original article, are K (as described earlier) and the number of degrees of freedom for mean square within groups (MS_{wg}). The test value can be calculated as follows:

$$t = \frac{|T_j - T_i|}{\sqrt{2MS_{wg/n}}} \tag{34}$$

where n is the number of observations in each of the groups. The mean square within group (MS_{wg}) is as we have defined it previously; T_j is the control group mean and T_i is the mean of, in order, each successive test group observation. Note that one uses the absolute value of the positive number resulting from subtracting T_i from T_J. This is to ensure a positive number for t.

Assumptions and Limitations

1. Dunnett's seeks to ensure that the type 1 error rate will be fixed at the desired level

by incorporating correction factors into the design of the test value table.

2. Treated group sizes must be approximately equal.

d. Williams' t Test.

Williams' t test is popular, although its use is quite limited in toxicology. It is designed to detect the highest level in a set of dose/exposure levels at which there is no significant effect: it helps find the NOEL. It assumes that the response of interest, such as the change in body weights, occurs only at higher levels and that the responses are monotonically ordered so that $X_0 \leq X_1 \ldots \leq X_k$. This is, however, frequently not the case, e.g., in the case of "U"-shaped dose–response relationships for essential nutrients. The Williams' technique handles the occurrence of such discontinuities in a response series by replacing the "offending value" and the value immediately preceding it with weighted average values. The test is also adversely affected by any mortality at high dose levels. Such mortalities "impose a severe penalty, reducing the power of detecting an effect not only at level K but also at all lower doses." Accordingly, it is not generally applicable in toxicology studies.

G. HYPOTHESIS TESTING ON MULTIVARIATE PARAMETERS

1. Analysis of Covariance

Analysis of covariance (ANCOVA) is a method for comparing sets of data that consist of two variables (treatment and effect, with the effect variable being called the "variate") when a third variable (called the "covariate") exists. This covariate can be measured but not controlled and has a definite effect on the variable of interest. In other words, analysis of covariance provides an indirect type of statistical control, allowing us to increase the precision of a study and to remove a potential source of bias.

One common example of this is in the analysis of organ weights in toxicity studies. We usually wish to evaluate the effect of dose or exposure level on the specific organ weights, but most organ weights also increase in proportion to increase in animal body weight. Because primary interest is not in the effect of the body weight covariate, it is measured to allow for adjustment. Care must be taken before using ANCOVA, however, to ensure that the underlying nature of the correspondence between the variate and covariate is such that it be relied on as a tool for adjustments.

The calculation is performed in two steps. The first is a type of linear regression between the variate Y and the covariate X. This regression, performed as described under the linear regression section, gives the following model:

$$Y = a_1 + \text{B}X + e,\tag{35}$$

where a is the intercept value for the y axis, b is the slope factor, and e is the statistical error term.

This model in turn allows us to define adjusted means ($\bar{Y}$ and X) such that $\bar{Y}_{1a} = \bar{Y}_1 - (\bar{X}_1 - X^*)$. If we consider the case where K treatments are being compared such that $K = 1, 2, \ldots k$ and we let X_{ik} and Y_{ik} represent the predictor and predicted values for each individual i in group k, we can let X_k and Y_k be the means. Then, we define the between-group (for treatment) sum of squares and cross products as follows:

$$T_{xx} = \sum_{k-1}^{K} n_k (\bar{X}_K - \bar{X})^2$$
$$T_{yy} = \sum_{k-1}^{K} n_k (\bar{Y}_K - \bar{Y})^2 \tag{36}$$
$$T_{xy} = \sum_{k-1}^{K} n_k (\bar{X}_k - \bar{X})(\bar{Y}_k - \bar{Y})$$

In a like manner, within-group sums of squares and cross products are calculated as

$$\sum_{xx} = \sum_{k=1}^{k} \sum_{i} (X_{ik} - X_k)^2$$
$$\sum_{yy} = \sum_{k=1}^{k} \sum_{i} (Y_{ik} - Y_k)^2$$
$$\sum_{xy} = \sum_{k=1}^{k} \sum_{i} (X_{ik} - X_k)(Y_{ik} - Y_k),$$

where i indicates the sum from all the individuals within each group and f is the total number of subjects minus number of groups.

$$S_{xx} = T_{xx} + \sum_{xx}$$
$$S_{yy} = T_{yy} + \sum_{xx}$$
$$S_{xy} = T_{xy} + \sum_{xy}$$

With these in hand, calculate the residual mean squares of treatments (St^2) and error (Se^2)

$$\text{St}^2 = \frac{\text{Tyy} - \frac{S^2xy}{Sxx} + \frac{\sum^2 xy}{\sum xx}}{lc - 1}$$
$$\text{Se}^2 = \frac{\left(\sum yy - \frac{\sum^2 y}{\sum xx} \right)}{f - 1} \tag{37}$$

These can be used to calculate an F statistic to test the null hypothesis that all treatment effects are equal:

$$F = \frac{\text{St}^2}{\text{Se}^2} \tag{38}$$

B represents the estimated regression coefficient of Y or X:

$$B = \frac{\sum xy}{\sum xx} \tag{39}$$

The estimated standard error for the adjusted difference between two groups can also be calculated:

$$\text{Sd} = \text{Se} \sqrt{\frac{1}{n_j} + \frac{1}{n_j} + \frac{(X_i - X_j)^2}{\sum xx}}, \tag{40}$$

where n_0 and n_1 are the sample sizes of the two groups, sd is the standard deviation, se the standard error, and X_i and X_j are pairs of values of the independent variable.

A test of the null hypothesis that the adjusted difference between the groups is zero can now be determined:

$$t = \frac{Y_1 - Y_0 - B(X_1 - X_0)}{\text{Sd}}. \tag{41}$$

The test value for the t is then looked up in the t table with $n - 1$ degrees of freedom. Although this is a complex procedure, computation is markedly simplified if all the groups are of equal size.

Assumptions and Limitations

1. The underlying assumptions for AN-COVA are fairly rigid and restrictive.

391

The assumptions include (a) the slopes of the regression lines of a Y and X are equal from group to group. This can be examined visually or formally (i.e., by a test). If this condition is not met, ANCOVA cannot be used. (b) The relationship between X and Y is linear. (c) The covariate X is measured without error. Power of the test declines as error increases. (d) There are no unmeasured confounding variables. (e) The errors inherent in each variable are independent of each other. Lack of independence effectively (but to an immeasurable degree) reduces sample size. (f) The variances of the errors within groups are equivalent between groups. (g) Measured data that form the groups are normally distributed. ANCOVA is generally robust to departures from normality.

2. Of the seven assumptions, the first four are the most important.

H. MODELING

The mathematical modeling of biological systems is an extremely large and vigorously growing area. Broadly speaking, modeling is the principal conceptual tool by which toxicologic pathology seeks to develop as a mechanistic science. In an iterative process, models are developed or proposed, tested by experiment, and refined in a continuous cycle. Such a cycle could also be described as two related types of modeling: explanatory (where the concept is formed) and correlative (where data are organized and relationships derived).

In toxicologic pathology, modeling is of prime interest in seeking to relate a treatment variable with an effect variable. The resulting model can then be used to predict values of the effect variable at values of the treatment variable, which have not been evaluated experimentally. Note that interpolative models can only accurately predict effects within the range experimentally derived data points, such as LD_{50} values. Models for extrapolation are used to predict effects where data cannot be obtained, such as low dose carcinogenesis probability. In such cases the model may readily predict an outcome that cannot be verified by

experiment. Models are also used to estimate how good our prediction is and, occasionally, simply to determine if a pattern of effects is related to a pattern of treatment.

For use in prediction, the techniques of linear regression, probit/logit analysis, (a special case of linear regression), moving averages (an efficient approximation method), and nonlinear regression (for dose–response data that do not fit a linear pattern and cannot be made to fit a linear pattern by mathematical transformation) are presented in this section. For evaluating the predictive value of these models, both the correlation coefficient (for parametric data) and Kendall's rank correlation (for nonparametric data) are given. Finally, the concept of trend analysis is introduced and a method presented.

Interpolation is the term used to describe efforts made to establish a pattern between several data points. This pattern may be in the form of a line or a curve. It is possible for any given set of points to produce an infinite set of lines or curves that pass near, for lines, or through, for curves, the data points. In most cases, the actual "real" pattern is not known so a basic principle of science—ACM's razor—is applied. This principle recognizes that the simplest explanation or, in this case, model, that fits the facts or data is the most likely correct explanation. A straight line is, of course, the simplest pattern to describe, so fitting the best line using linear regression is the most common model used in toxicologic pathology.

1. Linear Regression

Foremost among the methods for interpolating within a known data relationship is regression. Regression is the mathematical fitting of a line or curve to a set of known data points on a graph, and the interpolation or "estimation" of values along this line or curve in areas where there are no experimental data points. The simplest regression model is that of linear regression, which is valid when increasing the value of one variable changes the value of the related variable in a linear fashion, either positively or negatively, or when data can be transformed in such a way that transformed data show a linear relationship. Linear regression using the method of least squares will be addressed.

Given two sets of variables, x (e.g., mg/kg of test material administered) and y (e.g., percentage of animals so dosed that die), a solution is required for a and b in the linear equation $Y_i = a + bx_i$ [where the uppercase Y_i is the fitted value of y_i at x_i, and we wish to minimize $(y_i - Y_i)^2$]. The solution is as follows.

The linear equation:

$$Y_i = a + bx_i$$

where the uppercase Y_i is the fitted value of y_i at x_i, and we wish to minimize $(y_i - Y_i)^2$

$$b = \frac{\sum x_i y_i - n\bar{x}\bar{y}}{\sum x_1^2 - n\bar{x}^2}$$

$$\text{and} \quad a = \bar{y} - b\bar{x}$$

where a is the y intercept, b is the slope of the time, and n is the number of data points.

Note that in actuality, dose–response relationships are often not linear and instead either a transform to linearize the data or a nonlinear regression method must be used. Note also that the correlation test statistic (see correlation coefficient section) can be used to determine if the regression is significant and, therefore, the linear model is valid at a defined level of certainty.

A more specific test for significance is the linear regression analysis of variance. To do so, start by developing the appropriate ANOVA table, as described in Section VIIF4. Finally, determine the confidence intervals for the regression line. That is, given a regression line with calculated values for Y_i given x_i, within what limits at a 95% probability of certainty does the real value of Y_i lie? If the residual mean square in the ANOVA is given by s^2, the 95% confidence limits for a (denoted by A, the notation for the true—as opposed to the estimated—value for this parameter) can be calculated[2]:

---

[2]There are many excellent texts on regression, which is a powerful technique. These include Draper and Smith (1981) and Montgomery and Smith (1983), which are not overly rigorous mathematically.

$$t_{n-2} = \frac{a - A}{\sqrt{\dfrac{s^2(\sum x^2)}{n\sum x_i^2 - n^2\bar{x}^2}}} \tag{43}$$

Assumptions and Limitations

1. All the regression methods are for interpolation, not extrapolation. That is, they are valid only in the range that we have experimentally derived data not beyond. Note: extrapolation is common in attempting to determine effects beyond measured data. If such an extrapolation is made, the fact that this is a best guess must be given in the text and discussion as to the limitations of the prediction given.

2. The method assumes that data are independent and normally distributed and it is sensitive to outliers. The x axis (or horizontal) component plays an extremely important part in developing the least-square fit. All points have equal weight in determining the height of a regression line, but extreme x axis values unduly influence the slope of the line.

3. A good fit between a line and a set of data (i.e., a strong correlation between treatment and response variables) does not imply any causal relationship.

4. It is assumed that the treatment variable can be measured without error, that each data point is independent, that variances are equivalent, and that a linear relationship does not exist between the variables.

2. Probit/Log Transforms and Regression

Dose–response relationships are among the most common interpolation problems encountered in toxicologic pathology. As noted in the preceding section, these relationships are rarely simple so that a valid linear regression often cannot be made directly from raw data. The most common valid interpolation methods are based on probability ("probit") and logarithmic ("log") value scales, with percentage responses (death, tumor incidence, etc.) being expressed on the probit scale while doses (X_i) are expressed on the log scale.

There are two strategies for such an approach. The first is based on transforming data to these scales and then calculating a weighted linear regression on the transformed data. However, if one does not have access to a computer or a high-powered programmable calculator, it is not practical to assign weights to data. The second strategy requires the use of algorithms for the probit value and regression process and is extremely burdensome to perform manually.

An approach to the first strategy requires construction of a table with the pairs of values of x_i and y_i listed in order of increasing values of Y_i (percentage response). Beside each of these columns a set of blank columns remain so that the transformed values may be listed. Then the columns are added as described in the linear regression procedure. Log and probit values may be taken from any of a number of sets of tables in standard texts. The remainder of the table is then developed from the transformed x_i and y_i values (denoted as x_i' and y_i'). A standard linear regression is then performed.

The second strategy we discussed has been broached by a number of authors. All of these methods are computationally cumbersome. It is possible to approximate the necessary iterative process using the algorithms developed by Abramowitz and Stegun, but this process merely reduces the complexity to a point where the procedure may be readily programmed on a small computer or programmable calculator.

Assumptions and Limitations

1. The probit distribution is derived from a common error function, with the midpoint (50% point) moved to a score of 5.00.

2. The underlying frequency distribution becomes asymptotic as it approaches the extremes of the range. That is, in the range of 16 to 84%, the corresponding probit values change gradually—the curve is relatively linear. Beyond this range, however, they change ever more rapidly as they approach either 0 or 100%. In fact, there are no values for either of these numbers.

3. A normally distributed population is assumed, and the results are sensitive to outliers.

3. Nonlinear Regression

More often than not in toxicologic pathology, relationships between two variables are non-

linear, e.g., age and body weight. That is, a change in one variable (e.g., age) does not produce a directly proportional change in the other (e.g., body weight), but some relationship between the variables is apparent. If understanding such a relationship and being able to predict unknown points are of value, two options are available.

The first, which was discussed and reviewed earlier, is to use one or more transformations to make data linear. Once linear, a linear regression can be used. This commonly used approach has a number of drawbacks. Not all data can be suitably transformed. Sometimes the transformations necessary to achieve linearity require a cumbersome series of calculations. In addition, the resulting linear regression is not always sufficient to account for the differences among sample values. For example, there may be significant deviations around the linear regression line, i.e., a line may still not give us a good fit to data or do an adequate job of representing the relationship between data. In such cases, a second option can be used: fitting of data to some nonlinear function such as some form of curve. This is the general principle of nonlinear regression and may involve fitting data to an infinite number of possible functions. However, most often fitting curves to a polynomial function of the general form is used. As the number of powers of x increases, the curve becomes increasingly complex and more likely to fit a given set of data.

$$Y = a + bx + cx^2 + dx^2 + \ldots, \quad (44)$$

where x is the independent variable.

Plotting the log of a response, such as body weight, versus a linear scale of dose or stimulus, results in one of four types of nonlinear curves: *exponential growth, exponential decay, asymptotic regression*, and *logistic growth curve*. The following formulae [Eqs. (45–48)] describe these curves.

Formula for an exponential growth curve: $\log Y = A(B^x)$, e.g., growth curve for the log phase of a bacterial culture (45)

Formula for an exponential decay curve: $\log Y = A(B^{-x})$, e.g., radioactive decay curve. (46)

Formula for an asymptotic regression curve: $\log Y = A - B(p^x)$, such as a first-order reaction curve (47)

Formula for a logistic growth curve: $\log Y = A/(1 + Bp^x)$, e.g., a population growth curve. (48)

In all these cases A and B are constants while p is a log transform. These curves are illustrated in Fig. 14.

Iterative processes fit all four types of curves shown in Fig. 14. That is, best guess numbers are initially chosen for each of the constants and, after a fit is attempted, the constants are modified to improve the fit. This process is repeated until an acceptable fit has been generated. Analysis of variance or covariance can be used to objectively evaluate the acceptability of the choice.

Assumptions and Limitations

1. The principle of using least squares may still be applicable in fitting the best curve, if the assumptions of normality, independence, error-free measurement of the dose, and reasonably error–free measurement of response are valid.
2. Growth curves are best modeled using a nonlinear method.

4. Correlation Coefficient

The correlation procedure is used to determine the degree of linear correlation, or direct relationship, between two groups of continuous and normally distributed variables. Correlation indicates whether there is any statistical

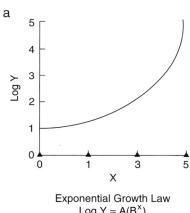

Exponential Growth Law
$\log Y = A(B^x)$

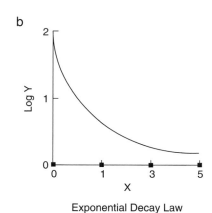

Exponential Decay Law
$\log Y = A(B^{-x})$

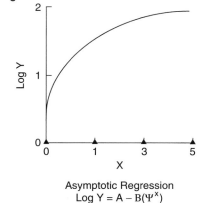

Asymptotic Regression
$\log Y = A - B(\Psi^x)$

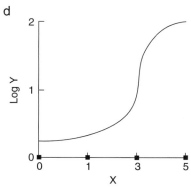

Logistic Growth Law
$\log Y = A/(1 + B\Psi^x)$

Figure 14. Common curvilinear curves.

relationship between the variables in the two groups. For example, liver weights of dogs on a feeding study may be correlated with their body weights. Thus, the correlation coefficient can be calculated between liver and body weights measured at necropsy to determine if there is some relationship. A formula for calculating the linear correlation coefficient (r_{xy}) is

$$r_{xy} = \frac{N\sum XY - (\sum X)(\sum Y)}{\sqrt{N\sum X^2 - (\sum X)^2}\sqrt{N\sum Y^2 - (\sum Y)^2}} \quad (49)$$

where X is each value for one variable (such as dog body weights in the example given earlier), Y is the matching value for the second variable (the liver weights), and N is the number of pairs of X and Y.

Once r_{xy} has been determined, it is possible to calculate t_r, which can be used for more precise examination of the degree of significant linear relationship between the two groups. This value is calculated as:

$$t_r = \frac{r_{zy}\sqrt{N-2}}{\sqrt{1 - r_{zy}^2}}. \quad (50)$$

It should be noted that this calculation is equivalent to r = sample covariance/ $(S_x S_y)$, as was seen earlier under ANCOVA.

The value obtained for r_{xy} can be compared to table values for the number of pairs of data involved minus two. If the r_{xy} is smaller at the selected test probability level the correlation is not significantly different from zero. There is no correlation. If r_{xy} is larger than the table value, there is a positive statistical relationship between the groups. Comparisons are then made at lower levels of probability to determine the degree of relationship. Note that if r_{xy} = either 1.0 or −1.0, there is complete correlation between the groups. If r_{xy} is a negative number and the absolute is greater than the table value, there is an inverse relationship between the groups. In other words, a change in one group is associated with a change in the opposite direction in the second group of variables.

Because the comparison of r_{xy} with the table values may be considered a somewhat weak test, it is perhaps more meaningful to compare

the t_r value with values in a t distribution table for N-2 degrees of freedom (df), as is done for the Student's t test. This will give a more exact determination of the degree of statistical correlation between the two groups. Note that this method examines only possible linear relationships between sets of continuous, normally distributed data.

Assumptions and Limitations

1. A strong correlation does not imply a causal relationship.[3]
2. The distances of data points from the regression line are the portions of the data not "explained" by the model. These are called residuals. Poor correlation coefficients imply high residuals, which may be due to many small contributions (variations of data from the regression line) or a few large ones. Extreme values (outliers) reduce correlation greatly.
3. X and Y are assumed to be independent as a null hypothesis. The test determines whether the dependent variable (Y) depends on the "independent variable (X).
4. r^2, the square of the correlation coefficient, is also called the coefficient of determination. It is a measure of the proportion of the variation of one variable determined by the variation of the other variable.

5. Kendall's Coefficient of Rank Correlation

Kendall's rank correlation, represented by τ, should be used to evaluate the degree of association between two sets of data when the nature of data is such that the relationship may not be linear. Most commonly, this occurs when data are not continuous and/or normally distributed. An example of such a situation is when an attempt is made to determine if there is a relationship between the number of hydra and their survival time in a test medium measured as a duration of hours (e.g., 1–2 hr, 2–3 hr). Both variables are discontinuous, yet a relationship probably exists as survival appears

[3]Feinstein (1979) has provided a fine discussion of the difference between correlation (or association of variables) and causation.

to decrease with time. Another common use of Kendall's rank correlation is to compare subjective scoring of lesions by two different toxicologic pathologists.

τ is calculated at $\tau = N/n(n-1)$, where n is the sample size and N is the count of ranks, calculated as $N = 4\sum^n C_i - n(n-1)$. If a second variable Y_2 is correlated exactly with the first variable Y_1, then the variates Y_2 should be in the same rank order as the Y_1 variates. However, if the correlation is less than exact the order of the variates, the rank order of Y_2 will not correspond entirely to that of Y. The quantity N measures how well the rank order of the second variable corresponds to the rank order of the first. It has a maximum value of $n(n-1)$ and a minimum value of $-n(n-1)$.

A table of data is created, and each of the two variables is ranked separately. Tied ranks are assigned as shown earlier under the Kruskal–Wallis test. From this point the original variates are disregarded and only ranks are used to complete the test. The ranks of one of the two variables are placed in rank order, from lowest to highest, paired with the rank values assigned for the other variable. If one, but not the other, variable has tied ranks, pairs are made with the variables without ties. The resulting value of τ will range from -1 to $+1$, as does the familiar parametric correlation coefficient, r.

Comment

1. A very robust estimator that does not assume normality, linearity, or minimal error of measurement.

6. Trend Analysis

Trend analysis is a collection of techniques dating back to the mid-1950s that have been employed in toxicology applications since the mid-1970s. These methods are a variation on the theme of regression testing. Trend analyses are used to determine whether a sequence of observations, taken over an ordered range of a variable (most commonly time), exhibit a pattern of change in another variable of interest, e.g., dosage or an exposure. For the purpose of illustration, time will be considered as the independent variable in the following discussion.

Trend corresponds to sustained and systematic variations over a long period of time. It is associated with the structural causes of the phenomenon in question, e.g., population growth, technological progress, new ways of organization, or capital accumulation. The identification of trend has always posed a challenging statistical problem. The difficulty is not one of mathematical or analytical complexity, but rather of conceptual complexity: one uses nonobservable variables. In this case, the extrapolation is made without support of measured data. Assumptions must be made on these latent, or unmeasured, variables as to their behavioral pattern. The trend is generally thought of as a smooth and slow movement over a long term. The concept of "long" in this connection is relative and what is identified as trend for a given series span might well be part of a long cycle once the series is considerably augmented. Often, a long cycle is treated as a trend because the length of the observed time series is shorter than one complete face of this type of cycle.

The ways in which data are collected in toxicologic pathology studies frequently serve to complicate trend analysis. This complication occurs because the features of the experimental design frequently artificially censor the length of time available for the phenomenon underlying a trend to be manifested. To avoid the complexity of the problem posed by a statistically vague definition, statisticians have resorted to two simple solutions. First, trend and cyclical fluctuations can be estimated together, calling this combined movement *trend cycle*. Second, the trend can be defined in terms of the series length, denoting it as the longest nonperiodic movement.

Within the large class of models identified for trend, we can distinguish two main categories, deterministic trends and stochastic trends. Deterministic trend models are based on the assumption that the trend of a time series can be approximated closely by simple mathematical functions of time over the entire span of the series.

397

These tests can be thought of as special cases of regression or correlation tests, in which association is sought between the observations and its ordered sample index. They are also related to ANOVA, except that the tests are tailored to be powerful against the subset of alternatives H_1 instead of the more general set $\{F_i \neq F_j, \text{some } i \neq j\}$. Different tests arise from requiring power against specific elements or subsets of this rather extensive set of alternatives.

The most popular trend test in toxicologic pathology is currently the Tarone trend test and is used by the National Cancer Institute (NCI) in the analysis of carcinogenicity data. A simple, but efficient alternative to this test is the Cox and Stuart test, which is a modification of the sign test. For each time point at which a measurement is made (such as the incidence of animals observed with tumors), a pair of observations is prepared: one from each of the groups we wish to compare.

In a traditional NCI bioassay this would mean pairing the control with low dose and low dose with high dose to explore a dose-related trend. Also, each time period observation in a dose group (except the first) with its predecessor is commonly compared to evaluate the time-related trend. When the second observation in a pair exceeds the earlier observation, a plus sign for that pair is recorded. When the first observation is greater than the second, a minus sign for that pair is used. A preponderance of plus signs suggests a downward trend, whereas an excess of minus signs suggests an upward trend. A formal test at an *a priori* selected confidence level can then be performed.

After defining the trend to test, first match the pairs as $(X_1 - X_{1+c}), (X_2, X_{2+C}), \ldots (X_{n'-c}, X_{n'})$, where $c = n'/2$ when n' is even and $c = (n' + 1)/2$ when n' is odd (where n' is the number of observations in a set). Comparing the resulting number of excess positive or negative signs against a sign test table then tests the hypothesis. Combination of a number of observations allows active testing for a set of trends, such as the existence of a trend of increasing difference between two groups of animals over a period of time.

Assumption and Limitation

1. Trend tests seek to evaluate whether there is a monotonic tendency in response to a change in treatment. That is, the dose–response direction is absolute: as dose goes up, the incidence of tumor increases. Thus the test loses power rapidly in response to the occurrences of "reversals," e.g., a low dose group with a decreased tumor incidence. There are methods that "smooth the bumps" of reversals in long data series. In toxicology, however, most data series are short, i.e., there are only a few dose levels.

Tarone's trend test is most powerful at detecting dose-related trends when tumor onset hazard functions are proportional to each other. For more power against other dose-related group differences, weighted versions of the statistic are also available.

In 1985, the United States *Federal Register* recommended that the analysis of tumor incidence data be carried out with a Cochran–Armitage trend test. The test statistic of the Cochran–Armitage test is defined as

$$T_{CA} = \sqrt{\frac{N}{(N-r))r}} \cdot \frac{\sum_{i=0}^{k}\left(R_1 - \frac{n_1}{N}r\right)d_1}{\sqrt{\sum_{i=0}^{k}\frac{n_i}{N}d_i^2 - \left(\sum_{i=0}^{k}\frac{n_i}{N}d_1\right)^2}}, \quad (51)$$

where dose scores are represented by d_i., the test statistic is represented by T, and the maximum likelihood estimator is represented by n/N.

Armitage's test statistic is the square of this term (T_{CA}^2). As one-sided tests are carried out for an increase of tumor rates, the square is not considered. Instead, the just-mentioned test statistic is used. This test statistic is asymptotically standard normal distributed.

Assumptions and Limitations

1. The Cochran–Armitage test is asymptotically efficient for all monotone alternatives, but this result only holds asymptotically.

2. Tumors are rare events; therefore, the binomial proportions are small. In this situation, approximations may become unreliable.

To address this potential unreliability, exact tests can be performed using conditional and unconditional approaches. In the conditional approach, the total number of tumors r is regarded as fixed. As a result the null distribution of the test statistic is independent of the common probability p. The exact conditional null distribution is a multivariate hypergeometric distribution. In contrast, the unconditional model treats the sum of all tumors as a random variable. Then the exact unconditional null distribution is a multivariate binomial distribution. the distribution depends on the unknown probability.

I. METHODS FOR THE REDUCTION OF DIMENSIONALITY

Techniques for the reduction of dimensionality are those that simplify the visual or numerical aspects of data to improve an understanding of patterns, while causing only minimal reductions in the amount of information present. These techniques operate primarily by pooling or combining groups of variables into single variables, but may also entail the identification and elimination of low information content, or irrelevant, variables.

Descriptive statistics, such as calculations of means and standard deviations, are the simplest and most familiar form of reduction of dimensionality. Other forms of reduction require the general conceptual tools of classification. *Classification* provides identities, quantities, similarities, and differences between groups of things that have more than a single linear scale of measurement in common. Classification is required for stratification of data. All classes essentially have to be mutually exclusive and mutually exhaustive so that data can be placed in only one class. Classification will be discussed further in the following section.

Multidimensional scaling (MDS) is a set of techniques for quantitatively analyzing simi-

larities, dissimilarities, and distances between data in a display-like manner. Nonmetric scaling is an analogous set of methods for displaying and relating data when measurements are nonquantitative, i.e., either categorical (nominal) or ordinal. In such a case, attributes or ranks describe the data. *Cluster analysis* is a collection of graphic and numerical methodologies for classifying things based on the relationships between the values of the variables that they share.

The final pair of methods for reduction of dimensionality, which will be addressed later in this chapter, are *Fourier analysis* and the *life table analysis*. Fourier analysis seeks to identify cyclic patterns in data and then either analyzes the patterns or the residuals after the patterns are taken out. Life table analysis techniques are directed at identifying and quantifying the time course of certain risks, such as death, or the occurrence of tumors.

1. Reduction of Dimensionality through Classification

Classification is both a basic concept and a collection of techniques, which are necessary prerequisites for further analysis of data when the members of a set of data are, or can be, each described by several variables. At least some degree of classification is necessary prior to any data collection (Table XVI). Classification enables subgrouping members of a group in accordance with a set of decision rules. Whether formally or informally, an investigator has to decide which characteristics are similar enough to be counted as the same and develop rules for governing collection procedures. Such rules can be simple as "measure and record body weights only of live animals on study" or as complex as that demonstrated by the expanded weighting classification procedure demonstrated later. Such a classification also demonstrates that the selection of which variables to measure will determine the final classification of data. Finally, classification needs to be balanced against the numbers of individuals within each class. As classes must be mutually exclusive and mutually exhaustive, excessive classification can reduce the number of individuals within the subgroups. The comical extent of such activity may result in each individual residing in a different class, thereby resulting in zero degrees of freedom for statistical analysis.

Classifications of data have two purposes: *data simplification*, which is also called a descriptive function, and *prediction*. Simplification is necessary because there is a limit to both the volume and the complexity of data that the human mind can comprehend and deal with conceptually. Classification allows us to name each group of data, hence these data are sometimes referred to as *nominal* data. Classification also permits creation of a summary of the data, i.e., assign individual elements of data to groups and to characterize the population of the group. Finally, it helps the scientist define the relationships between groups, i.e., develop taxonomy. An excellent example of such a classification scheme is given in Chapter 7.

Prediction, meanwhile, is the use of summaries of data and knowledge of the relationships between groups to develop hypotheses as to what will happen when further data are collected. Classification is necessary to predict risks *a priori* as required in risk characterization, part of the risk assessment and risk management process. For example, as more animals, or people, are exposed to an agent under defined conditions, a predicted outcome can be derived, e.g., number of tumors. By creating mutually exclusive classes, mechanisms can be investigated as to how such relationships develop.

Indeed, classification is the prime device for the discovery of mechanisms in all of science. A classic example of the use of classification was Darwin's realization that there were reasons, the theory of evolution, behind the differences and similarities in species. Earlier, this diversity led Linaeus to develop his initial modern classification scheme, or taxonomy, for animals.

2. Expanded Weighting Procedure

To develop a classification, one first sets bounds wide enough to encompass the entire range of data to be considered. This is typically done by selecting some global variables, which are variables every piece of data have in common, and limiting the range of each so that it just encompasses all the cases on hand. Then a set of local variables that serve to differentiate groups is selected. These variables have characteristics that only some of the cases have; others lack the characteristic. For example, the occurrence of certain tumor types, enzyme activity levels, or dietary preferences may be used to classify animals in an experiment.

Data are then collected, and a system for measuring differences and similarities is developed. Such measurements are based on some form of measurement of distance between two cases (x and y) in terms of each single variable scale. If the variable is a continuous one, then the simplest measure of distance between two pieces of data is the Euclidean distance ($d[x, y]$):

TABLE XVI
Example of Classification of Data from a Toxicologic Pathology Experiment

Decision criteria	Quantal output	Nominal (class output)
Is animal of desire species?	Yes/no	
Is animal member of study group?	Yes/no	
Is animal alive?	Yes/no	
Which group does animal belong to?		A. Control
		B. Low dose
		C. Intermediate dose
		D. High dose
What sex is animal?	Male/female	
Is the measured weight in acceptable range?		Yes/no

400

$$d(x, y) = \sqrt{(x_i - y_i)^2} \qquad (52)$$

For categorical or discontinuous data, the simplest distance measure is the matching distance, defined as

$$d(x, y) = \text{number of times } x_i \neq y_i.$$

After developing a table of such distance measurements for each of the local variables, some weighting factor is assigned to each variable. A weighting factor gives greater importance to those variables that are believed to have more relevance or predictive value. The weighted variables are then used to assign each piece of data to a group. The actual act of developing numerically based classifications and assigning data members to them is the realm of cluster analysis and is discussed later. Classification of biological data based on qualitative factors is a well-discussed area by authors who deal with both field and mathematical concepts.

Relevant examples of the use of classification techniques range from the simple to the complex. Toxicological pathologists grading the severity of lesions commonly use a simple classification of response. At the other end of the spectrum, mathematically based systems are used to classify data.

3. Multidimensional and Nonmetric Scaling

Multidimensional scaling is a collection of analysis methods for data sets that have three or more variables making up each data point. MDS displays the relationships of three or more dimensional extension of the methods of statistical graphics described previously.

MDS presents the structure of a set of objects from data that approximate the distances between pairs of the objects. Presented data contain similarities, dissimilarities, distances, or proximities. These data must be presented in such a form that the degree of similarities and differences between the pairs of the objects, each of which represents a real-life data point, can be measured and handled as a distance. The reader is referred back to the discussion of measures of distances under classifications. Similarity is a matter of degree. Objects with small differences among one another show a high degree of similarity, whereas objects are considered dissimilar if large differences exist.

In addition to the traditional human subjective judgments of similarity, data can be grouped based on an "objective" similarity measure, e.g., the difference in weight between a pair of animals. An index can be used to calculate similarity from multivariate data, e.g., the proportion of agreement in the results of a number of carcinogenicity studies. However, data must always represent the degree of similarity of pairs of objects.

A point in a multidimensional space represents each object or data point. These plots or projected points are arranged in this space so that the distances between pairs of points have the strongest possible relation to the degree of similarity among the pairs of objects. That is, two points that are close together represent two similar objects, and a pair of points that are far apart represent two dissimilar objects. The space is usually a two or three-dimensional Euclidean space but may be non-Euclidean and may have more dimensions.

MDS is a general term that includes a number of different types of techniques. However, all methods seek to allow geometric analysis of multivariate data. The forms of MDS can be classified according to the nature of the similarities in the data as qualitative, nonmetric (or quantitative), and metric MDS. MDS types can also be classified by the number of variables involved and by the nature of the model used. For example, in classical MDS there is only one data matrix, and no weighting factors are used. However, in replicated MDS, more than one matrix is used with no weighting. In weighted MDS, more than one matrix is used and at least some of the data are weighted.

MDS can be used in toxicologic pathology to analyze the similarities and differences between effects produced by different agent in an attempt to use an understanding of the mechanism underlying the actions of one agent to determine the mechanisms of the other agents. Algorithms and a good intermediate level presentation of MDS can be found in Davison (1983).

Nonmetric scaling is useful for the reduction of dimensionality. Nonmetric scaling uses a set of graphical techniques closely related to MDS. The primary objective of nonmetric scaling is to arrange a set of objects, which usually consist of a number of related observations, graphically in a few dimensions. This is done while retaining the maximum possible fidelity to the original relationships between members; i.e., values that are most different from each other are portrayed as furthest apart. This scaling is not a linear technique, as it does not preserve linear relationships, i.e., A is not shown as twice as far from C as B, even though its "value difference" may be twice as great. The spacing, or interpoint distance, is kept such that if the distance of the original scale between members A and B is greater than that between C and D, the distance on the model scale is greater between A and B than between C and D. Figure 10, presented earlier, uses a form of this technique in adding a third dimension by using letters to present degrees of effect on the skin.

This technique functions by taking observed measures of similarity or dissimilarity between every pair of M objects and then finding a representation of the objects as points in Euclidean space such that the interpoint distances "match," in some sense, the observed similarities or dissimilarities by means of weighting constants.

4. Cluster Analysis

Cluster analysis is a quantitative form of classification. It serves to help develop decision rules and then uses these rules to assign a heterogeneous collection of objects to a series of sets. This is almost entirely an applied rather than a theoretical methodology. The final result of cluster analysis is graphical display of classifications and a set of decision rules for the assignment of new members into the classifications.

The classification procedures are based on either density of population or distance between members. These methods can serve to generate a basis for the classification of large numbers of dissimilar variables. Examples of dissimilar variable include behavioral observations and compounds with distinct but related structures (i.e., homologs or analogs) and mechanisms of toxicity and to separate tumor patterns caused by treatment from those caused by old age.

There are four types of clustering techniques discussed in this chapter. In *hierarchical techniques*, classes are subclassified into groups, with the process being repeated at several levels to produce a tree that gives sufficient definition to the groups. In *optimizing techniques*, clusters are formed by optimization of a clustering criterion. The resulting classes are mutually exclusive where the objects are partitioned clearly into sets. In *density-* or *mode-seeking techniques*, clusters are identified and formed by locating regions in a graphical representation that contains concentrations of data points. In *clumping techniques*, a variation of density-seeking techniques are used in which assignment to a cluster is weighted on some variables so that clusters may overlap in graphic projections. We not that there are other methods, which are not discussed in this chapter. These methods are well described in the literature.

5. Fourier or Time Analysis

Fourier analysis is used most frequently as a univariate method for either simplifying data or for modeling. It can also be used as a multivariate technique for data analysis. In a sense, Fourier analysis is similar to trend analysis. It evaluates the relationship of sets of data from a different perspective. In the case of Fourier analysis, the approach resolves the time dimension variable in the data set. At the simplest level, Fourier analysis assumes that many events are periodic in nature, and the variation in other variables due to this periodicity can be removed using Fourier transforms. More powerful analysis can be done on Fourier-transformed data using the remaining (i.e., time-independent) variation from other variables. Unfortunately, when there may be several overlying cyclic time-based periodicities, or if time cycle event analysis is required, Fourier analysis may not be appropriate.

Fourier analysis allows one to identify, quantify, and remove the time-based cycles in data if necessary. The amplitudes, phases, and frequencies of data are evaluated by use of the Fourier transform.

6. Life Tables

Chronic *in vivo* studies are generally the most complex and expensive toxicity studies. Answers to multiple questions are sought in such a study, particularly if a material results in a significant increase in mortality or in the incidence of tumors in those animals exposed to it. The time course of these adverse effects is an essential part of the evaluation. The classic approach to assessing these age-specific hazard rates is by the use of life tables, also called survivorship tables.

It may readily be seen that during any selected period of time (t_i) there are a number of risks, or adverse events, that may affect an animal. These main adverse events usually considered are "natural death," death induced by a direct or indirect action of the test compound, and death due to occurrences of interest such as tumors. Of particular interest is whether, and when, the last two of these risks become significantly different from the "natural" risks, which are defined by events seen in the control group. Life table methods enable such determinations as the duration of survival, or time until tumors develop, and the probability of survival or the probability of developing a tumor, during any period of time to be made.

To use life table analysis, the interval length (t_i) for examination within the study must first be determined. As the interval is shortened, the information gained becomes more exact, but as interval length is decreased, the number of intervals increases and calculations become more cumbersome and less indicative of time-related trends because random fluctuations become more apparent. For a lifetime rodent study, an interval length of a month is commonly employed. Some life table methods, such as the *Kaplan–Meyer* table, display each new event, such as a death, as the start of a new interval.

Once the time interval length has been established, data are tabulated. A separate table is created for each group of animals, e.g., sex and dose level. The following columns are recorded in each table.

1. Interval of time selected (t_i).
2. Number of animals in the group that entered that interval of the study alive (I_i).
3. Number of animals withdrawn from study during the interval (such as those taken for an interim sacrifice or that may have been killed by a technician error) (ω_i).
4. Number of animals that died during the interval (d_i).
5. Number of animals at risk during the interval, $l_i = I_i - \frac{1}{2}\omega_i$, or the number on study at the start of the interval minus one half of the number withdrawn during the interval.
6. Proportion of animals that died $= D_i \frac{d_i}{l_i}$.
7. Cumulative probability of an animal surviving until the end of that interval of study, $P_i = 1 - D_i$, or one minus the number of animals that died during that interval divided by the number of animals at risk.
8. Number of animals dying until that interval (M_i).
9. Animals found to have died during the interval (m_i).
10. Probability of dying during the interval of the study $c_i = 1 - (M_i + m_i/l_i)$, or the total number of animals dead until that interval plus the animals discovered to have died during that interval divided by the number of animals at risk through the end of that interval.
11. Cumulative proportion surviving, p_i, is equivalent to the cumulative product of the interval probabilities of survival (i.e., $p_i = p_1.p_2.p_3 \ldots p_x$),
12. Cumulative probability of dying, C_i, equal to the cumulative product of the interval probabilities to that point (i.e., $C_i = c_1.c_2.c_3 \cdots c_x$).

403

Once the tables have been produced for each group in a study, the hypotheses that each of the treated groups has a significantly shorter duration of survival, or that individuals in the treated groups died more quickly, can be tested. Note that plots of total number of dead and alive animals will give one an appreciation of the data, but can lead to no statistical conclusions. There are many methods for testing significance in life tables, where the power of the analysis increases, as does the difficulty of computation [Eq. (53)].

First, the standard error of the K interval survival rate as:

$$S_K = P_k \sqrt{\sum_1^k \left(\frac{D_i}{l'_x - d_x} \right)}$$

The effective sample size (l_1) can be calculated in accordance with

$$l_1 = \frac{P(1 - P)}{S^2}$$

Compute the standard error of difference for any two groups (1 and 2) as

$$S_D = \sqrt{S_1^2 + S_2^2}$$

The difference in survival probabilities for the two groups is then calculated as

$$P_D = P_1 - P_2$$

The test statistic is then calculated as

$$t' = \frac{P_D}{S_D}$$

This is then compared to the z distribution table. If $t' > z$ at the desired probability level, it is significant at that level.

Life table analysis has become a mainstay in chronic studies. An example is the reassessment of the ED_{01} study, which radically changed interpretation of the results and understanding of underlying methods when adjustment for time on study was made. The increased importance and interest in the analysis of survival data have not been restricted to toxicology, but rather have encompassed all the life sciences. There are other general discussions regarding this subject for those with further interest.

J. META-ANALYSIS

Meta-analysis, meaning "analysis among," is being used increasingly in biomedical research to try to obtain a qualitative or quantitative synthesis of the research literature on a particular issue. The technique is usually applied to the synthesis of several separate but comparable studies. The process of systematic reviews and meta-analysis has three main components: (1) systematic review and selection of studies and (2) quantitative and (3) qualitative analyses.

1. Selection of Studies to be Analyzed: Systematic Reviews

The issue of study selection is perhaps the most problematic for those investigators doing meta-analysis. The criteria for selection may vary from project to project. However, there are several factors concerning selection that must be addressed before analyses commence. Each choice made by the investigator must be weighed carefully as to the likely effect of selection bias versus the perceived bias that the selection was designed to remove.

a. Use of the Gray Literature. The current dogma among many scientists is that only peer-reviewed literature is valuable for inclusion in reviews, and therefore by inference, systematic reviews. Should studies be limited to those that are peer reviewed or published? It is well known that negative studies, or those that report little or no benefit from following a particular course of action, are less likely to be published than positive studies. Therefore, the published literature may be biased toward studies with positive results, and a synthesis of these studies would give a biased estimate of the impact of pursuing some courses of action.

When a systematic review is planned, a plethora of industrial, academic, and government research papers have often been prepared that deal with the issue under consideration. Unfortunately, access to this gray literature is limited, although there are search engines now available for attempting to discover this unpublished information. These studies may give a less biased report on the topic in question; however, a number of these unpublished studies may be of lower quality than peer-reviewed materials. Sometimes poor research methods can produce reported results that underestimate the impact, hence providing an opposite bias to that described earlier.

b. Peer Review. As mentioned above, peer review is considered the primary method for quality control in scientific publishing. Should publications in a systematic review and meta-analysis be limited to peer-reviewed articles and, if so, what journals should be included or excluded? The choice of journal may be used as another filter based on the rigor of review and editor latitude given to fill the journal. Some investigators recommend that only those studies that are published in peer-reviewed publications be considered in meta-analysis. Although this may seem an attractive option, it might produce an even more highly biased selection of studies for systematic review.

c. Quality Control. Peer review is not the only method of providing quality control and quality assured data for meta-analysis. Additional quality control and assurance criteria may be used to select the best and most reliable data during systematic review. The rhetorical question we ask is should studies be limited to those that meet additional quality control criteria? If investigators, undertaking a systematic review, impose an additional set of criteria before including a study in the meta-analysis, the average quality of the studies used should be improved. Contrary to the quality issue is the concern about selection bias. In fact, by placing specific quality "filters" on data, the investigators may introduce more bias than created by the poor quality data. Moreover, different investigators may use different criteria for a "valid" study and therefore select a different group of studies for meta-analysis. The result is a possible conflicting output of the meta-analysis.

d. Study Design. Some investigators insist that systematic reviews be limited to randomized controlled studies. Such a limitation produces a variant of the potential bias described earlier. At one time, rigid quality standards

were more likely to be met by randomized controlled studies than by observational studies, but this is no longer necessarily the case. Observational methods are currently used to evaluate naturally occurring effects, particularly those that are uncommon. It is quite possible that more important issues, such as combining data from studies performed in different laboratories and using different strains of a single animal species, may result in more systematic error than the study design.

e. Methodology. Different methodologies can cause differing degrees of systematic bias on output data. This begs a question: should studies selected for use in meta-analysis be limited to those using identical methods? This limitation would mean using only separately published studies from the same laboratory in a limited time frame for which the methods were comprehensively monitored and determined to be identical. In practice, application of this filter would massively reduce the number of studies that could be used in the meta-analysis, whose power would therefore be decreased greatly. Accordingly, the user must understand the inherent differences between studies and exercise caution and judgement in selecting and rejecting them for use.

2. Pooled (Quantitative) Analysis

The main purpose of meta-analysis is to provide a quantitative assessment of the similarity of responses in a number of studies. The goal is to develop better overall estimates of the degree of benefit achieved by specific exposure and dosing techniques based on the combining, or pooling, of estimates found in the existing studies of the interventions. This type of meta-analysis is sometimes called a pooled analysis because the analyst pools the observations of many studies and then calculates parameters such as risk or odds ratios from the pooled data.

Because of the many decisions regarding inclusion or exclusion of studies, different meta-analyses might reach very different conclusions on the same topic. Even after the studies are chosen, there are many other methodological issues in choosing how to combine means and variances, e.g., what weighting methods should be used. Pooled analysis should report relative risks and risk reductions as well as absolute risks and risk reductions.

3. Methodological (Qualitative) Analysis

Sometimes the question to be answered is not how much toxicity is induced by the use of a particular exposure, but whether there is any biologically significant toxicity. In this case, a qualitative meta-analysis may be done, in which the quality of the research is scored according to a list of objective criteria. The analyst then examines the methodologically superior studies to determine whether the question of toxicity is answered consistently by them. This qualitative approach has been called methodological analysis or quality scores analysis. In some cases, the methodologically strongest studies agree with one another and disagree with the weaker studies. These weaker studies may be consistent with one another.

K. BAYESIAN INFERENCE

Sensitivity and specificity of a test are important to characterize to understand the accuracy and precision of data generated. Once a researcher decides to use a certain test to diagnose an illness, two important questions require answers. First, if the test results are positive, what is the probability that the researcher has uncovered the condition of interest? Second, if the test results are negative, what is the probability that the patient does not have the disease? Bayes' theorem provides a method to answer these two questions.

The English clergyman after whom it is named first described Bayes' theorem centuries ago. It is one of the most imposing statistical formulas in the biomedical sciences. Put in symbols more meaningful for researchers such as pathologists, the formula is as follows:

$$P(D \mid T+) = \frac{p(T+ \mid D+)p(D+)}{[p(T+ \mid D+)p(D+)] + [p(T+ \mid D-)p(D-)]} \quad (54)$$

where p denotes probability, D+ means that the animal has the effect in question, D− means

that the animal does not have the effect, T+ means that a certain diagnostic test for the effect is positive, T− means that the test is negative, and the vertical line (|) means "conditional upon" what immediately follows.

Most researchers, who have to address sensitivity, specificity, and predictive values, often do not wish to use Bayes' theorem. However, this is a useful formula. Closer examination of the equation reveals that Bayes' theorem is merely the formula for the positive predictive value.

The numerator of Bayes' theorem describes **cell a**, the true positive results, in a 2 × 2 table. The probability of being in cell a is equal to the prevalence multiplied by the sensitivity, where $p(D+)$ is the prevalence, i.e., the probability of being in the affected column, and where $p(T+ \mid D+)$ is the sensitivity, i.e., the probability of being in the top row, *given the fact of being in the affected column*. The denominator of Bayes' theorem consists of two terms, the first of which again describes **cell a**, the true positive results, and the second of which describes **cell b**, the false positive error rate. This rate can be represented by $p(T+ \mid D-)$, which is multiplied by the prevalence of unaffected animals, or $p(D-)$. True positive results (a) divided by true positive plus false positive results ($a + b$) give $a/(a + b)$, give the positive predictive value.

In genetics, an even simpler-appearing formula for Bayes' theorem is sometimes used. The numerator is the same, but the denominator is $p(T+)$. This makes sense because the denominator in $a/(a + b)$ is equal to all of those who have positive test results, whether they are true positive or false positive results.

1. Bayes' Theorem in the Evaluation of Safety Assessment Studies

In a population with a low prevalence of a particular toxicity, most of the positive results in a screening program for that lesion or effect would be falsely positive. Although this does not automatically invalidate a study or assessment program, it raises some concerns about cost effectiveness, which can be explored using Bayes' theorem.

An example to illustrate Bayes' theorem is a study employing an immunochemical stain-based test to screen tissues for a specific effect. This test uses small amounts of antibody, and the presence of an immunologically bound stain is considered a positive result. If the sensitivity and specificity of the test and the prevalence of biochemical effect are known, Bayes' theorem can be used to predict what proportion of the tissues with positive test results will have true positive results, i.e., truly showing the effect.

Figure 15 shows how the calculations are made. If the test has a sensitivity of 96%, and if the true prevalence is 1%, only 13.9% of tissues predicted showing a positive test result actually will be true positives.

Pathologists and toxicologists can quickly develop a table that lists different levels of test sensitivity, test specificity, and effect prevalence and shows how these levels affect the proportion of positive results that are likely to be true positive results. Although this calculation is fairly straightforward and is extremely useful, it seldom has been used in the early stages of planning for large studies or safety assessment programs.

2. Bayes' Theorem and Individual Animal Evaluation

Uncertainty concerning the exact cause of death of an animal is a problem that faces most toxicologic pathologists. Suppose a

Part 1. Initial data:

Sensitivity of immunological stain	= 96% = 0.96
False-negative error rate of the test	= 04% = 0.04
Specificity of the test	= 94% = 0.94
False-positive error rate of the test	= 06% = 0.06
Prevalence of effect in the tissues	= 01% = 0.01

Part 2. Use Bayes' theorem:

$$p(D+ \mid T+) = \frac{p(T+\mid D + p(D+)}{[p(T+\mid D+)p(D+)] + [PT+\mid D-)p(D-)]}$$

$$= \frac{(Sensitivity)(Prevalence)}{[(Sensitivity)(Prevalence)] + (False-positive\ error\ rate)(1-Prevalence)}$$

$$= \frac{(0.96)(0.01)}{[0.96)(0.01)] + [0.06)(0.99]} = \frac{0.0096}{0.0096 + 0.0594} = \frac{0.0096}{0.0690} = 0.139 = 13.9\%$$

Part 3. Use of a 2 x 2 table, with numbers based on the assumption that 10,000 tissues are in the study:

	TRUE DISEASE STATUS		
Test result	Affected (%)	Not affected (%)	Total (%)
Positive	96 (96)	594 (6)	690 (7)
Negative	4 (4)	9,306 (94)	9,310 (93)
Total	100 (100)	9.900 (100)	10,000 (100)

Positive predictive value = 96/690 = 0.139 = 13.9%

Figure 15. Use of Bayes' theorem or a 2 × 2 table to determine the positive predictive value of a hypothetical tuberculin-screening program.

toxicologic pathologist is uncertain about an animal's cause of death and has a positive test result, such as in the example given earlier. Even if the toxicologic pathologist knows the sensitivity and specificity of the test in question, interpretation is still problematic. In order to calculate the positive predictive value, it is necessary to know the prevalence of the particular true tissue/effect that the test is designed to detect. The prevalence is thought of as the expected prevalence in the population from which the animal comes. The actual prevalence is usually not known, but usually an estimate is attempted.

An example of such a situation is when a pathologist evaluates a male primate observed to have fatigue and signs of kidney stones. No other clinical signs of parathyroid disease are detected on physical examination. The toxicologic pathologist considers the possibility of hyperparathyroidism, s/he arbitrarily decides that its prevalence is perhaps 2%, reflecting that in 100 such primates, probably only 2 of them would have the disease. This probable disease prevalence is called the *prior probability*, reflecting the fact that it is estimated prior to the performance of laboratory tests. This probability is based on the estimated prevalence of a particular pathology among primates with similar signs and symptoms.

Although the toxicologic pathologist believes that the probability of hyperparathyroidism is low, s/he considers the serum calcium concentrations to "rule out" the diagnosis. Somewhat to his or her surprise, the results of the test were positive, with an elevated level of calcium of 12.2 mg/dl. S/he could order other tests for parathyroid disease, but some test results may be positive and some negative due to a number of reasons.

Under these circumstances, Bayes' theorem could be used to make a second estimate of probability, which is called the *posterior probability*, reflecting the fact that this determination is made after the test results are known. Calculation of the posterior probability is based on the sensitivity and specificity of the test that was performed, which in this case was elevated serum calcium, and on the prior probability,

which in this case was set at 2%. If the serum calcium test had a 90% sensitivity and a 95% specificity, a false positive error rate of 5% would be expected. Note that specificity plus the false positive error rate always equals 100%.

When this information is used in the Bayes' equation, as shown in Fig. 16, the result is a posterior probability of 27%. This means that the animal in question is now within a group of primates with a significant possibility of parathyroid disease. In Fig. 16, note that the result is the same when a 2 × 2 table is used, i.e., 27%. This is true because the probability based on the Bayes' theorem is identical to the positive predictive value.

In light of the 27% posterior probability, the pathologist decides to order a parathyroid hormone radioimmunoassay, even though this test is expensive. If the radioimmunoassay had a sensitivity of 95% and a specificity of 98% and the results turned out to be positive, the Bayes' theorem could again be used to calculate the probability of parathyroid disease. This time, however, the posterior probability for the first test (27%) would be used as the prior probability for the second test. The result of the calculation, as shown in Fig. 17, gives a new probability of 94%. Thus, the primate in all probability did have hyperparathyroidism.

The reader may be wondering why the posterior probability increased so much the second time. One reason was that the prior probability was considerably higher in the second calculation compared to the first (27% versus 2%) based on the fact that the first test yielded positive results. Another reason was that the specificity of the second test was high (98%), which markedly reduced the false positive error rate and therefore increased the positive predictive value.

VIII. Data Analysis Applications in Toxicologic Pathology

Having reviewed basic principles and provided a set of methods for the statistical handling of data, the remainder of this chapter addresses the practical aspects and difficulties encountered

Part 1. Beginning data:

Sensitivity of the first test	= 90%= 0.90
Specificity of the first test	= 95%= 0.95
Prior probability of disease	= 02%= 0.02

Part 2. Use Bayes' theorem:

$$p(D+ \mid T+) = \frac{p(T + \mid D + p(D+)}{[p(T + \mid D+)p(D+)] + [PT + \mid D-)p(D-]}$$

$$= \frac{(0.90)(0.02)}{[(0.90)(0.02) + (0.05)(0.98)]}$$

$$= \frac{0.018}{0.018 + 0.049} = \frac{0.018}{0.067} = 0.269 = 27\%$$

Part 3. Use of a 2 x 2 table:

	TRUE DISEASE STATUS		
Test result	Affected (%)	Not affected (%)	Total (%)
Positive	18 (90)	49 (5)	67 (6.7)
Negative	2 (10)	931 (95)	933 (93.3)
Total	20 (100)	980 (100)	1,000 (100.0)

Positive predictive value = 18/67 = 0.269 = 27%

Figure 16. Use of Bayes' theorem or a 2 × 2 table to determine posterior probability and positive predictive values.

in preclinical safety assessment in the field of toxicologic pathology.

Analyses of pathology data are well defined, although they may not necessarily use the best methods available. The use of statistical methodology is discussed in the remainder of this chapter. The aim of this section is to review statistical methods on a use-by-use basis and to provide a foundation for the selection of alternatives in specific situations. Meta-analyses and Bayesian approaches are not addressed in detail, but should be kept in mind.

A. BODY AND ORGAN WEIGHTS

Body weight and the weights of selected organs are usually collected in studies where animals are dosed with, or exposed to, a chemical. In fact, body weight is frequently the most sensitive indication of an adverse treatment effect. How to analyze these data best and in what form to analyze the organ weight data, such as absolute weights, weight changes, or percentages of body weight, have been the subject of great discussion.

Both absolute body weights and rates of body weight change are best analyzed by ANOVA followed, if called for, by a *post hoc* test. Body weight change is usually calculated as changes from a baseline measurement value, which is traditionally the animal's weight immediately prior to the first dosing with or exposure to test material. To standardize body

Part 1. Beginning data:

Sensitivity of the first test	= 95%= 0.95
Specificity of the first test	= 98%= 0.98
Prior probability of disease	= 27%= 0.27

Part 2. Use Bayes' theorem:

$$p(D+ \mid T+) = \frac{p(T + \mid D+ \; p(D+)}{[p(T + \mid D+)p(D+)] + [PT + \mid D-)p(D-]}$$

$$= \frac{(0.95)(0.27)}{[(0.95)(0.27) + (0.02)(0.73)]}$$

$$= \frac{0.257}{0.257 + 0.0146} = \frac{0.257}{0.272} = 0.9449^* = 94\%$$

Part 3. Use of a 2 x 2 table:

Test result/ True disease status	TRUE DISEASE STATUS		
	Affected (%)	Not affected (%)	Total (%)
Positive	256 (95)	15 (2)	271 (27.1)
Negative	13 (5)	716 (98)	729 (72.9)
Total	269 (100)	731 (100)	1,000 (100)

Positive predictive value = 256/271 = 0.9446* = 94%

*The slight difference in the results for the two approaches is due to rounding errors. It is not important biologically.

Figure 17. Use of Bayes' theorem or a 2 × 2 table to determine second posterior probability and second positive predictive values.

weight, no group should be significantly different in mean body weight from any other group, and all animals in all groups should lie within 2 SD of the overall mean body weight. Even if the groups were randomized properly at the beginning of a study, there is an advantage to performing the computationally slightly more cumbersome changes in body weight analysis. The advantage of this calculation is an increase in sensitivity because the adjustment of starting points, i.e., the setting of initial weights as a "zero" value, reduces the amount of initial variability. In this case, Bartlett's test is performed first to ensure the homogeneity of variance and the appropriate sequence of analysis follows.

If sample sizes are small or normality of data is uncertain, nonparametric methods, such as Kruskal–Wallis, may be more appropriate. The analysis of relative organ weights is a valuable tool for identifying possible target organs. How to perform this analysis is still a matter of some disagreement. Organ weight data, expressed as percentages of body weight, should be analyzed separately for each sex. Often, conclusions from organ weight data of males differ from those of females, hence separating these data by gender should always be done. Other factors, such as the stage of the reproductive cycle on uterine weight, may also influence organ weights. These factors must be taken into account both in the stratification of animals and in the interpretation of results.

The two alternative approaches to analyzing relative organ weights call for either calculating organ weights as a percentage of total body weight at the time of necropsy and analyzing the results by ANOVA or analyzing results by ANCOVA, with body weights as the covariates as discussed previously. A number of considerations should be kept in mind when this choice is made. First, one must recognize the difference between biological significance and statistical significance. By evaluating relative body weight, the significance of a weight change that is not proportional to changes in whole body weights must be determined. Second, the toxicologic pathologist now must interpret small changes while still retaining a similar sensitivity, i.e., the $p < 0.05$ level.

Several tools can be used to increase power of the analysis. One is to increase the sample size by increasing the number of animals and the other is to utilize the most powerful test available that is appropriate to the data. The number of animals used in the groups is presently under debate with respect to power of detecting a significant change. The power of statistical tests is important in the consideration of animal numbers.

In the majority of cases, except for the brain, the organs of interest change weight in proportion to total body weight, except in extreme cases of obesity or starvation. This change is the biological rationale behind analyzing both absolute body weight and the organ weight to body weight ratio. Analyses are designed to detect cases where this relative change does not occur. Analysis of data from several hundred studies has shown no significant difference in rates of weight change of target organs, other than the brain, compared to total body weight

for healthy animals in rats, mice, rabbits, and dogs used for repeated dose studies. The analysis of covariance is of questionable validity in analyzing body weight and related organ weight changes, as a primary assumption is the independence of treatment. In toxicologic pathology the assumption that the relationship of the two variables is the same for all treatments is not true.

In cases where the differences between the error mean squares are much greater during the analysis, the ratio of F ratios will diverge in precision from the result of the efficiency of covariance adjustment. These cases occur where either sample sizes are large or where the differences between means themselves are great. This latter case is one that does not occur in the designs under discussion in any manner that would leave analysis of covariance as a valid approach because group means are very similar at the beginning of the experiment and cannot diverge markedly unless there is a treatment effect. As discussed earlier, a treatment effect invalidates a prime underpinning assumption of analysis of covariance.

B. CLINICAL CHEMISTRY

A number of clinical chemistry parameters are commonly determined on the blood and urine collected from animals in chronic, subchronic, and, occasionally, acute toxicity studies. In the past, and currently in some places, the accepted practice has been to evaluate these data using univariate-parametric methods, primarily t tests and ANOVA. However, this is not the best approach.

First, biochemical parameters are rarely independent of each other; neither is the focus of inquiry limited to only one of the parameters. Rather, there are a number of parameters that change when toxicity is seen in specific organs. For example, simultaneous elevations of creatinine phosphokinase, γ-hydroxybutyrate dehydrogenase, and lactate dehydrogenase are strongly indicative of myocardial damage. In such a case, the clinical important of these findings is not limited to a significant elevation in one of these enzyme; all three must be con-

411

sidered together. Detailed coverage of the interpretation of such clinical laboratory tests can be found elsewhere.

Second, interaction occurs among parameters; therefore, each parameter is not independent. For example, serum electrolytes (sodium, potassium, and calcium) interact such that a decrease in one is frequently tied to an increase in one of the others.

Finally, either because of the biological nature of the parameter or the way in which it is measured, data are frequently skewed or not continuous. This skewness and discontinuous nature of data can be seen in some of the reference data for experimental animals, e.g., creatinine, sodium, potassium, chloride, calcium, and blood.

C. HEMATOLOGY

Much of what was said about clinical chemistry parameters holds true for the hematological measurements made in toxicology studies. Choosing the correct statistical test to perform should be evaluated by use of a decision tree until one becomes confident as to the most appropriate method(s). Keep in mind that sets of values and, in some cases, population distribution vary not only between species, but also between the commonly used strains of species. This means that "control" or "standard" values will "drift" over the course of only a few years.

Again, the majority of these parameters are interrelated and highly dependent on the method used to determine them. Red blood cell count (RBC), platelet counts, and mean corpuscular volume (MCV) may be determined using a device such as a Coulter counter to take direct measurements. The resulting data are usually stable for parametric methods. The hematocrit, however, may actually be a value calculated from the RBC and MCV values and hence is dependent on them. If the hematocrit is measured directly, instead of being calculated from the RBC and MCV, it may be compared using parametric methods.

Hemoglobin is directly measured and is an independent and continuous variable. However, the distribution of values is rarely normal, but rather may be a multimodal. This distribution probably occurs as a result of a number of forms and conformations of hemoglobin present, such as oxyhemoglobin, deoxyhemoglobin, and methemoglobin. Here a nonparametric technique such as the Wilcoxon rank-sum test is called for.

Consideration of the white blood cell (WBC) and differential counts leads to another problem. The total WBC is typically a normally distributed population amenable to parametric analysis. However, differential cell counts are normally determined by manually counting one or more sets of 100 cells each. The resulting relative percentages of neutrophils are then reported as either percentages or are multiplied by the total WBC count with the resulting "count" being reported as the "absolute" differential WBC. Such data where the distribution does not approach normality, particularly in the case of eosinophils, should usually be analyzed by nonparametric methods. It is widely believed that "relative" (%) differential data should not be reported because they are likely to be misleading.

Finally, it is rare for a change in any single hematological parameter to be clinically meaningful. Rather, because these parameters are so interrelated, patterns of changes in parameters should be expected if a real effect is present, and analysis and interpretation of results should focus on such patterns of changes. Classification analysis techniques often provide the basis for a useful approach to such problems.

D. INCIDENCE OF HISTOPATHOLOGIC FINDINGS

The last two decades have been increasing emphasis placed on the histopathologic examination of tissues collected from animals in subchronic and chronic toxicity studies, hence the development of the discipline of toxicologic pathology. The biological significance of a statistically significant finding is particularly important for the toxicologic pathologist to address. In most cases, a statistical evaluation is the only way to determine if what is seen in treated animals is different in number and severity from that seen in control animals. Expertise is required in cases where a lesion may be of such a rare type that the occurrence of only one or a few such in treated animals "raises a flag." Although tumor pathology is a major concern, nonneoplastic "sentinel" lesions are often of greatest use in determining possible mechanisms of action of the test article.

For statistical analysis, comparison of incidences of any one type of lesion between controls and treated animals is made using the multiple 2×2 χ^2 test or Fisher's exact test with a modification of the numbers of animals as the denominators. The special case of carcinogenicity bioassays is discussed later.

Grading of lesions as to severity results in ordinal data, which increase in the information content of data that should not be available by performing an analysis based only on the perceived quantal nature of a lesion being present or absent.

The traditional method of analyzing multiple, cross-classified data has been to collapse the N X R contingency table over all but two of the variables. Following this data condensation, a computation of some measure of association between these variables is undertaken. For an N-dimensional table, this results in $N(N-1)/2$ separate analyses. This method results in a crude filtered analysis, where if the data are inappropriate pooled yields a faulty understanding of the meaning of data. Although computationally more laborious, a multiway (N X R table) analysis should be utilized.

E. CARCINOGENESIS

Inferences about the potential human carcinogenicity of substances are based on experimental results obtained from a nonhuman species given the substance at a high dose or exposure level. The aim of this procedure is to predict the possibility and probability of occurrence of tumorogenesis in humans at much lower levels. An entire textbook could be devoted to examining the assumptions involved in this undertaking and review of the aspects of design and interpretation of animal carcinogenicity studies. Such detail is beyond the scope of this chapter.

The reader is referred to Gad (1998) for more detail.

In the past, the single most important statistical consideration in the design of carcinogenicity bioassays was based on a simple quantal response: cancer did or did not occur. Experiments were designed so that a sufficient number of animals were used so as to have a reasonable expectation of detecting an effect if one occurred. Although the primary objective was to determine whether the incidence of tumors was increased following exposure to the test article of interest, a much more complex model should now be considered to answer other questions pertinent to the extrapolation of experimental results in animals to make inferences about risks to human health.

The time to tumor, patterns of tumor incidence, effects on survival rate, and age at first tumor can now be evaluated. The rationale for including these factors lies in concerns associated with likely planned or unplanned exposure of humans to xenobiotic and naturally occurring substances and relatively small increases in the incidence of tumors over background would require the use of an impractically large number of test animals per group.

To illustrate this point, data are given in Table XVII. Here only 46 animals per group are required to show a 10% increase over a zero background, where the background included a rarely occurring tumor type. To detect a tenth of a percent increase above a 5% background, 770,000 animals per group would be needed! As dose increases the incidence of tumors, the response will also increase. This increase occurs until it reaches the point where a modest increase, e.g., 10%, over a reasonably small background level, e.g., 1%, could be detected using an acceptably small-sized group of test animals. Table XVII shows that 51 animals would be needed for such a situation. It can be seen that the number of animals required to demonstrate a 1/100,000 increase above a 25% background incidence would be very large.

There are, however, at least two potential difficulties that often occur in the group given

Shayne C. Gad and Colin G. Rousseaux

TABLE XVII
Average Number of Animals Needed to Detect a Significant Increase in the Incidence of an Event (Tumors, anomalies, etc.) over the Background Incidence (Control) at Several Expected Incidence Levels Using the Fisher Exact Probability Test ($p = 0.05$)

Background incidence	No. of animals[a]					
	0.01	0.1	1	3	5	10
0	46,000,000[a]	460,000	4,600	511	164	46
0.01	46,000,000	460,000	4,600	511	164	46
0.1	47,000,000	470,000	4,700	520	168	47
1	51,000,000	510,000	5,100	570	204	51
5	77,000,000	770,000	7,700	856	304	77
10	100,000,000	1,000,000	10,000	1,100	400	100
20	148,000,000	1,480,000	14,800	1,644	592	148
25	160,000,000	1,600,000	16,000	1,840	664	166

[a]Number of animals needed in each group: controls as well as treated.

the highest dose. First, mortally can be higher than other groups. There must be sufficient rodents surviving to the end of the study to allow for meaningful statistical analysis. Second, toxicologic pathologists must select the high dose level based only on the information provided by a subchronic or range finding study, usually 90 days in length. To predict carcinogenic effects across species, it is necessary that the metabolism and mechanism of action of the chemical at the highest level tested are the same as at the low levels where human exposure would occur. Unfortunately, selection of either too low a dose may make the study invalid for the detection of carcinogenicity or too high a dose, where toxicokinetics result in different metabolism, may seriously impair the use of the results for risk assessment.

There are several solutions to this problem of group size. One of these is the approach of the National Toxicology Program bioassay program, which is to conduct a 3-month range-finding study with sufficient dose levels to establish a level that significantly (10%) decreases the rate of body weight gain. This dose is defined as the maximum tolerated dose (MTD) and is selected as the highest dose. Two other levels, generally one-half MTD and one-quarter MTD, are selected for testing as the intermediate and low dose levels. In many earlier National Cancer Institute studies, only one other level was used.

The dose range-finding study is necessary in most cases, but the suppression of body weight gain is a scientifically questionable benchmark when establishing safety factors. Physiologic, pharmacological, or metabolic markers generally serve as better indicators of systemic response than body weight. Indeed, the toxicokinetic question raised earlier, where metabolic mechanisms for handling a compound at real-life exposure levels can be saturated or overwhelmed, bringing into play entirely artifactual metabolic and physiologic mechanisms. To make sure that the metabolic profile of the test article is the same as would be observed at lower doses, a series of well-defined acute and subchronic studies should be undertaken. These studies are designed to determine the "chronicity factor" and to study the onset of pathology. Such a series of studies can be more predictive for dose setting than body weight suppression. The regulatory response to questioning the appropriateness of the MTD as a high dose level has been to acknowledge that occasionally an excessively high dose is selected. The response also counters that using lower doses would seriously decrease the sensitivity of detection.

IX. Summary and Conclusions

We have attempted to highlight some of the issues that the toxicologic pathologist must

414

address during study design and data analysis. There are many more statistical models and experimental designs that have not been addressed in this chapter but can be seen in standard reference texts. Regardless of the methodology used, nothing surpasses common sense and remembering that statistical analysis is a tool to aid in understanding data rather than a prerequisite to data evaluation. The field of biostatistics is complex and may appear complicated to the untrained user, just as toxicologic pathology seems incomprehensible to a number of other scientists. For this reason we urge the reader to discuss the design and analysis of an experiment with a biostatistician *before* execution of the experiment. Similarly, we recommend that the toxicologic pathologist understand the assumptions of the statistical models that are being used and the ramifications of violating these assumptions. Finally, we recommend using the most powerful test appropriate to the form, quantity, and quality of the data.

ACKNOWLEDGMENT

The authors gratefully acknowledge the detailed review and suggestions performed by Dr. R. Brecher.

SUGGESTED READING

Abramowitz, M., and Stegun, I. A. (1964). "Handbook of Mathematical Functions," pp. 925–964. National Bureau of Standards, Washington, DC.

Anderson E. (1960). A Semigraphical method for the analysis of complex problems. *Technomet* 2, 387–391.

Anderson, S., Auquier, A., Hauck, W. W., Oakes, D., Vandaele, W., and Weisburg, H. I. (1980). "Statistical Methods for Comparative Studies." Wiley, New York.

Anderson, T. W. (1971). "The Statistical Analysis of Time Series." Wiley, New York.

Anscombe, F. J. (1973). Graphics in statistical analysis. *Am. Stat.* 27, 17–21.

Armitage, P. (1955). Tests for linear trends in proportions and frequencies. *Biometrics* 11, 375–386.

Beyer, W. H. (1976). "Handbook of Tables for Probability and Statistics." Chemical Rubber Co., Boca Raton, FL.

Beyer, W. H. (1976). "Handbook of Tables for Probability and Statistics." CRC Press, Boca Raton, FL.

Bickis, M. G. (1990). Experimental design. *In* "Handbook of in Vivo Toxicity Testing" (D. L. Arnold, H. C. Grice, and D. R. Krewski, eds.), pp. 113–166. Academic Press, San Diego.

Bliss, C. I. (1935). The calculation of the dosage-mortality curve. *Ann. Appl. Biol.* 22, 134–167.

Bloomfield, P. (1976). "Fourier Analysis of Time Series: An Introduction." Wiley, New York.

Box, G. E. P., and Tiao, G. C. (1973). "Bayesian Inference in Statistical Analysis." Addison-Wesley, Reading, MA.

Boyd, E. M. (1972). "Predictive Toxicometrics." Williams & Wilkins, Baltimore.

Boyd, E. M., and Knight, L. M. (1963). Postmortem shifts in the weight and water levels of body organs. *Toxicol. Appl. Pharm.* 5, 119–128.

Breslow, N. (1984). Comparison of survival curves. *In* "Cancer Clinical Trials: Methods and Practice" (M. F. Buse, M. J. Staguet and R. F. Sylvester, eds.), pp. 381–406. Oxford Univ. Press, Oxford.

Chambers, J. M., Cleveland, W. S., Kleiner, B., and Turkey, P. A. (1983). "Graphical Methods for Data Analysis." Wadsworth, Belmont.

Chernoff, H. (1973). The use of faces to represent points in K-dimensional space graphically. *J. Am. Stat. Assoc.* 68, 361–368.

Cleveland, W. S. (1985). "The Elements of Graphing Data." Wadsworth Advanced Books, Monterey, CA.

Cleveland, W. S., and McGill, R. (1984). Graphical perception: Theory, experimentation, and application to the development of graphical methods. *J. Am. Stat. Assoc.* 79, 531–554.

Cochran, W. F. (1954). Some models for strengthening the common Chi-square tests. *Biometrics* 10, 417–451.

Cochran, W. G., and Cox, G. M. (1975). "Experimental Designs." Wiley, New York.

Conover, J. W., and Inman, R. L. (1981). Rank transformation as a bridge between parametric and nonparametric statistics. *Am. Stat* 35, 124–129.

Cox, D. R. (1972). Regression models and life-tables. *J. Roy. Stat. Soc.* 34B, 187–220.

Cox, D. R., and Stuart, A. (1955). Some quick tests for trend in location and dispersion. *Biometrics* 42, 80–95.

Crowley, J., and Breslow, N. (1984). Statistical analysis of survival data. *Annu. Rev. Public Health* 5, 385–411.

Cutler, S. J., and Ederer, F. (1958). Maximum utilization of the life table method in analyzing survival. *J. Chron. Dis.* 8, 699–712.

Davison, M. L. (1983). "Multidimensional Scaling." Wiley, New York.

Diamond, W. J. (1981). "Practical Experimental Designs." Lifetime Learning Publications, Belmont, CA.

Draper, N. R., and Smith, H. (1981). "Applied Regression Analysis." Wiley, New York.

Duncan, D. B. (1955). Multiple range and multiple F tests. *Biometrics* **11**, 1–42.

Dunnett, C. W. (1955). A multiple comparison procedure for comparing several treatments with a control. *J. Am. Stat. Assoc.* **50**, 1096–1121.

Dunnett, C. W. (1964). New tables for multiple comparison with a control. *Biometrics* **16**, 671–685.

Dykstra, R. L., and Robertson, T. (1983). On testing monotone tendencies. *J. Am. Stat. Assoc.* **78**, 342–350.

Elandt-Johnson, R. C., and Johnson, N. L. (1980). "Survival Models and Data Analysis." Wiley, New York.

Engelman, L., and Hartigan, J. A. (1969). Percentage points of a test for clusters. *J. Am. Stat. Assoc.* **64**, 1647–1648.

Everitt, B. (1980). "Cluster Analysis." Halsted Press, New York.

Everitt, B. S., and Hand, D. J. (1981). "Finite Mixture Distributions." Chapman and Hall, New York.

Federal Register (1985). No. 50, Vol. 50. Washington, DC.

Federer, W. T. (1955). "Experimental Design." Macmillan, New York.

Feinstein, A. R. (1979). Scientific standards vs. statistical associations and biological logic in the analysis of causation *Clin. Pharmacol. Ther.* **25**, 481–492.

Finney, D. J., Latscha, R., Bennet, B. M., and Hsu, P. (1963). "Tables for Testing Significance in a 2 × 2 Contingency Table." Cambridge Univ. Press, Cambridge.

Finney, D. K. (1977). "Probit Analysis," 3rd Ed. Cambridge Univ. Press, Cambridge.

Gad, S. C. (1984). Statistical analysis of behavioral toxicology data and studies. *Arch. Toxicol. Suppl.* **5**, 256–266.

Gad, S. C. (1998). "Statistics and Experimental Design for Toxicologists." CRC Press, Boca Raton, FL.

Gad, S. C., and Chengelis, C. P. (1992). "Animal Models in Toxicology." Dekker, New York.

Gad, S. C., and Taulbee, S. M. (1996). "Handbook of Data Recording, Maintenance and Management for the Biomedical Sciences." CRC Press, Boca Raton, FL.

Gad, S. C., Reilly, C., Siino, K. M., and Gavigan, F. A. (1985). Thirteen cationic ionophores: Neurobehavioural and membrane effects. *Drug Chem. Toxicol.* **8**(6), 451–468.

Gallant, A. R. (1975). Nonlinear regression. *Am. Stat.* **29**, 73–81.

Garrett, H. E. (1947). "Statistics in Psychology and Education", pp. 215–218, Longmans, Green, New York.

Gehring, P. J., and Blau, G. E. (1977). Mechanisms of carcinogenicity: Dose response, *J. Environ. Pathol. Toxicol.* **1**, 163–179.

Gerbarg, Z. B., and Horwitz, R. I. (1988). Resolving conflicting clinical trials: Guidelines for meta-analysis. *J. Clin. Epidemiol.* **41**, 503–509.

Ghent, A. W. (1972). A method for exact testing of 2 × 2, 2 × 3, 3 × 3 and other contingency tables, employing binomiate coefficients. *Am. Mid. Natu.* **88**, 15–27.

Glass, L. (1975). Classification of biological networks by their qualitative dynamics. *J. Theor. Bio.* **54**, 85–107.

Gold, H. J. (1977). "Mathematical Modeling of Biological System: An Introductory Guidebook." Wiley, New York.

Gordon, A. D. (1981) "Classification." Chapman and Hall, New York.

Greenland, S. (1994). Invited commentary: A critical look at some popular meta-analytic methods. *Am. J. Epidemiol.* **140**, 290–296.

Grubbs, F. E. (1969). Procedure for detecting outlying observations in samples. *Technometrics* **11**, 1–21.

Hammond, E. C., Garfinkel, L., and Lew, E. A. (1978). Longevity, selective mortality, and competitive risks in relation to chemical carcinogenesis. *Environ. Res.* **16**, 153–173.

Harris, E. K. (1978). Review of statistical methods of analysis of series of biochemical test results. *Ann. Biol. Clin.* **36**, 194–197

Harris, R. J. (1975). "A Primer of Multivariate Statistics," pp. 96–101. Academic Press, New York.

Harter, A. L. (1960). Critical values for Duncan's new multiple range test. *Biometrics* **16**, 671–685.

Hartigan, J. A. (1983). Classification. *In* "Encyclopedia of Statistical Sciences" (S. Katz and N. L. Johnson, eds.), Vol. 2. Wiley, New York.

Haseman, J. K. (1977). Response to use of statistics when examining life time studies in rodents to detect carcinogenicity. *J. Toxicol. Environ. Health* **3**, 633–636.

Haseman, J. K. (1985). Issues in carcinogenicity testing: Dose selection. *Fundam App. Toxicol.* **5**, 66–78.

Hicks, C. R. (1982). "Fundamental Concepts in the Design of Experiments." Holt, Rinehart, and Winston, New York.

Hoaglin, D. C., Mosteller, F., and Tukey, J. W. (1983). "Understanding Robust and Explanatory Data Analysis." Wiley, New York.

Hollander, M., and Wolfe, D. A. (1973). "Nonparametric Statistical Methods," pp. 124–129. Wiley, New York.

Jackson, B. (1962). Statistical analysis of body weight data. *Toxicol. Appl. Pharmacol.* **4**, 432–443.

Kotz, S., and Johnson, N. L. (1982). "Encyclopedia of Statistical Sciences," Vol. 1. pp. 61–69. Wiley, New York.

Kowalski, B. R., and Bender, C. F. (1972). Pattern recognition, a powerful approach to interpreting chemical data. *J. Am. Chem. Soc.* **94**, 5632–5639.

Kraemer, H. C., and Thiemann, G. (1987). "How Many Subjects? Statistical Power Analysis in Research." Sage Publications, Newbury Park, CA.

Lee, E. T. (1980). "Statistical Methods for Survival Data Analysis." Lifetime Learning Publications, Belmont, CA.

Lee, P. N., and Lovell, D. (1999). Statistics for toxicology, *In* "General and Applied Toxicology" (B. Ballantyne, T. Marrs, and T. Syversen, eds.), 2nd Ed. pp. 291–302. Grove's Dictionaries, New York.

Lindley, S. V. (1971). Bayesian Statistics: A Review. SIAM, Philadelphia.

Litchfield, J. T., and Wilcoxon, F. (1949). A simplified method of evaluating dose effect experiments. *J. Pharmacol. Exp. Ther.* **96**, 99–113.

Loeb, W. F., and Quimby, F. W. (1999). "The Clinical Chemistry of Laboratory Animals," 2nd Ed. Taylor & Francis, Philadelphia, PA.

Marriott, F. H. C. (1991). "The Dictionary of Statistical Terms." Longman Scientific & Technical, Essex, England.

Martin, H. F., Gudzinowicz, B. J., and Fanger, H. (1975). "Normal Values in Clinical Chemistry." Dekker, New York.

Mendell, N. R., Finch, S. J., and Thode, H. C., Jr. (1993). Where is the likelihood ratio test powerful for detecting two component normal mixtures? *Biometrics* **49**, 907–915.

Mitruka, B. M., and Rawnsley, H. M. (1977). "Clinical Biochemical and Hematological Reference Values in Normal Animals." Masson, New York.

Montgomery, D. C., and Smith, E. A. (1983). "Introduction to Linear Regression Analysis." Wiley, New York.

Myers, J. L. (1972). "Fundamentals of Experimental Designs." Allyn and Bacon, Boston.

Peto, R., and Pike, M. C. (1973). Conservatism of approximation; (0 -E) 2/E in the log rank test for survival data on tumour incidence data. *Biometrics* **29**, 579–584.

Peto, R., Pike, M. C., Armitage, P., Breslow, N. E., Cox. D. R., Howard, S. V., Kantel, N., McPherson, K., Peto, J. and Smith, P. G. (1977). Design and analysis of randomized clinical trials requiring prolonged observations of each Patient. II. Analyses and examples. *B. J. Cancer* **35**, 1–39.

Peto, R., Pike, M., Day, N., Gray, R., Lee, P., Parish, S., Peto, J., Richards, S., and Wahrendorf, J. (1980). Guidelines for simple, sensitive significance tests for carcinogenic effects in long-term animal experiments. *In* "IARC Monographs on the Evaluation of the Carcinogenic Risk of Chemicals to Humans," pp. 311–346. International Agency for Research in Cancer, Lyon.

Pollard, J. H. (1977). "Numerical and Statistical Techniques." Cambridge Univ. Press, New York.

Portier, C., and Hoel, D. (1984). Type I error of trend tests in proportions and the design of cancer screens. *Comm. Stat. Theory Meth.* **A13**, 1–14.

Prentice, R. L. (1976). A generalization of the probit and logit methods for dose response curves. *Biometrics* **32**, 761–768.

Racine, A., Grieve, A. P., and Fluhler, H. (1986). Bayesian methods in practice: Experiences in the pharmaceutical industry. *App. Stat.* **35**, 93–150.

Ridgemen, W. J. (1975). "Experimentation in Biology," pp. 214–215. Wiley, New York.

Romesburg, H. C. (1984). "Cluster Analysis for Researchers." Lifetime Learning Publications, Belmont, CA.

Salsburg, D. (1980). The effects of life-time feeding studies on patterns of senile lesions in mice and rats. *Drug Chem. Tox.* **3**, 1–33.

Schaper, M., Thompson, R. D., and Alarie, Y. (1985). A method to classify airborne chemicals which alter the normal ventilatory response induced by CO_2. *Toxicol Appl Pharmacol.* **79**, 332–341.

Scheffe, H. (1959). "The Analysis of Variance." Wiley, New York.

Schmid, C. F. (1983). "Statistical Graphics." Wiley, New York.

Siegel, S. (1956). "Nonparametric Statistics for the Behavioral Sciences." McGraw-Hill, New York.

Sinclair, J. C., and Bracken, M. B. (1994). Clinically useful measures of effect in binary analyses of randomized trials. *J. Clin. Epidemiol.* **47**, 881–889.

Snedecor, G. W., and Cochran, W. G. (1980). "Statistical Methods," 7th Ed. Iowa State Univ. Press, Ames, IA.

Sokal, R. R., and Rohlf, F. J. (1994). "Biometry," 3rd Ed. Freeman, San Francisco.

SOT ED01 Task Force (1981). Reexamination of the ED01 study-adjusting for time on study. *Fundam. Appl. Toxicol.* **1**, 8–123.

Tarone, R. E. (1975). Tests for trend in life table analysis. *Biometrika* **62**, 679–682.

Tufte, E. R. (1983). "The Visual Display of Quantitative Information." Graphics Press, Cheshire, CT.

Tufte, E. R. (1990). "Envisioning Information." Graphics Press, Cheshire, CT.

Tufte, E. R. (1997). "Visual Explanations." Graphics Press, Cheshire, CT.

Tukey, J. W. (1977). "Exploratory Data Analysis." Addison-Wesley, Reading, MA.

Velleman, P. F., and Hoaglin, D. C. (1981). "Applications, Basics and Computing of Exploratory Data Analysis." Duxbury Press, Boston.

Weil, C. S. (1962). Applications of methods of statistical analysis of efficient repeated-dose toxicological tests. I. General considerations and problems involved. Sex differences in rat liver and kidney weights. *Toxicol. Appl. Pharmacol.* **4**, 561–571.

Weil, C. S. (1973). Experimental design and interpretation of data from prolonged toxicity studies. *In* "Proc. 5th

Int. Congr. Pharmacol.," Vol. 2, pp. 4–12. Beacon Press, San Francisco.

Weil, C. S. (1982). Statistical analysis and normality of selected hematological and clinical chemistry measurements used in toxicologic studies. *Arch. Toxicol. Suppl.* **5**, 237–253.

Weil, C. S., and Gad, S. C. (1980). Applications of methods of statistical analysis to efficient repeated-dose toxicologic tests. 2. Methods for analysis of body, liver and kidney weight data. *Toxicol. Appl. Pharmacol.* **52**, 214–226.

Young, F. W. (1985). Multidimensional scaling. *In* "Encyclopedia of Statistical Sciences" S. Katz, and N. L. Johnson, (eds.), Vol. 5. pp. 649–659 Wiley, New York.

Zar, J. H. (1974). Biostatistical Analysis, p. 50. Prentice-Hall, Englewood.

16

Preparation of the Report for a Toxicology/Pathology Study

Hugh E. Black

Hugh E. Black & Associates, Inc.
Sparta, New Jersey

I. Introduction

This chapter emphasizes the importance of preparing a clear concise final report for a toxicology study and discusses the potential impact of a poorly written report. It presents an outline of the typical information and level of detail that one expects to find in a final report for a repeat-dose toxicity study conducted under good laboratory practices. Examples are presented of how to organize study results that are easy for the reader to visualize and understand. These are contrasted with examples taken from actual study reports.

There are at least four important reasons for conducting a careful and thorough toxicology program for a new medicine: (1) to assure that the drug will not harm the patient to whom it is administered by the route, dose, and regimen to be administered, (2) to provide the physician who is taking the compound into man for the first time with some parameters he/she can monitor as indicators of developing toxicity, (3) to assure the sponsoring company that it is appropriate to proceed with the clinical development of the drug and to do so with an under-

standing of the drug's toxicity profile, and (4) to provide the regulatory reviewer the assurance that the toxicity of the compound has been evaluated thoroughly and that there is an acceptable safety margin for the use of the drug in the indication, by the route, and at the dose and regimen to be used in the clinic.

Many studies will be conducted and reported to create the toxicity profile and develop the safety margin for a new medicine. Data presented in the final report for a single study represent only one small piece of this information. In addition to the four reasons for conducting and reporting toxicity studies, the toxicology reports may be used for other purposes, depending on the client. When one considers the different reasons why potential clients may use the final report, it becomes obvious that the report for a single study is very different than an article for publication and therefore must be written very carefully and its results discussed relative to the results from other studies with the compound or other compounds in its class. There should be a minimum of speculation.

II. Clients

Who are the clients that may use the data presented and interpreted in toxicology report? The client may be an individual in upper management within the sponsoring corporation who has to decide to either continue assigning resources to the development of the new medicine or recommend that the project be stopped because of recent findings in toxicology. The client may be a reviewer in a regulatory agency somewhere in the world who has to make a decision on whether to recommend approval of the product. The client may be the lawyer(s) for a consumer who alleges he/she was injured by the product. The client may be the attorney(s) who is defending the company in the product liability suit. The client may be a scientist from an outside company that is considering buying or licensing the product. As part of the outside company's licensing and due diligence process it has its own scientific staff review the reports. Because of this broad spectrum of potential clients and the very different reasons why each may be reading the toxicology reports, the author(s) should keep in mind two things: (1) the impact their presentation/interpretation of data can have on the client and his/her decisions and (2) the subsequent impact the client's decisions can have on the project or their own company.

When the author is preparing the final report, he/she is "speaking" directly to the client, presenting the results of the study and giving his/her interpretation of data. He/she should keep in mind that the client could be reviewing the report several years after it was issued when neither the author nor other individuals who were involved with the study are with the company to answer questions or resolve concerns. Thus care must be taken to identify and resolve issues during the preparation of the document. The author should also consider the educational background, the first language, and the experience of the reader. The reader may be neither a toxicologist nor a pathologist. The reader may be using his/her second language to read and understand what is being reported. Further, the reader may be working with reports that have been translated into another language. For these many reasons the author should make every effort to make the report concise and clear and, in particular, to avoid long detailed descriptions. Ideally the results should be easy for the reader to visualize.

This can be accomplished by the use of text tables to present and highlight the significant compound-related findings. The text table can then be followed by a brief interpretation or comment that tells the reader why the information in the text table is important.

The author should also assure that the words are correct and the message being delivered is the message that was intended. An example of a sentence that may not convey the message the author thought it did is the following: "There were no other treatment-related lesions in the study." This write-off statement may be made to indicate to the reader that everything that was treatment related has been identified. However, the statement actually says, depending on where it is placed, all lesions described up to this point in the report were treatment related. Is that what the author intended to say?

III. Impact of a Poorly Written Report

There is no substitute for carefully constructed and conservatively interpreted final reports for toxicology studies in a regulatory submission. When a regulatory submission is filed by a corporation, it is with the intent that the review will be swift and that the documents will raise few questions and create no major issues with the reviewing agency.

Every time a report is approved to be issued, the author(s)/management should remind themselves of the negative, ripple effect that a poorly written report can have on the drug development process. Consider the impact on the company if it receives a letter from a regulatory agency declining to approve their product and concluding that a major preclinical toxicity study should be repeated before their product can be approved. Imagine further the consternation that results, if it is obvious that the conduct of the study and the data were acceptable, but the way the findings were presented and interpreted in the final report were the real issue.

At the point in the regulatory review process where the agency forwards to the sponsor written questions that identify issues in the toxicology/pathology report(s), it is too late. Questions from a regulatory agency can cause a tremendous upset within a company. They may be perceived to signal a possible delay in the approval and marketing of the product. A delay in approval represents a significant problem for a corporation that requires a stream of new products to maintain and increase its financial strength and to maintain a positive relationship with its investors. To answer questions submitted by a regulatory agency or to resolve issues or correct mistakes becomes an immediate, unplanned, high-priority project. To resolve the issues may require the diversion of significant amounts of financial and human resources away from ongoing high-priority projects. Reallocating resources to resolve issues for a product whose development is "complete" creates significant strains within an organization. It will almost surely lead to concern, if not outright anger, on the part of managers who are committed to meeting deadlines on current, high-priority projects. The tolerance of individuals who may have little or no understanding of the regulatory issues being responded to can be minimal; their willingness, however, to direct blame to the toxicologist or pathologist whose work has been challenged can be significant. The negative impact of this type of directed blame, whether warranted or not, should not be underestimated.

The cost of a poorly written toxicology/pathology report that results in an approval delay has a monetary value that can be calculated. If the drug is projected to have third-year sales of $120,000,000, then each month's delay in the approval costs the company a minimum of $10,000,000 in sales. This does not include the up-front expenses incurred to resolve the issue with the regulatory agency and does not include losses the company may have incurred to prepare the product for market launch on an optimistic projected approval date. Thus the financial cost to a corporation of poorly written

and interpreted toxicology/pathology reports can be very significant.

IV. Preparation of the Final Report for a Toxicology Study

The preparation of the final report that documents and interprets the results of a single study is often the most difficult step in bringing the study to a successful conclusion. However, all the effort to conduct an excellent study will quickly be undone if the same level of care is not applied to the preparation of the final report. Further, the study results are of little value to anyone if they are not carefully written up and issued as a final report. Within a large corporation, individual departments depend on one another to complete their work accurately, completely, and on time. Frequently they cannot initiate their own work until the results of studies conducted in another department have been completed and reported. An example is the dependence of the clinical studies department on the department of drug safety. The clinical department cannot initiate its studies in humans unless the preclinical toxicity studies have been completed, their findings evaluated, and their significance for humans understood.

Once a report for a toxicity study is signed and issued, the information and interpretations it contains move like a ripple on a pond. From the date it is issued the final report is beyond the control of the individuals who wrote it or the department in which it was generated. From the issue date forward, data and interpretations of that data become an official document of the sponsoring corporation and become a permanent part of the record for the compound. The report is available for review and use by other individuals in the company and becomes one of the products that will be used in the decision-making process as development of the compound progresses. When the corporation completes and forwards regulatory submissions or submits annual updates for the compound, information in the individual final toxicology reports moves out of the corporation's control and into the domain of the regulatory agency to which they were submitted.

V. Organization of the Report

Unfortunately, many final reports for toxicology studies are organized and assembled in a manner that minimizes the time and costs incurred by the laboratory that conducted the study. It would appear that in many cases neither the management of the company who conducted the studies nor the authors who prepared the final reports ever critically evaluated the organization, presentation of data, or ease of review of their products. Little consideration appears to be given to the needs of the client(s) who will ultimately read their reports and make decisions based on their contents. Neither the corporate management nor the individual authors seem to have taken into account the fact that their reports are the products the client/reviewer will use to evaluate their corporate or individual capabilities. Based on the organization and quality of the interpretation of many toxicology reports, particularly from contract organizations, one is led to believe that neither the management nor the authors have ever had to defend their work before a regulatory agency. For the sponsoring corporation, lack of attention to the quality of the reports submitted to them by contract laboratories for approval and acceptance can be a major, and sometimes costly, mistake.

Examples of data taken directly from final toxicology reports will be presented later to demonstrate the just-described points.

A. TITLE PAGE

What is in a title? Something as simple as a corporate format for preparing titles for toxicology reports can be very important in data and document organization and retrieval. To facilitate efficient organization of the reports for a compound and their easy retrieval from archives, it is ideal if the title includes the compound number, species, route of delivery, duration of dosing, any special dosing regimen, and information about the recovery period. The title may have

other information specific to the type of study or assay that was conducted, e.g., reproductive toxicity studies or mutagenicity studies.

An example of a title format for an *in vivo* repeat-dose toxicity study might be the following: OTS-556: 28-Day Intravenous Toxicity Study with a 14-Day Recovery in the Sprague–Dawley Rat.

A simple title like the example has several benefits. When it comes time to archive the report it permits the archivist to file the report under the compound number, OTS-556, and to place the report with the rat studies conducted by the intravenous route, after the acute study results and before the longer term studies. Thus, organization of the archives can be simplified and the retrieval of the report made simple. However, to be effective, this method of titling reports has to be followed throughout the department and must also be followed by contract laboratories conducting studies for the sponsor.

When a regulatory submission is being prepared, the careful selection of the title for each study, based on use of a predetermined, uniform department procedure, will facilitate development of a very logical and clear table of contents for the regulatory documents.

B. INFORMATION/SIGNATURE PAGE

A page in the front of the report should present pertinent information about the study. Examples of information about the study that can be summarized on one of the initial pages of the report include the following:

The name and address of the sponsor
The name and address of the laboratory that conducted the study
The study initiation date
The study completion date
The report issue date
The name of the study director
The name of the pathologist who read the slides
The signature of the study director
The signature of the pathologist
The signature of the senior manager of the laboratory or department that conducted the study

This information is important for the purpose of documenting responsibility for data and responsibility for its interpretation. Ready access to this information can be very important at some future date if there is a need to compare data in the report to control data developed in the same laboratory, at the same time, and in the same species and strain of animal. This information is also useful if there is a request, at some future time, to compare data being developed by a current method to data developed in the study by a previous method.

C. TABLE OF CONTENTS

The tables of contents presents in chronological order all the sections and subsections of the report, its tables and figures, and its appendices. To be useful to the reviewer, the table of contents for the final signed report should present the page numbers where specific information can be located. Some laboratories, for their own convenience, do not paginate the appendices and leave it up to the reviewer to find the page where data are located. In a multivolume report, searching for individual animal data in the appendices can be a very frustrating and irritating exercise.

D. QUALITY ASSURANCE STATEMENT

The quality assurance (QA) statement should include a list of the dates when different activities within a study were inspected, the dates the inspections were conducted, and the dates the results were reported to management. It should be signed by the individuals who conducted the QA inspections and countersigned by the manager of the QA area. Careful review of QA statements found in final toxicology reports can raise a reviewer's concerns about the quality/thoroughness of this work. Mistakes such as giving a date for reporting findings to management that precedes the date when the actual inspections were conducted does not do much to inspire confidence in how carefully the study was inspected.

E. SUMMARY

The summary section in a final toxicology report can be scanned readily by individuals who only want to know the significant results of the study. Consequently, the summary is frequently placed before the introduction of the study. For this reason, significant effort should be expended in the preparation of the summary for a report.

The summary should include a brief statement of the objective of the study followed by a concise description of the study design. The study design section should include the compound number, the species used, group sizes, doses studied, route of administration, and duration of dosing. An abbreviated summary of the methods should be followed by a more extensive summary of results. It should include information on any mortalities that occurred and any compound-related findings in the in-life portion of the study followed by postmortem results. A useful format is to present data by dose group beginning with the findings at the lowest dose followed by the findings in each of the higher dose groups. The summary should either end with an evaluation of data or be followed by a separate section titled evaluation.

F. EVALUATION

Evaluate for the reader, either as the last paragraph of the summary or in a section titled evaluation, the significant findings in the study. An evaluation of data *is not* a restatement of the significant findings. The points that can be addressed in the evaluation include the following:

a. how well the drug was tolerated clinically by the animals and at up to what multiple of the clinical dose
b. the significant information in the toxicokinetic data (were the AUCs dose proportional or dose related or was there evidence of accumulation)
c. the target organ(s) of toxicity
d. the "no-observed adverse effect level" (NOAEL)
e. the significance of the findings

Include literature references in the evaluation to support interpretations of findings, if appropriate, e.g., the findings were consistent with those induced by a glucocorticoid (reference).

G. BODY OF THE REPORT

1. Introduction

The introduction to most toxicology reports should be brief unless there is a specific reason to provide additional information for the benefit of the reviewer. The introduction can include a brief description of the compound, its pharmacologic activity, and its intended clinical indication. When the final report for a single study is incorporated into a regulatory submission, it is only one of the many toxicology reports that will be reviewed. Thus it is not necessary to keep restating or summarizing the findings from previous studies to set the stage for the study that is being reported. The last sentence of the introduction should be a clear statement of the *objective* of the study. An example of a simple statement of the objective would be as follows: "The objective of this study was to determine in the rat the toxicity of compound OTS-556 when administered orally daily by gavage for 21 days." If the objective of the study is either not stated or not stated clearly, it can leave the reviewer questioning why the sponsor initiated the study.

2. Methods

The methods used to conduct a study are presented in a very organized fashion.

a. The Test Article. Information about the test article includes its chemical name and structure, its purity and stability, the storage conditions used prior to and during use, the lot number (and manufacturer), and information on how the material was prepared for administration to the test species. Information is presented on how samples of test article for each dose group were collected, stored, and analyzed to assure the accuracy of the doses administered over the course of the experiment.

b. Test Animals. Information is presented on the species, age, and weight of the animals that were used, their supplier, and how they were quarantined/vaccinated (if appropriate) and acclimated to the laboratory environment. Documentation should include how the animals were housed, the types of caging, numbers of animals per cage, the number of air changes per hour, the temperature and humidity of the animal room, and the light cycle that was used. In addition, information regarding what the animals were fed and the methods used to feed and water them, possible contaminants in the feed and water, who developed data, and where actual assay data are located should be given.

c. Experimental Design. The supportive information just given is presented before the experimental design is outlined. The experimental design can be presented effectively as a text table that lets the reviewer visualize the organization of the study. An example of a text table that outlines the experimental design is presented in Table I. The experimental design is supported by the justification for the doses, route, and regimen of administration that were selected for the study.

When the reviewer has completed reading the experimental design section of the report, there should be no doubt in his/her mind about the design of the study. Unfortunately, that is not always the case. An example of a poorly written experimental design is presented in the section on things to avoid and is demonstrated in Table II.

d. Clinical Signs, Body Weights, Food Consumption, etc. How data were collected during the in-life portion of the study include information on how and how frequently clinical signs, body weights, and food consumption were determined. If ophthalmologic evaluations were

TABLE I
14-Day Subcutaneous Toxicity Study in the Rat
Study Design[a]

Compound (mg/kg)	Dose volume	Number of rats/group	
		Males	Females
Control[b]	2.0	5	5
0.03	2.0	5	5
0.8	2.0	5	5
1.0	2.0	5	5
2.0	2.0	5	5

[a]This simple clear study design provides the reviewer with the study number, doses, route of administration, duration of dosing, species, and numbers of animals/sex/dose.
[b]0.5% carboxymethyl cellulose.

TABLE II
28-Day Oral Toxicity Study in the Rat
Experimental Design[a]

Dose (mg/kg)	Males	Females
1.65	5	
1.98	5	5
2.38	5	5
2.85	5	5
3.42	5	5
4.10		5

[a]Experimental design table from a toxicology report that one suspects was created after the study was conducted.

conducted or electrocardiograms were obtained, information regarding how and when this information was collected is presented.

e. Toxicokinetic Data. If toxicokinetic or single time-point data were obtained, information about collection intervals, sample preparation, storage, and assay methods are presented.

f. Clinical Pathology Data. Toxicokinetic information is followed by a presentation of how clinical pathology data were collected, when the samples were collected, how they were collected, and how they were prepared. The specific parameters that were evaluated in hematology, clinical chemistry, and urinalysis and the method used to generate data for each of the parameters are listed.

g. Postmortem Data. Next, the methods of sacrifice, necropsy, and tissue collection and tissue evaluation are presented. These include a list of all the organs that were weighed, all tissues that were collected, and an outline of how the tissues were fixed and stored. The last of the postmortem methods is a listing of tissues that were evaluated microscopically and identification of the dose at which the tissues were evaluated.

If pathology data were peer reviewed, the methods used to conduct the review and the methods used to resolve differences in diagnosis between the study pathologist and the peer review pathologist are outlined.

h. Statistical Evaluation. The last item presented in the methods section is the statistical

methods that were used in the study and identification of the significance levels that were used to assess drug-related changes.

3. Results

The presentation of data in the results section of the report should follow, as close as possible, the sequence in which data were collected as outlined in the methods section.

a. Mortality. One of the first pieces of information to be presented early in the results section is mortality data. This information identifies the doses at which mortality occurred, presents the clinical signs that preceded death, and presents the gross and microscopic changes that were associated with death. This method of presentation may show that the findings in the animals that died were consistent with changes observed at certain doses in the animals terminated at the scheduled necropsy. Comparing the two sets of findings may indicate that early deaths probably were compound related. However, it may demonstrate the opposite, that the findings in animals that died were not similar to those in the animals that survived to the end of the study and the deaths were probably not related to administration of the compound.

b. Toxicokinetic Data. Toxicokinetic data may be presented very early in the results, possibly after the information on mortality. Toxicokinetic data provide the reviewer with a framework against which to compare the rest of the study results. Toxicokinetics may explain why the drug appeared to be very safe (compound was poorly absorbed) or why the findings showed a dose or possibly a sex relationship.

c. Clinical Observations, Body Weight, and Food Consumption. Clinical signs, body weight, and food consumption data are followed by results from ophthalmological evaluations and cardiovascular studies (if conducted). Clinical pathology data are presented (hematology, clinical chemistry, and urinalysis), followed by necropsy, organ weight, and microscopic findings. In presenting data from many of these parameters, text tables followed by a brief written description are very useful tools for presenting and interpreting compound-related data concisely. Text tables can present complex information that would be difficult to describe concisely and accurately. However, to be useful, the tables have to be constructed carefully and thoughtfully so they convey the correct message accurately. Text tables are not to be confused with or take the place of raw data tables or overall summary tables. Text tables are presented to give the reader a specific message.

Unfortunately, not all text tables are as clear to the reviewer as they were to their author. An example of how text tables can confuse the presentation of data is illustrated in Table III. Table III shows clinical observations that were included in a dermal toxicity report. It was intended to demonstrate the incidence of erythema observed at the site of application of the test material. However the way the table was constructed, made it impossible for the reviewer to determine the incidence of this observation. What was the incidence of erythema in this study? Similarly, graphs, if used to present complex data, visually, need to be constructed so they neither magnify nor conceal the significance of a finding.

d. Clinical Pathology Data. In the presentation of hematology and clinical chemistry data, text tables are a simple way to identify to the reviewer those parameters considered to reflect compound-related changes. Table IV is an example of a text table for clinical pathology

data. If there are individual values for certain parameters that are statistically significantly different than control, it is important to indicate how the author interprets these observations in the accompanying text. For example, "The values, though statistically significant, were still in the range for control values for the parameter and there was no evidence of a dose relationship to the observation."

e. Organ Weights. A brief written description of compound-related changes that occurred in organ weight data complemented by a text table that displays the compound-related changes is an effective way to present this information. The text table presents both absolute and relative weights, by sex, for the organs in which the weights were either higher or lower than the controls. The reviewer can see that both absolute and relative weights changed in the same direction and that both values were statistically significantly different than the controls. For weight changes that are of questionable significance, the points as to why they are not considered to reflect a compound-related change should be developed in the text.

Organ weight data taken from the final report of a toxicology study are presented in Table V. Table V permits the reader to visualize quickly data that the author(s) interpreted to reflect compound-related changes. To create Table V from the original report, it was necessary to review and select data from five pages of tables of organ weights. Tables V, VI, and VII are illustrated to demonstrate the effort a reviewer often has to make to confirm the interpretations of the author. Table VI is data found on page 44 of the report. Data for Table VII came from page 46 of the report (right half of absolute organ weights table—males) and from page 48 of the report (remainder of relative organ weights—males). No data indicating a compound-related effect were found on page 45 or 47 of the organ weight tables.

The amount of effort required on the part of the reviewer in this report to confirm an organ weight change can only serve to alienate the reviewer and certainly will not serve to develop confidence that the sponsor reviewed the report

TABLE III
One-Month Dermal Toxicity Study in Rabbit
Clinical Observations[a]

	Incidence of findings				
Group	1	2	3	4	5
Dose (mg/kg)	0	2	8	32	128
Number/group	3	3	3	3	3
Erythema					
None	3	3	3	3	3
Minimal	0	1	2	1	2
Mild	0	1	3	3	2
Moderate	0	0	0	1	3

[a]A clinical observation table from a dermal toxicity report that leaves the reviewer questioning what it means.

TABLE IV
OTS-556: 28-Day Oral Toxicity Study in Rat
Clinical Pathology Data[a]

	OTS-556 (mg/kg)									
	Males					Females				
	0	6	24	96	384	0	6	24	96	384
Number	10	10	10	10	10	10	10	10	10	10
Hematology										
WBCs (10^3/ml)	10.1	9.1	7.9*	8.7	8.1*	6.0	5.6	5.8	5.0	6.3
NEU (10^3/ml)	1.8	1.2	1.0*	1.2	1.3	1.0	0.9	0.8	0.7	0.9
LYM (10^3/ml)	7.9	7.5	6.4	7.0	6.3	4.7	4.5	4.7	4.1	5.1
RBCs (10^6/ml)	9.04	9.10	8.84	9.07	8.67*	8.66	8.51	8.54	8.59	8.50
Hct (%)	46.3	45.7	45.1	45.5	44.9	46.5	46.1	46.0	45.7	44.7*
Hgb (g/dl)	15.2	14.9	15.0	15.2	15.3	15.7	15.6	15.6	15.6	15.4
RET (%)	1.7	1.5	1.4	0.9*	1.7	0.7	1.2	1.0	1.0	1.2
MCV	51.2	50.2	51.1	50.2	51.9	53.8	54.2	53.8	53.2	52.7*
MCH	16.8	16.4	17.0	16.8	17.7*	18.1	18.3	18.2	18.2	18.1
MCHC	32.9	32.7	33.2	33.5	34.1*	33.7	33.8	33.9	34.1	34.4
APTT	18.1	18.1	17.6	17.6	17.1	17.0	16.7	16.7	15.7*	16.5
Serum biochemistry										
GOT (IU/liter)	114	105	92	99	101	117	111	90	109	125
GPT (IU/liter)	45	41	32	41	40	53	48	31*	35*	45
LDH (IU/liter)	2467	2555	2361	2190	2380	1923	1580	1618	1871	1549
ChE (IU/liter)	22	23	28*	27	33*	312	302	314	325	286
UN (mg/dl)	18.3	18.1	17.5	18.7	18.2	18.4	18.5	18.8	19.1	20.3
CRE (md/dl)	0.50	0.48	0.46	0.50	0.44*	0.55	0.50	0.54	0.51	0.49
A/G	1.15	1.11	1.23	1.17	1.30	1.54	1.69	1.66	1.70*	1.73*
TP (g/dl)	6.19	6.17	5.94*	6.02	5.77*	6.64	6.37	6.39	6.36	6.18
T CHO (mg/dl)	64	74	69	71	85*	82	83	78	88	83
Na (mEq/liter)	142	142	142	143	140*	140	114	141	141	140
P (mg/dl)	5.9	6.0	5.7	5.8	5.9	4.4	4.6	4.3	4.5	4.8
γ-globulin (g/dl)	0.21	0.14*	0.13*	0.14*	0.12*	0.23	0.18*	0.18*	0.17*	0.15*
β-1-globulin	1.04	1.05	0.99	0.98	0.95	1.05	0.96*	0.94*	0.95*	0.89*

[a]Example of a text table in a toxicology study that gives the reviewer an immediate overview of the changes observed in clinical chemistry parameters.
*$P < 0.05$ compared to control.

carefully. The system used to tabulate data in this particular report was clearly for the convenience of the laboratory that did the work and not for the client who will review and evaluate it.

f. Gross Observations. Presentation of a brief written description of the significant compound-related findings by dose administered, starting with the lowest dose in which a finding was observed, again provides the reviewer with a mental picture of the doses at which no gross pathologic changes occurred.

Including a text table that presents the gross observations by dose, sex, and incidence is a format that is easy to understand and presents the findings effectively. An example of a format that makes it easy to visualize gross or

Hugh E. Black

TABLE V
OTS-556: 13-Week Oral Toxicity Study in the Rat[a]

Dose group		Terminal body weight (g)	Thyroid		Heart		Liver		Spleen	
			g	%	g	%	g	%	g	%
0.0	Mean	309	0.021	0.0068	1.24	0.399	13.43	4.324	0.83	0.268
	SD	19	0.002	0.0007	0.10	0.020	1.75	0.306	0.05	0.022
	Number	10	10	10	10	10	10	10	10	10
0.3	Mean	315	0.015*	0.0047*	1.24	0.395	13.41	4.253	0.83	0.264
	SD	19	0.003	0.0007	0.11	0.018	1.22	0.203	0.10	0.019
	Number	10	10	10	10	10	10	10	10	10
3.0	Mean	303	0.016*	0.0052*	1.17	0.387	12.92	4.262	0.81	0.269
	SD	27	0.003	0.0006	0.10	0.026	1.50	0.168	0.08	0.025
	Number	10	10	10	10	10	10	10	10	10
30.0	Mean	276	0.018*	0.0066*	1.08*	0.39	15.29*	5.534*	0.69*	0.249
	SD	19	0.002	0.0010	0.10	0.21	1.36	0.369	0.06	0.015
	Number	10	10	10	10	10	10	10	10	10

Group mean organ weights (males)

[a]Example of a text table of organ weight data that gives the reviewer an immediate overview of significant changes that occured in both absolute and relative values.
*$P < 0.001$.

microscopic pathology data is presented in Table VIII.

g. *Microscopic Observations.* As with gross observations, presenting only a brief written description of the significant compound-related microscopic findings and accompanying it with a well-organized text table is an effective way to present complex observations. An example of a text table that will permit the reviewer to visualize the incidence of compound-related micro-

TABLE VI
13-Week Oral Toxicity Study in the Rat[a]

Absolute group mean organ weights
Dose (mg/kg) 0, 0.3, 3.0, 30.0

Group/sex		Terminal body weight (g) (page 44)	Thyroid (g) (page 44)	Heart (g) (page 44)	Liver (g) (page 44)	Spleen (g) (page 44)
1 M	Mean	309	0.021	1.24	13.43	0.83
	SD	19	0.002	0.10	1.75	0.05
	Number	10	10	10	10	10
2 M	Mean	315	0.015*	1.24	13.41	0.83
	SD	19	0.003	0.11	1.22	0.10
	Number	10	10	10	10	10
3 M	Mean	303	0.016	1.17	12.92	0.81
	SD	27	0.003	0.10	1.50	0.08
	Number	10	10	10	10	10
4 M	Mean	276**	0.018*	1.08*	15.29**	0.69*
	SD	19	0.002	0.10	1.36	0.06
	Number	10	10	10	10	10

[a]Table of absolute organ weights from one of five pages of organ weight tables in an issued toxicology report (page 44) (used to construct Table IV).
* $P < 0.01$.
** $P < 0.001$.

428

TABLE VII
13-Week Oral Toxicity Study in the Rat[a]

| | | Group mean relative organ weights Dose (mg/kg) 0, 0.3, 3.0, 30.0 | | | |
Group/sex		Thyroid (%) (page 46)	Heart (%) (page 46)	Liver (%) (page 48)	Spleen (%) (page 48)
1 M	Mean	0.0068	0.399	4.324	0.268
	SD	0.0007	0.020	0.306	0.222
	Number	10	10	10	10
2 M	Mean	0.0047*	0.395	4.253	0.264
	SD	0.0007	0.018	0.203	0.019
	Number	10	10	10	10
3 M	Mean	0.0052*	0.387	4.262	0.269
	SD	0.0006	0.026	0.168	0.025
	Number	10	10	10	10
4 M	Mean	0.0066*	0.390	5.534*	0.249
	SD	0.0010	0.021	0.369	0.015
	Number	10	10	10	10

[a]Table of relative organ weights from two of five pages of organ weight tables (pages 46 to 48) in an issued toxicology report (used to construct Table IV).
*$P < 0.01$.

TABLE VIII
OTS-556: 28-Day Oral Toxicity Study in the Rat
(Microscopic Observations)[a]

Dose (mg/kg) Sex	0		2.0		8.0		16.0	
	Male	Female	Male	Female	Male	Female	Male	Female
28-Day Necropsy Number	3	3	3	3	3	3	3	3
GIT								
Lymphoid atrophy								
Stomach					1/3	0/3	3/3	3/3
Duodenum							0/3	1/3
Jejunum							0/3	0/3
Ileum							3/3	3/3
Caecum							3/3	3/3
Colon							3/3	2/3
Mucosal atrophy								
Duodenum					2/3	2/3	3/3	3/3
Jejunum					2/3	2/3	3/3	3/3
Lymphoid atrophy								
Thymus							3/3	3/3
Mesenteric LN					1/3	1/3	3/3	3/3
Mandibular LN					0/3	1/3	3/3	3/3
Spleen							3/3	3/3
Bone marrow (femur)								
Atrophy							2/3	2/3
Bone marrow (sternum)								
Atrophy							3/3	3/3

[a]Example of a text table that quickly illustrates for the reviewer the distribution and incidence of microscopic changes that the pathologist determined to be compound related.

429

TABLE IX
One-Month Dermal Toxicity Study in the Rabbit[a]

	Microscopic changes in the skin				
Group	1	2	3	4	5
Dose (mg/kg)	0	2	8	32	128
Number/group	3	3	3	3	3
Intact/abraded					
Hyperkeratosis					
Minimal	0/0	3/2	2/2	1/3	3/3
Mild	0/0	0/1	1/1	2/0	0/0
Inflammation					
Minimal	1/0	1/3	1/3	1/2	2/3
Mild	0/0	1/1	1/0	1/1	1/0

[a]Example of a text table of microscopic observations taken from a dermal toxicity study that leaves the reviewer questioning its meaning.

scopic lesions by organ and dose group quickly is presented in Table VIII. As stated previously, careful preparation of the text table is necessary. Contrast the ease of review and evaluation of the dose-related findings in Table VIII with the microscopic observations presented in Table IX from a dermal toxicity final report.

The presentation of data using a format such as that in Table IX leaves the reviewer questioning its meaning. Further review and tabulation of individual animal data in the report from which Table IX was taken demonstrated that the incidence of microscopic findings was actually as presented in Table X. Note the marked difference reformatting the data had

on the reviewers understanding of what occurred in the study.

4. Discussion

A discussion of the results in a final report may not be necessary if changes have been interpreted at the time they were presented in the results section of the report. If a discussion is written, it should put the significant findings in the study in context for the reviewer. The discussion *should not be* a restatement of the results. Changes that reflect the known pharmacologic activity of the compound should be identified and referenced. If the findings were consistent for the class of compound, that should be stated and supported with a reference

TABLE X
One-Month Dermal Toxicity Study in the Rabbit[a]

	Microscopic changes in the skin									
	Intact					Abraded				
Group	1	2	3	4	5	1	2	3	4	5
Dose (mg/kg)	0	2	8	32	128	0	2	8	32	128
Number/group	3	3	3	3	3	3	3	3	3	3
Hyperkeratosis										
Minimal	0	3	2	1	3	0	2	2	3	3
Mild	0	0	1	2	0	0	1	1	0	0
Inflammation										
Minimal	1	1	1	1	2	0	3	3	2	3
Mild	0	0	1	1	1	0	0	0	1	0

[a]The same data as presented in Table IX but reformatted. Note the difference in the ease with which this table can be read and understood.

to the published literature. The consistency or difference of the results of the present study from those observed in previous studies should be pointed out to the reader. The specific studies with the compound to which the writer is referring must be identified clearly for the reader. When developing a discussion, do not include any speculation. A report for a toxicology study is not a publication. The writer must keep in mind the different ways a document of this type may eventually be used.

5. Conclusion

Points to be addressed in the conclusion of a final report include how well the drug was tolerated clinically by the animals and at up to what multiple of the clinical dose; the significant information in toxicokinetic data (were the AUC's dose proportional or dose related or was there evidence of accumulation); the target organ(s) of toxicity; the NOAEL; and the significance of the findings.

Literature references are included to support the conclusions, if appropriate, e.g., "findings were consistent with those induced by a glucocorticoid" (reference).

6. References

All publications or company reports referred to in the toxicology report should be referenced as they would be for a publication.

7. Summary Tables

Summary tables should present data in a format that facilitates review by the client. Thought should go into the titles as well as how data are organized and presented. The reviewer should not have to guess as to the data being presented. Presentation of the title on only the first page of a table that extends for a number of pages is not acceptable.

8. Appendices

Appendices contain the "raw data" that a reviewer can use to recreate summary data or confirm an observation, if necessary.

    toxicokinetics

week of death for each animal
individual body weights
individual food consumption
individual clinical signs for each animal to include the week of observation of each sign and a description of each sign and its subsequent course
individual clinical pathology values
individual organ weights, and organ/body weight ratio
individual gross pathology findings
individual histopathology findings
statistical methods references
certificate of analysis
ophthalmologist's signed report
cardiologist's signed report
pathologist's signed report
clinical pathologist's signed report
study protocol and protocol amendments
MSDS for test articles and vehicle
list of study deviations and statement by study director certifying integrity of study

H. THINGS TO AVOID IN PREPARING A FINAL REPORT

1. A Study Design That Is Difficult for the Reader to Understand

What was the experimental design in the following study? "In the preliminary study there were four males per group. Deaths were 2, 3, 4, and 4 in the 2.85-, 4.10-, 5.9-, and 7.08-mg/kg groups, respectively. In the main study, deaths occurred in 1/5, 0/5, 2/5, 4/5, and 5/5 males."

Based on the last sentence of the justification of the study design and the study design table, the reviewer is left questioning if the study design in the original protocol was as stated or if it evolved as data became available.

If the reviewer is not sure of the study design, as illustrated in Table II, he/she may also be skeptical of the findings presented in the results.

2. Presentation of Selected Results in the Methods Section of a Report

The findings in a study should not be presented in the methods section of a report. It has the effect of leading the reviewer to conclusions before the individual has read the results section.

The following example is presented where repeated reference to selected findings in the methods section of a report led a reviewer to conclude that the sponsor should rerun the study. Lost in all the discussion about 3/45 weanling animals (one of the three was a control) that died during the first 15 days on study was the fact this was a 6-month study. There were no deaths after day 15. The animals were dosed at up to 10 times the proposed clinical dose and there were no compound-related changes in clinical pathology, necropsy, organ weights, or microscopic findings at any dose in animals that survived to the terminal necropsy. Unfortunately, in the results section of the report, the authors also placed all emphasis on the three animals that died between days 1 and 15.

The following examples show how the author influenced the reviewer's thinking.

1. *Hematology.* No hematology parameters or clinical chemistry data were obtained from animals #3, #10, and #14 that died on days 4, 14, and 15, respectively. The following hematological parameters were determined at day 1 and weeks 4, 8, 16, and 24 (the individual parameters are listed).

2. *Organ weights.* No organ weights were obtained for dogs #3, #10, and #14 that died on days 4, 14, and 15, respectively. The following organs were weighted at the terminal necropsy: liver, kidney (and the remainder of the list is presented).

3. *Necropsy.* In addition to the tissues processed as outlined later, the mesenteric lymph node was collected from animal #3 that died on day 4; three sections of pancreas were collected from animal #10 that died on day 14 and three sections of pancreas and an additional section of the stomach were collected from animal #14 that died on day 15. The following tissues were collected at the terminal sacrifice (the list of tissues collected at necropsy is then provided).

There was a detailed description in the results section of the heroics that the laboratory veterinarian went to in an attempt to save animal #14, which the author failed to mention was a control animal.

3. Presentation in Results of Parameters Not Mentioned in the Methods Section

It is important to build credibility with the reviewer as he/she evaluates the results of a study. Do not present data in the results section without first indicating in the methods section that data were developed. It causes an immediate concern in the reviewer's mind as to whether other data may have been developed during the study and excluded arbitrarily from the report. Further, do not present data in a table or figure and then present the method used to develop it as a footnote to the table or figure. The level of detail that can be presented as a footnote to a table does not give sufficient detail to be convincing and credible. It makes the reader question the design of the original protocol, the quality control in the conduct of the study, and if there was some specific reason the author did not want the information included in the methods section of the report. Surprising the reader with unanticipated data does not inspire confidence in the report.

4. Do Not Irritate the Reviewer

The author(s) can unintentionally introduce material into a report that will irritate the reviewer. This includes only referring to the compound as the "test article" instead of using the compound number, referring to the dose groups by group number rather than by the dose administered, or referring to the test species as animals rather than the specific species that was used for the study. It is understood that these methods of presentation are convenient for the author(s) or for computerization of report preparation, but they can prove to be very awkward for the reviewer. They can force the reviewer to keep returning to the study design constantly to refresh his/her memory as to which group number refers to which dose of the compound being evaluated. Shortcuts such as these do not take into account the need of the client, usually the reviewer in a regulatory agency.

VI. Conclusion

Preparing the final report for a toxicology study can be the most difficult part of the study. The needs of the client must have priority in this process. The report is the product that will be used by the client(s) to make decisions. The report is also the tool used by the client to evaluate the capabilities of the laboratory where the study took place and the competence of the individuals who conducted it. The ultimate client, however, is the patient who will receive the compound as a medication in the treatment of his/her disease. It is that client that the author should always keep in mind.

PART C
Selected Topics in Toxicologic Pathology

Risk Assessment: The Changing Paradigm

Stephen K. Durham
Discovery Safety Optimization
Bristol-Myers Squibb PRI
Princeton, New Jersey

James A. Swenberg
Laboratory of Molecular Carcinogenesis and Mutagenesis
University of North Carolina
Chapel Hill, North Carolina

I. Introduction

When viewed in a broad context, veterinary pathologists and toxicologists participate in the risk assessment process on a daily basis. The pathologist, together with the input from his colleagues in toxicology, initially identifies the potential adverse effects of chemicals and drugs in laboratory animals, defines the dose–response of the effects, and then determines whether they are likely to express themselves in humans. Risk only occurs when both hazard and exposure exist, i.e., risk is the probability that a hazard will be expressed. In order to ascertain an accurate conclusion in the risk assessment process, broad scientific knowledge with biologically based mechanistic information is required. Mechanism helps to determine whether the hazard will develop in humans and may give quantitative information to suggest that risk is more or less likely to occur. It may also help identify subpopulations that are at greater or lessor risk. Thus, there is a critical need for a scientific understanding of mechanism to reduce the extent of uncertainty associated with the assessment of risk.

Several definitions are required to fully appreciate the risk assessment process. *Hazard*

identification entails the identification of agents with potential adverse effects such as carcinogenicity, neurotoxicity, and developmental toxicity. *Dose–response assessment* evaluates the conditions under which the agent might manifest the toxicity. *Exposure assessment* estimates the populations that might be exposed, the routes of exposure, and the magnitude, duration, and timing of such exposure. *Risk assessment* is the systematic, integration of the just-described data to characterize the potential for adverse effects on human health as a result of exposure to hazardous agents or situations. This type of assessment should carefully weigh the scientific evidence. It can be either qualitative or quantitative in nature and should ultimately include the potential magnitude of any risks and a description of the associated uncertainties in the conclusions and estimates. Risk assessment is not limited to human health applications, but is widely utilized by a number of nonmedical disciplines. Risk assessment is an entity that is distinct from risk management. *Risk management* is the decision-making process that formulates policy actions designed to reduce the probability that the hazard will be expressed. Different skill sets are required for risk assessment and risk management. In addition to evaluating risk estimates, risk managers must also consider statutory, economic, social, and political factors. The perception of risk and its impact varies greatly between societies. *Risk communication*, the process of disseminating comprehensible risk assessment and risk management information, is addressed in Chapter 18.

II. Traditional Risk Assessment

The ultimate objectives of the risk assessment process are to balance the risks and the benefits to an individual and to society, select acceptable levels of risk for that individual and society, and estimate residual risks and methods for risk reduction after implementation. There are major differences in the risk assessment of a drug and a chemical with widespread environmental exposure. In the case of the drug, the same individual that receives the benefit incurs the risk. In contrast, in the case of environmental exposure to a pesticide, the benefit is to the manufacturer and the user, whereas the risk resides in a different population. There are several key factors, and their associated assumptions and limitations, in traditional risk assessment (Tables I and II). A predominant problematic factor for the risk assessor during this process is the quality of the scientific data. A paradigm change that incorporates a broad scientific knowledge with biologically based, mechanistic information should enhance this aspect of risk assessment by increasing confidence in the accuracy of the assessment. As mentioned earlier, traditional risk assessment is composed of four major components: (1) hazard identification, (2) dose–response evaluation, (3) exposure assessment, and (4) risk characterization.

Hazard identification is a qualitative process utilized to identify the potential exposure and

TABLE I
Key Factors in Traditional Risk Assessment

Environmental or occupational exposure
Dose-related toxicologic responses in animal studies
Pharmacokinetic and toxicokinetic profiles in animal studies
Human epidemiological studies
Mathematical and statistical models

TABLE II
Assumptions and Limitations in Traditional Risk Assessment

High-dose studies used to predict low-dose effects
Assumption of genetic homogeneity in the population
Simple mathematical models representing complex anatomy and pharmacokinetics
Interspecies differences used a $10 \times$ safety factor
Gender-related differences ignored

nature of the adverse health effect in humans for a particular chemical. Adequate identification of a hazard incorporates numerous data sets, including structure–activity relationships, *in vitro* analyses, genotoxicity, metabolism, animal bioassays, and epidemiological data. The identification of numerous potential chemical hazards has occurred following the establishment of robust structure–activity data sets. The structural similarities between chemotypes, and their associated physical and reactive properties, represent important information in the early identification of potential hazards. The sensitivity (ability to identify true hazards) and specificity (ability to differentiate between true positives and negatives) from early computational (*in silico*) approaches evaluating carcinogenicity have been disappointing. However, modifications of these *in silico* toxicology programs have generated more promising results. The utilization of robust, validated *in vitro* tests provides an avenue for rapid and economical risk assessment. Genotoxicity data are among the most commonly used *in vitro* data. Likewise, information on metabolic activation and detoxication pathways, including species differences and dose–response relationships, is critical information that has an impact on the risk assessment. The incorporation of these data into biologically based pharmacokinetic models permits more accurate high-to-low dose and species-to-species extrapolation. It is important to recognize that reliance on tests whose outcomes include either false negatives or false positives can affect society adversely.

Animal bioassays, another tier in the hazard identification process, are a standard component of hazard identification. Animal carcinogenicity studies usually employ ~ 50 animals/sex/dose, but are being used to predict risks to large populations of humans. Thus, sensitivity is a major issue of concern. To maximize the ability to identify a potential human carcinogen, such animals are usually exposed to the maximum amount of test substance that is tolerated without inducing excessive toxicity. These high-dose exposures may alter the way a chemical is metabolized and result in conditions that do not occur at low exposures. Knowledge of such effects needs to be incorporated into dose–response modeling of data. The most appropriate rodent bioassays are usually those that evaluate exposure pathways of most relevance to humans. In the realm of carcinogenicity, a principal default assumption is that chemicals that induce tumors in animals are presumed to cause tumors in humans. Although this concept is the accepted standard default, it is widely recognized that there are exceptions. In the absence of adequate epidemiologic data in humans, animal carcinogenicity data must be used to identify potential hazards. Other major default assumptions in cancer risk assessment are that humans are assumed to be as sensitive as the most sensitive animal species and that the dose–response is assumed to be linear. Again, the default is needed in the absence of data, but should be replaced when appropriate data are available.

The most convincing evidence for risk in humans is derived from sound, well-conducted epidemiological studies that document a positive association between exposure and disease. Three major subtypes of epidemiological studies can be performed: cross-sectional, cohort, and case–control. Cross-sectional studies survey groups of humans to identify exposure to risk factors and incidence of disease; cross-sectional studies are not useful for establishing cause and effect relationships. Cohort studies select individuals based on their exposure to the hazard under study and are monitored prospectively for the development of disease. Case–control studies are retrospective in nature and select individuals based on disease status with comparison to disease-free individuals. Epide-

miological studies should be evaluated for robustness of detection, appropriateness of outcomes, verification of exposure, complete assessment of confounders, and general applicability of the outcomes to other populations at risk. Epidemiologists have identified criteria for evaluating data, including consistency and strength of data, specificity of the response, temporality of disease versus exposure, coherence of multiple data sets, dose–response, biological plausibility, and experimental support and analogy. It is through such a thorough evaluation of data that distinctions are made regarding causality versus association. To determine that a chemical or process is causally related to the induction of cancer in humans requires a robust data set. This conclusion is clearly different from a single observation of an association between exposure and some form of cancer. Such associations require further hypothesis testing and by themselves do not withstand the rigor required for causality.

There is an increasing shift from simple hazard identification to *hazard characterization*. Hazard characterization includes all of the parameters of hazard identification, but also brings in information on "under what conditions is the hazard present." This concept is important, as chemicals were often placed in a category or "box" early in the risk assessment process, and it was very difficult to remove them from that classification when additional data became available that demonstrated a lack of, or decreased relevance for, the end point for humans. It must be recognized that risk assessment of a given agent is an evolving process that changes as additional data are gathered. Using a weight-of-the-evidence approach that incorporates the best scientific understanding will provide the most accurate characterization of risk.

The second major component of risk assessment is the dose–response evaluation. *Dose–response evaluation* characterizes the relationship between exposure to an agent of concern and the incidence or severity of the adverse response in the exposed population qualitatively and quantitatively. Dose–response relationships normally characterize effect levels over a broad range of conditions, including acute, subchronic, and chronic effects. The no observed adverse effect level (NOAEL) is usually an important data point for evaluations of toxicity. During the characterization phase, margins of safety or exposure and therapeutic indexes are usually determined. Likewise, data can be evaluated to determine if the dose–response is linear or nonlinear. Typically for risk assessment purposes, human exposure data that can be used in the prediction of responses in human populations are extremely limited. Thus, the majority of biological responses to the test agent of concern are derived from animal bioassay data. A real dilemma is that risk assessors are usually interested in low-exposure concentrations that are often well below the experimental range of responses in animal bioassays. It is well understood that many effects of high-dose exposure do not occur at low exposures. Examples of this include saturation of detoxication and increases in cell proliferation associated with toxicity. Such effects can be incorporated into physiologically based models to predict low-dose effects more accurately. The utilization of low-dose extrapolation models coupled with animal-to-human hazard extrapolation methods largely constitute the predominant aspects of the dose–response assessment process. The incorporation of biologically based models whenever possible should reduce uncertainties.

Exposure assessment entails the determination of the source, amount, and duration of human exposure to the agent of concern. The determination of the relevant exposure pathways is crucial to this process. A confounding factor for exposure assessment is the broad variation in behavior and susceptibility. Marked variation in susceptibility largely resides in the genetic heterogeneity of the human population coupled with individual factors, such as behavioral traits. This represents an important area for future investigation.

More and more, data on blood and tissue concentrations of the chemical or drug, or biomarkers of exposure such as DNA or protein adducts, are being incorporated into the risk assessment process. Here, a large difference exists between pharmaceuticals and industrial or agrichemicals. Human data are usually available for the former group, but only occasionally available for the latter agents. Furthermore, human exposure is often within an order of magnitude of animal toxicity data for pharmaceuticals, but often three to six orders of magnitude lower for environmental exposures. Physiologically based pharmacokinetic models can incorporate much of this type of information and more closely approximate species differences in exposure and response.

Risk characterization predicts the frequency and severity of effects in the exposed population. The initial components of the risk assessment process are based on objectively examined, highly factual scientific data. As one proceeds through the process, rational judgement plays a much greater role, as the risk assessor has to address variability, uncertainty, and social policy that may conflict directly with objectivity. The current regulatory framework of this process was initiated in the middle of the 20th century, with the subsequent implementation of numerous federal laws related to exposures to toxic substances. In the past, hazard identification process largely focused on carcinogens, with numerous classification schemes from a variety of agencies, such as the Occupational Safety and Health Administration, International Agency for Research an Cancer, and U.S. Environmental Protection Agency (EPA). The regulatory agencies involved in this process usually rely on epidemiological and animal toxicology data. Infrequently, controlled clinical exposure data are also employed. More recently, greater attention has on noncancer end points, including developmental toxicity, reproductive toxicity, and neurotoxicity.

III. The Changing Paradigm

Within the past decade, there has been a substantial effort to move from the traditional default-based risk assessment paradigm to a science-based risk assessment process that utilizes mechanistic data more fully. This new paradigm is based on integrating additional knowledge on metabolism, toxicology, pathology, and mechanisms to improve the risk assessment process. For example, using a valid toxicokinetic model to predict exposures at the tissue, cell, or molecular level, rather than using a surface area correction for interspecies extrapolation of data, would more likely improve the accuracy of a risk assessment. Superficially, the expansion and inclusion of additional scientific information in this process should be readily accepted and reduce uncertainty. However, the utilization of this information has clearly added complexity to the process. The International Program on Chemical Safety and the EPA have developed a framework to assist in evaluating mechanistic data. This framework is based on the Bradford Hill criteria used to evaluate epidemiology data that were discussed previously. Basically, a mode of action for a given toxic response is postulated and key events in this process are identified. Data are then evaluated for dose–response, temporality, strength, consistency, and specificity of the key events and the toxic end point. The biological plausibility and coherence of data are reviewed and alternative modes of action are assessed. Based on the results of this framework analysis, the proposed mode of action is evaluated objectively. In addition, important data gaps, inconsistencies, and uncertainties are identified.

While there is little doubt that science-based risk assessment is desirable, it often creates confusion in the general public. When regulatory standards are lowered because greater risk was assumed using default-based risk assessment, environmentalists and members of the general public are concerned that the new regulations are "less protective of the public health." It is important that the scientific and regulatory communities point out that such default-based risk assessments have large uncertainties associated with estimated risks and that they are not known risks. The protection of public health is always the primary objective of risk assessment, but such protection is not without societal cost.

A more accurate risk assessment based on good science, rather than default-based risk assessment with great uncertainty, will both protect the public health and minimize costs of regulation to society. As long as the risk assessment process incorporates the uncertainty associated with the use of high-to low-dose extrapolation methods and interspecies extrapolation, there will always be room for improvement.

IV. Examples of Mechanistically Based Risk Assessment

A. $\alpha_{2\mu}$-GLOBULIN NEPHROPATHY

Initial concerns were raised following the development of $\alpha_{2\mu}$-globulin nephropathy and increased renal neoplasia in male rats following exposure to a diverse set of compounds in which humans are regularly exposed, including unleaded gasoline, D-limonene, 1,4-dichlorobenzene, tetrachloroethylene, decalin, and lindane. Acute to subacute $\alpha_{2\mu}$-globulin nephropathy in male rats is characterized by the presence of protein droplets in proximal tubular epithelium, the formation of granular casts, and the presence of scattered, regenerative tubules. The progression of this syndrome to the chronic stage is characterized by chronic progressive nephrosis, mineralization of the renal medulla, and a variable incidence of tubular adenoma or carcinoma. $\alpha_{2\mu}$-Globulin is synthesized in the liver under multihormonal control, including androgens, and is freely filtered by the glomerulus due to its low molecular weight (18,700 Da). Approximately one-half of the $\alpha_{2\mu}$-globulin is reabsorbed via endocytosis in the S2 segment of the proximal tubule, where it is hydrolyzed slowly. Many of the compounds or their metabolites bind reversibly to $\alpha_{2\mu}$-globulin and decrease the effectiveness of lysosomal proteases to break down the moiety, resulting in the characteristic protein droplet morphology. Mechanistic studies indicate that the genesis of renal tumors resides in tubular epithelial necrosis secondary to lysosomal overload, leading to a sustained increase in cell proliferation in the renal cortex, followed by the formation of preneoplastic to neoplastic foci. Additional studies documented that the key events leading to this nephropathy and associated neoplasia do not occur in male NBR rats, which lack $\alpha_{2\mu}$-globulin synthesis. In light of these mechanistic studies, humans were not considered to be at risk because they do not synthesize $\alpha_{2\mu}$-globulin. In addition, humans secrete less low molecular weight proteins (LMWP) in their urine as compared to rats, do not have LMWPs in the urine that are structurally similar to $\alpha_{2\mu}$-globulin, or bind to compounds that bind reversibly to $\alpha_{2\mu}$-globulin.

B. PEROXISOME PROLIFERATORS

Another example in which species-specific mechanisms lowered the assessment of human risk was the class of chemicals known as peroxisome proliferators. Rodents treated chronically with a variety of drugs and chemicals, including fibrate hypolipidemic drugs, herbicides, plasticizers, and solvents, develop a significant increase in the number and size of hepatocellular peroxisomes, induction of enzymes involved with β oxidation, and hepatocellular neoplasia. There are marked species differences in the response to peroxisome proliferators: mice and rats being highly responsive, hamsters intermediate, and dogs, rabbits, monkeys, and humans poor to nonresponders. The differential species response correlates directly with the number of hepatocellular peroxisome proliferator—activated receptor-α (PPAR-α) receptors; human liver only expresses 1–10% of the number of PPAR-α receptors present on rodent liver. Furthermore, the human peroxisome proliferator response element (PPRE) for acyl-CoA oxidase has a different sequence than the rat and is not activated by the ligand–heterodimer complex, whereas the rat PPRE is highly responsive. Other mechanistic studies have shed additional light on peroxisome proliferator-induced hepatocarcinogenicity. Sustained increases in hepatocellular proliferation are associated with the rapid development of neoplasia following exposure to the most potent agents, and tumor regression occurs following the withdrawal of the peroxisome proliferator.

The regression of liver tumors following the withdrawal of peroxisome proliferators is thought to be due to a reversal of a key event: the inhibition of apoptosis. Another pivotal study involved the PPAR-α receptor knockout mouse. Knockout and wild-type mice received the potent nongenotoxic peroxisome proliferator WY-14,643. Wild type, but not knockouts, had peroxisome proliferation, sustained increases in hepatocellular proliferation, and 100% incidence of hepatocellular tumors within a year. These studies elegantly documented that peroxisome proliferators require the PPAR-α receptor for the development of hepatocellular neoplasia and indirectly implied that humans were at minimal or no risk. As an example, no risk would be expected for humans exposed intravenously (IV) to small amounts of diethylhexylphthalate, a weak peroxisome proliferator that diffuses out of medical devices, such as IV administration units, because humans do not have a functional PPAR-α receptor and such intermittent exposures would not inhibit apoptosis or promote initiated cells.

C. BUTADIENE

Butadiene is an important industrial chemical that is a potent carcinogen in mice and a weak carcinogen in rats. Epidemiology studies have shown that workers in the styrene butadiene rubber (SBR) industry have an increased incidence of leukemia, whereas workers in the monomer industry do not. The presence of a potential confounder in the SBR studies, dimethyldithiocarbamate, may explain this difference. Butdiene is metabolized to three genotoxic epoxides, including epoxybutene, epoxybutane diol, and diepoxide. These differ in mutagenic potency by up to 200-fold, with diepoxide being by far the most mutagenic. Metabolism studies focused on epoxybutene and diepoxide and demonstrated that mice produced about 100 times more diepoxide than epoxybutene. Studies on the molecular dosimetry of DNA adducts demonstrated that the epoxybutane diol is responsible for the major DNA adduct of butadiene, N-7-trihydroxybutylguanine. These data suggest that the epoxybutane diol is formed by the rapid detoxication of the diepoxide by epoxide hydrolase. Epoxide hydrolase is the major pathway for detoxication in humans and rats, whereas glutathione is the major pathway in the mouse. These species differences may result in greater amounts of diepoxide in mice, resulting in much greater genetic insult.

Several molecular epidemiology studies have or are presently being conducted to evaluate biomarkers of exposure and genotoxicity. Hayes *et al.* (2000) demonstrated that trihydroxybutylvaline hemoglobin adducts correlated well with exposure of Chinese butadiene workers, but that none of the biomarkers for genotoxicity had exposure-related increases. Similar findings were demonstrated in a second molecular epidemiology study conducted in the Czech Republic (Albertini *et al.*, personal communication). Combining the knowledge from animal and human studies, it appears that the rat will be a better predictor of human risk than the mouse. Additional studies using biomarkers specific for diepoxide are necessary to confirm this.

V. Future Implications and Methodologies for Toxicology

The increased use of mechanistic data in risk assessment has clear implications for toxicologic research. There will be a substantial integration of mechanistic-based tools and approaches aimed at improving and expediting the risk assessment process (Table III). Special emphasis will be placed on genotyping of the human population and the utilization of surrogate biomarkers (Table III). These techniques have already yielded significant results. Genetic polymorphisms of drug-metabolizing enzymes in humans that could result in serious clinical consequences were among the first identified. The relationship between polymorphism of drug-metabolizing enzymes in humans and expression of p53 or clinical drug resistance in lung cancer has been underscored. These methodologies have also proven useful in the identification of at-risk genotypes regarding human glutathione transferase.

TABLE III
Tools to Improve and Expedite Mechanistic-Based Risk Assessment

Genotyping the human population
  Distribution of mutated genes in the affected population
  Identification of at-risk genotypes
  Distribution of genetic polymorphism for susceptibility
New biomarkers and improved methodologies
  Novel diagnostic and prognostic markers in biofluids
  DNA and protein adducts
  Improvement in biomonitoring assays detection of metabolites in biofluids or tissues
  Sensitive, high-throughput genotyping- and phenotyping-based assays
Predictive models and bioinformatics
  Physiological-based pharmacokinetic models incorporating relevant toxicity determinants
  Models that account for a higher level of anatomical complexity
  Improved mathematical models and statistical software
  Creation of relevant, detailed databases with data mining
  Neural networks to identify toxicophores and predict liabilities of novel chemotypes

Another exciting area for future research is the ability to test specific hypotheses using transgenic and knockout mice. If a particular metabolic pathway is hypothesized to play a critical role in the induction of the toxicity, that gene can be over- or underexpressed in a suitable transgenic animal. A prime example of this is the use of the PPARα knockout mouse in demonstrating the importance of this pathway in peroxisome proliferators.

The identification of relevant surrogate biomarkers will improve and expedite mechanistic-based risk assessment. The identification of specific markers, such as oncoproteins in biofluids and tissues, has proven useful from both a diagnostic and a prognostic perspective. The rapid expansion in the number of suitable surrogate markers has been accompanied by a marked improvement in biomonitoring assays, with the widely ranging activities from the detection of xenobiotics and their metabolites to the quantification of transcriptionally dependent genes. The advent of sensitive, high-throughput assays will result in the rapid screening of a large number of xenobiotics, while simultaneously elucidating the proposed mechanism of activity. The use of improved physiologically based pharmacokinetic models that identify and quantify the relevant physiological, biochemical, and molecular determinants of toxicity, coupled with additional models that account for a higher level of anatomical complexity, should prove of great value in mechanistic-based risk assessment. The incorporation of biomarkers of exposure and effect into both animal studies and molecular epidemiology studies will provide methods for validating such models and incorporating such mechanistic data into the risk assessment process.

The advent and utilization of virtual screening for risk assessment may accelerate our understanding of the process and the inherent dynamics of virtual systems. The creation of detailed databases containing all appropriate toxicity, exposure, biochemical, and molecular end points from animal and human studies will be necessary. Although the establishment and use of detailed databases are at the infancy stage, the value of their utility has already been recognized. Data mining should reveal relationships among chemotype, known toxicity, and human susceptibility. The use of neural networks will accelerate the identification of chemical substructures responsible for toxicity and predict the potential toxicity of new chemical entities. The incorporation of these various techniques, coupled with significant advances in computational systems and databases, should provide fruitful avenues in mechanistic-based risk assessment.

SUGGESTED READING

General

Faustman, E. M., and Omenn, G. S. (1996). Risk assessment. *In* "Casavett and Doull's Toxicology" (C. D. Klaazagen, ed, 5th ed., McCraw Hill, New York.) pp. 75–88.

National Research Council (NRC) (1983). "Risk Assessment in the Federal Government: Managing the Process." Committee on the Institutional Means for Assessment of Risks to Public Health, Commission on Life Sciences, National Academy Press, Washington, DC.

NRC (1994). "Science and Judgment in Risk Assessment." Committee on Risk Assessment of Hazardous Air Pollutants, Board on Environmental Studies and Toxicology, Commission on Life Sciences, National Academy Press, Washington, DC.

Traditional Risk Assessment

Ashley, J., and Tennant, R. W. (1994). Prediction of rodent careinogenicity for 44 chemicals: Results. *Mutagenesis* 9, 7–15.

EPA (1991). "Guidelines for Developmental Toxicity Risk Assessment," Notice 56, Federal Register, 63798–63826, 5 December.

EPA (1996). "Proposed Guidelines for Carcinogen Risk Assessment," Notice 61, Federal Register, 17959–18011, 23 April.

EPA (1996). "Guidelines for Reproductive Toxicity Risk Assessment," Notice 61, Federal Register, 56274–56322, 31 October.

EPA (1998). "Guidelines for Neurotoxicity Risk Assessment," Notice 61. Federal Register, 56274–56322, 14 May.

International Agency for Research on Cancer (IARC) (1982). "IARC Monographs on the Evaluation of the Carcinogenic Risk of Chemicals to Humans. Supplement 4, Chemicals, Industrial Processes, and Industries Associated with Cancer in Humans." IARC Monographs, Vols. 1–29, Lyon, France.

IARC (1994). "IARC Monographs on the Evaluation of Carcinogenic Risks to Humans. Some Industrial Chemicals," Vol. 60, IARC, Lyon, France.

Lave, L. B., and Omenn, G. S. (1986). Cost-effectiveness of short-term tests for carcinogenicity. *Nature* 324, 29–34.

Mathews, E. J., and Contrerra, J. F. (1998). A new highly specific method for predicting the carcinogenetic potential of pharmaceuticals in rodents using enhanced MCASE QSAR-ES software. *Regul. Toxicol. Pharmacol.* 28, 242–264.

Occupational Safety and Health Administration (OSHA) (1980). Identification, characterization, and regulation of potential occupational carcinogens. *Fed. Reg.* 45, 5002–5296.

Omenn, G. S., and Lave, L. B. (1988). Scientific and cost-effectiveness criteria in selecting batteries of short-term tests. *Mutat. Res.* 205, 41–49.

Report of the Surgeon General (1982). "The Health Consequences of Smoking." Department of Health and Human Services.

Examples of Mechanistically Based Risk Assessment

Borghoff, S. J., Short, B. G., and Swenberg, J. A. (1990). Biochemical mechanisms and pathobiology of alpha 2μ-globin nephropathy. *Annu. Rev. Pharmacol. Toxicol.* **30**, 349–367.

Cochrane, J. E., and Skopek, T. R. (1994). Mutagenicity of butadiene and its epoxide metabolites. I. Mutagenic potential of 1,2-epoxybutene, 1,2,3,4-diepoxybutane and 3,4-epoxy-1,2-butanediol in cultured human lymphoblasts. *Carcinogenesis* **15**, 713–717.

Delzell, E., Sathiakumar, N., Hovinga, M., Macaluso, M., Julian, J., Larson, R., Cole, P., and Muir, D. C. (1996). A follow-up study of synthetic rubber workers. *Toxicology* **113**, 182–189.

Dietrich, D. R., and Swenberg, J. A. (1991). The presence of alpha 2μ-globulin is necessary for d-limonene promotion of male rat kidney tumors. *Cancer Res.* **51**, 3512–3521.

Doull, J., Cattley, R., Elcombe, C., Lake, B. G., Swenberg, J., Wilkinson, C., Williams, G., and Van Gemert, M. (1999). A cancer risk assessment of di (2-ethylhexyl) phthalate: Application of the new US EPS risk Assessment Guidelines. *Regul. Toxicol. Pharmacol.* **29**, 327–357.

Environmental Protection Agency (EPA) (1986). "Guidelines for carcinogen risk assessment." *Fed. Reg.* **51**, 33992–34003.

Gonzales, F. J., Peters, J. M., and Cattley, R. C. (1998). Mechanism of action of the nongenotoxic peroxisome proliferators: Role of the peroxisome proliferator-activator receptor alpha. *J. Natl. Cancer Inst.* **90**, 1702–1709.

Hayes, R. B., Zhang, L., Yin, S., Swenberg, J. A., Xi, L., Wiencke, J., Bechtold, W. E., Yao, M., Rothman, N., Haas, R., O'Neill, J. P., Zhang, D., Wiemels, J., Dosemeci, M., Li, G., and Smith, M. T. (2000). Genotoxic markers among butadiene polymer workers in China. *Carcinogenesis* **21**, 55–62.

Himmelstein, M. W., Acquavella, J. F., Recio, L., Medinsky, M. A., and Bond, J. A. (1997). Toxicology and epidemiology of 1,3-butadiene. *Crit. Rev. Toxicol.*, **27**, 1–108.

Huber, W. W., Grasl-Kraupp, B., and Schulte-Hermann, R. (1996). Hepatocarcinogenic potential of di(2-ethylhexyl)phthalate in rodents and its implications on human risk. *Crit. Rev. Toxicol.* **26**, 365–481.

International Agency for Research on Cancer (IARC)/World Health Organization (WHO) (1995). IARC Technical Publication No. 24: Peroxisome proliferation and its role in carcinogenesis. Lyon, France.

Irons, R. D., and Pyatt, D. W. (1998). Dithiocarbamates as potential confounders in butadiene epidemiology. *Carcinogenesis* **19**, 539–542.

Koc, H., Tretyakova, N. Y., Walker, V. E., Henderson, R. F., and Swenberg, J. A. (1999). Molecular dosimetry of N-7 guanine adduct formation in mice and rats exposed to 1,3-butadiene. *Chem. Res. Toxicol.* **12**, 566–574.

Koivisto, P., Kipelainen, I., Rasanen, I., Adler, I. D., Pacchierotti, F., and Peltonen, K. (1999). Butadiene diolepoxide-and diepoxybutane-derived DNA adducts at N7-guanine: A high occurrence of diolepoxide-derived adducts in mouse lung after 1,3-butadiene exposure. *Carcinogenesis* **20**, 1253–1259.

Lehman-McKeeman, L. D., and Caudill, D. (1992). Alpha 2μ-globulin is the only member of the lipocalin protein superfamily that binds hyaline droplet inducing agents. *Toxicol. Appl. Pharmacol.* **116**, 170–176.

Lehman-McKeeman, L. D., and Caudill, D. (1994). D-Limonene induced hyaline droplet nephropathy in alpha 2μ-globulin transgenic mice. *Fundam. Appl. Toxicol.* **23**, 562–568.

Marsman, D. S., and Popp, J. A. (1994). Biological potential of basophilic hepatocellular foci and hepatic adenoma induced by the peroxisome proliferator, Wy-14,643. *Carcinogenesis* **15**, 111–117.

Peters, J. M., Cattley, R. C., and Gonzalez, F. J. (1997). Role of PPAR alpha in the mechanism of action of the nongenotoxic carcinogen and peroxisome proliferator Wy-14, 643. *Carcinogenesis* **18**, 2029–2033.

Roberts, R. A., James, N. H., Hasmall, S. C., Holden, P. R., Lambe, K., Macdonald, N., West, D., Woodyatt, N. J., and Whitcome, D. (2000). Apoptosis and proliferation in nongenotoxic carcinogenesis: Species differences and role of PPARalpha. *Toxicol. Lett.* **112–113**, 49–57.

Roberts, R. A., James, N. H., Woodyatt, N. J., Macdonald, N., and Tugwood, J. D. (1998). Evidence for the suppression of apoptosis by the peroxisome proliferator activated receptor alpha (PPAR alpha). *Carcinogenesis* **19**, 43–48.

Swenberg, J. A. (1993). Alpha 2μ-globulin nephropathy: Review of the cellular and molecular mechanisms involved and their implications for human risk assessment. *Environ. Health Perspect.* **101**(Suppl. 6), 39–44.

Swenberg, J. A., and Lehman-McKeeman, L. D. (1999). Alpha 2μ-urinary globulin-associated nephropathy as a mechanism of renal tubular cell carcinogenesis in male rats. *IARC Sci. Publ.* **147**, 95–118.

Thornton-Manning, J. R., Dahl, A. R., Bechtold, W. E., Griffith, W. C., and Henderson, R. F. (1997). Comparison of the disposition of butadiene epoxides in Sprague–Dawley rats and B6C3F$_1$ mice following a single and repeated exposures to 1, 3-butadiene via inhalation. *Toxicology* **123**, 125–134.

Woodyatt, N. J., Lambe, K. G., Myers, K. A., Tugwood, J. D., and Roberts, R. A. (1999). The peroxisome proliferator (PP) response element upstream of the human acyl CoA oxidase gene is inactive among a sample human population: Significance for species differences in response to peroxisome proliferators. *Carcinogenesis* **20**, 369–372.

Future Implications and Methodologies

Bailer, A. J., and Dankovic, D. A. (1997). An introduction to the use of physiologically based pharmacokinetic models in risk assessment. *Stat. Methods Med. Res.* **6**, 341–358.

Basak, S., Gute, B., Opitz, D., and Balasubramanian, K. (1999). Use of statistical and neural net methods in predicting toxicity of chemicals: A hierarchical QSAR approach. AAAI Spring Symposium on Predictive Toxicology of Chemicals: Experiences and Impact of AI Tool.

Gaido, K. W., Leonard, L. S., Lovell, S., Gould, J. C., Babai, D., Portier, C. J., and McDonnell, D. P. (1997). Evaluation of chemicals with endocrine modulating activity in a yeast-based steroid hormone receptor gene transcription assay. *Toxicol. Appl. Pharmacol.* **143**, 205–212.

Gross, A. S., Kroemer, H. K., and Eichelbaum, M. (1991). Genetic polymorphism of drug metabolism in humans. *Adv. Exp. Med. Biol.* **283**, 627–640.

Juge-Aubry, C. E., Hammar, E., Siegrist-Kaiser, C., Pernin, A., Takeshita, A., Chin, W. W., Burger, A. G., and Meier, C. A. (1999). Regulation of the transcriptional activity of the peroxisome proliferator-activated receptor alpha by phosphorylation of a ligand-independent trans-activating domain. *J. Biol. Chem.* **274**, 10505–10510.

Kawajiri, K., Eguchi, H., Nakachi, K., Sekiya, T., and Yamamoto, M. (1996). Association of CYP1A1 germ line polymorphisms with mutations of the p53 gene in lung cancer. *Cancer Res.* **56**, 72–76.

Molica, S., Mannella, A., Dattilo, A., Levato, D., Iuliano, F., Peta, A., Consarino, C., and Magro, S. (1996). Differential expression of BCL-2 oncoprotein and Fas antigen on normal peripheral blood and leukemic bone marrow cells. A flow cytometric analysis. *Haematologica* **81**, 302–309.

Morawski, K., Gabriel, A., Namyslowski, G., Ziolkowski, A., Pietrawska, V., and Steplewska, K. (1999). Clinical application of proliferating cell nuclear antigen, oncoprotein p53 and tumor front grading analysis in patients operated on for laryngeal cancer. *Eur. Arch. Otorhinolaryngol.* **256**, 378–383.

Nakanishi, Y., Kawasaki, M., Bai, F., Takayama, K., Pei, X. H., Takano, K., Inoue, K., Osaki, S., Hara, N., and Kiyohara, C. (1999). Expression of p53 and glutathione S-transferase-pi relates to clinical drug resistance in non-small cell lung cancer. *Oncology* **57**, 318–323.

Nuccetelli, M., Mazzetti, A. P., Rossjohn, J., Parker, M. W., Board, P., Caccuri, A. M., Federici, G., Ricci, G., and Lo Bello, M. (1998). Shifting substrate specificity of human glutathione transferase (from class Pi to class alpha) by a single point mutation. *Biochem. Biophys. Res. Commun.* **252**, 184–189.

Opitz, D. Basak, S., and Gute, B. (1999). Hazard Assessment Modeling: An Evolutionary Ensemble Approach. Genetic and Evolutionary Computation Conference (1643–1651), Orlando, FL.

Ritter, M. A., Furtek, C. I., and Lo, M. W. (1997). An improved method for the simultaneous determination of losartan and its major metabolite, EXP3174, in human plasma and urine by high-performance liquid chromatography with fluorescence detection. *J. Pharm. Biomed. Anal.* **15**, 1021–1029.

Roy, B., Dey, B., Chakraborty, M., and Majumder, P. P. (1998). Frequency of homozygous null mutation at the glutathione-s-transferase M1 locus in some populations of Orissa, India. *Anthropol. Anz.* **56**, 43–47.

Smith, R. L. (1986). Polymorphism in drug metabolism—implications for drug toxicity. *Arch. Toxicol. Suppl.* **9**, 138–146.

Tennant, R. W. (1991). The genetic toxicity database of the National Toxicology Program: Evaluation of the relationships between genetic toxicity and carcinogenicity. *Environ. Health Prospect.* **96**, 47–51.

Tucker, G. T. (1994). Clinical implications of genetic polymorphism in drug metabolism. *J. Pharm. Pharmacol.* **46**(Suppl 1), 417–424.

Wu, J. T., Astill, M. E., Gagon, S. D., and Bryson, L. (1995). Measurement of c-erbB-2 proteins in sera from patients with carcinomas and in breast tumor tissue cytosols: Correlation with serum tumor markers and membrane-bound oncoprotein. *J. Clin. Lab. Anal.* **9**, 151–165.

18

Principles of Risk Communication: Building Trust and Credibility with the Public

Ronald W. Brecher
GlobalTox International Consultants Inc.
Guelph, Ontario, Canada

Terry Flynn
Frontline Corporate Communications Inc.
Kitchener, Ontario, Canada

I. Introduction

Communicating sensitive, technical information to the public can be one of the most difficult challenges that a scientist faces today. This is especially true given the public's growing distrust of corporations, academic institutions, and government agencies charged with protecting the health and safety of our communities.

Since the mid-1980s, the science of risk communication has grown from a purely academic field of social science into a practice dominated by both public relations practitioners and technical risk experts. With our daily consumption of contradictory health, environmental, and safety news, it is now clear that this new field of communications will continue to enjoy exponential growth in years to come.

For those who have found themselves in the midst of a risk controversy, whether on a local scale or at an international level, it is obvious that risk communication is an essential pillar in the risk management process. Evidence obtained by scientific methods used in qualitative or quantitative risk assessments is not worth the paper that they are written on if the information cannot be communicated effectively to its intended stakeholder group. Furthermore, should the results of scientific risk assessments be the basis for policy decision making, the communication skills of the risk manager may be the critical factor in the eventual adoption of the policy.

To those that have had the good fortune of watching risk controversies from the sidelines or just on the evening news, this chapter is intended for you. The lessons learned from those that have been actively involved in risk communication form the basis of our discussions and recommendations. After all, our individual experiences as risk assessment and risk communication consultants have seen us at the center of some of North America's most recent risk controversies. These include, for example, the scientific, policy, and political issues around vinyl products; the question of the safety of phthalates in childrens' toys and medical

Handbook of Toxicologic Pathology, Second Edition
Volume 1

447

devices; the environmental justice movement; and the cleanup of a number of environmentally sensitive manufacturing sites.

The key to risk communication is timeliness. The analogies of horses escaping from corrals, genies out of bottle, or cats out of bags were never more true than in communicating risk. As will become evident, perception of risk is the reality of risk to the stakeholder. Good (or bad) risk communication has the ability to have an impact on perception and the actions taken to respond to them. So do not sit back and keep the process on track. If risk communication is new to you, consider it as an innovative way of helping you to manage events. Scientists have a critical role to play in risk controversies, as do activists, politicians, corporations, and the media. Do not be surprised if one of those groups disagrees with you and your opinion vehemently. Do not take these disagreements personally, they are just another part of the overall risk management process.

This chapter intends to give you the science and insights behind the field of communicating technical information during times of high concern and low trust. By understanding some of the behavioral issues behind the "facts" concerning risk, it will become apparent that communicating and managing risk-related issues require a proactive process.

II. The Risk Communication Perspective

Food safety, chemical contamination, air emissions, hazardous materials, chemical warfare material: just look through any newspaper or watch any newscast and you can be guaranteed that someone is claiming that their health, or the health of their community, has or is being affected by something or someone. In fact, in today's litigious, activist environment, class-action law suits, product boycotts, and political pressure have forced the withdrawal of a number of products and processes because the scientific and technical communities have not effectively communicated beneficial information to the public.

As mentioned previously, the purpose of this chapter is to provide the science and insights behind the field of communicating technical information during times of high concern and low trust. While considerable research has been conducted in the fields of risk communication and risk management on communicating with the public, the opportunity to build trust and establish credibility with the public goes beyond risk issues. In fact, the principles that underlie the science of risk communication can be used in the workplace, in community groups, during moments of crisis, and even in personal relationships. This chapter, however, will be limited to discussing how effective risk communication can enhance the credibility of your technical message and build trust in you as a source of information for the public.

III. Risk Communication and Public Involvement

The recognition of the important role of risk communication is a relatively new development in the context of risk management processes. No longer does the public accept that the identification, assessment, and management of risk are solely within the domain of the scientific community. In fact, following the tragic events of the chemical plant explosion in Bhopal, the oil spill off the coast of Alaska, and questions about the safety of our food supplies, the public has demanded, and won the right, to be involved in the environmental decision-making process.

Since 1986, the U.S. Environmental Protection Agency (EPA) has implemented a number of key laws and regulations that mandate the "community's right to know" about the potential hazards that may affect their health or their livelihoods. These regulatory requirements put the onus of responsibility of communicating risk issues on the companies and governmental agencies rather than on the public. No longer can corporate spokespeople simply say, "If you want that information, you'll have to get it yourself." The shoe is now clearly on the other foot, with the public telling both governments and industries: "We want the information and the law requires that you give it to us!"

As a result of these initiatives, industry and government have been forced to look at new and sometimes uncomfortable methods of communicating with the public. These efforts now include listening to the public; understanding the public's perception of risk issues; engaging in two-way dialogue with the public; and, finally, empowering the public to be involved in decisions that affect them.

In 1989, the risk communication research community, working with the National Research Council (NRC) and the EPA, developed a series of definitions to explain this new and emerging field. According to the NRC, "risk communication is an interactive process of exchange of information and opinions among individuals, groups, and institutions." The EPA spoke more specifically about the role of risk communications in the risk management process. They stated that risk communication is "any purposeful exchange of information and interaction between interested parties regarding health, safety, or environmental risks."

It is obvious from these definitions that the focus of communication with the public has shifted from the old, one-way style of communication, to the more involved, two-way symmetrical method of community involvement. To help individual communicators understand this shift, the EPA published their "seven cardinal rules of risk communication," which outlined the critical steps to effective dialogue with the public.

1. Accept and involve the public as a legitimate partner.
2. Listen to their concerns.
3. Be honest, candid, and open.
4. Coordinate and collaborate with credible sources.
5. Speak clearly and concisely with care and compassion.
6. Plan carefully and evaluate efforts continually.
7. Meet the needs of the media (where appropriate).

In 1998, the Food and Agriculture Organization (FAO) of the United Nations and the World Health Organization (WHO) conducted an expert consultation on risk communication. The consultation also published a series of goals of risk communication, similar to the "cardinal rules" of the EPA. These goals included:

1. To promote awareness and understanding of the specific issues under consideration during the risk analysis process, by all participants.
2. To promote consistency and transparency in arriving at and implementing risk management decisions.
3. To foster public trust and confidence in the safety of the food supply.
4. To strengthen the working relationships and mutual respect among all participants.
5. To exchange information on the knowledge, attitudes, values, practices, and perceptions of interested parties concerning risks associated with food and related topics.

In their report, the consultation "recognized that risk communication, being an integral part of risk analysis, is a necessary and critical tool to appropriately define issues and to develop, understand and arrive at the best risk management decisions."

IV. Challenges and Obstacles to Effective Risk Communication

Effective communications depend on the existence of a "common language" that can be understood by both the communicator and the audience. To understand any language, a listener and the receiver of the communications, must understand both the *meaning* of words and the *context* within which the words are used. These two factors, meaning and context, present the greatest obstacle for effective risk communication. The remainder of this section explores three key issues that complicate communications.

A. DATA VERSUS INFORMATION

Scientists are trained to deal effectively with data. Raw data are collected, organized, analyzed, and synthesized, ultimately leading an investigator to a conclusion about the meaning of the data. In other words, a "data" set is a collection of single observations, which, when synthesized, provides information.

The public is at a disadvantage compared to scientists when it comes to interpreting data. They often do not have the technical knowledge to synthesize data into information or even understand the meaning of a single datum. This can lead to misinterpretation of data or to the inappropriate focusing of attention on a single, uninterpreted, experimental result. More data may be perceived to mean "more concern." Therefore, the public should be provided with *information* in understandable language. It is important to avoid presenting data, particularly at the expense of providing information.

Effective communicators examine their data carefully and present it in a manner that provides information in language that is accessible to their audience. Accessibility of language is key here: information that is presented in unintelligible language does not impart knowledge, does not empower involvement in decision making, and may be perceived to be a tactic designed to hide or conceal important information from the audience.

B. THE PUBLIC'S EXPECTATIONS OF SCIENCE

In the past, the public came to expect science to be accurate, precise, definitive, and beneficial to society, and even wondrous. After all, in the last century or so, science and technology have allowed us to put people on the moon, to reduce suffering due to diseases such as polio, to reduce the infant mortality rate dramatically in developed countries, to extend the shelf life of foods through refrigeration, to increase the world's food supply through modern agriculture, and to reduce waterborne diseases through provision of clean drinking water.

However, the public is faced daily with news of scientific failures and impending threats.

Some examples are the "Challenger" space shuttle explosion, the emergence of "superbugs" resistant to multiple antibiotics, babies affected by thalidomide, the depletion of the Earth's protective ozone layer, desertification of land through too intensive agriculture, and chemicals in drinking water that may cause cancer. It is not surprising that, in the face of these "failures," the public has lost confidence in science.

At the same time, as people have serious doubts about the positive role of science in their lives, they often find that scientists are inaccessible or aloof. This is often a result of the inability or unwillingness on the part of scientists to use clear, simple language to explain what they do, how they do it, and what they have found. It is not surprising that scientists have difficulty in meeting the public's expectations of science: the public desires absolute answers and science can generally only identify likely and unlikely outcomes. Thus, scientists resist distilling information down to simple yes/no answers, preferring instead to present probabilities and theories, recounting all the evidence in support and against. This is an important disconnect in communications between technical experts and the public: the public desires simple and absolute answers, which science often cannot provide.

C. CONTRADICTORY EXPERT OPINIONS

The scientific method is rooted in hypothesis testing, in healthy debate that validates interpretations of data through experimentation, and through argument about alternative interpretations. Those interpretations that stand up to this rigorous scrutiny become established as the most plausible and become a platform for the further expansion of knowledge. Unfortunately, the public rarely has an opportunity to see this constructive collegial process and does not comprehend the difference among hypotheses (theories), validated peer-reviewed scientific proof, and opinion of individual scientists. Instead, the public's exposure to scientific debate often comes through the mass media in the form of diametrically opposed opinions from experts (and nonexperts) about issues that are of public concern, where there has been little attempt to separate "scientific fact" from "personal scientific opinion." This apparent inability of scientists to agree on how to interpret their results fuels the public's mistrust of science and decisions based on it. This mistrust is intensified when opinions come from experts representing specific interests, such experts may be seen as "hired guns."

V.   Perception and Acceptance of Risk

It is possible to identify a number of factors that affect the ways in which different people, under different conditions, perceive and are willing to accept risks. Perception of risk is a subjective process that is essential for survival. There are some common attributes of the risk agent that influence the perception of its acceptability. Some of the most important are outlined in this section.

A.   LIKELIHOOD (SIZE) OF THE ADVERSE EFFECT

The likelihood of a risk being realized as an adverse effect is one factor that affects how a risk is perceived. In many cases, risks that have a very small likelihood of affecting a person will be perceived to be less important than risks that are more likely to impact on that person ("It will never happen to me"). However, some extremely unlikely effects may be deemed unacceptable due to the other factors discussed later. To further complicate the matter, some relatively large risks (e.g., dying of a smoking-related illness or dying in a car accident) are perceived by many as being relatively acceptable.

B.   "DREAD" FACTOR

Risks that are not well understood by the public are often perceived as more severe and less acceptable than risks that are well understood. These poorly understood "risks" are often referred to as "dread" risks. This term highlights the role of fear in determining how people judge risks. Fear, arising in part from poor understanding of the nature of the risk, tends to make people less risk tolerant and more likely to deem a risk to be unacceptable, even when the likelihood of any person being impacted is very small.

C.   PERMANENT OR REVERSIBLE NATURE OF THE ADVERSE EFFECT

Different types of risk (i.e., cancer vs increased frequency of colds) are usually perceived differently and for obvious reasons. Most people are more willing to accept the risk of effects that are relatively minor and whose effects are reversible or temporary (e.g., colds). However, they are less likely to accept an increased risk of cancer, which is less reversible and leads more often to serious negative impacts on quality or length of life.

D.   VOLUNTARY ACCEPTANCE OF RISKS

People who make a deliberate choice to accept a risk tend to be more tolerant of that risk than people who have similar risks imposed upon them. For example, smokers knowingly accept a greatly increased risk of cancer and other serious diseases. Many nonsmokers are unwilling to be exposed to even small amounts of tobacco smoke for fear of these same diseases.

E.   WHO BENEFITS FROM ACCEPTANCE OF A RISK?

People who may benefit from accepting a risk tend to be more willing to accept that risk than people who do not. This becomes particularly important when the people who accept the risk (e.g., residents in an industrial area affected by industry emissions) are different from those who stand to reap the greatest benefit (the owners and operators of the industry). In this case, even very small risks may be completely unacceptable due to the lack of perceived benefits.

F.   JARGON AND TECHNICAL TERMS

Use of jargon and technical terms tends to make risks less acceptable. The negative perception of even relatively well-understood terms is illustrated by a survey conducted by Health Canada. One part of the survey examined word associations for the word "chemical."

451

While generally negative associations (such as "danger," "pollution," and "toxic") accounted for 518 of 1506 responses, only 10 distinctly positive responses were given. Names of chemical products ("medicines," "gasoline," etc.) were given about as often as the negative terms. Jargon tends to decrease the acceptability of risks for at least two possible reasons: lack of trust for a communicator who does not "speak to us in language we can understand" and the "dread" factor discussed earlier.

G. AGE AND SEX OF THE RISK TAKER

A study by Health Canada suggests that females are more likely to consider a risk as a "high risk" than males. This was the case for 37 of 38 risks evaluated in the survey (the exception was "heart pacemakers"). There are also differences in risk perception with age. In the Health Canada survey, younger respondents (under 30) tended to be more likely to characterize a risk as "high" than older respondents (55 and older) in the following categories related to substances in the environment or in drinking water: bottled water, PCBs or dioxin, tap water, waste incinerators, outdoor air quality, pesticides in food, and chemical pollution. However, older respondents tended to be more concerned than the under-30s for the following hazards: asbestos, high-voltage power lines, nuclear power plants and waste, and indoor air quality.

H. SOURCE OF INFORMATION

People's confidence in the source of information is likely to affect their perception of risk. If a source is considered credible, people may assume that the risk has been described fairly. However, when risk information comes from sources perceived as less credible, people may assume that the severity and amount of risk have been either under- or overstated. Looking at people who expressed either "a lot" or "fair" confidence in various information sources, Health Canada's survey suggests that people trust medical doctors the most, followed by federal government sources. People tended to have less confidence in news media and university

scientists, and even less confidence in friends and relatives and environmental groups. Confidence in provincial and municipal governments was still lower, with confidence in private industry being lowest of all the categories surveyed.

VI. Assessing the Issue: "Is There a Risk?"

"Risk" is the probability that a specific adverse effect will occur in an individual or a population exposed to a hazard. Risk depends on both intrinsic properties of the risk agent (i.e., the hazard) and extrinsic properties, namely the receptor (the individual or population at risk) and the conditions of exposure, including duration, magnitude, frequency, and route of exposure.

"Risk assessment" is a largely scientific process for developing inferences about risk. It follows the general paradigm shown in Fig. 1. This section discusses each of the components of risk assessment.

A. PROBLEM FORMULATION

Problem formulation is the process of defining all possible risk factors in the situation whose risks are to be assessed. In assessing risks associated with long-term exposure to chemicals in the environment or workplace or in evaluating risks associated with pharmaceuticals, the problem formulation step is essentially the same. This step involves developing a conceptual model that identifies the three necessary components for risk: a hazardous material(s), receptors, and pathways of exposure.

B. EXPOSURE ASSESSMENT

Exposure assessment involves developing a detailed understanding of exposure to the toxicant(s) of interest. Knowledge of the exposure routes (i.e., ingestion, inhalation, dermal, injection), frequency, duration and dose rate, and, of course, receptor characteristics (age, sex, health status, concomitant exposures to other toxicants, etc.) are all necessary for an evaluation of risk.

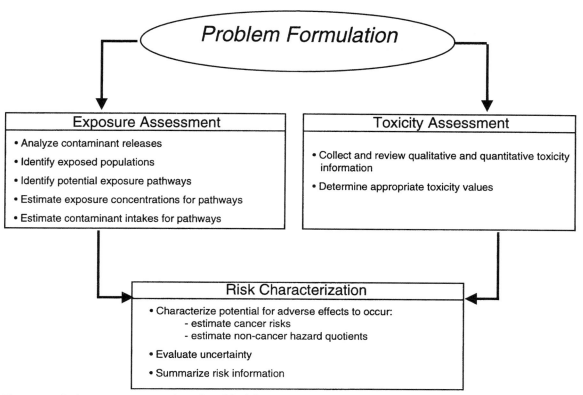

Figure 1. Risk assessment paradigm [modified from US EPA (1989)].

C. TOXICITY ASSESSMENT

The toxicity assessment portion of the risk assessment involves developing dose–response information for adverse effects of interest. In general, the most sensitive adverse effect (i.e., that adverse effect that is likely to occur at the lowest dose under the expected conditions of exposure) is identified as the "critical" effect. The critical effect is used to develop reference values that represent doses below which significant adverse effects are not expected under the anticipated exposure conditions. The logic used here is that if exposures are such that the critical effects cannot occur, other adverse effects, which occur only following more intense, prolonged, or frequent exposures, will not occur.

D. RISK CHARACTERIZATION

The risk characterization step marries the information obtained from the exposure and toxicity assessments to make qualitative and quantitative statements about risk and the conditions under which the risk may occur. In its simplest terms, and in an ideal world, risk characterization simply represents the use of exposure information to interpolate along the dose–response curve. However, this is oversimplistic; risk characterization usually involves more extrapolation than interpolation, and many types of extrapolation are required (inter- and intraspecies, high to low dose, etc.). It is the risk characterization that is used to answer the question posed in the title of this section: "Is there a risk?" Risk characterization defines the nature and degree of the risk under specific exposure conditions to the hazard in sufficient detail to allow the consideration of appropriate risk management options.

VII. How Can Risks Be Managed?

In essence, there are always at least three options in managing a risk, although not all are practical for a given risk: do nothing, allow the risk to remain; eliminate the risk by eliminating exposure altogether; or manage the risk by reducing exposure or by monitoring adverse effects.

Interestingly, the choice of option is often not directly related to either the magnitude of the risk or the severity of the adverse effect. Consider, for example, the relative acceptability of disease-causing smoking compared to the relatively unacceptable hypothetical risk of exposure to small amounts of disinfection by-products in drinking water. In some instances, traditional risk assessments may be able to demonstrate no plausible risk, and yet fear and distrust may demand some action to alleviate the perceived risk. Some of the factors that have an impact on the acceptability of risks have been discussed previously in this chapter.

The process of evaluating risk management options should consider risk assessment as a key source of information, but can rarely be based solely on risk assessment data. In the face of limited resources for managing health risks, decisions must be made about which risks should be managed at all, the technical and economic constraints impacting on the issue must be identified, and decisions must be made within the context of a particular regulatory climate. Finally, and perhaps most importantly, risk management decisions must take account of stakeholder views.

A. HOW DO PEOPLE FEEL ABOUT THE RISK?

At the two extremes, people may feel extreme outrage or apathy. Many others fall between these extremes and are concerned about the risk, but are open-minded to considering the issues and implications of the risks to themselves and their fellow citizens. People who feel very strongly about a risk are unlikely to change these beliefs and will tend to focus on information that supports their beliefs, whereas people whose beliefs are held relatively weakly are influenced more easily by the way in which risk information is presented. Thus, it is important to assess people's feelings in developing a

risk communication strategy. Some important determinants of how people feel about risk have been identified already. Additional questions to consider are also given.

1. Communications Legacy

What has been the experience of people in dealing with past risk issues and risk communicators? People who feel they have been treated poorly in the past may come to expect similar treatment in the future.

2. Cohesiveness of the Community

How cohesive is the community and how well do they work together on issues of general community concern? Communities that have come together on previous issues, risk related or other, often feel a greater sense of empowerment and involvement than those that are loose knit.

3. How Much Time Do People Have for Being Involved?

This question speaks to the issue of priorities. All people have constraints on their time and must somehow rank, or prioritize, issues. Any factor that influences the perception of risk may influence the priority of the issue and the amount of time and energy that people are prepared to dedicate to being involved in finding solutions.

4. What Are the Agendas (and Hidden Agendas) of the Stakeholders?

Stakeholders come to the issue table with different agendas, which are not always obvious. Stakeholders may adopt positions based not on the issue of interest *per se*, but on such grounds as setting (or not setting) precedents, "getting even" for a perceived past wrong, or being seen to adopt a stance that reflects the belief of the community. This can occur even when such beliefs are not supportable based on the available information surrounding the issue. A relatively well-defined local issue may play out in the context of broader regional, national, or international contexts within which

TABLE I
Methods for Involving Stakeholders in Issue Assessment and Resolution

Method	Benefit to stakeholder	Benefit to proponent	Comments/cautions
One-on-one meetings	Opportunity to speak privately, avoids fear of public speaking, on home territory	Reaches stakeholders who might otherwise not participate, demonstrates commitment and dedication to dialogue	Time-consuming and expensive. Spokesperson needs to be seen as honest, open, neutral, and qualified
Public meetings	Opportunity for community members to hear others' views and gain shared understanding. Opportunity to attract media attention	Gauge extent of concern about issue in the community; opportunity to identify most vocal issue leaders in the community.	Must be planned carefully, well publicized, and followed up. Provides an opportunity for nonlocal vested interests to exert influence over local concerns. Be prepared for media attention
Flyers/bulletins delivered to stakeholders	Opportunity to digest the information at a convenient time and in private. Provides a written record of commitments and progress that stakeholders can collect and review from time to time	Provides information to stakeholders who might otherwise not participate. Opportunity to make commitments in writing and then confirm they have been met	Can be perceived as impersonal and should contain information about how stakeholders can speak with someone to ask questions or identify concerns
Public comment periods on documents	Allows stakeholders to have meaningful input by giving them input into documents before they are finalized and putting their comments "on the record" for the issue	Allows a written record to be established of what issues were raised and how they were responded to	Public comment periods are only useful if a follow-up is available to stakeholders who comment. They should be able to verify that their comments were heard and considered
Making information accessible in local libraries, on the internet, news servers, and on-line discussion groups	Allows stakeholders to obtain and review the information of greatest interest to them and to solicit comments from other interested parties locally, regionally, nationally, and internationally	Seen as open and forthcoming	Once released, information cannot be retracted. Information that is available *only* on-line may be inaccessible to many stakeholders. Documents should not be removed from libraries to ensure a complete information set is always available
Mass media	Readily available and inexpensive. Media information tends to be focused and brief, can be taken in within a short time, and is usually quite nontechnical	Opportunity to reach a wide audience, including people who might not otherwise be interested in the issues	Media can influence risk perception (positive or negative) and change issue focus. Mass media is out of the control of the proponent; no assurance that most important information will be well communicated

the local issue is placed in the role of a "pawn." Information and perceptions arising from these larger scale contexts may override the information directly relevant to the issue at hand. Organizations or individuals who have not had prior involvement in local issues, but who have other vested interests may deliberately distort the concerns and beliefs of local stakeholders. The agendas of such organizations and individuals, although they purport to be in the interest of the local stakeholders, may be directed toward achieving a broader scale (i.e., regional, national, or international) impact.

B. INVOLVING STAKEHOLDERS IN ISSUE DEFINITION

Every person looks at information, however objectively, with some degree of subjectivity based on their past experience, upbringing, personal circumstances, and level of understanding. In order to ensure that the correct issue is assessed and managed, and that the most important (from the perspective of the stakeholders) information is disseminated, it is important to involve all stakeholders in issue definition. It is also imperative to maintain this involvement throughout issue assessment, evaluation and implementation of management options, and issue closure.

There are many ways to involve stakeholders. Each has benefits to the proponent (or "owner" of the issue) and the public and other stakeholders. Table I summarizes some methods for ensuring stakeholder involvement, highlighting benefits for both stakeholders and proponents. It should be stressed that no single method is likely to be adequate if used in isolation. Rather, a combination of methods should be selected based on the level of concern among stakeholders, the number, type, and geographic location of stakeholders.

VIII. Putting It All Together

In the end, the primary goal of any risk communication program is to provide the public with meaningful, relevant, and accurate information, in clear and understandable terms targeted to a specific audience. In so doing, risk communicators will have increased the public's awareness and understanding of the risk and what role they have in the overall risk management process. Effective risk communication will build trust and establish credibility, create opportunities for greater involvement, and may (although it is by no means guaranteed) provide a greater degree of agreement and consensus on the decisions to be made.

Unlike normal communication scenarios, the onus of responsibility to create awareness, establish understanding, and to finally ascertain a new level of appreciation rests with the communicating scientist or manager. No longer can one assume that "they get it" or that in fact it is "their fault that they just do not understand." Scientists, technicians, and managers must learn the new rules of this endeavor if they truly want to affect change, safeguard the public, and build a new understanding of the overall risk management process.

IX. Summary

In today's regulatory environment, the effective communication of scientific information with the public is one of the most important elements of the risk management process. Scientific, technical, and managerial personnel must develop an understanding of the dynamics of communicating during times of high concern and low trust in order to establish credibility and build trust with the public.

ACKNOWLEDGMENTS

Portions of the text and Fig. 1 have been reproduced from *Toxicologic Pathology* 25, 23–26 (1997), with permission of the Journal and the Society of Toxicologic Pathologists.

SUGGESTED READING

Covello, V., and Allen, F. (1988). "Seven Cardinal Rules of Risk Communication." Environmental Protection Agency, Washington, DC.
Covello, V., Slovic, P., and von Winterfeldt, D. (1988). "Risk Communication: A Review of the Literature." National Science Foundation, Washington, DC.
Covello, V. (1992). Risk communication: An emerging area of health communication research. In "Communication Yearbook 15" (S. Deetz, ed.), pp. 359–373. Sage Publications, Newbury Park.
Davies, C.J., Covello, V.T., and Allen, F.W. (eds.) (1987). "Risk Communication." Proceedings of the National Conference on Risk Communication, The Conservation Foundation, Washington, DC.
Fischoff, B. (1989). "Risk: A guide to controversy." Report of the Committee on Risk Perception and Communication, Commission on Social Sciences and Education. Appendix C, pp. 211–319. National Research Council, Washington, DC.
Frewer, L., Raats, M., and Shepherd, R. (1993). Modeling the media: The transmission of risk information in the British quality press. *J. Math. Appl. Bus. Indust.* 5, 235–247.
Frewer, L., Shepherd, R., and Sparks, P. (1994). The interrelationship between perceived knowledge, control

and risk associated with a range of food-related hazards targeted at the individual, other people and society. *J. Food Safety* **14**, 19–40.

Frewer, L.J., Howard, C., Hedderley, D., and Shepherd, R. (1996). What determines trust in information about food-related risks? Underlying psychological constructs. *Risk Anal.* **16**, 473–486.

Groth, E. (1991). Communicating with consumers about food safety and risk issues. *Food Technol.* **45**, 248–253.

Hathaway, S.C. (1993). Risk assessment procedures used by the Codex Alimentarius Commission and its subsidiary and advisory bodies. *Food Control* **4**, 189–201.

Kahneman, D., and Tversky, A. (1979). Prospect theory: An analysis of decision under risk. *Econometrica* **47**, 263–291.

McCallum, D.B., and Santos, S.L. (1995). Participation and Persuation: A Communication Perspective on Risk Management. *In* "Risk Assessment and Management Handbook for Environmental, Health and Safety Professionals." McGraw-Hill, New York.

Needleman, J. (1988). Sources and policy implications of uncertainty in risk assessment. *Stat. Sci.* **3**, 328–338.

Powell, D.A. (1996). Eat, drink and be wary, a risk communications workshop. International Association of Milk Food an Environmental Sanitarians annual meeting. Seattle, WA.

Powell, D. A., and Leiss, W. (1997). "Mad Cows and Mother's Milk: The Perils of Poor Risk Communications." McGill Univ. Press, Montreal.

Sandman, P.M. (1987). Risk communication: Facing public outrage. *EPA J.* **13**, 21–22.

Santos, S.L. (1990). Developing a risk communication strategy. J.A.W.W.A., November, p. 45–49.

Slovic, P. (1986). Informing and educating the public about risk. *Risk Anal.* **6**, 403–415.

Slovic, P. (1987). Perception of risk. *Science* **236**, 280–285.

Slovic, P. (1990). The legitimacy of public perceptions of risk. *J. Pest. Reform* **10**, 13–15.

U.S. EPA (1989). "Risk Assessment Guidance for Superfund: Human Health Manual" U.S. Environmental Protection Agency, Washington, DC.

19

Biomedical Devices and Biomaterials

Mary E. P. Goad
Department of Veterinary Pathology
Louisiana State University School of
Veterinary Medicine
Baton Rouge, Louisiana

Dale L. Goad
Department of Veterinary Anatomy and Cell Biology
Louisiana State University School of
Veterinary Medicine
Baton Rouge, Louisiana

I. Introduction

The purpose of this chapter is to describe and define the major biomaterials used as biomedical implants or biomedical devices in humans and animals and to discuss methods of assessing the anticipated and abnormal reactions associated with these implants. Biomedical implants are composed of a wide variety of materials ranging from inert elements to highly reactive chemicals or composites. Composite can refer to many things ranging from two or more forms of the same material used as a single implant to two or more totally different materials used as a single implant. Biomedical implants also span the range from a single known element, such as titanium, to living cells or tissues initially derived from the host organism. The definitions presented in this chapter are essential for an understanding of biomaterials and biomedical devices and implants. Definitions vary with each user and are different depending on the context and source. Understanding these definitions (as presented here) will help in the determination of appropriate analysis of the biomaterials and predic-

Handbook of Toxicologic Pathology, Second Edition
Volume 1
Copyright © 2002 by Academic Press
All rights of reproduction in any form reserved.

tions of possible pathology associated with them. This chapter will not cover host-versus-grant or graft-versus-host reactions anticipated with some implants and will concentrate on those materials and devices that are primarily synthetic or composite in nature and design. Definitions in this chapter are not all-inclusive or accepted by all biomaterial users.

II. Definition of Biomaterial and Biomedical Devices

A biomaterial is a single element or a compound, a composite or mixture of elements and synthesized or derived compounds used in the body to preserve, restore, or augment structure or function in the body. Examples of biomaterials range from titanium metal screws in bones to suture materials to implanted cells.

A biomedical device is a device used temporarily or permanently, externally or internally, to diagnose conditions or to preserve, restore, or augment structure or function in the body. Devices include clinical chemistry analyzers, contact lenses, MRI units, artificial hearts, syringes, needles, and breast implants.

Prosthetic devices are artificial structures designed to replace parts of the body. Artificial limbs, breast implants, and eyes are examples of prostheses.

These definitions, in part, are derived from the U.S. Food and Drug Administration (FDA) and the International Organization of Standardization (ISO) that regulates the testing and use of biomedical devices and biomaterials. The FDA defines medical devices based on their location relative to the body. Noninvasive devices include such apparatus as diagnostic kits or serum chemistry analyzers. External devices include electrocardiographs, stethoscopes, and ultrasound equipment. Internal or communicating devices range from lancets to indwelling catheters to implanted metal screws in the vertebrae. These are further subdivided by the FDA based on possible harmful effects, removal capabilities, and results of failures of the devices.

Biomaterials include any nonendogenous substances placed in the body to preserve, restore or augment structure or function. Nonendogenous is used rather than exogenous because many of the newer bioengineered biomaterials are derived from body tissues and fluids, including cells and tissue of the specific host or patient to be treated. Biomaterials can be temporary, lasting for seconds to months, or permanent. Permanent implants may remain in the body for the life of the implant or the life of the host or patient. Table I lists some of the major categories of biomaterials and their uses. Table I lists designations of temporary versus permanent; this designation is based on FDA and ISO criteria and not on the actual life of the implants or potential uses in the body.

A biomedical device, in this context, is a functional or structural entity composed of biomaterials and implanted in the body. The implant can be in contact with the surface only, can be completely implanted in the body with no external communication, or can be in the body with external communication. The FDA and ISO add confusion to these areas by also defining implants in certain areas of the body to be internal or external based on the ease of removal. Always remember to check with the regulatory agencies for their approved designation of the device before designing testing

TABLE I
Selected Examples of Biomaterial Types and Uses

Organ or tissue repaired or replaced	Biomaterials used
Bone	Allograft (human)
	Xenograft (bovine)
	Synthetic chemical (hydroxyapatite)
	Polymer (polymethylmethacrylate)
	Metal
	Pins, screws, plates (steel, titanium)
Joint	Metal (titanium)
	Polymer (methylmethacrylate)
	Plastic (PTFE)
	Ceramics
Dental alveoli	Bone substitutes
	Metal screws
Middle ear	Ceramics
	Bioglass
	Polymers, plastics
	Metals
Heart valves	Metals
	Polymers/plastics
	Xenograft (porcine, bovine)
	Composite (metal, polymer, and bovine)
Soft tissue/incision repair	Polymers/plastics
	Metals
Eye lenses	Polymers/plastics
	Bioglass
Biodelivery systems	Polymers/plastics
	Lipid vesicles
	Hydroxyapatite
	Alginate

protocols. Devices that can be removed, whether or not they are externally communicating or not, are considered to be potentially less problematic than those that cannot be removed. An example of this is dental devices. Bone substitute materials are used commonly in the dental alveoli to rebuild or augment diseased or absent bone, but because the oral cavity is easily accessible, oral implants of bone substitute materials are not held to the same testing standards as those implanted in the axial or appendicular skeleton.

A. TYPES OF BIOMATERIALS

The types of materials used as biomedical implants are as varied as the users' imagination.

Some of the more typical devices and materials are summarized in Table I. Many of the same compounds are used in many locations in the body for disparate purposes. Some of the more common biomaterials include metals, plastics, polymers, and products derived from cells and tissues. A detailed description of examples of these is included with the more specific uses to follow.

B. USES OF BIOMATERIALS

Biomaterials and biomedical devices have been used throughout history to diagnose and treat diseases. Until the last century, most biomaterials were limited to natural products as ivory, animal bones, wood, and other fibers from animals and plants. Metals were also used for limb replacements and to replace bones of the skull or chest as coverings over large openings. Metal was the primary material used for implants because it caused fewer reactions in the body than other materials that were implanted and because it could be molded or shaped into many applications and sizes such as thin, durable sheets and rods. The use and sources of implants have increased with an understanding of body reactions to these materials and our ability to control or limit those reactions.

The purpose of implanted biomaterials and biomedical devices is limited only by technology and imagination. Implants are used as grafts or additions in many tissues, especially bones and joints, to replace lost or damaged tissues, and to restore that tissue to normal structure and function. Implants are also used to augment or alter tissue or organ structure or function, such as insulin-releasing pumps or an artificial pancreas, or for cosmetic surgery to correct congenital defects or alter unpleasing physical appearances. Devices are also used to replace function for tissues still in the body that are nonfunctional or unable to support structure, such as in heart valve failure or Parkinson's disease. The implanted biomaterials covered in this chapter include those used for tissue defect and incision repair, repair of bones and joints, valves and vessel replacement, biodelivery systems, and some miscellaneous implants such as silicone gel breast implants (see Table I).

Depending on the qualities and function or structure desired, many different compounds of biological, synthetic, and elemental origin can be used as implants. Some of the properties considered when selecting a biomaterial for a specific structure or function include resorption, strength, flexibility, size, biocompatibility, and surfaces. These properties are the same ones to be considered when assessing biomaterials for safety and efficacy. Materials can be rapidly or slowly resorbable or nonresorbable. Strength can be related to tension, weight bearing, or ability to withstand normal pressures and stresses in the desired implant site. Flexibility characteristics can be based on the resorption, size, and strength and can be desirable or inappropriate. Surfaces can be rough or smooth. Size can be microscopic or as large or larger than normal gross structure such as limbs and joints. The most significant parameter that determines the host or patient's reaction at the tissue or cellular level is designated *biocompatibility* or the reaction of the body induced by the implant. This will be covered in more detail in the section on assessment of reactions to biomaterials.

III. Biomedical Devices

A. SOFT TISSUE DEFECTS AND INJURY REPAIR

Suture material and associated grids, sponges, and meshwork implants placed at the time of most surgeries are the most common and widely used biomaterials and implanted devices. Suture materials and other materials used in soft tissue repair fall into two basic categories: absorbable and nonabsorbable. Nonabsorbable materials include mainly metal and synthetic plastics such as stainless steel suture and staples, nylon sutures and meshes, and polytetrafluoroethylene (PTFE, Teflon or Gore Tex). These materials are used to create nonabsorbable implants, including polypropylene (Prolene, Marlex) and polyester (Mersilene).

Incision, defect, or hernia repair materials are assessed for their ability to withstand tearing, breaking pressures, tensions, their tensile strength and their ability to elicit a long-lasting fibrotic reaction, and their biocompatibility. For soft tissue repair, the surgeon often relies on the development of a fibrotic reaction to the implant. This fibrosis will not only keep the implant in the desired location, but will also add to the strength of the material. These materials must also be flexible and not cause pain. This is a major drawback of metal in soft tissue repair, and stainless-steel staples and sutures induce pain locally because they are hard and inflexible compared to the surrounding tissue. A more recent problem with metal implants is detection by metal-detecting devices used to keep out weapons.

Absorbable materials are absorbable or biodegradable because of their composition and because of the host or body reaction to those materials. With these materials, pain can be elicited due to the inflammatory reaction produced. The unique properties of the different absorbable materials are used to the surgeon's advantage. Bioabsorbable or biodegradable devices have expanded to include internal fixation devices such as pins, screws, suture material anchors, and bone conductive surfaces. These devices are designed to dissipate over a length of time governed by the choice of material.

Selection is based on length of time to resorption and intensity of the body's reaction to the material. Some absorbable implants are designed to last months or years. Control of the biomaterial resorption rate takes advantage of the body's reaction to the material. Implants that evoke continuous and intense acute inflammation may be resorbed or degraded more rapidly than those that evoke milder and more chronic responses.

Resorbable chromic gut is the standard material used to compare local tissue reactions for implant biocompatibility of most biomaterials for any use. That is, local tissue reaction and repair following implantation of chromic gut is the baseline for the characteristic intense response to implant biomaterial. Typically, chromic gut elicits an intense acute reaction most typical of a pyogranuloma. Depending on the site of implantation, chromic gut can be re-

sorbed, phagocytized, or dissipated in 7 to 10 days and can induce proportionately large pyogranulomas, which resolve as the gut is resorbed.

B. BONES AND JOINTS

For over 100 years surgeons have used various autogenous, allogenous, and xenogenic bone grafts to facilitate the healing of bone defects, especially large or nonunion defects (Table II). These sources of grafts have many risks, including viral transmission associated with allogenous grafts. These problems, along with needs for materials with different properties that can be used in a variety of applications, have been the impetus for intensive investigations and development of bone implants and bone substitute materials. Various authors have promulgated criteria for an ideal bone implant; however, these criteria may not be ideal for each type of application, e.g., criteria for ideal implants used in periodontal augmentation, long bone fracture repair, or arthroplasty procedures. Nonetheless, criteria espoused by various authors can be a useful rubric in evaluating bioimplants used in bone.

In general, the compounds used for bone and joint substitutes are the same used for middle ear replacements. Middle ears should not be resorbable, and compounds that might be resorbed would be poor choices for those applications.

Evaluation of bone implants can be reduced to this concept: the implant should react appropriately and adequately with a tissue in an application that is defined by the user. This aphorism is deceptively simple because the tissue response to a specific implant can be affected by (1) the surgical aspects of the implantation procedure, such as site of implantation, the load placed on the implant, the viability of bone and soft tissue around the implant, and the stability of fixation of the implant; (2) the chemical composition and physical characteristics of the implanted materials, including crystalline structure; and (3) the physical characteristics of the implant, such as porosity and texture. Comparison and assessments of bioimplants require rigorous experi-

TABLE II
Bone and Joint Implants

Material	Uses	Potential problems/lesions

Metals
  Stainless steel
  Cobalt chromium
	Joints
	Structural support Screws, Pins, External Fixation
		Corrosion
		Degradation
		Particle formation, wear
		Debris

Titanium	Bone replacement Prostheses	Hypersensitivity Foreign body reaction

Coral
  Processed natural coral
  Coralline
Hydroxyapatite
  Porous coralline ceramic
	Bone replacement
	Grout/filler
		Hypersensitivity
		Poor incorporation
		Foreign body reaction

Ceramics and glasses
  Solids (formed)
  Granules
  Plaster of Paris (PoP)
  Hydroxyapatites
	Bone replacement
	Grout/filler
		Foreign body reaction
		Poor incorporation
		Migration
		Exothermic (PoP)

Polymers/plastics	Cement/adhesive	Particle fromation, wear Debris
Polymethylmethacrylate (PMMA) PTFE Polyglycolic acids	Grout/filler Joints	Exothermic (PMMA) Loss of strength/incorporation Foreign body reaction Cement/adhesive failure

Grafts
  Exogenous
    Bovine
	Bone replacement	Hypersensitivity
		Foreign body reaction

mental controls and critical evaluation of the biology of the tissue, the materials, and surgical aspects of the implantation. Many of the details of materials science and surgical techniques are beyond both the scope and intent of this chapter. This chapter focuses on fundamentals of evaluation, some methodologies used in the evaluation of bone implants, and selected important aspects of bone biology that affect the interaction of the material with tissues.

1. Metal Implants

Metals are used as joints, internal support and fixation structures, and externally communicating fixation devices. Metals used as implants are considered biocompatible insofar as they usually incite little tissue reaction in short-term applications. However, metals other than gold or platinum are not inert. Gold and platinum, however, provide little or no structural support. Metals used in orthopedic implants

undergo degradation by electrochemical corrosion, wear, and by the combined actions of these processes. Metal corrosion products and particles have both local and potential systemic effects in the host.

Three metal alloy systems are used for orthopedic implants: stainless steel, cobalt–chromium, and titanium alloys. Stainless-steel alloys contain mainly iron along with chromium (17–24%), nickel (11–13%), molybdenum (2–3%), and manganese (2 or 4–6%). Cobalt–chromium alloys are composed primarily of cobalt and chromium (19–30%) with variable amounts of nickel (1 up to 9–11%) and iron (<1 up to 3%). Cobalt–chromium–molybdenum alloys contain molybdenum (5–7%, 9–10) and either low (<1%) or high (30–37%) nickel. Titanium is used either as commercially pure titanium, which contains some iron and carbon (< 1% each), or as an alloy termed Ti-6A1-4V, which contains aluminum (6%) and vanadium (4%).

Corrosion of implanted metals involves multiple factors that act in concert to facilitate the breakdown of the metals. Oxidation reactions on the surface release two potentially reactive species: metal ions and electrons. Metal ions in solution form metal oxides and other chemical species that may be soluble or form precipitates. The insoluble products can either adhere to the surface of the metals or can migrate away from the surface of the metal. Formation of a film of metal oxides on the entire surface of metal prevents additional oxidation and reduction reactions and corrosion of the metal. Various passivation processes enhance formation of a metal oxide film on the surface of metals. The cobalt and titanium alloys form a passive oxidation film spontaneously and rapidly in the presence of biologic fluids and an undisturbed film is a barrier to corrosion. Disruption of the passive film allows renewed corrosion to occur with additional release of metal ions until the passive film is reestablished. More profound corrosion can occur at sites of micromotion between components (fretting). Repeated or ongoing abrasion allows oxidation reactions with release of metal ions, formation of metal oxides, local consumption of oxygen, and a fall in pH. Galvanic corrosion, which occurs when dissimilar metals are in direct contact while in an electrolyte solution, causes enhanced corrosion of the more reactive metal and passivation of the less reactive metal. Although uncommon, it can occur when stainless-steel cerclage wire comes into direct contact with less reactive alloys, such as cobalt–chromium.

2. Toxic Effects of Metals

Metal particles released from a joint prosthesis can have effects at sites distant from the implant. In a postmortem evaluation of 123 patients who had either stainless-steel or cobalt–chromium joint implants, metal particles were found in lymph nodes draining the limb as well as in distant lymph nodes, liver, spleen, and bone marrow. Some of the granulomatous response to metal particles has been ascribed to a cell-mediated immune response. Necrosis was also observed in lymph nodes that drained

limbs that had implants with prominent wear. These data suggest that released particles have the potential for systemic effects.

Certain metals elicit typical hypersensitivity reactions in some individuals. These include mercury, gold, platinum, beryllium, chromium, and nickel. Fortunately for people with implants, these are most typically seen with skin contact and not with implants in bone or soft tissue.

3. Metals and Carcinogenicity

Metals known to be carcinogenic in humans include nickel, arsenic, beryllium, and hexavalent chromium. Metallic nickel in human implant use has not been definitively associated with tumor induction, but reports of humans who have developed sarcomas at the sites of joint prosthesis implantation, as well as concerns over possible carcinogenicity of metals released from the implants, have led to both prospective studies in animals and retrospective studies on human patients with implants. No positive associations could be identified between implants and carcinogenicity in these studies. No increased risk for development of malignant bone tumors at the sites of implants was found in several large epidemiological studies conducted in Finland and Denmark. However, there were discordant results in the Danish and Swedish studies concerning risks for development of tumors of prostate and kidney. Animal studies of metal-associated tumors have identified the physical form of the metal as well as the length of time in sites as factors contributing to tumor prevalence. In rats, a single injection of metal powder or wear debris from titanium or cobalt–chromium did not lead to development of any tumors by the end of 24 months, although sarcomas developed in joints of animals injected with nickel, a carcinogenic metal not found in implants but used in the study as a positive control. In a different study in rats, tumors developed at sites of loose metal implants but not in well-fixed implants. Thus, tumors at the implant sites were likely related to the foreign body reaction rather than the metal implant itself. Taken together with results from epidemiological studies in humans, there is an absence of convincing evidence that metal implants lead to tumor development at the sites of implants.

4. Wear Debris

Wear debris refers to particles of material ranging from submicron to several microns in size that separate from the implant. Wear debris comes from frictional wear of articulating components (metals, polythylene linings, or ceramic, depending on the prosthesis) and potentially from the bone–implant interface. Particles of hardened adhesive used to secure cemented implants and previously generated wear debris can exert an abrasive action in the articulating components and act to generate more wear debris. Even in a well-functioning prosthesis the potential number of particles released into the joint space is estimated to be in the range of millions, to tens of billions of particles per year.

Potential consequences of wear debris include cytoxicity, foreign body reactions, and hypersensitivity reactions. Cobalt metal particles have been observed to be toxic to synoviocytes maintained in culture. Small particles (<5–$10\,\mu m$) of wear debris undergo phagocytosis by macrophages, whereas giant cells surround larger particles, leading to granulotanous inflammatory (foreign body) reaction. Macrophages produce proinflammatory cytokines [tumor necrosis factor, interteukin (IL)-1, IL-6] and inflammatory mediators (prostaglandins) that enhance the reaction and can stimulate bone resorption around the implant.

Detection and identification of wear particles can be made by several microscopic methodologies. Polyethylene particles are intensely birefringent under polarized light. An alternative method that is less specific is staining of sections with Oil Red O. In H&E-stained sections, ceramic debris appears as brownish-red granules and metal debris appears as black deposits. At the ultrastructural level, analysis of samples by inductively coupled atomic emission spectrophotometry can be used to identify the presence of specific metal ions (presence of free metal ions in tissue).

5. Cement Disease or Particle Disease

The term "particle disease" has replaced the term "cement disease." The original observation was associated with the use of polymethylmethacrylate (PMMA) adhesives to fix the implants to bone. In addition to the exothermic reaction (heat generated by the hardening of the adhesive) and associated local necrosis and other problems with their use, these adhesives are not resorbed. Regions of osteolysis surrounding failed implants contained abundant PMMA debris. Associated lesions range from increased macrophages to a marked granulomatous response to severe fibrosis. Fractures of the PMMA "mantle," as well as the surrounding bone, have been reported.

6. Definitions and Terms Used in the Evaluation of Interactions of Bone Implants and Bone Substitutes

Several terms are used in evaluation of bone implants, but few have a definition that is both unambiguous and universally accepted. Thus, the following is a list of operational definitions for the terms. These have been collated and collected from the current literature.

Osseointegration was originally defined as "direct contact between living bone and implant as observed on the light microscopic level." Osseointegration is currently often used as a general term denoting intimate contact between bone and an implant, by which definition it encompasses many other nonspecific terms used to describe the bone–implant interface, including biointegration, bone ingrowth, and bone bonding. ***Biointegration*** has been used to refer to "controlled interactions" between the tissue and the implant. ***Bone ingrowth*** is used to denote the formation of bone in irregular or porous surfaces of an implant that are made porous by various means (sintering, coatings). The quality of implant fixation is often based on an assessment of bone ingrowth. ***Bone bonding*** suggests an intimate association between the implant and the bone. While these terms come under the general category of osseointegration, they do not necessarily imply true contact between the bone and full implant. The presence of an intervening layer of fibrous connective tissue between bone and implant would suggest the presence of a foreign body reaction or a consequence of the use of surgical adhesives (i.e., methylmethacrylate) and would not be osseointegration.

Bioactivity has been defined as the property of the implant to elicit a host response; however, the definition is not a value definition in that the response could be beneficial or deleterious. Many implants can evoke a foreign body reaction. Classification of this reaction would not truly fit the working definition of bioactive and would not really meet the criteria for being bioinert. The most unambiguous classification would be to call it what it is: a foreign body reaction.

The effects of bone substitutes or bone graft substitutes on bone formation can be classified into three categories that are not mutually exclusive: ***osteoconductive, osteoinductive***, and ***osteogenic***. Osteoconductive refers to the ability of a material to act as a scaffold upon which the host's cells form new bone. Osteoconduction is an active process whereby fibrovascular tissue invades the implant and there is formation of capillaries and migration of osteprogenitor cells into the implant. The vascular component and cellular migrations are essential for osteoconduction. Thus, osteoconductive activity of an implanted material is determined by (1) characteristics of the material or material surface, (2) proximity of the material to bone when implanted, (3) viability of the bone tissue, and (4) stability of the implant in bone. Therefore, the assessment of bone implants must include an appreciation and evaluation of factors that affect osteoconduction.

Osteoinductive refers to the ability of the implant to stimulate or induce new bone formation from the host's tissues. This is exemplified by implants in which growth factors such as bone morphogenic proteins (BMPs) are combined with the implanted material. Osteogenic describes implants in which cells that have the capacity to form bone, such as bone marrow cells, are introduced along with the implanted material. Thus, these implants have the capacity to form bone.

Biodegradable refers to the capacity of an implant to undergo *in vivo* degradation, which can be by chemical, enzymatic, or cell-mediated mechanisms. The processes most relevant to bone substitute materials are (1) phagocytosis mediated by macrophages, osteoclasts, or both and (2) dissolution. The amount and rate of resorption of bone substitute materials are variable and depend on the material as well as other processes, such as ingrowth of bone into the implant and the body inflammatory response to the implant.

7. Bone Substitute Materials

Bone substitute materials encompass a complex array of materials and forms of materials both natural and synthetic. The host response to bone substitute materials is influenced by the physiochemical nature of the material at the time of implantation, including the chemical composition of the material, heat treatment (i.e., sintered or non-sintered), the form (solid or granules), porosity, temperature of formation (exothermic reactions); by the surgical technique (stability of fixation); and by viability of the tissue surrounding the implant.

Bone substitute materials can be combined with metals, polymers, other fibers (e.g., collagen), or other bone substitute materials or agents (e.g., BMPs) to generate composites that have more optimal properties than those of the individual components, such as added strength or stability or partial resorption. Implanted materials, particularly biodegradable materials or polymers in the implants, have the potential to deliver pharmacologic agents (such as antibiotics) or osteogenic proteins (such as bone morphogenic proteins) that would enhance the healing of bone defects and modify the host responses to the implant. More intriguing is the possibility of gene therapy in conjunction with bone substitutes, especially with the observation that naked DNA adsorbed to the implant or an attached polymer can be taken up by local cells and expressed transiently. This could lead to more sustained production of osteogenic factors in the defect site than would occur by incorporation of the protein in the material. All of these strategies can change the properties of the implant and alter the host response to the tissue. Porosity is a key determinant for ingrowth of bone into an implant. The pores must be of sufficient size to allow the invasion of both cells and new blood vessels, there must be interconnected pores to allow the blood vessels to penetrate the implant, and there must be enough porosity (volume of the material composed of pores) that tissues can grow into the implant. Unfortunately, increased porosity is associated with diminished mechanical strength. Thus, the use of porous materials is restricted to applications in which there is no load or one in which the loads are taken away from the implant. However, if the porous portions of the implant are replaced by bone, the implanted area has the potential to regain the mechanical strength of bone.

8. Coralline Bone Substitutes

These bone substitutes are derived from the exoskeletons of marine corals that form interconnecting porous structure with calcium carbonate in a crystalline structure called aragonite. Coralline materials used in bone include (1) natural corals, in which the organic materials have been removed from the corals without and preimplantation modification of the mineral component, although a layer of calcium phosphate forms on the surfaces in vivo; (2) coralline hydroxyapatite in which calcium carbonate is converted to hydroxyapatite by a hydrothermal exchange reaction; and (3) a coralline porous ceramic in which the conversion to hydroxyapatite is restricted to the surfaces.

The biologic response to coralline bone substitute is influenced by the coral porosity and mineral content. The pore size and the degree of porosity vary between species of corals. Implantation of corals with greater porosity is associated with enhanced ingrowth of bone and resorption of the implant. The calcium phosphate layers of coral facilitate the inter-

action of bone with the implant. Hydroxyapatite and calcium carbonate in the aragonite structure are resorbed, but heat can convert the calcium carbonate to the calcite form, which is poorly resorbed. Thus, the form of the mineral can affect the biologic response.

Nacre is the mother-of-pearl layer derived from the marine oyster *Pinctada maxima* and consists of calcium carbonate in the form of aragonite crystals. Nacre is bioactive, and implants in sheep had formation of new bone at the interface without any intervening fibrous connective tissue and without any resorption of the implant. In this study, no inflammatory cells were present in material that had been implanted for 10 months.

9. Ceramics, Glasses, and Ceramic Glasses

By English usage definitions, ceramic refers to a product made from nonmetallic mineral that is heated to a high temperature, and porcelains are a high grade of ceramics usually containing much silicates. Glasses are formed when a mixture cools without formation of crystals and are often made of silicates. Ceramics used in bone implants can be divided into two functional categories: bioinert and bioactive. These terms do not refer to the biocompatibility or resorption characteristics of these implants.

a. Bioinert Ceramics. Bioinert ceramics, such as alumina and zirconia, are hard and brittle with a high surface finish, low frictional moment, and low wear. These ceramics are not degraded *in vivo* and are used to construct gliding components of joint prostheses and nondegradable screws. Despite low wear characteristics, frictional wear of a joint prosthesis generates wear particles that can cause granulomatous foreign body reactions in the periprosthetic tissue. Brittleness of these ceramics leads to fracture and failure of the implants and subsequent pathology from that failure.

b. Bioactive Glasses. Bioactive glasses are composed of SiO_2, CaO_2, P_2O_5, and Na_2O, but in proportions that are different from stable soda–lime–silica glasses used in nonbiologic applications. The glasses can be converted into a glass–ceramic by the addition or formation of crystals within the glass itself. Both bioglasses and bioactive glass–ceramics have surfaces on which hydroxycarbonate apatite (HCA) precipitates and crystallizes within an hour of implantation. The HCA crystals provide a base for adsorption of components of the extracellular matrix and subsequent interactions with cells. The biologic response to bioactive glasses and glass–ceramics involves attachment of bone; however, interactions between the bioglasses and bone are restricted to the surface. There is neither ingrowth of bone into the glasses nor is there any resorption. The relative bioactivity of the bioglasses for bone and for soft tissue relates to the composition of the bioglasses, which is a major determinant of their bioactivity. Thus, the relative selectivity of bonding between bioglasses and bone versus soft tissue can be manipulated by alterations in their composition. Al_2O_3 can diminish bioglass bonding to bone and may negatively influence mineralization of bone.

c. Bioactive Ceramics.

Bioactive ceramics include hydroxyapatite, tricalcium phosphate, and biphasic ceramics that contain a mixture of hydroxyapatite and tricalcium phosphate. These compounds are sintered (heated to a high temperature) to form a ceramic. The ceramics are prepared as blocks that are manufactured to be porous. After sintering, the porous ceramics can be used either as porous blocks or crushed and sieved to yield granules within a specific size range that can be used as bone filler material.

The resorbability of a ceramic is affected by its physiochemical state, including the material itself, the crystallinity or density of the ceramic, the proportion of hydroxyapatite and tricalcium phosphate in biphasic ceramics, the porosity, and the size of granules used (in bone fillers). Hydroxyapatite ceramics are generally more stable than tricalcium phosphate, which is degraded too rapidly for osteoconduction to occur. This disparity can be overcome in part by mixing hydroxyapatite and tricalcium phosphate (often in a ratio of 60:40) to create biphasic ceramics with more predictable rates of degradation. The resorption of hydroxyapatite

is inversely related to crystallinity or denseness of the material, i.e., dense or highly crystalline hydroxyapatite ceramics persist without appreciable degradation, whereas material that is less crystalline or amorphous is more resorbable. Smaller particle size can also apparently increase bioactivity and resorption.

Ceramic materials do not evoke an immunologic response, necrosis, or infiltration by neutrophils or lymphocytes. The injectable materials (granular bone fillers) elicit a foreign body reaction with infiltrates of mononuclear and multinucleated giant cells that engulf small ceramic particles. Fibrous connective tissue may be a component of the tissue response to ceramic implants; however, the material alone may not be the stimulus. For example, Dupraz and colleagues found that particles of biphasic calcium phosphate injected into cylindrical bone defects that had been drilled into the distal femurs of rabbits elicited a foreign body reaction with phagocytic cells but without fibrous encapsulation. In a dog study with diaphyseal ulnar defects stabilized with intramedullary pins and filled with test materials, bone formed at sites that had been filled with cancellous bone in the presence or absence of biphasic calcium ceramic. However, nonunions with intervening fibrous connective tissue present at the defect site occurred in four of six dogs in which the defects had been filled with biphasic calcium ceramic alone. The apparent discordant results from these studies illustrate the complexity of interpretation of the tissue response to bioceramics and biomaterials. These studies were conducted in different species, in sites that had very different loading conditions, and with materials that may not have been identical in composition or particle size. In addition, a fibrous connective tissue response elicited by micromotion at the defect site cannot be excluded in dogs that developed nonunions.

10. Calcium Sulfate (Plaster of Paris)

Calcium sulfate is a bone substitute that has been used intermittently over the last 100 years. When mixed with water it forms a hard crystalline structure in an exothermic reaction.

It is biocompatible and resorbable. Recent medical grades of calcium sulfate yield material with more homogeneous crystal structure, porosity, and predictable resorbability, which is about 30–60 days. Long-term implants are not associated with inflammation; however, the exothermic reaction prevents the addition of labile components such as cytokines.

11. Hydraulic Cements

Hydraulic cements are calcium phosphate preparations that after mixing and injection in liquid form undergo spontaneous curing *in situ*. The meaning of cements in this context is more like the word "grout" in that the calcium phosphate mixture acts as filler and a medium for other components rather than as an adhesive. The term "cement" has been used to refer to adhesives used to adhere implants to bone as well as to bone substitute materials that are injected as a liquid and then solidify *in situ*.

12. Composite Materials

Composites are composed of multiple different materials. The advantage of composites is that the benefits of the individual components can be exploited while minimizing their disadvantages. Currently, there is an expansion in the development of composites that are can be used as bone substitute materials as well as scaffolding for cells as a part of tissue engineering. Some composites consist of collagen, cellulose, or other polymer matrix or carrier mixed with calcium phosphate ceramics to create injectable bone substitutes (bone cement).

C. HEART VALVES AND VESSELS

Heart valves are commonly replaced when they do not function because of congenital or acquired defects. In general, congenital defects are detected early in a patient's life and may require periodic replacements of the prosthetic valves. Acquired defects, which may occur at any time in life, generally require fewer replacements of the valves. Replacement heart valves have been in use since the 1950s. The major problem with implanted valves is structural fail-

ure due to processes such as fatigue rupture of the leaflets, degradation, calcification, and thrombosis.

Heart replacement valves are historically either metal or mechanical valves, usually synthesized from a composite of metals and plastics or polymers or bioprosthetic valves (i.e., valves derived from animals, usually pigs as well as valves made from bovine pericardium) (Table III). The newest classes of valves are composites of the mechanical and bioprosthetic types, and bioengineered valves that may contain tissues and cells from the patient. The reaction of the body and local heart tissue to the implanted valve is both the main determinant of choice of valve used and the cause of valve failure.

1. Mechanical Valves

Mechanical heart valves such as the Bjork–Shiley valve induce coagulation, leading to thrombi and emboli at and around the valve. This requires continued use of anticoagulation therapy in the patient to prevent undesired coagulation leading to thrombosis.

2. Bioprosthetic

Porcine bioprosthetic valves, including the Hancock and Carpentier-Edwards valves, are harvested from pig hearts with sizes corresponding to the patients' hearts. Mineralization or calcification of the prosthesis and adjacent tissues is the major problem with porcine valves and bovine pericardial valves. Treatment of the valves with glutaraldehyde and other fixatives tends to decrease the mineralization. Younger patients tend to develop calcification more frequently than older patients. Medication or intercurrent disease, such as renal failure, also increases the risk of valve mineralization.

TABLE III
Examples of Replacement Heart Valves

Mechanical—Metal	Bjork–Shiley
Bioprosthetic	Hancock
Porcine valves	Carpentier–Edwards
Bovine valves	
Bovine pericardium	

Porcine valves are sometimes subject to degradation and failure because of the same reasons that the initial or native valve failed, including bacterial diseases, thrombosis and stenosis, or insufficiency. Valve leaflet failure may also occur because of degradation and tearing of the tissues. Other valves from animals include those fashioned from pericardium of bovine or porcine origin and mounted on metal or plastic or polymer stents and scaffolding.

3. Bioengineered Valves

The newest type of heart valve and vessel replacement is the bioengineered valve or vessel created by the synthesis of biodegradable polymer scaffolds covered with cells grown from the patient. These valves have been used successfully in sheep and calves and have characteristics more similar to native valves than mechanical, synthetic, or bioprosthetic valves.

4. Vessels

a. Stents. Stents are fairly rigid devices used to provide support for hollow, usually tubular, structures that are being held in one position. The tubular stent structure is usually anastomosed or secured in place, and patency of the structure must be maintained because they usually support tubes that fluid flows. Stents are the rigid support in the base of heart replacement valves or the wall of implants for vessels, esophaguses, urethras, ureters, and other tubular organs. They are typically made of nonabsorbable materials such as metal, polyethylene, or polypropylene.

The major contributions to stent failure are the sutures or cements used to keep them in place until the tissue around the stent heals and the nature of the biomaterial compared to that of the surrounding tissues. Ruptures and leakage may occur at the suture sites until healing occurs; however, these sites must be of equal strength and flexibility as the tissue they are placed into. The biomaterial used for the stent must also be of the same pliability, strength, flexibility, and durability as the tissue it is used to replace. If it is not, then it may induce rup-

tures above or below it or it may fail because it cannot resist the same changes as the native tissues. This is why temporary devices may be used along with permanent ones so that end-to-end healing may occur prior to allowing the local pressures on the implanted materials.

D. SILICONE IMPLANTS

Silicon is an element usually found in nature as silica (silicon dioxide or SiO_2). Silica is a component of sand and glass; crystalline silica is quartz. Other forms of silica include talc, feldspar, mica, vermiculite, and asbestos. Silicon is required for the development and maintenance of connective tissues and is found in highest concentrations in tissues with large amounts of connective tissue, including large arteries, ligaments and tendons, bone and cartilage, and dental enamel. Silicon provides links within and between glycosaminoglycans and their respective proteins. Silicone and silicones are compounds with some or all of the carbons replaced by silicon. Silicone gel is used as a material for breast implants, and silicone is used as a component of tubing, delivery devices, and packaging.

Silicone gel and saline packaged in rubber or plastic are used to enhance or augment the breast and other parts of the body. Craniofacial reconstruction requires the use of a wide variety of soft tissue replacements, and surgeons often select silicone gels because they mimic the softness and pliability of normal tissue, which is especially important around the head and neck. The use of silicone gel in breast implants has been a source of controversy and litigation due to suggestions that the leakage of silicone gel from implants may be associated with the development of autoimmune disorders in women with these implants. Overall, because of the desirable properties of silicone gels, they are still considered good tissue replacements but are used less frequently because of the associated nonscientifically based liability issues.

In general, adverse reactions to breast implants, whether filled with gel or with saline, that are reported to and by the FDA are the same as for every other surgical procedure. Reported problems with breast implants include hematomas, surgical site and implant site contraction, and fibrosis due to excess scar tissue, incision healing failure or dehiscence, implant rupture with leakage of contents, and inflammation around the implant. Implant failure usually implies significant adverse reactions or rupture of the implant with leakage of contents, and these events may require repeated surgical procedures. However, breast implants are not considered "lifetime" implants and may be removed, replaced, or repaired several times.

Retrospective and prospective controlled scientific studies, including many reviewed by the U.S. FDA, show no significant increased risk of autoimmune or immune-mediated diseases in women with silicone gel breast implants when compared to women without implants.

Reactions of the body to silicon-containing compounds that are dispersed or free in the body typically initiate granulomatous reactions. Talc granules, as an example, especially talc from surgical gloves or other devices, can induce local or disseminated foreign body granulomas, which can remain at the surgical site or spread throughout the body.

Silicone and silicates may leach out of the silicone tubing into the body, and drugs or compounds kept in silicone packaging may also contain leached silicon. Prior to the breast implant controversy, this silicone was considered nontoxic and was thought to elicit no, or very little, host or tissue response.

E. BIOENGINEERED IMPLANTS AND DELIVERY SYSTEMS

Biomaterials and devices for the delivery of substances range from simple tubing or catheters implanted from the external surface into the organ or vessel of interest to local implants of materials that are impregnated with a substance that is released over time. Materials used for sustained release either bind the drug or substance or are degraded and gradually release the drug. Many of the biodegradable bone substitutes are also used as biodelivery systems because hydroxyapatite binds proteins and cyanoacrylates can be mixed with many sub-

stances. These types of devices rely on the dissolution or degradation of the implant to deliver the drug or substance.

Most of the implants that are currently derived from autografts, xenografts, and synthetic materials may be replaced in the near future with engineered materials that are composites of the host and synthetic scaffolding. Some of these implants will have the same problems as the synthetic implants. For the most part, these implants will more closely mimic autografts; however, these should still be subject to the same evaluations and problems as any other biomaterials. Articular cartilage, auricular, and nasal cartilage, skin, vessels, and valves are some of the host cell-derived tissue implants currently in use or under development. Other bioengineered implants are being developed from animal sources because the human or animal patient has nonfunctional tissue. Some of these include pancreatic islets, hepatocytes, and DOPA-producing brain nuclei.

Many of the current biodelivery devices have bioengineered components. Examples of these include polyethylene tubes containing pancreatic islet cells, alginate beads with bone or cartilage cells, collagen sponges with chondrocytes, and PTFE mesh containing hepatocytes.

IV. Safety Evaluation of Biomaterials and Devices

A. ASSESSMENT OF LESIONS

Most lesions associated with biomedical devices and biomaterial implants are factors that affect foreign body reaction of varying severity. The types of foreign body reactions differ with location of the implant, the local tissue trauma, exposure to blood and bodily fluids, and the patient's (host) responses. Foreign body reactions and inflammation may be undesirable or may be advantageous and required to elicit a desired fibrotic reaction around the implant.

The typical foreign body reaction to implanted materials is a granuloma or granulomatous inflammation (Fig. 1). The center of the granuloma or granulomatous inflammation usually consists of necrotic debris and larger pieces of the implant or the entire implant. Depending on the material, most degradable implants have an adjacent layer of neutrophils or heterophils surrounded by a mixture of lymphocytes and macrophages often interspersed with multinucleated giant cells and fibroblast and an outer layer of fibrous connective tissue (Fig. 2). This description is of a "neat" or tidy arrangement. With materials that disintegrate rapidly or break into many small particles, the granuloma is seen more often as central implant particles interspersed with macrophages, lymphocytes, fibrous connective tissue, and scattered neutrophils. As the reaction resolves with time, the leukocytes are no longer a main component of the reaction process and the primary observation is fibrosis directly around the implant. This is especially true of nonabsorbable implants. The exact nature and timing of the reaction and healing process varys considerably from one material to another. Implants that elicit intense purulent reactions in one site of the body may elicit little or no reaction in the intended location. Implants for which significant peri-implant fibrosis is desirable may have resolution and loss of fibrous connective tissue over time. Intriguing new animal models include implants encased in screened or enclosed compartments with little or no direct contact with the animal's blood or bodily fluids, suggesting that any tissue reaction in the chambers is a direct effect of the implanted material.

Over time, usually days to weeks, most acute inflammatory reactions resolve to less severe responses. Of concern is a continued neutrophil or heterophil infiltrate. Reactions that continue to have significant numbers of neutrophils along with the foreign body reaction and fibrosis usually have some other process involved. This continued intensity of neutrophil infiltrates is usually a result of breakdown of the implant into fragments that elicit cytokines and thus neutrophils or, more commonly,

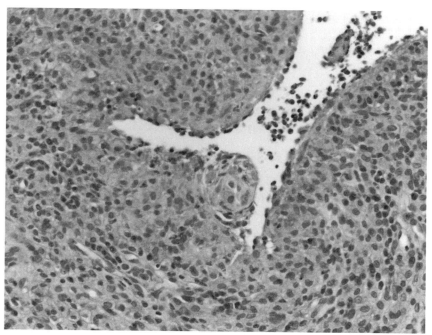

Figure 1. Section of tissue from the edge around an implanted polymer and metal device. This section was collected 23 days postimplantation. Tissue consists primarily of fibrous connective tissue with infiltrates of lymphocytes and macrophages. By 23 days, most peri-implant tissue should have no neutrophils (20×; H&E).

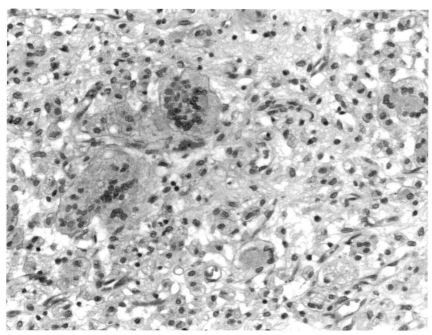

Figure 2. Several large multinucleated giant cells are present in the tissue surrounding a metal and polymer-implanted device. This is a fairly typical foreign body reaction with foreign body multinucleated giant cells (20×, H&E).

contamination of the implant. The most common contaminant of implanted biomaterials that induces neutrophilic infiltrates is endotoxin. Because of the nature of many biomaterials, sterilization can be problematic and removal of endotoxins may be difficult. Irradiation or gas sterilization (ethylene oxide) does not remove all endotoxins, especially those formed prior to sterilization.

Clinical assessment of the animal and human patients is essential. Intense granulomatous or other inflammatory reactions around implants are often not associated with pain or illness or altered host function. A grossly or microscopically intense inflammatory reaction that is essentially subclinical may be less severe of a reaction than one with pronounced inflammatory changes that cause pain or functional deficits.

This is why each biomaterial must not only be tested according to FDA guidelines, but also under prediction conditions in the tissue and site of intended use and for the life span of the implant or patient. Motion, even micromotion,

at the implant site may alter the inflammatory processes or the desired healing around the implant.

The optimal methods used to assess degree of reaction, severity of reaction, ingrowth, incorporation, or any cellular of tissue response visible by light or electron microscopy are by morphometry or measurement of the parameter evaluated. Single specimen evaluations from each implanted animal may be acceptable for qualitative descriptions of the type of inflammation or tissue reaction but are not adequate to evaluate growth of tissue or degrees of implant resorption, movement, or alteration. With the assistance of statisticians, the investigator must determine the appropriate site, size, and number of tissue evaluations to be performed to yield meaningful results.

Selection of the appropriate animal model for efficacy testing is more difficult than the justification for the appropriate animal model for safety testing. An example of this is bone substitute materials. Intervertebral or spinal bone grafts have been performed in dogs,

473

sheep, goats, and monkeys. Many investigators believe that only animals that support themselves in the upright position are appropriate; however, the FDA considers that goats are sufficiently "upright" because they often walk on their hind legs only.

Scientific judgment must be used. The most scientifically appropriate tests of efficacy or failure may not be the tests required by the FDA. Stress and pressure testing with analytical instruments such as the Instron for structural stability and implant strength after the implants has been *in vivo* may not be appropriate for implants designed to resorb or not designed to provide structural support.

B. CARCINOGENICITY

Implants intended to function for the life of the patient that do not resorb and cannot be removed easily must also be assessed for carcinogenicity. Carcinogenicity studies for biomaterials must be designed carefully and must take into consideration previous testing of components of the devices. The selection of species is very important. Rats of almost any strain are very susceptible to the development of sarcomas at the implant site. The numbers of animals per treatment group must be statistically meaningful and the background prevalence of tumors in the selected strain must be well documented.

PTFE, which is considered inert and noncarcinogenic, can induce sarcomas in rats if implanted subcutaneously. Granules of almost any nondegradable compound can also induce sarcomas in rats. The two types of implants with mostly anecdotal data to support the premise of tumor induction are silicone breast implants in women and metal bone or joint implants in dogs and humans. Tests of implanted silicone gel and metals in rats have shown an association with sarcomas, but no more than implantation of any other nonresorbable implant. Reports of sarcomas at the site of metal implants in bones are all retrospective and in both animal and human patients, not test subjects.

The physical form of implants also significantly influences the type of inflammatory reaction and the induction of tumors in rodents. Finely ground materials, meshes with a lot of surface area, and particles tend to be associated with the induction of inflammation followed by resolution in rats regardless of the implant site. Materials that have large surface areas tend to induce little active inflammation with more prominent fibrosis and then neoplasia rather than chronic inflammation. These implants also tend to be associated with more mutations and DNA strand breaks than particulates. Thus, the most consistent finding in biomaterial implant studies in rodents is that large implants with large surface areas are more often associated with the induction of tumors, usually sarcomas at the site. These tumors may be due to a physical effect of the implant that induces DNA lesions and mutations leading to carcinogenesis.

Assessment of biomedical devices and biomaterials must meet criteria to prove that (1) they work (2), they are safe, and (3) they will or will not fail. Most important is the prediction of failure or adverse effects of the device. These assessments depend on (1) the purpose of the implant (2), the site of implantation (3), the method of implantation (4), the defined life span of the implant, and (5) predictions of failure based on previous devices and on *in vitro* assays. Assays and animal models should be justified based on scientific hypotheses and specific aims and not FDA requirements alone. The battery of standard FDA biocompatibility studies should be the starting point to aid decision making about additional tests needed to prove or verify safety or efficacy.

The purpose or intended use of the implant must be specifically defined in order to select the most appropriate annual model. Issues considered when selecting animal models include implant physical characteristics such as size, shape, strength, flexibility, and durability of the biomedical device as well as the site of implant in the animal model. Rodents may be inappropriate animals because they are too small, just as dogs may not have the appropriate physiology or anatomy. Pigs and sheep are often selected because they have anatomy and organ size comparable to humans. However, the specific function of the implant and the type of use must be taken into account. For example, most animals do not place most of their body weight on their rear legs. Rabbits are often used as bone substitute models, but rabbits have atypical calcium metabolism compared to humans and carnivores.

The current trend is to select an animal model with the same defect or problem as the patient population for which the implant is intended. For example, insulin infusion devices should be tested in diabetic animals. The optimal diabetic animals would be those with the same type of diabetes mellitus as the intended human population.

C. FDA AND ISO GUIDELINES

Analysis of biomaterials is based on two broad categories as defined by the FDA and ISO, which are efficacy and safety. Efficacy is narrowly defined by U.S. FDA as whether a device or biomaterial performs as specified in detail by the manufacturer ("proof of concept"). The specific use of the implant must be described in detail as to the indication for use and the patient population. Efficacy for the producer of the biomaterial may be defined more broadly. Most biomaterial developers envision many uses of their product and test the material in all possible forms and phases.

The FDA and the ISO specify safety tests for biomedical devices and biomaterials. The requirements are similar to but less stringent than the toxicity testing required for drugs and food additives. FDA testing guidelines for biomedical devices, including biomaterials, are outlined in Title 21 of the Code of Federal Regulations (21 CFR). The guidelines for each type of device and implant are not listed specifically in 21 CFR. More detailed guidance is provided by FDA memoranda and brochures and by following previous submissions (available by the Freedom of Information Act or FOI) to the appropriate section of the FDA. The most commonly used source of information for biocompatibility testing for the FDA is the "Tripartite Agreement" guideline memor-

andum, which can be found on the FDA website. This has been modified with incorporation of many of the ISO guidelines to cover those requirements also.

The FDA bases much of biomaterial and biomedical device safety and efficacy assessments on "predicate" devices, which are devices of similar design, construction, or composition used for similar purposes. Thus, it is very important for implant manufacturers to always compare the reactions of their material to materials already in clinical use. This may be done using the actual predicate device or material in head-to-head testing or by literature reviews. The FDA makes the final judgement as to whether a compound or material is a device or a drug and also determines the minimal preclinical and clinical efficacy and toxicity or safety testing required. Most biomedical materials and devices are reviewed by the Center for Devices and Radiological Health, Office of Device Evaluation in Rockville, Maryland. Other branches of the FDA may review some devices, especially bioengineered materials.

In general, the location of a device or implant relative to the body, the length of time it contacts the body, and its specific use will determine the tests required by the FDA. Body contact is divided into surface devices, external communicating devices, and completely implanted devices. The surface devices may contact skin, mucosal membranes, and breached or compromised surfaces. External communicating devices include those that are indirectly in the path of blood, those that communicate directly with tissue (including subcutis and tissue fluids), bone, or dentin, and those that communicate directly with circulating (vascular) blood. The times defined by the FDA and ISO include limited (up to 24 hr), prolonged (24 hr to 30 days), and permanent (greater than 30 days).

The standard battery of FDA/ISO safety tests includes *in vitro* cytotoxicity, genotoxicity, pyrogenicity (*Limulus* amebocyte assays), and hemolysis testing. *In vivo* tests include dermal sensitization in guinea pigs, topical or intracutaneous irritation in rabbits, acute systemic toxicity (usually in mice IV or IP), subacute or subchronic toxicity, and implantation in rabbits (intramuscular and/or subcutaneous). These assays are usually performed on "extracts" of the material or implant device and not using the actual device or material itself. Tests considered to be supplementary and dependent on the nature of the implanted device include chronic toxicity, biodegradation, reproductive/developmental toxicity, and carcinogenicity. The choice of species used for each of the *in vivo* tests may be different and may depend on the implant itself as well as the typical reaction of the selected species. Thus with devices the selection of a rodent and nonrodent species, as with drugs, is not automatic. This is especially true where the large size of the implant may prevent studies in rodents.

The FDA provides guidance documents and some protocols on their internet site (www.fda.gov/cdrh), but a complete understanding of the biomaterials to be tested and the desired use of those materials must be determined by the manufacturer of the devices and not solely by the FDA or the ISO.

For many biomaterials, further testing of the material or device falls somewhere between efficacy and safety. Sufficient testing for device or material failure depends on the intended use. For example, the FDA requires more efficacy tests and tests for failure of devices and material used in and around vertebrae than for devices used in and around the appendicular skeleton. Efficacy testing for implanted metal valves or joints requires testing until failure not only determined with appropriate pressures and stresses, but also to determine implant life spans once they are in place in a patient.

SUGGESTED READING

Bloomfield, P., Wheatley, D., Prescott, R., and Miller, H. (1991). Twelve-year comparison of a Bjork-shiley mechanical heart valve with porcine bioprostheses. *N. Engl. J. Med.* **324**, 573–579.

Böstman, O., Hirvensalo, E., Mäkinen, J., and Rokkanen, P. (1990). Foreign-body reactions to fracture fixation implants of biodegradable synthetic polymers. *J. Bone Joint Surg.* **72-B**, 592–596.

Bostrum, M., Saleh, K., and Einhorn, T. (1999). Osteoinductive growth factors in preclinical fracture and long bone defects models. *Orthop. Clin. North Am.* **30**, 647–658.

Bouchard, P., Black, J., Albrecht, B., Kaderly, R., Galante, J., and Pauli, B. (1996). Carcinogenicity of CoCrMo (F-75) implants in the rat. *J. Biomed. Mater. Res.* **32**, 37–44.

Boyan, B., Hummert, T., Dean, D., and Schwartz, Z. (1996). Role of material surfaces in regulating bone and cartilage cell response. *Biomaterials* **17**, 137–146.

Brawer, A. (1998). Silicon and matrix macromolecules: New research opportunities for old diseases from analysis of potential mechanisms of breast implant toxicity. *Med. Hypoth.* **51**, 27–35.

Case, C., Langkamer, V., James, C., Palmer, M., Kemp, A., Heap, P., and Solomon, L., (1994). Widespread dissemination of metal debris from implants. *J. Bone Joint Surg.* **76-B**, 701–712.

Constantz, B., Ison, I., Fulmer, M., Poser, R., Smith, S., Van Wagoner, M., Ross, J., Goldstein, S., Jupiter, J., and Rosenthal, D. (1995). Skeletal repair by in situ formation of the mineral phase of bone. *Science* **267**, 1796–1799.

Cornell, C. (1999). Osteoconductive materials and their role as substitutes for autogenous bone grafts. *Orthop. Clin. North Am.* **30**, 591–598.

Doorn, P., Campbell, P., and Amstutz, H. Metal versus polythylene wear particles in total hip replacements. *Clin. Orthop. Rel. Res.* **329S**, 206–216.

El-Ghannam, A., Ducheyne, P., and Shapiro, I. (1999). Effect of serum proteins on osteoblast adhesion to surface-modified bioactive glass and hydroxyapatite. *J. Orthop. Res.* **17**, 340–345.

Gerszten, P. (1999). A formal risk assessment of silicone breast implants. *Biomaterials* **20**, 1063–1069.

Glower, D., Landolofo, K., Cheruvu, S., Cen, Y., Harrison, J., Bashore, T., Smith, P., Jones, R., Wolfe, W., and Lowe, J. (1998). Determinants of 15-year outcome with 1,119 standard Carpentier-Edwards porcine valves. *Ann. Thorac. Surg.* **66**, S44–S48.

Hollinger, J., Brekke, J., Gruskin, and Lee, D. (1996). Role of bone substitutes. *Clin. Orthop. Rel. Res.* **324**, 55–65.

Howie, D., Rogers, S., McGee, M., and Haynes, D. (1996). Biologic effects of cobalt chrome in cell and animal models. *Clin. Orthop. Rel. Res.* **329S**, 217–231.

Hubbell, J. (1999). Bioactive biomaterials. *Curr. Opin. Biotechnol.* **10**, 123–129.

Hyde, J., Chinn, J., and Phillips, R., Jr. (1999). Polymer heart valves. *J. Heart Valve Dis.* **8**, 331–339.

James, S., Pogribna, M., Miller, B., Bolon, B., and Muskhelishvili, L. (1997). Characterization of cellular re-

19. Biomedical Devices and Biomaterials

sponse to silicone implants in rats: Implications for foreign-body carcinogenesis. *Biomaterials* **18**, 667–675.

Jamieson, W., Marchand, M., Peletier, C., Norton, R., Pellerin, M., Dubiel, T., Aupart, M., Daenen, W., Holden, M., David, T., Ryba, E., and Anderson, W. (1999). Structural valve deterioration in mitral replacement surgery: Comparison of Carpentier-Edwards supra-annular porcine and perimount pericardial bioprostheses. *J. Thorac. Cardiovasc. Surg.* **118**, 297–305.

Karesh, J. (1998). Biomaterials in ophthalmic plastic and reconstructive surgery. *Curr. Opin. Opthal.* **9**, 66–74.

Kienapfel, H., Sprey, C., Wilke, A., and Griss, P. (1999). Implant fixation by bone ingrowth. *J. Anthroplasty* **14**, 355–368.

Klinge, U., Klosterhalfen, B., Conze, J., Limberg, W., Obolenski, B., Öttinger, P., and Schumpelick, V. (1998). Modified mesh for hernia repair that is adapted to the physiology of the abdominal wall. *Eur. J. Surg.* **164**, 951–960.

Listgarten, M. (1996). Soft and hard response to endosseous dental implants. *Anat. Rec.* **245**, 410–425.

MacNeill, S., Cobb, C., Rapley, J., Glaros, A., and Spencer, P. (1999). In vivo comparison of synthetic osseous graft materials. *J. Clin. Periodontal.* **26**, 239–245.

Mayer, J., Jr., Shin'oka, T., and Shum-Tim, D. (1997). Tissue engineering of cardiovascular structures. *Curr. Opin. Cardiol.* **12**, 528–532.

Mericle, R., Kim, S., Lanzino, G., Lopes, D., Wakhloo, A., Guterman, L., and Hopkins, L. (1999). Carotid artery angioplasty and use of stents in high-risk patients with contralateral occlusions. *J. Neurosurg.* **90**, 1031–1036.

Mueller, E., and Regnault, W. (1998). Replacement heart valves and performance standards. *J. Heart Valve Dis.* **7**, 125–129.

Panduranga Rao, K., and Shanthi, C. (1999). Reduction of calcification by various treatments in cardiac valves. *J. Biomater. Appl.* **13**, 238–268.

Plenk, H., Jr. (1998). Prothesis-bone interface. *J. Biomed. Mater. Res.* **43**, 350–355.

Rubash, H., Sinha, R., Shanbhag, A., and Kim, S. (1998). Pathogenesis of bone loss after total hip arthroplasty. *Orthop. Clin. North Am.* **29**, 173–186.

San Millán Ruíz, D., Burkhardt, K., Jean, B., Muster, M., Martin, J., Bouvier, J., Fasel, J., Rüfenacht, D., and Kurt, A. (1999). Pathology findings with acrylic implants. *Bone* **25**, 85S–90S.

Schwartz, Z., and Boyan, B. (1994). Underlying mechanisms at the bone-biomaterial interface. *J. Cell Biochem.* **56**, 340–347.

Shors, E. (1999). Coralline bone graft substitutes. *Orthop. Clin. North Am.* **30**, 599–613.

Sittinger, M., Perka, C., Schultz, O., Häupl, T., and Burmester, G. (1999). Joint cartilage regeneration by tissue engineering. *Z. Rheumatol.* **58**, 130–135.

Smith, S., Estok, D., III, and Harris, W. Total hip arthroplasty with use of second-generation cementing techniques. *J. Bone Joint Surg.* **80-A**, 1632–1640.

Steflik, D., Corpe, R., Young, T., and Buttle, K. (1998). In vivo evaluation of the biocompatibility of implanted biomaterials: Morphology of the implant-tissue interactions. *Implant. Dent.* **7**, 338–350.

Steflik, D., Corpe, R., Lake, F., Young, T., Sisk, A., Parr, G., Hanes, P., and Berkery, D. (1998). Ultrastructural analyses of the attachment (bonding) zone between bone and implanted biomaterials. *J. Biomed. Mater. Res.* **39**, 611–620.

Tay, B., Patel, V., and Bradford, D. (1999). Calcium sulfate- and calcium phosphate-based bone substitutes. *Orthop. Clin. North Am.* **30**, 615–623.

Walker, P., and Gold, B. (1996). The tribology (friction, lubrication and wear) of all-metal artificial hip joints. *Clin. Orthop. Rel. Res.* **329S**, 4–10.

Yoshii, E. (1997). Cytotoxic effects of acrylates and methacrylates: Relationships of monomer structures and cytotoxicity. *J. Biomed. Mater. Res.* **37**, 517–524.

20

Biotechnology and Its Products

Anne M. Ryan
Department of Pathology
Pfizer Global Research and Development,
Groton, Connecticut

Timothy G. Terrell
Vistagen Inc.
Burlingame, California

I. Introduction
II. Biopharmaceuticals
III. Safety Evaluation of Biopharmaceuticals
IV. Summary and Conclusions
Suggested Reading

I. Introduction

Recent scientific advances in molecular biology, recombinant DNA technology, and monoclonal antibody production have led to the development of a new class of therapeutic agents, biopharmaceuticals, for the treatment of both human and veterinary disease. These novel therapeutic agents are produced by recombinant DNA technology, which involves the cloning and expression of a specific gene followed by large-scale production of the purified protein for therapeutic use. Bacteria such as *Escherichia coli* can be used to produce nonglycosylated recombinant human proteins; if glycosylation is critical to protein function, eukaryotic (mammalian or insect-derived) cells are used to produce fully glycosylated human proteins for clinical use. Recombinant DNA technology also has the advantage of producing purified proteins with greater yield and lower cost than the more traditional methods of protein production from animal tissues or human cadavers.

The first biopharmaceutical for human use, recombinant human insulin (rhinsulin), was approved by the Food and Drug Administration (FDA) in 1982 for patients with diabetes mellitus. Originally developed to replace missing or defective endogenous proteins, biopharmaceuticals have since expanded to include product classes such as hormones (erythropoietin and growth hormone), blood products (factor VIII, tissue plasminogen activator), cytokines (interferons, interleukins, colony-stimulating factors), and human and murine monoclonal antibodies. The current clinical applications for biopharmaceuticals are diverse (Table I). Although today's biopharmaceuticals are derived from genes of known function, recent advances in genomics and large-scale cloning have identified thousands of novel genes. These represent a wealth of biopharmaceutical candidates for future development, once their biological functions have been determined.

Although many biotechnology products are proteins or polypeptides that are used primarily as therapeutics, recombinant DNA technology has also facilitated the development of synthetic vaccines (such as rabies, hepatitis B, diptheria) and DNA and RNA probes for diagnostic use. Monoclonal antibodies (mAbs) are important reagents in the manufacture of biopharmaceuticals (e.g., to purify proteins) and are also integral to diagnostic assays (RIA, ELISA). Because of their epitope specificity, mAbs can also be used therapeutically, either to target individual cell types or to neutralize secreted proteins. When conjugated to a radioisotope, a chemotherapeutic agent, or a toxin, mAbs can be used for diagnostic imaging or ablation of a specific cell type.

TABLE I
Clinical Applications of Biopharmaceuticals

Clinical application	Biopharmaceutical examples
Replace genetic or acquired deficiency of endogenous factor	GH-growth hormone EPO-anemia, decrease transfusions
Augment cell activation for therapeutic effects	IL-2-immunotherapy for cancer IFNs-antiviral effects
Facilitate procedures or treatments	GM-CSF-PBPC mobilization, decrease neutropenia posttransplant
Substitute recombinant factor to avoid	
Immunogenicity (heterologous protein)	Recombinant insulin
Contamination (infectious agents)	GH, factor VIIa, factor IX
Target specific cells to minimize side effects	mAb for cancer immunotoxins

In recent years, both large, more traditional pharmaceutical companies and small biotechnology firms have made considerable financial and intellectual investments in the research and development of products derived from biotechnology processes, with the hope of developing novel therapeutic strategies to treat cancer and inherited diseases. In addition, continued developments in biotechnology provide powerful reagents and new molecular techniques to dissect complex disease pathways and to identify novel molecular targets, ultimately leading to the development of new therapeutics.

Biopharmaceuticals represent a special class of medicinal products, being complex, high molecular weight molecules; as such, they cannot be fully defined by conventional physical and chemical tests, and require specialized immunological, biochemical, and bioassay techniques to quantitate biological activity. Many future therapeutics will not be simple organic molecules but will be protein or gene based, including antisense oligonucleotides, ribozymes, and gene therapy. Although designed to mimic/regulate intracellular pathways or to replace endogenous proteins, these complex therapeutics still need to be evaluated for safety and efficacy. In addition, special animal models, including transgenic and knockout mice, may provide a

better understanding of the consequences of over- or underexpression of specific gene products on disease onset and progression. Some of these animal models can also be exploited to evaluate the pharmacology, efficacy, and toxicology of these new biotherapeutics.

The development of biopharmaceuticals has provided new challenges for the toxicologic pathologist. In general, recombinant human proteins can be antigenic in animals and have species-specific pharmacological effects, making traditional rodent-based safety assessment programs inappropriate for evaluating these agents. In addition, because of their large molecular weight, biopharmaceuticals require novel delivery systems, as the oral route of administration (commonly used for small molecule drugs) is inappropriate for protein-based therapeutics.

II. Biopharmaceuticals

Recombinant DNA technology has given us the ability to manipulate, construct, modify, or otherwise "engineer" genetic material to produce desired characteristics. Biotechnology is the adaptation of these genetically engineered organisms to industrial processes to produce new and useful protein products in sufficient quantities to be clinically useful. Biotechnology is now used routinely to produce novel and highly complex therapeutics, diagnostic agents, and vaccines. Biotechnology has led to the development of products that were previously not feasible, that are more specific and thus less toxic (i.e., targeted to only tumor cells), and that can be manufactured economically in large quantities. Often, biopharmaceuticals are developed for use against diseases in which no other effective therapy exists.

Biotechnology-based therapeutics have increased from fewer than 5 Investigational New Drug Applications (IND) submitted to the FDA in 1980 to 327 in 1998. In 1999, there were more than 50 approved biotechnology products on the market, over half of which were marketed by large pharmaceutical companies. Of the 6000 or so drugs in preclinical

c. Ribozymes and Aptamers. Ribozymes are small RNA structures that catalytically cleave covalent bonds in target DNA. They can inhibit gene expression in a sequence-specific manner and have the therapeutic potential to eliminate mRNA in cancer and viral diseases. There is a small amount of preclinical safety data at this point, and the safety profile appears promising. Aptamers are single- or double-stranded nucleic acids capable of binding proteins or other small molecules. In contrast to ribozymes, binding is based on shape recognition, not sequence. As therapeutics, aptamers may have a wide range of protein targets, including transcription factors, extracellular proteins, and cell surface molecules.

5. Drug Delivery Issues with Biopharmaceuticals

Most proteins are inherently unstable. As pharmaceuticals, they must be formulated, stabilized, and delivered. Because proteins are often large macromolecules, they possess multiple functional groups and have three-dimensional structures, all of which affect stability. Teritary structure is important for biologic or pharmacologic activity. As biopharmaceuticals, the formulations must be biocompatible and stable, either in solution or in a lyophilized state.

Because tertiary structure is critical for biologic and pharmacologic activity, recombinant human proteins are generally administered parenterally, usually by intravenous bolus injection or continuous infusion. Intramuscular or subcutaneous administration can be used for either local delivery (e.g., administration of a vascular growth factor to ischemic skeletal muscle) or to provide systemic exposure following lymphatic uptake of the protein. Because the intramuscular and subcutaneous routes of administration can be accompanied by local degradation of the protein with subsequent loss of activity, proteins administered by these routes may be more immunogenic and less efficacious than those delivered by intravenous injection.

Oral administration is usually not attempted due to generally poor absorption (it is difficult to transport these large molecules across biological membranes in the absence of specific ligand–receptor binding), proteolysis by digestive enzymes in the upper gastrointestinal tract, "first pass" liver metabolism, and slow absorption. In general, oral absorption will not correlate with bioavailability due to protein degradation/denaturation. Alternative routes of administration (e.g., nasal, pulmonary, and transdermal) are being investigated for protein biopharmaceuticals. Of these, the lung appears to be most promising for systemic delivery due to large blood volume:surface area. Small peptides are transported more easily across the alveolus than large proteins, but absorption following protein aerosolization is a complex function of particle size (which influences the site of deposition), concentration, charge, molecular conformation, and interaction with the pulmonary epithelium.

Efforts to improve the biological half-life of proteins have included chemical modification, conjugation to hydrophilic polymers such as polyethylene glycol (PEG), and incorporation of proteins into biodegradable polymers or liposomes. While conjugation to PEG does not stimulate immunogenicity, slow-release formulations can have increased immunogenicity due to body temperature-induced protein denaturation or aggregation.

C. RECENTLY APPROVED BIOPHARMACEUTICALS

As an indication of the breadth of current biopharmaceuticals, Table V lists examples of recent FDA approved biopharmaceuticals arranged by general product type (recombinant proteins, mAbs, immunotoxins, fusion proteins, and vaccines). Selected examples of some of these products are described. Additional information on these and other approved biopharmaceuticals can be found at the FDA website (www.fda.gov/cber/products.htm).

1. Rituximab

Rituxin is approved for patients with relapsed or refractory low-grade or follicular B-cell non-Hodgkin's lymphoma (NHL). It is a chimeric murine–human IgG1$_k$ mAb against CD20 that

TABLE V
FDA-Approved Biopharmaceuticals

Generic name	Trade name	Indication (protein or target)
Becaplermin	Regranex	Diabetic ulcers (rhPDGF-BB)
IFNA-2a	Roferon A	CML, Kaposi's sarcoma
IFNA-2b	Intron A	Hepatitis B and C; follicular lymphoma
IFNA-n1	Wellferon	Chronic hepatitis C
IFNAcon-1	Infergen	Chronic hepatitis C
IFNB-1a	Avonex	Multiple sclerosis
IFNB-1b	Betaseron	Multiple sclerosis
IFNG-1b	Actimmune	Chronic granulomatous disease
Dornase α	Pulmozyme	Cystic fibrosis (DNA)
Reteplase	Retavase	AMI (plasminogen activator)
Alteplase	Activase	Ischemic stroke (plasminogen activator)
Imiglucerase	Cerezyme	Gaucher's disease (β-glucocerebrosidase)
Filgrastim	Neupogen	Neutropenia, PBC mobilization (G-CSF)
Sargramostim	Prokine	Neutropenia (GM-CSF)
Aldesleukin	Proleukin	Metastatic renal cell carcinoma, melanoma (IL-2)
Oprelvekin	Neumega	Platelet enhancement (IL-11)
Epoetin α	Epogen/Procrit	Anemia (EPO)
Factor VIIa	NovoSeven	Hemophilia A and B
Factor IX	Benefix	Hemophilia B
Abciximab	ReoPro	Inhibit platelet aggregation (GPIIbIIIa)
Rituximab	Rituxan	B-cell non-Hodgkin's lymphoma (CD20)
Daclizumab	Zenepax	Acute renal transplant (CD25)
Basiliximab	Simulect	Acute renal transplant (CD25)
Palivizumab	Synagis	Respiratory synctial virus
Infliximab	Remicade	Crohn's disease (TNFα)
Trastuzumab	Herceptin	Breast cancer (HER-2)
Denileukin difitox	Ontak	Cutaneous T-cell lymphoma (CD25)
Etanercept	Enbrel	Rheumatoid arthritis (TNF)
Lyme disease vaccine	LYMErix	Lyme disease (OspA)
Rabies vaccine	RabAvert	Rabies (pre-and postexposure)
Diptheria/tetanus toxoid and pertussis vaccine	Certiva	Diptheria, tetanus, and pertussis
Rotavirus vaccine	RotaShield	Rotavirus

is expressed on the surface of normal and malignant B lymphocytes. Rituximab is produced in Chinese hamster ovary suspension cultures and is purified by affinity and ion-exchange chromatography followed by inactivation of any contaminating viruses. Following intravenous administration, rituximab binds specifically to the CD20 antigen on pre-B and mature B lymphocytes and B-cell NHL; rituximab does not bind to hematopoietic stem cells, pro-B cells, plasma cells, or other normal tissues. The Fc domain mediates B-cell lysis *in vitro*, suggesting complement-dependent cell lysis and antibody-dependent cellular toxicity as possible mechanisms of action. Cell lysis is also suggested by infusion-related symptoms (hypotension, bronchospasm, and angioedema) in some patients (which resolve following a reduction in the infusion rate) and the rapid and sustained depletion of circulating and tissue-based B cells. B-cell recovery begins approximately 6 months post infusion, with return to normal B-cell levels around 12 months.

2. Daclizumab

Zenepax is administered prophylactically in conjunction with immunosuppressive drugs to prevent acute organ rejection in renal transplant patients. It is a humanized IgG1 mAb that binds to the CD25 subunit of the IL-2 receptor (IL-2R) expressed on the surface of activated lymphocytes. Daclizumab functions as an IL-2R antagonist, preventing IL-2 binding and inhibiting the activation of T lymphocytes and the subsequent cellular immune response involved in allograft rejection. Although cellular immunity is inhibited following Daclizumab administration, humoral immunity is not affected, as evidenced by the development of nonneutralizing anti-idiotype antibodies in 8% of the patients. Increased susceptibility to viral or bacterial infections was not observed in clinical studies. Basiliximab (Simulect) is a chimeric IgG1$_k$ mAb against the same epitope and is approved for a similar indication.

3. Becalpermin

Regranex gel is approved for the topical treatment of lower extremity diabetic neuropathic ulcers in patients with adequate blood supply. The active ingredient is becaplermin (rhPDGF-BB), which is produced by the insertion of the gene for the PDGF B chain into the yeast *Saccharomyces cerevisiae* and formation of a homodimer joined by disulfide bonds. Becaplermin promotes the chemotactic recruitment and proliferation of cells involved in wound repair, enhancing the formation of granulation tissue. With topical administration, systemic bioavailability is low; however, because it is a growth factor, becaplermin is contraindicated in patients with cutaneous tumors at the site of application. In preclinical studies, exposure of rat metatarsals to becaplermin produced periosteal hyperplasia, subperiosteal bone resorption, exostosis, fibroplasia, and mononuclear cell infiltration, consistent with the ability of PDGF to stimulate connective tissue growth.

4. Palivizumab

Synagis is approved for prophylaxis of lower respiratory tract disease due to respiratory synctial virus (RSV). It is a humanized IgG1$_k$ mAb directed against the A epitope of the F protein of RSV. Palivizumab has neutralizing and fusion-inhibitory activity against RSV and is indicated for prevention of serious lower respiratory tract disease caused by RSV in pediatric patients. For registration, safety and efficacy were established in infants with bronchopulmonary dysplasia and infants with a history of prematurity.

5. Infliximab

Remicade is indicated for the treatment of patients with active or fistulating Crohn's disease. It is a chimeric IgG1$_k$ mAb that binds with high affinity to the soluble and transmembrane forms of human TNFα to inhibit TNFα receptor binding. Infliximab inhibits the biological effects of TNFα such as the induction of proinflammatory cytokines (IL-1 and IL-6), enhancement of leukocyte migration, activation of neutrophil and eosinophil function, and induction of acute phase and other liver proteins. Cells expressing transmembrane TNFα bound by infliximab can be lysed by complement or effector cells. Infliximab does not neutralize TNFβ (lymphotoxin α), a related cytokine that binds the same receptor as TNFα. In patients with Crohn's disease, infliximab reduces the number of inflammatory cells in the lamina propria that express TNFα and IFNG. Patients also have decreased levels of serum IL-6 and C-reactive protein. Infusion-related reactions (fever, chills, urticaria, dyspnea, and hypotension in the 2-hr post infusion period) are more common in those patients who develop human antichimeric antibodies (HACA); concurrent immunosuppressive therapy can decrease the incidence of infusion-related reactions as well as the development of HACA. Because TNFα mediates inflammation and modulates the immune response, infliximab treatment can be associated with an increased incidence of infections or abscesses. Infliximab has been approved for use in combination with methotrexate for patients with rheumatoid arthritis.

6. Trastuzumab

Herceptin is approved for metastatic breast cancer patients whose tumors overexpress the human epidermal growth factor receptor 2 (HER-2) protein. Trastuzumab is a humanized IgG1$_k$ mAb that binds selectively with high affinity to the extracellular domain of the HER-2. Produced in Chinese hamster ovary suspension culture, Herceptin mediates antibody-dependent cellular toxicity (ADCC) on HER-2 overexpressing cancer cells. HER-2 protein overexpression is present in 25–30% of breast cancers and can be diagnosed by immunohistochemistry using fixed sections of tumor. Trastuzumab administration is associated with an increased incidence of cardiac dysfunction, particularly in those patients receiving anthracyclines. Fever and/or chills can be observed in some patients during the first infusion, but this does not appear to be associated with immunogenicity, as human antihuman antibodies (HAHA) occur in ~1% of patients.

7. Denileukin Diftitox

Ontak is a recombinant DNA-derived fusion protein produced in *E. coli*. It consists of the amino acid sequences for diptheria toxin fragments A and B fused to the human IL-2 sequence. Denileukin diftitox directs the cytotoxic action of diptheria toxin to cells expressing IL-2R. Approved for use in patients with cutaneous T-cell lymphoma, Ontak binds to CD25, the high-affinity IL-2R subunit, to inhibit protein synthesis and kill activated T and B lymphocytes, activated macrophages, and malignant cells expressing CD25. Low titer antibodies that cross-react with the diptheria toxin domain (presumably due to prior diptheria immunization) can be observed in naïve patients. However, development of antidenileukin diftitox antibodies postdosing can alter subsequent Ontak PK (increased clearance and decreased

systemic exposure). The presence of antibodies is independent of the development of acute hypersensitivity-type reactions and vascular leak syndrome observed in some patients following denileukin diftitox infusion.

8. Etanercept

Enbrel is a fusion protein consisting of the extracellular ligand-binding domain of the human TNF receptor (TNFR) linked to the Fc region of human IgG1. It is produced by recombinant DNA technology in a Chinese hamster ovary expression system and is approved for the treatment of patients with moderately to severely active rheumatoid arthritis. Etanercept is a soluble dimeric form of the p75 TNFR; it can bind two TNF molecules [either TNFα or TNFβ (LTα)] to inhibit the interaction of TNF with its cell surface receptor. This renders TNF biologically inactive and reduces the expression of cell adhesion molecules such as E-selectin and ICAM-1 and decreases serum IL-6 and MMP-3 levels. However, cells expressing transmembrane TNF that bind Enbrel are not lysed. Anti-TNF therapy with either infliximab or etanercept has been associated with the formation of autoimmune antibodies (antinuclear, anti-dsDNA, anticardiolipin). Non neutralizing antibodies to etanercept develop in ~15% of patients, but these are not associated with adverse events.

D. TOXICOLOGIC PATHOLOGY FINDINGS WITH BIOPHARMACEUTICALS

Compared to more traditional pharmaceuticals that undergo xenobiotic metabolism through several different biotransformation pathways with varying metabolic profiles in animals and human (see Chapter 2), recombinant protein-based therapeutics are metabolized by proteolysis and excreted as small peptides and amino acids. Consequently, the histopathologic lesions associated with the administration of biopharmaceuticals are generally not as extensive as those that can be observed in toxicology studies with small molecules. Histopathologic findings in safety studies of biopharmaceuticals may be limited to local effects at the injection site (ranging from formulation-induced irritation to perivascular neovascularization or fibrosis following the leakage of intravenously administered rhVEGF or rhPDGF at the injection site). If the biopharmaceutical is immunogenic, immune complex disease, lymphoid aggregates at the injection site, or generalized lymphoid hyperplasia may be observed. More complicated histopathologic changes may result from receptor antagonism (with loss of normal signaling capability) or receptor induction on nontarget tissues, producing unexpected results. Supraphysiologic doses or exaggerated pharmacology can result from the administration of large doses (relative to the amount of endogenous protein) or from the systemic delivery of a factor that normally acts at a specific "local" site.

The absence of histopathologic lesions should not lead the toxicologic pathologist to automatically assume that the biopharmaceutical is "safe." The absence of histopathologic lesions could reflect the presence of neutralizing antibodies (which would decrease systemic exposure, and therefore the toxicity of the molecule) or indicate that the study was performed in a species in which the molecule was not bioactive.

The toxicologic pathologist has an advantage when interpreting the pathogenesis of lesions observed with biopharmaceuticals. There is generally a wealth of information on the normal biology of the factor and its role in disease. Because many of these recombinant protein drugs act as ligands, most of the effects of biopharmaceuticals, both desirable and adverse, are receptor mediated. In addition to direct receptor inhibition or stimulation, these biopharmaceuticals can also have effects on related or nontarget tissues (e.g., B-cell depletion following rituximab administration). Because many biopharmaceuticals affect complex biologic processes or signaling cascades, it is important for the pathologist to discriminate between enhanced physiologic or pharmacologic effects and toxicity of the molecule.

An example of enhanced physiologic effects seen with the administration of biopharmaceuticals is the physeal dysplasia observed in young adult cynomolgus monkeys following rhuMAb-VEGF administration. rhuMAbVEGF is a humanized IgG1 mAb directed against VEGF that is currently being developed as an antiangiogenic agent for the treatment of solid tumors. Twice-weekly administration of rhuMAbVEGF for either 4 or 13 weeks resulted in the complete inhibition of capillary growth, manifested as the absence of the normal invasion of metaphyseal blood vessels into the physis. In contrast, mature, quiescent blood vessels were not affected by rhuMAbVEGF administration. Inhibition of metaphyseal capillary proliferation resulted in an imbalance between chondrocyte proliferation and the normal vascular invasion, chondrocyte loss, and trabecular bone formation. As a consequence, there was increased thickening of the physis with degeneration of the cartilage matrix. The physeal dysplasia was completely reversible with resumption of capillary proliferation at the end of the treatment period.

Because rhuMAbVEGF was bioactive only in nonhuman primates, mechanistic studies were performed in mice using a soluble VEGF receptor fusion protein (Flt-IgG). These studies demonstrated that VEGF-mediated capillary invasion was an essential regulator of growth plate morphogenesis. VEGF was absolutely required for chondrocyte death, chondroclast function, extracellular matrix remodeling, capillary proliferation, and bone formation at the physis. VEGF was also shown to be critical for the vascular proliferation associated with organogenesis and postnatal organ maturation, as well as physiologic angiogenesis (ovulation and menstruation), but was not required for the maintenance of existing vasculature. These mechanistic studies on the consequences of VEGF inhibition (either by rhuMAbVEGF or Flt-IgG), coupled with an understanding of the biology of normal and pathologic angiogenesis, demonstrated that the morphologic changes observed in the rhuMAbVEGF preclinical safety program represented an enhanced physiologic, rather than a toxic, response.

Because the effects of growth factors and cytokines in toxicity studies are often due to exaggerated pharmacologic effects, the species specificity of a biopharmaceutical can influence histopathologic findings. This is best illustrated with rhGM-CSF and the rhIFNs, which are bioactive in a limited range of species. rhGM-CSF induces proliferation and differentiation of myeloid precursors in several nonhuman primates (Rhesus, cynomolgus, and marmoset), but has no biological activity in rodents. rhGM-CSF also activates monocytes and granulocytes; at high doses, proinflammatory cytokines released by these cells produced widespread serosal, hepatic, and injection site inflammation in Rhesus monkeys. Increased numbers of circulating granulocytes were also associated with thrombotic events, a finding similar to that observed with high doses of rhG-CSF. These preclinical studies in Rhesus monkeys were predictive of adverse events observed in the clinic. However, preclinical safety studies performed only in rodents would have been misleading because, in this case, rats and mice are nonresponsive to the effects of rhGM-CSF.

In humans, the principal dose-limiting toxicities with IFNs consist of a flu-like syndrome (fever, chills, myalgia, arthralgia, and headache). Hematological toxicities include leukopenia, anemia, and thrombocytopenia. Safety studies with rhIFNG in rats did not demonstrate any evidence of toxicity, consistent with the lack of homology between rodent and human IFNG. Safety studies in nonhuman primates, however, demonstrated generalized systemic toxicity characterized by fever, lethargy, anorexia, and changes in hematology and chemistry parameters similar to those observed in humans. Although the cynomolgus monkey has a decreased level of sensitivity of rhIFNG relative to human, the toxicity of rhIFNs can be characterized in nonhuman primates if the doses are high enough. While nonresponsive species may have utility in testing for nonspecific toxic effects (formulations, contaminants, etc.), they are not predictive of the toxicity related to the biological activity of the molecule. Although early safety studies with biopharmaceuticals were performed (usually unknowingly) in nonresponsive species,

safety testing is now usually done only in species in which the molecule exhibits pharmacologic activity. The improved purity of biopharmaceuticals has also obviated the need for testing in nonresponsive species.

Although many recombinant human therapeutics have activity and can therefore be assessed for safety and efficacy in nonhuman primates, they are still heterologous proteins, which can be immunogenic in nonhuman primates. The formation of neutralizing antibodies can also influence the toxicity profile, either by decreasing bioavailability or pharmacodynamic (PD) effects (secondary to enhanced clearance and/or decreased systemic exposure) or by the formation of circulating immune complexes, which can deposit in tissues. Diminished toxicity, coinciding with the development of neutralizing antibodies, was observed with rhIFNG, rhIFNA, rhIL-1, rhIL-3, and rhIL-6. Glomerular lesions (proliferative glomerulonephritis with increased mesangial matrix) suggestive of immune complex disease (but negative for immune deposits in the basement membrane by electron microscopy) were observed in nonhuman primate studies with rhIFNG and rhIL-12.

Histopathologic findings secondary to antigen cross-reactivity have been observed in several *Pseudomonas* exotoxin (PE) and ricin A immunotoxin studies. This cross-reactivity may result from ectopic expression of the antigen or from an immunologically related epitope on cells other than those of the expected target tissue. *In vitro* tissue screens to identify cross-reacting epitopes or additional target organs should be performed for all immunotoxin and mAb products early in preclinical development. Hepatocellular toxicity was observed following intravenous immunotoxin (HER-2-PE, IL-4-PE) administration to nonhuman primates, and pancreatic toxicity was observed following administration of a murine mAb-PE conjugate to dogs. Ricin A immunotoxins have been reported to cause degeneration and necrosis of synovial membranes, liver, and tongue in rats and demyelination and Schwann cell neuropathy in humans.

The histopathologic findings following administration of a biopharmaceutical may not reflect the effects of that molecule, but rather the consequences of activation of a downstream signaling molecule. This is best exemplified by rhIL-12, an immunomodulatory cytokine with broad antitumor and antiviral effects. Preclinical safety studies of rhIL-12 in responsive species (guinea pigs, squirrel monkeys, cynomolgus monkeys, and chimpanzees) demonstrated a spectrum of hematopoietic, hepatic, pulmonary, and intestinal effects similar to those observed in human clinical trials. IL-12 activates natural killer and T lymphocytes, resulting in the synthesis and release of IFNG. Because the histopathologic findings associated with rhIL-12 administration were similar to those observed with rhIFNG, mechanistic studies were performed using the homologous protein, recombinant murine IL-12 (rmIL-12), in IFNG receptor knockout mice. Because these mice lack the IFNG receptor, they are nonresponsive to IFNG and therefore only manifest the toxic effects of IL-12. Use of the homologous protein in this murine model enabled the direct toxic effects of IL-12 to be separated from those indirect toxic effects due to IFNG induction. This model demonstrated that the observed biologic and toxic effects of rhIL-12 in humans and nonhuman primates were secondary to IL-12-mediated IFNG induction and secretion.

III. Safety Evaluation of Biopharmaceuticals

The purpose of the preclinical safety program for biopharmaceuticals is identical to that for small molecule drugs. The goals of safety assessment are to (1) identify an initial safe starting dose and subsequent dose escalation scheme for the clinic, (2) identify potential target organs of toxicity and determine the reversibility of these toxicities, (3) identify biomarkers that can be use to monitor toxicity in the clinic, and (4) identify clinical subpopulations at risk for toxicity. Preclinical safety evaluation studies are designed to provide a sufficient understanding of the pharmacology (both PK and PD) and toxicity prior to the initiation of studies in humans. The ability to identify potential adverse effects critical to the design of human clinical trials can minimize these adverse effects.

A. REGULATORY RESOURCES

More than 85% of biopharmaceuticals are regulated through the Center for Biologics Evaluation and Research (CBER) at the FDA. This branch of the FDA is charged with the scrutiny and oversight of "conventional" biologics (blood and blood products, vaccines, and allergens) and biotechnology products (recombinant proteins, mAbs and antigenic peptides for tumor vaccines). CBER is also responsible for the regulation of "novel" biotechnology products, such as gene therapy, engineered or xenotransplanted tissues, and nucleic acid-based diagnostic reagents and therapies. Other biotechnology-derived products, such as antisense theapies, synthetic peptides smaller than 40 amino acids, and recombinant hormones, are regulated through the other branch of the FDA, the Center for Drug Evaluation and Research (CDER). Further information about these branches and their regulatory responsibilities can be found at the FDA website (www.fda.gov).

The use of recombinant DNA methods for generating human therapeutics does not require any more extensive toxicologic studies for product registration than small molecules. In fact, because of issues of immunogenicity and species specificity, the safety assessment program may be truncated. However, as one might expect, biotechnology-derived products have created new issues related to the manufacture and testing of these products for human use. These have been addressed in a series of approximately 20 "Points to Consider" documents, which are available through the CBER website (www.fda.gov/cber/guidelines.htm). Because of the wide variety of biopharmaceuticals, their varied mechanisms of action, and their attendant diversity of potential therapeutic indications, these documents do not reflect specific regulatory requirements, but provide general principles, rather than inflexible rules, for the testing of biopharmaceuticals. The safety assessment of biopharmaceuticals is approached on a "case-by-case," science-based approach that takes into consideration the specific structure, pharmacology, kinetics, and known biologic properties of the molecule.

As part of an effort to promote international harmonization of regulatory requirements, industry and regulatory representative from the European Union, Japan, and the United States have participated in the International Conference on Harmonization of Technical Requirements for Registration of Pharmaceuticals for Human Use (ICH). This group has also produced several guidelines relevant to the safety evaluation and quality of biopharmaceuticals; these can be found at the ICH website (www.ifpma.org/ich1.html).

Table VI provides some examples of the types of CBER and ICH documents relevant to the safety evaluation of biopharmaceuticals. These guidelines and guidances address some of the issues inherent in the safety testing of biotechnology products, namely: (1) the identification of a biologically or pharmacologically relevant animal species, (2) the implication of antibody formation on toxicity testing, (3) issues surrounding toxicology studies traditionally conducted for small molecules (specifically, genotoxicity, reproductive toxicity, and carcinogenicity studies), and (4) the use of alternative

means of assessing toxicity such as the use of homologous proteins, transgenic animals, and animal models of disease.

B. STUDY DESIGN ISSUES

The primary objectives of the safety evaluation program for a biopharmaceutical are to (1) identify dose limiting and target organ toxicity and evaluate potential reversibility; (2) estimate potential adverse clinical reactions; (3) understand the dose–activity relationship; and (4) correlate route and schedule with activity and toxicity. Additional studies may be needed to determine the mechanism of action, to facilitate future clinical development for additional indications, or to support labeling claims. The preclinical studies should be designed to mimic as closely as possible the route of exposure, treatment schedule, and duration of treatment that will be used in the clinic. Because many biopharmaceuticals are bioactive in a limited number of species, careful selection of the most appropriate animal species is required to adequately characterize the adverse effects of the biopharmaceutical, which frequently are manifested as exaggerated pharmacology. An understanding of the biology of the molecule, the species specificity and tissue distribution of the receptor (or other pharmacologic target), and the cross-reactivity of the recombinant protein for nontarget tissues are critical to the design and interpretation of animal studies used to predict human safety.

The safety program should include studies that demonstrate the extent of species specificity of the molecule, the time course and consequences of antibody formation (if any), and the influence of route of administration, formulation, and dose schedule on the PK and toxicology. While multidose studies should ideally support the duration of the proposed clinical plan, the development of neutralizing antibodies will negate any effects of continued dosing so it is seldom meaningful to dose beyond this point. In addition to traditional PK, toxicological, clinical, and histopathological end points in multidose studies, *in vivo* local tolerance and safety pharmacology studies and *in*

TABLE VI
Regulatory Guidelines and Guidances for Biopharmaceuticals

GLP regulations

CBER guidelines and guidances (www.fda.gov/cber/ guidelines/htm)
  "Points to Consider" in the . . .
    Production and testing of new drugs and biologicals produced by recombinant DNA technology (1992)
    Characterization of cell lines to produce biologicals (1993)
    Manufacturing and testing of monoclonal antibody products for human use (1997)
ICH guidelines (www.ifpma.org/ich5.html)
  S6—Preclinical safety evaluation of biotechnology-derived pharmaceuticals
  Q5—Quality of biotechnology products
FDA guidance documents

vitro tissue cross-reactivity and hemolytic potential studies may be needed.

Some of the factors influencing the design of preclinical safety studies are summarized in Table VII. The "biology" of the molecule, the proposed clinical indication, and the proposed clinical plan should always dictate the preclinical strategy. For preclinical toxicity testing, the selection of the appropriate test species is critical. This can be based on comparable pharmacologic activity, the expression and tissue distribution of the target receptor, or the phylogenetic conservation of protein and receptor between the test species and humans. Due to the restricted bioactivity of many recombinant proteins, these studies are usually performed in nonhuman primates and are limited to a single species. (There is no specific requirement for the

use of two species—one rodent, the other non-rodent—for biologics.) Because of the expense involved in nonhuman primate studies, group sizes are small (usually four to six/sex/group). Doses are selected to provide information on the dose–response relationship; overall exposure, rather than the actual dose, is chosen to mimic anticipated human exposure in the clinic. PK or PD end points are correlated with toxicity in the test species, and once available in humans, exposure data are used to compare human and animal toxicity. Toxicology and exposure data should be generated in the same animal species and can even be measured in the same study, especially in nonhuman primate studies where blood volume is adequate for both assessments.

While toxicity in the test species generates the safety factors for the clinic, it may not always be possible to reach the maximum tolerated dose (MTD) with a biopharmaceutical. This may be due to the limited solubility of the test material or to limitations on dose volume (intravenous administration) or bioavailability (subcutaneous route). As discussed earlier, the lack of significant toxicity does not mean that the biopharmaceutical is "safe." In the absence of an identified MTD, it is important to confirm pharmacological activity in the high-dose animals; otherwise, the absence of toxic effects could reflect poor bioavailability, PK, or the development of neutralizing antibodies.

In addition to the identification of an appropriate test species, the other critical parameter for the preclinical safety assessment of biopharmaceuticals is the immunogenic potential of the recombinant material. A number of factors can influence immunogenicity, including (1) intrinsic properties of the protein (i.e., analogues versus heterologous proteins); (2) the form of the protein (e.g., conjugation to drugs, toxins, PEG, or creation of fusion proteins generating new antigenic determinants); (3) formulation, and (4) product-related impurities (e.g., aggregates, fragments or chemically modified/oxidized proteins). These can be either directly immunogenic or act as an adjuvant in the dosing solution. As discussed previously, regimen

TABLE VII
Factors Influencing the Design of the Preclinical Safety Program for Biopharmaceuticals

Homology to endogenous protein
  Amino acid sequence
  Tertiary structure
  Glycosylation
  Mutants or variants
  Immunogenicity
Scientific rationale
  Physiological or pharmacologic properties (site of action)
  Potency assays
  Receptor characteristics
  Scientific literature
  In vitro and *in vivo* studies
  Experience with related molecules or with murine homologues
Proposed clinical indication
  Replacement vs prophylaxis vs diagnosis
  Magnitude of exposure relative to endogenous protein
  Patient population
  Acute vs chronic therapy
  Single agent or combination therapy
Proposed clinical plan
  Dose
  Route
  Schedule
Identification of suitable (reactive) animal species
  Sequence homology of ligand and receptor with human sequences
  Receptor expression and tissue distribution similar to humans
  In vitro and *in vivo* bioactivity similar to humans
  Immunogenicity of the molecule in test animal species
Clinically relevant end points
  Biomarkers for clinical monitoring

factors such as dose, route, and frequency of administration can induce immunogenicity. In addition, host factors including MHC haplotype, autoimmune disease, existing antibodies to bacterial products (Diptheria toxoid, etc.), and the use of concurrent medications can influence immunogenicity. For example, the incidence of HACA antibody formation is decreased in infliximab-treated Crohn's disease patients treated with corticosteroids compared to patients receiving infliximab alone.

Toxicokinetic studies should include an evaluation of the antibody response to the biopharmaceutical. Ideally, animals should be naïve to recombinant human proteins prior to the initiation of the study. If this is not possible, serologic screening for cross-reacting proteins that interfere with PK assays and determination of preexisting antibody titers should be performed at baseline. During the course of the study, it is important to sample animals (as a minimum, after the first and last dose) to determine if antibodies are elicited and to characterize the time course and nature (binding vs neutralizing) of the response. Antibody formation can limit the planned study duration because neutralizing antibodies eliminate the biological activity of the recombinant human protein.

Other consequence of antibody formation that could complicate preclinical safety studies include (1) cross-reactivity with endogeneous proteins (e.g., MGDF-induced antibodies to endogeneous TPO, producing thrombocytopenia), (2) immune complex formation with the potential to deposit complexes in tissues, (3) injection site reactions and systemic infusion-related reactions (e.g., anaphylaxis), and (4) effects on PK. Antibody formation and removal of protein–antibody complexes from the circulation can result in decreased bioavailability or changes in the initial volume of distribution. Nonneutralizing antibodies can increase bioavailability due to increased size (and consequently, decreased clearance) of the complexes.

Although antibody formation may impact the design and interpretation of animal toxicokinetic studies, it is not always predictive of immunogenicity in humans. Murine mAbs have a higher incidence of antibody formation than either chimeric or humanized mAbs (50–80% HAMA vs 1–15% HACA or HAHA response), but there is no clear correlation between antibody development to the biopharmaceutical and molecular weight, glycosylation status, or homology to the endogenous protein. Only a small proportion of the antibodies are neutralizing, and the incidence of adverse effects associated with antibody development is also low. In addition to local (injection site) or systemic (anaphylaxis) hypersensitivity, other types of adverse effects noted in humans following the administration of biopharmaceuticals have included flu, vascular leak syndrome (aldesleukin, rhIL-12, rhIL-2), cytokine release syndrome (rhIFNs and rhILs), first-dose effects (rhGM-CSF), and Fc-mediated effects such as complement activation and ADCC (rituximab) and infusion-related cardiopulmonary reactions (infliximab). Approaches to managing these adverse effects have included pretreating with acetaminophen and/or corticosteroids, decreasing the infusion rate (rituximab), or administrating a priming dose (IL-12).

C. OTHER STUDIES

Highly immunogenic proteins or proteins with a restricted choice of reactive species (e.g., a humanized mAb cross-reactive only with chimpanzee) may be studied in rodents after cloning of the homologous rodent protein. However, inferences of safety and therapeutic index in humans must be made with caution, as the distribution, activity, and clearance of these proteins may not be analogous to the human protein. The use of homologous species has been demonstrated with proteins such as IFNG, IL-12, and anti-VEGF (Flt-IgG) for both safety and mechanism of action studies.

Transgenic models can also be considered when there is no relevant animal for a human-specific mAb and the study of homologous proteins is not suitable. However, it is important to have accurate information on the distribution of the epitope, its density, turnover, expression, and activity in such transgenic animals. There is no point in testing a humanized antibody against a human growth factor in a transgenic mouse unless the growth factor binds the murine receptor or the transgenic mouse also expresses the human receptor. Transgene expression must also be targeted with the appropriate promoter, and expression must be at physiologic levels for these studies.

For immunotoxins and mAb products, immunohistochemical studies are performed on a panel of frozen human tissues to rule out cross-reactivity with epitopes other than the target antigen. Generally, tissues from three unrelated donors are screened; in addition, tissues from several nonhuman species can be screened to identify the most relevant animal for toxicology testing. For human tissues, the test antibody should be labeled directly to prevent the binding of secondary reagents to endogenous human immunoglobulins. After direct labeling, the bioactivity of the test antibody should be verified. Other approaches to circumvent endogenous immunoglobulins in the test tissue include, for example, the use of primary antibody–secondary antibody-preformed complexes as an immunohistochemical reagent.

The relevance and value of conducting classical carcinogenicity bioassays with biopharmaceuticals have been debated. Usually conducted in rodents, these studies may not be possible if the species is nonresponsive to the molecule; in addition, the development of neutralizing antibodies may preclude long-term dosing. The decision to conduct a 2-year bioassay will be determined on a case-by-case basis and is dependent on, for example, the specific properties of the molecule, its indication, the target population, and duration of use indication (such as chronic use for a nonlife-threatening condition). Genomic integration or induction of cell proliferation are two properties of biopharmaceuticals that might require further characterization of long-term effects. Other approaches to assess carcinogenic potential, such as the ability of a growth factor to increase tumor burden or metastasis *in vivo* or to stimulate the growth of transformed cells *in vitro*, need to be explored further.

Because large molecular weight proteins are unlikely to react with DNA and other chromosomal material, genotoxicity is generally of little value. There is no evidence that recombinant proteins or mAbs are metabolized differently from endogenous proteins or that they are genotoxic. Initially, genotoxicity testing was performed to demonstrate that bacterial impurities associated with recombinant protein production were not clastogenic or mutagenic. With improved methods of synthesis and purification, and more sensitive techniques to detect impurities, the need for genotoxicity testing has declined. However, genotoxicity testing might be appropriate to determine the toxicity of conjugates or organic linkers in the molecule or to assess potential contaminants or impurities in the product.

Generally, reproduction/development tests for small molecule drugs are performed in rat and rabbit. These tests monitor fertility, reproductive performance, potential for fetal malformations, and toxicity during both perinatal and postnatal periods. However, because of species-specificity issues with biopharmaceuticals, nonhuman primates may well be the only suitable choice for reproductive toxicology testing. The cost, animal availability, lack of historical databases, and seasonal breeding status of some human primates may, however, hamper studies in these animals. Situations in which reproductive toxicology studies may be suitable include evidence of gonadal binding or immunosuppressive potential. For some biotherapeutics (e.g. angiogenesis inhibitors), reproductive toxicology findings can be anticipated based on the biological activities of the molecule, leading to the exclusion of infants and women of childbearing age for nonlife-threatening indications.

IV. Summary and Conclusions

Advances in recombinant DNA technology have led to the development of a new class of therapeutic compounds, biopharmaceuticals. Over the past two decades, numerous biotechnology-based drugs have been approved as novel treatments for either diseases in which no other effective treatment was available or as adjuncts to existing therapies. One of the advantages of biopharmaceuticals is that by utilizing specific receptor–ligand interactions, they can be targeted to individual cell types, eliminating many of the side effects associated with the administration of nontargeted therapies. However, this specificity comes at a price, as the species-specific nature of most of these molecules complicates the design and interpretation of the preclinical safety program.

As with small molecule drugs, the proposed clinical indication and development plan for a biopharmaceutical dictate the design of the preclinical safety assessment program. Ideally, preclinical toxicology studies should mimic the proposed clinical protocol with respect to route, schedule, and duration of dosing. In addition, factors such as the purity, activity, and potency of the molecule can impact or confound the interpretation of toxicology studies.

However, in contrast to small molecule drug development, the safety evaluation of biopharmaceuticals is a more customized approach, tailored to what is known about the biology of the molecule, the disease target, and the anticipated pharmacological effects. Rather than a prescribed set of standard studies to be performed ("box-checking"), the specific preclinical safety program is designed on a "case-by-case" basis to directly address issues (either known or anticipated) for the specific biopharmaceutical.

The two most important issues to be addressed in the safety evaluation of recombinant human therapeutics are (1) the selection of an appropriate (reactive) test species and (2) the immunogenicity of the molecule in the test species and in humans. Both of these factors influence the design, interpretation, and relevance of the preclinical toxicity program. Because biopharmaceuticals are usually protein-based drugs, toxicity testing in a pharmacologically nonresponsive species is generally uninformative, unless the protein has been modified in some way (e.g., chemical linkers, conjugation to immunotoxins) that may result in a chemical-based, rather than receptor-mediated,

toxicity. Administration of protein-based therapeutics may be immunogenic in the test species or in humans; the development of neutralizing antibodies can alter exposure and may impact the duration of safety studies in traditional toxicology species. The development of neutralizing antibodies and the formation of immune complexes in heterologous test species can confound the interpretation of safety studies; therefore, the consequences of immunogenicity need to be discriminated from actual toxic effects of the molecule itself.

SUGGESTED READING

Growth Factors, Colony-Stimulating Factors, and Hormones

Buckel, P. (1996). Recombinant proteins for therapy. *Trends Pharmacol. Sci.* **17**, 450–456.
Cebon, J., Lieschke, G., Bury, R., and Morstyn, G. (1992). The dissociation of GM-CSF efficacy from toxicity according to route of administration: A pharmacodynamic study. *Br. J. Haematol.* **80**, 144–150.
Danilenko, D. (1999). Preclinical and early. clinical development of keratinocyte growth factor, an epithelial specific tissue growth factor. *Toxicol. Pathol.* **27**, 64–71.
Dempster, A. M. (1995). Pharmacological testing of recombinant human erythropoietin. *Drug Dev. Res.* **35**, 173–178.
Di Marchi, R. D., Chance, R. E., Long, H. B., Shields, J. E., and Slieker, L. J. (1994). Preparation of an insulin with improved pharmacokinetics relative to human insulin through consideration of structural homology with insulin-like growth factor-1. *Horm. Res.* **41**(Suppl 2), 93–96.
Froesch, E. R., and Hussain, M. (1994). Recombinant human insulin-like growth factor-1: A therapeutic challenge for diabetes mellitus. *Diabetologia* **37**(Suppl. 2), S179–S185.
Fussenegger, M., Bailey, J. E., Hauser, H., and Mueller, P. P. (1999). Genetic optimization of recombinant glycoprotein production by mammalian cells. *Trends Biotechnol.* **17**, 35–42.
Hayes, T., and Cavagnaro, J. (1992). Progress and challenges in the preclinical assessment of cytokines. *Toxicol. Lett.* **64/65**, 291–297.
Johnson, C. W., Nachtman, J. P., Cimprich, R. E., Moon, H. L., Mills, S. E., Beckendorf, J., Levine, B. S., Long,

R. C., and Fuller, G. B. (1993). Clinical and histopathological effects of M-CSF in laboratory animals. *In* "International Review of Experimental Pathology; Cytokine-Induced Pathology: Interleukins and Hemopoietic Growth Factors" (G. W. Richter and K. E. Solez, eds.), 34 Part A, pp. 189–204. Academic Press, San Diego.

Keller, P., and Smalling, R. (1993). Granulocyte colony stimulating factor: Animal studies for risk assessment. *In* "International Review of Experimental Pathology; Cytokine-Induced Pathology: Interleukins and Hemopoietic Growth Factors" (G. W. Richter and K. Solez, eds.), 34 Part A, pp. 173–188. Academic Press, San Diego.

Knight, E., Oldman, J., Mohler, M., Liu, S., and Dooley, J. (1998). A review of nonclinical toxicology studies of becaplermin (rhPDGF-BB). *Am. J. Surg.* **176**, 55S–60S.

Le Grand, E. (1998). Preclinical promise of becaplermin (rhPDGF-BB) in wound healing. *Am. J. Surg.* **176**, 48S–54S.

McCabe, R., Childs, A., Reynolds, D., and Johnson, D. (1998). Exposure-based safety evaluation of recombinant human macrophage colony-stimulating factor (M-CSF) in cynomolgus monkeys. *Toxicol. Sci.* **43**, 61–67.

Murray, K. M., and Dahl, S. L. (1997). Recombinant human tumor necrosis factor receptor (p75): Fc fusion protein (TNFR:Fc) in rheumatoid arthritis. *Ann. Pharmacother.* **31**, 1335–1338.

Prow, D., and Vadhan-Raj, S. (1998). Thrombopoietin: Biology and potential clinical applications. *Oncology* **12**, 1597–1604.

Remick, D. G., and Kunkel, S. L. (1993). Pathophysiologic alterations induced by tumor necrosis factor. *In* "International Review of Experimental Pathology; Cytokine-Induced Pathology: Interleukins and Hemopoietic Growth Factors" (G. W. Richter and K. Solez, eds.), 34 Part B, pp. 7–25. Academic Press, San Diego.

Robison, R. L., and Myers, L. A. (1993). Preclinical safety assessment of recombinant human GM-CSF in rhesus monkeys. *In* "International Review of Experimental Pathology; Cytokine-Induced Pathology: Interleukins and Hemopoietic Growth Factors" (G. W. Richter and K. Solez, eds.), 34 Part A, pp. 149–172. Academic Press, San Diego.

Schuh, J., and Morrissey, P. (1999). Development of a recombinant growth factor and fusion protein: lessons for GM-CSF. *Toxicol. Pathol.* **27**, 72–77.

Siegel, J., Gerrard, T., Cavagnaro, J., Cohen, R., and Zoon, K. (1995). Development of biological therapies for oncologic use. *In* "Biologic Therapy in Cancer" (V. De Vita, S. Hellman, and S. Rosenberg, eds.), pp. 879–890. Lippincott, Philadelphia.

Ulich, T., del Castillo, J., Senaldi, G., Kinstler, O., Yin, S., Kaufman, S., Tarpley, J., Choi, E., Kirley, T., Hunt,

P., and Sheridan, W. (1996). Systemic hematologic effects of PEG-rHuMGDF-induced megakaryocyte hyperplasia in mice. *Blood* **87**, 5006–5015.

Winter, M. (1997). Preclinical safety assessment of the recombinant TNF receptor-immunoglobulin fusion protein. *Clin. Immunol. Immunopathol.* **83**, 21–24.

Interferons and Interleukins

Anderson, T., Hayes, T., Powers, G., Gately, M., Tudor, R., and Rushton, A. (1993). Comparative toxicity and pathology associated with administration of recombinant IL-2 to animals. *In* "International Review of Experimental Pathology; Cytokine-Induced Pathology: Interleukins and Hematopoietic Growth Factors" (G. Richter and K. Solez, eds.), 34 Part A, pp. 57–77. Academic Press, San Diego.

Anderson, T. D., Arceo, R., and Hayes, T. J. (1993). Comparative toxicity and pathology associated with administration of recombinant HuIL-1-alpha to animals. *In* "International Review of Experimental Pathology; Cytokine-Induced Pathology: Interleukins and Hemopoietic Growth Factors" (G. W. Richter and K. Solez, eds.), 34 Part A, pp. 9–36. Academic Press, San Diego.

Bouchard, P., Dorner, A., Goldman, S., Schaub, R., Keith, J., Timony, G., Larsen, G., and Warner, G. (1998). Preclinical safety assessment of recombinant human interleukin-11. Proceedings of the annual meeting of the Society of Toxicologic Pathologists, Vancouver, BC. [Abstract]

Burke, F., and Balkwill, F. R. (1996). Cytokines in animal models of cancer. *Biotherapy* **8**, 229–241.

Car, B., Eng, V., Schnyder, B., LeHir, M., Shakhov, A., Woerly, G., Huang, S., Aguet, M., Anderson, T., and Ryffel, B. (1995). Role of interferon-gamma in IL-12 induced pathology in mice. *Am. J. Pathol.* **147**, 1693–1707.

Car, B. D., Eng, V. M., Lipman, J. M., and Anderson, T. D. (1999). The toxicology of interleukin-12: A review. *Toxicol. Pathol.* **27**, 58–63.

Dean, J. H., Cornacoff, J. B., Barbolt, T. A., Gossett, K. A., and La Brie, T. (1992). Preclinical toxicity of IL-4: A model for studying protein therapeutics. *Int. J. Immunopharmacol.* **14**, 391–397.

Gunn, H. (1997). Immunogenicity of recombinant human interleukin-3. *Clin. Immunol. Immunopathol.* **83**, 5–7.

Harada, Y., and Yahara, I. (1993). Pathogenesis of toxicity with human-derived interleukin-2 in experimental animals. *In* "International Review of Experimental Pathology; Cytokine-Induced Pathology: Interleukins and Hemopoietic Growth Factors" (G. W. Richter and K. Solez, eds.), 34 Part A, pp. 37–55. Academic Press, San Diego.

Kammueller, M., and Ryffel, B. (1997). Extrapolation of experimental safety data to humans: The interleukin-6 case. *Clin. Immunol. Immunopathol.* **83**, 15–17.

Klug, S., Neubert, R., Stahlmann, R., Thiel, R., Ryffel, B., Car, B., and Neubert, D. (1994). Effects of recombinant IL-6 (rhIL-6) in marmosets (*Callithrix jacchus*). *Arch. Toxicol.* **68**, 619–631.

Leach, M. W., Snyder, E. A., Sinha, D. P., and Rosenblum, I. Y. (1997b). Safety evaluation of recombinant human interleukin-4. I. Preclinical studies. *Clin. Immunol. Immunopathol.* **83**, 8–11.

Leonard, J., Nebenn, T., Kozitza, M., Quinto, C., and Goldman, S. (1996). Constant subcutaneous infusion of rhIL-11 in mice: Efficient delivery enhances biological activity. *Exp. Hematol.* **24**, 270–276.

Leonard, J., Sherman, M., Fisher, G., Buchanan, L., Larsen, G., Atkins, M., Sosman, J., Dutcher, J., Vogelzang, N., and Ryan, J. (1997). Effects of single-dose interleukin-12 exposure on interleukin-12 exposure on interleukin-12-associated toxicity and interferon gamma production. *Blood* **90**, 2541–2548.

Loy, J., Davidson, T., Berry, K., Macmaster, J., Danle, B., and Durham, S. (1999). Oncostatin M: Development of a pleiotropic cytokine. *Toxicol. Pathol.* **27**, 151–155.

Quesniaux, V. F. J., Mayer, P., Liehl, E., Turner, K., Goldman, S. J., and Fagg, B. (1993). Review of a novel hematopoietic cytokine, interleukin-11. *In* "International Review of Experimental Pathology; Cytokine-Induced Pathology: Interleukins and Hemopoietic Growth Factors" (G. W. Richter and K. Solez, eds.), 34 Part A, pp. 205–214. Academic Press, San Diego.

Reiner, G., Ronneberger, H., and Hintz-Obertreis, P. (1993). Comparative toxicity of *Escherichia coli* and yeast rhIL-3 in cynomolgus and Rhesus monkeys. *In* "International Review of Experimental Pathology; Cytokine-Induced Pathology: Interleukins and Hemopoietic Growth Factors" (G. W. Richter and K. Solez, eds.), 34 Part A, pp. 119–147. Academic Press, San Diego.

Ryffel, B., Car, B., Woerly, G., Weber, M., DiPadova, F., Kammuller, M., Klug, S., Neubert, R., and Neubert, D. (1994). Long term interleukin-6 administration stimulates sustained thrombopoiesis and acute phase protein synthesis in a small primate-the marmoset. *Blood* **83**, 2093–2101.

Ryffel, B., Mihatsch, M., and Woerly, G. (1993). Pathology induced by interleukin-6. *In* "International Review of Experimental Pathology; Cytokine-Induced Pathology: Interleukins and Hemopoietic Growth Factors" (G. W. Richter and K. Solez, eds.), 34 Part A, pp. 79–89. Academic Press, San Diego.

Ryffel, B., and Weber, M. (1995). Preclinical safety studies with recombinant human interleukin 6 (rhIL-6) in the primate *Callithrix jaccus* (Marmoset): Comparison with studies in rats. *J. Appl. Toxicol.* **15**, 19–26.

Sarmiento, U., Riley, J., and Knack, P. (1994). Biologic effects of recombinant human interleukin-12 in squirrel monkeys (*Sciurus saimiri*). *Lab. Invest.* **71**, 862–873.

Soda, H., Raymond, E., Sharma, S., Lawrence, R., Cerna, C., Gomez, L., Schaub, R., Von Hoff, D., and Izbicka, E. (1999). Recombinant human interleukin-11 is unlikely to stimulate the growth of the most common solid tumors. *Anti-Cancer Drugs* **10**, 97–101.

Sreevalasan, T. (1995). Biologic therapy with interferon alpha and beta: Preclinical studies. *In* "Biologic Therapy of Cancer" (V. De Vita, S. Hellman, and S. Rosenberg, eds.), pp. 347–364. Lippincott, Philadelphia.

Terrell, T., and Green, J. (1993). Comparative pathology of recombinant murine interferon gamma in mice and recombinant human interferon gamma in cynomolgus monkeys. *In* "International Review of Experimental Pathology; Cytokine-Induced Pathology: Interleukins and Hemopoietic Growth Factors" (G. Richter and K. Solez, eds.), 34 Part B, pp. 73–101. Academic Press, San Diego.

Wolfgang, G., McCabe, R., and Johnson, D. (1998). Toxicity of subcutaneously administered recombinant human interleukin-2 in rats. *Toxicol. Sci.* **42**, 57–63.

Monoclonal Antibodies

Alegre, M. L., Lenschow, D. J., and Bluestone, J. A. (1995). Immunomodulation of transplant rejection using monoclonal antibodies and soluble receptors. *Digest. Dis. Sci.* **40**, 58–64.

Bodmer, M., Fournel, M. A., and Hinshaw, L. B. (1993). Preclinical review of anti-tumor necrosis factor monoclonal antibodies. *Crit. Care Med.* **10**(Suppl.), S441–S446.

Casadevall, A. (1999). Passive antibody therapies: Progress and continuing challenges. *Clin. Immunol.* **93**, 5–15.

Gerber, H. P., Hillan, K. J., Ryan, A. M., Keller, G. A., Rangell, L., Wright, B. D., Radtke, F., Aguet, M., and Ferrara, N. (1999). VEGF is required for growth and survival in neonatal mice. *Development* **126**, 1149–1159.

Gerber, H. P., Vu, T. H., Ryan, A. M., Kowalski, J., Werb, Z. and Ferrara, N. (1999). VEGF couples hypertrophic cartilage remodeling, ossification and angiogenesis during endochondral bone formation. *Nature Med.* **5**, 623–628.

Green, L., and Jakobovits, A. (1998). Regulation of B cell development by variable gene complexity in mice reconstituted with human immunoglobulin yeast artificial chromosomes. *J. Exp. Med.* **188**, 483–495.

Klingbeil, C., and Hsu, D.-H. (1999). Pharmacology and safety assessment of humanized monoclonal antibodies for therapeutic use. *Toxicol. Pathol.* **27**, 1–3.

Panchagnula, R., and Dey, C. S. (1997). Monoclonal antibodies in drug targeting. *J. Clin. Pharm. Therap.* **22**, 7–19.

Peterson, N. (1996). Recombinant antibodies: Alternative strategies for developing and manipulating murine-derived monoclonal antibodies. *Lab. Anim. Sci.* **46**, 8–13.

Revillard, J. P., Robinet, E., Goldman, M., Bazin, H., Latinne, D., and Chatenoud, L. (1995). *In vitro* correlates of the acute toxic syndrome induced by some monoclonal antibodies: A rationale for the design of predictive tests. *Toxicology* **96**, 51–58.

Ryan, A., Eppler, D., Hagler, K., Bruner, R., Thomford, P., Hall, R., Shopp, G., and O'Neill, C. (1999). Preclinical safety evaluation of rhuMAbVEGF, an anti-angiogenic humanized monoclonal antibody. *Toxicol. Pathol.* **27**, 78–86.

Sandborn, W. J., and Hanauer, S. B. (1999). Antitumor necrosis factor therapy for inflammatory bowel disease: A review of agents, pharmacology, clinical results, and safety. *Inflamm. Bowel Dis.* **5**, 119–133.

Vaswani, S., and Hamilton, R. (1998). Humanized antibodies as potential therapeutic drugs. *Ann. Allergy Asthma Immunol.* **81**, 105–115.

Weiner, L. (1999). An overview of monoclonal antibody therapy of cancer. *Sem. Oncol.* **26**, 41–50.

Wellstein, A., Sale, E. B., Chung, H. C., Fang, W. J., Smith, R. V., Colley, K. C., and Czubayko, F. (1995). Growth factors as targets in tumor therapy. *Int. J. Pharmacogen.* **33**(Suppl.), 35–47.

Yang, X. D., Corvalan, J. R., Wang, P., Roy, C. M., and Davis, C. G. (1999). Fully human anti-interleukin-8 monoclonal antibodies: Potential therapeutics for the treatment of inflammatory disease states. *J. Leukocyte Biol.* 401–410.

Emerging Therapeutics

Cohen, J. (1991). Oligonucleotides as therapeutic agents. *Pharmacol. Therap.* **52**, 211–225.

Crooke, S. (1992). Therapeutic applications of oligonucleotides. *Annu. Rev. Pharmacol. Toxicol.* **32**, 329–376.

Graham, M. J., Crooke, S. T., Monteith, D. K., Cooper, S. R., Lemonidis, K. M., Stecker, K. K., Martin, M. J., and Crooke, R. M. (1998). *In vivo* distribution and metabolism of a phosphorothioate oligonucleotide within rat liver after intravenous administration. *J. Pharmacol. Exp. Therap.* **286**, 447–458.

Henry, S., Stecker, K., Brooks, D., Monteith, D., Conklin, B., and Bennett, C. F. (2000). Chemically modified oligonucleotides exhibit decreased immune stimulation in mice. *J. Pharmacol. Exp. Therap.* **292**, 468–479.

Henry, S., Templin, M., Gillett, N., Rojko, J., and Levin, A. (1999). Correlation of toxicity and pharmacokinetic properties of a phosphorothioate oligonucleotide designed to inhibit ICAM-1. *Toxicol. Pathol.* **27**, 95–100.

Hughes, J., Raper, S., Wivel, N., Tazelar, J., Baker, C., Chirmule, N., and Wilson, J. (1998). Preclinical safety evaluation of adenoviral and AAV vector to be used in human gene transfer. Proceedings of the annual meeting of the Society of Toxicologic Pathologists, Vancouver, BC. [Abstract]

Monteith, D., and Levin, M. (1999). Synthetic oligonucleotides: The development of antisense therapeutics. *Toxicol. Pathol.* **27**, 8–13.

Monteith, D. K., Horner, M. J., Gillett, N. A., Butler, M., Geary, R., Burckin, T., Ushiro-Watanabe, T., and Levin, A. A. (1999). Evaluation of the renal effects of an antisense phosphorothioate oligonucleotide in monkeys. *Toxicol. Pathol.* **27**, 307–317.

Morrissey, R., Patrick, J., Bordens, R., and Horvath, C. (1997). Preclinical studies of SCH 58500, a replication-deficient adenoviral vector expressing the human p53 gene. *Toxicologist* **36**, 183.

Nagel, K. M., Holstad, S. G., and Isenberg, K. E. (1993). Oligonucleotide pharmacotherapy: An antigene strategy. *Pharmacotherapy* **13**, 177–188.

Parker, S., Vahlsing, H., Serfilippi, L., Franklin, C., Doh, S., Gromkowski, S., Lew, D., Manthorpe, M., and Norman, J. (1995). Cancer gene therapy using plasmid DNA: Safety evaluation in rodents and non-human primates. *Hum. Gene Ther.* **6**, 575–590.

Parker, S. E., Vahlsing, H. L., Lew, D., Martin, T., Hall, B., Kornbrust, D., and Norman, J. (1999). Cancer gene therapy using plasmid DNA: Pharmacokinetics and safety evaluation of an IL-2 plasmid DNA expression vector in rodents and nonhuman primates. *BioPharm* **12**, 18–24.

Pilaro, A., and Serabian, M. (1999). Preclinical development strategies for novel gene therapeutic products. *Toxicol. Pathol.* **27**, 4–7.

Seigfried, W. (1993). Perspective in gene therapy with recombinant adenoviruses. *Exp. Clin. Endocrinol.* **101**, 7–11.

Verdier, F., and Descotes, J. (1999). Preclinical safety evaluation of human gene therapy products. *Toxicol. Sci.* **47**, 9–15.

Wilson, J. (1996). Adenoviruses as gene delivery vehicles. *N. Engl. J. Med.* **334**, 1185–1187.

Zhang, W., Alemany, R., Wang, J., Koch, P., Ordonez, N., and Roth, J. (1995). Safety evaluation of Ad5CMV-p53 *in vitro* and *in vivo*. *Hum. Gene Ther.* **6**, 155–164.

Zwacka, R. M., and Dunlop, M. G. (1998). Gene therapy for colon cancer. *Hematol. Oncol. Clin. North Am.* **12**, 595–615.

Immunotoxins

Chiron, M. F. (1997). Recombinant immunotoxins and chimeric toxins for a targeted therapy in oncology. *Bull. Cancer* **84**, 1135–1140.

Haggerty, H., Warner, W., Comereski, C., WM, P., Mezza, L., Damle, B., Siegall, C., and Davidson, T.

(1999). BR96 sFv-PE40 immunotoxin: Nonclinical safety assessment. *Toxicol. Pathol.* **27**, 87–94.

King, C., Fisher, P., Rando, R., and Pastan, I. (1996). The performance of e23(Fv)PEs, recombinant toxins targeting the erbB-2 protein. *Sem. Cancer Biol.* **7**, 79–86.

Kreitman, R. J. (1999). Immunotoxins in cancer therapy. *Curr. Opin. Immunol.* **11**, 570–578.

Puri, R. (1999). Development of a recombinant interleukin-4-*Pseudomonas* exotoxin for therapy of glioblastoma. *Toxicol. Pathol.* **27**, 53–57.

Westwood, F., Jones, D., and Aldridge, A. (1996). The synovial membrane, liver and tongue: target organs for a ricin A-chain immunotoxin (ZD0490). *Toxicol. Pathol.* **24**, 477–483.

Safety Evaluation of Biopharmaceutical

Black, L., Bendele, A., Bendele, R., Zack, P., and Hamilton, M. (1999). Regulatory decision strategy for entry of a novel biologic therapeutic with a clinically unmonitorable toxicity into clinical trials: Pre-IND meetings and a case example. *Toxicol. Pathol.* **27**, 22–26.

Braun, A., Gassmann, R., Kraus, K., Lorenzi, G., and Weigel, U. (1996). Special considerations concerning regulatory requirements and drug development for peptides and biotech products in the EU. *Pharm. Acta Helvetiae* **71**, 447–458.

Cavagnaro, J. (1992). Science-based approach to preclinical safety evaluation of biotechnology products. *Pharm. Engin.* **12**, 33–32.

Cavagnaro, J. (1997). Preclinical safety assessment of biological products. *In* "Biologic Development: A Regulatory Overview" (M. Mathieu, ed.), pp. 21–36. PAREXEL International Corporation, Waltham, MA.

Claude, J. (1992). Difficulties in conceiving and applying guidelines for the safety evaluation of biotechnology-produced drugs: some examples. *Toxicol. Lett.* **64/65**, 349–355.

Dayan, A. D. (1995). Safety evaluation of biological and biotechnology-derived medicines. *Toxicology* **105**, 59–68.

Green, J., and Terrell, T. (1992). Utilization of homologous proteins to evaluate the safety of recombinant proteins-case study: recombinant human interferon gamma (rhIFNG). *Toxicol. Lett.* **64**, 321–327.

Griffiths, S., and Lumley, C. (1998a). Non-clinical safety studies for biotechnology-derived pharmaceuticals: Conclusions from an international workshop. *Hum. Exp. Toxicol.* **17**, 68–83.

Griffiths, S., and Lumley, C. (1998b). "Safety Evaluation of Biotechnology-derived Pharmaceuticals: Facilitating a Scientific Approach." Kluwer Academic, Boston.

Hayes, T. (1991). Interpretation of toxicological data from responsive and nonresponsive species. *In* "Preclinical Evaluation of Peptides and Recombinant Proteins" (A. Sundwall, L, Ekman, H. Johansson, B. Sjoberg, and I. Sjoholm, eds.), pp. 49–56. Skogs Grafiska AB, Sweden.

Hayes, T., and Cavagnaro, J. (1992). Progress and challenges in the preclinical assessment of cytokines. *Toxicol. Lett.* **64/65**, 291–297.

Henck, J., Hilbish, K., Serabian, M., Cavagnaro, J., Hendrickx, A., Agnish, N., Hung, A., and Mordenti, J. (1996). Reproductive toxicity testing of therapeutic biotechnology agents. *Teratology* **53**, 185–195.

Pilling, A. (1999). The role of the toxicologic pathologist in the preclinical safety evaluation of biotechnology-derived pharmaceuticals. *Toxicol. Pathol.* **27**, 678–688.

Revillard, J. P., Robinet, E., Goldman, M., Bazin, H., Latinne, D., and Chatenoud, L. (1995). *In vitro* correlates of the acute toxic syndrome induced by some monoclonal antibodies: A rationale for the design of predictive tests. *Toxicology* **96**, 51–58.

Serabian, M., and Pilaro, A. (1999). Safety assessment of biotechnology-derived pharmaceuticals: ICH and beyond. *Toxicol. Pathol.* **27**, 27–31.

Terrell, T., and Green, J. (1994). Issues with biotechnology products in toxicologic pathology. *Toxicol. Pathol.* **22**, 187–193.

Thomas, J. (1995). Recent developments and perspectives of biotechnology-derived products. *Toxicology* **105**, 7–22.

Thomas, J., and Myers, L. (1993). "Biotechnology and Safety Assessment." Raven Press, New York.

Woerly, G., and Ryffel, B. (1993). The use of receptor assays for the rapid selection of an appropriate animal species for the preclinical investigations of human interleukins. *In Vitro Toxicol.* **6**, 67–79.

21

Endocrine Disruptors

Paul S. Cooke
Department of Veterinary
Biosciences
University of Illinois
at Urbana-Champaign
Urbana, Illinois

Richard E. Peterson
School of Pharmacy and
Environmental Toxicology Center
University of Wisconsin
Madison, Wisconsin

Rex A. Hess
Department of Veterinary
Biosciences
University of Illinois
at Urbana-Champaign
Urbana, Illinois

I. Introduction

There has been growing concern in recent years that a variety of natural and synthetic chemicals could be producing serious health effects in humans and other species by mimicking or inhibiting the actions of endogenous hormones. Public attention was originally drawn to the idea that environmental chemicals could disrupt the endocrine system of wildlife by the publication of Rachel Carson's "Silent Spring" in the 1960s. This book described deleterious reproductive effects of the then-commonly used insecticide, dichlorodiphenyltrichloroethane (DDT), on birds and other wildlife. However, the first published evidence for environmental disruptors had actually appeared more than a decade earlier, when it was reported that consumption of a certain type of clover disrupted reproduction in sheep. Both of these reports involved chemicals that were estrogenic in that they acted through estrogen receptors to either mimic or antagonize the normal actions of estro-

gens. Because of the critical effects of estrogens on female reproduction and its ability to also induce abnormalities in male reproductive systems, studies in the endocrine disruptor area were initially centered on estrogenic effects of environmental chemicals. The subsequent identification of a very large number of chemicals that act, at least partially, by binding the estrogen receptor, coupled with the widespread environmental distribution of certain of these chemicals (e.g., DDT), has resulted in a continuing focus on endocrine disruptors that act by altering signaling through the estrogen receptor. However, in recent years, there has been a rapid increase in information concerning the ability of various chemicals to mimic or inhibit the actions of other hormones (e.g., androgens, progestins, thyroid hormone). It is now clear that although endocrine disruptors that function as estrogens and/or antiestrogens are the most common, endocrine disruption is a phenomenon that can potentially affect any hormonal system.

While evidence exists for adverse effects of endocrine disruptors on wildlife populations, there is as yet only limited evidence that links environmental exposure to these substances and adverse effects on human health. Dioxins and polychlorinated biphenyls (PCBs) are emerging as an exception to this generalization because of the increasing number of epidemiology studies that have been and are continuing to be conducted on them. Nevertheless it has been suggested that exposure to endocrine-disrupting chemicals may be responsible for a possible decline in human sperm production and increases in other male reproductive problems, such as testicular cancer. Even those who believe that there have been no deleterious effects on humans from past and present exposure to endocrine disruptors would at least acknowledge the potential for such harm. This emphasizes the critical nature of this topic and the necessity to more clearly understand compounds that function as endocrine disruptors so that we can more definitively evaluate their health effects in humans and wildlife.

This chapter reviews the historical development of work on endocrine disruption, and attempts to provide a concise description of the state of our present knowledge as it regards the ability of chemicals to disrupt a number of hormone systems. In addition, the potential for these compounds to affect animal and human health is discussed, as are potential future research directions in this area.

II. Mechanisms of Endocrine Disruption

The process by which hormones are produced in an endocrine organ, released into the circulation, transported to target tissues, and then bind to receptors in target cells to affect their subsequent activity is obviously extremely complex and closely regulated. Each step of this process for any hormone signaling system is potentially vulnerable to disruption by an external agent (Fig. 1). Indeed, there are known examples of endocrine disruption that result from effects at a wide variety of sites of action encompassing almost all aspects of hormone production, transport, and action.

One of the most obvious mechanisms by which a compound may function as an endo-

crine disruptor is by having toxic effects on an endocrine organ(s) and subsequently altering the production of that hormone. A compound can also disrupt hormone synthesis by a specific effect on an endocrine organ, rather than by causing generalized toxicity. An example of this type of mechanism is the effects of some isoflavones on thyroid peroxidase, an enzyme that is essential for the normal synthesis of thyroid hormones by the thyroid gland. Similarly, steroid hormones are synthesized from cholesterol by an elaborate enzymatic pathway, and compounds that either increase or decrease levels of steroidogenic enzymes would have the potential to produce alterations in the hormone production of those cells.

Compounds that alter the metabolism and breakdown of hormones also have the potential to function as endocrine disruptors. One example of this indirect mode of action is illustrated by the effects of PCBs on thyroid hormone levels, as detailed in Section IV,E.

One of the most common mechanisms by which a compound can function as an endocrine disruptor is by having affinity for and binding to endogenous hormone receptors. The compounds may then mimic the action of the natural hormone, or antagonize it, as explained later. This mode of action is typified by the large number of natural and man-made chemicals that can bind to estrogen receptor α (ERα), but a number of compounds that are capable of binding to the androgen receptor have also been described.

A compound that has affinity for one receptor may also function as an endocrine disruptor by changing the expression levels of other hormone receptors and/or responsiveness to these hormones. This mode of action is well illustrated by the report that the exposure of developing rodent fetuses to low levels of exogenous estrogens results in subsequent alterations in the production of prostate androgen receptors and eventual changes in prostate size.

There also are compounds that bind to the aryl hydrocarbon receptor (AhR) and function as endocrine disruptors. The most striking and environmentally relevant example of this type

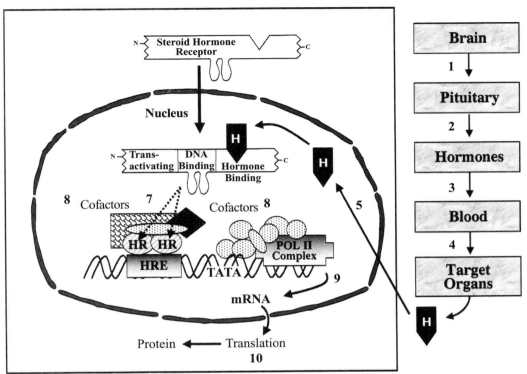

Figure 1. Potential sites of action for chemicals that disrupt steroid hormone signaling. The schematic diagram of the production, transport, and cellular mechanism of action of a typical steroid hormone illustrates that many aspects of this process can potentially be altered by endocrine-disrupting chemicals. A chemical could have effects on the hypothalamus, other brain areas, or the pituitary to alter the levels of trophic pituitary hormones that regulate the activity of a steroidogenic organ (1 and 2). A chemical can have direct effects on the steroidogenic organ to alter hormone production (3) or could alter blood levels by altering transport and binding to transport proteins or catabolism of the circulating hormone. A chemical can mimic or antagonize the binding of the endogenous ligand to its receptor (5) and could potentially affect other processes, such as the movement of receptor from the cytoplasm to the nucleus (6). A chemical could inhibit receptor dimerization or the binding of the liganded hormone receptor to the DNA (7) or could alter the binding of cofactors and the initiation of transcription (8). Additional modes of action, such as altering the transport or stability of the mRNA produced in response to hormonal stimulation (9) or the translation of the mRNA into protein (10), are also possible.

of compound is 2,3,7,8-tetrachlorodibenzo-*p*-dioxin (TCDD). As explained in detail in the section on AhR agonists, TCDD disrupts a variety of endocrine pathways, but substantial work is still needed to clarify how these effects are induced.

It is sometimes difficult to discern from the literature whether a chemical causes a direct endocrine effect on the target organ evaluated or if the observed effects are indirect. For example, early studies suggested that boric acid-induced testicular atrophy was due to indirect

effects through the hypothalmo–pituitary–gonadal axis because there was no effect of boric acid on Leydig cell steroidogenesis *in vitro*. However, further studies in treated animals revealed that there was an increase in follicle-stimulating hormone and a decreased ability of the testis to produce testosterone in response to hormonal stimulation. Thus, it was concluded that the effect was testicular and that the hormonal changes were secondary. However, it is reasonable to ask if endocrine-disrupting chemicals should be classified as such only if they show direct effects on endocrine organs or cells that synthesize hormones.

Another difficulty in assessing health risks from endocrine disruptors is that effects may not be apparent until long after exposure. Diethylstibestrol (DES) is one of the best examples of a chemical that can produce developmental effects that are not detected until adulthood, both in humans and in experimental animals, and in males as well as females. In adult males, epididymal granulomas are found following *in utero* DES exposure.

It is sometime difficult to accurately assess effects of an endocrine disruptor because the observed effects may be secondary to the primary effect. An example that demonstrates target organ pathology inducing secondary effects on a primary endocrine organ is the fungicide benomyl. This fungicide is often listed as an endocrine disruptor, primarily because it causes male infertility, testicular atrophy, and elevation of intratesticular testosterone and androgen-binding protein. However, the primary target that is involved in causing testicular atrophy is the efferent ductules, not the testis. Within a few hours after treatment with either benomyl or its metabolite, carbendazim, the efferent ductules become occluded, causing fluid to accumulate in the rete testis and to back up into the testis. Thus, secondary damage to the testis due to pathological changes in the efferent ductules is the ultimate cause of testicular atrophy and the elevation in intratesticular testosterone. Therefore, it is reasonable to conclude that while some compounds are reproductive toxicants they are not necessarily endocrine disruptors. Proper identification of endocrine disruptors will require the analysis of more than one or two end points and may depend on an understanding of the sequence of organ pathology.

III. Target Organs

The major potential targets for environmental endocrine disruption are the reproductive, neurological, thyroid, and immune systems. Other endocrine organs, such as stomach, pancreas, kidney, and adrenals, are also potential

targets, but less is known about their susceptibility. Carcinogenicity is often included as a separate toxicological end point of endocrine disruption, but a major portion of this research comes from the study of mechanisms associated with breast, prostate, and other reproductive cancers. Therefore, it is possible to include cancer and tumor formation as end points under each target organ system. In all animals, the class of chemical will determine which organ system is the primary target. However, major differences are found when comparing mammalian and fish species. For example, in mammalian species, estrogenic compounds will have their major effects on the reproductive organs and the mammary gland; but in fish, it is possible that the most demonstrable effect will be estrogenic chemical induction of vitellogenin production in the liver. Therefore, target organs that are endocrine responsive will vary depending on the class of vertebrate and type of chemical. For a more detailed analysis of each organ system, the reader should consult the separate chapters elsewhere in this text. Tables I–V provide a partial listing of target organs, potential endocrine-disrupting effects, and suspect chemicals. The mechanisms of effect are not known for all of these compounds and some may be acting through indirect pathways. It should be noted that controversies exist in the literature for some chemicals and effects have been disputed in others.

IV. Classes of Compounds with Endocrine-Disrupting Activity

A. ESTROGENS

1. Chemicals with Known Estrogenic Actions

The topic of environmental estrogens or xenoestrogens has been a major focus in toxicology for many years, stemming primarily from the first reported animal model for DES exposure that exhibited both male and female reproductive abnormalities and the early literature documenting estrogenic effects of DDT. The importance of steroid hormones, particularly estrogens, in the study of endocrine disruptors

TABLE I
Male Reproductive System, Organ Targets, and Reported Effects of Endocrine-Disrupting Chemicals

Organ	Reported effects	Chemicals
Developmental effects	Pseudohermaphrodite vaginal pouch	Procymidone, vinclozolin, di(2-ethylhexyl)phthalate (DEHP)
	Hypospadia	Hydroxyflutamide, procymidone, vinclozolin, finasteride, DEHP
	Microphallus/cleft phallus	DES, procymidone, vinclozolin
	Decreased anogenital distance	vinclozolin, linuron, p,p' DDE, dibutyl phthalate, procymidone, DEHP
Testis	Cryptorchidism or delayed testicular descent	DES, TCDD, hydroxyflutamide, procymidone, vinclozolin
	Tubular atrophy	TCDD, vinclozolin, linuron, boric acid, dibutyl phthalate
	Decreased testis weight	DES, octyphenol phenoxylate, octylphenol, butyl benzyl phthalate, boric acid, DEHP
	Decreased testosterone	TCDD, heptachlor, boric acid, N-nitroso-N-ethylurea, PCBs, ethane dimethanesulfonate, lindane, dibromoacetic acid, phthalate esters, hexachlorocyclohexane
	Cancer	Procymidone, pronamide, lacidipine, lansoprazole, ammonium perfluorooctanoate, acrylamide, γ-oryzanol
Rete testis	Cancer	DES
Efferent ductules	Dilation, decreased epithelial height	Genistein, octylphenol, bisphenol-A
Epididymis	Cysts–granulomas/abnormal development/function	DES, linuron, dibutyl phthalate, procymidone, phosphamidon, ethane dimethanesulfonate (EDS), epichlorohydrin, TCDD, DEHP, α-chlorohydrin, cadmium, chloroethylmethanesulphonate, dibromo-chloropropane, benomyl, carbendazim
Sperm	Decreased sperm production, ejaculated numbers	TCDD, DES, 4-octyphenol, butylbenzyl phthalate, dibutylphthalate, vinclozolin, p,p' DDE
Prostate	Cancer/growth or weight changes/abnormal development/absent prostate	Bisphenol-A, TCDD, p,p' DDE, coke oven emissions, cadmium, N-hydroxy-3,2'-dimethyl-4-amino biphenyl, procymidone, N-methyl-N-nitrosourea, hydroxyflutamide, 3,2'-dimethyl-4-aminobiphenyl

cannot be ignored due to their influence in the regulation of reproductive physiology and especially for their role in development. Estrogens and xenoestrogens are the most widely studied of the potential endocrine disruptors, as discussed in Section I. They range from numerous synthetic chemicals, such as the well-known PCBs, which have both estrogenic and antiestrogenic properties depending on the commercial mixture or congener being studied, to a wide variety of natural compounds found in the foods that we eat (Table VI). A search of the National Library of Medicine database using Medline reveals the rapid growth of research in the area of "environmental estrogens" (Table VI).

A compound is designated as estrogenic or as a xenoestrogen if it has the ability to mimic the ability of estradiol to bind to estrogen receptors and induce responses typical of estrogen. In certain scenarios, these compounds may exert antiestrogen effects. There are now two recognized ERs, ERα and ERβ, which complicates the study of environmental estrogens. Because the overall homology between the two ERs is only about 50%, there is a strong possibility that different tissue expressions of these ERs and different ligand-binding affinities may reflect differences in species and target organ responses to synthetic estrogens and antiestrogens. Differences in ERα and β binding are now clearly evident. The binding of 17β-estradiol (E_2) is

TABLE II
Female Reproductive System, Organ Targets, and Reported Effects of Endocrine-Disrupting Chemicals

Organ	Reported effects	Chemicals
Ovary	Cancer	DES, procymidone, vinclozolin, iprodione, captan
	Change hormone concentrations	Ketoconazole, methoxychlor, heptachlor, di-(2-ethylhexyl)phthalate
	Ovarian atrophy	Methoxychlor, difluoromethylornithine, TCDD
	Oocyte abnormalities/anovulation	Kepone, methotrexate, DDT, PCBs
	Abnormal cyclicity/persistent estrus	DES, atrazine, simazine, cyanazine, methoxychlor, kepone, o,p'-DDT, chloroquine,
	Cancer, carcinoma	DES, 1,2,3-trichloropropane, 2-dimethylhydrazine, chloroethane, bromoethane, N-ethyl-N'-nitro-N-nitrosoguanidine, N-methyl-N-nitrosourea, methotrexate, ethylenethiourea
	Endometriosis/cysts	DES, TCDD, PCBs, s-triazine herbicide, tamoxifen, toremifene, pentachlorophenol, triallate
	Inhibit implantation, increase resorptions	Methoxychlor, alloxan, PCBs, nitric oxide, phthalates, tributyltin chloride, ketoconazole, carbon tetrachloride, cabergoline, monothiosemicarbazone compounds,
Vagina	Cancer/malformation, altered development	DES, dinaline, TCDD
Mammary gland/breast	Cancer/abnormal development	DES, chlorotriazine, benzene, methylnitrosourea, dinaline, tetrachlorobiphenyl, ethylene oxide, ethylenethiourea, 1,3-butadiene, dimethylhydrazine, trichloropropane, 7,12-dimethylbenz[a]anthracene, dichlorvos, 2-amino-1-methyl-6-phenylimidazo[4,5-b] pyridine, atrizine, chlormadione acetate, N-ethyl-N-nitrosourea, captan, nalidixic acid, methylene chloride, diol epoxides, nitrofurazone, 1,2-dibromoethane, 1,2-dichloroethane, glycidol, sulfallate, TCDD

equivalent between the two ERs. However, large differences exist in binding affinities for synthetic estrogens and phytoestrogens. DES has a much greater affinity for ERα, whereas 4-OH-tamoxifen has a stronger affinity for ERβ. All of the phytoestrogens bind with higher affinity to ERβ than to ERα. This dichotomy in ER binding also appears to extend to the environmental estrogens, as bisphenol A has a K_i of 195 nM for ERα and a K_i of 35 nM for ERβ. Further studies are required to determine the cellular and physiological processes regulated by ERβ.

TABLE III
Central Nervous System, Organ Targets, and Reported Effects of Endocrine-Disrupting Chemicals

Organ	Probable effects	Chemicals
Brain/hypothalamus	Change in sexual behavior/defeminization/ demasculinization	Methoxychlor, DES, PCBs, kepone, DDT, zearalenone, o,p'-dicofol, alkylphenols, TCDD, vinclozolin, perinatal estradiol, or zearalenone
Pituitary	Cancer	Hexane, DES, taltirelin tetrahydrate, chronic 17 β-estradiol, atrazine, ethylene thiourea, γ-oryzanol, dinaline, oxytetracycline, captan, nalidixic acid
	Changes in hormone concentrations	Vinclozolin, procymidone, DES, PCBs, methoxychlor, TCDD, 1,2-dibromo-3-chloropropane, boric acid, oxolinic acid, trifluralin, lindane, dimethoate, trifluralin, triallate, lead acetate

TABLE IV
Reported Effects of Endocrine-Disrupting Chemicals on the Thyroid Gland and Immune System

Organ	Reported effects	Chemicals
Thyroid gland	Cancer, tumors, intrafollicular hyperplasia, goiter	DDT, DDE, DES, chlordane, heptachlor, mirex, dieldrin, 2,4-diaminoanisole sulfate, amitrole, diniconazole, N,N'-diethylthiourea, 4,4'-thiodianiline, 2-chloro-N-(2,6-diethylphenyl)-N-(methoxymethyl)acetamide, clofentezine, mancozeb, etridiazole, N-octyl bicycloheptene dicarboximide, terbutryn, triadimefon, trifluralin, ethylene thiourea, metiram, oryzalin, bromacil, 2,3,5,6-tetrachloro-1,4-benzenedicarboxylic acid dimethyl ester, ethiozin, ethofenprox, fenbuconazole, fipronil, toxaphene, N-octyl bicycloheptene dicarboximide, pronamide, pyrethrins, pyrimethanil, thiazopyr, γ-oryzanol, N-bis (2-hydroxypropyl) nitrosamine, phytoestrogens
	Changes in hormone concentrations	PCBs, TCDD, carbofuran, trifluralin, thiazopyr, chlorpyrifos, dimethoate, methoxychlor, pentachlorophenol, lindane, metribuzin, 2,4-dichlorophenoxyacetic acid, 1-methyl-3-propylimidazole-2-thione, food color FDC Red No. 3, thiocarbamide, toxaphene, diniconazole, diethofencarb
Immune system	Immunosuppression/thymic atrophy	Lindane, aldicarb, methomyl, triazine, meso-2,3-dimercaptosuccinic acid, bis(tri-n-butyltin) oxide, 17 β-estradiol, malathion, methyl parathion, dimethoate, TCDD, methylcholanthrene, pyrimethamine, PCBs, lead, cadmium

TABLE V
Chemicals with Known or Suspected Estrogenic Activity[a]

Endogenous estrogens
  Estradiol
  Estrone
  Estriol
Industrial and agricultural chemicals
  Bisphenol-A
  Chlordane
  Chlordecone (Kepone)
  DDT, DDE (also listed as antiandrogen)
  Dieldrin
  Endosulfans
  Lindane
  Methoxychlor
  Nonylphenol carboxylylate
  Nonylphenol ethoxylate
  p-Nonylphenol
  p-Octylphenol

Phthalate esters
PCBs
p-tert-Butylphenol
Toxaphene
Drugs
  Diethylstilbestrol (DES)
  Tamoxifen
  Zearalanone
Phytoestrogens
  Coumesterol
  Equol
  Enterodiol
  Enterolactone
  Flavones, flavonols, favanones, lignans
  Genistein, daidzein, isoflavones
  Indolo[3,2-b]carbazole

[a]Although these chemicals are classified as estrogenic, their relative potency and ER-binding affinities vary widely. For example, compared to estradiol, p-nonylphenol has a relative potency of 0.000003. Also see an extensive list with references in National Research Council (1999).

Experimental evaluation of environmental endocrine disruptors has occurred using a variety of *in vitro* and *in vivo* techniques to show estrogenic activity. For a complete and thorough discussion of this area, the reader is referred to a report by the National Academy of

TABLE VI
Results of a National Library of Medicine Online Search for the Word Combination "Environmental Estrogen"

Years	Total number of articles published	Emphasis of research titles
1966–1970	9	Effects of light and heat on reproduction; one reference to PCBs
1971–1975	27	Effects of light and heat; first references to DES
1976–1980	63	More references to DES; emphasis on breast cancer and estrogens
1981–1985	78	Increased number of DES references; emphasis on diets
1986–1990	144	Greater emphasis on estrogen receptors; cancer; first reference to phytoestrogens; effects of estrogen on greater number of organs; first references to TCDD; Lindane
1991–1995	351	First reference to "xenoestrogens"; first use of "environmental estrogens" in a title; increased reference to PCB, Ah receptor; emphasis on biomarkers for estrogens; first mention of phthalate plasticizers as environmental estrogens; first mention of E Screen[a]; first presentation of the estrogen hypothesis for declining sperm counts
1996–1999	519	Increased number of chemicals evaluated; bisphenol-A referenced; increased use of in vitro testing; more aquatic species; large increase in number of end points; debates over significance of topic appear for the first time; emphasis on mechanisms of toxicity; first use of the words, "endocrine disruptor"

[a] A tissue culture bioassay to assess estrogenicity of a chemical.

Science on the these compounds and the variety of methodologies that have been used to determine that a compound is estrogenic.

Although not all environmental estrogens will be considered here, data for bisphenol-A (BPA) will be presented in some detail to illustrate the type of information that has been developed for environmental estrogens and the variety of species and experimental approaches that have been used. This will illustrate the difficulty in accurately assessing the hazards that such compounds pose in the environment. BPA is a well-recognized environmental estrogenic chemical that is used extensively in polycarbonate plastics, acrylic resins, dental sealants, and many common everyday products. Although the potency of BPA is approximately 1/1,000th to 1/5000th that of E_2, it has been shown to elicit estrogenic responses. At doses of 40–45 μg/day, BPA had a similar efficacy as estradiol for increasing prolactin release in the Fisher 344 rat. BPA also caused a large increase in prolactin gene expression through estrogen response element (ERE) activation in vitro in a pituitary cell line transfected with a reporter gene. BPA also induced progesterone receptor mRNA and protein to levels similar to estradiol

exposure, but did not change cell proliferation in the human endometrial cell line ECC-1. Using a human breast cancer cell line, BPA at concentrations at or above 10^{-6} M significantly increased cell proliferation, similar to that seen with 10^{-9} M estradiol. Other effects of BPA on female reproduction include increased uterine weight, premature vaginal opening, and persistent vaginal cornification following treatment of immature mice.

There are also estrogenic effects of BPA on the developing male. In utero exposure produces early and delayed effects on the male reproductive system. A treatment of 2 to 20 μg/kg during development causes an increase in prostate weight when the male reaches adulthood, an effect similar to that seen with DES and methoxychlor. A study by Fisher and colleagues found early effects of BPA and other estrogenic compounds (DES, ethinyl estradiol, tamoxifen, octylphenol, and genistein). With treatments between 2 and 18 days postnatally, most of these chemicals caused either an increase or a decrease in testis weight on days 18–75. Treatments that caused an increase in testis weight are interesting in light of the discovery that ERα in the efferent ductules is necessary for normal reabsorption of rete testis fluid in the male tract. In that study, the ERα knockout mouse showed luminal dilation in efferent ductules, rete testis, and seminiferous tubules, suggestive of fluid accumulation. Dilation of the rete testis was also observed with perinatal exposures to BPA, DES, and ethinyl estradiol. Decreases in testis weight and daily sperm production were also found with perinatal treatments using the estrogenic chemicals 4-octylphenol, DES, and butyl benzyl phthalate. In conclusion, evidence shows that compounds such as BPA are environmental estrogens and have effects on the male and female reproductive systems of laboratory animals, particularly during reproductive system development. However, it is difficult to establish whether this compound is a human health risk.

Aroclors are complex mixtures of different PCB congeners that were produced commercially. Certain of these PCB mixtures were discovered to be estrogenic even though the highly potent coplanar PCB congeners contained in them are antiestrogenic. In other words, the estrogenic properties of some PCB mixtures outweigh the antiestrogenic properties of the coplanar PCB congeners that they contain. This is an important point. It illustrates that large concentrations of less potent estrogenic PCB congeners in a mixture can overwhelm the effects of small concentrations of very potent antiestrogenic PCB congeners. Exposure of female rats to Aroclor 1221 greatly shortens the time to vaginal opening, induces a state of persistent vaginal estrus, and causes anovulation by 6 months of age. These effects are consistent with Aroclor 1221 being estrogenic, and the PCB congeners in Aroclors that are responsible for the estrogenic effects of the mixtures are now being identified. PCB 1, PCB 4, PCB 52, and PCB 155 were found to be estrogenic by some investigators. In addition, Soto and co-workers tested 18 PCB congeners for estrogenicity *in vitro* using the MCF-7 cell-based E-SCREEN assay and found that PCB 21, PCB 48, PCB 61, PCB 75, and PCB 136 were positive for estrogenic activity, whereas 13 other PCB congeners and Aroclor 1221 were

negative. One of the more significant outcomes of this research was the finding that none of the PCB congeners found to be estrogenic in the just-described studies is an AhR agonist.

Activity of these estrogenic PCBs is considered to result from their ability to bind ER and initiate transcription of estrogen-responsive genes. These estrogenic PCB congeners and certain hydroxylated PCB metabolites have been discovered to bind ER with highest affinity when they have at least two *ortho* chlorines, a structural feature that is incompatible with AhR agonist (TCDD-like) activity. Thus, the estrogenic activity of these PCBs and their hydroxylated metabolites is not mediated by binding AhR and activating the AhR signaling pathway. Hydroxylated metabolites of certain PCB congeners have also been discovered to exert estrogenic effects by a mechanism that does not involve binding ER. Kester and co-workers found that some hydroxylated PCBs are potent inhibitors of estrogen sulfotransferase. This enzyme is critical for sulfation and eventual inactivation of E_2. This inhibitory effect on estrogen sulfotransferase may result in increased E_2 bioavailability in estrogen target tissues and represents a new mechanism for the estrogenicity of hydroxylated PCBs of which we were previously unaware.

2. Human Health Risks

Although there is limited evidence that xenoestrogens disrupt human physiological systems, the one exception is DES, which has been studied extensively in animal models as well as in humans exposed to this compound. The effects of the potent synthetic estrogen DES on development and function of the reproductive tract illustrate a pathological response to a chemical that binds the estrogen receptor. DES was used as a prescription drug from the 1940s to the 1970s in women having a history of difficult pregnancies. In the male offspring, and in experimental animals exposed to DES during development, there are a wide variety of pathological responses. These include cryptorchid testis, testicular atrophy, epididymal cysts, sperm abnormalities, sperm granulomas, adenocarcinoma of the rete testis, prostatic inflammation, and other changes that could affect fertility and male reproductive function. One interesting discovery has been the persistence of Müllerian duct remnants in the male, which apparently interferes with the development of the male reproductive tract. A precise biochemical mechanism to account for this abnormal development is lacking. However, Sato and colleagues demonstrated that DES exposure *in utero* induces an early appearance of estrogen receptor in the male tract and that this appearance is coincident with an increase in cell division. Thus, it appears that DES may be acting directly on the developing ductal tissues. One hypothesis would be that blind-ending tubules are formed, which become filled with stagnant sperm, leading to epididymal sperm granulomas. DES stimulation of cell division in the mesonephric tubules may also lead to abnormal growth of the excurrent ducts.

In female offspring of women treated with DES during pregnancy, the first major discovery was the development of a rare form of vaginal cancer, clear cell adenocarcinoma, in the young women as they entered puberty. However, the full effects of DES exposure in women may not have reached its peak, as DES daughters are just now entering an age during which breast cancer and reproductive tract neoplasms and dysfunction commonly appear. In the female mouse exposed to DES during development, there are clear patterns of abnormal development that parallel the human, such as the presence of adenocarcinoma of the vagina. Other abnormalities, such as mammary tumors, uterine adenocarcinoma, endometrial gland hyperplasia, and prolactinomas, could be predictive of long-term problems in aging women exposed to DES *in utero*. Therefore, major human health concern remains for DES exposures that occurred nearly 50 years ago. This concern is justified based on the mouse DES model, which has been available since the 1970s.

For many years, PCBs and DDT have been suspected to be inducers of breast cancer in humans. However, epidemiology studies have found no correlation between serum concentrations of PCBs and an increased risk of breast cancer. Thus, a gap remains between clearly established data from animal studies showing chemically induced mammary gland carcinogenesis and the potential of human breast cancer following exposure to environmental estrogens. Evidence shows that some organochlorine compounds act as antiestrogens. As an antiestrogen, these chemicals could inhibit the growth of breast and endometrial cancers. An Italian study found that a group of women accidentally exposed to high levels of TCDD in 1976 had a lower incidence of breast cancer and no increase in deaths due to breast cancer. While such a finding illustrates the potential benefit of developing antiestrogens based on an Ah receptor (AhR) mechanism of action, the same Italian studies show increased risk for digestive, ovarian and bone cancers, and melanoma in the women exposed to TCDD.

Although the epidemiological findings for PCB effects on breast cancer are inconsistent across various studies, this does not lessen the impact of reports clearly showing that children are exposed to high levels of PCBs *in utero* and in breast milk. The most disturbing results are those that show learning impairment in children exposed to PCBs *in utero*.

Chlordecone was once widely used as a pesticide. It now serves as one of the best examples of an environmental estrogen having effects in men. Studies of human exposure have led to the conclusion that this compound can decrease sperm counts and induce abnormal changes in sperm morphology. Although data for chlordecone exposure in man and animal experiments support the hypothesis that environmental estrogens could lead to a decline in human sperm concentrations, a controversy over this issue still exists in the scientific community.

3. Species Differences and Applicability of in Vitro Data

Data indicating that a particular compound is estrogenic have frequently come from work with one species or one *in vitro* screening system. A crucial and controversial question for establishing the risks that environmental estrogens pose for both humans and wildlife is to establish what data showing estrogenicity in one species potentially means for other species, and to also establish how *in vitro* results demonstrating estrogenicity translate into potential risks for animals and humans *in vitro*. There are well-known species differences in susceptibility to various toxicants, even among closely related species. Furthermore, Spearow and co-workers demonstrated large differences (more than 16-fold) in the susceptibility of various strains of mice to endocrine disruption of testicular development by estrogen. Therefore, if reliable data are available showing estrogenic effects of a compound in one species, must the effects be established in each species? Conversely, does a lack of an effect in one species necessarily mean that the compound will also lack effects in another species? The potential pitfalls of either approach are clear. If we assume that a compound does have estrogenic effects in all species, based on results with one sentinel species, the potential for errors if there is substantial species variation in the responsiveness to these compounds is obvious. Conversely, to argue that effects need to be demonstrated in each species is impractical due to the obvious cost burden.

Likewise, does the ability of a test compound to show weak affinity for binding to purified estrogen receptor *in vitro* translate to real potential for harm for an animal *in vivo*? Does the ability of a compound to show estrogenic activity based on its stimulation of proliferation in the estrogen-responsive MCF-7 cell line translate into demonstrable risks for an animal *in vivo*? Questions concerning the extrapolation of *in vitro* results to different species and the ability of *in vitro* results to be extrapolated to *in vivo* situations further complicate the important task of assessing the risks of these compounds and are likely to be highly contentious no matter what approach is adopted. Although the consideration of species differences and applicability of *in vitro* data to animals *in vivo* is included in this section, the basic questions have relevance and applicability to all types of

compounds that are potentially disrupting any endocrine system and must be considered on a case-by-case basis.

B. ANDROGENS AND ANTIANDROGENS

The majority of research in the area of endocrine disruptors was initially focused on estrogenic chemicals, but recent work has indicated that other endocrine systems are also vulnerable to disruption by a variety of environmental chemicals. Androgens are critical for differentiation of the developing male reproductive system and play essential roles in the subsequent development and adult function of the testis, prostate, epididymis, and other male reproductive organs. Although environmental chemicals can potentially act at many levels to disrupt androgenic signaling (e.g., direct actions on Leydig cells to decrease or increase activities of steroidogenic enzymes, actions on the kidney and liver to alter catabolism and excretion of androgens, decreases or increases in the activity of 5α-reductase, the enzyme that converts testosterone to its more active metabolite, dihydrotestosterone), present evidence indicates that one of the critical mechanisms of action may involve environmental chemicals that have affinity for the androgen receptor and can directly affect androgenic signaling by this mechanism. The fungicide vinclozolin was the first compound identified that worked in this manner. Vinclozolin was reported to induce a variety of antiandrogenic effects in developing males. The mechanism of this effect was subsequently elucidated when it was shown that the two major metabolites of vinclozolin, M1 and M2, could compete strongly for androgen receptor binding (although the parent compound vinclozolin has only very limited activity in this regard) but they do not activate subsequent transcriptional steps as the normal androgenic ligands would. Similarly, *p,p'*-DDE, a very persistent metabolite of DDT that is widely distributed in the environment, is not an estrogen but does bind androgen receptor and inhibit androgen-induced transcriptional activity. The widely used insecticide methoxychlor appears to be another chemical that acts by a similar mechanism in that a metabolite of methoxy-chlor, HPTE, is a competitive inhibitor of androgen receptor binding.

Sohoni and Sumpter have used *in vitro* yeast-based assays to examine androgenic and anti-androgenic activities of a variety of environmental chemicals of current interest; their results showed that other chemicals previously shown to act as environmental estrogens, such as bisphenol A and butyl benzyl phthalate, were also antiandrogenic. Interestingly, another compound with documented estrogenic activity, nonylphenol, was found to be a weak androgen agonist using the yeast system, although it is not clear if it would exhibit those properties in animals *in vivo*. Results have also indicated that other environmental chemicals, such as di(*n*-butyl) phthalate (DBP) and diethylhexylphthalate (DEHP), can disrupt male rat reproductive development and function in a manner similar to antiandrogens. Because DBP and its biologically active metabolite did not bind the androgen receptor *in vitro*, it is an example of an environmental antiandrogen that disrupts androgen-regulated male sexual differentiation through a mechanism apparently distinct from the other antiandrogens described previously.

In summary, there is a growing list of environmental compounds that function as antiandrogens by binding the androgen receptor without activating transcription. Some of these compounds are also estrogenic, but not all environmental estrogens are antiandrogenic, and there is at least one example of an environmental estrogen that also functions as a weak androgen, at least *in vitro*. The recent description of an antiandrogen that does not appear to interact with the androgen receptor further illustrates the complexity of this area and the need for further study to understand the mechanisms of action of these chemicals. Information on whether environmental antiandrogens cause adverse health effects in humans or wildlife is limited. Two studies suggest that exposure to an antiandrogenic DDT metabolite is associated with shortened lactation in humans.

C. EFFECTS OF ENDOCRINE DISRUPTORS ON PROGESTERONE SIGNALING

Substantial evidence suggests that endocrine disruptors may affect both progesterone production and progesterone receptor (PR) expression. Coplanar PCBs can decrease serum progesterone concentrations in females. The AhR agonist TCDD has also been reported to decrease plasma progesterone levels, suggesting that the PCBs might inhibit progesterone production through an AhR-mediated mechanism. However, other studies have not reported changes in progesterone following PCB treatment. The variety of species and dosing regimens used in these studies makes it hard to interpret the different results and suggests that effects of PCB exposure on circulating progesterone levels need to be established more definitively.

Estrogenic endocrine disruptors also have the capacity to alter the levels of expression of PR, and thus affect normal progesterone signaling in this manner. Estrogen is the major regulator of the magnitude of PR expression in reproductive organs such as the vagina and uterus. Estrogen normally increases PR, and effects of estrogen on PR expression are primarily mediated by ERα. Therefore, environmental chemicals that are estrogenic and can signal through ERα would also be expected to modulate PR expression. Indeed, increases in PR in the mink in response to PCB treatment have been reported. Likewise, environmental compounds with antiestrogenic effects would also be expected to modulate PR expression and therefore affect progesterone signaling.

D. DISRUPTION OF ENDOCRINE HOMEOSTASIS THROUGH OTHER STEROID RECEPTORS

The past decade has witnessed the use of the techniques of molecular biology to identify a wide variety of receptors for which no ligand was initially known. The elucidation of the functions of these orphan receptors and their natural ligands will almost certainly be accompanied by the discovery of natural or man-made compounds that can interact and signal through these orphan receptors. Therefore, it is likely that the list of endocrine disruptors, as well as the types of effects ascribed to them, will continue to grow in the coming years.

An example of this is the discovery of pregnane X receptors (PXR), new members of the nuclear hormone receptor superfamily, and the subsequent discovery that PCBs can act as an agonist for this receptor. Following the initial discovery of PXR, it was found that several steroid hormones, such as progesterone, pregnenolone, the antiandrogen cyproterone acetate, and synthetic glucocorticoids and antiglucocorticoids, bind to PXR and modulate the expression of cytochrome P450 3A genes in the liver. Activation of this receptor may be involved in modulating hepatic cytochrome P450 activity in response to endogenous dietary or hormonal signals and thus may be important in steroid hormone metabolism. PCBs, as well as other endocrine-disrupting chemicals, such as phthalic acid and nonylphenol, have been shown to bind and activate PXR. Thus, environmental endocrine disruptors such as PCBs may affect steroid hormone metabolism through PXR, indicating not only direct endocrine-disrupting effects through PXR agonist activity, but also the possibility of secondary effects on a wide variety of steroid hormones due to altered metabolism.

E. DISRUPTORS OF THYROID HORMONE HOMEOSTASIS

1. Mechanism of Action

A variety of natural and man-made chemicals can alter thyroid hormone levels. Among the most important are the environmentally ubiquitous PCBs, which can produce decreases in circulating thyroxine (T_4) of as much as 80–90%. TCDD also produces decreased T_4 concentrations. However, triiodothyronine (T_3) concentrations are not decreased following TCDD treatment, and there is evidence that TCDD-treated rats are not functionally hypothyroid because they do not show alterations in liver enzymes and other parameters typically associated with hypothyroidism. In addition, some

pesticides such as linuron or decomposition products of pesticides such as ethylenethiourea also produce hypothyroidism, and a variety of coal-derived pollutants have been shown to have antithyroid activities. Finally, the consumption of a diet low in iodine results in goiter and, in more severe cases, hypothyroidism in humans. Therefore, the dietary content of an essential nutrient such as iodine can also function as an environmental endocrine disruptor.

Environmental agents that produce hypothyroidism, such as PCBs and TCDD, appear to do so by altering transport, metabolism, and/or degradation of the thyroid hormone. These compounds increase levels of hepatic UDP-glucuronosyltransferase, which catalyzes glucuronidation of T_4 and ultimate excretion of T_4-glucoronide in bile; therefore, increases in this enzyme result in decreased circulating T_4. In addition, some hydroxylated PCB metabolites compete with T_4 for transthyretin, the plasma thyroid hormone transport protein. Certain PCB congeners actually have greater affinity for transthyretin than does T_4 itself, which causes enhanced displacement of T_4 from its carrier protein. Because bound T_4 is not removed from circulation but unbound is, PCB binding to transthyretin results in increased unbound T_4 and enhanced removal of T_4 from the circulation.

The ability of PCBs to compete for transthyretin binding, along with structural similarities between PCBs and thyroid hormones, led to speculation that PCBs may bind to thyroid hormone receptors. Thus, PCBs may act at the thyroid receptor in addition to their other effects, but this remains unproven.

2. Human Health Effects

A critical question is whether exposure of humans to PCBs, TCDD, or other environmental chemicals can produce deleterious effects in humans due to their effects on thyroid hormones. There is some evidence linking these environmental chemicals to changes in thyroid hormone levels and subsequent neurological effects of altered thyroid homeostasis. Two

Dutch studies have found that levels of PCBs and TCDD in breast milk were correlated with decreases in thyroid hormones in both the mother and offspring. Children of mothers exposed to high levels of PCBs through the consumption of PCB-contaminated cooking oil during pregnancy in the Yusho incident in Japan and Yu-Cheng incident in Taiwan have intellectual deficits. In addition, a series of studies in both the United States and Europe have suggested that environmental exposures to PCBs prenatally can affect neurological development, although not all studies in this area have found neurological changes as a result of PCB exposure. The critical role of thyroid hormones in neurological development suggests an obvious link between the observed effects of PCBs on thyroid hormone levels and neurological development. However, no one has yet proven a causative link between PCB effects on thyroid hormones and their effects on neurological development, although this remains an area of active investigation.

F. ARYL HYDROCARBON RECEPTOR AGONISTS

In laboratory mammals, TCDD exposure causes a wide variety of adverse health effects, including developmental and reproductive toxicity, and it appears that the vast majority of effects of TCDD are mediated by binding to the AhR. Although it is generally agreed that AhR binding is necessary for manifestation of TCDD effects and that TCDD exposure can modulate estrogen and androgen signaling and disrupt thyroid hormone homeostasis, it is not clear in all cases how TCDD exerts its endocrine-disrupting effects. Certain coplanar PCBs that also activate AhR signaling pathways can mimic both antiestrogenic and antiandrogenic effects of TCDD. The effects of TCDD and coplanar PCBs on thyroid hormone homeostasis were discussed in a separate section because a number of compounds can affect thyroid hormone homeostasis by mechanisms that do not involve AhR. This section considers antiestrogenic and antiandrogenic actions of AhR agonists.

1. AhR Agonists Can Function as Antiestrogens

TCDD has been shown to act as an antiestrogen in a number of model systems. For example, it inhibits estradiol-induced increases in uterine wet weight in mice and rats and interferes with estradiol-induced increases in rat uterine peroxidase activity and rat uterine epidermal growth factor receptor-binding activity level. The mechanism of these effects may involve TCDD-induced decreases in estrogen receptor protein levels and consequent decreases in binding activity, both of which have been observed in the uterus and liver. However, antiestrogenic effects of TCDD exposure may also be due to TCDD interference in the process by which the liganded estrogen receptor binds DNA, and this could also be a crucial component of the antiestrogenic TCDD effect.

Increases in estradiol metabolism in a breast cancer cell line have also been observed, although *in vivo* studies have in general failed to link increased estradiol metabolism with TCDD exposure, suggesting that it does not make a critical contribution to the antiestrogenic effects of TCDD *in vivo*.

The antiestrogenic effects of TCDD appear to result from interference with processes believed to be mediated by the classical estrogen receptor ERα. The discovery of a second form of ER, ERβ, further complicates analysis of the antiestrogenic actions of TCDD. The role of ERβ is not yet understood, and it is not clear if TCDD will also inhibit actions mediated by this second form of ER. In summary, although TCDD is known to be antiestrogenic in several model systems, its mechanism for producing this effect remains to be definitively determined.

In addition to the estrogenic effects of certain PCB congeners and/or their hydroxylated metabolites, discussed in Section IV,A,1, some PCBs and hydroxy-PCBs can also inhibit the effects of endogenous estrogens and function as antiestrogens. Seven PCBs have been shown to produce antiestrogenic effects (PCBs 77, 126, 169, 155 *in vivo* and *in vitro*, PCBs 105, 114, and 156 *in vitro* only), while another two (PCBs 37 and 81) have predicted antiestrogenic properties. In addition, a series of hydroxy-PCBs have antiestrogenic activity. Like the antiestrogenic effects of TCDD, the antiestrogenic effects of these PCB congeners are thought to be mediated by the AhR. Coplanar PCBs, which function as AhR agonists, are normally the PCB congeners with demonstrated or predicted antiestrogenic activity, but at least one higher chlorinated noncoplanar congener (PCB 155) has demonstrated antiestrogenicity both *in vitro* and *in vivo*.

2. AhR Agonists Can Function as Antiandrogens

Treatment of adult male rats with an overtly toxic dose of TCDD decreases circulating androgen concentrations due to decreased LH-stimulated testosterone production by the testis and other Leydig cell effects. Similarly, treatment of young rats with the coplanar PCB 77 leads to decreased circulating testosterone levels at 35 and 70 days of age. It has also been found that prenatal treatment of rats with either Aroclor 1254, which contains coplanar PCBs with AhR agonist activity, or a reconstituted mixture of PCB congeners that simulates the congener mixture found in human milk caused decreased testosterone levels during adulthood.

In utero and lactational exposure of male rats to low doses of TCDD decreases accessory sex organ weights, delays preputial separation, decreases epididymal and ejaculated sperm numbers, partially demasculinizes sexual behavior, partially feminizes sexual behavior, and partially feminizes the regulation of LH secretion. The manifestation of these effects would be consistent with decreased testicular androgen production and/or circulating androgen concentrations, but neither of these parameters has been shown to be significantly affected, either perinatally or at later times, by *in utero* and lactational TCDD exposure. The possibility remains, however, that the androgenic deficiency-like syndrome that follows *in utero* and lactational TCDD exposure could be the result

of interference with androgen receptor signaling at or beyond the androgen receptor.

Administration of an androgen receptor antagonist such as flutamide, the fungicide vinclozolin, or the DDT metabolite *p,p'*-DDE to male rodents during perinatal development can result in decreased testis, epididymis, and accessory sex organ weights, delayed preputial separation, decreased daily sperm production, and decreased caudal epididymal sperm number. However, with developmental antiandrogen exposure, the decreases in daily sperm production and caudal epididymal sperm number stem from a high incidence of seminiferous tubule atrophy and, in some cases, a failure of the testis to descend, while this does not occur with TCDD exposure. Effects of antiandrogen and TCDD exposure on sexual behavior, the volume of certain hypothalamic nuclei associated with sexual behavior, and the regulation of LH secretion are qualitatively similar. In contrast, antiandrogen exposure but not TCDD exposure decreases relative anogenital distance, causes sterility, feminizes external genitalia, produces hypospadias with cleft prepuce, and results in nipple formation.

In some respects, effects of *in utero* and lactational TCDD exposure resemble those of *in utero* exposure to the 5α-reductase inhibitors. However, as with antiandrogen exposure, *in utero* exposure of male rats to finasteride results in feminization of external genitalia, hypospadias with cleft prepuce, and nipple formation, effects that are not observed in response to *in utero* and lactational TCDD exposure. In addition, 5α-reductase inhibition significantly decreases relative anogenital distance, while TCDD exposure usually does not. These discrepancies cannot be explained by different windows of sensitivity for effects of 5α-reductase inhibition nor can they be explained by different dose–response curves for effects of 5α-reductase inhibition so it is unlikely that TCDD-induced inhibition of 5α-reductase activity could explain effects on prostate growth and preputial separation, and the exact mechanism of the antiandrogenic actions of TCDD remain unclear.

3. Can Aryl Hydrocarbon Receptor Agonists Produce Adverse Health Effects in Humans?

A relationship between TCDD exposure and adverse outcomes is suggested by various epidemiologic studies. An increased risk of cancer is associated with a TCDD body burden in humans of 109–7000 ng/kg. Reduced birth weights and delayed developmental milestones occur at a maternal body burden of 2130 ng of TCDD equivalents (TEQs)/kg. These body burdens are greater than the background body burden of the TCDD-like polychlorinated dibenzo-p-dioxins (PCDDs), polychlorinated dibenzofurans (PCDFs), and PCBs in people that was estimated in 1995 to be 9–13 ng TEQs/kg body weight and is about half that range today. Nevertheless, a lower birth weight, poorer neurologic condition, and lower psychomotor scores have been associated with maternal body burdens of about 16 ng TEQ/kg, which are just above background. Also, background level dioxin exposure in humans has been associated with an increased prevalence of diabetes. Taken together, these findings suggest that TCDD and related compounds are capable of producing adverse health effects at near background body burdens in humans.

Results of laboratory animal studies support this interpretation. Treatment of pregnant rats with a single dose of TCDD of 64 ng/kg (Holtzman strain) or 50 ng/kg (Long Evans strain) on gestational day 15 caused significant reductions in sperm counts in male offspring in adulthood. The 50 ng/kg dose resulted in a maternal body burden of 27 ng/kg of TCDD on gestational day 21, a few times higher than the background body burden in people, and a TCDD body burden in the rat fetus on gestational day 21 of only 4.3 ng/kg. Thus, adverse developmental effects of TCDD can also be produced in animals at near background human body burden levels. Because epidemiologic studies demonstrate that animals and humans are generally similar in their response to TCDD, these findings suggest that the current margin of exposure of humans to TCDD and related compounds is probably not adequate.

G. PHYTOESTROGENS

1. Effects Mediated through ERα

For many years, the majority of research on endocrine disruptors has been focused on man-made chemicals such as DDT, PCBs, and dioxins, which are global environmental contaminants and have well-documented endocrine effects. However, not all endocrine disruptors are man-made, and not all endocrine disruptors are necessarily deleterious to human health. There is a significant literature extending back almost 50 years that documents the effects of phytoestrogens, which are defined as estrogenic compounds of plant origin. In recent years, there has been substantial interest in the potential for these compounds to exert broad beneficial effects on human health, based on a variety of studies using epidemiological, in vitro, and in vivo approaches.

Over 300 plants that have estrogenic activity have been identified, although only about half of these plant species are consumed routinely by humans or livestock. A variety of isoflavonoids, lignans, and other compounds have been shown to have estrogenic activity. However, the vast majority of the research activity has focused on coumestrol, which is found in high concentrations in certain types of clover, and genistein and daidzein, which are most abundant in soy, but are also found at lower levels in other foods.

The first literature on the effects of phytoestrogens dates back to the 1940s, when sheep in Australia developed a variety of reproductive problems, including decreased fecundity. The problem was eventually found to result from the consumption of clover (Trifolium subterraneum) by the sheep, although it was a decade later when the phytoestrogens in clover were actually identified.

An extensive literature suggests that phytoestrogens from soy may have effects on human health. People in Far Eastern countries, who consume diets rich in soy, have lower incidences of prostate cancer, heart disease, osteoporosis, and menopausal symptoms than residents of Western countries. In addition, studies of women in Japan and Singapore have reported a 30–60% decrease in premenopausal breast cancer in women consuming high levels of soy. Similarly, consumption of tofu by Asian-American women was associated with a decrease in both premenopausal and postmenopausal breast cancer. The benefits of soy on breast cancer have not been seen universally, however, and a Chinese study reported no link between soy consumption and either premenopausal or postmenopausal breast cancer.

Although the mechanism by which soy consumption is associated with decreased susceptibility to these diseases is not clear, the phytoestrogens found in soy may play a major role in its health benefits. For example, Anthony and colleagues showed that a diet containing soy as the major protein source reduced coronary artery atherosclerotic lesions by 90% in monkeys as compared to those given a diet containing casein and lactalbumin as protein sources. However, when the phytoestrogens were extracted from the soy, it was much less effective in inhibiting atherosclerosis.

Genistein and daidzein were previously available only in relatively low levels in food, but products containing high levels of genistein and daidzein are now sold as health supplements, based on their potential role in lessening major human diseases. Similarly, coumestrol is now marketed as a natural estrogen supplement that can lessen menopausal symptoms in women and has a variety of beneficial effects in postmenopausal women due to its estrogenic properties. These compounds can now be obtained in dietary supplements in quantities greater than would ever be obtained in food, suggesting that humans consuming these supplements will be exposed to levels of genistein, daidzein, and other soy constituents at levels that are not obtained naturally.

Of greatest concern may be the effects on human infants consuming high levels of soy. Setchell and co-workers have shown that plasma levels of genistein and daidzein in infants drinking soy milk were 10-fold greater than those in adults consuming a high soy diet and that levels of soy isoflavones in these infants were up to 22,000 times higher than levels of estradiol during early life. There clearly are potential beneficial effects of phytoestrogens, but the fact that these chemicals are from natural sources does not eliminate the possibility that they could be harmful in excessively large amounts or that they could be contraindicated for certain people based on age or disease status (e.g., women who have estrogen-responsive breast cancer). Because substantial numbers of adults are beginning to ingest large amounts of these substances regularly and because soy milk is used extensively to feed infants that cannot tolerate normal milk, it is imperative that we develop a more complete understanding of the potential effects of phytoestrogens.

As discussed previously, estrogens are the major endocrine regulator of female reproduction, play critical roles in the etiology and growth of breast, endometrial, cervical, and vaginal cancer, and also have at least a permissive role in diseases such as endometriosis. ERα is the critical ER for the vaginal and uterine effects commonly associated with estradiol treatment, while the role of ERβ in the female reproductive tract is not yet established. Genistein, daidzein, coumestrol, and other compounds that act as phytoestrogens bind ERα, although their affinity for ERα and their ability to induce transcription of estrogen-responsive genes are very low compared to the major endogenous estrogen, E_2. For example, although estimates of the ability of genistein to mimic the effects of E_2 on ERα vary depending on the test system, Kuiper and co-workers reported that genistein had approximately 1/4000th of the potency of E_2 for stimulating the transcription of genes through the ERα receptor. Despite the low estrogenic potency of genistein, it is potentially capable of exerting major physiological effects due to its high concentrations in some human diets. Asian diets that are high in soy may result in daily consumption of 1 mg of isoflavones/kg body weight, and plasma concentrations of 1 μM have been reported in Japanese consuming a high soy diet.

In addition to functioning as an ERα agonist, genistein may also act as an ERα antagonist in certain situations, which may also be crucial for its health benefits. For example, in menopausal women where E_2 levels are low, genistein may ameliorate the effects of the E_2 deficiency on bone loss and menopausal symptoms by acting as a weak agonist for ERα. Conversely, in premenopausal women, genistein may occupy a significant fraction of ERα receptors, thereby attenuating the stimulation due to the high endogenous levels of E_2 in these women, and produce a lower estrogen response than would occur if these receptors bound E_2. This appears to be a significant factor in the ability of genistein to prevent breast cancer. Thus, genistein can act either as an agonist or as an antagonist, depending on the hormonal environment, and both effects can be beneficial.

2. Can Phytoestrogens Affect Signaling though ERβ?

ERβ is widely expressed in the male and female reproductive tract, vascular system, heart, brain, and other estrogen target organs, and ERβ is frequently expressed in estrogen-dependent tumors. Therefore, although its role in normal tissue and the development and progression of certain tumors remain to be established, ERβ may be an important regulator of estrogenic responses in both normal and pathological tissue. Despite extensive data documenting the interaction of phytoestrogens such as genistein, coumestrol, and daidzein with ERβ, it is unknown if these chemicals can interact with ERβ in vivo to induce physiological effects. This critical lack of information results from the fact that ERβ was discovered only in the late 1990s, and that despite the presence of high levels of ERβ in some reproductive organs such as prostate and the expression of significant levels in all others, no reproductive functions of ERβ have been identified.

Although it still is unclear which effects of estrogen may involve ERβ, studies indicate that genistein may act preferentially through ERβ.

Genistein has low affinity for binding to ERα (only 4% that of E_2), but genistein has high binding affinity for ERβ (87% of that for E_2). The increased binding affinity of genistein for ERβ suggests that this phytoestrogen might act preferentially through ERβ, but a critical test is whether genistein binds ERβ and initiates transcription. Kuiper and colleagues investigated the estrogenic activity of genistein and other phytoestrogens in a transient gene expression assay. In this assay, ERβ cDNA and an estrogen-dependent reporter gene who transfected into human cells and then the ability of E_2 to induce transcription was measured by examining reporter gene induction in response to E_2, genistein, or other phytoestrogens. Interestingly, genistein was more effective than E_2 in this system. Most other natural and synthetic estrogens had similar abilities to induce transcription through ERα or ERβ, but the strong ability of genistein to induce transcription through ERβ contrasted with its modest ability to do so through ERα, suggesting genistein acts preferentially through ERβ.

It has not been possible to determine whether phytoestrogen actions in vivo may be mediated in part by ERβ due to the lack of known effects mediated by ERβ. One difficulty in identifying ERβ-mediated effects is that normal animals express both ERα and ERβ, making it difficult to attribute any E_2 effect to ERβ. The availability of the ERα knockout (αERKO) mouse, along with the development of the ERβ knockout (βERKO) mouse, should provide useful tools to determine which effects of phytoestrogens, if any, are mediated through ERβ.

3. Human Health Effects of Soy Mediated through Endocrine Modulation

Although epidemiological studies suggest human health benefits from the consumption of soy and phytoestrogens such as genistein, the effects of these compounds are not firmly established. This is an area of increasing research focus because the consumption of dietary supplements containing extremely high levels of soy protein or phytoestrogens derived from soy or other sources by humans is presently occurring. Such consumption of these compounds, which are far in excess of what would be obtained in representative human diets, may be premature until we develop a better understanding of how these compounds act, when they may be useful, and when they may not be advisable.

V. Exposure to Endocrine Disruptors: Are There Risks?

A. WILDLIFE POPULATIONS

Endocrine disruption among wildlife populations has been suspected since the 1960s, beginning with the use of the organochlorine pesticide DDT. DDT was finally banned in most developed countries in the 1970s because its metabolite p,p'-DDE and the contaminating pesticide isomer o,p'-DDT were thought to be estrogenic. These insecticides, along with other chlorinated hydrocarbon pesticides, are lipophilic and capable of accumulating in body and egg fat of birds, fish, amphibians, mammalian wildlife, domestic animals, and humans. Thus, these chemicals enter the food chain and are stored primarily in the body fat and are passed on to subsequent generations or to higher levels within the food chain. Numerous abnormalities and endocrine disorders have been reported from exposure to these estrogenic (and, in some cases, antiandrogenic) chemicals. These anomalies include avian egg shell thinning; feminization or demasculinization of birds, fish, reptiles, and mammals; reduced gonad size; reduced egg size; decreases in fertility or hatching; disruption of thyroid function; weakened immune system; skewed sex ratios; and cryptorchidism.

One of the best known examples of endocrine disruption in a wildlife population is the alligator living in Florida's Lake Apopka. In 1980, there was a chemical spill from a nearby company, which contaminated the lake with a mixture of dicofol, DDT, and DDE. Numerous endocrine abnormalities were observed in the population of alligators: demasculinized male genital system resulting in small phalluses; abnormal testes, decreased levels of hormones;

relative increase in estrogen in both males and females; abnormal ovaries; decreased hatching; increased mortality rate of hatchlings; and a 90% decline in the number of juvenile alligators from 1980 to 1987. Dr. Lou Guillette and co-workers at the University of Florida were the first to recognize this pattern of endocrine disruption as a potential problem of environmental estrogen contamination. This hypothesis has since been modified to include the new finding that certain effects of DDT are mediated in part through antiandrogenic actions of its persistent metabolite p,p'-DDE (see previous section).

Another important focus in the 1990s has been the effects of endocrine disruptors on fish reproduction. This topic was brought to light with the report that synthetic estrogens from the use of birth control pills (ethinyl estradiol) were appearing in river waters in the United Kingdom. Hermaphrodite fish were also being caught in lagoons near sewage treatment plants. Therefore, experiments were performed by placing control male fish in selected pools downstream from suspect sewage sites. Vitellogenin can be used as a sensitive as an estrogen biomarker, as it is normally synthesized in the liver of female fish in response to estrogen and used in the formation of egg yolk, but is not produced in males unless they have been exposed to estrogens. Researchers found vitellogenin expression in the male fish, where it would not normally be expected to occur, indicating that the effluents from sewage treatment plants were contaminated with estrogen-like chemicals. In addition to ethinyl estradiol, synthetic alkylphenols, natural plant sterols, and organochlorines have been associated with these contaminated waterways. In conclusion, wildlife species have functioned as sentinels for potential endocrine-disrupting contaminants in our environment, although it is not clear if the chemical exposures that have deleterious effects on wildlife populations represent a significant threat to human health.

B. HUMAN HEALTH

Evidence shows that human exposure to DES, TCDD and related AhR agonists, DDT, or

DDE can lead to the development of adverse human health effects, particularly through developmental deficits. Other examples of environmental endocrine disruption in humans are lacking. However, that is not to say that concern for endocrine disruptors does not apply to humans. Rather, it is difficult to assess human health risk from an evaluation of laboratory animal and human health effects data when there is a general paucity of exposure data on human body burdens of mixtures of potential environmental endocrine-disrupting chemicals, particularly in women of childbearing age. Humans have been exposed directly to high levels of DES and to certain organochlorines, and documented effects included reproductive tract cancers, abnormal development of the reproductive tract, and thyroid alterations. Thus, future work must address this concern and our lack of understanding on how best to extrapolate experimental data to human health risk.

Although there may be relatively few examples of environmental endocrine disruptors affecting humans directly, there are several circumstantial concerns that have stirred scientific inquiry and debate, as well as extensive lay press coverage. The most popular is the reported decline in human sperm counts. This report, along with a string of studies showing potential environmental effects on penis development and increases in the incidence of cryptorchidism and testicular cancers, led to the formal presentation of the hypothesis that exposure *in utero* to chemicals having estrogen-like activity could account for these purported abnormalities in male reproduction. This hypothesis has stirred no less than a worldwide debate among scientists as well as news reporters. Good arguments are presented in favor of this conclusion, including new studies among Frenchmen, whereas other studies provide evidence that argues against a global decline in sperm counts. Thus, from epidemiological data, it may be impossible to conclude that sperm counts are declining worldwide due to environmental endocrine disruptors, but the weight of evidence strongly suggests that declines are occurring in a region-specific manner.

However, experimental animal data have clearly established pathophysiological mechanisms to account for chemical-induced reductions in sperm counts.

Another major concern is the discovery that dramatic increases in testicular cancer in men less than 50 years of age have occurred in several countries. The differences between countries is dramatic, with Denmark exhibiting the highest incidence with nearly 25 cases per 10,000 men. It may be argued that such an increase in testicular cancer is more likely due to environmental factors because the increases are so specific to geographic locations. Another compelling argument is the fact that testicular cancer has a strong association with cryptorchidism, which is one of the most recognized effects of estrogenic compounds on the male reproductive tract during development.

It has also been tempting to link the rising incidence of prostate cancer on environmental factors, although an expansion in detection through screening may also be a factor in the reported increase. However, one study in Canada did show a weak but significant correlation between the number of acres sprayed with herbicides in 1970 and risk of prostate cancer mortality. Prostate cancer has also been associated with long-term exposure to coke oven emissions, which contain coal tar volatiles and polycyclic aromatic hydrocarbons. Thus, although much of the evidence for endocrine disruptor effects in humans may be circumstantial, data suggest that long-term exposures to some chemicals may increase the chances of cancer in the male reproductive system.

Finally, the potential link between breast cancer and environmental chemical exposures cannot be ignored. In fact, it was this specific concern that led to the current law requiring the Environmental Protection Agency (EPA) to develop a screening and testing strategy for the detection of endocrine disruptors. Although a recent epidemiology study does not show correlation between PCB exposure and risk for breast cancer, the weight of other evidence has been sufficiently strong to warrant the formation of a major program at Cornell University titled,

"Breast Cancer and Environmental Risk Factors in New York State." Their internet website provides one of the most thorough discussions on this topic (http://www.cfe.cornell.edu/bcerf/default.t). The potential roles that diet, estrogens, and exposures to pesticides and alcohol play in establishing the risk for breast cancer are carefully analyzed. There is concern that current animal models may not be appropriate for screening environmental chemicals for induction of mammary tumors. For example, the herbicide atrazine induces mammary tumors in the Sprague–Dawley rat, a strain that has a high rate of spontaneous mammary tumors, but not in the Fisher 344.

VI. Techniques for Screening Endocrine Disruptors

In the early 1990s, the U.S. EPA was concerned about the potential for chemicals to act as endocrine disruptors and began to discuss endocrine screening methods. The complexity of designing screening methods that are capable of detecting endocrine disruption is easily recognized by the large number of end points that are now considered evidence for estrogenicity. In 1996 the EPA formed a scientific committee called (Endocrine Disruptor Screening and Testing Advisory Committee; EDSTAC) under the Federal Advisory Committee Act for the purpose of advising the EPA on the screening and testing of pesticides and chemicals for their potential to disrupt the endocrine system. Two acts of Congress were passed in 1996: the Food Quality Protection Act and amendments to the Safe Drinking Water Act, which required the EPA to develop the screening and testing strategy by August 1998 and to implement screening and testing by August 1999. A final report by the committee can be found at the following internet site: http://www.epa.gov/oscpmont/oscpendo/. Many of the concepts found in this report and the screening methods adopted by the EPA are worthy of evaluation.

The congressional act required the EPA to "develop a screening program, using appropriate validated test systems and other scientifically relevant information, to determine whether certain substances may have an effect in humans that is similar to an effect produced by a naturally occurring estrogen, or other such endocrine effect as the Administrator may designate." The EPA basically accepted the recommendations of the EDSTAC report, which found agreement to include the testing for androgens, antiandrogens, and thyroid hormone effects, in addition to screening for estrogens and antiestrogens. A general definition of an endocrine disruptor was accepted by EDSTAC: "an exogenous chemical substance or mixture that alters the structure or function(s) of the endocrine system and causes adverse effects at the level of the organism, its progeny, populations, or subpopulations of organisms, based on scientific principles, data, weight-of-evidence, and the precautionary principle."

The conceptual framework of the committee's recommendations is seen in the final report. It basically establishes tiers for screening, testing, and hazard assessment after an initial sorting using existing data. A compound that does not enter tier 1 or 2 is placed in a "hold" category. After the initial sorting of data, it will be necessary to set priorities on chemicals entering the tier 1 phase of testing. Priority will be based on (1) prior testing using "high throughput prescreening" that will detect hormonal activity for biological effects-related information; (2) exposure-related information; and (3) specially targeted compartments, i.e., chemicals having widespread exposure at the national level, chemical mixtures, and naturally occurring nonsteroidal estrogens such as mycotoxins.

The high throughput prescreening method will detect hormone receptor-binding affinity and transcriptional activation by incorporating rapid instrument technologies with the use of *in vitro* assays. To reduce the overwhelming load of such a screen, the EDSTAC recommended the testing of only chemicals produced in an amount equal to or greater than 10,000 pounds per year and all pesticides (approximately 15,000 chemicals). Receptor-binding assays of biochemical preparations containing the hormone receptor will determine binding as a function of the test chemical concentration. However, receptor binding alone does not correlate with effects on gene expression, be they positive or negative. Thus, transcriptional activation assays using cells *in vitro* will also be employed. These assays utilize a hormone receptor and a reporter gene construct (such as luciferase) that upon binding of the chemical (ligand) to the receptor–ligand complex can result in DNA transcription and subsequent production of the marker protein mRNA. The EPA has the responsibility of validating these assays and determining the feasibility of performing these rapid screens on a large number of diverse chemicals.

The tier 1 screening assays recommended include three *in vitro* [estrogen receptor (ER) binding/transcriptional activation assay, androgen receptor (AR) binding/transcriptional activation assay, and steroidogenesis assay with minced testis] and three *in vivo* (rodent 3-day uterotrophic assay, rodent 20-day pubertal female assay with thyroid evaluation, and rodent 5 to 7-day castrated male rat hershberger assay) mammalian assays and two *in vivo* nonmammalian assays (frog metamorphosis assay and fish gonadal recrudescence assay).

Possible alternative assays, recommended by EDSTAC, include *in vitro* placental aromatase assay, *in vivo* rodent 14-day intact adult male assay with thyroid evaluation, and *in vivo* Rodent 20-day thyroid/pubertal male Assay.

Positive controls for these assays would be E$_2$, diethylstilbestrol, testosterone, or thyroxine. It was recommended that the route of exposure should be decided based on that which is "most realistic for detecting potential endocrine activity" for the tier 1 screen.

For tier 2, the assays would be based on an "exposure route(s), which approximates the ecologically relevant exposure pathway, dependent on the test species and fate of the chemical in the environment." The tier 2 screening battery recommended *in vivo* studies. Proposed are a two-generation reproductive toxicity study using mammalian species and multigeneration tests

using other taxonomic groups, including birds, amphibians, fish, and invertebrates. These other tests would involve avian reproduction; fish life cycle; mysid life cycle; and amphibian development and reproduction. Another type of mammalian reproduction test or a one-generation test could substitute for the two-generation mammalian reproduction study.

In summary, the EPA will be using the recommendations of the EDSTAC report to establish screening methods for the detection of chemicals that disrupt estrogen, androgen, and thyroid hormone function. Proposed is a tier system with an initial sorting and priority setting based on published effects and data collected from a high-throughput prescreening system. Specific screening methods recommended ranged from *in vitro* receptor-binding assays to *in vivo* rodent, bird, frog, fish, and invertebrate assays.

VII. Conclusions, Controversy, and Questions

In conclusion, it appears that wildlife data provide the strongest support for environmental chemicals having the potential to act as endocrine disruptors. The sparseness of human epidemiological data is of concern to many biological scientists, especially in light of the "weight of evidence" that is provided by wildlife data that have been published to date. The topic of endocrine disruption is not becoming more simple to understand, but rather more complex. For example, we now must consider the interaction of two estrogen receptors, ERα and ERβ, which have the same affinity for the most common estrogen, 17β-estradiol, but exhibit differences in binding affinities for environmental estrogens, such as genistein and bisphenol-A. Some have argued that the normal intake of natural and environmental antiestrogens would counteract the potentially harmful endocrine disruptors that humans are exposed to during their lifetime. However, until we obtain more information regarding the actual concentrations of these chemicals in human tissues at critical times during development and reproductive function, it is difficult to speculate further on this topic. Finally, because the endocrine system is highly dependent on the function of the nuclear hormone superfamily of steroids, it will be necessary for future environmental studies to take into consideration the numerous coregulators that exist with tissue-specific distributions. Such coregulators have the potential to determine the sensitivity of endocrine target cells to the diverse types of environmental endocrine disruptors and could, in the future, even change the way we screen for such chemicals.

SUGGESTED READING

General

Peterson, R. E., Cooke, P. S., Kelce, W. R., and Gray, L. E. (1997) Environmental endocrine disruptors. *In* "Comprehensive Toxicology" (I. G. Sipes, C. A. McQueen, and A. J. Gandolfi, eds.), Vol. 10, pp. 181–197. Pergamon Press, New York.

Sharpe, R. M. and Skakkebaek, N. E. (1993). Are oestrogens involved in falling sperm counts and disorders of the male reproductive tract? *Lancet* **341**, 1392–1395.

Mechanisms of Endocrine Disruption

Crisp, T. M., Clegg, E. D., Cooper, R. L., Wood, W. P., Anderson, D. G., Baetcke, K. P., Hoffmann, J. L., Morrow, M. S., Rodier, D. J., Schaeffer, J. E., Touart, L. W., Zeeman, M. G., and Patel, Y. M. (1998). Environmental endocrine disruption: An effects assessment and analysis. *Environ. Health Perspect.* **106**(Suppl. 1), 11–56.

Fail, P. A., Chapin, R. E., Price, C. J., and Heindel, J. J. (1998). General, reproductive, developmental, and endocrine toxicity of boronated compounds. *Reprod. Toxicol.* **12**, 1–18.

Hansen, L. G. (1998). Stepping backward to improve assessment of PCB congener toxicities. *Environ. Health Perspect.* **106**(Suppl. 1), 171–189.

Hess, R. A., Moore, B. J., Forrer, J., Linder, R. E., and Abuel-Atta, A. A. (1991). The fungicide benomyl (methyl 1-(butylcarbamoyl)-2-benzimidazolecarba-

mate) causes testicular dysfunction by inducing the sloughing of germ cells and occlusion of efferent ductules. *Fundam. Appl. Toxicol.* **17**, 733–745.

McLachlan, J. A., Newbold, R. R., and Bullock, B. (1975). Reproductive tract lesions in male mice exposed prenatally to diethylstilbestrol. *Science* **190**, 991–992.

Nakai, M., Hess, R. A., Moore, B. J., Guttroff, R. F., Strader, L. F., and Linder, R. E. (1992). Acute and long-term effects of a single dose of the fungicide carbendazim (methyl 2-benzimidazole carbamate) on the male reproductive system in the rat. *J. Androl.* **13**, 507–518.

Roman, B. L., and Peterson, R. E. (1998). Developmental male reproductive toxicology of 2,3,7,8-tetrachlorodibenzo-p-dioxin (TCDD) and PCBs. *In* "Reproductive and Developmental Toxicology" (K. S. Korach, ed.), Vol. 24, pp. 593–624. Dekker, New York.

vom Saal, F. S., Timms, B. G., Montano, M. M., Palanza, P., Thayer K. A., Nagel, S. C., Dhar, M. D., Ganjam, V. K., Parmigiani, S., and Welshons, W. V. (1997). Prostate enlargement in mice due to fetal exposure to low doses of estradiol or diethylstilbestrol and opposite effects at high doses. *Proc. Natl. Acad. Sci. USA* **94**, 2056–2061.

Target Organs

Pelissero, C., Flouriot, G., Foucher, J. L., Bennetau, B., Dunogues, J., Le Gac, F., and Sumpter, J. P. (1993). Vitellogenin synthesis in cultured hepatocytes; an *in vitro* test for the estrogenic potency of chemicals. *J. Steroid Biochem. Mol. Biol.* **44**, 263–272.

Reiter, L. W., DeRosa, C., Kavlock, R. J., Lucier, G., Mac, M. J., Melillo, J., Melnick, R. L., Sinks, T., and Walton, B. T. (1998). The U.S. federal framework for research on endocrine disruptors and an analysis of research programs supported during fiscal year 1996. *Environ. Health Perspect.* **106**, 105–113.

Classes of Compounds with Endocrine-Disrupting Activity

Adlercreutz, H. (1998). Human health and phytoestrogens. *In* "Reproductive and Developmental Toxicology" (K. Korach, ed.), pp. 299–371. Dekker, New York.

Allen, J. R., Barsotti, D. A., Lambrecht, L. K., and Van Miller, J. P. (1979). Reproductive effects of halogenated aromatic hydrocarbons on non-human primates. *Ann. N.Y. Acad. Sci.* **320**, 419–425.

Anthony, M. S., Clarkson, T. B., Bullock, B. C., and Wagner, J. D. (1997). Soy protein versus soy phytoestrogens in the prevention of diet-induced coronary artery atherosclerosis of male cynomolgus monkeys. *Arterioscler. Thromb. Vasc. Biol.* **17**, 2524–2531.

Astroff, B., and Safe, S. (1990). 2,3,7,8-Tetrachlorodibenzo-p-dioxin as an antiestrogen: Effect on rat uterine peroxidase activity. *Biochem. Pharmacol.* **39**, 485–488.

Bertazzi, P. A., Zocchetti, C., Guercilena, S., Consonni, D., Tironi, A., Landi, M. T., and Pesatori, A. C. (1997). Dioxin exposure and cancer risk: A 15-year mortality study after the "Seveso accident." *Epidemiology* **8**, 646–652.

Bitman, J., and Cecil, H. C. (1970). Estrogenic activity of DDT analogs and polychlorinated biphenyls. *J. Agric. Food Chem.* **18**, 1108–1112.

Bjerke, D. L., Brown, T. J., MacLusky, N. J., Hochberg, R. B., and Peterson, R. E. (1994). Partial demasculinization and feminization of sex behavior in male rats by *in utero* and lactational exposure to 2,3,7,8-tetrachlorodibenzo-p-dioxin is not associated with alterations in estrogen receptor bindingor volumes of sexually differentiated brain nuclei. *Toxicol. Appl. Pharmacol.* **127**, 258–267.

Bjerke, D. L., and Peterson, R. E. (1994). Reproductive toxicity of 2,3,7,8-tetrachlorodibenzo-p-dioxin in male rats: Different effects of *in utero* versus lactational exposure. *Toxicol. Appl. Pharmacol.* **127**, 241–249.

Bjerke, D. L., Sommer, R. J., Moore, R. W., and Peterson, R. E. (1994). Effects of *in utero* and lactational 2,3,7,8-tetrachlorodibenzo-p-dioxin exposure on responsiveness of the male rat reproductive system to testosterone stimulation in adulthood. *Toxicol. Appl. Pharmacol.* **127**, 250–257.

Chen, Y., Guo, Y. L., Hsu, C. C., and Rogan, W. J. (1992). Cognitive development of Yu-Cheng ("oil disease") children prenatally exposed to heat-degraded PCBs. *JAMA* **286**, 3213–3218.

Couse, J. F., Curtis, S. W., Washburn, T. F., Lindzey, J., Golding, T. B., Lubahn D. B., Smithies, O., and Korach K. S. (1995). Analysis of transcription and estrogen insensitivity in the female mouse after targeted disruption of the estrogen receptor gene. *Mol. Endocrinol.* **9**, 1441–1454.

Couse, J. F., Lindzey, J., Grandien, K., Gustafsson, J.-A., and Korach K. S. (1997). Tissue distribution and quantitative analysis of estrogen receptor-alpha (ERalpha) and estrogen receptor-beta (ERbeta) messenger ribonucleic acid in the wild-type and ERalpha-knockout mouse. *Endocrinology* **138**, 4613–4621.

DeVito, M. J., Birnbaum, L. S., Farland, W. H., and Gasiewicz, T. A. (1995). Comparisons of estimated human body burdens of dioxinlike chemicals and TCDD body burdens in experimentally exposed animals. *Environ. Health Perspect.* **103**, 820–831.

DeVito, M. J., Thomas, T., Martin, E., Umbreit, T. H., and Gallo, M. A. (1992). Antiestrogenic action of 2,3,7,8-tetrachlorodibenzo-p-dioxin: Tissue specific regulation of estrogen receptor in CD-1 mice. *Toxicol. Appl. Pharmacol.* **113**, 284–292.

Ecobichon, D. J., and MacKenzie, D. O. (1974). The uterotropic activity of commercial and isomerically-pure chlorobiphenyls in the rat. *Res. Commun. Chem. Pathol. Pharmacol.* **9**, 85–95.

Fingerhut, M. A., Halperin, W. E., Marlow, D. A., Piacitelli, L. A., Honchar, P. A., Sweeney, M. H., Greife, A. L., Dill, P. A., Steenland, K., and Suruda, A. J. (1991). Cancer mortality in workers exposed to 2,3,7,8-tetrachlorodibenzo-p-dioxin. *N. Engl. J. Med.* **324**, 212–218.

Fiolet, D. C. M., Cuijpers, C., and Lebret, E. (1997). Exposure ot polychlorinated organic compounds and thyroid hormone plasma levels of human newborns. *Organohalogen Compounds* **34**, 459–465.

Fisher, J. S., Turner, K. J., Brown, D., and Sharpe, R. M. (1999). Effect of neonatal exposure to estrogenic compounds on development of the excurrent ducts of the rat testis through puberty to adulthood. *Environ. Health Perspect.* **107**, 397–405.

Gallo, M. A., Hesse, E. J., MacDonald, G. J., and Umbreit, T. H. (1986). Interactive effects of estradiol and 2,3,7,8-tetrachlorodibenzo-p-dioxin on hepatic cytochrome P-450 and mouse uterus. *Toxicol. Lett.* **32**, 123–132.

Gellert, R. J. (1978). Uterotrophic activity of polychlorinated biphenyls (PCB) and induction of precocious reproductive aging in neonatally treated female rats. *Environ. Res.* **16**, 123–130.

Geyer, H. J., Rimkus, G. G., Scheunert, I., Kaune, A., Schramm, K.-W., Kettrup, A., Zeeman, M., Muir, D. C. G., Hansen, L. G., and Mackay, D. (2000). Bioaccumulation and occurrence of endocrine-disrupting chemicals (EDCs), persistent organic pollutants (POPs), and other organic compounds in fish and other organisms including humans. *In* "The Handbook of Environmental Chemistry" (B. Beek, ed.), pp. 1–166, Springer-Verlag, Berlin.

Gray, L. E., Jr., Kelce, W. R., Monosson, E., Ostby, J. S., and Birnbaum, L. S. (1995). Exposure to TCDD during development permanently alters reproductive function in male Long Evans rats and hamsters: Reduced ejaculated and epididymal sperm numbers and sex accessory gland weights in offspring with normal androgenic status. *Toxicol. Appl. Pharmacol.* **131**, 108–118.

Gray, L. E., Jr., Ostby, J. S., and Kelce, W. R. (1994). Developmental effects of an environmental antiandrogen: The fungicide vinclozolin alters sex differentiation of the male rat. *Toxicol. Appl. Pharmacol.* **129**, 46–52.

Gray, L. E., Ostby, J. S., and Kelce, W. R. (1997). A dose-response analysis of the reproductive effects of a single gestational dose of 2,3,7,8-tetrachlorodibenzo-p-dioxin (TCDD) in male Long Evans Hooded rat offspring. *Toxicol. Appl. Pharmacol.* **146**, 11–20.

Gray, L. E., Jr., Wolf, C., Lambright, C., Mann, P., Price, M., Cooper, R. L., and Ostby, J. (1999). Administration of potentially antiandrogenic pesticides (procymidone, linuron, iprodione, chlozolinate, p,p'-DDE, and ketoconazole) and toxic substances (dibutyl- and diethylhexyl phthalate, PCB 169, and ethane dimethane sulphonate) during sexual differentiation produces diverse profiles of reproductive malformations in the male rat. *Toxicol. Indust. Health* **15**, 94–118.

Guzelian, P. S. (1976). Fourteen workers exposed to pesticide kepone are probably sterile, researchers report. *Occup Health Safety Lett.* **6**, 2.

Hany, J., Lilienthal, H., Sarasin, A., Roth-Harer, A., Fastabend, A., Dunemann, L., Lichtensteiger, W., and Winneke, G. (1999). Developmental exposure of rats to a reconstituted PCB mixture or Aroclor 1254: Effects on organ weights, aromatase activity, sex hormone levels, and sweet preference behavior. *Toxicol. Appl. Pharmacol.* **158**, 231–243.

Hess, R. A., Bunick, D., Lee, K. H., Bahr, J., Taylor, J. A., Korach, K. S., and Lubahn, D. B. (1997). A role for oestrogens in the male reproductive system. *Nature* **390**, 509–512.

Hurst, C. H., DeVito, M. J., Woodrow Setzer, R., and Birnbaum, L. S. (2000). Acute administration of 2,3,7,8-tetrachlorodibenzo-p-dioxin (TCDD) in pregnant Long Evans rats: Association of measured tissue concentrations with developmental effects. *Toxicol. Sci.* **53**, 411–420.

Huisman, M., Koopman-Esseboom, C., Fidler, V., Hadders-Algra, M., van der Paauw, C. G., Tuinstra, L. G., Weisglas-Kuperus, N., Sauer, P. J., Touwen, B. C., and Boersma, E. R. (1995). Perinatal exposure to polychlorinated biphenyls and dioxins and its effect on neonatal neurological development. *Early Hum. Dev.* **41**, 111–127.

Huisman, M., Koopman-Esseboom, C., Lanting, C. I., van der Paauw, C. G., Tuinstra, L. G., Fidler, V., Weisglas-Kuperus, N., Sauer, P. J., Boersma, E. R., and Touwen, B. C. (1995). Neurological condition in 18-month-old children perinatally exposed to polychlorinated biphenyls and dioxins. *Early Hum. Dev.* **43**, 165–176.

Jacobson, J. L., and Jacobson, S. W. (1996). Intellectual impairment in children exposed to polychlorinated biphenyls in utero. *N. Engl. J. Med.* **335**, 783–789.

Jansen, H. T., Cooke, P. S., Porcelli, J., Liu, T. C., and Hansen, L. G. (1993). Estrogenic and anti-estrogenic actions of PCBs in the female rat: In vitro and in vivo studies. *Reprod. Toxicol.* **7**, 237–248.

Kelce, W. R., Gray, L. E., and Wilson, E. M. (1998). Antiandrogens as environmental endocrine disruptors. *Reprod. Fertil. Dev.* **10**, 105–111.

Kester, M. H. A., Bulduk, S., Tibboel, D., Meinl, W., Glatt, H., Falany, C. N., Coughtrie, M. A. H., Bergman, A, Safe, S. H., Kuiper, G. G. J. M., Schuur, A. G., and Visser, T. J. (2000). Potent inhibition of estrogen sulfotransferase by hydroxylated PCB metabolites:

A novel pathway explaining the estrogenic activity of PCBs. *Endocrinology* **141**, 1897–1900.

Kliewer, S. A., Lehmann, J. M., Milburn, M. V., and Wilson, T. M. (1999). The PPARs and PXRs: Nuclear xenobiotic receptors that define novel hormone signaling pathways. *Recent Prog. Horm. Res.* **54**, 345–367.

Korach, K. S., Sarver, P., Chae, K., McLachlan, J. A., and McKinney, J. D. (1988). Estrogen receptor-binding activity of polychlorinated hydroxybiphenyls: Conformationally restricted structural probes. *Mol. Pharmacol.* **33**, 120–126.

Koopman-Esseboom, C., Morse, D. C., Weisglas-Kuperus, N., Lutkeschipholt, I. J., Van der Paauw, C. G., Tuinstra, L. G., Brouwer, A., and Sauer, P. J. (1994). Effects of dioxins and polychlorinated biphenyls on thyroid hormone status of pregnant women and their infants. *Pediatr. Res.* **36**, 468–473.

Krege, J. H., Hodgin, J. B., Couse, J. F., Enmark, E., Warner, M., Mahler, J. F., Sar, M. Korach, K. S., Gustafsson, J. A., and Smithies, O. (1998). Generation and reproductive phenotypes of mice lacking estrogen receptor beta. *Proc. Natl. Acad. Sci. USA* **95**, 15677–15682.

Kuiper, G. G., Carlsson, B., Grandien, K., Enmark, E., Haggblad, J., Nilsson, S., and Gustafsson, J. A. (1997). Comparison of the ligand binding specificity and transcript tissue distribution of estrogen receptors alpha and beta. *Endocrinology* **138**, 863–870.

Kuiper, G. G., Enmark, E., Pelto-Huikko, M., Nilsson, S., and Gustafsson, J. A. (1996). Cloning of a novel receptor expressed in rat prostate and ovary. *Proc. Natl. Acad. Sci. USA* **93**, 5925–5930.

Kuiper, G. G., Lemmen, J. G., Carlsson, B., Corton, J. C., Safe, S. H., van der Saag, P., van der Burg, B., and Gustafsson, J. A. (1998). Interaction of estrogenic chemicals and phytoestrogens with estrogen receptor beta. *Endocrinology* **139**, 4252–4263.

Kurita, T., Lee, K-J., Cooke, P. S., Taylor, J. A., Lubahn, D. B., and Cunha, G. R. (2000). Paracrine regulation of progesterone receptor by estradiol in female reproductive tract. *Biol. Reprod.* **62**, 821–830.

Longnecker, M. P., and Michalek, J. E. (2000). Serum dioxin level in relation to diabetes mellitus among Air Force veterans with background levels of exposure. *Epidemiology* **11**, 44–48.

Lucier, G. (1991). Humans are a sensitive species to some of the biochemical effects of structural analogus of dioxin. *Environ. Toxicol. Chem.* **10**, 727–735.

Mably, T. A., Bjerke, D. L., Moore, R. W., Gendron-Fitzpatrick, A., and Peterson, R. E. (1992). *In utero* and lactational exposure of male rats to 2,3,7,8-tetrachlorodibenzo-p-dioxin. 3. Effects on spermatogenesis and reproductive capability. *Toxicol. Appl. Pharmacol.* **114**, 118–126.

Mably, T. A., Moore, R. W., Goy, R. W., and Peterson, R. E. (1992). *In utero* and lactational exposure of male rats to 2,3,7,8-tetrachlorodibenzo-p-dioxin. 2. Effects on sexual behavior and the regulation of luteinizing hormone secretion in adulthood. *Toxicol. Appl. Pharmacol.* **114**, 108–117.

Mably, T. A., Moore, R. W., and Peterson, R. E. (1992). *In utero* and lactational exposure of male rats to 2,3,7,8-tetrachlorodibenzo-p-dioxin. 1. Effects on androgenic status. *Toxicol. Appl. Pharmacol.* **114**, 97–107.

Masuyama, H., Hiramatsu, Y., Kunitomi, M., Kudo, T., and MacDonald, P. N. (2000). Endocrine disrupting chemicals, phthalic acid and nonylphenol, activate Pregnane X receptor-mediated transcription. *Mol. Endocrinol.* **14**, 421–428.

McLachlan, J. A., Korach, K. S., Newbold, R. R., and Degen, G. H. (1984). Diethylstilbestrol and other estrogens in the environment. *Fundam. Appl. Toxicol.* **4**, 686–691.

McLachlan, J. A., and Newbold, R. R. (1987). Estrogens and development. *Environ. Health Perspect.* **75**, 25–27.

Moore, R. W., Potter, C. L., Theobald, H. M., Robinson, J. A., and Peterson, R. E. (1985). Androgenic deficiency in male rats treated with 2,3,7,8-tetrachlorodibenzo-p-dioxin. *Toxicol. Appl. Pharmacol.* **79**, 99–111.

Moore, M., Mustain, M., Daniel, K., Chen, I., Safe, S., Zacharewski, T., Gillesby, B., Joyeux, A., and Balaguer, P. (1997). Antiestrogenic activity of hydroxylated polychlorinated biphenyl congeners identified in human serum. *Toxicol. Appl. Pharmacol.* **142**, 160–168.

Mylchreest, E., Sar, M., Cattley, R. C., and Foster, P. M. D. (1999). Disruption of androgen-regulated male reproductive development by di(n-butyl) phthalate during late gestation in rats is different from flutamide. *Toxicol. Appl. Pharmacol.* **156**, 81–95.

National Research Council (1999). "Hormonally Active Agents in the Environment." National Academy Press, Washington, DC.

Olea, N., Pulgar, R., Perez, P., Olea-Serrano, F., Rivas, A., Novillo-Fertrell, A., Pedraza, V., Soto, A. M., and Sonnenschein, C. (1996). Estrogenicity of resin-based composites and sealants used in dentistry. *Environ. Health Perspect.* **104**, 298–305.

Patandin, S., Koopman-Esseboom, C. K. E., de Ridder, M. A. J., Weisglas-Kurperus, N., and Sauer, P. J. J. (1998). Effects of environmental exposure to polychlorinated biphenyls and dioxins on birth size and postnatal growth. *Pediatr. Res.* **44**, 538–545.

Pesatori, A. C., Consonni, D., Tironi, A., Zocchetti, C., Fini, A., and Bertazzi, P. A. (1993). Cancer in a young population in a dioxin-contaminated area. *Int. J. Epidemiol.* **22**, 1010–1013.

Rogan, W. J., Gladen, B. C., Hung, K. S., Koong, S. L., Shih, L. Y., Taylor, J. S., Wu, Y. C., Yang, D., Ragan, N. B., and Hsu, C. C. (1988). Congenital poisoning by polychlorinated biphenyls and their contaminants in Taiwan. *Science* **241**, 334–336.

Roman, B. L., Sommer, R. J., Shinomiya, K., and Peterson, R. E. (1995). *In utero* and lactational exposure of the male rat to 2,3,7,8-tetrachlorodibenzo-p-dioxin: Impaired prostate growth and development without inhibited testicular androgen production. *Toxicol. Appl. Pharmacol.* **134**, 241–250.

Safe, S. H. (1995). Modulation of gene expression and endocrine response pathways by 2,3,7,8-tetrachlorodibenzo-p-dioxin and related compounds. *Pharmacol. Ther.* **67**, 247–281.

Schmitt, C. J., Zajicek, J. L., May, T. W., and Cowman, D. F. (1999). Organochlorine residues and elemental contaminants in U. S. freshwater fish, 1976–1986: National Contaminant Biomonitoring Program. *Rev. Environ. Contam. Toxicol.* **162**, 43–104.

Setchell, K. D., Zimmer-Nechemias, L., Cai, J., and Heubi, J. E. (1997). Exposure of infants to phytooestrogens from soy-based infant formula. *Lancet* **350**, 23–27.

Sharpe, R. M., Fisher, J. S., Millar, M. M., Jobling, S., and Sumpter, J. P. (1995). Gestational and lactational exposure of rats to xenoestrogens results in reduced testicular size and sperm production. *Environ. Health Perspect.* **103**, 1136–1143.

Shiverick, K. T., and Muther, T. F. (1983). 2,3,7,8-Tetrachlorodibenzo-p-dioxin (TCDD) effects on hepatic microsomal steroid metabolism and serum estradiol of pregnant rats. *Biochem. Pharmacol.* **32**, 991–995.

Sohoni, P., and Sumpter, J. P. (1998) Several environmental oestrogens are also anti-androgens. *J. Endocrinol.* **158**, 327–339.

Soto, A. M., Lin, T. M., Justicia, H., Silvia, R. M., and Sonnenschein, C. (1992). An "in culture" bioassay to assess the estrogenicity of xenobiotics (E-Screen). In "Chemically Induced Alterations in Sexual and Functional Development: The Wildlife/Human Connection" (T. Colborn and C. Clements, eds.), pp. 295–309. Princeton Scientific Publishing Co., Princeton, N. J.

Soto, A. M., Sonnenschein, C., Chung, K. L., Fernandez, M. F., Olea, N., and Serrano, F. O. (1995). The E-SCREEN assay as a tool to identify estrogens: An update on estrogenic environmental pollutants. *Environ. Health Perspect.* **103**(Suppl. 7), 113–122.

Spearow, J. L., Doemeny, P., Sera, Robyn, Leffler, R., and Barkley, M. (1999). Genetic variation in susceptibility to endocrine disruption by estrogen in mice. *Science* **285**, 1259–1261.

Steinmetz, R., Brown, N. G., Allen, D. L., Bigsby, R. M., and Ben-Jonathan, N. (1997). The environmental estrogen bisphenol. A stimulates prolactin release *in vitro* and *in vivo*. *Endocrinology* **138**, 1780–1786.

Stewart, P., Darvill, T., Lonky, E., Reihman, J., Pagano, J., and Bush, B. (1999). Assessment of prenatal exposure to PCBs from maternal consumption of Great Lakes fish: An analysis of PCB pattern and concentration. *Environ. Res.* **80**, S87–S96.

Truelove, J. F., Tanner, J. R., Langlois, I. A., Stapley, R. A., Arnold, D. L., and Mes, J. C. (1990). Effect of polychlorinated biphenyls on several endocrine reproductive parameters in the female rhesus monkey. *Arch. Environ. Contam. Toxicol.* **19**, 939–943.

Vincent, D. R., Bradshaw, W. S., Booth, G. M., Seegmiller, R. E. and Allen, S. D. (1992). Effect of PCB and DES on rat monoamine oxidase, acetyl-cholinesterase, testosterone, and estradiol ontogeny. *Bull. Environ. Contam. Toxicol.* **48**, 884–893.

Welshons, W. V., Nagel, S. C., Thayer, K. A., Judy, B. M., and Vom Saal, F. S. (1999). Low-dose bioactivity of xenoestrogens in animals: Fetal exposure to low doses of methoxychlor and other xenoestrogens increases adult prostate size in mice. *Toxicol. Indust. Health* **15**, 12–25.

Wetzel, L. T., Luempert, L. G., III, Breckenridge, C. B., Tisdel, M. O., Stevens, J. T., Thakur, A. K., Extrom, P. J., and Eldridge, J. C. (1994). Chronic effects of atrazine on estrus and mammary tumor formation in female Sprague-Dawley and Fischer 344 rats. *J. Toxicol. Environ. Health* **43**, 169–182.

Wolff, M. S., and Toniolo, P. G. (1995). Environmental organochlorine exposure as a potential etiologic factor in breast cancer. *Environ. Health Perspect.* **103**(Suppl. 7), 141–145.

Wu, A. H. (2000). Diet and breast carcinoma in multi-ethnic populations. *Cancer* **88**, 1239–1244.

Exposure to Endocrine Disruptors: Are There Risks?

Auger, J., and Jouannet, P. (1997). Evidence for regional differences of semen quality among fertile French men. Federation Francaise des Centres d'Etude et de Conservation des Oeufs et du Sperme humains. *Hum. Reprod.* **12**, 740–745.

Belisle, A. A., Reichel, W. L., Locke, L. N., Lamont, T. G., Mulhern, B. M., Prouty, R. M., DeWolf, R. B., and Cromartie, E. (1972). Residues of organochlorine pesticides, polychlorinated biphenyls, and mercury and autopsy data for bald eagles, 1969 and 1970. *Pestic. Monit. J.* **6**, 133–138.

Brucker-Davis, F. (1998). Effects of environmental synthetic chemicals on thyroid function. *Thyroid* **8**, 827–856.

Carlsen, E., Giwercman, A., Keiding, N., and Skakkebaek, N. E. (1992). Evidence for decreasing quality of semen during past 50 years. *Br. Med. J.* **305**, 609–613.

Colborn, T., vom Saal, F. S., and Soto, A. M. (1993). Developmental effects of endocrine-disrupting chemicals in wildlife and humans. *Environ. Health Perspect.* **101**, 378–384.

Costantino, J. P., Redmond, C. K., and Bearden, A. (1995). Occupationally related cancer risk among coke oven workers: 30 years of follow-up. *J. Occup. Environ. Med.* **37**, 597–604.

Fisch, H., Goluboff, E. T., Olson, J. H., Feldshuh, J., Broder, S. J., and Barad, D. H. (1996). Semen analyses in 1,283 men from the United States over a 25-year period: No decline in quality. *Fertil. Steril.* **65**, 1009–1014.

Fry, D. M. (1995). Reproductive effects in birds exposed to pesticides and industrial chemicals. *Environ. Health Perspect.* **103**(Suppl. 7), 165–171.

Fry, D. M., and Toone, C. K. (1981). DDT-induced feminization of gull embryos. *Science* **213**, 922–924.

Guillette, L. J., Jr., Crain, D. A., Rooney, A. A., and Pickford, D. B. (1995). Organization versus activation: The role of endocrine-disrupting contaminants (EDCs) during embryonic development in wildlife. *Environ. Health Perspect.* **103**(Suppl. 7), 157–164.

Guillette, L. J., Jr., and Guillette, E. A. (1996). Environmental contaminants and reproductive abnormalities in wildlife: Implications for public health? *Toxicol. Indust. Health* **12**, 537–550.

Morrison, H., Savitz, D., Semenciw, R., Hulka, B., Mao, Y., Morison, D., and Wigle, D. (1993). Farming and prostate cancer mortality. *Am. J. Epidemiol.* **137**, 270–280.

Nakagawa, R., Hirakawa, H., Iida, T., Matsueda, T., and Nagayama, J. (1999). Maternal body burden of organochlorine pesticides and dioxins. *JAOAC Int.* **82**, 716–724.

Potosky, A. L., Miller, B. A., Albertsen, P. C., and Kramer, B. S. (1995). The role of increasing detection in the rising incidence of prostate cancer. *JAMA* **273**, 548–552.

Sharpe, R. M. (1993). Declining sperm counts in men: Is there an endocrine cause? *J. Endocrinol.* **136**, 357–360.

Skakkebaek, N. E., Berthelsen, J. G., Giwercman, A., and Muller, J. (1987). Carcinoma-*in-situ* of the testis: Possible origin from gonocytes and precursor of all types of germ cell tumours except spermatocytoma. *Int. J. Androl.* **10**, 19–28.

Sumpter, J. P. (1998). Xenoendorine disruptors: Environmental impacts. *Toxicol. Lett.* **102–103**, 337–342.

Toppari, J., Larsen, J. C., Christiansen, P., Giwercman, A., Grandjean, P., Guillette, L. J., Jr., Jegou, B., Jensen, T. K., Jouannet, P., Keiding, N., Leffers, H., McLachlan, J. A., Meyer, O., Muller, J., Rajpert-De Meyts, E., Scheike, T., Sharpe, R., Sumpter, J., and Skakkebaek, N. E. (1996). Male reproductive health and environmental xenoestrogens. *Environ. Health Perspect.* **104**(Suppl. 4), 741–803.

Zitko, V., and Choi, P. M. (1972). PCB and p,p'-DDE in eggs of cormorants, gulls, and ducks from the Bay of Fundy, Canada. *Bull. Environ. Contam. Toxicol.* **7**, 63–64.

Paul S. Cooke, Richard E. Peterson, and Rex A. Hess

Techniques for Screening Endocrine Disruptors

Ashby, J., Odum, J., Tinwell, H., and Lefevre, P. A. (1997). Assessing the risks of adverse endocrine-mediated effects: Where to from here? *Regul. Toxicol. Pharmacol.* **26**, 80–93.

Bergeron, R. M., Thompson, T. B., Leonard, L. S., Pluta, L., and Gaido, K. W. (1999). Estrogenicity of bisphenol A in a human endometrial carcinoma cell line. *Mol. Cell. Endocrinol.* **150**, 179–187.

Calabrese, E. J., Baldwin, L. A., Kostecki, P. T., and Potter, T. L. (1997). A toxicologically based weight-of-evidence methodology for the relative ranking of chemicals of endocrine disruption potential. *Regul. Toxicol. Pharmacol.* **26**, 36–40.

Cook, J. C., Kaplan, M. A., Davis, L. G., and O'Connor, J. C. (1997). Development of a Tier I screening battery for detecting endocrine-active compounds (EACs). *Regul. Toxicol. Pharmacol.* **26**, 60–68.

O'Connor, J. C., Frame, S. R., Biegel, L. B., Cook, J. C., and Davis, L. G. (1998). Sensitivity of a Tier I screening battery compared to an *in utero* exposure for detecting the estrogen receptor agonist 17 beta-estradiol. *Toxicol. Sci.* **44**, 169–184.

Soto, A. M., and Sonnenschein, C. (1999). Estrogens, xenoestrogens, and the development of neoplasms. *In* "Endocrine Disruptors" R. K. Nazi, ed., pp. 125–163. CRC Press, Boca Raton, FL.

Conclusions, Controversy, and Questions

Cooper, R. L., and Kavlock, R. J. (1997). Endocrine disruptors and reproductive development: A weight-of-evidence overview. *J. Endocrinol.* **152**, 159–166.

22

Radiation and Heat

Stephen A. Benjamin
College of Veterinary Medicine and
Biomedical Sciences
Department of Pathology
Colorado State University
Fort Collins, Colorado

Fletcher F. Hahn
Lovelace Respiratory Research Institute
Albuquerque, New Mexico

Barbara E. Powers
College of Veterinary Medicine and
Biomedical Sciences
Department of Pathology
Colorado State University
Fort Collins, Colorado

Donna F. Kusewitt
Department of Veterinary Biosciences
The Ohio State University
Columbus, Ohio

I. Introduction

This chapter discusses the pathological mechanisms associated with exposure to ionizing radiation, ultraviolet (UV) radiation, and heat (hyperthermia), as they are not only important as injurious agents in our environment, but also are used for therapeutic or cosmetic purposes. Thus, the pathologist is often required to recognize the pathological changes resulting from these agents, either alone or as complications of other disease problems. Radiation toxicology is a vast science itself and has engendered many volumes devoted to it. This chapter is not meant to be an all-inclusive listing of every organ system and type of radiation or radionuclide that can cause injury. The basic approach is to present an overview, addressing basic mechanisms of radiation and hyperthermic injury and how these relate to the pathological changes seen by the morphologist.

Handbook of Toxicologic Pathology, Second Edition
Volume 1
Copyright © 2002 by Academic Press
All rights of reproduction in any form reserved.

The increasing use of diagnostic and therapeutic irradiation and hyperthermia in medical practice makes it important for the pathologist to be familiar with their effects. In clinical medicine, for example, the morphological changes caused by therapeutic ionizing radiation often complicate postmortem evaluation of tissues from both veterinary and human patients. This is often further complicated by the fact that individuals are treated with combinations of ionizing radiation, other physical agents including heat, and toxic chemotherapeutic drugs. The potential for accidental exposures to ionizing radiation, such as nuclear accidents, also stresses the importance of the pathologist being familiar with lesions produced by radiation. Finally, the effects of ultraviolet radiation on skin are a well-known and important health concern.

We will concentrate on the effects of radiation and heat alone, rather than concerning ourselves with interactive effects. Understanding the basic nature of radiation or heat injury can help separate such effects when combined injury is present. This chapter addresses ionizing and ultra-violet radiation as separate entities due to some basic differences in the nature of their actions.

A. SOURCES AND OCCURRENCE

1. Ionizing Radiation

The greatest contributors to ionizing radiation exposure to all living systems are natural sources (see Table I). These include (1) external exposures from radioactive materials in the earth and from cosmic radiation from space occurring naturally and (2) internal exposures from naturally occurring radionuclides deposited in the body. Although these exposures account for well over half of the total population dose, the average dose to individuals is relatively small. Our discussions of radiation injury are predicated on effects of much larger radiation doses; therefore, we are more concerned with those sources that are more likely to result in significant pathological changes.

a. External Radiation. Medical exposures to ionizing radiation constitute the second largest source of exposure to the human population and the largest to man-made radiation. The majority of such exposures are for diagnostic purposes. Diagnostic X-rays for both medical and dental diagnosis far exceed any other categories of exposure. Fluoroscopy is used much less now than it was several decades ago. Most diagnostic procedures result in doses to patients that are far below those necessary for the

production of any acute biological injury. The risk to an individual from diagnostic exposure with respect to such health problems as cancer induction is small, but can be quantified on a population basis. Occupational doses to personnel administering diagnostic and therapeutic procedures can be considerably higher.

From the standpoint of significant acute tissue injury, therapeutic irradiation is a major factor. Most therapeutic regimes involve the delivery of high radiation doses to localized regions of the body, resulting in much tissue injury, despite the goal of limiting injury while maximizing tumor control. External beam radiation therapy can be administered by linear and particle accelerators, γ ray sources, and specialized orthovoltage X-ray machines.

The production and use of nuclear energy contribute to the overall radiation exposure of the population, but to a much lesser degree than medical sources. Nuclear weapons testing has contributed to environmental contamination with a variety of short- and long-lived radionuclides, although with the reductions of atmospheric testing, this contribution is now relatively small worldwide. While the contribution of nuclear power generation to the population dose is quite small, events such as the 1986 disaster at Chernobyl in the Soviet Union underscore the potential for nuclear accidents leading to injurious doses to many individuals. There is also the potential for persons employed in the nuclear industry to accumulate biologically significant radiation doses due to small-scale accidents such as those recently experienced in Japan. External partial or whole body exposures are certainly a factor with respect to nuclear power; however, the actual deposition of radionuclides in the body is also of concern.

b. Internally Deposited Radionuclides. Sources of the typical internally deposited radionuclides (internal emitters) can be classified into five major groups: natural sources, technologically enhanced natural sources, occupational exposures, nuclear reactions associated with nuclear weapons or nuclear power production, and medical sources.

TABLE I

Ionizing Radiation Contributions to U.S. Population Exposures

Sources	Percent	
	Total	Individual
Natural	82	
Radon		55
Internal radionuclides		11
Cosmic		8
Terrestrial		8
Anthropogenic	18	
Medical		15
Consumer products		3
Occupational		<1
Fallout		<1
Nuclear power		<1

Naturally occurring radionuclides in air, food, and water contribute to the background radiation dose. These radionuclides come from minerals in the earth's crust and gain entrance to the body by inhalation or ingestion. Perhaps the most important, as far as health effects are concerned, is radon. The short-lived decay products of ^{220}Rn and ^{222}Rn are considered to contribute significantly to lung cancer incidence.

Some radionuclides can be concentrated (technologically enhanced sources) and may be a potential problem. An example is the manufacture of widely used consumer products, such as special building materials, luminous watches, and smoke detectors that contain radionuclides.

Occupational exposures can potentially result in a relatively high deposition of radionuclides in the body, as exemplified by two specific occupational exposure situations. Groups of underground miners, particularly uranium miners, have been exposed to relatively high concentrations of radon and radon decay products with subsequent increase in the incidence of lung cancer. Radium dial painters in the early 1900s were exposed to ^{224}Ra by ingestion, resulting in the induction of bone sarcomas. Studies of these occupational exposure situations have provided the basic data on the response of people to irradiation from internal emitters.

Certain elements, primarily uranium or plutonium, can be induced to fission by the absorption of neutrons. These nuclear reactions can occur in a nuclear weapon or in a nuclear power reactor. Many fission product radionuclides are produced during nuclear fission, resulting in a wide range of radiation types, half-lives, and energies. Fallout consists primarily of long-lived fission product radionuclides, such as ^{137}Cs and ^{90}Sr.

Exposures resulting from nuclear power production are low for the general population, but can be high in accident situations. In addition, some portions of the nuclear fuel cycle, such as uranium mining and milling and nuclear waste disposal, could result in significant exposures for workers in the industry. Concern exists for accidental exposure of larger populations from potential accidents during the shipping of nuclear wastes. Important radionuclides in the nuclear fuel cycle are fission product radionuclides, such as radioiodine, ^{144}Ce, ^{90}Sr, and the α-emitting transuranic elements of nuclear fuels, such as plutonium.

A number of internal emitters are used in nuclear medicine and radiation therapy. One radionuclide of interest is radioiodine, used in the diagnosis and treatment of thyroid disorders. Of historical interest is the radiographic contrast medium Thorotrast, which contained large amounts of thorium.

2. Ultraviolet Radiation

The sun is the most common source of ultraviolet radiation exposure to humans and other animals. The electromagnetic radiation emitted by the sun extends over a wide range from very long wavelengths, e.g., radio waves, to very short wavelengths, e.g., cosmic rays. This range includes ultraviolet radiation with wavelengths of 100–400 nm. Total global ultraviolet irradiance is composed of the radiation transmitted directly through the atmosphere and the scattered radiation. The global ultraviolet irradiance and spectral distribution depend on a number of factors. These included the thickness of the stratospheric ozone layer, which in combination with other atmospheric molecules completely absorbs ultraviolet radiation below 290 nm (UV-C); solar elevation, which is influenced by season and latitude; the altitude above sea level; solar zenith angle; cloud cover; local air pollution; and ground reflectivity.

Common artificial sources of biologically effective UV radiation can be classified into the general categories of direct and fluorescent gas discharge sources, incandescent sources, and lasers. Radiation emitted by a gas discharge results from the passage of an electric current through a gas. Types of direct gas discharge arcs include low- and high-pressure mercury arcs, high-pressure xenon arcs, metal halide lamps, and flashtubes. Most of the power emitted from low-pressure mercury arcs is of a wavelength of 253.7 nm. High-pressure mercury arcs emit a broader range of UV radiation than low-pressure mercury arcs and are used in industrial photochemical reactors, in printing, and in phototherapy of skin diseases. High-pressure xenon arcs emit radiance with a spectral distribution similar to that of the sun above the stratosphere. Their uses are similar to those of mercury arcs. Metal halide lamps are high-pressure mercury lamps with metal halide additives, which are used extensively in phototherapy and cosmetic tanning. In the confined-arc flashtube, a brief avalanche of high-velocity the electrons passing between the electrodes excites the gas. Flashtubes produce different optical spectra depending on the gas (xenon, krypton, argon, neon, etc.) used within the tube. Xenon flashtubes are used commonly in photography, visual beacons, printing, flash photolysis, and laser excitation.

Fluorescent lamps consist of an electric arc discharge source, mercury vapor in an inert gas at low pressure, and a coating of fluorescent material (phosphor) on the inner surface of a glass tube. The phosphor converts shorter wavelength UV radiation into longer wavelength radiation (UV or visible light). Fluorescent lamps are used commonly in phototherapy and for tanning.

An incandescent source is one that emits radiation primarily because of its temperature. Quartz halogen lamps are one type of incandescent source used commonly for lighting. Oxyacetylene, oxyhydrogen, and plasma torches, incandescent sources used in arc welding, are common causes of UV radiation eye and skin damage. Lasers have been developed that emit beams of monochromatic UV radiation. These UV lasers are primarily research tools.

3. Hyperthermia

Heat, or hyperthermia, is used in physical therapy and cancer therapy. Three basic heating patterns, with peak temperatures in different locations of the body, are used clinically. These patterns are local or superficial hyperthermia, deep or regional hyperthermia, and systemic or whole body hyperthermia. Heating modalities include use of heated water, hot paraffin, hot moist air, warmed blood perfusion, shortwave diathermy, infrared radiation, microwave and radio frequency waves, ultrasound, and convection whole body hyperthermia.

Heat stroke is a manifestation of pathologic systemic hyperthermia. Temperatures sufficient to cause heat stroke can be reached by strenuous physical exercise in a high external environmental temperature, by heat from the surrounding media (as in experimental models of hyperthermia), or by endogenous heat caused by high metabolic heat production (fever).

II. Ionizing Radiation

A. NATURE AND ACTION OF IONIZING RADIATION

1. Types

Ionizing radiation can be separated into *electromagnetic* and *corpuscular* or particulate types. Electromagnetic radiation includes X and γ rays that are part of the electromagnetic spectrum and have characteristic short wave lengths. They consist of streams of energetic photons that can interact with tissues. γ rays tend to have shorter wavelengths and higher energies than X rays. X rays originate outside the nucleus of atoms, whereas γ rays originate from unstable atomic nuclei. Both are highly penetrating radiation and have generally similar interactions with matter.

Particulate radiation is also produced by radioactive decay of unstable nuclei and includes α and β particles and neutrons, among others. α particles consist of two protons and two neutrons. They carry a double positive charge and are relatively massive (8000 times heavier than electrons). Their mass and charge account for their highly ionizing and poorly penetrating nature in tissue, respectively.

β particles are electrons that have a small mass and a single negative charge. They are formed from the conversion of a neutron to a proton in the nucleus. Because of the small mass and electrical charge, they have a greater range of penetration in tissues but much less ionizing power than α particles.

Neutrons are uncharged particles consisting of an electron and a proton. Their mass gives them considerable energy and, because of the lack of charge, they penetrate tissues readily.

Other particles of potential interest include electrons, positrons (positively charged particles of identical mass to electrons), protons, and a variety of heavy particles that can be accelerated to higher energy artificially. These can be of importance in radiotherapy. Most of the effects with which we will be concerned, however, will relate to the electromagnetic and the first three particulate radiations mentioned. Injury from other types of radiation will be similar in nature but will differ in degree of damage per dose delivered.

2. Radiation Biophysics

The quantitation of radioactivity, radiation exposure, and radiation dose are important to an understanding of radiation effects. The International System of Units (SI) for describing special quantities of radiation is now used; however, much of the literature still contains the units of the older system. Thus, the equivalency of both systems will be described.

The SI unit of expression of radioactivity is the Becquerel (Bq), which equals one disintegration per second. The older term, the curie (Ci), equals 3.7×10^{10} disintegrations per second or 3.7×10^{10} Bq. The roentgen (R) is a unit of exposure applied to X and γ radiation. It is a measure of ionization in air, and 1 R equals 2.58×10^{-4} coulomb/kg of air. The SI unit, the Grey (Gy), replaces the rad as the unit of absorbed dose. The Gy equals 1 J/kg in any medium and is equal to 100 rads. For practical usage, especially when describing low doses, 1 cGy equals 1 rad.

Linear energy transfer (LET) is the average amount of energy lost per unit track length in tissue by a particular type of radiation. Low LET radiation includes β particles, X rays, and γ rays, where the distance between ionizing events is large on the scale of a cellular nucleus. High LET radiation includes α particles and neutrons, where the distance between ionizing events is much smaller.

Factors such as dose and LET play an important role in determining the nature and degree of radiation injury. Also important is the period of time over which radiation dose is delivered to the tissues. Dose rate is defined as the absorbed dose delivered per unit time. Dose protraction refers to a situation where radiation is delivered continuously over a relatively long period of time. This is common when various radionuclides are deposited in and remain in tissues, undergoing decay in those locations. Dose fractionation is a method of administering radiation in which discrete doses are given at defined intervals. This allows for repair of radiation damage between the fractions, reducing tissue injury. This is an important therapeutic principle. Cumulative dose is the total dose to a tissue or organism that results from repeated or protracted exposure.

The distribution or localization of dose is a critical factor in radiation injury. Injury is present only in those cells and tissues that have been subjected to radiation exposure. This disregards secondary effects from injury to an exposed organ, e.g., hormonal imbalances due to pituitary destruction.

3. External Radiation and Internal Emitters

a. External Radiation. External irradiation can be defined as radiation entering the body and tissues from some source outside the body. This could be from a point source, such as an X-ray machine or linear accelerator, or a more generalized exposure, such as cosmic irradiation. Exposures can be partial or whole body, again depending on the nature of the source, distance, and shielding. The type of radiation is important in determining the radiation dose; i.e., the specific energy and penetration of tissue are factors. External exposures can be of either electromagnetic or particulate types. Biological effects are basically dependent on the dose delivered, the dose rate, dose fractionation, and the portions of the body exposed.

b. Internal Emitters.

i. Definition Radionuclides that are deposited within the body and that deliver radiation doses to various organs and tissues are

533

typically called internal emitters. The biological effects of internal emitters depend on dose, dose rate, the organ specificity of the radionuclide, and the radiosensitivity of the organ affected. Dosimetry aspects of internal emitters depend on the chemical nature, solubility, half-life, type of radioactive decay, tissue of incorporation, and metabolic fate of the radionuclide.

Internal emitters usually localize in one or a few organs and frequently result in prolonged irradiation in these local sites. These two factors, i.e., dose localization and protraction, frequently cause the effects of internal emitters to differ in time of onset, severity, and dose response from those seen with brief external exposures.

ii. Emissions Radiation from internal emitters includes α or β particles and other particulate radiation, including neutrons, as well as X and γ rays. The type of emission has important implications in the production of biological effects. For example, α emitters are much more effective in producing biological damage than β emitters, as will be discussed.

iii. Chemical form The chemical form of internal emitters is important because it determines the solubility of the radionuclide. The solubility, in turn, is a key determinant of absorption into the body and translocation within the body. Relatively soluble radionuclides are readily absorbed and translocated to internal organs based on the elemental nature of the radionuclide. Insoluble radionuclides are retained at the site of initial deposition.

iv. Metabolism Once radionuclides enter the body and systemic circulation, they follow the metabolic pathway dictated by their elemental nature. Some are excreted rapidly through the kidney or liver whereas others are sequestered in specific organs and released only slowly. The internal emitters of most interest translocate primarily to bone, liver, thyroid, or the whole body (Table II). The retention time of internally deposited radionuclides is described by the effective half-life, or the time for the radioactivity in the body to be reduced by one-half. Two components make up the effective half-life: the physical half-life and the biological half-life.

TABLE II
Target Organs for Some Important Internally Deposited Radionuclides

Radionuclides	Organs
Halogens	
Iodine	Thyroid
Alkali metals	
Cesium	Whole body
Alkaline earths	
Radium	Bone
Strontium	Bone
Lanthanides	
Cerium	Lung, bone, liver
Actinides	
Plutonium	Lung, liver, bone

The physical half-life is the time required for the radionuclide to be reduced to one-half its original activity. The biological half-life is the time it takes for the concentration of a stable isotope to be reduced by one-half in a tissue or organ.

v. Chemical class Several different radionuclides are of interest because of their potential for exposure of animals or humans and their potential harmful effects. The following radionuclides are discussed later with respect to their involvement in tissue injury.

Radioiodine, particularly ^{131}I, has widespread use in medical diagnostics and therapeutics and is abundant in the radionuclide inventory of an operating nuclear power reactor or in weapons fallout. ^{131}I is primarily a β emitter with some low-energy γ emissions. The short physical half-life of 6 days means that ^{131}I is only a factor in weapons fallout or reactor accidents at short times after the event. Significant human exposures have occurred because of the accident at Chernobyl and from atmospheric nuclear weapons testing. The normal food chain to humans and animals contributes to the hazard because radioiodine is concentrated in milk and, ultimately, the thyroid glands. Radioiodines are also used for diagnosis and therapy of thyroid diseases.

^{137}Cesium, an alkali metal, is a significant component of radioactive fallout and in releases from nuclear reactor accidents. ^{137}Cs and its decay product ^{137}barium emit energetic β and γ radiation and have a physical half-life of 30 years. As a metabolic homologue of potassium, cesium is uniformly distributed in the body and results in whole body irradiation.

Radium is an alkaline earth and more is known about its dosimetry and biological effects in animals and humans than about any other internal emitter. Radium and its isotopes are metabolic analogs of calcium and, when absorbed, are deposited in bones. Radium is present in soil, minerals, foodstuffs, groundwater, and many building materials. Although α, β, and photon radiation are released in radium decay, α particles are the most abundant and significant for the production of biological effects.

The second alkaline earth element of interest is strontium, which is abundant as ^{90}Sr in fission products from nuclear reactions. ^{90}Sr, with its decay products, is a β emitter with a physical half-life of 28 years. Strontium is a metabolic analog of calcium and is absorbed readily into the circulation and deposited in bone.

A number of radioisotopes of the lanthanide series of elements are produced during nuclear reactions. The radioisotopes of cerium, however, are of primary interest because of their abundance in fission products of a nuclear power reactor. ^{144}Ce has a physical half-life of 285 days. It decays with energetic β emissions. Cerium is poorly absorbed from the intestine but once in circulation, deposits almost equally in liver and bone.

Actinide elements include uranium and all those with higher atomic numbers. Actinide elements are similar chemically and all are radioactive. They tend to be poorly absorbed from the intestinal tract, are concentrated in liver and osteoid tissue, and are slowly excreted in the feces. Plutonium is particularly important because of its biological effects and potential for population exposure. ^{239}Pu is used in nuclear weapons and is produced in nuclear power reactors. ^{239}Pu has a physical half-life of 24,400 years and is an α emitter. Another radioisotope of plutonium, ^{238}Pu, has a physical half-life of 86.4 years and is 230 times more radioactive per

unit mass than ^{239}Pu. Because of its high specific activity, ^{238}Pu is used as a heat source to power thermoelectric devices used in cardiac pacemakers and space vehicles.

Radon is a noble gas produced by the decay of ^{226}Ra. Radon, in turn, decays by α emission to a series of solid short-lived radionuclides collectively referred to as radon decay products. Two of these are α emitters. ^{226}Ra is present in soils and rocks. As radon forms, it can leave the soil or rock and enter surrounding air or water. Radon concentration can be increased by the presence of a rich radium source or by low ventilation. Examples of these situations are underground mining of ores containing radium and homes built on land containing high concentrations of radium (uranium mine tailings).

Thorium is widely distributed in the environment. It has a physical half-life of 1.4×10^{10} years and decays by emission of an α particle, resulting in a series of radioactive decay products. The primary importance of thorium is its high density and atomic number that led to its use as an early radiographic contrast agent in commercially prepared Thorotrast, a 20% colloidal solution of thorium dioxide. Because of its colloidal characteristics, Thorotrast was ultimately deposited in the fixed phagocytic cell system in liver, spleen, and bone marrow.

vi. Routes of entry Radionuclides may enter the body by four routes: ingestion followed by gastrointestinal absorption; inhalation followed by pulmonary retention or translocation to the circulation; percutaneous absorption; or injection through wounding. The last two are relatively unimportant and occur only in special or occupational situations.

Radioactive materials are most likely to be ingested when they are contaminants in food or water. Direct radiation effects on the gastrointestinal tract generally are not significant because the normal ingesta in the gastrointestinal tract absorbs much of the radiation dose from α or β emitters and critical cells are protected by their location deep in the intestinal crypts.

The absorption of radionuclides from the intestinal tract is a much more significant factor than direct irradiation of the intestinal tract. Radionuclides are absorbed to varying degrees depending on their solubility. Some radionuclides may be discriminated against during absorption in favor of their normal metabolic analog; e.g., calcium is absorbed in favor of strontium.

The inhalation mode of exposure has long been recognized as being of major importance for certain radioactive materials, particularly in occupational or accidental situations. Radioactive materials important for inhalation hazards may be in a gaseous or particulate form, with the latter being more usual. After inhalation, deposition of these particles in the lung is determined by particle characteristics (particle size, shape, and density), respiratory tract anatomy (airway dimensions, numbers and angles of airway branching), and by respiratory patterns (volume and frequency, nasal versus oral).

Once particles are deposited in the lung, they may be cleared to the circulation, transported up the trachea and swallowed, or transported to local lymph nodes. Particles that deposit on ciliated airways are translocated out of the lung by mucociliary action within 1 day. Insoluble particles that deposit deep in the lung may be retained with a biological half-time of years. The cytotoxicity of some highly radioactive particles may be sufficient to prolong the retention of the particles in the lung. Solubility is a key factor in the retention of radionuclides in the lungs. Soluble materials translocate readily from the lung to the blood, where, based on their elemental characteristics, the radionuclides are carried to tissues or organs. For example, inhaled strontium in ionic form is translocated within a matter of minutes from lung to bone. Strontium made insoluble by incorporation in aluminosilicate particles is retained in the lung with an effective half-life of about 5 years.

vii. Dose localization Radiation doses from internal emitters are usually calculated as the average dose to the target organ. It is determined by integrating the amount of radioactivity in the organ over the retention time of the radionuclide in the organ. Radiation doses from internal emitters are not easily measured

directly. Direct radioactivity counting of the whole body or of radioactivity in body excretions must be used with mathematical models to calculate radiation doses to organs.

One complication in dose calculations is the fact that, in some situations, the radionuclide is not distributed evenly throughout the organ. The prime example of this is the initial localization of many bone-seeking radionuclides on bone surfaces, resulting in higher doses to those bone surfaces. In these cases, the effective radiation dose to critical bone-forming cells can be five times the average radiation dose to the entire bone.

B. MECHANISMS OF IONIZING RADIATION INJURY

1. Interaction of Ionizing Radiation with Biological Materials

The biological effect of ionizing radiation is partly due to the indirect result of free radicals produced in water and partly due to the direct ionization of biological molecules. For low LET radiation, such as X or γ rays, the indirect action predominates. As radiation quality changes to high LET, the direct action becomes more important. Because living material consists of 70–90% water, the radiolysis of water is of considerable importance. However, from a biological standpoint, whether a molecule is damaged directly through the absorption of the radiation energy or indirectly through the radiolysis of water with free radical injury is immaterial for the purposes of our discussion.

The distribution of ionizing events within the cell is important in relation to specific biological targets. The probability of ionization occurring within a given target volume is critical for the development of specific biological effects. Theoretically, some critical or sensitive part of the cell must be damaged ("hit") in order to produce some recognizable degree of injury. It is possible that a single target must be hit more than once, or that two different target sites must be hit, in order to produce biological damage.

The number of damaging events or "sublesions" caused in a cell is proportional to the absorbed dose of radiation and its spatial or temporal delivery. Theoretically, if two sublesions are spatially and temporally close they can interact, causing a more permanent lesion and a recognizable biological effect. Thus, it is evident that with low LET radiation at low doses the ionizing events will be scattered with many sublesions not close enough in time or space to one another to interact. As the dose increases, the sublesions will become more frequent and closely spaced, interaction more common, and recognizable biological effects more frequent. When the radiation has high LET, even at low doses, the ionizations are relatively close together in time and space and the sublesions can interact more readily. Complicating the picture is the fact that radiation injury to the cell is repairable. Thus, even sublesions that are produced in close proximity may not interact if a sufficient time passes between their production to allow repair of the initial injury.

These considerations can account for the various manifestations of differing responses to different types of radiation and radiation delivery schemes. At similar total doses, high LET radiation causes considerably more measurable injury to cells and tissues than low LET radiation. The spreading of a similar total dose over a longer period of time reduces the effect of low LET radiation because there is more time for the repair of sublesions prior to interaction. For high LET radiation, the effect of protraction or fractionation is much less because the original sublesions would have been produced close in time and space and the interaction likelihood would have been quite high. Thus, for low LET radiation, induction of a biological effect at relatively low dose rates may require a higher total dose to achieve the same effect as irradiation of the same tissue at a high dose rate. For high LET radiation, the effect is more independent of dose rate.

Relative biological effect (RBE) is a factor used to compare the biological effectiveness of a radiation dose from different types of radiation under given conditions. A standard reference low LET radiation of low biological effectiveness, i.e., ^{60}cobalt γ rays, is used for comparison and assigned a RBE value of 1.0. Using this scale, high LET radiation have RBE values of greater than 1.0. Although RBE varies with the LET, it also varies with the total dose, dose rate, target tissue or cell, and the end point under evaluation.

2. Subcellular and Cellular Effects of Ionizing Radiation

Despite the vast amount of study of the mechanisms of ionizing radiation injury, an absolute understanding of all the subcellular targets has not been determined. Despite the fact that many chemical bonds can be deleteriously affected by radiation, it often takes enormous doses (thousands of cGy) to get substantial inactivation of biological systems such as respiratory enzymes, partly due to the redundancy that exists in such systems. Such doses are far in excess of what is needed to produce significant cell death. In fact, mean lethal doses to most cell types are on the order of hundreds of cGy. It is clear that many subcellular structures, such as mitochondria, lysosomes, and cell membranes, can be damaged and can lead to cellular changes. However, another more sensitive target is needed to explain the range of biological effects seen.

Most of the significant effects of ionizing radiation from cell killing to carcinogenesis and, logically, genetic effects appear to be related to injury to DNA. While radiation can cause a variety of DNA lesions, including DNA base alterations, DNA–DNA and DNA–protein cross links, and single and double strand breaks, double strand breaks are implicated as being of primary importance. Ionizing radiation induces relatively large-scale structural damage in DNA, often resulting in the loss of entire genes or groups of genes from aberrations such as deletions, rearrangements, and recombinations, rather than point mutations.

A phenomenon recognized only in the past decade is radiation-induced genomic instability. Genomic instability has been characterized as the increased rate of acquisition of alterations in the mammalian genome. The loss of genome stability has long been recognized as a hallmark of cancer cells and carcinogenesis. Genomic instability can be reflected in changes in mutation rates, gene expression, and chromosomal destabilization in the offspring of irradiated cells. Many pathways and genes regulate the stability of the normal genome, and the mechanisms that lead to genomic instability are not known. Both low and high LET radiation can induce genomic instability and delayed genomic effects in irradiated cells. Delayed effects that have been described include delayed mitosis-linked death, delayed mutation, and delayed chromosome instability. The latter resembles the chromosomal changes seen in tumor cells. That delayed effects represent truly inherited phenomena is supported by the fact that most direct mutations seen after ionizing radiation are large deletions, whereas the great majority of delayed mutations are point mutations.

Repair of radiation-induced cell injury is a critical biological phenomenon. Complex enzyme systems are important in the repair of radiation-induced DNA lesions. Such repair has been shown to occur within minutes to hours after injury. On a molecular level, much radiation-induced DNA injury is sublethal and is fully repaired. A cell can accumulate an amount of damage that is potentially lethal and still survive, as shown by the fact that a variety of treatments given after irradiation can modify the survival characteristics of a cell population. For example, changing the proliferation kinetics of a cell population to allow more time for repair before division can reduce lethality under certain conditions. As well as normal repair, abnormal repair or misrepair can take place and contribute to more permanent DNA lesions. It is clear that some of the benefits of temporal protraction or fractionation of irradiation can be related to DNA repair. The longer the time between the production of DNA sublesions, the greater the probability that repair will take place before formation of another sublesion capable of interacting with the first. Differences in biological responses between low and high LET radiation also are

related, and repair is less effective after high LET exposures.

In addition to DNA repair, the state of the DNA with respect to replication is of great importance in determining the sensitivity of cells to radiation injury. Effects such as delay of the progression of irradiated cells through the cell division cycle, the production of chromosome aberrations, and cell killing vary with the stage of the cell cycle at exposure.

Cell cycle delays from irradiation may occur at all stages of the cell cycle. Sensitivity is progressively greater moving from G_1 to S to early G_2. Cells irradiated in late G_2, after protein synthesis necessary for mitosis has taken place, or in M, usually complete division without delays unless the doses are very large. Disturbances of cell kinetics can play a role in tissue regeneration and repopulation and the development of morphological lesions.

The stage of the cell cycle can also affect cell killing. Cells in mitosis show the greatest radiosensitivity, which might relate to the highly condensed state of the DNA, limiting access by DNA repair enzymes to the damaged sites. Cell cycle delays from irradiation at earlier cell cycle stages (G_1, S, and early G_2) would allow more time for repair, reducing sensitivity to cell killing. The hypersensitivity of some G_0 cells to killing and delay is unique and is discussed later.

Chromosome damage is one of the most obvious subcellular changes recognizable after radiation exposure. Although there is a reasonable correlation between chromosome breaks and the reproductive failure and death of the cell, this is not an absolute relationship. Many karyotypic changes allow cell survival and even proliferation, as in neoplasia. A complete discussion of radiation-induced chromosome aberrations is beyond the scope of this chapter; however, a few points are worth noting. Interphase irradiation leads to two types of changes. Early in interphase (G_1) before DNA synthesis and duplication, damage is to whole chromosomes with identical lesions on both chromatids. Irradiation after duplication (G_2) causes effects in single chromatids. Irradiation during synthesis (S) can cause both types of lesions depending on the stage of replication for specific chromosomes. In general, the G_2 stage is the most sensitive for the induction of chromosome aberrations. Aberrations include a variety of types such as breaks, deletions, rings, translocations, dicentrics, and acentrics seen at the subsequent mitosis. Some of these gross aberrations are incompatible with survival of the cells.

Cell killing plays a central role in the understanding of radiation injury because so much of the tissue damage seen by the pathologist is dependent on it. Even other effects, such as carcinogenesis, are dependent on survival of the damaged cells to allow expression. While changes such as pyknosis, karyorrhexis, and karyolysis are no different in cells injured by radiation than in those damaged by other causes, two types of radiation-induced cell death recognized are related to the time of exposure in the cell cycle and the kinetics of cell reproduction. Sufficient irradiation during interphase of the cell cycle results in cell death, but usually this requires a much larger dose of radiation than the second form, mitosis-linked death (also called reproductive death). Some cell types, such as lymphocytes and serous salivary gland cells, undergo interphase death even at very low doses of radiation through the induction of apoptosis. In contrast, mitosis-linked death occurs as a result of the attempt of the cell to divide after irradiation. It is related to the inability of the cell to undergo reproduction and, to some degree, to chromosome abnormalities, although other mechanisms may also play a role. Mitosis-linked death is highly dependent on the cell population being studied. Cell death occurs more quickly in rapidly proliferating populations, such as bone marrow, than in slowly proliferating tissues, such as liver. Thus, cellular kinetics of various organs play a critical role in determining pathological responses.

3. Cell and Tissue Radiosensitivity to Ionizing Radiation

The frequency of cell division generally is inversely proportional to the degree of differentiation of a cell population. This correlates well with cell radiosensitivity; the least differentiated and most actively proliferating populations have the greatest sensitivity. There are, however, exceptions to this rule; the lymphocyte is one of the best examples. It is critical to understand that cell radiosensitivity is a relative concept. It is not only dependent on the cell involved but on the choice of the biological effect to be evaluated. For example, the response of an intracellular enzyme system to irradiation may differ from that for lethality.

Using the criterion of mitosis-linked cell death after radiation exposure, we can draw some general conclusions relating to sensitivity. The most sensitive populations are the relatively undifferentiated or primitive cells that are rapidly dividing and whose progeny may undergo subsequent differentiation. Stem cells of the hematopoietic system, crypt epithelium of the intestine, primitive spermatogonia, and epidermal basal cells, all continuously proliferating populations, are examples.

The next most sensitive group is also made up of cell types that divide frequently, but undergo differentiation between divisions. As they become more differentiated, their radiosensitivity decreases. Examples of such cells would be the committed erythroid and myeloid progenitors of the hematopoietic system and the intermediate spermatogonia. The various multipotential connective tissue cells, which do not divide frequently but may do so in response to a variety of stimuli, are intermediate in terms of their radiosensitivity. Fibroblasts, endothelium, and other mesenchymal cells fall in this category.

The relatively long-lived cell populations, which do not normally undergo much division except in response to stimuli such as loss of significant numbers of cells in an organ, are of low radiosensitivity. This group includes many well-differentiated epithelial parenchymal cells such as those of the liver, kidney, and endocrine glands.

The least radiosensitive populations are those cells that normally do not divide or have lost that capability. They are highly differentiated cells, such as neurons or skeletal muscle cells, or end-stage cells in a differentiation pathway, such as polymorphonuclear leukocytes or spermatozoa. Figure 1 depicts the relationships between radiosensitivity and differentiation for some of the hematopoietic cells of the bone marrow.

The efficiency of ionizing radiation-induced cell death is thought, as mentioned previously, to be related to double strand breaks in DNA, and differences in radiosensitivity between cells are largely related to differences in DNA repair. Another factor is mode of cell death. For example, lymphoid and hematopoietic cells, which have a high radiosensitivity to cell killing, undergo apoptosis, whereas cells with low sensitivity undergo necrosis after irradiation. Even within lymphoid and myeloid cell lines differences in radiosensitivity correlate with the rapidity of induction of apoptosis. In some cases, this can be correlated with differences in the status of the *p53* gene, which is important in the induction of apoptosis. For example, hematopoietic cell lines with the wild-type p53 protein are more sensitive to radiation-induced apoptosis than cells with mutant protein. It is also important to recognize that the degree of injury, in this case the total radiation dose, can affect the mode of cell death. Cells that may undergo apoptosis after mild injury may undergo necrosis when insulted with more severe damage of the same type.

It is appropriate to briefly discuss the relationships between oxygenation of cells and radiosensitivity. It is generally true that the presence of increased concentrations of dissolved oxygen increases the sensitivity of cells to ionizing radiation compared with lower oxygen concentrations or hypoxic conditions. Increased sensitivity due to a higher oxygen concentration relates to most of the common biological manifestations of damage, such as division delay, gene mutations, and chromosome aberrations. The mechanisms involved implicate the formation of free radicals, including the superoxide ion, as important. That radiosensitivity can be reduced by the use of compounds, which lower the cellular concentrations of free radicals, such as glutathione and other thiol-containing molecules, supports this. In a practical sense, this can be important for the radiotherapist treating a variety of malignancies that can show considerable local hypoxia, making them less sensitive to radiation-induced cell killing. Tumor hypoxia is considered to be a major cause of failure of radiotherapy for cancer.

4. General Tissue and Organ Effects of Ionizing Radiation

In terms of radiation effects at the level of tissues, organs, and the whole organism, such effects have been classified in several different ways. Traditionally, we speak of "somatic"

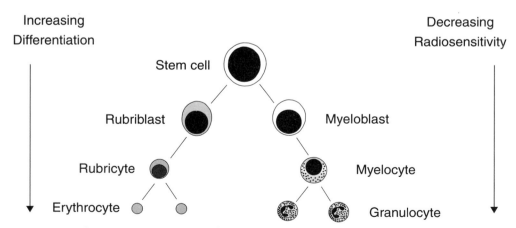

Figure 1. Schematic representation of the relationship between differentiation and radiosensitivity in selected hematopoietic cell lines of the bone marrow.

effects, those that are manifested in the exposed individual, or "hereditary" effects, those manifested in the descendants of the exposed individual. In this chapter we are restricting discussions to somatic effects; however, it should be remembered that injury to the genetic material is still involved in most radiation injury.

An important determinant of understanding both acute and late-occurring injury in any tissue is the ability to recognize the critical target cells that are originally injured and later result in specific pathological changes. It does not always follow that the most radiosensitive cells for acute effects are the same targets that result in late-occurring effects. Whether specific acute effects are predictive for late effects, including cancer induction, is also not a given.

The sensitivity of specific cell types is defined after acute exposure and short time periods of observation. Short-term acute effects are generally dependent on early specific cell killing. Necrosis leading to atrophy in continuously proliferating tissues requires relatively small doses, whereas in slowly dividing tissues, larger doses are needed. As doses increase, however, a more indirect mechanism comes into play. This includes radiation effects on stromal tissues, which can affect the parenchymal cells secondarily. For example, higher radiation doses to the bone marrow affect not only the proliferating hematopoietic cells, but also the stromal microenvironment, which is critical for supporting normal hematopoiesis. In many organs, when doses are high enough to cause significant injury to the microvasculature, late-occurring effects may be a result of the slow development of ischemic conditions. Tissue atrophy can also be the result of indirect effects, such as the radiation-induced loss of tissues or organs that produce a humoral factor that may be necessary for the maintenance of some other tissue. Radiation has also been shown to initiate the release or activation of growth factors and cytokines that may profoundly affect late effects and tissue structure.

Thus, the response of a particular tissue or organ to ionizing radiation injury is dependent on multiple factors, including the cell populations involved and their characteristics, the nature of the radiation insult, and the general and local host environment. Table III lists some of the important factors.

5. Fine Vascular and Connective Tissue Effects of Ionizing Radiation

Changes in the supporting tissues, including the vasculature and connective tissues, play an important role in the pathogenesis of radiation-induced injury in many organs. This is true for the most immediate acute responses seen as well as for various late effects occurring months to years later. The changes seen in vascular and connective tissues after irradiation are not pathognomonic and can be seen after many other types of injury. After recovery from early lesions involving direct radiosensitivity of an organ's parenchymal populations, late-occurring stromal responses are even less specific. Vascular responses tend to be important throughout the entire course of a tissue's response to irradiation, whereas connective tissue responses become more important with increasing time.

A simplified scheme addressing the role of vascular and connective tissues in radiation injury is presented in Table IV. Early responses to radiation injury, occurring within hours of exposure, are mainly related to increased vascular permeability due to endothelial damage, with cell killing playing a minor role. Intermediate time changes (days to months) are related to

TABLE III
Factors Affecting Tissue and Organ Radiation Responses

General factors	Specific attributes
Characteristics of cell populations	Mixtures of cell types in the tissue
	Specific radiosensitivity of parenchymal cells
	Cell proliferation kinetics of tissue
	Ability of cell to repair sublethal damage
Radiation exposure	Total dose delivered
	Time course of dose delivery
	Radiation quality (LET)
Environmental factors	Specific hormone and growth factor levels
	Cell and tissue oxygenation

TABLE IV
Phases of Radiation Injury

Phase	Time	Characteristic changes
Early	Hours	Endothelial injury Increased vascular permeability
Intermediate	Days – months Days Weeks – months Months	Mitosis-linked cell death GI epithelium Parenchymal tissues Endothelium
Late	Months – years	Vascular occlusion Parenchymal atrophy Interstitial fibrosis

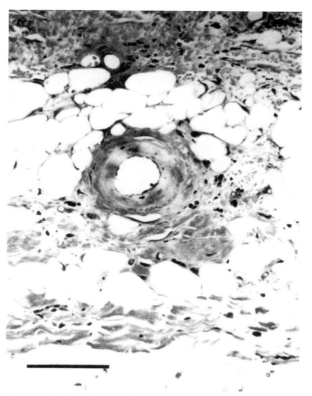

Figure 2. Small arteriole showing medial necrosis and hyalinization, as well as mild perivascular fibrosis in a dog given a single dose of 3500 cGy electrons 1 year earlier. Hematoxylin and eosin (H&E) stain. Bar: 100 μm.

cell killing, primarily mitosis-linked death. Late effects are related to more chronic injury to the vasculature and the development of excessive fibrosis.

The radiosensitivity of the endothelial cell is purported to be intermediate between the bone marrow stem cell and the intestinal epithelial stem cell. After most irradiations, however, mitosis-linked cell death plays only a minimal role in early injury because the turnover time of endothelium is quite long—on the order of months. Within hours of irradiation of a tissue, the endothelium has such changes as swelling, vacuolization, a few necrotic cells, and opening of intercellular junctions. There is an initial narrowing of the lumens of the very small vasculature that can contribute to local ischemia or thrombosis. The other early changes are essentially those of the acute inflammatory response. Endothelial injury itself can be responsible for triggering the acute inflammatory response. The compensatory endothelial hyperplasia that follows can further compromise vascular lumens and blood flow.

Although connective tissue proliferation is not characteristic of the early pathological changes, there is activation of fibroblastic cells that can begin the organization of the fibrinous exudates resulting from the inflammation. TGF-β is activated after irradiation in a variety of organs and tissues and likely plays a role in late-occurring fibrosis. The development of more chronic vascular lesions is characterized by degenerative vascular changes (Fig. 2) and by fibroblast proliferation and excess collagen deposition. The latter takes the form of arteriocapillary fibrosis, and interstitial and septal fibrosis of organs. As the early radiation reaction progresses, the plasma leakage results in connective tissue deposition in the perivascular interstitial tissues (Fig. 3). This process, once started, can progress slowly for years and, ultimately, result in significant thickening of the vascular wall as well as the perivascular interstitial tissues. All these changes are more severe with increasing doses. Whereas this fibrous connective tissue deposition occurs slowly, the turnover of these tissue elements is also slow, so this represents a long-lasting, often permanent, injury.

With time, the progression of small vessel fibrosis causes progressively more interference with the local circulation with significant diminution of blood flow to part or all of an

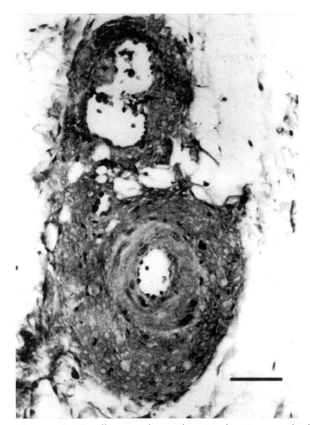

Figure 3. Small arteriole and vein showing marked perivascular fibrosis in a dog given 4400 cGy electrons in 400-cGy fractions 1 year earlier. H&E stain. Bar: 50 μm.

organ. The buildup of connective tissue around the vessels increases this ischemia, further, which causes a greater diffusion barrier to the passage of oxygen and nutrients to the tissue. The end result is that even organs that may have recovered from the initial parenchymal injury may have a secondary loss of parenchyma and gradual atrophy due to the slowly developing vascular lesions. Many noncarcinogenic late effects have this vascular lesion as their primary pathogenesis.

6. Ionizing Radiation Carcinogenesis

The carcinogenic effect of ionizing radiation is well known. For radiation, as well as other carcinogenic agents, the first critical event in neoplastic induction (initiation) appears to involve changes in DNA that are transmitted to daughter cells, representing a cellular "heritable" trait. These may be direct changes such as point mutation or, in the case of ionizing radiation, more commonly larger DNA lesions. As with other carcinogenic agents, radiation carcinogenesis may involve abnormal activation of oncogenes or inactivation or deletion of tumor suppressor genes. Carcinogenesis is a multistage process with initiation followed by events that allow the transformed cells to proliferate ("promotion") and undergo further phenotypic change to more malignant states ("progression").

Ionizing radiation is often referred to as a "complete" carcinogen. It can cause initiation by its ability to damage DNA in a susceptible cell. It can also act as a promoter by causing local tissue damage, which results in cell proliferation as part of repair and by its immunosuppressive nature, which might allow already initiated cells to escape putative "immunosurveillance" mechanisms. Through its DNA-damaging and clastogenic actions, ionizing radiation can further alter phenotypic characteristics of already developed neoplasms, thus affecting neoplastic progression.

Recent research has focused on the possible role of genomic destabilization in radiation carcinogenesis. As noted, chromosomal instability has long been considered a hallmark of carcinogenesis, and the process of progression is commonly associated with increasing karyotypic abnormalities. It has been proposed that the induction of genetic instability is the initial step in radiation carcinogenesis, especially when critical genes such as *p53* are mutated. It has been demonstrated that loss of normal *p53* function greatly increases the susceptibility to radiation-induced neoplasia in rodents. In a mouse model of breast carcinogenesis, *p53* mutations appeared to arise in the progeny of irradiated cells rather than being induced directly. These mutations were point mutations rather than the larger deletions usually associated with direct radiation exposure. Further, C57BL/6 mice that are relatively resistant to mammary carcinogenesis are also resistant to development of radiation-induced instability as evaluated by delayed chromosomal aberrations, and BALB/c mice that were sensitive to carcinogenesis were also sensitive to radiation-induced instability. These findings support the concept that genomic instability can be linked as an early event in radiation-induced cancer leading to secondary mutations (such as those in *p53*) at later times. The future of this research path would appear to be fruitful, not only for radiation-induced cancer, but also for cancer research in general.

Ionizing radiation can cause an increase in the incidence of neoplasms in an irradiated population and can also cause an earlier appearance of neoplasms, i.e., an age-related increase in tumors that would have appeared in a population at a later time. Identification of a neoplasm as radiation induced is difficult, if not impossible, in the individual patient. Clinically and morphologically, radiation-induced neoplasms are indistinguishable from those spontaneous tumors that would be seen in a population from any other cause. Recognition of radiation-induced neoplasms is by statistical evaluation of exposed populations rather than by morphological means in individuals. In such populations, radiation-induced tumors are considered to be those that appear in statistically significant excess in an exposed population compared with some control population. The suspicion that a particular neoplasm might be radiation induced can be supported by knowledge that an organ or tissue has received a significant radiation dose and that the particular type of tumor has been associated with radiation exposure in the past.

Several biological factors are of particular importance with respect to radiation carcinogenesis, including age at exposure, gender, genetic background, and the specific tissue or organ exposed. Age at exposure has been referred to as perhaps the single most important modifying factor with respect to the carcinogenic response in humans. In general, the younger the individual at the time of irradiation, the greater the risk for cancer induction. While there are some exceptions to this rule with respect to specific types of cancer, this age-related sensitivity extends even back to the

fetal period. While there has been controversy over the unusually high sensitivity of the fetus, both human epidemiological data and animal studies have supported this finding. Epidemiological studies have reported increased risk for childhood cancer, particularly leukemias, after prenatal diagnostic irradiation. Beagle dogs have been reported to show increased risk for neoplasia both early in life and throughout the life span after prenatal and early postnatal exposures. One possible pathogenesis is the presence of greatly increased cell proliferation in the growing fetus and immature individual that would create an overall environment for the promotion of neoplasia. Another explanation for the increased lifetime risk is the longer latent period available for the expression of cancers when exposures occur early in life.

Gender is also an important factor in radiation carcinogenesis. Females have an overall greater risk of radiation-induced neoplasia. In part, this is explained by the induction of breast cancer because the breast is one of the most sensitive tissues to radiation-induced cancer. Breast cancer incidence does not totally explain the greater risk of neoplasia in females, however, as hormonal balance plays a role in other cancer types. For example, in the mouse, leukemias are more frequent in females because estrogen has a promoting effect on these tumors.

Genetic background affects radiation carcinogenesis as evidenced by the great differences in types of cancers seen in different species and different strains within species. Radiation-induced cancer is considered to be imposed as an augmentation to the natural background incidence in any species, thus there is an increase in the types of tumors already seen, rather than induction of totally unique neoplasms.

Finally, the type of tissue or organ is a critical factor, as there is great variation in the sensitivity of different tissues to radiation carcinogenesis. The bone marrow, the thyroid gland, and the breast are considered to be the most sensitive tissues to radiation. The lung has a somewhat lower but still significant sensitivity. Risk to human populations must take into account not only the inherent sensitivity of the tissue, but also the natural incidence of spontaneous disease, as the rate of radiation-induced tumors is dependent on the spontaneous incidence, either as an additive or as a multiplicative factor. Thus, diseases such as breast and lung cancer, both of which have a very high spontaneous incidence along with significant sensitivity to induction by radiation, are of concern for human health. While leukemia and thyroid cancer have lower background incidences, their extremely high sensitivity also makes them of particular concern.

C. RESPONSE TO INJURY INDUCED BY IONIZING RADIATION

1. *Hematopoietic and Lymphoid Systems*

a. General Reaction to Ionizing Radiation Injury. Normal functioning of hematopoietic tissues involves complex balances between stem cell renewal and differentiation and development of more mature cell types, and regulation by the stromal microenvironment and extracellular growth factors. This is true for both bone marrow and lymphopoietic tissues. The various cells of the hematopoietic system are among the most sensitive in the body to ionizing radiation. There are some very significant differences between the responses of lymphoid cells and the other cell types of the hematopoietic series, which will be discussed separately.

The population of pluripotential stem cells of the bone marrow, which give rise to erythroid, myeloid, lymphoid, monocytic, and megakaryocytic cell lines, has a high turnover and is highly radiosensitive. The more differentiated committed progenitor cells of these lines are less radiosensitive. As the cells in these lines move toward terminal differentiation, they become progressively less sensitive. This is an important factor in understanding the pathological effects seen after acute whole body radiation exposure. Although the entire population of stem cells and committed progenitors is sensitive, there is evidence of heterogeneity in sensitivity among the different progenitor cell subsets.

Erythroid cells have greater sensitivity to destruction than myelomonocytic and megakaryocytic cells. Little is known about the lymphoid cell precursors in the bone marrow, and lymphocytes outside the marrow represent a special case. The various nonhematopoietic and stromal components of the marrow, including fibroblasts, adipocytes, endothelium, and endosteum, traditionally have been considered to have a lesser degree of radiosensitivity than the hematopoietic elements. However, recent research has suggested that under some conditions the stromal sensitivity can be as great or greater than that of hematopoietic cells. The stroma forms a critical inductive microenvironment, without which normal hematopoiesis cannot take place. The stroma is not simply supportive in nature but plays a determinative role in growth and differentiation. Stromal injury can play an important role in the genesis of some late radiation effects.

After an acute whole body radiation exposure at the LD_{50} dose, there is a delay of cycling of the proliferating bone marrow stem and progenitor cell compartments. After this delay, a wave of cell division follows with a large amount of mitosis-linked death. About 1 day later, bone marrow necrosis is present as evidenced by pyknotic and karyorrhectic nuclei and phagocytosis of cell debris. At this time, many of the more mature differentiated cells remain intact. Because these cells are relatively radioresistant, they continue to mature and are ultimately exported to the peripheral blood. This further depletion leads to a hypoplastic marrow by about 3 days after irradiation. Necrosis continues as the remaining stem and progenitor cells cycle and undergo mitosis-linked death.

These bone marrow changes are reflected in lowering of the peripheral blood cell counts, but this is delayed. The time of appearance of these cell decrements is basically determined by the life span of the various blood cells and can differ among species. Because of the much shorter life span of the granulocytes and platelets (on the order of a few days to a week or so), severe granulocytopenia and thrombocytopenia are seen relatively early when compared with the occurrence of anemia. The latter is delayed because of the longer life span of erythrocytes, which is on the order of 3 months. Granulocytopenia is actually preceded by a lymphocytopenia that develops immediately after irradiation, reaching a maximum at day 1 postexposure. This timing is due to the high sensitivity of lymphocytes to interphase death, which occurs rapidly and is not dependent on cell division. Thus, the timing of the development of various cell decrements in the blood, i.e., lymphopenia, granulocytopenia, thrombocytopenia, and anemia, represents not just the inherent sensitivity of the cell lines, but also their life span. Because of the slow turnover of the stromal cell population, mitosis-linked death is minimized, as is acute injury to this compartment.

This sequence of events results in what is referred to as the "hematopoietic syndrome." The severity of the changes is directly dependent on the dose, as well as on the species irradiated. Species differences in radiosensitivity as measured by the $LD_{50/30}$ for acute whole body radiation can range up to twofold; for example, from 200 to 300 cGy in the dog to 600 cGy or greater in rodents. Several explanations have been suggested as to the mechanisms of this species variation, including differences in kinetics of hematopoiesis, differences in concentrations of stem cells per kilogram body weight, and differences in intrinsic sensitivity of the hematopoietic precursors.

Because resistance to infection is dependent on both functional granulocytes and normal immune function, radiation-induced panleukopenia leaves the individual susceptible to severe and often fatal infections. The susceptibility to infection can be compounded by thrombocytopenia, resulting in severe hemorrhage. Anemia is much less a problem after acute exposures; however, it can be of importance after chronic exposure. Other later occurring changes observed in the bone marrow include hematopoietic atrophy and myelofibrosis (Fig. 4).

Internally deposited radionuclides can be of concern if they deliver significant radiation

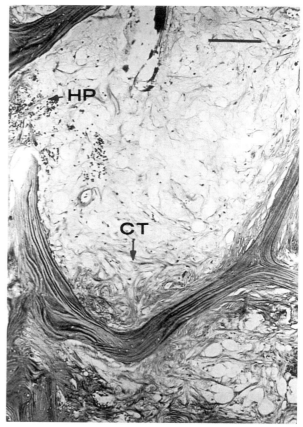

Figure 4. Hematopoietic atrophy and myelofibrosis in a dog 5 years after a single dose of 3500 cGy electrons to the bone. There are few hematopoietic cells (HP) and increased fibrous connective tissue (CT) in the bone marrow. H&E stain. Bar: 100 μm.

doses to the bone marrow. For example, the potassium analog ^{137}Cs distributes throughout the body and its high-energy γ emission results in whole body exposure that can cause the acute hematopoietic syndrome. Bone-seeking radionuclides such as ^{144}Ce, ^{90}Sr, or ^{239}Pu partially or preferentially deposit in bone and irradiate the adjacent marrow. Such internal emitters can also cause hematopoietic depletion at very high doses, but are more usually associated with the development of hematopoietic and bone neoplasms at lower doses and later times.

Whereas it is customary to refer to the lymphocyte as a highly radiosensitive cell, it is critical to remember the diversity within the lymphoid cell population. There are differences in the radiosensitivities of thymocytes and peripheral lymphocytes as well as significant differences among the peripheral cells themselves. B lymphocytes are recognized as having a greater radiosensitivity than T lymphocytes. Various subclasses of T lymphocytes have different radiosensitivities. Suppressor or cytotoxic T lymphocyte populations are more sensitive than helper-inducer cells, although even here there can be variations depending on further subclasses evaluated, species, and other factors. Natural killer cells seem to be more radioresistant than other lymphocytes. Finally, the basic radiosensitivity of lymphocytes is dependent on their state of differentiation and activation. With respect to immune responses, primed B or T cells have much decreased radiosensitivity. The highly radiosensitive lymphocyte undergoes interphase death with all the morphological and physiological characteristics of apoptosis. Evidence shows that lymphoid cells have a deficient ability to repair sublethal radiation-induced DNA injury, which adds to their overall sensitivity.

b. Radiation Leukemogenesis. External exposures to relatively high doses of radiation are necessary to cause the acute effects discussed. However, even low doses can be associated with the development of hematopoietic neoplasia. The hematopoietic system is one of the most sensitive to the induction of malignancies. In humans, there is clear association of irradiation with myeloid leukemias (both acute and chronic forms) and with acute lymphoid leukemia. In animals, the mouse develops primarily thymic lymphomas and some myeloid leukemias after irradiation. Irradiated dogs develop myeloproliferative disorders, including myeloid leukemias, as well as lymphomas. Rats develop myeloid leukemias, and swine developed lymphomas after irradiation.

The pathogenesis may well differ to some degree among species. In the mouse, many factors can affect radiation leukemogenesis. Dose rate plays an important role in leukemogenesis from low LET radiation, whereas it is not a factor after high LET exposures. Gender of the animals can be important. Female mice are more sensitive to the induction of thymic lymph-

omas, whereas male mice are more sensitive to the induction of myeloid leukemia. Experimentally, estrogens will enhance murine thymic lymphoma induction whereas androgens will inhibit it. Age at exposure plays an important role in both animals and humans, with leukemia sensitivity decreasing with an individual's age. In some species, including humans, the fetus appears to be particularly sensitive to leukemia induction.

For many years, a viral agent has been associated with radiation leukemogenesis in the mouse and, because of this, much attention has been given to the pursuit of a similar etiology in other species. There is no question that certain murine viruses are associated with radiation-induced leukemias; however, viruses are not always found and it may not be a universal phenomenon.

Radiation-induced acute myeloid leukemia (AML) in the highly sensitive CBA mouse is a good example to illustrate the pathogenesis of leukemia development. Murine AML is consistently associated with radiation-induced chromosome number two (2) rearrangement in pluripotential hematopoietic cells. Chromosome number two lesions are reported only in radiation-induced myeloid leukemia and not in spontaneous cases. Cytogenetic analyses reveal that large numbers of chromosome number two aberrations can be seen only days after irradiation, but that only a small percentage of these cells survive as clones and progress to leukemia. Factors such as treatment with corticosteroids or induction of inflammatory responses can promote leukemia induction. It has been shown that chromosome number two contains specific radiosensitive "hot spots" for aberration formation, accounting for the specificity of aberrations. Deregulation of the interleukin-1β gene located on the altered chromosome number two adjacent to the break site has been suggested as playing a role in the process.

Another example for illustrating some basic pathogenetic mechanisms relating to radiation-induced bone marrow injury and leukemogenesis is the chronically irradiated dog (Fig. 5). In this model, beagles were exposed to whole body

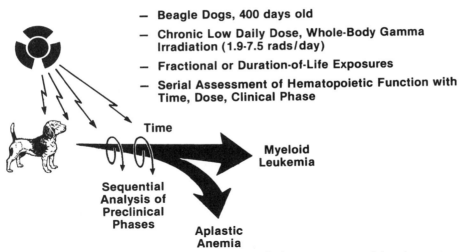

— **Beagle Dogs, 400 days old**

— **Chronic Low Daily Dose, Whole-Body Gamma Irradiation (1.9-7.5 rads/day)**

— **Fractional or Duration-of-Life Exposures**

— **Serial Assessment of Hematopoietic Function with Time, Dose, Clinical Phase**

Figure 5. Primary feature of a chronic radiation leukemogenesis model in the canine. Dogs were serially assessed for clinical phasing and hematopoietic function throughout the radiation exposure period. Reproduced from Seed (1987), with permission.

^{60}Co γ radiation at relatively low daily doses (1.9–7.5 cGy/day) for a major portion of their life span. On the basis of survival and pathological changes, two groups of dogs were recognized in the study (Fig. 6). One was a "radiosensitive," aplastic anemia-prone (AA-prone) group with a short survival. The other was a "radioresistant," long-surviving group that did not develop aplastic anemia. Within the radioresistant group were two subgroups: one myeloid leukemia-prone (ML-prone) and a second that did not develop anemia or leukemia. This dichotomy tells us much about the pathological responses of the bone marrow to long-term irradiation. The major difference between these groups was their ability to recover from or repair hematopoietic injury, with AA-prone dogs having a deficient recovery ability.

In AA-prone dogs, the marrow cellularity was progressively depleted with continuing exposure over time. In contrast, ML-prone dogs had an initial decline in marrow cellularity like the AA-prone dogs, but at about 200–300 days of exposure the bone marrow cell loss slowed, stabilized, and then underwent partial recovery (Fig. 7). Recovery was associated with the appearance of specific clones of radioresistant progenitors. This ability to recover from the acute phase injury, however, put the animal at risk for the later development of myeloproliferative disorders, including leukemia. Radioresistant dogs that were not AA or ML prone had hematopoietic recovery kinetics that was intermediate between the other two. There was a general hypertrophy of the stromal supporting elements in the later stages of leukemia development. In a few dogs, significant myelofibrosis accompanied the other changes.

c. Lymphoid Tissues. A detailed discussion of the effects of ionizing radiation on the immune response is beyond the scope of this chapter; however, it can be seen from its severe lymphocytolytic character that ionizing radiation must have equally severe depressant effects on immune function. Relating to the sensitivity of various lymphocyte subsets, this is a complex problem and depends on the timing of

RESPONDING SUBGROUPS

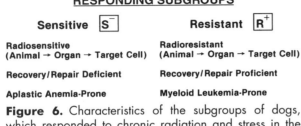

Sensitive $\boxed{S^-}$ **Resistant** $\boxed{R^+}$

Radiosensitive
(Animal → Organ → Target Cell)

Radioresistant
(Animal → Organ → Target Cell)

Recovery/Repair Deficient

Recovery/Repair Proficient

Aplastic Anemia-Prone

Myeloid Leukemia-Prone

Figure 6. Characteristics of the subgroups of dogs, which responded to chronic radiation and stress in the chronic radiation leukemogenesis model. Reproduced from Seed (1987), with permission.

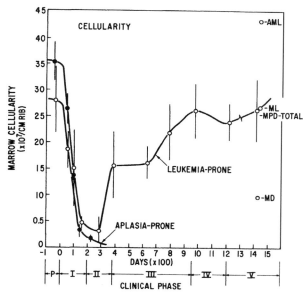

Figure 7. Sequential change in bone marrow cellularity with time of chronic irradiation and relationship to preclinical and clinically evident disease in dogs with aplastic anemia (AA prone) or myeloid leukemia (ML prone). Reproduced from Seed (1987), with permission.

irradiation with respect to antigen exposure, dose, and many other factors. For example, primary responses are more radiosensitive than anamnestic responses relating, at least in part, to the greater resistance of primed antigen-stimulated cells. Dose is a factor because exposure to very low doses of radiation (up to 25 cGy) can actually augment immune responses. This has been attributed to the killing of an exquisitely radiosensitive population of T suppressor lymphocytes, thus allowing increased responsiveness.

Much as is seen in the peripheral blood, lymphoid tissues such as lymph node and splenic white pulp undergo changes in a matter of hours after irradiation. Initial morphological findings include necrosis and cell debris from the death of the lymphocytes with a general lymphoid depletion occuring in several days. It takes high doses (thousands of cGy) to affect the filtration capacity of the nodes and to lead to stromal fibrosis and atrophy.

The thymus has a unique response to acute irradiation, which is intimately associated with bone marrow function. Cortical thymocytes are highly sensitive to both irradiation and corticosteroids, whereas the medullary thymocytes are resistant to both. In contrast, the stromal elements are considered radioresistant. It takes high doses of radiation to reduce the thymus to an atrophic-fibrosed organ. The usual response to a moderate dose is a biphasic recovery curve. In rodents, acute whole body doses of several hundred cGy cause an initial decrease in thymic weight due to thymocyte loss, with recovery by 5–12 days due to proliferation of a radioresistant intrathymic population of thymocytes. A secondary decrease in thymic weight occurs shortly thereafter, apparently due to a reduced influx of thymocyte precursors from the irradiated bone marrow. About 20 days after irradiation, a secondary recovery begins as the bone marrow recovers and precursors again circulate to the thymus. At lower doses (<200 cGy) or with bone marrow shielding, the secondary atrophy does not occur because there is insufficient injury to the bone marrow precursors.

One other unusual effect of internally deposited radionuclides is worth mentioning. Dogs that have inhaled relatively insoluble particles of α- or β-emitting radionuclides retain these in the lung for long periods with some translocation of the particles to the tracheobronchial lymph nodes. These dogs develop a lymphocytopenia that is both dose and dose rate dependent. Apparently, this is due to the continuous irradiation of lymphocytes as they circulate through the lung in the peripheral blood. Ultimately, the dogs can develop lymphoid depletion in the various distant peripheral lymph nodes as well. The tracheobronchial nodes themselves can become completely atrophic and fibrotic and can be the site of radiation-induced neoplasms. This effect is somewhat analogous to the effects of extracorporeal irradiation of blood.

2. Respiratory System

a. General Reaction to Ionizing Radiation Injury.
Irradiation of the respiratory tract can result in either early or late morphologic effects. Early histologic effects involve degeneration

and inflammation and occur within weeks to months of irradiation, with the onset being dependent on dose. This time course of reaction in the lung is delayed when compared with other organ systems, such as bone marrow or intestine, because of differences in cytokinetics among these organs. Late visible effects are fibrosis and neoplasia, which may be seen years after exposure.

The possible association between early and late injuries is a matter of debate. Radiation pneumonitis and pulmonary fibrosis have been studied extensively because of their importance as untoward results of thoracic irradiation for cancer therapy. There are several schools of thought on the pathogenesis and association of early and late radiation injury in the lungs. Early effects have been related to cytotoxic damage to alveolar type II cells or endothelial cells. Surfactant release by damaged alveolar type II cells has been suggested as a predictor of developing radiation pneumonitis. In studies with laboratory animals, there is a strong correlation between increased surfactant release and lethal pulmonary injury.

One late effect of irradiation, pulmonary fibrosis, may come about in one of several ways. One explanation is that damage to small vessels eventually leads to ischemic degeneration of the parenchymal cells and to fibrosis. Another explanation is that radiation damage to the slowly proliferating epithelial cells of the parenchyma results in loss of these cells and, ultimately, fibrosis.

The type of cell affected and the cytokinetics are of great importance in considering the reaction of the lung to irradiation. Turnover time of the alveolar epithelium appears long, and that of the endothelium is exceedingly long (>100 days). The alveolar type II cell has been shown to be the progenitor cell of the alveolar epithelium and has a turnover time of more than 28 days. Type I cells turn over in about 100 days, whereas airway epithelial turnover ranges from 2 to 10 days.

Using data regarding cell kinetics, it is tempting to speculate that the early radiation effects in the deep lung are due to damage to alveolar type II cells and that late nonneoplastic effects are due to irradiation of the endothelium. In this scheme, early and late effects could progress independently. A second speculation is that both early and late effects are the result of vascular injury and inflammation. A number of studies have shown that vascular injury with increased microvascular permeability occurs early after exposure. This injury causes leakage of plasma proteins into the interstitium and onto the alveolar surfaces. This could be related to the injury of endothelial cells and their subsequent death and depletion.

b. Radiation Pneumonitis and Pulmonary Fibrosis. Irradiation of the lung, as occurs in radiation therapy or from inhaled radionuclides, can induce a clinically significant radiation reaction. The acute syndrome is called radiation pneumonitis and can be divided into three phases: latent phase, exudative phase, and acute pneumonitis phase. The extent and time of appearance of each phase are related to radiation dose, with a single dose of 800–2000 cGy of external thoracic irradiation being required for the syndrome to be apparent. With multiple small fractions or protracted irradiation, higher doses are required to produce the same effect.

i. Latent phase The latent phase generally lasts at least 3–4 weeks. During this time, there is scant morphological evidence of injury with light microscopy, but ultrastructural lesions can be seen. There is little agreement among various investigators as to what the initial or most important ultrastructural lesions are in this latent phase. Most report ultrastructural changes in endothelial cells and evidence of increased capillary permeability, but this is not uniformly the case. Others demonstrate alterations in type I or type II alveolar epithelial cells. The contradictory findings in the latent phase syndrome are among the factors preventing the clarification of the pathogenesis of the radiation pneumonitis syndrome.

ii. Exudative phase The exudative phase is generally seen 3–10 weeks after a single high dose of radiation and is characterized by protein-rich deposits in the alveoli with evidence of alveolar epithelial and endothelial cell damage.

Death may occur during this phase with sufficiently high radiation doses (single dose that is greater than 2000 cGy). Hyaline membrane formation is reported in humans and is seen in dogs, but rarely in laboratory rodents. Many investigators report major changes in vascular and mechanical properties of the lung that begin in the exudative phase.

iii. Acute pneumonitis The acute pneumonitis phase occurs 2–18 months after exposure. The lesion in acute radiation pneumonitis is an interstitial pneumonia characterized by infiltration of the alveolar septa with monocytes, lymphocytes, and a few neutrophils, and accumulation of fibrin, macrophages, and a few neutrophils in the alveoli. Alveolar type II cells are increased in number and size. One characteristic finding in humans and dogs, but not in rodents, is the presence of atypical hypertrophic type II cells with enlarged nucleoli and a high nuclear to cytoplasmic ratio (Fig. 8). Alveolar septal fibrosis also may be present and is more prominent in dogs and primates than in rodents.

iv. Pulmonary fibrosis Pulmonary fibrosis and pulmonary neoplasia are the major late effects of pulmonary irradiation. A role for fibroplasia in neoplastic induction is often suggested but not proven. In some situations, fibroplasia, neoplasia, and inflammation occur simultaneously. Neoplasia can occur at much smaller radiation doses than required to produce radiation pneumonitis or pulmonary fibrosis; thus inflammation and fibrosis are not necessary in neoplastic induction but may promote it. Radiation-induced early inflammation probably contributes to late fibrosis, based on analogy with the course of inflammation in other tissues. Inflammation may not be a necessary component, however, for fibrosis to develop.

Pulmonary fibrosis may occur from 6 months to several years after lung irradiation. In humans, localized doses greater than 2000–3000 cGy result in significant fibrosis, although mild fibrosis has been reported after doses of about 500 cGy. In radiation therapy involving the lung, fibrosis is a common sequel, but the

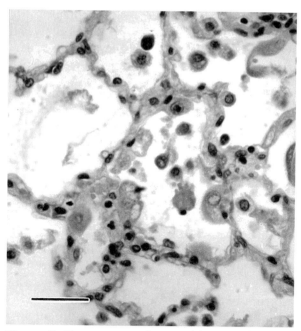

Figure 8. The presence of atypical hypertrophic type II epithelial cells is frequent in radiation pneumonitis in most species. H&E stain. Bar: 37 μm.

clinical signs are usually minimal with only mild deterioration of pulmonary function, partly due to the reserve of unirradiated lung volume. Biochemical and histologic evidence of fibrosis may be present as early as 2 months after exposure. Fibrosis may progress over a period of 1 to 2 years and then reach a state of stability.

Results of studies of mice exposed to external thoracic irradiation have demonstrated a two-phased radiation reaction: an early phase at about 16 weeks after exposure, related to pneumonitis, and a late phase at about 36 weeks after exposure, related to fibrosis. Fractionation of the dose can mitigate the pneumonitis phase, but not the fibrosis phase. The implications are that the mechanisms for these two reactions are separate and different. Although these studies are provocative, the phenomenon has only been demonstrated in mice. In addition, biochemical changes in collagen were not separated into two phases of injury.

Another study using mice demonstrated the role of type I alveolar cells in radiation-induced pulmonary fibrosis. Butylated hydroxytoluene was used to cause type I cell death concurrently with a low dose of thoracic irradiation. When given together, the two treatments were synergistic in producing fibrosis. If given in sequence separated by 6 days, however, no fibrosis was produced. This study suggests that alveolar re-epithelialization may be an important factor in preventing pulmonary fibrosis.

Acute and late effects in the respiratory tract are seen in humans and animals exposed to internally deposited radionuclides, although very few human have been exposed to sufficient amounts of internally deposited radionuclides to cause such lesions. The histologic changes are the same as those resulting from external thoracic irradiation, but the syndrome differs significantly in the time of onset, severity, and spectrum of lesions at any given time after initial inhalation. These differences are related to the tremendous variations in total dose, dose rate, and dose distribution in the lung that can be the result of inhaled particulate radionuclides. Very high radiation doses can be delivered to the lung, but the time span over which this occurs may be days to years. Radionuclides with long effective half-lives in the lung can irradiate the lungs for much of the lifetime of the animal. In such cases, there is blending of the phases of early and late radiation reactions (Fig. 9).

Irradiation of the lungs from internally deposited α-emitting particles can result in severe focal lesions. These focal lesions may not compromise pulmonary function, as the tissue between the foci is relatively unaffected. Figure 10 illustrates focal fibrosis, inflammation, and alveolar macrophage accumulation around numerous α-emitting particles. The fibrosis is concentrated around the particles and generally does not form in a septal pattern.

v. Vascular lesions Another effect of irradiation of the lungs is the induction of vascular lesions. Similar lesions are seen after irradiation from external sources or internally deposited β-emitting radionuclides. The most striking changes are vasculitis and fibrinoid necrosis involving bronchial and pulmonary vessels. Vasculitis is seen most commonly in small muscular

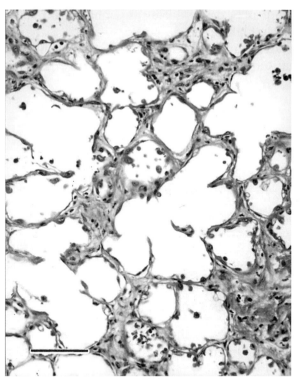

Figure 9. Interstitial pneumonia with septal fibrosis caused by a long-lived β-emitting radionuclide, ^{90}Sr, deposited in the lung. H&E stain. Bar: 100 μm.

arterioles, but veins and venules may also be involved. Progressive vascular inflammation leads to extensive intimal proliferative lesions and fibromuscular hypertrophy with eventual fibrous accumulation around blood vessels, obliterative intimal and medial thickening, and luminal narrowing. In large elastic arteries, there is a segmental subintimal proliferation of fibroelastic tissue. Such changes constitute the morphological basis for the observed increased pulmonary vascular resistance and development of cardiac dilation and hypertrophy, which reflect pulmonary hypertension.

c. Respiratory System Neoplasia. Neoplasms of the nasal cavity or paranasal sinuses can be induced with internally deposited α or β emitters. Cancer of the paranasal sinuses of the mastoid bone has long been associated with the skeletal deposition of radium. Radium-exposed persons have developed epidermoid, mucoepidermoid, and adenocarcinomas of these tissues.

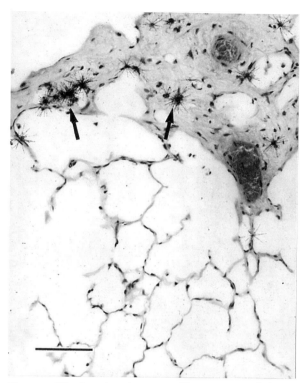

Figure 10. Focal pulmonary fibrosis caused by an α-emitting radionuclide, ^{239}Pu, deposited in the lung. Radioactive particles are shown as "stars" in this autoradiograph (arrows). H&E stain. Bar: 100 μm.

The cells at risk for producing paranasal sinus carcinomas are the epithelial cells lining the nasal cavity and sinuses, but the mode of irradiation is a matter of speculation. Studies of persons who ingested radium salts while painting watch dials lend support to the idea that radon gas in the expired air is the source of the radiation exposure rather than irradiation directly from the radium in the bone. This is supported by results of dosimetric studies, which demonstrate that the target mucosal cells lie outside the range of α particles coming from radium in the bones. Further, beagle dogs that inhaled radon also developed sinus and nasal cancers, whereas beagle dogs injected with radium did not.

β-emitting radionuclides have been associated with the induction of nasal carcinomas in beagle dogs. A majority of these cancers were squamous cell carcinomas of the respiratory epithelium of the nasal cavity (Figs. 11 and 12), although adenocarcinomas of the nasal cavity and squamous cell carcinomas of the frontal sinuses have also been observed. Most of these neoplasms have been recorded in studies with inhaled soluble β emitters that are bone-seeking radionuclides (^{91}Y, ^{144}Ce, ^{90}Sr). Following inhalation, these radionuclides were translocated from the respiratory tract to the bone. This resulted in a variable period of nasal mucosal irradiation from the initial deposition in the upper respiratory tract (Fig. 13) and a longer period of exposure from radionuclide in the underlying bone. This dual irradiation appears to be much more effective in producing cancers than either exposure route alone.

Results of epidemiologic and experimental studies show that lung cancer incidence can be increased in humans and animals exposed to external or internal radiation. Epidemiologic studies of such populations as the externally exposed A bomb survivors, radiologists, and patients treated with X-irradiation for ankylosing spondylitis have shown an increased risk of lung cancer. There is nothing specific about the types of lung neoplasms found in these populations; the spectrum of neoplasm types is similar to that seen in unexposed populations. External whole body or thoracic irradiation increases lung neoplasm incidence in mice, rats, and hamsters. In mice, the neoplasm types are those normally seen in that particular strain, whether they are adenomas or adenocarcinomas. Squamous cell carcinomas have been reported in both rats and Syrian hamsters.

The association of radon and radon decay product exposure with human lung cancer has been the subject of many epidemiologic studies of underground miners. The lung cancer risk associated with exposure to radon decay products depends on the cumulative radiation dose, age, and time since exposure. The major confounding factor in lung cancer risk in radon-exposed miners is cigarette smoking. Several analyses of epidemiologic data have attempted to clarify the combined effects of smoking and radon decay product exposure. Most evidence points to a more than additive

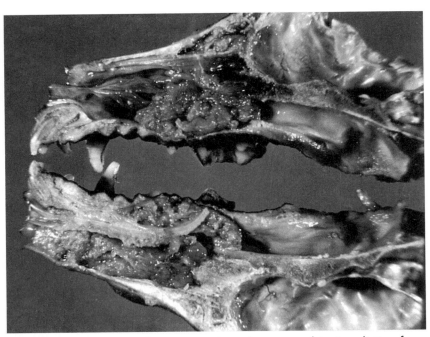

Figure 11. Squamous cell carcinoma in a dog exposed to β radiation from inhaled $^{144}CeCl_2$. The neoplasm filled the right nasal cavity and was locally invasive. Reproduced from Benjamin *et al.* (1979), with permission.

effect of the combined exposure, and most likely a multiplicative effect. It is now suggested that radon inhalation may also be a significant factor in lung cancer risk for the general population.

The specific histopathologic cell types of lung cancer in exposed miner populations are not unusual, but there is a difference in the percentages of the different lung cancer types among miners and those who do not mine. With few exceptions, the cancers in miners have been classified as squamous cell carcinoma, small cell carcinoma, adenocarcinoma, or large cell carcinoma of the bronchus, whereas in cigarette-smoking miners, there is an excess of small cell carcinomas. Data for nonsmoking miners are sparse and conflicting and do not support an excess of small cell carcinomas.

Numerous studies have been conducted with laboratory animals exposed to radon decay products to help sort out the complexities of radon carcinogenesis. The lung cancer types seen in these studies, however, were not the same as those seen in the radon-exposed miner population. Many of the neoplasms in both rats and dogs were bronchioloalveolar carcinomas or papillary adenocarcinomas in the peripheral lung rather than the bronchial tree. Small cell carcinomas, a type not reported as occurring spontaneously in laboratory animals, have not been induced by radon. The radiation dose is delivered primarily to the bronchial epithelium by radon and radon decay products; thus, this discrepancy in location and type of carcinomas between laboratory animals and humans is one of the current enigmas of respiratory carcinogenesis.

Neoplasms of the peripheral portions of the lung are the most significant sequelae following the inhalation of relatively insoluble radioactive particles that primarily deposit in and irradiate the deep lung. Numerous studies with laboratory animals have been conducted to determine the dose–response relationships for inhaled particulate radionuclides and to determine important factors that influence the dose relationship.

Lung cancers were the major radiation-induced cause of late deaths in animals that

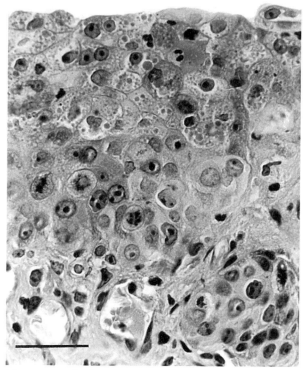

Figure 12. Early squamous cell carcinoma in the turbinate of a dog exposed to β radiation from inhaled $^{144}CeCl_2$ showing numerous mitoses and keratohyaline granule formation. This indicates the nasal turbinate epithelial origin of these neoplasms. H&E stain. Bar: 40 μm. Reproduced from Benjamin *et al.* (1979), with permission.

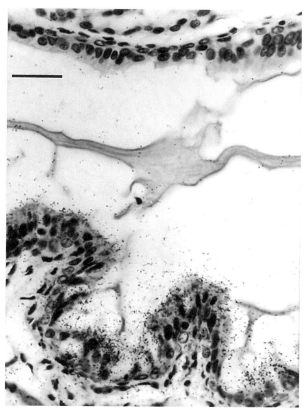

Figure 13. Autoradiograph of turbinate epithelium from a dog killed 8 days after exposure to $^{144}CeCl_2$. Exposed silver grains show the focally heavy concentration of radionuclide associated with the epithelium. H&E stain. Bar: 50 μm. Reproduced from Benjamin *et al.* (1979), with permission.

inhaled β-emitting radionuclides in forms sufficiently insoluble to be retained for long periods in the lungs. Such radionuclides include the β emitters ^{90}Y, ^{91}Y, ^{144}Ce, and ^{90}Sr when inhaled in fused aluminosilicate particles. Hemangiosarcomas were observed in dogs, mice, and rats at cumulative doses greater than 35,000 cGy to lungs. These neoplasms originated in the lungs, but metastasized widely and were uniformly and rapidly fatal. Aside from such studies, primary hemangiosarcomas of the lung are a virtually unheard of spontaneous neoplasm in any species.

At lower radiation doses, carcinomas of the lung predominated over hemangiosarcomas. The carcinomas included bronchioloalveolar carcinomas (Fig. 14), papillary adenocarcinomas, squamous cell carcinomas, and adenosqua-

mous carcinomas. While the carcinomas frequently invaded locally or metastasized within the lung and to draining lymph nodes, they rarely metastasized out of the thorax.

Another aspect of the pathogenesis of lung neoplasms induced by inhaled β-emitting radionuclides is the influence of radiation dose rate. Studies have demonstrated that a brief high dose rate exposure over 2.5 days is about three times more effective for neoplastic induction as the same total radiation dose delivered at lower dose rate over 500 days.

Inhaled α-emitting radionuclides are potent inducers of pulmonary neoplasia as well as late-occurring radiation pneumonitis and pulmonary fibrosis. Inhaled α-emitting radionuclides are more effective in producing pulmonary

555

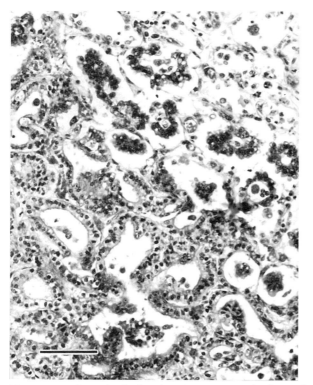

Figure 14. Bronchioloalveolar carcinoma in the lung of a dog exposed to β radiation from insoluble ^{144}Ce. H&E stain. Bar: 75 μm.

neoplasms than inhaled β-emitting radionuclides. Increased numbers of lung neoplasms have been observed in rats with cumulative doses to the lungs as low as 10 cGy with maximum incidences at cumulative doses of about 2000 cGy. One of the primary questions related to inhaled α-emitting radionuclides is the influence of spatial distribution of the dose in the lungs. Data support the concept that a uniform dose to the lungs is more hazardous than the same dose delivered to a very small fraction of the total lung tissue. This is important because of the high degree of concern over the potential carcinogenic risk from single plutonium particles in the environment that might deliver very high but localized radiation doses.

The morphological types of neoplasms induced by inhaled α-emitting radionuclides have been studied in rats, dogs, mice, Syrian hamsters, and baboons. In rats, a number of morphological types are reported, including bronchioloalveolar adenoma and carcinoma, papillary adenocarcinoma, squamous cell carcinoma, adenosquamous carcinoma, and hemangiosarcoma. Similar to the situation with β-emitting radionuclides, hemangiosarcomas in rats are the result of high radiation doses, occur at relatively early times after exposure, and originate from the peripheral portions of the lung. Squamous cell carcinomas are also generally associated with high radiation doses. Where high radiation doses are accumulated, radiation-induced pulmonary neoplasms often are found in association with radiation pneumonitis and pulmonary fibrosis, as well as type II epithelial cell hyperplasia and squamous metaplasia. It has been suggested that this environment of continuing epithelial degeneration and repopulation creates a promoting environment for the carcinogenic process. Immunohistochemical studies in rats have shown that the vast majority of plutonium-induced lung tumors have phenotypic features of type II cells.

Gene alterations have been studied in radiation-induced lung cancers in both humans and laboratory animals. Mutations of *p53* and the K-*ras* protooncogene are common genetic defects in human lung cancer. A rare *p53* codon 249 mutation has been reported in 31% of a series of large cell and squamous cell carcinomas from uranium miners, but infrequently in adenocarcinomas from these miners. Results suggest that there is a histological tissue-type specificity for the codon 249 mutation in individuals exposed to high levels of radon and radon daughters. A similar association of *p53* mutation and tumor type has not been found in radiation-induced lung tumors in animals.

A high mutation frequency of the K-*ras* gene, 46%, is associated with Pu-induced lung cancers of various phenotypes in rats. In addition, hyperplastic epithelium and adenomas express a similar mutation frequency of K-*ras* mutations. In contrast, less than 3% of X-ray-induced lung cancers contain an activating K-*ras* mutation, even though a more sensitive assay was used. Thus, activation of the K-*ras* gene in X-ray-associated tumors is a rare and probably a late event in rats, possibly stemming from genomic instability during tumor progression. The relatively high mutation frequency in Pu-induced lung tumors may relate to the large local energy deposition from the high LET particles.

Using immunohistochemical staining, *p53* gene alterations are found only in squamous cell carcinomas of the lung of rats. Relatively few of these carcinomas are positive, 7% of the Pu-induced tumors and 18% of the X-ray-induced tumors. A more definitive, single-stranded conformational polymorphism, analysis of *p53* gene alterations, verified that few radiation-induced lung tumors have *p53* mutations. Thus, the *p53* gene appears to be involved only in the genesis of a few radiation-induced lung tumors, those with a squamous phenotype, in rats.

An assay for methylation of *p16* exon one in radiation-induced lung tumors showed a high incidence of hypermethylation, regardless of type of exposure (X or plutonium α irradiation). A methylation-specific polymerase chain reaction (PCR) technique was used to detect aberrant methylation of the CpG island in the *p16* gene. Of the 15 lung cancers examined, 80% were hypermethylated, thus implicating CpG island methylation as a major mechanism for inactivating this tumor suppressor gene in lung tumors of rats.

A potential sequence of events in plutonium-included lung neoplasia in rats is shown in Fig. 15. The scheme undoubtedly applies to all α emitters deposited in the lung. The low LET radiation may have a slightly different sequence based on the differences in the localized radiation dose around particles in the lung and the cells irradiated. The relation of this scheme to radiation-induced lung cancer in humans is more problematic. Although *p53* and K-*ras* gene mutations are found frequently in human lung cancer, the relationship of these changes to inducing agents is poorly understood.

3. Alimentary System

a. General Reaction to Ionizing Radiation Injury.
The radiation sensitivity of the alimentary tract varies with the type of epithelium and glandular structures present and the degree and nature of the vascularization. The radiosensitivities for mitosis-linked cell death of epithelium from highest to lowest are the small intestine, esophagus, stomach, colon, and rectum. The primary determinant of the small intestinal response is the high sensitivity of the generative crypt epithelium, which has a turnover rate two to six times than that of other regions in the gastrointestinal tract. The high vascularity of this absorptive region also contributes to the sensitivity. The sensitivity of the basilar epithelium of the esophagus, the next most rapidly dividing mucosal population,

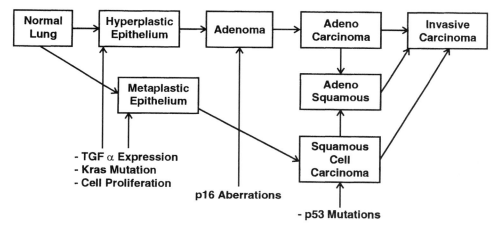

Figure 15. Potential sequence of events in plutonium-induced lung neoplasia in rats.

makes the esophagus an organ of concern for radiotherapists.

Parenchymal cells of the liver, including hepatocellular and bile duct epithelium, are relatively radioresistant because these cells turn over slowly. Further, the sinusoids of the liver are lined, not only by endothelium, but by marrow-derived phagocytic cells (Kupffer cells) that are also relatively resistant to ionizing radiation.

As with any organ, depending on dose and delivery schedules, significant damage can be produced in any portion of the alimentary system, but, for the purposes of discussion of mechanisms, we will limit ourselves to the intestine, esophagus, and liver.

b. Small Intestine. Progenitor cells at the base of mucosal crypts are the most sensitive in the intestine because of their high turnover. While the pathological changes in the intestine can be seen within the first 24 hr of irradiation, related clinical signs are dependent on the exact renewal times of the surface epithelium. This can vary with species and is somewhat faster for small rodents than for humans and nonhuman primates. The overall degree of change is dependent not only on the dose of radiation, but also on whether the exposure is localized to portions of the intestine or whole body. Acute doses of 700–1500 cGy will lead to the sequence of changes described next.

Pathological changes in the first 24 hr consist of the usual initial mitotic delay, followed by a wave of mitosis-linked cell death in the crypts. The more differentiated surface epithelium is relatively radioresistant and has few lesions at this point. After the first day, normal differentiation and migration of the mucosal epithelium up the villi toward the tips continue and there is loss of senescent cells from the surface. There is no replacement of these cells because of the stem cell depletion, so major portion of the epithelium is denuded. There is also significant shortening of the crypts and villi. The few remaining crypt cells are hypertrophied and pleomorphic. The combination of the loss of the absorptive epithelium and the decrease in overall absorptive surface area of the mucosa leads to a malabsorption situation. Edema and acute inflammation in the mucosa complicate this further. Endothelial swelling and thrombosis obliterate the abundant capillary loops, which complicate the initial injury. Exudation adds to the general loss of fluid through the intestine.

Clinical signs associated with these early lesions include diarrhea, dehydration, and progressive electrolyte and fluid imbalances. There is often intercurrent infection. This complex of signs and lesions is referred to as the gastrointestinal syndrome. In humans, it usually occurs in about a week when the mucosal changes reach a maximum. In individuals who receive whole body exposures, the associated pancytopenia is also significant at this time. The concurrent development of the hematopoietic syndrome, with its granulocytopenia and lymphocytopenia, can lead to severe secondary infections because of a combination of increased access of microorganisms through the damaged mucosal barrier and depressed immune and inflammatory responses. Death can ensue from a combination of these various factors.

After about 3–4 days, there is a resurgence of epithelial repopulation unless there has been total destruction of the stem cells. After 700 cGy, there is significant proliferation, whereas following 2000 cGy, there is relatively little recovery and the mucosa remains atrophic. At the lower doses, there is sometimes a mucous metaplasia with large numbers of goblet cells. At the higher doses, ulceration becomes a significant feature of the lesions. As the repopulation of the intestinal mucosa progresses, there is often retention of the senescent epithelium on the villous surfaces due to a lack of cell replacement from below. Thus, a syncytium of atypical epithelium can form over the mucosal surface. If the local injury has been severe enough, full recovery of the mucosa may never occur and, in fact, some aspects of the changes can be progressive.

Ulcerative lesions would certainly appear to relate to the vascular damage. Vascular lesions include fibrinoid necrosis and, in chronic lesions, hyaline thickening and vacuolization of the vessel walls. Intimal, medial, and adventitial fibrosis are chronic lesions. This longer term interference with the microcirculation is important in the genesis of late effects. Besides the vasculature, fibrosis can occur at all levels of the intestinal wall from the mucosa to the serosa. Fibrosis can lead to abdominal adhesions that can be a significant complication in patients recovering from abdominal radiotherapy.

c. Esophagus. Although the esophagus is less radiosensitive than the intestine, it is important to the radiotherapist because of its location in common treatment fields. The germinal basilar epithelium is the radiosensitive target population, and the differentiating squamous layers and the glandular epithelium are relatively resistant. The response is similar to that of epidermis but, because of the tubular structure, the results are more severe. A single dose of 2000 cGy causes an early acute esophagitis, followed in about 2 weeks by sloughing of the esophageal mucosa with ulceration. Regeneration of mucosa occurs by 3 weeks and is accompanied by considerable fibrosis. Fibrosis is most marked in the submucosa but can extend into the muscularis. Submucosal mucous glands atrophy.

At later times, vascular injury results in secondary mucosal atrophy and increases the deposition of connective tissue further. As the collagen matures, it contracts and stenosis results. Even in individuals who survive the early radiation-induced changes, the slower process caused by the arteriocapillary injury can be a source of continuing difficulty.

d. Liver. Acute, severe liver injury generally occurs only after very high external radiation doses upwards of 1500–2000 cGy. The acute phase, seen 3–6 months postirradiation, is associated with a form of veno-occlusive disease with progressive centrilobular obstruction due to centrilobular fibrosis but little inflammation. This progresses to chronic radiation hepatitis characterized by obliteration of the centrilobular veins, parenchymal cell loss, and collapse and distortion of the lobular architecture. Peri-

portal fibrosis and biliary hyperplasia may be seen as well.

Hepatic neoplasms have been associated with internally deposited radionuclides in both humans and animals. Hepatic neoplasms are reported in human patients injected with the radiographic contrast medium Thorotrast, a colloidal suspension of thorium dioxide, an α emitter. When injected intravenously, it is retained in organs with large numbers of fixed phagocytic cells such as the liver, spleen, lymph nodes, and bone marrow. The late lesion observed most frequently after Thorotrast injection is fibrosis. This fibrosis can be local, at the site of injection, or diffuse in the organs where the Thorotrast is deposited. In the liver, the most common lesion is the atrophy of hepatocytes adjacent to Thorotrast deposits with rupture of trabeculae and fibrosis producing a pattern of pseudolobulation. Development of malignant neoplasms is the most severe consequence of Thorotrast exposure. These include hepatocellular carcinomas, cholangiocellular carcinomas, and sarcomas, including hemangiosarcomas. The hemangiosarcomas deserve special mention because of the high frequency (>30%), compared with their low frequency (1%), in the normal human population. Thorotrast also causes hepatic hemangiosarcomas and carcinomas in mice, rats, and rabbits.

Point mutations in the *p53* gene have been found in a high percentage of Thorotrast recipients who developed liver cancer, mostly of bile duct and blood vessel origin. Accompanying tissues without tumors from these patients also had *p53* mutations, but at a much lower frequency than in the tumors. The distribution pattern of the point mutations was significantly different between nonneoplastic and tumor tissues. These results support the idea that *p53* mutations are important in the genesis of Thorotrast-induced tumors, but that these point mutations are probably secondary to genomic instability induced by irradiation.

Plutonium deposited in the liver will induce hepatic neoplasia in dogs, deer mice, and grasshopper mice. These species were chosen for study because, unlike the usual laboratory rodent species, they have a prolonged retention of actinide elements in the liver, much like humans. In dogs that inhaled ^{238}Pu dioxide, a radionuclide that is slowly translocated to the liver, hepatic neoplasms were divided equally between sarcomas (fibrosarcomas, neurofibrosarcomas, and undifferentiated sarcomas) and biliary neoplasms, including carcinoids. Few hepatocellular carcinomas and no hemangiosarcomas were observed. In contrast, dogs injected with soluble ^{239}Pu had primary hepatic neoplasms, but the most frequent were bile duct adenomas (62%) and bile duct carcinomas (21%). Only two fibrosarcomas were observed. The reasons for the different responses in these two studies are uncertain because the type of radiation was similar, but may relate to the rate of dose delivery. The injected radionuclide was delivered in one bolus to the liver, whereas the inhaled material was translocated from the lungs to the liver over several months, thus protracting the dose. A common feature in both studies was the relatively long latent period for these canine neoplasms. Few were noted earlier than 8 years after exposure, and the average was about 11 years after exposure. This latent period probably reflects the relatively long life span of hepatic cells and the low mitotic activity in the liver.

Hepatic degeneration and fibrosis were noted before liver neoplasms appeared in these dogs. These changes were more pronounced in studies of injected plutonium. Soluble plutonium was carried initially to the hepatocytes and then, after cell necrosis, to the fixed phagocytic cells. Evidence of hepatocyte death was detected by increased serum activity of alanine aminotransferase. The enzyme activity increased in a dose-related fashion, within a few years after exposure. The significance of hepatocellular necrosis in the pathogenesis of the hepatic neoplasms is uncertain. Studies of intravenously injected α- and β-emitting liver-seeking radionuclides in the Chinese hamster demonstrated that increased cell division caused by partial hepatectomy could serve to promote an increased incidence of hepatocellular and mesenchymal hepatic neoplasms. The cell death

would alter both the rate of cell proliferation and the dose distribution of the irradiation by causing more hepatocellular plutonium to be shifted to the phagocytic cells.

Hepatic degeneration and neoplasia are important late sequelae of irradiation of the liver with the β emitter ^{144}Ce. Dogs exposed by inhalation of ^{144}Ce chloride received significant radiation doses to the liver because of translocation of the soluble radionuclide from the lungs to the liver. Hepatic degeneration and necrosis often were severe, resulting in the death of the animal within 3 years of exposure. The reason for the greater severity of the hepatocellular degeneration of necrosis with ^{144}Ce than with plutonium is the more uniform radiation dose from the β-emitting cerium compared with the local irradiation from the α-emitting plutonium. Hepatic neoplasms developed in dogs exposed to ^{144}Ce about 4 years after inhalation exposure. Most of these were hepatic hemangiosarcomas (Fig. 16), but several cholangiocarcinomas and hepatocellular carcinomas were also present. In addition, biliary cysts and cystadenomas were found related to hepatic degeneration in dogs with high radiation doses.

4. Skeletal System

a. General Reaction to Ionizing Radiation Injury. The adult skeletal system is considered to be relatively resistant to irradiation; however, many changes may develop in bones that are not detected clinically. Serious complications often do not develop until months to years after radiation exposure and may be expressed as osteopenia and osteonecrosis that may lead to pathological fracture and septic osteonecrosis. The growing or immature skeletal system is more sensitive to irradiation and this sensitivity is manifested as disturbances in growth. Radiation injury to healing bone can result in delayed union and nonunion of fractures. There is debate about whether the effects of irradiation on bone are due to direct effects on individual bone cells or on the vasculature of bone.

Radiographic changes observed after irradiation of mature bone include decreased densities,

560

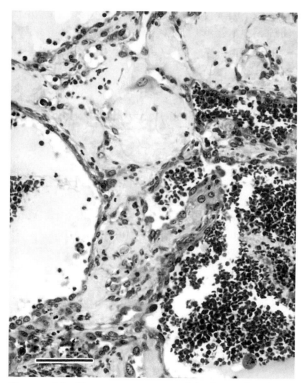

Figure 16. Hemangiosarcoma of the liver of a dog exposed to β radiation from $^{144}CeCl_2$ deposited in the liver. H&E stain. Bar: 50 μm.

pathological fractures, coarsening of the trabecular pattern, irregular cortical thickening and thinning, osteolysis, and sclerotic areas. Such changes take months to years to develop and are detectable at doses of 4200–4500 cGy given in 20-cGy fractions. Radiographic procedures, however, can only detect changes when there has been at least a 30% loss of mineral density in bone. Histologic changes seen after irradiation in all species include loss of osteocytes from their lacunae, loss of osteoblasts, decreased osteoclasts, periosteal fibrosis, and bone marrow fibrosis. Osteoblasts are believed to be more sensitive to radiation than osteoclasts, which are terminally differentiated nonmitotic cells that resorb bone. A single dose of 1000 cGy destroys osteoblasts in rabbit femurs whereas 2000 cGy destroys osteoclasts. Therefore, bone resorption tends to be spared more than formation, with the resultant effect of decreased bone mass. Metaplastic new bone for-

mation may be observed in the bone marrow, primarily along the endosteal surfaces. Vascular changes such as obliterative endarteritis, periarteritis, intimal proliferation, medial hyalinization and necrosis of arterioles, perivascular fibrosis, and, occasionally, thrombosis are often reported. Reduction of blood flow to irradiated bone has been documented experimentally, but this is not as consistent as loss of bone cells.

Areas of necrotic bone are susceptible to secondary infections. When this develops after irradiation, it is referred to as septic osteoradionecrosis (Fig. 17). Usually at least 5000 cGy in fractions is needed to cause this effect. For example, a high susceptibility of the mandible to necrosis following irradiation has been ascribed primarily to its poor blood supply, leading to

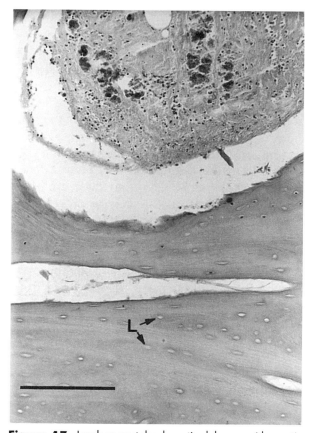

Figure 17. Lumbar vertebral cortical bone with septic osteoradionecrosis from a dog 5 years after receiving 4700 cGy electrons. There is loss of osteocytes from lacunae (L), loss of osteoblasts lining bone surfaces, and a mass of necrotic debris and bacteria (top). H&E stain. Bar: 100 μm.

poor healing and inflammation. There is increased tooth decay due to changes in salivary pH resulting from radiation-induced salivary gland injury and damage to mucous membranes. All of these factors contribute to the increased risk of the mandible to septic infection.

The clinical manifestations of irradiation of the immature or growing skeletal system are growth disturbances. Growth disturbances observed most commonly in humans are a reduction in height, scoliosis, and deformities of the facial bones. These changes are seen at relatively low doses, indicating a greater sensitivity of the growing skeleton than the mature skeleton to irradiation. Significant growth arrest may be seen in children under 1 year of age with doses of 1000 cGy. The sensitivity to irradiation decreases with increasing age but is not necessarily proportional to growth rate. Growth retardation is well documented in developing rodents and dogs.

In growing rodents, histological changes are seen within the physis a few days after irradiation. These changes include a decrease in the number of mitoses, pyknosis of nuclei of cells in the proliferative and hypertrophic zones, and a decrease in the number of osteoblasts and cartilage cells. Mild histologic changes may be seen at doses as low as 400 cGy but these are often transient. At doses of 1200 cGy or more, swollen and enlarged cells and enlarged lacunae are seen in the zone of calcified cartilage. Cartilage columns are often aligned irregularly with irregular areas of calcification and ossification. Chondroblasts appear to be more sensitive than osteoblasts, as cartilage proliferation is inhibited at doses of 1800 cGy while osteoid production and mineralization continue. Resorption of cartilage may be irregular and deficient. The relative importance of the sensitivity of individual bone and cartilage cells in the growing physis and the fine vasculature in the expression of radiation damage is poorly understood. It also is not clear whether growth retardation associated with very low whole body radiation doses (50–200 cGy) is related to direct bone injury, to general endocrine metabolic disturbances, or to both.

Irradiation can cause delayed union or nonunion of healing fractures. Radiographically, callus formation is inhibited and microangiograms show a decrease in the degree of vascularity. In mice irradiated 24 hr before fracture of the femur, the dose that inhibited callus formation in 50% of the animals 50 days after fracture was 1750 cGy. In studies of bone regeneration in rabbits, 500 cGy caused a 17% decrease in bone regeneration, whereas 1500 cGy caused a 76% decrease. Histologically, there was decreased bone formation, but no lesions were observed in the vasculature, suggesting that the effects of irradiation were due to the effects on osteogenic cells rather than the vasculature. Other studies in rats noted decreased new bone formation, increased fibrous tissue and cartilage formation, and decreased new vessel formation, suggesting that the effects of irradiation on healing bone are a combination of damage to osteoblasts and vessels.

External beam irradiation can also induce bone tumors, especially osteosarcomas, as has been reported in humans, dogs, monkeys, and mice. Most tumors develop after doses greater than 2000 cGy and occur 2 to 5 years after irradiation.

b. Skeletal Injury from Internal Emitters. A number of radionuclides deposit in bone after entry into the body. Table V shows some of the important bone-seeking radionuclides. Two factors affect radiation microdosimetry in bone: emission type and chemical localization. β-emitting radionuclides deliver a more uniform dose to the bone than α emitters because of the greater tissue penetration of the β particles. Radionuclides that are "volume seekers" (such as alkaline earths) deposit initially on all bone surfaces, but return quickly (<1 day) to

TABLE V
Important Bone-Seeking Radionuclides

Radionuclide	Type emission	Distribution in bone
Strontium 90	β	Volume
Plutonium 238, 239	α	Surface
Radium 224, 226, 228	α	Surface

the blood. Subsequently, there is a long-term exchange of ions between blood and bone volume that produces a diffuse labeling of the bone with radionuclide. In contrast, radionuclides that are "surface seekers" (such as the transuranic elements and rare earths) deposit on all bone surfaces, including periosteal, endosteal, and trabecular surfaces, and on surfaces of haversian and volkman canals. They remain there until they are removed by resorption of the bone. In adults, a few surface deposits are buried by apposition of new bone. In growing bone, continued apposition of new bone ultimately buries most of this activity within the volume of the bone.

An important factor in radiation injury to bone is the organization of the tissue and the spatial relationship of the cells to the radioactive material. Irradiation of various bone cells is relatively uniform by volume seekers. However, there is a greater radiation dose delivered to those cells closest to the bone surfaces by surface seekers. These cells include endosteal cells, osteoblasts, and osteoclasts, among others. Dose localization is more important for α-emitters than β emitters because of the much shorter range of α particles in tissue.

i. Nonneoplastic lesions Nonneoplastic lesions of bone can occur after high doses from internal emitters. Injury and death of bone cells and overlying mesenchymal cells can occur with radiation doses as low as 75 cGy given in 12 hr. Vascular damage can have a marked chronic effect in the bone with ischemia and infarction resulting in devitalized bone and pathological fractures. More subtle changes in the vascular supply can disturb the mineral metabolism at the bone surface so the remaining bone is mineralized excessively. Endosteal or periosteal fibrosis may occur, which may be in conjunction with vascular changes, or may be found with no apparent association with other lesions. The relative mix of these changes of vascular damage, osteonecrosis, and osteofibrosis varies depending on the radionuclide involved, the radiation dose, and the exposure regime. Protracted radiation exposures from α-emitting radionuclides seem more effective than β

emitters in producing these nonneoplastic lesions.

ii. Skeletal neoplasia Bone neoplasms have been induced in a variety of laboratory animals with a number of internally deposited α-emitting radionuclides. Bone neoplasms are a major delayed effect of bone-seeking α emitters in dogs. ^{226}Ra given by injection results in osteosarcomas primarily, but fibrosarcomas, chondrosarcomas, and hemangiosarcomas are also induced. Many tumors exhibit a combination of fibroblastic, chondroblastic, and osteoblastic components. Bone sarcomas induced by ^{226}Ra occur mostly in the long bones, but no tumors are found in the ribs, scapula, or sternum.

A model for the pathogenesis of ^{226}Ra-induced bone sarcomas arising in cortical bone has been developed based on studies of exposed humans and beagles (Fig. 18). A hyaline material accumulating in the adventitia of haversian vessels leading to the occlusion of haversian canals is the initial lesion. Progressive vascular occlusion leads to ischemia and death of osteons, thus stimulating an increase in the bone remodeling process. As long as vascular perfusion is maintained, the bone resorption phase of remodeling continues because resorption is mediated by osteoclasts, relatively radioresistant cells that have a hematopoietic origin and are formed out of the area of irradiation. However, bone formation in the remodeling unit is impaired because the locally derived radiosensitive osteoprogenitor cells cannot be formed in areas of heavy irradiation. Thus, the cortical bone remodeling unit is "uncoupled," and the bone resorption proceeds more rapidly than bone formation. Uncoupling results first in small and, later, in large porosities in the bone. These cavities are filled with proliferating mesenchymal tissue. This irradiated mesenchyme forms atypical bone or fibrous tissue resembling fibrous dysplasia, ossifying fibroma, or osteoblastoma. The increased remodeling activity and other changes described lead to the proliferation of osteogenic progenitor cells, osteoblasts, and mesenchymal cells, essentially creating an environment of neoplastic promotion. High radiation doses to these cells in

563

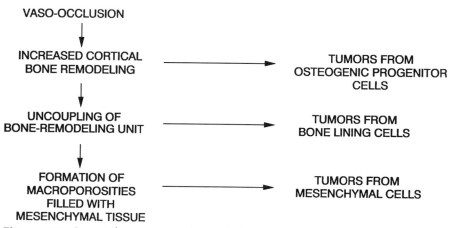

Figure 18. Potential sequence of morphologic events in radium-induced bone neoplasia.

such a promoting environment would lead to a high incidence of neoplasms. Here the more primitive osteogenic progenitors could give rise to a variety of mesenchymal neoplasms, including chondro- and osteosarcomas. Osteoblasts would give rise to osteogenic neoplasms only. Mesenchymal cells would be likely to give rise mostly to mesenchymal neoplasms, such as fibrosarcomas.

Plutonium deposited in bone results in osteosarcomas that are slow growing and seldom metastasize. The distribution of neoplasms among various bones is interesting because there is a relatively high incidence of neoplasms in the trabecular bone of the vertebrae and proximal humerus and a relatively low incidence in the long bones. This distribution contrasts with that of radium-induced neoplasms, which are found mainly in the cortical bone. Differences in the degree of initial radionuclide deposition on trabecular bone surfaces and the rate of trabecular bone turnover appear to be critical factors in the distribution of osteosarcomas induced by plutonium and radium.

^{90}Sr is an important bone-seeking, β-emitting radionuclide because of its abundance following the fissioning of nuclear fuels. Dogs fed ^{90}Sr from the time they were *in utero* until 540 days of age, during skeletal formation and growth, developed bone neoplasms as early as 6 years of age. The neoplasms were primarily osteosarco-

mas, although several hemangiosarcomas and one liposarcoma of bone were also attributed to radiation exposure. More neoplasms were found in the compact bone than in the trabecular bone. The one exception was the relatively large number of lesions and neoplasms in the mandible. This increase was related to the high concentration of strontium in the teeth, laid down in early life and maintained there for the lifetime of the dog. Although some lesions similar to those described for radium-induced injury were seen, a pathogenesis that includes increased remodeling, uncoupling of the bone remodeling unit, and osteodystrophy would not appear to be the sole pathway to neoplasia. In other studies with inhaled or injected ^{90}Sr, no radiation osteodystrophy has been associated with bone neoplasms. Few neoplasms occurred in the vertebra, femur, humerus, and all cancellous bone, and numerous neoplasms occurred in the skull, scapula, and ribs. This different pattern of location of neoplasms from those induced by radium suggests a different pathogenesis. The fact that both α- and β-emitting radionuclides can induce bone sarcomas and, depending on the chemical nature and even the mode of administration, can result in significant differences in neoplasm localization underscores the complexity of the overall processes relating to radiation injury and carcinogenesis.

5. *Nervous System*

a. General Reaction to Ionizing Radiation Injury. The brain, spinal cord, and peripheral nerves are sensitive to radiation injury, with the effects depending on age at exposure and radiation dose. Because of their critical function, these tissues are often dose-limiting structures for therapeutic irradiation. Neurons are assumed to be resistant to the effects of irradiation because they are terminally differentiated cells that do not divide. The role of the astrocyte in radiation injury to the central nervous system is not known. Oligodendrocytes and Schwann cells are slowly proliferating, but radiosensitive, cells. Vascular supply in the nervous system is also radiosensitive, as it is in other organs. The type of lesions in the nervous system and time to development of lesions depend on the dose of radiation received and the size of the dose per fraction. The difference in lesion type and latent period has been proposed to be a reflection of damage to the different cell or tissue types, i.e., the oligodendrocytes or Schwann cells or the microvasculature. However, the role of the vasculature in the pathogenesis of radiation damage to the nervous system has been shown to dominate.

b. Brain. The response of the brain to irradiation is divided into three phases: acute reactions, early delayed reactions, and late delayed reactions. Acute reactions occur during the course of radiation treatment using single doses of 1000 cGy or more. Doses above this are often fatal and the lesion is principally massive edema. The early delayed reaction occurs a few weeks to months after irradiation and is often transitory. In humans, it is expressed clinically as somnolence. Rarely, the reaction may be fatal. Histologically, areas of demyelination, loss of oligodendrocytes, gliosis, and minimal vascular lesions are seen. Lesions are thought to reflect damage to oligodendrocytes and the myelin formed by them. The onset and time of recovery from these signs correspond to oligodendrocyte turnover time.

Segmental demyelination and nodal widening occur in nerves within 2 weeks of irradiation

and remyelination begins after 2 months. This suggests that transient demyelination is a factor in the early delayed reaction. Also, there is an early transient increase in tumor necrosis factor (TNF)-α and interleukin-1 in mouse brain within 24 hr after 2500 cGy, which may contribute to vascular leakage.

The late delayed reaction of the brain to irradiation occurs several months to years after exposure and is often fatal. This syndrome can have an acute onset that is characterized histologically by massive coagulation necrosis and hemorrhage, typical of infarction. The onset also may be slowly progressive, characterized by cerebral atrophy. The white matter is affected more than the gray matter, and the topography of the lesions suggests vascular damage. Histologically, vascular damage, such as hyaline thickening of blood vessel walls, fibrinoid necrosis, thrombosis, perivascular fibrosis, and endothelial proliferation, is often observed. In humans, doses of 6000 cGy in 200-cGy fractions approach the threshold for delayed brain necrosis. In rat brains, vascular damage, as measured by blood flow, breakdown of the blood–brain barrier, endothelial cell hypertrophy, and cell loss, is observed at 2000–3000 cGy in single doses and precedes necrosis of white matter. In dogs, 3–9 months after 1100–3000 cGy as a single dose, brain lesions are characterized by areas of white matter edema with variable amounts of demyelination, swollen axons, small areas of coagulation necrosis of the white matter, and fibrinoid necrosis of blood vessels. In some brains, large areas of coagulation necrosis of the white matter are associated with necrosis of vessels and axons and areas of hemorrhage and mineralization. There is also an increase in TNF-α at 2–3 months after 2500 cGy in mice, which persists until 6 months.

c. Spinal Cord. The radiation response of the spinal cord is similar to that of the brain and is divided into an early delayed reaction and a late reaction. The early delayed reaction occurs weeks to months after irradiation and is transient. In humans, this clinical syndrome is expressed as transient paresthesia or numbness and is believed to be due to transient demyelination and later remyelination. Increased vascular permeability with resultant edema may contribute to the early transient signs.

The late reaction occurs months to years after irradiation, with the latent period depending on the dose. Higher radiation doses cause earlier developing lesions. This reaction is often permanent and may be fatal. Some cases in humans appear to be slowly progressive whereas others develop rapidly. Lesions include areas of demyelination and focal white matter necrosis with swollen axons, gliosis, and lipid-laden macrophages. Hemorrhage, thrombosis, and fibrinoid necrosis of vascular walls are seen (Fig. 19). A dose of 5000 cGy in 200-cGy fractions approaches the tolerance of the spinal cord to irradiation. There is also a volume effect

for spinal cord tolerance, as smaller volumes require higher doses to produce lesions. In dogs, lesions of white matter necrosis, massive hemorrhage, and parenchymal atrophy occur 6 to 18 months after irradiation with an ED_{50} of 5700 cGy in 400-cGy fractions to a 20-cm length, compared with an ED_{50} of 6880 cGy for a 4-cm length. In mice and rats, white matter necrosis develops earlier, preceded by decreased blood flow, while at later times, hemorrhagic infarction and telangiectasis are seen in some animals (Fig. 20).

Studies using boron neutron capture in rodents limited radiation doses to the endothelial cells and produced lesions identical to those seen with X rays, indicating that endothelial cells are key target cells for the lesions of white matter necrosis. Furthermore, although a

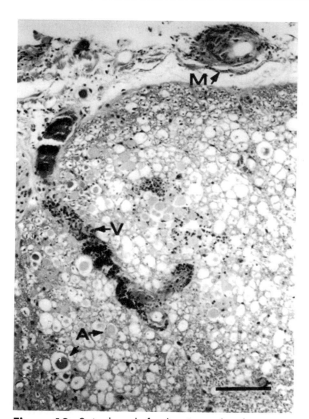

Figure 19. Spinal cord of a dog 3 months after receiving 7600 cGy electrons in 400-cGy fractions. White matter necrosis is characterized by severe vacuolar change with many swollen axons (A). A penetrating small vessel (V) is necrotic and occluded, and a meningeal artery (M) is partially occluded. H&E stain. Bar: 100 μm.

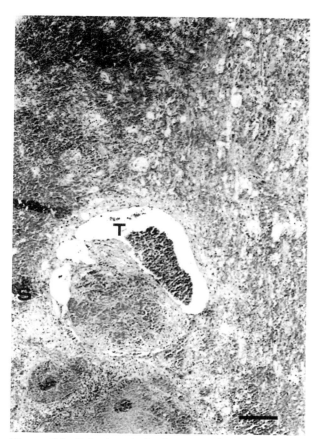

Figure 20. Spinal cord of a dog 5 months after receiving 7600 cGy electrons in 400-cGy fractions. Centrally is an area of telangiectasis (T) surrounded by necrotic and hemorrhagic white matter. Bar: 200 μm.

reduction in oligodendrocyte number occurs, these changes are not related to the development of white matter necrosis or clinical signs. Cytokines such as interleukin-1 and TNF-α are increased after irradiation and may contribute to endothelial cell and oligodendrocyte cytotoxicity, and may cause astrocyte proliferation.

d. Peripheral Nerves. The peripheral nervous system is considered to be more resistant to the effects of irradiation than the central nervous system. Peripheral neuropathies usually develop months to years after exposure to doses of 6000 cGy in 200-cGy fractions. Histologically, there is endoneurial, perineurial, and epineurial fibrosis with loss of nerve fibers, capillaries and small vessels (Fig. 21). Dogs given 1500–4750 cGy as a single dose to

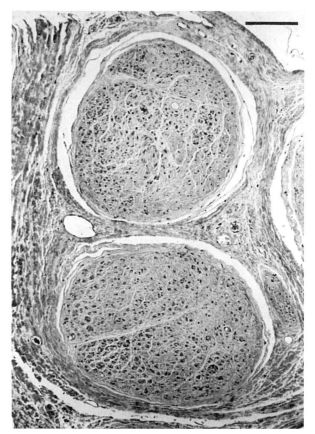

Figure 21. Femoral nerve from a dog 2 years after receiving 3200 cGy electrons. There is marked endoneurial, perineurial, and epineurial fibrosis, and nerve fibers are decreased in number and myelin is reduced. H&E stain. Bar: 100 μm.

peripheral nerves have neuropathies as early as 4 months after the higher doses and as late as 2 years after the lower doses. At the higher doses, there is fibrinoid necrosis and disruption of small vessels associated with coagulation necrosis of the entire nerve bundle. Fibers at the periphery of the nerve bundle, where the blood supply is better, may be spared.

The pathogenesis of radiation damage to peripheral nerves is likely related primarily to vascular effects as indicated by this sparing of nerve fibers at the nerve bundle periphery, loss of microvascular density, and fibrosis throughout. The complete loss of fibers rather than only demyelination also indicates a vascular effect, as Schwann cell injury should result in demyelination and not complete fiber loss.

6. Eye

a. General Reaction to Ionizing Radiation Injury. Because the eye contains some unique components that vary greatly in their structure, function, and sensitivities to ionizing radiation injury, a general discussion of reaction to injury is not appropriate and the critical components are addressed individually.

b. Retina. The neural cells of the retina are similar, in many respects in their response to irradiation, to the cells of the central nervous system. The mature retina is a specialized neural end organ and is relatively insensitive to direct radiation effects. However, this tissue is sensitive to the indirect effects caused by radiation injury to its vascular supply. To cause significant retinal lesions in the adult, cumulative doses of 1000 cGy are required. In humans, this is usually delivered in therapeutic fractions of about 200 cGy. The latent period for retinal changes can be 1 or more years. Visual deterioration is associated with, and the result of, progressive obliteration of the retinal vasculature, often with focal occlusion, hemorrhages, telangiectasis, and microaneurysms (Fig. 22). The retinal injury can produce lesions varying from focal atrophy to full thickness necrosis.

The developing retina is particularly sensitive to irradiation. The developing neuroblastic retinal cells are highly radiosensitive and undergo

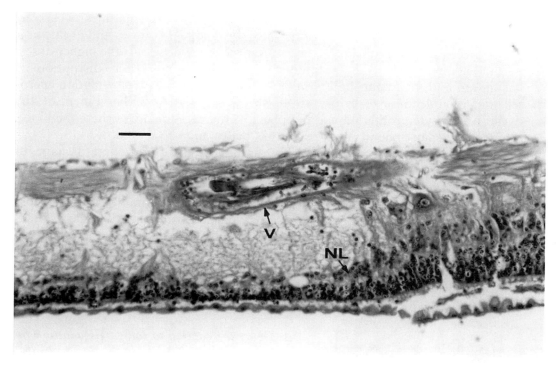

Figure 22. Retinal degenerative vasculopathy in a therapeutically irradiated adult dog. Retinal nuclear layers (NL) are mostly lost or degenerating. There is separation of the vascular wall (V) by a dissecting inflammatory exudate. H&E stain. Bar: 25 μm. Reproduced from Ching *et al.* (1990), with permission.

necrosis shortly after exposure to very low doses. In the dog, acute doses as low as 10 cGy of γ radiation can cause necrosis, although the dose must equal 100 cGy to produce more than transient injury. Doses of 100 cGy and above can result in permanent damage to the retina. Characteristic morphological changes include disorganization and atrophy of the various retinal nuclear layers, as well as retinal folds and rosettes (Fig. 23). In many animals, especially in those irradiated at doses of 200 cGy and above, these lesions are followed by a progressive retinal atrophy accompanied by retinal vascular attenuation (Figs. 24 and 25). Because these vascular lesions occur at much smaller doses than in the adult, it suggests an increased sensitivity of the developing vasculature as well. Whether the progressive atrophy is due entirely to the vascular changes or to some direct residual effect on the retinal neural cells is not known.

c. Lens. Cataracts are well-known sequelae to exposure by ionizing radiation. The lens is relatively radiosensitive, with a dose threshold of about 200 cGy of low LET radiation necessary to produce visually impairing lenticular opacities in humans. The threshold for high LET radiation is much lower and depends on the type of radiation and pattern of delivery. The severity of radiation-induced cataracts is dose dependent and the latency is related inversely to dose. The young lens has a greater radiosensitivity than the mature lens.

Evidence suggests that the critical target cells for cataracts induced by low doses are germinative epithelial cells at the lenticular equator. These cells proliferate regularly, either renewing themselves or undergoing differentiation to lens fibers. One day after irradiation, abnormal mitosis and mitotic delay occur in this cell population. The injured, but viable, epithelium appears to be important because those cells

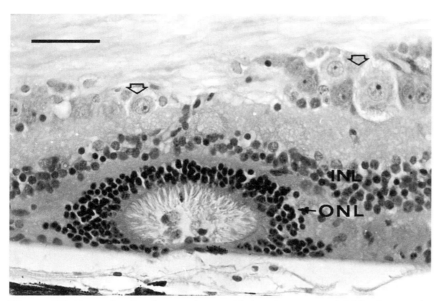

Figure 23. Tapetal retina from a 4-year-old dog that received 160 cGy γ radiation at 55 days of gestation. There is a typical dysplastic rosette with outer nuclear layer cells (ONL) arranged around a central space that contains degenerate rod and cone-like structures. The thickness of the inner nuclear layer (INL) is variable. Ganglion cells (arrows) are relatively unaffected. The same dog is shown in Figs. 24 and 25. H&E stain. Bar: 50 μm. Reproduced from Schweitzer *et al*. (1987), with permission.

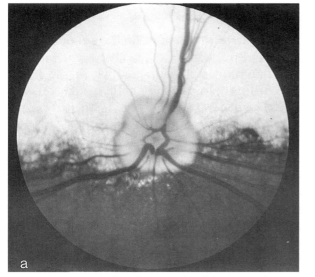 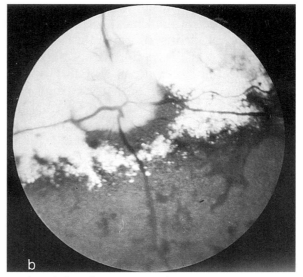

Figure 24. (a) Fundic photograph of the retina from a nonirradiated dog showing normal vascularity. (b) Fundic photograph from a 4-year-old dog that received 160 cGy γ radiation at 55 days of gestation. There is marked vascular attenuation evident. Reproduced from Schweitzer *et al*. (1987), with permission.

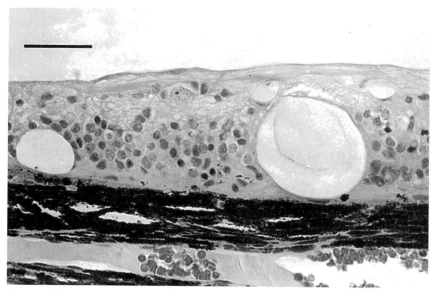

Figure 25. Nontapetal retina from a 4-year-old dog that received 160 cGy γ radiation at 55 days of gestation. The cysts are atrophic remnants of rosettes. There are scattered nuclei but no discernable nuclear layers or photoreceptor segments. H&E stain. Bar: 50 μm. Reproduced from Schweitzer *et al.* (1987), with permission.

that are killed do not produce abnormal lens fibers. The injury to lenticular epithelium interferes with the orderly formation and replacement of lens fibers. There is also interference with the migration of epithelium and differentiating fibers to the lenticular poles and the posterior aspect of the lens. Aberrant cells and degenerate cell debris also migrate to the posterior part of the lens, ultimately adding to cytoarchitectural alterations and loss of lens transparency in this region. At very high radiation doses, there can be damage to transport mechanisms in the cells on the anterior surface of the lens, which can also lead to cataract formation. Histological changes are characterized by the disorganization of lens epithelium and fibers, retention of nuclei, and posterior migration of nuclei and bladder cells (Fig. 26).

d. Other Ocular Tissues. Within 1 month of irradiation, corneal epithelial atrophy occurs associated with blepharitis and keratoconjunctivitis. With time, these lesions become less severe and more chronic. Chronic keratitis, and "dry eye," is a relatively common lesion seen after irradiation and is probably due to damage

to the highly sensitive serous lacrimal glands. Serous gland cells undergo interphase death after irradiation. Late occurring vascularization and fibrosis of the cornea can lead to severe and permanent opacity.

7. Cardiovascular System

a. General Reaction to Ionizing Radiation Injury. The response of the cardiovascular system to irradiation includes reactions of the heart, pericardium, aorta, and smaller diameter vessels. The general reaction of the microvasculature in radiation injury was discussed earlier. The heart is considered to be relatively resistant to the effects of irradiation because heart muscle cells do not divide. However, late developing effects on the vasculature of the heart may lead to compromised cardiac function, often years after radiation exposure. There is a slightly increased risk of cardiac deaths in humans treated for Hodgkin's disease and breast cancer when significant portions of the heart are included in the treatment field. Reactions also develop in the pericardium, resulting in pericardial effusions or fibrosis that can restrict heart function.

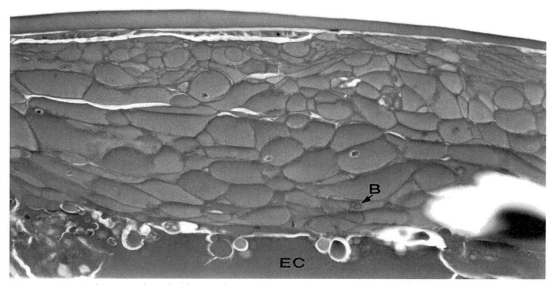

Figure 26. Radiation-induced subcapsular and cortical cataract in a therapeutically irradiated dog. Lens fibers have degenerated into large nucleated forms or bladder cells (B) or nonnucleated globular forms. The deeper cortex has degenerated into an eosinophilic coagulum (EC). H&E stain. Bar: 100 μm. Reproduced from Ching *et al.* (1990), with permission.

The effects of irradiation on the aorta and large arteries can result in serious complications, such as vessel rupture and infarction of dependent tissues.

b. Heart. Studies of the effects of irradiation on the hearts of rats, rabbits, and dogs have been reported. One month after fractionated doses of 3600–5200 cGy, there is a transient increase in heart weight and wall thickness primarily due to mild but diffuse inflammatory edema. After 3 months, mesothelial cell hypertrophy becomes pronounced. Significant changes may occur in the microvasculature during this time period, including endothelial cell swelling and thinning, cytoplasmic blebbing, loss of organelles, formation of lamellar bodies, obliteration of capillary lumens, and occasional thrombosis. At later times, there is slowly progressive perivascular, subendocardial, and subepicardial fibrosis. Interstitial fibrosis can be severe in the hearts of rabbits and humans, but not dogs or rats, after irradiation. A progressive decrease in capillary density and endothelial alkaline phosphatase staining is also seen. Nine to 12 months after exposure, thinning of the heart wall and large focal areas of myofiber loss are seen. Empty sarcolemmal sheaths and a mild influx of macrophages characterize these areas, but fibrosis is variable, depending on the species. Cardiac muscle fibers around these areas often have vacuolization typical of myocytolysis (Fig. 27). These foci of fiber loss are considered to result from damage to the microvasculature, arterioles, or larger arteries, as these lesions are similar to those that develop after ischemia. Intimal proliferation of coronary arteries that leads to significant narrowing of the vessel lumens may be seen near foci of fiber loss, giving further evidence that myocytolytic lesions have a vascular basis.

Along with differences in radiation-induced interstitial fibrosis, another species peculiarity is the apparent extreme radiosensitivity of the right atrial wall of the canine heart. Within 1 month of irradiation, the right atrial myocardium becomes hemorrhagic, which is followed by inflammation. By 12 months after irradiation, the right atrial myocardium is severely shrunken and, histologically, is characterized

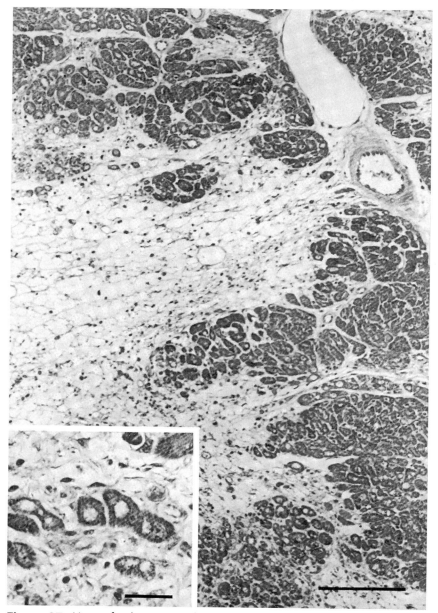

Figure 27. Heart of a dog 1 year after receiving 5200 cGy electrons in 400-cGy fractions. There is loss of muscle fibers with remnants of sarcolemmal sheaths and vacuolization of myofibers (myocytolysis). Myocytolysis is shown in the inset. Masson's trichrome stain. Bar: 100 μm; inset bar: 25 μm. Reproduced from McChesney *et al.* (1988), with permission.

by hemorrhage, fibrosis, and myofiber degeneration and necrosis. Two years or more after irradiation, hemangiosarcomas may develop in the irradiated tissue. While the left atrial wall shows some similar lesions, the changes are much less severe. This right atrial lesion has also been seen in dogs whose hearts have received radiation exposures from radionuclides deposited and retained in the lung. The sensitivity of the right atrial myocardium in the dog is of unknown pathogenesis and has not been seen in other species. Interestingly, the right atrial wall is a common site for the occurrence of spontaneous hemangiosarcomas in the dog.

c. Pericardium. The pericardium responds to irradiation in two general phases. One to 3 months after irradiation, there is hypertrophy of the mesothelial cell lining, dilated vessels, edema, and an infiltration of lymphocytes, plasma cells, and a few neutrophils. Effusions can occur after acute 1500-cGy doses. If severe, they can result in cardiac tamponade and death. More often, the effusion regresses slowly while the pericardium slowly thickens due to fibrosis. This late developing pericardial fibrosis can lead to constrictive pericarditis.

d. Blood Vessels. The radiation response of the aorta is characterized by intimal proliferation consisting of subendothelial nodular masses or plaques of collagenous connective tissue admixed with smooth muscle and elastin fibers (Fig. 28). This intimal proliferation increases with increasing dose given in 200- to 300-cGy fractions. If given as a single dose, intimal proliferation increases up to 1500 cGy and then decrease progressively at higher doses. Similar lesions can be observed after mechanical removal of the endothelial cell layer and are due to migration of a pluripotent smooth muscle-type cell from the tunica media, with subsequent production of collagen and elastin. Adventitial fibrosis is another characteristic radiation-induced lesion. Three or more years after single doses of 3500 cGy or above, there can be near total obstruction of the aortic lumen by thrombosis, disruption of the internal elastic lamina, disruption of elastic fibers in the media, medial fibrinoid necrosis and hyalinization, and the development of dissecting aneurysms (Fig. 29). These lesions tend to be more severe at the point where branch arteries leave the aorta, where there is more turbulent blood flow and, hence, more stress.

Early endothelial cell damage by irradiation probably leads to intimal proliferation. A variety of growth factors, such as basic fibroblast growth factor, platelet-derived growth factor, and TGF-β, are involved in the pathogenesis of the vascular injury. Damage to the vasovasorum with vascular leakage may lead to progressive adventitial fibrosis. The combination of intimal proliferation, fibrosis of the adventitia, and damage to the vasovasorum may compromise the nutrient and oxygen supply to the media and result in medial necrosis. These would predispose the aorta to thrombosis and

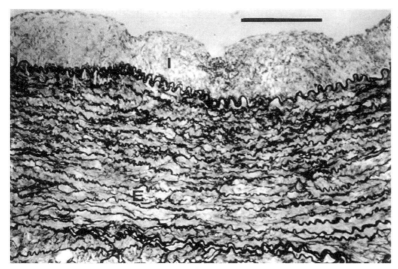

Figure 28. Canine aorta 5 years after exposure to 6000 cGy electrons in 200-cGy fractions. There is reduplication of the internal elastic lamina (E) and subendothelial nodular intimal (I) proliferation of fibrous connective tissue and elastin. Verhoeff–van Gieson stain. Bar: 100 μm.

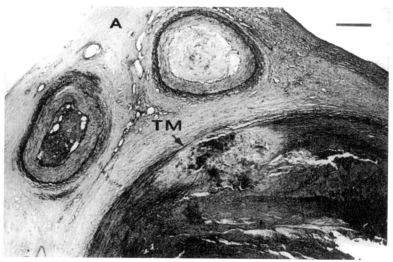

Figure 29. Aorta of a dog 5 years after exposure to 5500 cGy electrons. The aorta and branch arteries are thrombosed and there is disruption of the tunica media (TM) of the aorta. Adventitial fibrosis (A) is marked. Masson's trichrome stain. Bar: 300 μm. Reproduced from Gillette *et al*, (1989), with permission.

disruption. Smaller arteries and arterioles show lesions similar to that of the aorta, but they appear at earlier times after irradiation and at lower doses. Such lesions in smaller arteries and arterioles may be responsible for many of the later developing injuries seen after irradiation in a variety of organs and tissues. Small and large veins are resistant to irradiation, except those veins of the liver and intestine, which can become occluded by collagen fibrils and thrombi. Lymphatics are considered radioresistant.

8. Urinary System

a. General Reaction to Ionizing Radiation Injury. Irradiation of the urinary system may involve damage to the kidneys, ureters, and urinary bladder. The kidney is a radiosensitive organ that is often a limiting factor when giving radiation therapy involving the abdomen. Radiation nephropathy may develop months to years after irradiation. Clinically, radiation nephropathy is manifest by proteinuria, oliguria, azotemia, anemia, and the presence of casts in the urine. Renal tubular epithelium and glomerular endothelial cells appear to be the most radiosensitive populations. Radiation damage to the ureter can result in stricture formation and subsequent hydronephrosis, whereas radiation damage to the urinary bladder can cause fibrosis and loss of function.

b. Kidney. The pathogenesis of radiation nephropathy in dogs was studied by sequential renal biopsy every 2 weeks after a single dose of 1500 cGy. At 3 weeks after irradiation, there was a mild vacuolar change in renal tubular epithelial cells. This lesion progressed to degeneration and a reduction of total tubular epithelial cell volume by 50% at 9 weeks after exposure (Fig. 30). Evidence of tubular regeneration, characterized by enlarged basophilic flattened cells lining tubules, was evident 5 weeks after irradiation and resulted in a recovery of tubular epithelium to 80% of normal volume by 11 weeks. However, by 13 weeks, the renal tubular epithelium volume started to decrease again and reached a level of 15% of normal volume by 24 weeks. As the percentage of renal tubular epithelium decreased there was a corresponding increased in interstitial connective tissue. Blood vessel lesions were characterized by an early thickening of the medial and intimal layers of small arteries and arterioles.

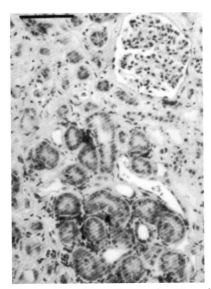

Figure 30. Kidney from a dog 9 weeks after exposure to 1500 cGy electrons. There is extensive tubular atrophy, representing an approximate 50% decrease in tubular epithelium. The interstitium is increased. Masson's trichrome stain. Bar: 100 μm. Reproduced from Hoopes *et al.* (1985), with permission.

Fibrinoid necrosis and fibrosis of the media accompanied progressive perivascular fibrosis. The glomerular volume remained unchanged, but marked thickening of the juxtaglomerular arteries was associated with loss of some glomeruli as early as 3 weeks after irradiation. Glomerular and periglomerular sclerosis was seen at later times. These results suggest that irradiation affects both vasculature and tubular epithelium. The earliest loss of tubular epithelium may be due to a direct effect of irradiation. After epithelial repopulation, the second wave of depopulation may be related to a decreased vascular supply.

In contrast, in mice, renal tubular damage was thought to be due to a slow loss of irradiated parenchymal cells rather than to injury to blood vessels. The thickening of the tunica media and intima of arteries was felt to be secondary to the tubular epithelial damage. Still other investigators have suggested that the initial lesions of radiation damage occur in the glomeruli. Irradiation of the kidneys of mice, pigs, and monkeys produced early thickening of glomerular capillary walls beginning at 6 weeks.

These changes progressed to replacement of the glomerular tuft by amorphous eosinophilic material consisting of basement membrane fragments, collagen, and fibrin thrombi in capillary lumens at 9 and 12 months after irradiation. In contrast, tubular atrophy and stromal fibrosis was not seen before 4 months and was not as severe as the glomerular lesions. In pigs after a 980-cGy single dose, there was early leukocyte adhesion to glomerular capillaries, followed by endothelial cell swelling, microthrombi formation, and increased capillary permeability. At 12 weeks, there was exudation, mesangial proliferation, and sclerosis with a resultant decreased glomerular filtration rate. Most evidence suggests a key role for the microvasculature in both glomerular and tubule damage. There is also a role for TGF-β as this has been shown to be increased in mesangium after irradiation.

c. Ureter. Histological lesions after irradiation of the ureter in the rat and dog consist of early thinning and degeneration of the urothelium, which progresses to ulceration and inflammation by 2–6 months after irradiation. Later lesions consist of focal areas of urothelial thinning and cystic degeneration alternating with areas of hyperplasia and polypoid proliferation. Varying degrees of fibrosis of the lamina propria and adventitia can extend into the muscle wall. There is sometimes muscular hypertrophy associated with strictures due to fibrosis. Ureteral stricture can lead to hydronephrosis. Vascular lesions consist of adventitial fibrosis, fibrinoid necrosis of the media, intimal proliferation, and decreased microvascular volume. These changes occur at single doses of 3000 cGy and above. The volume or length of ureter irradiated affects the dose required to cause strictures.

d. Urinary Bladder. Radiation damage to the urinary bladder has been studied in mice and dogs. Transitional epithelium of the urinary bladder normally has a slow turnover rate, which increases after injury. In humans, acute radiation cystitis is transitory and usually mild. Chronic radiation cystitis develops months to years later and can result in severe hemorrhage

and blood loss. After doses of 3000 cGy to
the canine urinary bladder, initial submucosal
edema, petechiae, and lymphocytic infiltration
are followed after 3–6 months by vacuolization
of the epithelial cells, multifocal ulceration,
submucosal and smooth muscle fibrosis, and
fibrinoid degeneration and intimal fibrosis of
submucosal arterioles. Squamous metaplasia
of the epithelium may occur. The submucosal
and muscle fibrosis is thought to cause increased urinary frequency and decreased bladder volume that is evident clinically. Urinary
frequency and decreased bladder volume are
both dose-related changes in mice. Submucosal
fibrosis has been proposed to be secondary to
surface ulceration and perhaps related to vascular lesions. Similar lesions are observed in
humans after urinary bladder irradiation.

9. Genital System

a. General Reaction to Ionizing Radiation Injury. The effects of irradiation on the testes are
most striking in the highly sensitive differentiat-
ing spermatogonia, which are affected by only
20 cGy in rodents. After irradiation, testicular
sperm counts remain constant for 20 days and
then decrease to a minimum at 29 days. The
constant sperm counts until 20 days indicate
that the spermatocytes and spermatids are relatively resistant to irradiation. The decrease in
sperm at 29 days indicates that spermatogonia
have the highest sensitivity, as this is the time
they would normally have become sperm. After
this time, sperm counts may increase again, indicating recovery of stem cell spermatogonia.
However, at fractionated doses above 600 cGy,
there is often incomplete recovery of sperm production, indicating residual damage to stem
cells. Humans and nonhuman primates take
much longer to regenerate spermatogenic cell
populations than rodents. Leydig cells and Sertoli cells are much less sensitive to irradiation
than spermatogonia. Histologically, irradiated
testes have absent sperm, rare spermatogonia,
thickened basement membranes of seminiferous
tubules, and vascular sclerosis.

Radiation damage to the ovary is dependent
on the age of the ovum and the development of
the granulosa cell layers. Oocytes with few
layers of granulosa cells are more radiosensitive
than oocytes with more layers. This finding
suggests that injury to the oocyte may be indirect with the granulosa cells being being the
target, possibly because the granulosa cells
play a supportive role for the oocyte. In some
species this may not be true. Radiation-induced
ovarian fibrosis and progressive vascular sclerosis also may contribute to ovum death. The
mature ovary may tolerate doses of 2000 cGy
before permanent sterility is observed. Because
all primary ovarian follicles are formed at birth,
in utero irradiation can have marked effects on
the developing ovary. Doses to the fetus in the
100- to 200-cGy range can cause a marked reduction of follicles in the postnatal animal.

10. Integumentary System

a. General Reaction to Ionizing Radiation Injury. Radiation injury to the skin includes the
reaction of the stratified keratinizing epidermis,
the connective tissue dermis with vascular and
nervous tissue components, and the adnexa,
including hair follicles, sebaceous glands, and
sweat glands. The epithelium and some hair
follicles are in a constant state of cell turnover
as basal cells divide, mature into keratinocytes,
and slough from the surface. This rapidly dividing population of basal cells is sensitive to irradiation and is responsible for some of the acute
reactions seen during therapeutic irradiation.
Late reactions of fibrosis, atrophy, necrosis,
and telangiectasia occur months to years after
irradiation.

The early reaction of the skin to irradiation is
a transient erythema within hours of exposure
to 1500–2000 cGy in fractions. The capillaries
of the dermis become dilated and have increased permeability within 24 hr. Within 1
week of irradiation, a more prolonged erythema
occurs. This erythema is dose dependent, and
the time to development depends on the species
and the site irradiated. During this time, there is
depletion of the basal cell layer of the epidermis, which, if severe enough, can lead to ulceration. In the pig, there is an initial decrease in
proliferation in the basal cell layer leading to a

decrease in cell density of the epidermis. Degeneration and necrosis of the basal cells may also be seen. Proliferation and cell density start to return toward normal 2 weeks after exposure. In the dermis, capillaries may still be dilated, and perivascular edema and inflammatory cell infiltrates are common. Also present at this early stage are endothelial cell swelling, proliferation, necrosis, and, occasionally, microthrombosis. This first acute skin reaction is the result of a combination of epithelial and dermal responses, but the epithelial responses are probably the most significant. Also during this time there is increased TGF-β expression in the suprabasal layers of the skin and in the dermis, which peaks at 14 days after 2000–5000 cGy. The increase persists until 30 days after irradiation.

The acute reaction of the skin usually regresses and the skin returns to normal. However, if the dose is high enough, a second wave of skin reaction occurs. In the pig, this second reaction is characterized by erythema and dermal necrosis and occurs 2–4 months after irradiation. It is thought to be primarily a result of damage to the microvasculature. In the dermis, the density of endothelial cells decreases starting 1 month after irradiation, and nuclear pyknosis and loss of cell nuclei of endothelial cells increase progressively. Capillary density in the dermis decreases and focal edema is present. Blood and lymphatic flow are decreased at 9–12 weeks after irradiation. Increased TGF-β expression is recognized at 3 months and peaks at 9 months after irradiation.

At 1 year or more after irradiation, medial necrosis of arterioles and small arteries in the deep dermis and telangiectasis of the upper dermis may occur. Fibroblasts decrease in number by 3 months after irradiation and the maximum reduction is seen at 6 months. This corresponds to a decreased dermal thickness that is greatest at 6 months. Remaining dermis is fibrosed. The overlying epidermis may be thinned to one cell layer or, in some cases, may become completely necrotic and ulcerated. Although this second later reaction of the skin to irradiation is thought to be due to changes in the dermal vasculature, some investigators think that the vascular changes are secondary to changes in the epidermis. It is likely that the TGF-β increase seen also contributes to the late fibrosis.

Irradiation induces melanocytes in the skin to increase melanosome production, which results in hyperpigmentation. However, high radiation doses can destroy melanocytes, which then results in hypo- or depigmentation. Langerhans cells, which are derived from bone marrow precursors and take part in immune responses in the epidermis, may decrease in number in mouse skin 8–12 days after 2000 cGy but then return to normal numbers as cells migrate in from the blood. At 19 and 20 months after irradiation, a second decrease in the number of Langerhans cells occurs that is thought to be due to damage to the blood vessels and connective tissue in the dermis inhibiting the replacement of cells.

Hair follicles react in a manner similar to the epidermis. Early damage to the hair follicles is probably a result of damage to the basal cells and results in hair loss. As hair follicle proliferative activity is normally cyclic, the extent of radiation damage to the hair and the extent of alopecia depend on the stage of cycle the hair follicle was in when irradiated. Later developing, more permanent, damage to the hair follicle may be secondary to changes in dermal microvasculature and progressive fibrosis. Sebaceous glands appear to be quite radiosensitive and decrease in number within 3–4 weeks of irradiation. Sweat glands are less sensitive and do not decrease in number until 3–4 months after irradiation. At lower doses the glands may regenerate. Permanent atrophy of these glands is often accompanied by early periglandular infiltrates of lymphocytes and plasma cells and fibrosis. The pathogenesis of the effects of irradiation on these glands is not well understood.

While the skin is not considered to be a sensitive tissue with respect to ionizing radiation-induced carcinogenesis, both squamous cell and basal cell carcinomas can be induced in humans and animals with high enough doses.

11. Thyroid Gland

a. General Reaction to Ionizing Radiation Injury. The thyroid is susceptible to radiation exposure because it concentrates radioiodine and because it is commonly incorporated in therapeutic radiation fields. Because the thyroid follicular epithelium has a long turnover time (on the order of 1 to 2 years), injury can be delayed until cells undergo mitosis-linked death after acute radiation doses. The sensitivity of thyroid follicular epithelium is related to the dose of radiation with a possible lower threshold between 200 and 400 cGy for acute injury. The pituitary axis can compensate for a considerable degree of thyroid injury with increases in thyroid-stimulating hormone (TSH) production.

^{131}I therapy for thyrotoxicosis at radiation doses on the order of 5000 cGy and above is associated with destruction of the thyroid gland and hypothyroidism characterized by chronic inflammation, fibrosis, and atrophy. In humans, the occurrence of hypothyroidism relates to radiation dose, but also to the prior status of antithyroid antibodies in irradiated patients, there being a correlation between the occurrence of thyroid autoantibodies and the development of hypothyroidism.

Also reported is that hyperthyroidism associated with autoimmune disease can be induced by ionizing radiation exposure. Treatment of goiter with ^{131}I can be associated with increased serum levels of TSH receptor antibodies and hyperthyroidism. It has been suggested that irradiation could lead to a release of antigen from the damaged thyroid with the subsequent production of antibodies that stimulate the TSH receptors eliciting thyroid hyperactivity.

b. Thyroid Neoplasia. The thyroid gland is well known to be among the most sensitive tissues to the carcinogenic effects of ionizing radiation in both humans and animals. In humans, epidemiologic studies of irradiated populations, including atomic bomb survivors and children exposed for diverse conditions, suggest that there is an increased risk for thyroid cancer at doses as low as 10 cGy or less. Both external radiation exposures and exposures to ^{131}I have been associated with increased risk, although it is considered that external radiation is relatively more carcinogenic on a per dose basis because of the higher dose rates for most external exposures compared to that related to radioiodine decay. The exact difference in RBE between X rays and ^{131}I is the subject of some considerable debate. This is important because the U.S. population received a significant exposure to ^{131}I resulting from the years of atmospheric testing of nuclear weapons. An average thyroid dose of about 2 cGy to the population collectively was estimated, with many individuals receiving doses above 10 cGy. Even small differences in the estimates of the effectiveness of ^{131}I in inducing cancer would have a significant impact on the overall risk estimates of the United States for radiation-induced thyroid cancer.

Beyond dose and dose rate, a number of factors influence ionizing radiation-induced thyroid cancer. Women are known to have a higher risk than men, although this sex difference is not consistent between species. Of particular importance, age at exposure is a modifying factor in thyroid carcinogenesis. Data suggest a doubling of risk for persons exposed during childhood or adolescence and a similar increased risk has been seen in beagles irradiated as juveniles and in immature rodents.

From a mechanistic standpoint, it is of interest to examine the role of TSH in thyroid carcinogenesis. Elevated levels of TSH have been shown to increase the incidence of thyroid neoplasia in multiple species, including increased risk after irradiation. Treatment with goitrogens, partial thyroidectomy, and hypothyroidism have all been demonstrated to increase radiation-induced thyroid cancer. It is thought that reduced levels of circulating thyroid hormone lead to a compensatory increase in TSH that, in turn, stimulates the proliferation of remaining thyroid epithelium, essentially acting as a promoter for cells initiated by the irradiation.

III. Ultraviolet Radiation

A. NATURE AND ACTION OF ULTRAVIOLET RADIATION

Ultraviolet radiation includes wavelengths of electromagnetic energy between 10 and 400 nm, thus bridging the gap between ionizing radiation (X rays) and visible light. By convention, UV radiation is subdivided into extreme UV (10–120 nm), far UV (120–200 nm), UV-C (200–280 nm), UV-B (280–320 nm), and UV-A (320–400 nm) regions. Sunlight includes all UV wavelengths; however, the earth's atmosphere attenuates sunlight by processes of absorption and scattering, screening out UV wavelengths shorter than 280 nm. Because of this screening, biologically relevant wavelengths of UV include only the UV-A and portions of the UV-B regions of the spectrum. Removal of short wavelength UV is due primarily to stratospheric ozone. Focal thinning of the stratospheric ozone layer has been observed in the spring near the South Pole and is attributed to ozone destruction catalyzed by free chlorine released from man-made chlorofluorocarbons. It is predicted that global decreases in stratospheric ozone will ultimately result in increased UV exposure and associated adverse health effects.

When UV interacts with matter, it behaves as though composed of particles (termed "photons"). The energy of a photon is transferred to the electron of an atom or molecule, resulting in an excited state. The electronic excitation energy is then dissipated by releasing the energy as heat or light, by losing an electron to form a free radical or ion, by using the energy to drive chemical reactions with other molecules, or by undergoing fragmentation. For a molecule or atom to absorb photons of a given wavelength, it must have electrons in appropriate energy levels. Thus, not all molecules absorb all UV wavelengths. A molecule that absorbs a given UV wavelength is a "chromophore" for that wavelength. UV doses are expressed as energy per unit area, typically as Joules/m^2. The biological effects of UV depend not only on the total energy of UV absorbed, but also on the wavelength of that energy. The "action spectrum" expresses the functional relationship between biological effect and wavelength for a given UV dose. Action spectroscopy can help identify the UV chromophore ultimately responsible for initiating a given biological response. For example, as shown in Fig. 31, the action spectrum for UV-induced skin cancer indicates that the most effective wavelengths are those that can penetrate the skin and damage DNA, suggesting that DNA is a major chromophore for this response.

B. MECHANISMS OF ULTRAVIOLET RADIATION INJURY

Biologically important cellular targets for UV include DNA, RNA, proteins, and lipids. Because carbohydrates do not absorb light above 230 nm, they are unaffected by UV radiation reaching the earth's surface. UV effects on biological molecules may be direct or

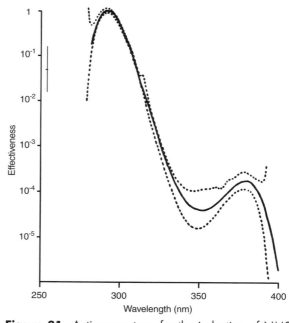

Figure 31. Action spectrum for the induction of NMSC skin cancer in hairless albino (SKH-1) mice (solid line). The χ^2 is 13.4 with 7 degrees of freedom. Dashed curves indicate the accuracy of this curve (χ^2 increased by 1). The efficacy of wavelengths in the 280- to 320-nm range suggests that DNA, which receives maximal direct damage at 260 nm, is a major chromophore for NMSC. Reproduced from de Gruijl et al. (1993), with permission.

photosensitized. In photosensititivity reactions, UV-activated intermediate compounds such as free radicals actually mediate UV effects. Most UV-A-induced cellular damage is due to the formation of activated oxygen species, such as peroxides, superoxide anion, and hydroxyl radical. Pyrimidines in nucleic acids (maximum absorption at 260 nm) appear to be more sensitive to direct UV damage than purines. Pyrimidine dimers are the most numerous pyrimidine lesions; (6–4) adducts form much less frequently. Cyclobutane pyrimidine dimers can form between any two adjacent pyrimidines, but (6–4) adducts form only at TC, CC, and TT pairs. These DNA photoproducts appear to be responsible for many of the adverse cellular effects of UV, including cell death and mutation.

Unlike pyrimidines, purines are fairly insensitive to direct photochemical interactions but do undergo photosensitized reactions. Because of the short half-life and relative abundance of RNA, the effects of RNA photoproducts are difficult to assess. The only amino acids that are excitable by UV are tryptophan, tyrosine, and cysteine, with maximal absorption at 280 nm for tryptophan and tyrosine and absorption over a broad range of UV-B wavelengths for cysteine. Tryptophan is the major chromophore of proteins. When tryptophan absorbs UV, the indole ring is photoionized to form a neutral indolyl radical and a hydrated electron. Reactions of the indolyl radical subsequently form a variety of products, including potent photosensitizers. The hydrated electron is scavenged by oxygen to form the superoxide radical ion. Cysteine and tyrosine can undergo direct or sensitized photolysis. In the case of cysteine, interchain disulfide bridges may thus be split. Methionine, histidine, cysteine, and tryptophan can be photooxidized to cause protein denaturation. Lipids do not absorb UV above 290 nm, with the exception of the vitamin D precursor 7-dehydrocholesterol, and are thus not susceptible to direct UV damage. However, photosensitized oxidation of lipids is an important mechanism for UV-induced changes in biological membrane function.

Photoreactivation, nucleotide excision repair, or postreplication repair may repair DNA photoproducts. Photoreactivation of pyrimidine dimers and (6,4) photoproducts is an error-free repair system catalyzed by specific photolyases that recognize and bind to the appropriate photoproduct, absorb long-wavelength visible light, and use the absorbed energy to drive the enzymatic monomerization of the photoproduct. While most species appear to possess a (6,4) photolyase, placental mammals seem to lack a pyrimidine dimer photolyase. Excision repair acts on a variety of bulky DNA adducts, such as photoproducts, to introduce single-strand nicks on either side of the adduct, to remove a short segment of the DNA strand containing the lesion, and to resynthesize the missing DNA using the remaining strand as a template.

Excision repair is accurate, but not error free. *Xeroderma pigmentosum*, a recessive human disorder, results from an inability to carry out efficient excision repair of DNA photoproducts. Disruption of any of several genes in the excision repair pathway can account for the phenotype. In the last few years, several excision repair genes have been cloned and characterized, and construction of knockout mice lacking some of these genes has yielded excellent models of *xeroderma pigmentosum*. Postreplication repair is not as well understood as nucleotide excision repair. It is a more error-prone repair system based on recombination. Both misrepair of DNA photoproducts and the presence of noninformative dipyrimidine photoproducts during replication may give rise to mutations. Signature UV mutations include C to T transitions and CC to TT tandem mutations at dipyrimidine sites.

Adverse cellular effects of UV include cell death (characteristically by apoptosis), cell cycle arrest, mutation, and altered gene expression. DNA damage plays a major role in initiating these responses; however, activation of cytoplasmic signaling pathways also contributes to some UV effects. The protein product of the *p53* tumor suppressor gene is an important mediator of UV-induced cell cycle arrest and apoptosis. Exposure to UV results in rapid and prolonged nuclear accumulation of the P53 protein. UV-induced G_1 arrest requires P53-dependent transcription of the $p21^{WAF1/CIP1}$ gene. The pathway linking P53 stabilization and apoptosis has not been elucidated and it is currently the subject of intense investigation.

The "UV response" is an ordered sequence of alterations in gene expression similar to that induced by many growth factors. The genes activated include those for a variety of transcription factors, cytokines and growth factors, and proteases. UV is believed physically to activate growth factor receptors on cell surfaces in a ligand-independent manner. The epithelial growth factor (EGF) receptor appears to be particularly important in mediating UV responses. Receptor stimulation, in turn, leads to the activation of cytoplasmic signaling pathways, including the mitogen-activated protein kinase cascade. Both cytoplasmic signaling pathways and DNA damage responses initiated by UV ultimately modulate the activity of transcription factors, particularly AP-1, P53, and NFκB, that coordinately regulate the expression of many genes.

C. RESPONSE TO INJURY INDUCED BY ULTRAVIOLET RADIATION

1. Skin

Most incident UV-B and UV-C radiation is absorbed in the epidermis by keratin of the stratum corneum, epidermal melanin, and keratinocyte DNA. In contrast, UV-A can penetrate to and be absorbed in the dermis.

a. Acute Skin Responses. Acute skin responses to UV include the edema, erythema, and desquamation that characterize sunburn. Action spectroscopy indicates that UV-B and UV-C are considerably more effective than UV-A in eliciting these changes. Edema and erythema are due to vascular changes in the dermis. UV-A, UV-B, and UV-C induce erythema responses with different time courses. UV-A induces a short-lived immediate increase in vascular permeability followed, after 2–8 hr, by a delayed response. UV-B-induced erythema

peaks at 6–24 hr after exposure and then fades gradually; a second peak is sometimes seen at about 48 hr.

Early phase erythema is responsive to non-steroidal anti-inflammatory compounds, but not to antihistamines. Late phase erythema does not response to either. UV-C-induced erythema is maximal at 8 hr and fades over the next day or two. Inflammatory mediators released from both the epidermis and dermal mast cells appear to stimulate vascular changes. A transient perivascular inflammatory cell infiltrate is seen in UV-exposed skin. A common measure of skin responsiveness to UV is the "minimal erythemal dose" (MED). The MED is the lowest UV dose required to stimulate, on previously unexposed skin, just perceptible erythema 24 hr after exposure. In experimental animals, measurement of skin thickness (edema) can also be used to determine MED.

UV-induced cell death in the epidermis is maximal at about 24 hr after exposure. Cell death occurs by *p53*-dependent apoptosis, and apoptotic epidermal cells are termed "sunburn cells" (Fig. 32). In hematoxylin and eosin-stained sections, they have pyknotic nuclei and deeply eosinophilic, homogeneously stained cytoplasm. UV exposure also stimulates a later phase of epidermal hyperplasia and parakeratosis with desquamation, peaking a few days to a week after exposure.

The epidermal melanocyte synthesizes melanin and donates it to surrounding epithelial cells. In humans, an epidermal melanin unit consists of one melanocyte surrounded by approximately 36 keratinocytes. Melanocytes synthesize both brown to black eumelanin and light brown to red pheomelanin. Constitutive skin color is due to genetically determined melanin levels, whereas facultative skin color is the UV- or pituitary hormone-induced increase in melanin pigmentation above constitutive skin color. In humans, an increase in epidermal melanin, which absorbs and scatters radiation over a broad spectral range, is the major adaptive response to UV exposure. Facultative skin color in response to UV exposure can be due to "immediate" or "delayed" tanning.

581

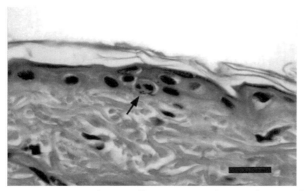

Figure 32. Sunburn cell (arrow) in the epidermis of *Monodelphis domestica* exposed 32 hr previously to a UV dose of 500 J/m² UV-B (approximately 0.75 MED). Note the homogeneous appearance of the cytoplasm and the pyknotic and fragmented nucleus of the sunburn cell. Removing pyrimidine dimers by photoreactivation reduced the number of sunburn cells markedly in the UV-exposed skin of this animal, implicating DNA damage as the initiating lesion. H&E stain. Bar: 20 μm. Photograph courtesy of Dr. R. D. Ley (University of New Mexico).

Immediate tanning (immediate pigment darkening, Mierowsky phenomenon) occurs within minutes of UV exposure and reaches a maximum in about an hour. UV-A wavelengths are more effective than UV-C or UV-B in producing immediate tanning, although visible light can also induce the phenomenon. Immediate tanning is caused by the photooxidation of preformed melanin, migration of melanosomes from the cell body to the cell processes of melanocytes, increased transfer of melanosomes from melanocytes to epidermal cells, and changes in the distribution of melanosomes within keratinocytes. There is no change in the size of melanosomes or the number of melanocytes. In delayed tanning, however, there is an increase in both the number and the size of functional melanocytes, accompanied by increased melanosome synthesis, increased size and melanization of melanosomes, and increased transfer of melanosomes from melanocytes to keratinocytes. Delayed tanning becomes visible approximately 72 hr after UV exposure and increases for several days thereafter. All UV wavelengths, as well as blue visible light, can induce delayed tanning, but UV-B is the most effective portion of the spectrum. The

skin of the trunk of many nonalbino rodents is unpigmented, with melanocytes restricted to hair follicles, therefore, few rodents tan in response to UV exposure.

b. Chronic Skin Reactions. In humans, chronic exposure to UV causes photoaging and skin cancer. Photoaging is characterized grossly by laxity, roughness, sallowness, irregular hyperpigmentation, and telangiectasia. Microscopic changes include increased deposition and degeneration of elastic fibers (elastosis) (Fig. 33), decreased insoluble collagen, increased glycosaminoglycans, chronic dermal inflammation, and focal epidermal hyperplasia and dysplasia (solar keratosis). Solar keratosis and elastosis have been reproduced in hairless mice. UV-B is considerably more effective than UV-A in inducing photoaging in this animal model.

c. Photosensitivity. Photosensitizers are endogenous or exogenous compounds that are activated readily by UV or visible light and, once activated, induce an adverse cutaneous response. UV-A is the most effective of the UV spectral ranges in eliciting photosensitization reactions. Exogenous photosensitizers may reach the skin by topical or systemic routes. Most photosensitizers are unsaturated tricyclic aromatic rings in linear arrangement, many

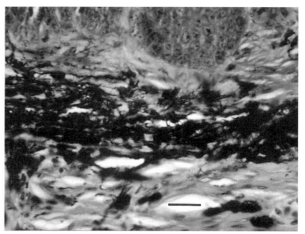

Figure 33. UV-B-induced solar elastosis in the skin of a hairless mouse. Dense tangled aggregates of thickened elastic fibers are located in the dermis. Luna's stain. Bar: 30 μm. Reproduced from Kligman *et al.* (1985), with permission.

have a lone pair of electrons not involved in bonding, and most are fluorescent. Efficient photosensitizers include coal tar derivatives, chlorothiazides, porphyrins, phenothiazines, sulfonamides, and tetracyclines. Photosensitivity can manifest as phototoxicity or photoallergy, and many chemicals that are phototoxins may also act as photoallergens.

Phototoxic reactions are characterized grossly by erythema, and sometimes edema, occurring during or immediately after exposure. Variable degrees of desquamation and hyperpigmentation follow. Microscopically, intracellular edema in the epidermis and necrosis of keratinocytes are seen and there is little dermal involvement. Phototoxicity is believed to be due to the formation of excited triplet states, free radicals, and peroxides. These damage cell membranes to cause release of lysosomal contents and mast cell degranulation. The severity of the reaction is proportional to the dose of photosensitizer or UV. Phototoxicity does not require an allergic response.

Photoallergy, however, involves a circulating antibody or a cell-mediated immune response. Thus, photoallergy differs from phototoxicity in requiring an incubation period after first exposure to the photosensitizer and repeated exposure to light or UV in previously sensitized individuals. The response is not linearly dose related. Photoallergy is characterized clinically by immediate erythema and urticaria or by delayed papular or eczematous dermatitis on sun-exposed skin. There is usually a dense lymphocytic infiltrate in the dermis, and epidermal spongiosis or vesicle formation may occur. The urticaria is associated with the degranulation of mast cells at the site of UV exposure, increased numbers of eosinophils, and release of neutrophil chemotactic factors.

Several mechanisms for the photoallergic reaction have been proposed. First, absorption of radiant energy by the photosensitizing molecule may lead to formation of a photohapten that binds to a carrier macromolecule in the skin to form a photoantigen. Second, radiation may alter a tissue protein to allow it to serve as a carrier for the photosensitizer or its photoproduct, thus forming an antigenic carrier–hapten complex. Finally, radiation in the presence of a photosensitizer may alter a tissue component to transform it into a tissue antigen.

2. Eye

UV wavelengths less than 315 nm are largely absorbed in the cornea and conjunctiva. With acute UV exposure, photoconjunctivitis and photokeratitis can develop following a latent period of 30 min to 12 hr and last up to 48 hr. Clinical signs include photophobia, lacrimation, blepharospasm, and scleral and conjunctival vasodilation. Microscopically, edema and an acute inflammatory cell infiltrate are seen. In severe cases, blistering and ulceration of corneal and conjunctival epithelium and edema of underlying stroma may occur. Repair of DNA damage and replacement of lost cells in the corneal epithelium are very rapid. With chronic UV exposure in experimental animals, neovascularization of the cornea may develop.

In vitro studies in several species, including humans, and in vivo studies in laboratory animals have provided considerable information about UV effects on the lens. The lenses of diurnal animals such as humans contain yellow pigments that effectively absorb 300–400 nm light. In addition, chromophores such as riboflavin and tryptophan can also absorb these wavelengths, leading to the formation of free radicals. These highly reactive compounds can trigger a variety of chemical reactions, including the formation of singlet oxygen, lipid peroxidation, protein cross-linking, and enzyme inactivation. The epithelium and outer portion of the lens sustain the major direct damage. Adverse UV effects on the lens include DNA damage to epithelium, decreased sodium–potassium ATPase activity, disruption of actin filaments, aggregation and breakdown of crystallins, and alterations in the oxidation–reduction balance (decreased glutathione levels, increased mixed disulfides, and decreased -SH groups). Swelling, degeneration, and loss of anterior lens epithelium; swelling and disruption of lens fibers; and formation of amorphous protein aggregates are seen microscopically.

583

Grossly, yellowing of the lens and the development of lens opacities are seen and, ultimately, cataracts are formed. Loss of visual acuity is due both to increased light scattering by and increased autofluorescence of altered lens components.

In general, the retina is protected from the effects of UV by the lens. However, in animals without yellow lens pigments, in aphakic animals and humans, and in those exposed to extremely high levels of UV, UV radiation in the 300- to 400-nm range can cause irreversible retinal degeneration and atrophy.

3. Immune System

UV is an immunosuppressive agent. Acute or chronic low-dose UV exposure inhibits both tumor rejection and the development of contact hypersensitivity. UV-induced skin tumors are highly antigenic and are rejected when transplanted into syngeneic mice. However, if the recipient mice are pretreated with UV-B, the transplanted tumors are not rejected. This tolerance is specific for UV-induced tumors; chemically induced tumors and skin allografts are rejected normally. Contact hypersensitivity is a cell-mediated immune response elicited by skin application of a sensitizing dose of hapten followed, days or weeks later, by cutaneous challenge with the hapten. When the sensitizing hapten is applied either to UV-B-irradiated or to unirradiated skin of mice that were immunized in an irradiated area, little response is seen upon challenge. This suggests that immunosuppression is both local and systemic in nature. As for tumors, hapten tolerance is specific. Both for tumors and for haptens, specific UV-induced tolerance can be transferred adoptively with splenic suppressor T cells, suggesting that maintenance of tolerance is an active process.

In all species, the major antigen-presenting cell of the skin is the bone marrow-derived Langerhans cells, a specialized epidermal dendritic cell capable of presenting antigen to Th_1 and Th_2 helper T lymphocytes. In addition, the mouse has dendritic epidermal T cells ($\gamma\delta T$ cells), and both human and mouse have dermal dendritic cells that can present antigen to suppressor T-cell populations. Epidermal and dermal dendritic cells capture antigen in the skin and migrate via lymphatics to regional lymph nodes where they present antigen to the appropriate T lymphocytes.

UV irradiation impairs the function of antigen-presenting cells both by direct UV effects on the cells themselves and by the production of soluble mediators that act indirectly on the cells. Candidate mediators include prostaglandins, cytokines, and urocanic acid, a component of the stratum corneum that isomerizes in response to UV from the *trans* form to the immunosuppressive *cis* isomer. The exact mechanism by which antigen presentation is downregulated has not been elucidated. In UV-exposed skin, Langerhans cells appear contracted, with a loss of dendritic processes and decreased ATPase and major histocompatibility class II antigen reactivity. Evidence suggests that UV may do more than physically deplete or functionally inactivate Langerhans cells; it may convert these cells from immunogenic to tolerogenic antigen-presenting cells that induce anergy.

Keratinocytes constitutively express rather low levels of cytokines, neuroendocrine hormones, and other immunomodulatory molecules. However, as shown in Table VI, UV exposure dramatically increases the production of a variety of these substances. The role of these molecules in UV-induced immunosuppression is under investigation in a number of laboratories. In the case of contact hypersensitivity, considerable evidence suggests that keratinocyte-derived TNF-α is an important mediator of UV-B effects. Furthermore, UV-induced degranulation of dermal mast cells releases interleukin-1, TNF-α, and histamine.

UV exposure can exacerbate a variety of human diseases, including herpes simplex dermatitis and systemic lupus eythematosus. Presumably, these effects are mediated via immune suppression, although the precise mechanisms have not been identified. The fact that UV is so potently immunosuppressive has raised fears that ozone depletion and increased UV exposure will increase the risk of infectious disease worldwide.

TABLE VI
Immunomodulatory Molecules Released from UV-Exposed Keratinocytes

Modulator	Effects
Interleukin 1α (IL-1α)	Fever, induction of acute-phase proteins; cytokine induction in several cell types; T lymphocyte chemotaxis; costimulation of B lymphocytes; stimulation of mediator production and cytotoxic activity by macrophages; increased ICAM-1 and ELAM-1 expression by vascular endothelium
Interleukin 6 (IL-6)	Fever, induction of acute-phase proteins; costimulation of T-cell proliferation, stimulation of natural killer and cytotoxic T-cell activity; B-cell differentiation, proliferation, immunoglobulin production
Interleukin 8 (IL-8)	Neutrophil, basophil, lymphocyte chemotaxis; neutrophil enzyme release
Interleukin 10 (IL-10)	Inhibitor of $T_h 1$ effector function and IL-1, IL-2, IFN-γ, GM-CSF, TNFα production; thymocyte and mast cell costimulation; inhibitor of antigen presentation by macrophages and B cells
Tumor necrosis factor-α (TNFα)	Cachexia, fever, hemorrhagic necrosis of tumors; neutrophil, eosinophil, macrophage, fibroblast activation; ICAM-1 expression by vascular endothelial cells; costimulation of B and T cells; stimulation of MHC I and II antigen expression on various cells
Granulocyte/macrophage colony-stimulating factor (GM-CSF)	Nonspecific stimulation of hematopoietic cell proliferation; stimulation of neutrophil, eosinophil, macrophage function; inhibition of neutrophil migration; induction of phagocytosis, eicosanoid production, and antibody-dependent cell-mediated cytotoxicity by macrophages
Interleukin 3 (IL-3)	Nonspecific stimulation of hematopoietic cell proliferation; induction of phagocytosis by macrophages
Basic fibroblast growth factor (bFGF)	Proliferation of multiple cell types; angiogenesis
Transforming growth factor α (TGF-α)	Keratinocyte proliferation
Nerve growth factor	Poorly characterized effects on hematopoietic cell differentiation and immune cell function
α Melanocyte-stimulating hormone	Antagonism of IL-1 and TNFα effects; stimulation of natural killer cell activity; reduction in MHC class I antigen expression; modulation of IgE synthesis
Adrenocorticotropic hormone	Modulation of IgE synthesis
Prostaglandins ($E_2, F_{2α}$)	Increased vascular permeability, vasodilation; neutrophil chemotaxis

4. Ultraviolet Radiation Carcinogenesis

a. Epidemiologic Evidence. Evidence for the role of sunlight in nonmelanoma skin cancer (NMSC) in humans (basal cell and squamous cell carcinomas) is based on a number of observations. First, people with light skin color are more susceptible to NMSC than those pigmented more heavily. Second, the frequency of NMSC in light-skinned people increases near the equator where solar radiation is high. Third, those who spend much of their time outdoors have a higher incidence of NMSC than those staying mostly indoors. Fourth, NMSC develops predominantly on sun-exposed parts of the body. Fifth, *xeroderma pigmentosum* patients unable to repair DNA photoproducts develop NMSC in sun-exposed areas at a frequency much greater than DNA repair-proficient individuals. Finally, NMSC can be produced in mice by chronic UV-B irradiation. Although sun exposure contributes to the development of melanoma in humans, its exact role is unclear. In the last few decades, there has been an alarming increase in the number of NMSC and melanomas among light-skinned populations throughout the world, leading some scientists to postulate an emerging epidemic of skin cancer.

b. Animal Models. Species and strains vary considerably in their susceptibility to UV-induced skin cancer. These differences are due largely to variables such as pigmentation, hair coat, and thickness of the stratum corneum. Mice appear to be the experimental animals most susceptible to UV carcinogenesis. Hairless SKH-1 mice are widely used for photobiology studies. Advantages of these mice are that they do not require shaving, are unpigmented, and have a relatively normal immune system; however, a limitation is that the mice are not inbred. Furthermore, UV exposure alone does not cause melanomas in mice or other commonly used experimental animals, although a combination of chemical carcinogen and UV is effective. For this reason, a variety of unusual animal models susceptible to UV-induced melanoma, such as the marsupial *Monodelphis domestica* and *Xiphophorus* fish, have been used to study the relationship between UV exposure and melanoma. With the advent of new strains of genetically altered mice, a host of new murine models are becoming available, including mice that are highly susceptible to melanoma, heterozygous and homozygous *p53* knockout mice, and murine models of *xeroderma pigmentosum*.

c. Mechanisms. Animal studies indicate that UV is a complete skin carcinogen. UV is an initiator by virtue of its mutagenic capability, a promoter due to its ability to alter gene expression and thus stimulate proliferation, and it drives tumor progression by a combination of its mutagenic and growth-promoting activities. As indicated in Fig. 31, the most effective wavelengths for UV-induced NMSC in the hairless mouse are those in the UV-B range, with peak activity at 293 nm. This action spectrum implicates DNA as the primary chromophore for NMSC. UV-A (340 nm) can induce NMSC in hairless mice, but it is 10,000-fold less effective than UV-B. In general, changes in fluence rate or interval between doses do not alter the shape or slope of the NMSC incidence curve, but may affect the latent period.

Studies indicate that the *p53* tumor suppressor gene provides significant protection against UV-induced NMSC. UV-induced DNA damage is a potent inducer of wild-type P53 protein. P53 induces cell cycle arrest in cells with damaged DNA, thus permitting repair of minor DNA damage and stimulating apoptosis of cells too badly damaged for effective repair. This eliminates genetically altered and potentially transformed cells from the skin. When *p53* is mutationally inactivated or deleted, dele-

terious mutations accumulate in UV-exposed keratinocytes, leading to the development of NMSC. More than 90% of UV-induced NMSC in the human and in the hairless mouse have mutationally inactivated *p53* genes. Mutations are concentrated in exons 5–8 of the *p53* gene. Most are missense point mutations arising on the nontranscribed strand of DNA. Most *p53* mutations in NMSC are hallmark UV mutations, C to T and CC to TT, at dipyrimidine sites, suggesting that UV is the proximate carcinogen for these tumors.

d. Skin Neoplasms. Chronic natural or experimental exposure to UV leads to the development of hyperplastic and neoplastic skin lesions in a variety of animal species. In many cases, hyperplastic lesions appear to serve as precursors for neoplastic lesions. Actinic keratoses in humans appear to give rise to squamous cell carcinoma. In the hairless mouse, foci of epidermal hyperplasia can evolve into sessile or pedunculated papillomas, and squamous cell carcinomas may arise in those papillomas (Fig. 34). With continued UV exposure, squamous cell carcinomas in the hairless mouse progress to increasingly invasive and anaplastic tumors (Fig. 35).

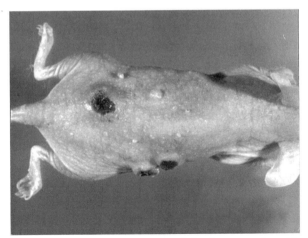

Figure 34. Gross appearance of skin lesions induced by chronic UV exposure in a hairless mouse. A number of pedunculated papillomas and three ulcerated squamous cell carcinomas are visible. Lesions arise and evolve independently. Photograph courtesy of Dr. V. E. Reeve (University of Sydney).

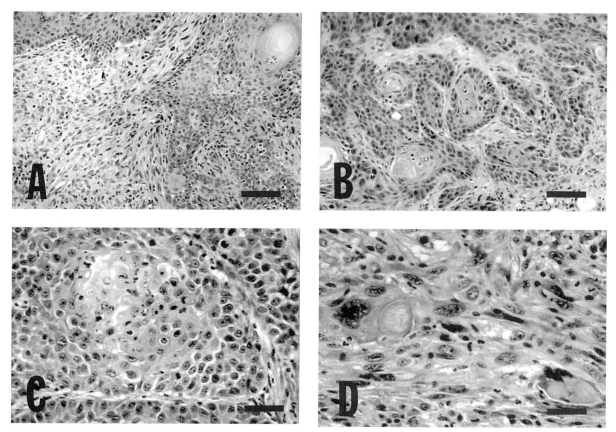

Figure 35. (A–D) Progression of UV-induced squamous cell carcinoma in a hairless mouse; each tumor is more aggressive and less differentiated than the previous. (A) Minimally invasive tumor and dermal fibroplasia. H&E stain. Bar: 200 μm. (B) More infiltrative tumor. H&E stain. Bar: 100 μm. (C) Individually keratinized cells in an aggressive tumor. H&E stain. Bar: 50 μm. (D) Marked anaplasia in a deeply invasive tumor. H&E stain. Bar: 50 μm. Photographs courtesy of Dr. V. E. Reeve (University of Sydney).

The behavior of UV-induced squamous cell carcinomas in humans and experimental animals is similar. Although clearly malignant and locally invasive, these tumors rarely metastasize. Squamous cell carcinoma in the unpigmented skin of dogs, the pinna of white cats, and the vulva of cattle and goats has been linked to natural sunlight exposure. Keratoacanthomas are invaginated keratin-filled masses lined by thickened epithelium that develop in humans and in some experimental animals in response to UV. In humans, these tumors are self-limiting and undergo involution, whereas in experimental animals, they appear to be capable of giving rise to squamous cell carcinomas. Basal cell tumors similar to those caused by sunlight in humans rarely arise in experimental animals; however, a murine model of basal cell carcinoma, the *Patched* knockout mouse, has been developed.

The only human sarcoma clearly associated with sunlight is the atypical fibroxanthoma of the elderly. However, chronic UV exposure in haired mice and in *M. domestica* can induce dermal fibrosarcomas and hemangiosarcomas, and sunlight exposure has been proposed as a cause of hemangiosarcoma in the sparsely haired skin of dogs (Fig. 36). Some UV-induced spindle cell tumors of the dermis in mice may represent anaplastic squamous cell carcinomas, and carcinosarcomas or "collision tumors" have been described. A number of models for

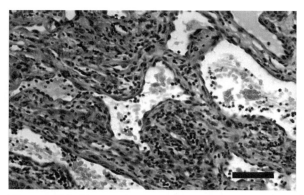

Figure 36. Hemangiosarcoma in unpigmented and sparsely haired skin of a dog. These tumors are associated with sunlight exposure. Note the cavernous spaces filled with erythrocytes. H&E stain. Bar: 75 μm. Photograph courtesy of Dr. J. P. Thilsted (New Mexico State University).

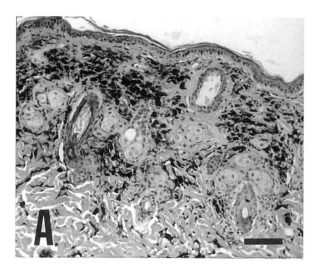

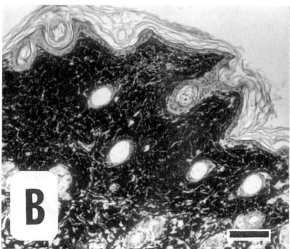

Figure 37. (A) Melanocytic hyperplasia. (B) Melanoma. These lesions in the skin of *Monodelphis domestica* were induced by chronic low-dose UV-B exposure. Melanocytic hyperplasia is a precursor of melanoma. H&E stain. Bar: 100 μm. Reproduced from Kusewitt *et al*. (1993), with permission.

human melanoma have been or are being developed, but none is entirely satisfactory.

Chronic UV exposure induces benign and malignant melanomas and the precursor lesion of melanocytic hyperplasia in *M. domestica* (Fig. 37). Genetically altered mice that develop a high incidence of melanoma have also been created; however, these mice tend to succumb very rapidly to metastatic disease, making them difficult to work with. Furthermore, in both mice and *Monodelphis*, melanomas arise in the dermis and show little or no junctional activity, unlike the situation in humans. Studies in the fish *Xiphophorus* have yielded some interesting and controversial results, suggesting that UV-A as well as UV-B may contribute to melanoma induction by sunlight. Melanomas associated with natural sunlight exposure in animals include perineal melanomas of gray horses and melanomas of the ears in Angora goats.

e. Ocular Neoplasia. In humans, squamous cell carcinoma of the conjunctiva is rare. It occurs with increased frequency in the tropics and in *xeroderma pigmentosum* patients, establishing a link with solar UV. Early papillary lesions are often found in association with chronic inflammation and stromal collagen degeneration. Squamous cell carcinoma of the eye is a serious economic problem in some breeds of cattle. The disease in cattle is clearly related to cumulative solar exposure, with pigmentation,

genetic background, and viral infection also playing a role in the disease. The neoplasms develop from plaques and papillomas to carcinoma *in situ* and, ultimately, invasive squamous cell carcinoma.

Squamous cell carcinoma of the conjunctiva has been associated with sunlight exposure in dogs. In mice exposed chronically to UV, ocular squamous cell carcinomas develop less frequently than corneal fibrosarcomas and hemangioendotheliomas. Precursor lesions include epithelial hyperplasia, neovascularization, and fibroplasia. Virtually all *M. domestica* exposed chronically to UV develop corneal fibroplasia and neovascularization that evolve into mesenchymal tumors of the cornea. It has also been observed that intraocular melanoma in humans has a higher incidence in those with blue eyes and in those living in the southern versus northern United States, suggesting a possible link to UV exposure.

IV. Hyperthermia

A. CLINICAL USE OF HYPERTHERMIA

Hyperthermia, alone or in combination with other treatment modalities such as ionizing radiation, has been used for cancer therapy. Use of hyperthermia depends on the increased heat sensitivity of malignant cells compared to normal cells. While normal tissue responds to moderate hyperthermia, 42–43°C, by increasing blood flow up to 10 times normal, many neoplasms, in the range of 41–42°C, show an initial increase in blood flow followed by a decrease or stasis within 1 to 2 hr. This difference in flow gives normal tissues a greater cooling capacity than tumor tissue. Therefore, the temperature tends to rise more in tumor than normal tissue, causing selective tumor necrosis. Tumor cell survival is further compromised by the hypoxic, acidic, and relatively nutrient-poor microenvironment of tumors. Hyperthermia enhances cell killing by ionizing radiation both additively and synergistically. The "thermal enhancement ratio" is the ratio of radiation dose producing a given effect to the reduced radiation dose required to produce the same effect in combination with heat.

B. MECHANISMS OF HYPERTHERMIA-INDUCED INJURY

Cell death in response to hyperthermia occurs 1 to 2 days after exposure. The fraction of cells surviving hyperthermia is not only a function of the absolute temperature, but also of the duration of hyperthermia. Based on *in vitro*, laboratory animal, and clinical studies, it appears that for each 1° rise in tissue temperature above 42°C, the time required for an equivalent effect is halved. Vascular changes play an important role in hyperthermia effects. In normal tissue, below 40°C, heating causes active hyperemia and vasodilation, with a resultant increase in tissue oxygen tension. However, at temperatures above 42°C, microcirculation to the heated tissue collapses and tissue oxygen tension decreases. At the same time, the cellular metabolic rate increases 10–15% for reach 1° increase in temperature. When the metabolic demands of the cells can no longer be met by the blood flow, heat injury begins. It is characterized microscopically by pyknosis, karyorrhexis, and coagulation of cytoplasm.

At the molecular level, heat alters weak molecular interactions, including hydrogen bonds, ionic interactions, and hydrophobic interactions, to induce conformational change in and destabilization of macromolecules. Membrane fluidity is increased due to changes in lipids, and denaturation of proteins alters the function of vital cellular components, including membrane and cytoskeletal proteins and essential enzymes. Hyperthermia increases K^+ efflux, increases Ca^{2+} and H^+ influx, uncouples oxidative phosphorylation, causes translational arrest, alters mitotic spindle function, inhibits DNA synthesis, and delays ligation of newly synthesized DNA. Because of its effects on the mitotic spindle, hyperthermia can cause polyploidy, chromosome aberrations, and death in S phase. Although dividing cells are particularly heat sensitive, hyperthermia-induced cell death does not require cell division. Heat radiosensitizes some tumors, presumably by enhancing nuclear protein binding, thus restricting DNA accessibility for repair enzymes and inhibiting the repair of radiation-induced DNA damage.

Studies *in vitro* and *in vivo* have shown that both neoplastic and normal cells and tissues develop resistance to repeated hyperthermic episodes. "Acute thermotolerance" is produced by a single prior sublethal heat exposure. It develops within several hours and decays over a few days. "Chronic thermotolerance"

589

develops after prolonged continuous heating. Induction of heat shock proteins is believed to be responsible for acute thermotolerance. These highly conserved acidic proteins ordinarily serve as molecular chaperones that supervise the folding of other cellular proteins. Under conditions of heat stress, they suppress irreversible protein unfolding, thus preventing protein aggregation. Chronic thermotolerance, however, can occur without increased cellular levels of heat shock proteins. "Acclimatization" is the response of an organism to multiple exposures to a warm environment over several days and is characterized by systemic adaptations (lower core temperature, reduced heart rate, decreased metabolic rate, and increased sweating) that increase heat dissipation.

C. RESPONSE TO INJURY INDUCED BY HYPERTHERMIA

The responses of normal tissues to hyperthermia are discussed. Hyperthermic damage to normal tissue occurs with heat stroke, high fever, lightning strike, and burns.

1. Reaction of Specific Organs and Tissue to Hyperthermia

a. Alimentary System. Investigations of hyperthermic damage to the mouse small intestine indicate that the mucosa is very thermosensitive. Nonproliferating villous enterocytes are more susceptible to thermal injury than crypt cells. After heating the intestine to 41.5°C for 1 hr, histologic examination 2 hr later revealed swollen villous enterocytes, loss of microvilli, extrusion of cells from the villous tips, a pleomorphic inflammatory infiltrate in the lamina propria, and collapse of the villous stroma. Stromal damage, especially edema and microvascular injury, may contribute to the epithelial injury.

In both animals and humans, liver enzyme values increase with temperatures above 42°C. Electron microscopic studies have shown increased numbers of autophagocytic vacuoles and dilation of both the Golgi apparatus and the endoplasmic reticulum following hyperthermic treatments in humans and rats. Liver damage is frequently a feature of heat stroke.

Elevations of alanine aminotransferase (ALT), (aspartate aminotransferase (AST), and lactic dehydrogenase (LDH) occur within 24 hr of heat stroke in humans and experimental models of heat stroke in dogs and rats. Histopathologic changes include dilation of central and portal veins, congestion of centrilobular sinusoids, degeneration or necrosis of centrilobular hepatocytes, and cholestasis. Ultrastructural studies show ballooning or flattening of hepatocellular microvilli, breaks in hepatocyte plasma membranes, vesiculation of the endoplasmic reticulum, detachment of ribosomes, and swelling of mitochondria.

b. Musculoskeletal System. The thermosensitivity of cartilage has been studied by measuring growth inhibition and necrosis of the tails of infant mice or rats. Heating the tails at 43°C for 1 hr induced stunting but not necrosis in about 10% of the animals, whereas heating at 44°C for 1 hr produced necrosis in more than 50% of the animals. Clamping the blood supply caused the infant rat tail to become much more thermosensitive, equivalent to a threefold increase in heating time or a temperature increase of 1.5°C.

The effects of 30 min at 40–48°C have been examined in pig muscle. One day after treatment, minimal myocyte necrosis was present in muscle heated to 43°C, whereas up to 30% of the muscle fibers were necrotic in muscle heated to 44–46°C. In areas of muscle heated above 46°C, edema, numerous inflammatory cells, hemorrhage, and coagulation necrosis of more than 30% of the muscle fibers were seen. One month after treatment, there was myofiber regeneration and focal fibrosis in muscle heated to 46–47°C. In tissue heated above 47°C, there was severe fibrosis and abscessation. Hyaline degeneration and necrosis of skeletal muscles have been observed in humans following heat stroke.

c. Nervous System. Localized heating of brain tissue in rats and cats using interstitial microwave antennae or ultrasound, respectively, has shown similar histologic results. Edema formation in both gray and white matter can occur in tissues held at 42°C for 50–70 min. Neuronal cell lysis occurs at temperatures greater than 43°C. Disruption of myelin tracts in the white matter is evident at brain temperatures of 43.0–43.5°C. Brain tissues in victims dying of heat stroke are grossly swollen. Histopathologic changes include degeneration and necrosis of neurons in the cerebral cortex, basal ganglia, and Purkinje cell layer.

d. Eye. The avascular lens dissipates heat poorly and can reach high temperatures. Microwave exposures can produce cataracts in rabbits, but the same exposures produce facial burns but no cataracts in monkeys.

e. Cardiovascular System. Whole body hyperthermia at 41°C for 20 min can cause cardiac damage in rats. Lesions reported include edema, vacuolization, hyperemia, subepicardial and subendocardial cell necrosis, inflammation, and interstitial fibrosis. There have been several reports of disseminated intravascular coagulopathy during whole body hyperthermia. It is not known if the consumption of coagulation factors occurs directly due to heating of the blood or in response to substances released from heat-damaged tumor or normal tissue. Hemorrhage due to fibrinolysis, hypofibrinogenemia, and thrombocytopenia secondary to intravascular clotting is also seen frequently in human or experimental animals dying of heat stroke. Focal necrosis of myocardial fibers is seen in heat stroke.

f. Urinary System. Mouse kidney exposed to local hyperthermia in the range of 41–45°C for 35 min has foci of subcapsular tubular necrosis with a neutrophilic response and minimal calcification 1 week after exposure. After 4 weeks, the zone of necrosis and calcium deposits remains, but the neutrophils are absent. The kidneys are quite resistant to damage during systemic hyperthermia treatment when electrolyte balance and fluid balance are maintained. This resistance to damage is probably due to high renal blood flow. Patients suffering from heat stroke as a result of physical exertion and insufficient fluid intake may exhibit anuria or oliguria and elevated blood urea nitrogen. Proteinuria, renal casts, and tubular degeneration are sometimes seen.

g. Genital System. One of the more sensitive organs to mild hyperthermia is the testis. In most mammals, even the thermal environment of the abdominal cavity will inhibit normal testicular development. Heating rat testes to 43°C for 15 min results in damage to transitional and late pachytene stages; spermatogonia are more heat resistant. As heating is extended to 30 min, damage involves all spermatocyte and early spermatid stages. Sertoli cells undergo vacuolar degeneration secondary to germinal epithelial damage. Leydig cells are not affected by this hyperthermic treatment. After about 3 weeks, rat testes will recover from this mild damage. In rabbits, the minimal scrotal temperature at which testicular damage occurs is 40°C. At that temperature, more than 100 hr of treatment are required for seminiferous tubule degeneration to occur.

h. Integumentary System. Local application of heat can result in cutaneous burns. A temperature of 70°C or higher for several seconds in humans causes complete transepidermal necrosis, although a temperature of 50°C for periods of 10 min may not cause serious damage. Cutaneous burns are divided into three categories: the first-degree burn, in which damage is limited to the outer layer of epidermis without significant dermal damage, other than erythema and mild edema; the second-degree burn, in which the epidermis is necrotic with vesicle and bulla formation, but with dermal sparing; and the third-degree burn, in which both the dermis and the epidermis are damaged and the skin surface is charred or coagulated.

Early microscopic evidence of mild thermal injury is nuclear and cytoplasmic swelling. More severe injury, as with second-degree burn, results in the rupture of nuclear membranes, pyknosis, and granular or homogeneously coagulated keratinocyte cytoplasm. In mild injury, dermal capillaries are dilated and there is interstitial edema. In severe injury, there may be coagulation of blood vessels and little evidence of exudation, except at the margins of the burn. The dermal collagen loses its fibrillar structure and becomes a homogeneous gel.

591

In pigs, subcutaneous fat heated to 40–48°C for 30 min develops a neutrophilic inflammatory infiltrate by 24 hr after treatment. In subcutaneous tissues heated to 45°C, the inflammation resolves without residual injury. One month after treatment, subcutaneous tissues heated to 46–47°C contain giant cells and prominent fibroplasia. In sites heated above 47°C, chronic panniculitis is accompanied by foci of necrosis and abscesses.

SUGGESTED READING

Ionizing Radiation

General

Committee on the Biological Effects of Ionizing Radiation (BEIR V) (1990). "Health Effects of Exposure to Low Levels of Ionizing Radiation." National Academy Press, Washington, DC.
Committee on the Biological Effects of Ionizing Radiation (BEIR IV) (1988). "Health Risks of Radon and Other Internally Deposited Alpha-Emitters." National Academy Press, Washington, DC.
Conklin, J. J., and Walker, R. I. (eds.) (1987). "Military Radiobiology." Academic Press, Orlando, FL.
Fajardo, L. F. (1982). "Pathology of Radiation Injury." Masson Publishing, New York.
Gossner, W., Gerber, G. B., Hagen, U., and Luz, A. (eds.) (1986). "The Radiobiology of Radium and Thorotrast." Urband and Schwarzenberg, München.
Hendry, J. H., Potten, C. S., Moore, C. V., and Hume, W. J. (eds.) (1986). Assays of normal tissue injury and their cellular interpretation: Proceedings of the 12th L. H. Gray conference. *Br. J. Cancer* **53**, Suppl. VII.

Nature and Action of Ionizing Radiation

Harley, N. H. (1996) Toxic effects of radiation and radioactive materials. *In* "Casarett and Doull's Toxicology: The Basic Science of Poisons" (C. D. Klaasen, ed.), pp. 773–800. McGraw-Hill, New York.

Mechanisms of Ionizing Radiation Injury

Altman, K. I., and Gerber, G. B. (1983). The effect of ionizing radiations on connective tissues. *Adv. Radiat. Biol.* **10**, 237–304.
Hall, E. J. (2000). "Radiobiology for the Radiobiologist," 5th Ed. Lippincott, Philadelphia.

Harms-Ringdahl, M., Nicotera, P., and Radford, I. R. (1996). *Mutat. Res.* **366**, 171–179.
Lee, L. M., Abrahamson, J. L. A., Kandel, R., Donehower, L. A., and Bernstein, A. (1994). Susceptibility to radiation-carcinogenesis and accumulation of chromosomal breakage in p53 deficient mice. *Oncogene* **9**, 3731–3736.
Little, J. B. (1993). Cellular, molecular, and carcinogenic effects of radiation. *Hematol. Oncol. Clin. North Am.* **7**, 337–352.
Nygaard, O. F., Sinclair, W. K., and Lett, J. T. (1992). "Effects of Low Dose and Low Dose Rate Radiation." Advances in Radiation Biology, Vol. 16. Academic Press, San Diego.
Ullrich, R. I. (1998). Radiation-induced instability and its relation to radiation carcinogenesis. *Int. J. Radiat. Biol.* **74**, 747–754.
Wright, E. G. (1998). Radiation-induced genomic instability in haemopoietic cells. *Int. J. Radiat. Biol.* **74**, 681–687.

Response to Injury Induced by Ionizing Radiation

Belinsky, S. A., Middleton, S. K., Picksley, S. M., Hahn, F. F., and K. J., Nikula. (1996). Analysis of the K-ras and p53 pathways in X-ray induced lung tumors in the rat. *Radiat. Res.* **145**, 449–456.
Benjamin, S. A., Boecker, B. B., Cuddihy, R. G., and McClellan, R. O. (1979). Nasal carcinomas in beagles after inhalation of relatively soluble forms of beta-emitting radionuclides. *J. Natl. Cancer Inst.* **63**, 133–139.
Benjamin, S. A., Lee, A. C., Angleton, G. M., Saunders, W. J., Miller, G. K., Williams, J. S., Brewster, R. D., and Long, R. I. (1986). Neoplasms in young dogs after perinatal irradiation. *J. Natl. Cancer Inst.* **77**, 563–571.
Benjamin, S. A., Lee, A. C., Angleton, G. M., Saunders, W. J., Mallinckrodt, C. H., and Keefe, T. J. (1998). Mortality in beagles irradiated during prenatal and postnatal development. I. Contribution of non-neoplastic diseases. *Radiat. Res.* **150**, 316–329.
Benjamin, S. A., Lee, A. C., Angleton, G. M., Saunders, W. J., Mallinckrodt, C. H., and Keefe, T. J. (1998). Mortality in beagles irradiated during prenatal and postnatal development. II. Contribution of benign and malignant neoplasia, *Radiat. Res.* **150**, 330–348.
Benjamin, S. A., Saunders, W. J., Lee, A. C., Angleton G. M., Stephens, L. C., and Mallinckrodt, C. H. (1997). Non-neoplastic and neoplastic thyroid disease in beagles irradiated during prenatal and postnatal development, *Radiat. Res.* **147**, 422–430.
Bouffler, S. D., Meijne, E. I. M., Morris, D. J., and Papworth, D. (1997). Chromosome 2 hypersensitivity and clonal development in murine radiation acute myeloid leukemia. *Int. J. Radiat. Biol.* **72**, 181–189.

Casarett, G. W. (1980). "Radiation Histopathology," Vols. I and II. CRC Press, Boca Raton, FL.

Ching, S. V., McChesney, S. L., Powers, B. E., Roberts, S. M., Gillette, E. L., and Withrow, S. J. (1990). Radiation induced ocular injury in the dog: A histological study. *Int. J. Radiat. Oncol. Biol. Phys.* **19**, 321–328.

Coggle, J. E., Lambert, B. E., and Moores, S. R. (1986). Radiation effects in the lung. *Environ. Health Perspect.* **70**, 261–291.

Committee on Thyroid Screening Related to I-131 Exposure and Committee on Exposure of the American People to I-131 from the Nevada Atomic Bomb Tests (1999). "Exposure of the American People to Iodine-131 from Nevada Nuclear Bomb Tests: Review of the National Cancer Institute Report and Public Health Implications." National Academy Press, Washington, DC.

DeGroot, L. J. (1988). Radiation and thyroid disease. *Baillieres Clin. Endocrinol. Metab.* **2**, 777–791.

Gillette, E. L., Powers, B. E., McChesney, S. L., Park, R. D., and Withrow, S. J. (1989). Response of aorta and branch arteries to experimental intraoperative irradiation. *Int. J. Radiat. Oncol. Biol. Phys.* **17**, 583–590.

Greenberger, J. S. (1991). Toxic effects on the hematopoietic microenvironment. *Exp. Hematol.* **19**, 1101–1109.

Hahn, F. F., and Lundgren, D. L. (1992). Pulmonary neoplasms in rats that inhaled Cerium-144 dioxide. *Toxicol. Pathol.* **20**, 169–178.

Hahn, F. F., Muggenburg, B. A., and Boecker, B. B. (1996). Hepatic neoplasms from internally deposited $^{144}CeCl_3$. *Toxicol. Pathol.* **24**, 281–289.

Herbert, R. A., Stegelmeier, B. L., Gillett, N. A., Rebar, A. H., Carlton, W. W., Singh, G., and Hahn, F. F. (1994). Plutonium-induced proliferative lesions and pulmonary epithelial neoplasms in the rat: Immunohistochemical and ultrastructural evidence for their origin from type II pneumocytes. *Vet. Pathol.* **31**, 366–374.

Hoopes, P. J., Gillette, E. L., and Benjamin, S. A. (1985). The pathogenesis of radiation nephropathy in the dog. *Radiat. Res.* **104**, 406–419.

Law, M. P. (1985). Vascular permeability and late radiation fibrosis in mouse lung. *Radiat. Res.* **103**, 60–76.

Lett, J. T., and Altman, K. I. (eds.) (1987). "Relative Radiation Sensitivities of Human Organ Systems." Advances in Radiation Biology, Vol. 12. Academic Press, Orlando, FL.

Lett, J. T., and Altman, K. I. (eds.) (1990). "Relative Radiation Sensitivities of Human Organ Systems, Part II." Advances in Radiation Biology, Vol. 14. Academic Press, San Diego.

Lett, J. T., and Altman, K. I. (eds.) (1987). "Relative Radiation Sensitivities of Human Organ Systems, Part III." Advances in Radiation Biology, Vol. 12. Academic Press, San Diego.

Maxon, H. R. (1985). Radiation-induced thyroid disease. *Med. Clin. North Am.* **69**, 1049–1061.

Maxon, H. R., and Saenger, E. L. (1996). Biological effects of radioiodines on the human thyroid gland. In "Werner and Ingbar's, The Thyroid: A Fundamental and Clinical Text" (L. E., and Braverman and R. D. Utiger, eds.), 7th Ed., pp. 342–351. Lippincott-Raven, Philadelphia.

McChesney, S. L., Gillette, E. L., and Powers, B. E. (1988). Radiation-induced cardiomyopathy in the dog. *Radiat. Res.* **113**, 120–132.

Morgan, W. F., Day, J. P., Kaplan, M. I., McGhee, E. M., and Limoli, C. L. (1996). Genomic instability induced by ionizing radiation. *Radiat. Res.* **146**, 247–258.

Muggenburg, B. A., Guilmette, R. A., Mewhinney, J. A., Gillett, N. A., Mauderly, J. L., Griffith, W. C., Diel, J. H., Scott, B. R., Hahn, F. F., and Boecker, B. B. (1996). Toxicity of inhaled $^{238}PuO_2$ in beagle dogs. *Radiat. Res.* **145**, 361–381.

National Cancer Institute (1997). "Estimated Exposures and Thyroid Doses Received by the American People from Iodine-131 in Fallout Following Nevada Atmospheric Nuclear Bomb Tests." U. S. Department of Health and Human Services, National Institutes of Health, Bethesda, MD.

National Council on Radiation Protection and Measurements (NCRP) (1985). Induction of thyroid cancer by ionizing radiation. NCRP Report No. 80, Bethesda, MD.

Northdurft, W. (1991). Bone marrow. In "Medical Radiology: Radiopathology of Organs and Tissues" (E. Scherer, Ch. Streffer, and K.-R. Trott, eds.), pp. 113–169. Springer-Verlag, Berlin.

Powers, B. E., Beck, E. R., Gillette, E. L., Gould, D. H., and LeCouter, R. A. (1992). Pathology of radiation injury to the canine spinal cord. *Int. J. Radiat. Oncol. Biol. Phys.* **23**, 539–549.

Schweitzer, D. J., Benjamin, S. A., and Lee, A. C. (1987). Retinal dysplasia and progressive atrophy in dogs irradiated during ocular development. *Radiat. Res.* **111**, 340–353.

Seed, T. M. (1987). Structure-function relationships in radiation-induced cell and tissue lesions: Special references to the contribution of scanning electron microscopy and hematopoietic tissue responses. *Scanning Electron Micros.* **1**, 255–272.

Special Issue (1988). Workshop on low dose radiation and the immune system. *Int. J. Radiat. Biol.* **53**.

Taylor, G. N., Lloyd, R. D., Mays, C. W., Angus, W., Miller, S. C., Shabestari, L., and Hahn. F. F. (1991). Plutonium- or americium-induced liver tumors and lesions in beagle dogs. *Health Phys.* **61**, 337–347.

Thompson, R. C. (1989). "Life Span Effects of Ionizing Radiation in the Beagle Dog." Pacific Northwest Laboratory, Battelle Memorial Institute, Richland, WA.

Thompson, R. C., and Mahaffey, J. A. (eds.) (1986). "Life Span Radiation Effects Studies in Animals: What Can They Tell Us?" U.S. Department of Energy, Washington, DC.

White, D. C. (1975). "An Atlas of Radiation Histopathology." National Technical Information Service, Springfield, VA.

Williams, E. D. (1991). Biologic effects of radiation on the thyroid. *In* "Werner and Ingbar's, The Thyroid" (L. E. Braverman and R. D. Utiger, eds.), pp. 421–436. Lippincott, Philadelphia.

Ultraviolet Radiation

General

Kohen, E., Santus, R., and Hirschberg, J. G. (1995). "Photobiology." Academic Press, San Diego.

Young, A. R., Björn, L. O., Moan, J., and Nultsch, W. (eds.) (1993). "Environmental uv Photobiology." Plenum Press, New York.

Mechanisms of Injury

Brash, D. E. (1997). Sunlight and the onset of skin Cancer. *Trends Genet.* **13**, 410–414.

De Gruijl, F. R., Sterenborg, H. J. C. M., Forbes, P. D., Davies, R. E., Cole, C., Kelfkens, G., ven Weelden, H., Slaper, H., and van der Leun, J. C. (1993). Wavelength dependence of skin cancer induction by ultraviolet irradiation of albino hairless mice. *Cancer Res.* **53**, 53–60.

Friedberg, E. C., Walker, G. C., and Siede, W. (1995). "DNA Repair and Mutagenesis." American Society for Microbiology Press, Washington, DC.

Herrlich, P., Sachsenmaier, C., Radler-Pohl, A., Gebel, S., Blattner, C., and Rahmsdorf, H. J. (1994). The mammalian UV response: Mechanism of DNA damage induced gene expression. *Adv. Enzyme Regul.* **34**, 381–395.

Invited Review (1996). Photocarcinogenesis: Mechanisms, models, and human health implications. *Photochem. Photobiol.* **63**, 355–447.

Tyrrell, R. M. (1996). Activation of mammalian gene expression by the UV component of sunlight: From models to reality. *BioEssays* **18**, 139–148.

Response to Injury

Altmeyer, P., Hoffman, K., and Stücker, M. (eds.) (1997). "Skin Cancer and UV Radiation." Springer-Verlag, Berlin.

Bissett, D. L., Hannon, D. P., and Orr, T. V. (1989). Wavelength dependence of histological, physical, and visible changes in chronically UV-irradiated hairless mouse skin. *Photochem. Photobiol.* **50**, 763–769.

Harber, L. C., and Bickers, D. R. (1981). "Photosensitivity Diseases: Principles of Diagnosis and Treatment." Saunders, Philadelphia.

Kligman, L. H., Akin, F. J., and Kligman, A. M. (1985). The contributions of UVA and UVB to connective tissue damage in hairless mice. *J. Invest. Dermatol.* **84**, 272–276.

Kligman, L. H., and Kligman, A. M. (1981). Histogenesis and progression of ultraviolet light-induced tumors in hairless mice. *J. Natl. Cancer Inst.* **67**, 1289–1297.

Krutmann, J., and Elmets, C. A. (eds.) (1995). "Photoimmunology." Blackwell Science, Oxford.

Yaar, M., and Gilchrest, B. A. (1998). Aging versus photoaging: Postulated mechanisms and effectors. *J. Invest. Dermatol. Symp. Proc.* **3**, 47–51.

Hyperthermia

General

Hahn, G. M. (1982). "Hyperthermia and Cancer." Plenum Press, New York.

Hornback, N. B. (1984). "Hyperthermia and Cancer: Human Clinical Trial Experience." CRC Press, Boca Raton, FL.

Myerson, R. J., and Emami, B. (1993). Normal tissue effects of hyperthermia in conjunction with radiotherapy. *Adv. Radiat. Biol.* **15**, 195–215.

Overgaard, J. (ed.) (1985). "Hyperthermic Oncology," Vols. I and II. Taylor and Francis, London.

Response to Injury Induced by Hyperthermia

Buchner, J. (1996). Supervising the fold: Functional principles of molecular chaperones. *FASEB J.* **10**, 10–19.

Moseley, P. L. (1994). Mechanisms of heat adaptation: Thermotolerance and acclimatization. *J. Lab. Clin. Med.* **123**, 48–52.

Song, C. W. (1984). Effect of local hyperthermia on blood flow and microenvironment: A review. *Cancer Res.* **44** (Suppl. 10), 4721s–4730s.

Storm, F. K. (ed.) (1983). "Hyperthermia in Cancer Therapy." Hall Medical Publishers, Boston.

Streffer, C. (1985). Metabolic changes during and after hyperthermia. *Int. J. Hypertherm.* **1**, 305–319.

23

Nutritional Toxicologic Pathology

Elizabeth H. Jeffery
*Department of Food Science and
Human Nutrition
University of Illinois at
Urbana-Champaign
Urbana, Illinois*

Matthew A. Wallig
*Department of Veterinary
Pathobiology
University of Illinois at
Urbana-Champaign
Urbana, Illinois*

M. E. Tumbleson
*Department of Veterinary
Biosciences
University of Illinois at
Urbana-Champaign
Urbana, Illinois*

I. Introduction

Dietary components traditionally are divided into macronutrients and micronutrients, shown in Table I. Macronutrients, which make up the bulk of the diet and provide energy, include lipids, carbohydrates, and protein. Fiber, while originally identified as that which is indigestible, is now known to be digested partly by colonic microflora, resulting in short chain fatty acids that can provide an important energy source in the colon. Micronutrients include both vitamins and minerals, the latter being divided into major minerals, such as calcium (Ca) and potassium (K), and trace elements, such as copper (Cu). The list of elements still fluctuates as new evidence emerges, supporting or opposing their essentiality. The element fluorine (F) is a good example of this. Although F does not appear essential for full growth, the American Dental Association supports a role for F in maintaining dental health. In contrast, a study from the National Toxicology Program suggests that even less than 1 ppm F, the dose provided in many municipal water supplies, has an adverse

effect on bone health in a segment of the population.

Nutrients not only play an essential role in optimal growth of the organism, but reverse the biochemical and pathological lesions of deficiency diseases, the characteristic nature of which can be used to diagnose specific nutritional imbalances. The dose required for optimal growth can be used to calculate the recommended dietary allowance (RDA). The Food and Nutrition Board of the National Research Council of the National Academy of Sciences has set RDAs for 15 different age and gender groups, including pregnant and lactating women. While the end point for production of "optimal growth" appears quite clear cut, determining the dose needed to overcome a deficiency disease becomes a matter of interpretation. For example, if the RDA of a nutrient is to be based on an end point with a sliding scale such as plasma cholesterol, it is necessary to define the "normal" cholesterol level. Clearly a decision as to which end points to include, and what values to place upon them, becomes confounded by the defined parameters of a normal healthy body.

The Food and Nutrition Board does not extend its area of concern to the potentially adverse effects of doses of nutrients that greatly

*Handbook of Toxicologic Pathology, Second Edition
Volume 1*

595

TABLE I
Summary of Vitamin Toxicities

Vitamin	Toxic dose[a]	Biochemical basis of toxicity[b]	Clinical manifestations[c]
A	$2–5 \times 10^6$ IU/day (acute)	Redifferentiation of epithelium into more complex forms (general mucoid)	Hyperirritability, dizziness, vomiting, diarrhea, erythema (acute)
	$1–2 \times 10^5$ IU/day (chronic)	Periosteal proliferation of bone, loss of cortical bone	Dermatitis, pruritis, double vision, headache, osteoporosis, exostoses (chronic)
D	$> 5 \times 10^5$ IU/day	Excessive uptake of calcium and phosphorus from the GI tract and reabsorption of calcium from bone and renal ultrafiltrate	Widespread deposition of hydroxyapatite in tissues, especially the kidney, leading to renal failure and pulmonary calcinosis
		Depression of tissue vitamin K concentrations	Bleeding tendencies
E	300–3000 IU/day	Depression of thromboxane production, ↓ generation of prostaglandins and leukotrienes	Impaired wound healing
K	5–25 μg/day	↑ generation of free radicals via redox recycling	Hemolysis
		Osmotic malabsorption in GI tract	Diarrhea, nausea, cramps
C	>1 g/day	↑ conversion to oxalic acid and ↑ excretion in urine (selected individuals)	Oxalate urolithiasis
Thiamine	>900 mg/day	Neuromuscular dysfunction	Headache, convulsions, paralysis, cardiac arrhythmias
Riboflavin	Not defined	Not defined	Not defined
		Vasodilation	Pruritis, headache
Niacin	>100 mg/day (oral) >25 mg/day (iv)	Abnormal liver function (cholestasis)	GI disturbances (duodenal ulcer), cholestatic liver disease
Pyridoxine	$>2–6$ g/day (over prolonged period)	Demyelination of peripheral sensory nerves, sensory nerve tracts in CNS	Progressive ataxia, loss of sensation in digits, tongue, and lips
Biotin	Not determined	Impaired estrogen and progesterone synthesis	Impaired reproductive performance in females
		Hypersensitivity reactions	Allergic reactions
Folic acid	>15 mg/day	Nephrotoxicity (tubular)	Renal failure
		Neurotoxicity	Malaise, irritability, depression, sleep disturbances
Cobalamin	Not determined	Not defined	Not defined

[a]Doses based on human data, not yet established for most animals.
[b]Based on both human and animal data.
[c]Mainly based on human data.

exceed the RDA. However, the availability of vitamin and mineral supplements on the market today permits ready opportunity for excess intake, and resulting overdose. Some nutrients have specific biological effects at doses in excess of the RDA, and most have nonspecific toxic effects if the dose is sufficiently large. A good example of a nutrient with a specific, pharmacologically useful effect at a higher dose is niacin, used to depress elevated plasma cholesterol levels. This effect is unrelated to the effect of niacin as a vitamin and requires gram quantities rather than the milligram quantities needed for vitamin action. Even at the optimal pharmacological dose of niacin one starts to see toxicity. Toxicity includes flushing and pruritis in response to unregulated prostaglandin production, which can be allayed by the use of aspirin prior to ingestion of these massive doses of niacin. If the dose is raised still further, frank toxicity ensues. For many minerals, ingestion of a great excess competitively inhibits the uptake of other minerals, precipitating a secondary nutritional deficiency. For example, molybdenum (Mo) excess produces Cu deficiency, and manganese (Mn) excess produces iron (Fe) deficiency anemia. In chronic Zinc (Zn) overdose, first Cu deficiency is seen, and if the excessive intake persists, Fe deficiency develops, both deficiencies due to the competitive inhibition of intestinal uptake by Zn.

The concept of nutrient overdose, so apparent to the pharmacologist and toxicologist, rarely has been addressed through nutritional research or food regulatory channels. For food additives such as the antioxidants butylated hydroxytoluene (BHT) and butylated hydroxyanisole (BHA), the concern for potential toxicity is recognized and regulated carefully. A few dietary components that are nutrients at low dose are recognized as particularly toxic or even carcinogenic at higher doses. For noncarcinogenic compounds, results of dose–response studies are used to calculate a no observable adverse effect level (NOAEL) or lowest observable adverse effect level (LOAEL). Determination of safe and appropriate dietary levels (acceptable daily intake, ADI) is carried out by dividing the experimental value by 100. This calculation is based on the belief that there is a threshold below which no toxicity occurs and takes into account possible variation in sensitivity among humans and the species tested, as well as among different genders and/or ages. An example of a nutrient that has been found to be toxic at higher doses is sodium (Na). The LOAEL leading to hypertension is considered to be 60 g/day. The ADI, if set two orders of magnitude below this, would be 0.6 g/day. However, many apparently healthy individuals take in 10 g/day or more, suggesting that the "1/100" safety margin used to calculate the ADI is larger than necessary.

This exaggerated safety calculation may go far in explaining the dichotomy that has risen for a number of trace elements, where the calculated ADI is of similar magnitude to the RDA.

Selenium is an extreme example of this dichotomy, where inclusion in the diet (at no less than 0.04 ppm) is recommended to avoid deficiency diseases, even though higher doses have proven carcinogenic. The RDA for selenium (Se) is 55 μg/day for women and 70 μg/day for men; however, the Environmental Protection Agency (EPA) has set the maximum contaminant level in drinking water at 10 μg/liter, even though the average daily consumption of water is only 2 liters! Thus the safety limit sits below the RDA. For nonnutrient carcinogens, the Delaney clause of 1954 required that no amount of a carcinogen is acceptable as a food additive, based on the assumption that there is no threshold for carcinogens. As the sensitivity of our methods for measurement of contaminants, such as pesticides, has increased, the Delaney clause has become more and more difficult to uphold. Today a tolerable increment in the risk for cancer has been set at that dose causing an increase in cancer risk of 10^{-6} per lifetime. Keeping these issues in mind, this chapter provides a brief overview of some biochemical and pathological lesions of nutrient deficiencies and excesses.

II. Macronutrients

A. PROTEINS

1. Deficiency

Protein deficiency usually is combined with carbohydrate/fat (i.e., energy) deficiency. When energy (i.e., carbohydrate) is the predominant limiting factor, the condition is termed marasmus in humans. When protein is the predominant limiting dietary factor, kwashiorkor is the resulting disease syndrome, a condition with more ominous consequences, as visceral as well as somatic protein reserves are depleted. This leads not only to wasting of muscle but also to atrophy of internal organs. Plasma protein concentrations decrease in kwashiorkor, leading to generalized edema in addition to generalized wasting, serous atrophy of visceral and peripheral fat stores, anemia, abnormal bone growth, endocrine atrophy, and skin lesions. In domestic and laboratory animals, generalized edema may not be evident, but serous atrophy of fat, visceral organ atrophy, anemia, poor hair coat, and predisposition to infectious disease are prominent features of protein and/or protein/ carbohydrate malnutrition. Changes attributable to protein malnutrition can be subtle and difficult to assess in a qualitative fashion histologically. Changes such as atrophy of fat can be discerned as an increase in myxomatous tissue with a high ground substance in places where fat normally would be found, but other changes, such as atrophy of cells within organs, can be more difficult and sometimes impossible without ancillary techniques such as organ-to-body weight ratios and morphometry.

However, there is another side of the coin with regard to moderate protein restriction that apparently is connected to the incidence of chronic diseases such as cancer and longevity. In relation to cancer, there are many definitive studies where scientists have utilized protein underfeeding and food restriction to reduce incidence and/or susceptibility to cancer. Suboptimal protein intakes generally have inhibited spontaneous and chemically induced tumor growth as well as the growth of transplantable tumors. However, increasing protein intake increases carcinogen-metabolizing capacity and hence may be protective in a different way. The evidence for protein restriction as a major means of preventing cancer, although compelling, is far from unequivocal, and the complicated interactions among protein, carbohydrate, and fat intake leading to promotion or prevention of cancer have yet to be discerned.

a. Excess. Protein excess seldom is of pathological relevance in most species except in the context of individual amino acids, as in most cases, excessive protein is degraded, individual amino acids are deaminated, and the carbon backbones enter the Krebs cycle or gluconeogenic pathways. Dietary management of patients with chronic renal failure continues to be challenging; excessive protein intake appears not only to increase the renal lesion rate of development of uremia but also to be deleterious to growth and nutritional status. One exception to this general rule that excess dietary

protein is not harmful to an animal with adequate renal function is in male rats, where dietary protein in excess of maintenance after maturity is the key component in the disease chronic progressive nephropathy, an almost universal problem in the typical rat colony (Chapter 33). The basic pathophysiologic change caused by excessive dietary protein is an enhancement of glomerular filtration rate, increased glomerular intracapillary pressure, and the subsequent leakage of proteins into the mesangium, where they accumulate in deposits that eventually compromise overall glomerular function, leading to tubular dysfunction and loss and finally to renal failure. Therefore, there is a growing consensus that protein should be limited to just that required for maintenance in adult rat diets.

2. Amino Acids

a. Deficiency. Deficiencies of specific amino acids are rare, although many diets can be relatively deficient in certain groups of amino acids. For example, many corn-based diets are limited in lysine and tryptophan content, whereas peanut and soy-based diets are often low in methionine content. General signs of amino acid deficiency are similar to those of kwashiorkor.

Arginine is one amino acid in which a deficiency can result in disease, particularly in the canine, which as an adult seems to have a requirement for this amino acid, normally not essential in adults of other mammalian species. The major manifestation is hyperammonemia, probably due to an inability to deaminate amino acids in the urea cycle. This ultimately leads to neurologic dysfunction and death.

Taurine, 2-aminoethanesulfonic acid, derived from cysteine, is a free intracellular amino acid that generally is synthesized in sufficient quantities in all species except the cat, which must obtain additional taurine from the diet. This additional requirement may be due to the fact that the cat must rely exclusively on taurine for the conjugation of bile acids and will deplete its taurine stores to perform that function at the expense of other pathways. The principal lesion that develops initially in cats with taurine deficiency is progressive central retinal degeneration, characterized by degeneration of the photoreceptor portions of first cones and then rods. Eventually the entire retina is involved. The mechanism of the degeneration is unknown but maintenance of photoreceptor membrane appears to be involved. Dilative cardiomyopathy has also been linked to subclinical taurine deficiency in cats, although the mechanism is unclear. Taurine deficiency disease has not been reported in other species.

b. Excess. Growth rate and food intake are depressed in rats fed a low protein diet to which a large excess of one indispensable amino acid has been added. The addition of excessive amounts of individual amino acids at concentrations that are disproportionate to appropriate ratios in which they are required for normal growth causes a depression in food intake and growth in addition to any toxicity specific to the particular amino acid in question. Food intake depression occurs soon after animals are fed the imbalanced diet. Dopamine metabolites may be involved in this adverse feeding response. These apparently are altered in amino acid imbalanced diets. Inclusion of excess methionine or tryptophan in rat diets produces a severe depression of food intake and growth. Feeding excess amounts of methionine or N-acetyl-L-methionine also results in retarded growth rates in rats. When administered to adult rats either parenterally or per os, tyrosine, causes a depletion of essential amino acids in the cerebral cortex.

Although essential for cats and important in many metabolic pathways (e.g., bile acid conjugation), taurine, produces oxidants and toxic substances in many tissues, including brain, retina, myocardium, skeletal muscle, liver, platelets, and leukocytes. However, excessive taurine intake is rare and unlikely to be encountered in nonexperimental conditions unless large quantities of taurine-rich animal protein are consumed.

An excess of dietary leucine retards rat growth rates. Dietary excess of leucine may be a precipitating factor in pellagra (niacin deficiency) when tryptophan is limiting and unable to meet a part or all of the requirements for the synthesis of nicotinamide nucleotides. When the intake of nicotinic acid is only marginally adequate so that there is considerable reliance on the synthesis of nicotinamide nucleotides from tryptophan, even a modest excess of leucine in the diet may precipitate pellagra. Also, rat diets containing high levels of threonine and tyrosine increase dietary tryptophan requirements.

Phenylalanine is an amino acid with high toxic potential (i.e., impairment of sulfatide formation in rat brains). However, the likely mechanism of phenylalanine toxicity involves inhibition of entry into the brain of large neutral amino acids. Phenylalanine toxicity is not a concern for most species except for humans, in which phenylketonuria, an inborn error of metabolism resulting from a lack of phenylalanine hydroxylase, has a relatively high incidence in certain Caucasian populations. Because only about one-half of phenylalanine in children is utilized for protein synthesis, any inborn error in the alternative pathways of metabolism (usually the tyrosine pathway) can result in hyperphenylalaninemia and accumulation of toxic intermediates. Mental retardation that results from phenylalanine excess may be due to a combination of impaired lipid synthesis and altered neurotransmitter synthesis.

Lysine is a major constituent of hyperalimentation solutions and is known to inhibit tubular reabsorption of protein. Both lysine and aminoglycoside antibiotics are nephrotoxic, and, when the two are combined, toxicity is additive. Lysine competes with aminoglycosides for a common receptor site on the proximal tubular brush border. Lysine is known to inhibit proximal tubular reabsorption of protein, an effect that promotes the formation of obstructive tubular casts. Also, excessive lysine is toxic to pancreatic acinar cells in the rat, with mitochondrial accumulation of calcium identified as an early abnormality, resulting in the release of cytochrome c from the electron transport chain and activation of the mitochondrial permeability transition. Subsequently, focal areas of oncotic necrosis develop, leading to pancreatitis.

In similar fashion to lysine, excessive doses of dietary arginine to rats induce acute necrotizing pancreatitis. Large doses of arginine depress polyamine biosynthesis and thus inhibit the synthesis of nucleic acid and protein. Excess arginine selectively destroys acinar cells while leaving other pancreatic cell types intact. As might be expected, rats fed an excess of arginine have reduced growth rates.

B. CARBOHYDRATES

1. Deficiency

The generalized deficiency of carbohydrates is of little consequence in most species, provided adequate lipids, proteins, vitamins, minerals, and micronutrients are present in the diet. Many carnivores do not even require a carbohydrate source in the diet. Absolute or relative carbohydrate deficiency in ruminants, usually associated with starvation or inanition, can lead to ketosis and fatty liver. This is particularly true during late pregnancy or lactation, when demand for glucose to nourish the rapidly developing late-term fetus (or fetuses) and to synthesize lactose for milk production is high. This results in excessive mobilization of fat and the formation of ketone bodies to meet the demands of other tissues in the body for energy. The deficiency of readily available glucose due to the peculiarities of ruminant carbohydrate metabolism sets in motion a complicated series of events that ultimately leads to severe fatty liver, even to the point of hepatic dysfunction and death.

Fatty liver in cats probably has a somewhat similar pathogenesis but this is not yet fully understood, although a relative carbohydrate deficiency that results when an obese cat abruptly stops eating probably has a role in triggering the excessive mobilization of peripheral fat stores that overwhelms the capacity of the liver to process the fat, leading to its storage.

Fatty liver in diabetes mellitus has a similar pathogenesis to fatty liver in ruminants, only in this case the glucose deficiency is due to the inability of peripheral tissues to take up glucose, leading to the mobilization of peripheral fat stores and dependence on the liver to process vast amounts of fat for the production of ketone bodies.

Severe caloric deficiency, whether due to insufficient carbohydrates or to combined carbohydrate–protein deficiency, leads to fairly typical changes across nonprimate species. These include wastage (atrophy) of musculature and serous atrophy of fat in the diaphyseal bone marrow and perirenal and renal pelvic fat depots in the coronary grooves of the heart and the abdominal mesentery. Thymic atrophy is a frequent finding in neonatal animals as well. In very small animals, serous atrophy may not be readily apparent but will instead manifest itself merely as a complete absence of visceral fat, including the epididymal fat pads in male rodents. Many animals, especially the young, are prone to viral and bacterial infections and often will have manifestations of infectious disease, particularly pneumonia.

2. Excess

Although it is difficult, if not impossible, to produce carbohydrate toxicity in the classical sense (excluding obesity), toxic responses to specific carbohydrates under certain situations, often when there is an inherited deficiency in a carbohydrate metabolizing enzyme, have been reported. An example of a toxicity from feeding a particular carbohydrate is the work done at the University of Illinois in the 1950s. In these studies it was determined that sucrose and fructose are toxic for neonatal piglets. Sucrose toxicity is a result of a low activity of intestinal sucrase (a disaccharidase) in the gut of young pigs. Therefore, neither glucose nor fructose is available as a energy source. Earlier, Cori and coinvestigators reported that during the first week of life, neonatal pigs absorb fructose intact; however, they are not able to phosphorylate the fructose. Consequently, this hexose is not catabolized to trioses for energy utilization. As a result, animals experience diarrhea and limited growth. Another example of a toxic response to a specific carbohydrate is the inability of the Fischer 344 and other rat strains to metabolize efficiently high concentrations (50% or greater) of sucrose in the diet, leading to fatty liver within 6–12 weeks. The lesions are typical of hepatic lipidosis in other species and may be the result of enhanced fatty acid synthesis with a concomitant reduction in apolipoprotein synthesis, triggered by the exaggerate conversion of sucrose to acetate. This finding, among others, has led to substantial changes in the dietary formulations for laboratory rodents in recent years.

Many neonatal mammals are unable to digest lactose to galactose and glucose due to a lack of intestinal lactase leading to malabsorption and diarrhea. Some human infants do not have the enzymes needed for galactose catabolism (e.g., galactose-1-phosphate uridyl transferase and UDP-glucose-4-epimerase); therefore, they experience a resultant toxicity syndrome characterized by vomiting, diarrhea, failure to thrive, icterus, brain damage, and cataracts. The specific mechanism of toxicity is unclear; the end result is fatty liver, cataract formation, edema and gliosis in the brain, and gonadal dysfunction. Cats develop cataracts (opacification of the lens) as a result of a buildup of galactitol, from an alternative pathway of galactose catabolism. The enzyme UDP-glucose-4-epimerase has an absolute requirement for nicotinamide adenine dinucleotide (NAD). Therefore, a dietary excess of leucine, which increases the requirement for tryptophan, which is necessary for *in vivo* synthesis of nicotinamide nucleotides, in conjunction with aberrant galactose metabolism may result in toxicity. It has been reported that excess dietary galactose results in food refusal by adult rats. Unlike lactose intolerance, due to intestinal malabsorption, galactose-induced flavor avoidance may be due to incomplete postabsorptive metabolism.

C. FATS

Even though dietary fat is important in the sense that certain fatty acids are essential for many species and that lipids are needed as carriers for the absorption of certain essential nutrients (such as the fat soluble vitamins), fat is not essential as a nutrient unless carbohydrate and protein are limiting as energy sources. In reality, in industrially developed countries, a dietary excess of fat has led to an "epidemic" of obesity, with all its unwanted consequences. In one sense, obesity is a toxicity; in another sense, it is a metabolic problem.

1. Deficiency

Whereas deficiencies of certain essential fatty acids, particularly linoleic, linolenic, and arachidonic acids, can be induced under experimental conditions, naturally occurring fatty acid deficiency is rare and requires a long time to develop. For most mammalian species, linoleic acid is essential, whereas for the other two, there is considerable species variability in essentiality. Fatty acid deficiency may occur if biliary or pancreatic dysfunction leads to the impairment of fat digestion and absorption, which may also lead to deficiencies of fat-soluble vitamins. Fatty acid deficiencies typically manifest themselves as skin abnormalities, including scaling and dermatitis, leading to dehydration and failure of wounds to heal.

2. Excess

There are numerous references to the enhancement of carcinogenesis resulting from the ingestion of high fat diets. However, there is considerable confounding evidence when high fat intakes and low carbohydrate intakes are taken into account; therefore, the issue of separating high fat intake from high caloric intake has yet to be resolved. In studies with experimental animals, feeding diets high in fat produced enhanced carcinogenesis. Generally, increased tumor incidence is observed in skin, lung, colon, liver, and/or pancreas when diets contain high levels of specific polyunsaturated fatty acids. Increasing dietary fat concentration increased the incidence and multiplicity of mammary cancers in a wide variety of carcinogen-induced, radiation-induced, spontaneous, transplantable, and metastatic rodent models. The effect of dietary fat on mammary tumor promotion may depend on the specific characteristics and peculiarities of the model under

Elizabeth H. Jeffery, Matthew A. Wallig, and M. E. Tumbleson

investigation. Experimental design often is predicated on the addition of a particular fat to a purified diet that is fed to animals; however, this does not account for the variety of fats, from numerous sources, ingested by human beings. Little or no effect of ethanol consumption on blood lipids of human subjects consuming a low-fat diet has been found. Decreases in cardiovascular disease risk factors typically observed with moderate ethanol intake may not be evident in individuals consuming a low-fat diet. Therefore, changes in risk factors associated with a low-fat diet and moderate ethanol consumption do not appear to be additive.

D. FIBER

Dietary fiber is the sum of polysaccharides and lignin that are not digested by the endogenous secretions of the gastrointestinal tract (6I). Dietary fiber includes substances not broken down by digestive enzymes and includes not only cellulose and lignin, but also hemicellulose, pectins, gums, and mucilages. Fiber may be divided into soluble and insoluble. Soluble fiber can be metabolized by the microflora of the lower gut in nonruminants, whereas insoluble fiber, or roughage, generally is nondigestible. However, this nondigestible fiber serves to retain water in the lumen of the lower gut and enhance the passage of ingesta. The vogue of "roughage" in humans has been incited before, namely in the 1920s and 1930s, only to fade into the sunset as conflicting concepts about therapeutic benefits of "soft" diets arise. The chemical constitution of fiber is not homogeneous. Cellulose, hemicelluloses, pectin, and lignin are present in varying percentages in various types of diets. Fermentation of different fiber constituents by fecal flora differs from substance to substance and depends on relative amounts of individual components. Short chain fatty acids, such as butyric acid, released by the fermentation of fiber in the lower GI tract provide not only energy to colonic epithelium but also serve as important mediators of cellular differentiation in this portion of the gut.

Dietary fiber possesses underappreciated antitoxic effects. Diets high in fiber reduce gut transit time; therefore, the length of exposure of harmful substances to the intestinal mucosa is lessened. Also, fiber has the ability to retain water, resulting in reduced concentrations of carcinogens so the effect on intestinal mucosa is reduced. Insoluble fiber undergoes minimal change in the digestive tract and primarily affects digestion by increasing stool bulk and promoting laxation.

An increased intake of water-insoluble fiber may result in bound mineral elements; therefore, ingestion of large amounts of fiber may interfere with intestinal absorption. Hypomagnesemic patients have a higher intake of total dietary fibers, which correlates with hypomagnesemic status. Theoretically, a loss of calcium and thus the development of osteoporosis might be expected under these conditions. Fibers may reduce and delay mono-saccharide absorption, thus reducing the postprandial hyperglycemic phase, which can affect patients with insulin-dependent diabetes mellitus. The reduction in absorption of minerals and vitamins could, in theory, have adverse nutritional consequences, particularly in populations eating diets inherently deficient in these nutrients, e.g., in developing countries or fastidious, health food conscious communities where diets may be marginal in micronutrients but high in fiber. The ingestion of dietary fiber may affect drug absorption either directly or by reducing gastric emptying or inhibiting mixing in the small intestine.

A potential hazard of increased fiber intake in the elderly is the formation of bezoars, dense masses of seeds, skins, and other fiber-containing plant parts. Normal aging leads to lower gastric acidity, creating an environment conducive of bezoar formation. Add to this factor the poor chewing of plant foods by individuals with teeth missing or ill-fitting dentures and the conditions for compaction stomach compaction are enhanced. Bowel obstruction by phytobezoars, large conglomerations of indigestible vegetable fiber, has been reported in humans who consume abnormally high amounts of fiber such as bran.

602

III. Micronutrients

A. VITAMINS

1. Vitamin A

a. Deficiency. Severe vitamin A deficiency, although virtually unknown in Western countries, is still a disease of high morbidity in many underdeveloped countries. Severe vitamin A deficiency is the second most prevalent nutritional disease in humans behind protein-calorie deficiency. Marginal deficiency is another matter, however, and may be more common than generally is thought, mainly because standard methods for assessing vitamin A status often do not take into account the varying activities and potencies of the various provitamin forms of vitamin A (e.g., carotenoids).

Deficiency disease begins to manifest itself when daily intake is less than 70% of the RDA (5000 IU for humans) for long periods of time. Such situations can occur when there is an insufficient intake of fresh vegetables and fruits. They also can occur in cases of severe protein deficiency, where the synthesis of retinol-binding protein is essential for the transport of vitamin A to peripheral tissues. Poor dietary intake associated with prolonged illness is a common cause of deficiency. Because vitamin A absorption is dependent on bile, pancreatic enzymes, dietary lipids, and chylomicron formation, long-standing gastrointestinal disease with malabsorption or maldigestion can result in deficiency. Liver damage (e.g., secondary to alcoholism) can also lead to deficiency because >90% of the body's stores of this vitamin are present in the liver. In addition, the liver is responsible for producing the binding protein necessary for transport to peripheral tissues.

The main pathophysiologic effect of deficiency that underlies most of the outward lesions is squamous metaplasia of pseudostratified columnar epithelium. This reflects the essential role of vitamin A in the differentiation of mucus-secreting, ciliated, and noncornified epithelium. The metaplastic epithelium eventually cornifies and loses any ciliary structures as well as any mucus-secreting cells. The most common and perhaps the earliest outward manifestation of deficiency is night blindness (nyctalopia) followed by keratinization of the conjunctival epithelium and lacrimal glands, leading to "dry eye" or xerophthalmia. Both conditions are reversible in the early stages if the deficiency is reversed. If deficiency persists, however, perforation of the cornea and permanent loss of vision occur. Likewise, retinal lesions, although less obvious, are manifested by the degeneration of rods, ultimately leading to atrophy of the entire retina. Unlike corneal lesions, retinal lesions and associated nyctalopia are not due to impaired differentiation but rather due to the role of 11-*cis*-retinal, a biologically active form of vitamin A, in the formation of rhodopsin, the light-sensitive pigment essential for night vision.

Keratinization is not confined to the eye in vitamin A deficiency, however, and squamous metaplasia with secondary loss of function are also present in genitourinary, upper respiratory, and gastrointestinal tracts. Impaired mucociliary clearance in the respiratory tract and malabsorption/maldigestion in the GI tract due to metaplastic changes in absorptive epithelium may be responsible in large part for the increased susceptibility to respiratory infections and diarrhea noted in severely deficient individuals. Squamous metaplasia of glandular ducts, e.g., in the pancreas and salivary glands (Fig. 1), is also common. Skin also can be affected, especially in domestic animals, with hyperkeratosis and hyperplasia leading to raised plaques on the skin. This change apparently is due to an overproduction of basal cells in the epidermis, leading to the death of overlying epithelial cells and replacement with keratinizing squamous cells. Immune function is also affected, with impaired functions of lymphocytes and macrophages. Bone development and maintenance are frequently abnormal, for vitamin A is required for the normal functioning of osteoclasts. The subsequent imbalance between osteoclast and osteoblast function leads to the formation of excessive cancellous bone, often leading to the narrowing of nerve foramina and resultant nerve dysfunction. Odontoblast

Elizabeth H. Jeffery, Matthew A. Wallig, and M. E. Tumbleson

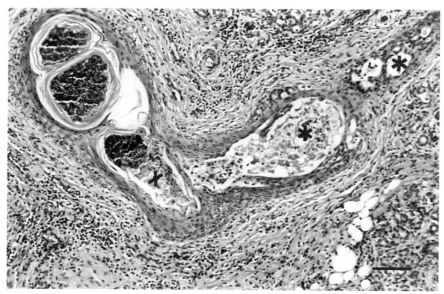

Figure 1. Vitamin A deficiency. Photomicrograph of salivary gland from a lamb illustrating squamous metaplasia of the salivary ducts (*) and surrounding inflammatory response. Keratin and cellular debris fill the ducts. Hematoxylin and eosin. Bar: 25 µm.

and ameloblast function may also be affected, leading to defective tooth formation. Perhaps the most definitive manifestations of deficiency are impaired growth and death, which can occur fairly rapidly after overt signs of deficiency develop, especially in the young. A significant inverse correlation exists in tropical and subtropical countries between vitamin A intake and mortality in children. A similar relationship has been shown between diarrhea and intake.

The link between vitamin A deficiency and cancer is not clear at this point, although experimental evidence in rodents would suggest that there is an enhanced susceptibility to cancer in deficient individuals. There is accumulating epidemiological evidence for a link between smokers with low intakes of vitamin A and increased chances for carcinoma of the lung.

b. Excess. The toxicity of vitamin A (hypervitaminosis A) is manifested in two forms: acute and chronic. In acute toxicity, adult humans become intoxicated when eating an excess of marine fish livers. Proforms of the vitamin, such as the carotenoids, generally are not toxic, even at very high doses, although an un-

pleasant yellow or orange hue may discolor the individual consuming excessively high doses. Neonates are more sensitive to toxic effects and can become acutely intoxicated at much lower doses. Generally, signs are vomiting, diarrhea (in neonates), and redness of the skin. In humans, headache, hyperirritability, and bulging fontanelles (in infants) commonly are manifest. Symptoms generally subside in a few days with no permanent side effects if no further vitamin is ingested.

Chronic hypervitaminosis A is much more common and insidious and is generally associated with self-prescribed oversupplementation by humans or improperly mixed diets in domestic animals. Aqueous preparations of vitamin A are most prone to overdose, as absorption is better and there is less loss in the feces than with traditional oil-based preparations. Symptoms are variable and may not necessarily correlate with blood levels or even dosage above a certain point.

Toxicity at the cellular level is manifested by the redifferentiation of simple types of epithelium into more complex forms, including mucous epithelium. Accompanying this is decreased cohesion among epithelial cells in the skin. Accordingly, most humans report skin changes such as pruritis, erythema, and dermatitis with bleeding and cracking of the skin, especially around lips and gums, as well as hair loss and nosebleeds. Double vision and headache are frequent, probably due to the increased cerebrospinal fluid pressure due to the blockage of fluid outflow. In domestic animals there can be narrowing of the spinal canal and braincase due to bony changes. These changes are the result of increased proliferation of periosteal bone and bone near the growth plate. The bone initially becomes thicker and then less dense, weaker, and more prone to fracture as the osteoblasts become dysfunctional and die. Enlargement of the liver has been reported due to an accumulation of vast numbers of vitamin A-laden Ito cells and swelling of vitamin A-laden hepatocytes, with ultimate loss of function and liver failure. There is evidence that vitamin A can also be teratogenic, apparently because of its role in inducing programmed cell death at the appropriate time in mesenchymal and epithelial development in the fetus, particularly the face, ears, eyes, digits, and brain. Epidemiologic evidence for teratogenicity, however, is still sparse.

Vitamin A toxicity in domestic animals generally is restricted to cats consuming large amounts of bovine liver. The effect is mainly on bone and apparently results from weakening of the bone at points of stretching or tension where ligaments and tendons attach. Fractures are most frequent in the neck and thoracic spine and in upper forelimbs, probably due to contortions associated with grooming. Fractures lead to bony callous formation; callouses then impinge on nerves leaving the spinal canal as well as impair bending of the spine, with the end result being a stiff-necked, painful animal. In dogs, and cats as well, vitamin A excess in young animals can result in osteoporosis and destruction of growth plates, leading to dwarfism, elongation of tuberosities on long bones, rotation of the epiphyses of long bones, and pathological fractures. Similar bony lesions occur in growing chickens and turkeys.

Vitamin A has interactions with several other nutrients, particularly iron. Supplementation of vitamin A to individuals with iron deficiency anemia maximizes erythropoiesis and enhances iron mobilization from the liver during iron repletion, especially in individuals with prolonged vitamin A deficiency. An attempt has been made to link vitamin A and zinc deficiencies because zinc-deficient animals are often vitamin A deficient as well, even when adequate dietary vitamin A is provided. Therefore, vitamin A deficiency may be due to the decreased food intake associated with zinc deficiency rather than a direct effect on vitamin A metabolism itself. There is experimental evidence in rats that excess dietary selenium decreases hepatic vitamin A storage, possibly potentiating a marginal vitamin A deficiency.

2. Vitamin D

a. Deficiency. Vitamin D, the "sunshine" vitamin, is not commonly associated with either deficiency disease or toxicity, but the consequences of either deficiency or excess, when they do occur, are serious, often irreversible, and even life-threatening. Vitamin D deficiency is seldom encountered today, although the role of "occult" deficiency in the elderly currently is being investigated. Historically, vitamin D deficiency results from three factors: insufficient exposure to sunlight (decreased conversion of plasma cholesterol to vitamin D_3, the first step in active synthesis), inadequate dietary intake in lieu of sunlight, or chronic renal disease leading to impaired conversion of the inactive monohydroxy form of D_3 (formed in the liver) to the active dihydroxy form. Occasionally, GI disease can cause deficiency. In recent years, vitamin D deficiency has been implicated in osteomalacia in patients receiving long-term total parenteral nutrition; occult vitamin D deficiency has been identified in postmenopausal women with hip fractures, with increased healing and decreased recurrence in those supplemented with the vitamin.

Major manifestations of deficiency are rickets in the young and osteomalacia in the adult. Although these conditions traditionally are associated with vitamin D deficiency, similar changes occur in dietary Ca or phosphorus (P) deficiency, although the biochemical mechanisms may differ. Characteristic features of rickets are enlargement of the metaphyseal regions of long bones with bending or bowing of the diaphyses and softening of the osseous matrix. Microscopically there is thickening and disorganization of the cartilaginous growth plate, with delayed ossification, retention of cartilage, and widening of the plate transversely. The osteoid that does get deposited is unmineralized, and the marrow often is fibrous rather than hematopoietic. Osteomalacia in adults occurs by similar mechanisms but results in different lesions because the growth plate is no longer present; the primary change is an increase in the deposition of unmineralized osteoid, resulting in a progressive thickening (and softening) of the diaphyseal portions of long bones and thickening of flat bones. The unmineralized bone is resistant to the action of osteoclasts; therefore, the osteoid accumulates progressively.

b. Excess. Toxicity (hypervitaminosis D) is rare in both humans and domestic animals. In humans and domestic animals, clinical signs are similar to those of renal failure. In animals, often the first sign is a dead animal or one in terminal stages of kidney failure. The manifestations of vitamin D toxicity are due to the primary effect of vitamin D on the small intestine, leading to increased synthesis of calcium-binding protein. This results in excess absorption of Ca (and P) from the gut. Also, there is reabsorption of Ca (as well as P) by the kidney and from resorption of bone, especially if the patient survives the initial onset of toxic signs. This massive uptake of calcium and phosphorus leads initially to profound hypercalcemia and hyperphosphatemia, which may return to normal over time as the excess Ca and P (as phosphate) precipitate out as hydroxyapatite in peripheral tissues. Ca deposition is most severe in the kidney (Fig. 2); affected individuals usually die of renal failure. The tunica media of arteries are prone to calcification, as are myocardium and skeletal muscle, all tissues with a high Ca turnover and which also have a high phosphorus content. The deposition of Ca salts in the joint capsules may occur in long-standing cases; pulmonary calcification with deposition of mineral in alveolar walls is a common lesion in young dogs (Fig. 3).

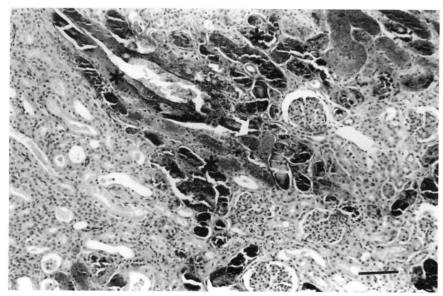

Figure 2. Vitamin D toxicity. In this section of kidney from a dog there is extensive tubular mineralization (*). Hematoxylin and eosin. Bar: 25 μm.

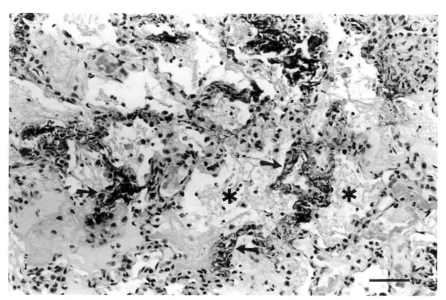

Figure 3. Vitamin D toxicity. There is extensive mineralization of the alveolar septa (arrows) in a lung from a dog. Hematoxylin and eosin. Note the fibrinous exudate within alveolar spaces (*). Bar: 25 μm.

Unique bone lesions, considered by some to be pathognomonic for vitamin D toxicosis, are characterized by initial rarefaction of spongy bone due to increased osteoclastic activity, followed by the deposition of intensely basophilic, disorganized fibrillar matrix. This defective matrix is produced by osteoblasts and is deposited on both endosteal and periosteal surfaces as well as on trabecula. The matrix becomes mineralized at some point well after its deposition by osteoblasts.

Under most circumstances, vitamin D toxicity is not a concern, but certain disease states can lead to a predisposition to vitamin D toxicity even when ingestion is slightly above recommended levels. In humans with chronic mycobacterial infections or certain chronic inflammatory conditions involving large numbers of activated macrophages, cytokines can be produced that result in increased bone resorption and hypercalcemia. Vitamin D exacerbates the situation by promoting absorption of calcium from the intestine. Renal failure patients being treated with vitamin D itself or vitamin D analogs, such as 1α-hydroxy-vitamin D, can become intoxicated. In domestic animals, there are three major causes of hypervitaminosis D;

overzealous supplementation of diet with vitamin D, ingestion of rodenticides containing cholecalciferol (vitamin D_3), and ingestion of plants containing cholecalciferols (*Cestrum, Solanum*).

The interactions of vitamin D with Ca, P, and parathyroid hormone are complex and often seemingly paradoxical. Secondary hyperparathyroidism is a common feature of vitamin D deficiency, further exacerbating the osteomalacia associated with the decreased intestinal and renal absorption, although the parathyroid hormone also stimulates the increased renal conversion of monohydroxy to the active dihydroxy form of the vitamin. Low dietary Ca, as well as low dietary P, will also enhance the renal conversion of the monohydroxy form to the dihydroxy form.

3. Vitamin E

a. Deficiency. Vitamin E (α-tocopherol) has attracted a large amount of attention in the popular press in recent years as the "antiaging" vitamin and has been linked to protection against cancer, as well as a whole host of other positive effects. Biochemically, vitamin E performs the antioxidant role in cell membranes

607

that vitamin C and the glutathione/glutathione peroxidase/glutathione reductase system perform in the cytosol by lodging in cell membranes and protecting unsaturated lipids from free radical peroxidation. Deficiency diseases associated with insufficient vitamin E consumption often respond to selenium supplementation as well as vitamin E; the precise etiology of these diseases often is complex and only partially understood. In some cases, the deficiency may be relative in the sense that increased dietary polyunsaturated fatty acids, which are prone to lipid peroxidation, may increase the requirement for vitamin E. In these cases a deficiency state occurs even if the individual is consuming otherwise adequate doses of the vitamin. Many of the well-known diseases associated with vitamin E deficiency in humans and domestic animals, such as Keshan disease (necrotizing cardiomyopathy followed by fibrosis) in humans and white muscle disease (nutritional myopathy), hepatosis dietetica (hepatic necrosis), and mulberry heart disease (dietetic microangiopathy), can also occur in dietary Se deficiency and are discussed in that section of this chapter. There are, however, several defi-

ciency syndromes that respond to vitamin E supplementation alone and/or which can be produced in situations of "pure" vitamin E deficiency. The primary cellular effects in skeletal muscle and myocardium are swelling of mitochondria, dissolution of myofibrils, fragmentation of sarcoplasmic reticulum, and degeneration of the sarcolemma, leading to cell swelling, hyalin change, and oncotic necrosis of the affected cell. Precipitation of Ca salts is a frequent occurrence as the cell dies (Fig. 4).

In humans, there is a syndrome in which there is loss of large myelinated axons in portions of the spinal cord associated with chronic malabsorption syndromes from exocrine pancreatic insufficiency or chronic cholestasis. This has been linked to lack of vitamin E absorption and subsequent occult deficiency. Accumulation of lipofuscin, the "wear and tear" pigment, has also been observed in these deficiency conditions. In animals, a steatitis consisting of yellow, firm, subcutaneous, and abdominal deposits of ceroid-laden necrotic adipocytes, surrounded by neutrophils and macrophages, has been reported in cats, mink, horses, pigs, and rats due to high dietary polyunsaturated

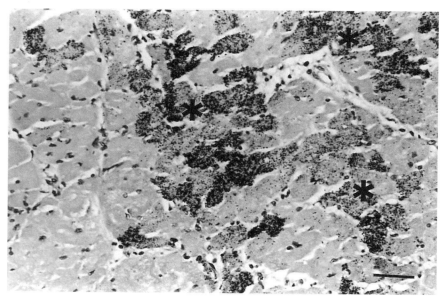

Figure 4. Vitamin E/selenium toxicity. Photomicrograph of the myocardium of a monkey in which there is acute myocardial necrosis with extensive mineralization (*). Hematoxylin and eosin. Bar: 25 μm.

lipids in the face of low dietary vitamin E consumption. Encephalomalacia in the cerebellum triggered by necrosis of vascular endothelium in the brain and axonal degeneration in the brain stem and spinal cord has been reported in chicks, rats, dogs, and monkeys with vitamin E deficiency. Testicular atrophy and aspermatogenesis are additional conditions connected with vitamin E deficiency in rats and guinea pigs, as is fetal resorption reported in rats and mice.

b. Excess. Unlike its mineral counterpart, Se, vitamin E is relatively nontoxic; what toxic effects do occur typically are reversible. Toxic effects reported in humans include headache, nausea, fatigue, and double vision, with severe muscle weakness, gastrointestinal disturbances, and elevated serum creatine kinase, but these symptoms are primarily anecdotal in nature. Rare and subtle but nevertheless serious physiological effects have also been identified. The most critical is the depression of prothrombin levels and increased clotting time in patients undergoing anticoagulant therapy or deficient in vitamin K, apparently because excessive vitamin E impairs vitamin K utilization, either through competitive absorption or prevention of oxidation. Another possibility is quenching of the endoperoxide intermediates during thromboxane production. Hemorrhagic tendencies have been shown experimentally in rats and mice, in both cases associated with a suppression of vitamin K-dependent reactions. Impaired wound healing has been reported as a consequence of hypervitaminosis E, probably because excess vitamin E may impair membrane turnover essential for macrophage activation and generation of prostaglandins and leukotrienes.

4. Vitamin K

a. Deficiency. The sole function of vitamin K that has been identified to date is as a cofactor in the posttranslational modification of factors II, VII, IX, and X of the clotting cascade, mediating selected carboxylation of glutamic acid residues necessary for these factors to function. It is difficult to achieve a deficiency of vitamin K unless an individual's intestinal microflora (source of vitamin "K2") are eliminated or disrupted (e.g., prolonged oral antibiotic therapy) and ingestion of fruits or vegetables (source of vitamin "K1" or phylloquinone) is inadequate. Impaired lipid absorption due to chronic intestinal disease or cholestasis may contribute to deficiency, as with the other lipid-soluble vitamins. Ingestion by cattle of sweet clover hay (*Meliotus* spp.), containing coumarin, a substance that frequently undergoes further chemical rearrangement to form dicoumarol, results in a potent vitamin K antagonism that over the course of a month or so results in severe hemorrhagic tendencies, including uncontrolled bleeding from nose and mouth, extensive subcutaneous and intramuscular bleeding from the slightest trauma, and bleeding into joints and abdominal organs as well as in the endocardium. Dicoumarol is the active component of warfarin, used not only as a rat poison but therapeutically in cardiac patients with thrombotic tendencies or postoperatively to prevent the hypercoagulation of blood. Such use in actuality produces a relative but regulated vitamin K deficiency that must be monitored carefully and assessed in relation to the patient's dietary intake of vitamin K-containing fruits and vegetables.

b. Excess. It is almost impossible to become intoxicated by vitamin K via the diet because an individual cannot consume enough plant or animal material to achieve toxic levels. Trouble arises, however, when an individual is treated parenterally with synthetic vitamin K (menadione or Vitamin "K3"). Toxicity is associated *not* with the function of vitamin K as a cofactor, but with its biochemical structure as a quinone, making it possible to undergo redox recycling to generate free radicals, resulting in hemolysis. Adults rarely have problems with vitamin K toxicity, although some can develop a hypersensitivity to injectable K3 (i.e., menadione). Acute tubular necrosis has been reported in horses treated with high doses of menadione.

Perhaps the greatest cautionary note for humans regarding vitamin K is for those being treated with vitamin K antagonists to prevent thrombosis. Ingestion of vitamin K-rich vegetables (especially cruciferous vegetables) can lead to reversal of the vitamin K antagonism (with subsequent thrombosis) if the dose of antagonist is not adjusted accordingly. Scientists have identified a Ca/vitamin K interaction in pigs; high levels of dietary Ca interfered with vitamin K-dependent clotting mechanisms. This was overcome with vitamin K supplementation.

5. Vitamin C

Water-soluble vitamins present a somewhat different picture toxicologically from fat-soluble ones, as their toxicokinetics are not the same. Water-soluble vitamins tend not to accumulate in tissues, partly because they are not lipid soluble, allowing them to be filtered out of plasma and excreted in the urine. For this reason, it is hard to "saturate the system" with these vitamins. No organ takes them up and stores them, and any excess is excreted into the urine. Therefore, toxicities of water-soluble vitamins, when they occur, tend to be acute in nature and will regress rapidly if the patient survives the episode.

a. Deficiency. Vitamin C has a variety of functions, the most important from a deficiency disease standpoint is its role in hydroxylation reactions, in particular the hydroxylation of proline in collagen to stabilize its helical structure. Vitamin C also serves as a water-soluble antioxidant in a variety of vitamin and mineral-dependent metabolic pathways and as a quencher of cytosolic free radical reactions. Vitamin C is a vitamin only in guinea pigs, Indian fruit bats, and primates; all other mammals, birds, reptiles, and amphibians can synthesize their own vitamin C. Deficiency is present only in primates and guinea pigs and is associated with diets poor in fruits and/or leafy green vegetables. "Scurvy" (or "scorbutus") is the hallmark feature of vitamin C deficiency, taking 1 month (guinea pigs) to several months (primates) to become manifest after elimination from the diet. Lesions of deficiency are classic and consist of gingivitis with hemorrhage and loosening of teeth, subperiosteal hemorrhages, and abnormal ossification characterized by calcification without ossification at growth plates (with resultant pathologic fractures; Fig. 5). Poor wound healing is another hallmark feature of vitamin C deficiency.

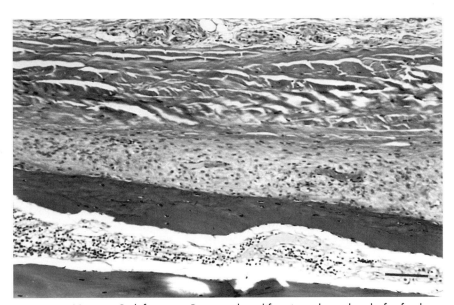

Figure 5. Vitamin C deficiency. Periosteal proliferation along the shaft of a long bone from a macaque. Hematoxylin and eosin. Bar: 25 μm.

b. Excess. After megadoses of vitamin C, acute toxicity does not appear to occur, although long-term high doses (generally above 1 g/day in humans) have been associated with GI disturbances such as nausea, diarrhea, and abdominal cramps, probably due to the osmotic effect of having a large bolus of slowly absorbed carbohydrate present in the gut. Perhaps of more import is that megadoses of vitamin C can cause an increase in the excretion of oxalic acid into the urine, which can precipitate as oxalate uroliths. This does not occur in most individuals, where this pathway of vitamin C metabolism is a minor one; however, there are those unfortunate few who have extremely efficient enzymes in their oxalate conversion pathway and urolithiasis can occur with doses of 1 to 2 g/day over the course of weeks to months.

Although humans can tolerate enormous doses of vitamin C, adverse effects can occur in individuals with predisposing conditions. Excessive vitamin C can actually raise oxygen requirements for normal cell function, resulting in a loss of high-altitude resistance in individuals taking megadoses of the vitamin. Excessive vitamin C increases the requirement for vitamin E, probably because the extra vitamin E is required to counteract the prooxidant behavior of vitamin C at high concentrations. Excessive vitamin C is dangerous to individuals with hemochromatosis, for vitamin C increases the uptake of Fe and therefore enhances the likelihood of liver or heart damage in affected individuals. Vitamin C can enhance the turnover of bone and cause extensive remodeling of bone, which may not be desirable in elderly individuals. Individuals with chronic renal disease may not be able to excrete the increased acid load associated with megadoses of vitamin C and suffer from acidosis.

6. The B Vitamins

a. Thiamine (Vitamin B₁).

i. Deficiency Thiamine was the first of the B vitamins to be discovered, and the results of its deficiency are well known, although its role in several diseases in domestic animals has been at times controversial and unclear. Thiamine is essential for several key metabolic reactions, among those reactions linking the glycolytic pathway and the Kreb's cycle, reactions within the Kreb's cycle itself and as a cofactor in the hexose monophosphate shunt. Thiamine is also essential for the maintenance of axonal membranes. Overt deficiency disease in humans can manifest itself as "beriberi". In "wet" beriberi, the initial abnormality is peripheral vasodilation. This eventually leads to overload of the heart and bilateral failure with resultant edema. The "dry" form, however, leads to nonspecific peripheral neuropathy, with demyelination and loss of function. A unique neurological form of thiamine deficiency, Wernicke–Korsakoff syndrome, is observed most often in prolonged deficiency, especially in alcoholics, and is the result of hemorrhage with necrosis of neurons in the paraventricular regions of the thalamus, midbrain, medulla, and cerebellum. Thiamine deficiency is an ever present concern in elderly individuals or the chronically ill, where food intake may be insufficient to meet daily thiamine requirements.

The counterpart of Wernicke–Korsakoff in domestic animals has been termed Chastek paralysis, first described in cats, foxes, and mink consuming raw fish rich in thiaminase. The lesions are similar in morphology and distribution as those in humans, although cerebral cortical gray matter may be involved as well. Myocardial lesions have also been described. Ruminants, whose microflora normally produce ample amounts of thiamine, may suffer deficiency upon consumption of thiaminase-rich plants such as bracken fern or horsetail.

ii. Excess Thiamine has been characterized as nontoxic in both humans and domestic animals, but relatively recently there have been reports of toxicity associated with megadose consumption. Dizziness and flushing are the most noteworthy signs; these regress soon after ingestion is stopped. Administration of thiamine parenterally can also lead to toxicity in humans if it is administered at doses several hundred times the RDA of 1 to 1.5 mg. There are important neuromuscular effects, including headache and convulsions, paralysis, and cardiac arrhythmias.

b. Riboflavin (Vitamin B₂).

i. Deficiency Riboflavin is an essential component of flavin mononucleotide and flavin adenine dinucleotide (FAD), which are cofactors in a variety of integral oxidation reactions, including those in the Kreb's cycle, monoamine oxidation, and several mitochondrial reactions. Deficiency, when encountered, is usually in combination with deficiencies of other B vitamins and a result of inadequate intake of food in general, as in alcoholics, the elderly, and the chronically debilitated. In domestic animals, deficiency is rare; ruminants receive their riboflavin from rumenal microflora and therefore do not require a dietary source. In humans and in animal models of the deficiency, the most consistent lesions are conjunctivitis with neovascularization and opacity, oral inflammation, dermatitis with alopecia and scaling, normocytic hypochromic anemia, and neuropathy (especially in chicks). The most noteworthy lesion at the cellular level is typified by changes in mitochondria in some species (e.g., the mouse), in which mitochondria are enlarged; in other species there is a decrease in mitochondrial volume and internal surface area.

ii. Excess To date, toxicity associated with high doses of riboflavin has not been characterized, and it appears that transport from the intestine into the body is saturated easily, making it difficult to achieve excessively high doses via the oral route. Also, riboflavin is eliminated very rapidly into the urine, again making it difficult to achieve high levels by parenteral routes.

c. Niacin.

i. Deficiency Niacin is an integral component of nicotinamide adenine dinucleotide (NAD) and nicotinamide dinucleotide phosphate (NADPH) and as such has an essential role in key cellular reactions such as electron transport, reduction, and dehydrogenation. Deficiency disease, termed "pellagra," occurs in humans and pigs when diets rich in corn are consumed. Chronic alcoholics may also be deficient. Niacin deficiency generally occurs in combination with other B vitamin deficiencies so that sorting out the various effects and relating them to deficiencies of the various vitamins may be difficult. In both humans and pigs, deficiency is characterized by a variety of signs, including anemia, bilaterally symmetrical dermatitis with hyperkeratosis, dermal fibrosis and alopecia, diarrhea due to atrophy of gastrointestinal epithelium, and nervous disorders characterized by degenerations of neurons in the brain and corresponding degeneration in associated tracts in the spinal cord. In dogs, ulcerative oral lesions have been reported, leading to the common name for the disease, "blacktongue."

ii. Excess Niacin toxicity has become a concern recently in Western countries as megadoses (3 to 10 mg/day) of the vitamin have been used to treat certain disease states in humans, particularly schizophrenia and atherosclerosis. Administration of niacin but *not* nicotinamide will result in flushing of skin due to vasodilation in most patients, even at doses as low as 100 mg orally or 20 mg intravenously. This is accompanied by pruritis, headache, and GI disturbances. Long-term, high doses of niacin have been linked to abnormal liver function and even to chronic cholestatic liver disease with jaundice at doses of 750 mg per day. Gout and duodenal ulcers have also been connected to high doses of niacin. Experimentally, lesions in mice are minimal; in poultry there is growth retardation with shorter than normal legs and coarse feathering.

d. Pyridoxine (Vitamin B₆).

i. Deficiency Pyridoxine is an essential cofactor for a large series of reactions involved in protein and amino acid metabolism, including transmination, decarboxylation, deamination, racemation, phosphorylation, and cleavage of cystathionine to cysteine in the methionine pathway. In humans, however, subclinical pyridoxine deficiency is a common occurrence in alcoholics, chronically ill patients, or infants fed poorly formulated milk products. Pyridoxine deficiency is similar in presentation to niacin deficiency in both humans and animals, with chronic dermatitis, oral inflammation, peripheral neuropathy, and, in some case, convulsions, especially in young calves, puppies, piglets, and rats. Cats may suffer renal tubular necrosis with oxalate accumulation. An additional feature of deficiency is a hypochromic microcytic anemia. Pyridoxine can be depleted in individuals being treated with certain drugs such as isoniazid, estrogens, and penicillamine.

ii. Excess Until recently, pyridoxine was considered to be nontoxic, even at doses 10 to 500 times greater than the RDA. Large doses of pyridoxine have been used to treat autism, schizophrenia, and even Down's syndrome, and there is some evidence that high doses are helpful in carpal tunnel syndrome, although this has been attributed to the toxicity of the vitamin masking the symptoms. Pyridoxine has been used to treat premenstrual syndrome; it was under these conditions that toxic effects first were seen. The toxicity of pyridoxine in humans is neurologic in nature at doses above 2 to 6 g/day during a 5- to 40-month period. There is a symmetrical, progressive ataxia, loss of sensation in the distal extremities, lips, and tongue, and a loss of sense of joint position and vibration, with the central nervous system and motor function not affected. The loss of sensation often is not reversible. Pyridoxine neurotoxicity has been confirmed in dogs and rats at doses of 50 to 300 mg/kg/day and is characterized by the demyelination of peripheral sensory nerves and nerve roots, with eventual axonal degeneration and demyelination of sensory tracts in the spinal cord.

e. Biotin.

i. Deficiency Biotin is a cofactor in carboxylation reactions and is distributed widely in plant and animal foods. Biotin deficiency is difficult to attain and is seldom encountered, but has been associated with diets excessively rich in eggs, where the avidin in egg white complexes to biotin to make it unabsorbable. When it occurs, under natural or experimental conditions, there is reproductive failure and marked teratogenesis in the young. Dermatitis with alopecia, hypopigmentation, and hyperkeratosis has been reported. A low biotin status in chicks in the face of high choline levels in the diet can exacerbate fatty liver and kidney syndrome.

ii. Excess Toxicity due to biotin is virtually nonexistent. However, experimental evidence in rats is suggestive that high doses may affect reproductive female performance by interfering with estrogen and progesterone biosynthesis. Dietary levels of biotin four times higher than required for optimal growth have improved foot health and improved hair coat in swine and have enhanced reproductive performance in poultry.

f. Folic Acid (Folate).

i. Deficiency Folic acid, in the form of tetrahydrofolate, is necessary for methyl transfer reactions, which in turn are essential for purine and pyrimidine synthesis. Folate is very important for rapidly growing or high turnover tissues with a high rate of cell division, especially important in bone marrow and GI mucosal turnover. Although not as common as iron deficiency, folate deficiency is of concern for the elderly, those with chronic GI disease, epileptics on anticonvulsant drugs, women taking contraceptives, alcoholics, and especially pregnant women, in whom occult folate deficiency is frequent during the second trimester of pregnancy. In overt folate deficiency, there is macrocytic anemia followed eventually by a decrease in circulating granulocytes and platelets. Neurological signs occur late in the course of deficiency. Pregnant women with poor initial folate stores often are overtly deficient by the time of parturition. In recent decades an association has been made between low folate in early pregnancy and neural tube defects, particularly spina bifida, leading to recent recommendations that during early pregnancy women use folate supplementation to prevent these defects. Folate status is key in maintaining homocysteine at normal levels. Low folate status is associated with high homocysteine levels in plasma and tissues, a well-known risk factor for coronary heart disease. Experimentally, folate deficiency can be induced in cats and monkeys.

ii. Excess Folate toxicity is very rare, but with the recent advent of megadose therapies using B vitamins, adverse reactions to folate have been reported. Many of the reactions appear to be hypersensitivity reactions rather than true toxic reactions, occurring at doses of 15 mg/day or higher. However, in laboratory animals, folic acid can be nephrotoxic at doses as low as 25 mg/kg body weight, with irreversible damage to the renal tubules. Neurotoxicity has been observed as well, with spasms, rotating movements, and increased aggressiveness. In humans, 15 mg folate/day or more can cause malaise, irritability, depression, and altered sleep patterns.

Folate has a complex interrelationship with cobalamin, which is necessary for the conversion of tetrahydrofolate to methyltetrahydrofolate, the cofactor that serves as the methyl donor in the conversion of homocysteine to methionine. Excess folate can compensate for a relative lack of cobalamin by conserving methionine, thereby preserving the methyl donor pathway for use in DNA and RNA synthesis. This will reverse anemia of B_{12} deficiency but will not reverse the neurodegeneration associated with vitamin B_{12} deficiency.

g. Cobalamin (Vitamin B_{12}).

i. Deficiency Cobalamin requires cobalt (Co) for function and, as hydroxycobalamin, is an essential cofactor in known reactions, the methylmalonyl CoA mutase, the key step for shunting propionate into the Krebs cycle. Its other role, as methylcobalamin, together with methyltetrahydrofolate, is a cofactor in methionine synthase. Individuals with chronic GI disease are prone to acquiring deficiency disease. Cobalamin deficiency has two forms, one that is identical to folate deficiency (i.e., macrocytic anemia), although the exact mechanism whereby the deficiency translates into a folate deficiency is disputed. The second, and most serious due to irreversibility, is a form of cobalamin deficiency termed subacute combined degeneration observed in both humans and monkeys. Psychiatric signs of unclear pathogenesis are present, but there is also neurological degeneration, characterized by myelinic vacuolation of axons in both ascending and descending tracts (especially of the pyramidal tracts). The combination of lesions in both ascending and descending tracts is a characteristic feature of cobalamin deficiency. Peripheral nerves are also involved.

ii. Excess The toxicity of cobalamin has not been described and little investigated to date. There is little evidence that it is toxic.

B. MINERALS

1. Major Minerals

a. Calcium.

i. Homeostasis and deficiency Ca is the most abundant divalent cation in the body, constituting 1–2% of body weight. While 99% of body Ca is found in the bone, maintenance of extracellular (10^{-3} M) and intracellular (10^{-7} M) Ca is so vital that if intake of Ca is compromised, bone will demineralize before development of hypocalcemia. Typically only about 30% of ingested Ca is absorbed. However, a small decrease in serum Ca triggers the PTH/calcitriol-dependent upregulation of absorption from the gut and decreased urinary excretion. If the diet remains low in Ca, the chronic hyperparathyroidism that results leads to loss of bone mineral density with fibrous osteodystrophy in adults and rickets in growing individuals. The lesions are the same as those of vitamin D excess (see earlier discussion). Osteomalacia is most pronounced in vertebrae, mandible, and the proximal and distal ends of the long bones, areas rich in trabecular bone, which turns over far more rapidly than cortical bone of long bone shafts. Diets high in protein or fiber can cause chronic Ca loss: the former through increased renal clearance of Ca and the latter through lumenal chelation of Ca and subsequent decreased absorption from the gut. Unless severe, these conditions are compensated for by increased uptake and decreased clearance, respectively. Acute Ca loss can occur in the presence of a chelator such as EDTA, precipitating convulsions, tremor, and tetany. For this reason, EDTA chelators typically are administered as the Ca salt. Ca, P, and Mg metabolism are related intimately, in that high dietary phosphate and low dietary Mg can lead to hypocalcemia. Thus all three conditions result in the same pathological condition:

renal failure, with loss of bone Ca and osteomalacia.

ii. Excess If dietary Ca is permitted to rise above 1%, daily food intake decreases, fecal weight increases, and growth is retarded. In one experiment, rats fed a 2% Ca lactate diet exhibited a sharp decrease in food intake, and growing rats (60 g at starting) died within the 15-day experimental period. Both protein and fat absorption are decreased by elevated dietary Ca. The mechanism is unknown and, while it has been linked to the decrease in intestinal pH following the ingestion of inorganic Ca salts, it is not clear that organic Ca salts cause any pH change, even though they also disrupt nutrient absorption. Experimental diets high in Ca alone or in both Ca and P cause renal tubular calcification, commencing at the corticomedullary junction and progressing throughout the inner cortex. Initial deposits of Ca salts are present in the lumen of the descending portion of the proximal tubule rather than intracellularly. This progresses to loss of brush borders with intracellular deposits appearing after extensive lumenal calcification. In the absence of concomitant increases in P, a high Ca diet leads to phosphate deficiency due to chelation and precipitation in the gut. Phosphate deficiency then leads to vitamin D production. Therefore, in many species, rather than renal calcification, excess Ca produces osteopetrosis due to inhibition of osteoclastic activity by vitamin D. High dietary Ca also aggravates Mg deficiency.

b. Phosphorus.

i. Homeostasis and deficiency Under normal circumstances, most (70 to 80%) dietary P (as phosphate) is absorbed regardless of the dose, and regulation is by excretion in urine or feces, which in most cases is extremely efficient, especially by the kidney. In dietary P deficiency, seen most commonly in ruminants, vitamin D production is increased and is associated with development of a mild hypercalcemia. While this is thought to trigger a compensatory decrease in renal P excretion, the same change in renal P excretion is seen in parathyroidectomized animals, casting doubt on the mechanism of regulation of P excretion. If uncompensated, hypophosphatemia results in osteomalacia, cardiomyopathy, and a decrease in erythrocyte adenosine triphosphate (ATP) levels, precipitating an oxidative state and hemolytic anemia.

ii. Excess The RDA for P (as phosphate) is 800 mg/day, but no adverse effects are observed even when P intake is raised to 2000 mg/day. Although this high P intake decreases Ca intake, renal clearance of Ca is decreased to compensate. However, in experimental animals, when the P (as phosphate) to Ca ratio is raised above 1:2 for an extended period of time, secondary hyperparathyroidism results in osteomalacia and fibrous osteodystrophy, most obvious in the mandible. The use of orthophosphates and polyphosphates, both as animal feed additives and as food additives to perform numerous functions in the food industry, including acidifiers, emulsifiers, leavening agents, and water binders, has led to a high dietary intake of phosphate in the Western world. This is of particular concern in relation to the high intake of phosphate in sodas that are so popular in America today. Although humans are relatively tolerant of a dietary imbalance in Ca and P, whether the persistent Ca:P imbalance in most Western diets and the resulting hyperparathyroidism is causative in the osteoporosis of old age seen in Western society is open to question and a public health issue with important financial and emotional implications. The high P level of cow's milk has been suggested as causative in a hypocalcemic tetany seen in some infants drinking cow's milk.

Sudden, acute hyperphosphatemia from excessive pharmacologic administration of phosphates can cause such a rapid decrease in plasma Ca that tetany results. The common response to chronic hyperphosphatemia is a mild hypocalcemia with hypercalciuria, which occasionally produces renal mineralization and, ultimately, renal failure. While this hypocalcemia causes fibrous osteodystrophy (Fig. 6), intracellular Ca actually rises, producing pathological calcification, particularly in heart and kidney. In rats fed a normocalcemic diet of 0.6% Ca, raising dietary P to 1.2% precipitated renal and aortic calcification. Therefore

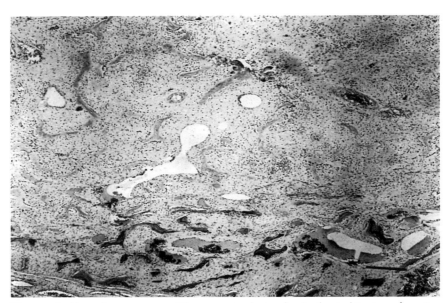

Figure 6. Phosphorus excess. Fibrous osteodystrophy in the turbinates of a pig. Note the exuberant proliferation of fibrous tissue with minimal production of osteoid. Hematoxylin and eosin. Bar: 25 μm.

pharmacologic use of P salts to lower blood Ca should only be undertaken with great caution.

Of related interest is the toxicology of elemental P, having caused the death of numerous children working in match factories in the 19th century. Following ingestion, P causes burns around the mouth, leading to vomiting and abdominal pains with a black diarrhea exuding a white vapor, the "smoking stool syndrome." This is followed by cardiac collapse due to myocardial damage or, if the victim survives, latent systemic damage to liver, heart, kidneys, and the central nervous system (CNS). The most apparent of these lesions is in the liver, with fatty change and necrosis in periportal regions due to a direct action of P on hepatocytes.

c. Magnesium.

i. Homeostasis and deficiency Whole body Mg is found 60–65% in bone, ~30% in muscle, and only 1% in the extracellular fluid. The body load of Mg is regulated by excretion/reabsorption in the renal proximal tubule and the ascending arm of the loop of Henle. It appears to be both filtered at the glomerulus and possibly secreted into the proximal tubule. The RDA is 4.5 mg/day, with about 30% of this being ab-

sorbed. High dietary levels of Ca and/or P (as phosphate) depress Mg absorption. Chronic hypomagnesemia is associated with abnormal neuromuscular function, including spasticity, convulsions, tremor, and tetany, and a hypocalcemia that does not respond to Ca feeding. Ruminants are particularly sensitive to Mg deficiency, which is known as winter tetany, grass staggers, or wheat pasture poisoning and is common in early lactation. Rats, however, respond very differently to Mg deficiency, with hypercalcemia, not hypocalcemia as seen in other species. There is a decrease in plasma Mg in myocardial heart disease, and while it is not clear whether this is causative or secondary, hypomagnesemia is associated with myocardial damage and arterial hypertension. In addition, chronic hypomagnesemia appears to be related to cancer mortality, particularly lymphoma. One possibility is that enhancement of both cardiac heart disease and carcinogenesis is due to a loss of antioxidant capacity in chronic Mg deficiency.

ii. Excess In humans, hypermagnesemia typically is associated with the pharmacological use of Mg salts, rather than dietary excess. In animals, hypermagnesemia is seen most frequently as a result of misformulation of diets. In hypermagnesemia, Mg competes successfully with Ca, producing vasodilation for which it is used clinically in eclampsia. CNS depression has been seen in infants born to mothers receiving Mg for more than 24 hr. Early signs of hypermagnesemia in animals are feed refusal and diarrhea. Hypermagnesemia also affects the peripheral nervous system. It is thought to interfere with the release of acetylcholine, producing a curare-like action on the neuromuscular junction, and CNS depression. Because cathartics and antacids can elevate plasma Mg, their use can lead to hypotension, CNS depression, respiratory depression, and finally death, particularly in renal insufficiency when Mg excretion is compromised. In areas of Minnesota, the Dakotas, and Montana, where Mg levels in the water can increase to 1% naturally, this is associated with muscular weakness in both humans and animals. Appetites are depressed and chronic exposure results in bone loss. Many of the adverse effects of excess Mg can be attenuated by Ca administration. Experimentally, 0.3% Mg appears to show no toxicity in sheep, while raising the level even to 0.8% has been associated with diarrhea, decreased feed intake, and decreased growth rate. Poultry, horses, and cows responded in a similar fashion. Intravenous infusion of large amounts of Mg (40 mg/kg body weight as Mg sulfate) to cattle and horses produces disruption of motor function, respiratory paralysis, and cardiac arrest.

d. Sodium/Chloride/Potassium.

i. Homeostasis and deficiency
Plant foods do not provide sufficient Na or chloride (Cl) for optimal animal health. Consequently, from early times, humans have sought a home where not only food and water are in abundance, but where there is a ready source of salt. Because salts must be added to animal feeds, deficiencies and toxicoses have been associated with incorrect mixing of diets. Extracellular fluid has as its major cation Na, whereas K is the major cation in intracellular fluid. Na, Cl, and K are absorbed fully and regulated primarily by urinary excretion, although sweat and diarrhea can contribute to excessive losses under certain circumstances. Homeostasis is lost in renal disease, when body Na, Cl, and water content increase, and in Addison's disease, when decreased aldosterone production permits excretion of Na to increase over intake, slowly leading to volume contraction, hypotension, shock, collapse, and death. Salt deficiency is accompanied by a salt craving (licking of rocks in animals) followed by a loss of appetite and signs of dehydration. Signs of K deficiency are weakness, lethargy, and cardiac arrhythmia leading to death. Either increasing or decreasing the plasma K level disrupts depolarization across the cell membrane. The signs and symptoms of hyper- and hypokalemia are therefore similar, both being due to the disruption of myocardial function.

ii. Excess
Salt restriction is found to lower blood pressure in many hypertensives, suggesting but not proving that excess salt will increase blood pressure. In contrast to Na, dietary K is related inversely to blood pressure. The mechanism is unknown, although it may be secondary to changes in blood Na, as urinary Na and K excretion are inversely related. In the Western world, blood pressure increases with age. The potential health benefit from lowering NaCl intake (or raising K) as one ages is not clear. Animals can withstand very large doses of NaCl, provided adequate water is made available. Cattle given water containing 12 g NaCl or more per liter exhibited anorexia, decreased water intake, weight loss, and finally collapse. In sheep, 13 g NaCl/liter caused decreased reproductive rates, poor weight gain in lambs, some diarrhea, and an increase in mortality. Swine have been given as much as 30 g/liter in water with no obvious adverse effects. However, 6 or 8% NaCl in the diet will precipitate staggering, weakness, paralysis, and histopathological changes in the liver. Four or 5% NaCl in the diet causes reduced weight gain, diarrhea, and increased mortality in poultry. The greatest risk for toxicity is in ruminants, pigs, and poultry. Lesions develop as a result of the inability of the cerebrospinal fluid to maintain ionic equilibrium with extracellular fluid,

leading to cerebral edema and inflammation characterized by the accumulation of eosinophils in Virchow–Robins spaces and necrosis of neurons in the cerebral cortex, especially in swine.

The relationship between intra- and extracellular K dictates the potential difference across the cell membrane, and thus controls the threshold for depolarization. If hyper- or hypokalemia develops acutely, the relationship between intra- and extracellular K is disrupted. In hyperkalemia the resting membrane potential may increase even to normal threshold for depolarization so that depolarization is permanent and repolarization cannot occur. Alternatively, in hypokalemia the potential difference is so great across the cell membrane that normal stimuli may not raise the resting potential to threshold, and depolarization is blocked. However, if the change in plasma K is slow, there is an accompanying partial reequilibration of intracellular K, and the relationship between intra- and extracellular K is maintained. Thus while chronic changes in extracellular K are accompanied by similarly directed changes within the cell, acute changes in extracellular K, such as from massive cell destruction during a hemolytic crisis, are not reflected immediately by changes within the cell and can be life-threatening.

A decrease in plasma pH is associated with an efflux of K from the cell, and thus metabolic acidosis can result in elevated plasma K, followed by excretion and subsequent hypokalemia. In cattle, the addition of 1 or 2% KCl to the diet (0.5 to 1% K) improves weight gain. However, chronic dietary intake at even mildly elevated K levels (2 to 5% KCl) can lead to Mg depletion and depressed weight gain. When dietary K is increased further, to 6% K, muscle weakness and stumbling, atrial flutter, tachycardia, and edema finally result in cardiac arrest. In cattle, early signs of hyperkalemia can look like grass staggers and can be associated with recent applications of high K fertilizer to grazing pastures. Intraperitoneal or intravenous injections of KCl have been used to produce rapid death by cardiac arrest; 0.3 g/kg being fatal within 15 or 30 min in rabbits.

e. Sulfur.

i. Homeostasis and deficiency Unlike plants, animals have no direct requirement for sulfur (S), but rather for the S-containing metabolic intermediates, methionine, biotin, and thiamine. Methionine is metabolized to many essential components in the body. Animals use inorganic S for the production of sulfate esters and in mucopolysaccharide synthesis. Ruminants, but not nonruminants, can utilize inorganic S in place of methionine because the rumenal flora can synthesize methionine.

ii. Excess S intoxication during industrial exposure is well documented, as are respiratory toxicities associated with oxides of S in air pollution. In contrast, dietary S excess has been ignored until recently, probably because of the low toxicity of ingested S. Cows fed excess S have anorexia, weight loss, and depression. Ruminants suffer S toxicoses more often when S-reducing microflora proliferate under conditions of high dietary sulfate or low dietary fiber, leading to very high levels of toxic sulfides and sulfites, responsible for necrotic lesions seen in brains of cows and sheep. While still considered of unknown etiology, and disputably associated with thiamine deficiency, polioencephalomalacia nevertheless can be precipitated by high dietary S. Characterized by laminar cerebrocortical necrosis with sparing of the white matter, polioencephalomalacia is of economic importance in areas of intense cattle and sheep farming, linked to overproduction of hydrogen sulfide in the rumen.

Pathological changes are not limited to CNS, but include constipation or diarrhea, emphysema, and hepatic necrosis. Acute massive doses of inorganic S are also associated with colic, a red/brown urine, and fecal H_2S with diarrhea in horses and with twitching, restlessness, and diarrhea in cattle. A dietary level of 0.4% S as sulfate is considered the maximum tolerable level in cattle. Sheep appear essentially unaffected by a high S diet unless given massive doses such as 60 g S per animal, when they too exhibit colic, depressed attitude, dyspnea, and foul breath. Excess methionine, considered the most toxic of amino acids, causes weight loss and splenic hemosiderosis in rats, but these effects are related directly to methionine rather than to S *per se*. Metabolism of other minerals, including Ca, P, Mo, Mn, Mg, and Zn, may be affected adversely at very high dietary S. For example, excess S will precipitate Cu deficiency due to Cu–S complex formation. High S has also been reported to interfere with Se uptake and can replace P in bone, leading to "sulfur rickets."

2. Trace Minerals

a. Chromium.

i. Homeostasis and deficiency The requirement for chromium (Cr) was first recognized in the 1950 as a "glucose tolerance factor" present in porcine kidney. Chromium has since been shown to stimulate the action of insulin, thereby playing a role in the regulation of carbohydrate metabolism. Requirements for Cr in lipid metabolism, lowering serum cholesterol, or in RNA synthesis are equivocal. The percentage absorption of trivalent Cr, 0.5 to 3% of an oral dose of $CrCl_3$, is more typical of absorption values reported for xenobiotic metals such as cadmium (Cd) or lead (Pb) than for a required mineral such as Fe. These absorption data and the equivocal nature of research evaluating a role for Cr in metabolism may well be indicative of the fact that many investigators may have used models that were not effectively Cr deficient and therefore the addition of Cr was without effect. During the last three decades, reported tissue levels of Cr have decreased three orders of magnitude, as both analytical methods and protection of samples from contamination during analysis have improved. This improvement in analytical technique can be expected to lead to more definitive studies on Cr deficiency.

ii. Excess Trivalent Cr, shown to be mutagenic in subcellular systems, is absorbed so poorly as to be considered nontoxic. Conversely, inhaled hexavalent chromate is associated with a number of toxicities, including allergic dermatitis, skin, nasal septum, and lung cancer. The carcinogenic form is thought to be trivalent Cr, formed by cellular reduction of the hexa-

valent form. Because a chromium picolinate supplement given to swine is considered to improve growth and percentage of muscle, chromium picolinate has come onto the market as a dietary supplement, carrying a similar promise of more lean mass and less fat in humans. This has not been borne out in clinical studies (i.e., individuals taking 6 to 10 times the recommended dose have presented with weight loss, anemia, thrombocytopenia, hemolysis, liver dysfunction, and renal failure). Cessation of the supplement has reversed all these changes within a year. Whether these adverse effects are due entirely to Cr alone, or to the salt, has been questioned and requires additional study.

b. Cobalt.

i. Homeostasis and deficiency Cobalt is not required as the free metal for incorporation into enzymes or other intermediary metabolites, but is required as a part of cobalamine (see earlier discussion). Therefore, there is no uptake requirement and no need for Co to be stored in the body other than as a cobalamin store. Analytically defined "Co deficiency" can be attenuated with cobalamin injections. Dietary Co is not available for cobalamin synthesis in many species, although it can be given to ruminants and horses, who host GI microbes that are able to synthesize cobalamin and to incorporate Co into the newly synthesized molecule. Enzootic marasmus, a wasting disease of sheep and cattle in Western Australia; "bush sickness," an anemia seen in cattle in certain areas of New Zealand; and other similar disorders are related to low soil Co in the area. Co deficiency has also been reported infrequently in the United States. This deficiency can be relieved by the use of Co-containing fertilizers, feeding Co directly, or feeding cobalamin.

ii. Excess Acutely, Co causes vasodilatation, producing flushing in humans and seen as bright pink ears in mice. When sheep were administered excess Co chronically (5 to 10 mg/kg), they developed anemia due to interference with Fe absorption: Ingested Co is absorbed via the Fe uptake system and excreted in urine. Rats and nonruminants given 200 or 250 ppm Co develop polycythemia with an associated hyperplasia of the bone marrow and reticulocytosis. Co formerly was used as an antifoaming agent in certain European beers, where as little as 8 mg/day (5 liters of beer) resulted in polycythemia, leading to increased hematocrit and thus increased blood viscosity, and ultimately to myocardial degeneration and necrosis with heart failure. Thyroid epithelial hyperplasia and colloid depletion have also been reported. Co cardiomyopathy has been modeled successfully in the dog using a high Co, low protein, and low thiamine diet. Animals can be somewhat protected from Co toxicity by feeding a high protein, particularly high methionine, diet.

c. Copper.

i. Homeostasis and deficiency The redox chemistry of Cu makes it particularly useful in electron transfer reactions. Copper is present at 1 to 2 μg/g in human tissues, with kidney and then liver having the highest concentrations, while the skeleton claims the greatest amount: ~40% of total body Cu. Plasma Cu is 1.05 μg/ml. There is no RDA for Cu, although requirements are considered to be 1.5 to 3 mg/day for humans, 4 to 5 ppm for swine and poultry, and 8 to 10 ppm in ruminants. Copper is absorbed primarily in the duodenum, 55 to 75% by a saturable system, so that excess Cu is absorbed at far lower rates. Under normal conditions, Cu is stored to a very minor extent and is regulated by excretion. While Cu is normally secreted into the intestine via saliva, pancreatic juices, and bile, a substantial portion of this is reabsorbed rather than lost in the feces. Absorption is depressed in the presence of excess Zn or Cd, possibly due to mucosal induction of a Cu-binding protein, metallothinein. Menke's disease, a Cu deficiency disease, has been linked to altered Cu transport in the gut mucosal epithelium.

Copper deficiency is occassionally seen in human infants, but rarely, if ever, in human adults. In animals, Cu deficiency can be due to low Cu soils, but occurs more frequently as a result of Mo excess in the presence of S, as these three elements are thought to combine in the rumen to form an unabsorbable triple complex. Cu deficiency has been found responsible for

ovine enzootic ataxia (swayback), bovine falling disease, aortic rupture in swine and turkeys, wool and hair depigmentation, and anemia. The basic neurologic lesion is bilaterally symmetrical demyelination with degeneration and loss of white matter in both spinal cord and cerebral cortex (Fig. 7). Deficiency results in a lessened capacity to carry out cellular respiration, leading to loss of energy. In the absence of normal Cu/Zn superoxide dismutase activity, lipids are oxidized and, in the absence of normal dopamine hydroxylase, catecholamine levels are disrupted. In addition, elasticity of membranes is lost due to the loss of lysyl oxidase activity, leading to erythrocyte fragility and other vascular lesions, such as an increased risk for aneurysms and loss of angiogenesis. Lysyl oxidase is also involved in collagen cross-linking during bone formation, and loss of activity leads to skeletal abnormalities. Microcytic, hypochromic anemia develops in Cu deficiency, probably associated with a loss of ceruloplasmin-dependent reduction of Fe, necessary for transfer onto transferrin. Chronically, Cu deficiency leads to a depressed immune response, hypercholesterolemia, with glucose intolerance and diabetes-like symptoms due to the formation of sugar alcohols.

ii. Excess Cu is not considered to be highly toxic in most species, although sheep are sensitive; they will exhibit a sudden onset hemolytic crisis, often weeks after they have commenced to accumulate Cu. Species variation in sensitivity is partly due to Cu–S interactions and the difference in S handling between ruminants and nonruminants. Sheep may also have a greater imbalance between rates of uptake and excretion of Cu.

In many species exposed to a large chronic excess of dietary Cu, it will accumulate asymptomatically in hepatocyte lysosomes, being released when the lysosomes become overloaded, resulting in oxidative damage and necrosis. As hepatocyte concentrations exceed 300 ppm, hepatocytes begin to degenerate, releasing Cu into the blood, which, due to uptake by erythrocytes, can result in hemolysis. Besides the resulting anemia, liver disease, and jaundice,

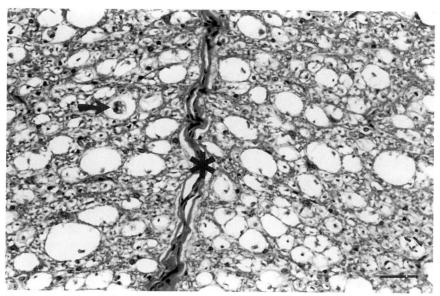

Figure 7. Copper deficiency. White matter degeneration in the spinal cord of a lamb. There is degeneration and loss of axon in white matter tracts on either side of the ventral median sulcus (*). A macrophage (arrow) is present within a dilated axonal space. Hematoxylin and eosin. Bar: 10 μm.

hemoglobin nephrosis occurs, seen as a "gun metal black" renal lesion (Fig. 8), characteristic of Cu toxicity. In addition to liver and erythrocytes, other tissues such as kidney, intestine, and brain can accumulate Cu and exhibit Cu-dependent oxidative damage. Brain, particularly the basal ganglia, is sensitive to accumulation and oxidative damage in humans. Canada geese ingesting pond water high in Cu sulfate develop necrosis of the proventriculus and gizzard.

Extensive liver damage occurs in humans with Wilson's disease, a genetic disorder that causes Cu accumulation. Long Evans "cinnamon rats" and dogs (particularly Bedlington terriers) have genetic defects that lead to the accumulation of Cu within hepatic lysosomes. As copper accumulates to excessive levels within lysosomes, rupture of the affected organelles eventually occurs, with subsequent necrosis of the hepatocyte, leading ultimately to an ongoing cycle of necrosis, inflammation, and fibrosis followed by more hepatocellular necrosis, etc. Cirrhosis is frequently the final outcome. Wilson's disease is treated in part by the administration of excess Zn, which is thought to interfere with Cu absorption. However, chelators are required to normalize Cu levels in these individuals. The defect appears to be in the transporter that carries Cu from hepatocytes into bile. As with Cu excess in normal individuals, excess Cu accumulates in lysosomes until lysosomal overload results in the abrupt release of Cu into the hepatocyte cytosol, leading to oxidant stress and hepatic necrosis. The resultant inflammation leads to cirrhotic changes.

d. Iodine.

i. Homeostasis and deficiency Iodine (I) is absorbed fully from stomach and colon and is taken up almost exclusively by the thyroid, although it can be found in kidney, salivary gland, and, to a lesser extent, in stomach, skin, mammary gland, placenta, and ovary. In the thyroid, I_2 is both stored and incorporated into the hormone thyroxine, necessary for the growth and regulation of metabolic rate and body temperature. Thyroxine and its active metabolite, triiodothyronine, are circulating hormones that, when metabolized, release their I_2 for excretion via urine, milk, and, to a lesser extent, feces and sweat. The ability of the

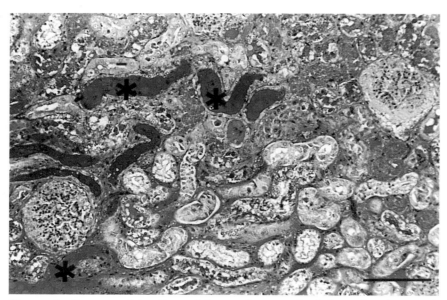

Figure 8. Copper toxicity. Hemoglobin nephrosis in the kidney of a sheep with massive hemolysis due to excessive copper ingestion. Tubules containing hemoglobin pigment (*) are dilated, and the epithelium is atrophied or sloughed. Hematoxylin and eosin. Bar: 50 μm.

thyroid gland to concentrate iodine is at once a blessing and a curse. It is a blessing in that intermittent sources of I_2 can be retained for synthesis during times of dietary deficiency. It is a curse in that episodic exposure of I_2-deficient individuals to a high I_2 source can lead to toxic accumulations of I_2 within a goiter. This is because during the time of deficiency the gland alters its metabolic baseline to compensate for the deficiency by increasing its efficiency of uptake. On the brighter side, it is also the unique power of the thyroid to accumulate I_2 that permits the use of radioiodine as a successful drug in the treatment of hyperthyroidism.

Iodine deficiency is associated with decreased fertility, disruption of embryonic and postnatal development, and increased fetal and perinatal mortality. Fetal deficiency results in neurological damage known as cretinism and includes spastic dysphagia and severe mental retardation. The major lesion of I_2 deficiency in both newborn and adult is hyperplasia of thyroid follicles and hypertrophy of individual follicular cells, with colloid production. Goiter often develops when I_2 is restored to the diet after a period of deficiency due to the overproduction

of colloid by a more efficient uptake by the compensated epithelium. In the Western world, I_2 deficiency has not been a problem since table salt fortification with potassium iodide was initiated. However, because of the uneven distribution of I_2 within the earth's crust, I_2 deficiency continues to be an important health problem in underdeveloped countries, readily discernible as thyroid goiters that can grow to become grossly disfiguring, causing obstruction to nearby organs, including trachea, larynx, and esophagus. Because thiocyanate competitively inhibits I_2 uptake into the thyroid, a marginally I_2-deficient diet containing cyanogenic glycosides, such as those found in cassava, can produce overt I_2 deficiency. Endemic neurological and neuromuscular abnormalities are common in areas of the world that are low in I_2 and depend on cassava as a major starch source. Fertility and survival of both livestock and the human population are affected adversely.

ii. Excess I_2-replete individuals are tolerant of high levels of I_2, shown by the fact that I_2 is used therapeutically in asthma to counter viscous bronchial secretions. In animals, I_2 is used therapeutically to treat foot rot and soft tissue

622

lumpy jaw in cattle, as well as for teat dips and udder washes for sanitizing. However, individuals who are marginally or overtly I_2 deficient are very sensitive to even moderate doses of I_2 and can develop thyrotoxicosis, particularly those who already have a nodular goiter. Because overt signs of thyrotoxicosis, such as exophthalmus, may not always be evident, weight loss, muscle weakness, and tachycardia may go undetected until the situation is life-threatening, particularly for individuals with underlying cardiac heart disease. Iodism can occur even in livestock fed the high end of "safe" dietary I_2 levels during long periods of time. The lesions, including weight loss, anorexia, lethargy, lacrimation, and scaly skin, mimic those of hypothyroidism, as excessive I_2 will inhibit the secretion of thyroid-stimulating hormone from the pituitary and actually lead to the decreased production of thyroxine. Maximum tolerable doses appear to be 50 ppm for most species, although horses are more sensitive and 5 ppm is suggested as a maximum. Excessive doses of I_2 given to experimental animals have caused decreased egg laying in chickens, loss of appetite, anemia, anorexia, and vomiting, leading to prostration, coma, and death. Goiters (thyroid hyperplasia) may also form in a number of animals. Upon autopsy, fatty deposits and areas of necrosis can be observed in liver, kidney, and mucosa of the GI tract. There are reports of retinal changes in dog, rabbit, and guinea pig.

e. Iron.

i. Homeostasis and deficiency Iron deficiency is the most common nutritional deficiency in humans, both within the United States and worldwide, producing microcytic anemia with concomitant low energy, impaired intellectual performance, and failure to maintain body temperature. Resistance to infection appears to be decreased, although the relationship between Fe deficiency and immunity has not been defined. Men store 30 to 40% of absorbed Fe, whereas women only store 10 to 15% due to loss of blood during menses and utilization of Fe during pregnancy and lactation, putting them at risk for Fe deficiency. Infants and young children have high Fe requirements because they are growing rapidly, and neonates frequently depend on milk for nutrition, which is a poor source of Fe. Infants born prematurely are at particular risk for Fe deficiency anemia, as neonates normally accumulate Fe stores during the third trimester. The body Fe load is regulated by Fe uptake, which depends on dietary content and form of Fe, in addition to body Fe status and erythrocyte synthetic rate (erythrocytes contain approximately two-thirds of body Fe). Iron absorption is regulated by the intestinal mucosal cells, with separate uptake systems for heme and nonheme iron, the former being more bioavailable by three- or fourfold. Environmental Pb toxicosis is often associated with Fe deficiency. This is due partly to the enhanced uptake of Pb by the Fe uptake system, which is unregulated in Fe deficiency, but also partly environmental, with those in the lower socioeconomic bracket often being both Fe deficient and living in a Pb-contaminated environment. Among domestic animals, young pigs, often raised in confinement with no access to soil, are especially prone to Fe deficiency and must be supplemented via injections.

ii. Excess Excess Fe produces depressed feed intake and growth rate. The lowest dose with an adverse effect is 500 ppm in calves, poultry, and sheep, although one group suggested that lambs receiving as little as 210 ppm Fe can exhibit diarrhea after only 1 month. Swine appear to have no adverse effects at doses as high as 3000 ppm, although body weight gain and feed intake are depressed at 5000 ppm Fe and signs of P deficiency appear. High Fe levels interfere with P, Cu, and vitamin E metabolism so that chickens can tolerate high Fe levels (1600 ppm) if Cu levels are raised. Iron excess in premature infants low in vitamin E rapidly produces oxidative damage in erythrocytes, leading to hemolytic anemia.

Hemorrhagic necrosis of the gastrointestinal tract, with bloody vomitus and black stools, are characteristic pathological signs of acute ingestion of excess Fe. This can be associated with elevated serum Fe, vascular congestion of multiple organs, anorexia, oliguria, diarrhea, hypothermia, metabolic acidosis, shock, and death. Hereditary hemochromatosis, a genetic abnormality in Fe uptake, causes Fe accumulation in various parenchymal cells, producing hepatic cirrhosis, arthritis, diabetes, and heart failure. Because there is no excretory system for Fe, the only treatment for Fe overload is phlebotomy or Fe chelation. The possibility that a nutritional Fe overload may be associated with increased risk for either cancer or cardiac heart disease has been raised, but further studies did not support either claim.

f. Manganese.

i. Homeostasis and deficiency Manganese, a name derived from the Greek word for magic, has long been recognized as essential for full growth and normal reproduction. Absorbed freely throughout the GI tract, Mn homeostasis appears to be regulated by excretion. Dietary aluminum (Al), Fe, and phytate are reported to slow absorption. This supports the suggestion that Mn may share the same uptake system as Fe and Al, although there are no data to support this proposal. Studies do show that Mn shares the transferrin system with Fe and Al for transport in blood. Ethanol has been found to increase the body load of Mn, possibly through the upregulation of Mn-dependent superoxide dismutase (Mn-SOD). Dietary Mn deficiency is rare, but can be a particular problem in grazing cattle, swine, and poultry, resulting in skeletal abnormalities and defective lipid and carbohydrate metabolism in addition to adverse effects on growth and reproduction. Manganese-deficient pigs have short, thick limbs, curvature of the spine, and swollen and enlarged joints due to the defective synthesis of ground substance in developing cartilage. Both osteoblast and osteoclast activities are depressed, aggravating defective bone development. Ataxia develops in animals that are deficient *in utero* due to the calcification of otoliths, cartilaginous structures in the inner ear. Pancreatic abnormalities, including hypoplasia, and depressed insulin synthesis and secretion can be corrected by feeding Mn. Ultrastructural changes in Mn deficiency, including an altered integrity of cell membranes,

swollen and irregular endoplasmic reticulum, and elongated mitochondria with stacked cristae, are considered a result of disrupted lipid metabolism.

ii. Excess Excessive Mn exposure in humans, typically derived from industrial dusts or contaminated water, can interfere with Fe uptake and transportation, producing Fe deficiency anemia. CNS abnormalities are seen, including hyperirritability, violent acts, hallucinations, and incoordination. Permanent damage occurs in the extrapyramidal system, producing symptoms similar to those of Parkinsonism. Also, like Al, Mn has been implicated in some cases of amyotrophic lateral sclerosis. Dietary Mn appears to have little adverse effect below 1000 ppm unless Fe levels are low. In one study it was reported that hemoglobin levels were depressed by as little as 125 ppm Mn in the diet. Interestingly, when Fe levels were increased to 400 ppm, even 2000 ppm Mn had no adverse effect on hemoglobin levels. Neurological abnormalities, including a transient paralysis of the extremities, have been reported only infrequently in animals receiving excess dietary Mn, where depressed growth, abnormal reproduction, and anemia are more typical.

g. Molybdenum.

i. Homeostasis and deficiency Molybdenum is required for three enzymes: sulfite oxidase, aldehyde oxidase, and xanthine oxidase; the recommended intake is 0.075 to 0.25 mg/day. Knowledge about Mo metabolism is sparse and relatively recent. Although Mo was shown to be essential in the 1950s, the first case of a human deficiency, secondary to Crohn's disease, was reported only in the 1980s. Molybdenum absorption appears to be in excess of 90%, occurring in the stomach and throughout the GI tract. Following uptake, Mo concentrates in the liver and kidney, from where it is excreted into both urine and bile. In the laboratory, signs of deficiency include high plasma methionine, high urinary sulfate, and increased sensitivity to sulfite toxicity, associated with abnormal S metabolism. In addition, experimentally Mo-deficient animals produce high urinary xanthine and hypoxanthine due to low xanthine oxidase activity, interrupting uric acid production. When similar disturbances in S and uric acid metabolism, associated with mental retardation, were seen in a patient on prolonged total parenteral nutrition (TPN), Mo treatment reversed the disorder. Deficiency can also be precipitated by dietary inclusion of tungsten, a Mo antagonist. Because bacterial nitrate reductase is Mo dependent, tolerance to dietary nitrate poisoning can be induced in sheep by including tungsten in the diet. However, while Mo deficiency may prevent nitrate poisoning, other manifestations of Mo deficiency not yet defined could be precipitated by such treatment. For example, there are unconfirmed reports that some New Zealand sheep developed xanthine calculi associated with Mo deficiency. Knowledge is still missing in the area of Mo deficiency disorders.

ii. Excess Molybdenum toxicity occurs when animals graze on plants growing on high Mo soils. Ruminants are most susceptible to Mo toxicity. Signs of toxicity are due mostly to a secondary Cu deficiency, with growth depression and anemia, anorexia, diarrhea, and posterior weakness with spinal cord degeneration, as described previously (Fig. 7). Unrelieved, animals become emaciated and finally die. Sheep have "crimping" or curling of wool and loss of wool pigmentation. Molybdenum toxicosis can be reversed by Cu supplementation. Humans exposed through industry or in areas with high natural Mo levels such as Armenia have elevated plasma uric acid levels and an increased incidence of gout.

h. Selenium.

i. Homeostasis and deficiency Se may be incorporated into the diet as inorganic selenium (selenite), seleno methionine, or selenocysteine. Eventually all are converted to selenite from whence, after conversion to selenophosphate, Se can be incorporated into proteins and RNA. A Se-deficient, torula yeast diet will precipitate hepatic necrosis and reproductive failure in rats, pancreatic dystrophy and exudative diathesis in chicks, hepatosis dietetica in swine, and white muscle disease in young lambs. While all of these syndromes can be reversed by feeding Se, Se requirements vary inversely with vitamin E and S amino acid status of the animal, and many Se deficiency syndromes can be diminished or even abolished by treatment with vitamin E. Thus Se deficiency uncomplicated by vitamin E status, while it can be defined in the laboratory, is not unraveled so easily in farm animals. Humans living in Se-low districts of China exhibit a cardiomyopathy termed Keshan's disease that can be corrected by feeding Se. A similar myopathy is seen in horses and nonhuman primates. Se may be anticarcinogenic if given at slightly greater doses than those required for full growth. However, epidemiological studies within the United States have not found any relationship between toenail Se status and cancer rates in women. The Finish government, in 1984, decided to incorporate Se into fertilizers, which lead to a dramatic increase in body Se loads. However, cancer mortality rates have not changed. At even higher levels, Se is positively carcinogenic.

ii. Excess Foraging of seleniferous plants can lead to toxicosis, termed selenosis. The hallmark of selenosis is the shedding of hair and sloughing of hoofs. Some seleniferous plants disrupt vision and produce stumbling and respiratory failure. These "blind staggers" probably are due to alkaloids in the plants rather than to Se. However, lameness, with malformation of hoofs, loss of hair, and emaciation are reproducible under experimental conditions by feeding Se and therefore are thought to be due to chronic exposure to raised levels of Se. While the response to severe Se excess varies among species, the most common outcome is hemorrhagic enteritis and myocardial hemorrhage. The latter leads to myocardial degeneration, cardiac insufficiency, and subsequent congestion and edema in visceral organs. In addition, reproduction can be affected adversely or diffuse hemorrhage may be found in the lungs. Fatty change, necrosis, and hemorrhage are evident in the liver, kidney, and pancreas. In pigs and horses, degeneration of gray matter of the spinal cord can develop, with necrosis of neurons, cavitation, and necrosis in ventral horn areas (Fig. 9).

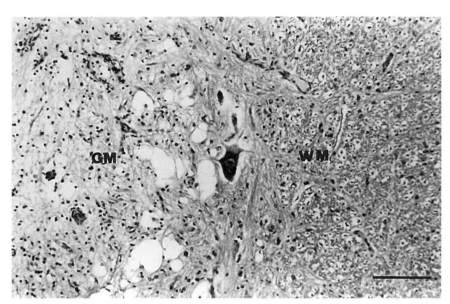

Figure 9. Selenium toxicity. Polioencephalomalacia in the gray matter (GM) of the ventral horn in the spinal cord of a pig, characterized by degeneration and loss of nerve cell bodies. White matter (WM) is unaffected. Hematoxylin and eosin. Bar: 25 μm.

i. Zinc.

i. Homeostasis and deficiency Unlike most other divalent cations, Zn has no redox chemistry. However, Zn is a strong Lewis acid, permitting it to bind well to thiolate and amine electron donors within the cell: Zn is >95% intracellular. Zinc homeostasis is regulated by both absorption (greatest in the jejunum in humans) and excretion (pancreatic secretion and direct secretion along the entire length of the gut). Plasma Zn, normally 1 μg/ml, can fluctuate greatly with intake and with stresses. Fasting is associated with hyperzincemia due to the release of Zn from muscle, while infection is associated with hypozincemia. In pancreatitis, Zn absorption is decreased and urinary excretion of Zn is increased. As a counterpoint to this, Zn deficiency produces changes in the exocrine pancreas, including loss of zymogen granules with the appearance of lipid droplets and prominent lysosome-like bodies. Even before a decrease in tissue concentration is evident, Zn deficiency causes a reduction in growth, associated with a reduction in food intake, termed Zn-related anorexia. This anoretic growth retardation has the effect of permitting Zn levels to remain more nearly normal. In contrast, if a rat is force fed a Zn-deficient diet, it continues to grow, plasma Zn levels fall, and the animal soon dies. Zinc deficiency is characterized not only by depressed appetite and retarded growth, but by skin lesions, immune deficiency, skeletal abnormalities, and impaired reproduction. Chronic Zn deficiency in humans is manifest as dwarfism and sexual immaturity, and even acute deficiency rapidly produces characteristic symmetrical skin lesions, prevalent around the facial orifices in humans but over sparsely haired areas as well in other species. The primary lesion of the skin that appears to underlie the skin condition in most species is acanthosis with parakeratosis and accumulation crusts of parakeratotic cellular debris on epidermal surfaces. This "acrodermatitis enteropathica" is especially common in Zn-deficient swine and is typically associated with infection, due to loss of immune function. It has also been reported in dogs, cats, and ruminants. While Zn deficiency has been linked to thymic atrophy and loss of immune function, the biochemical lesion is unknown. Fetal zinc deficiency results in severe alteration of normal bone formation and, in birds, abnormal feathering. Zinc deficiency is teratogenic in all species evaluated.

Zinc deficiency is not common and usually is caused either by a dietary component that has decreased Zn bioavailability, such as phytate, or by a GI disorder disrupting absorption such as alcoholism, cirrhosis, malabsorption, or pancreatitis. Soy-based foods or infant formulas are high in phytate and can precipitate Zn deficiency. Very high pharmacologic doses of Fe or Ca can interfere with Zn absorption, but within the normal dietary range, other minerals are without effect on Zn homeostasis. For the toxicologist, one should remember that EDTA chelation therapy in Pb-intoxicated patients, while given as the Ca salt in order to avoid Ca deficiency, can also deplete the body of Zn.

ii. Excess Zn toxicity is not encountered under normal dietary conditions. Acute Zn toxicity results in gastric distress, nausea, and disorientation. Emesis occurs with >150 mg. High Zn levels, like Zn deficiency, can cause immunocompromise and decreased feed intake. Examination of chronically Zn-intoxicated chickens revealed loss of feather pigmentation, feed refusal, and weight loss, possibly associated with defective pancreatic acinar cell function. Decreased bone mineralization and bone and joint deformities have been reported in several species, particularly swelling of the epiphyseal region of the long bones in horses, associated with lameness. These effects are considered to be associated with Zn-induced Cu deficiency due to a metallothionein/Cu interaction, leading to hypochromic anemia. This anemia is not due to Fe deficiency, as Fe can be seen accumulated in sideroblasts. However, if Zn intoxication persists, interference with both Cu and Fe absorption occurs, leading to a true Fe deficiency anemia. Interestingly, swine, unlike other species, exhibit no anemia and no decrease in circulating Cu levels. For most species, 1000 ppm Zn is associated with decreased tissue levels of Cu, Fe, and Mn, in addition to decreased utilization of Ca and P. Establishing a "maximum safe level" of Zn in

the diet is complicated by the interaction of Zn with dietary components such as phytate. In a purified casein-based diet, even 125 ppm Zn proved adverse to Japanese quail, whereas in regular diets, maximum tolerable levels appeared to vary between 300 for sheep to 1000 for most species, including swine and chickens, possibly dependent on differences in Zn bioavailability from different feeds.

Metal workers have been reported to suffer from metal fume fever, associated with inhalation of oxides of Zn and other metals. Symptoms include nausea, cough, headache, fever, and GI and muscle pain, and are thought to be allergenic, most often encountered on Mondays, after a 2-day weekend. Thereafter tolerance rebuilds and symptoms resolve.

IV. Dietary Contaminants

The "problem" of pesticides and other contaminants in the diet is a complex and controversial one, especially for human diets. Much attention has been focused on estimating an acceptable daily intake for humans, a judgement based on the no observed adverse effect level for a particular compound. The calculation of a NOAEL is based on determining the dose threshold in the most sensitive test or assay in the species most sensitive to the compound in question, with an additional "safety factor" multiplied into the equation. The calculation of an ADI is complicated by a variety of things, one of which from the nutrition aspect is the fact that children consume more food on a body weight basis than adults and that neonates and females of reproductive age have other considerations that must be taken into consideration when making the calculation. In the context of estimating ADIs for "contaminants" in the diet, it must be remembered that fruits and vegetables contain carcinogens "naturally" themselves, yet overall consumption of such foods consistently has been identified in epidemiologic and experimental studies as "beneficial."

Regarding pesticides, much of the current research has been focused on carbamates and organophosphates, with much debate centered around which rodent assay should take precedence when determining NOAEL and which uncertainty factor should be used for estimating the ADI—the rodent uncertainty factor of 100X or the human-based uncertainty factor of 10X. Complicating the debate is the observation that not all carbamates or organophosphates have the same mechanism of action, requiring modification of old or the development of new assays. Some scientists have concluded that covalently bound pesticide residues in foods (e.g., edible animal tissues) are either not bioavailable or nonreactive in their covalently bound form and hence of little concern to humans. Much of the evidence to date has been nebulous or inconclusive that low levels of pesticides in the diet result in a cancer risk to humans. Many of the pesticides (e.g., chlorinated hydrocarbons) that have been shown to be carcinogenic in rodent assay systems have yet to be shown to be associated with cancer in humans, and mix studies, using mixtures of common pesticides at levels that might be encountered realistically in the diet, have been negative for oxidative DNA damage in rodents, with the exception of diphenylamine and chlorothalonil.

Of more relevance to the toxicologic pathologist is the contamination of diets used to feed animals in experimental situations. Harmful naturally occuring substances, as well as man-made contaminants, have been found in commercial animal diets during the past decades. This is a more important problem, perhaps, when "natural" ingredients are used, the composition of which may vary considerably from batch to batch. This is particularly true when using plant material that may have widely varying concentrations of phytochemicals, depending on growth conditions, variety of plant grown, and processing for dietary inclusion. Furthermore, the problem of pesticide contamination is sometimes not considered when purchasing materials for inclusion in the dietary formulations.

In addition, certain nutrients assume new or exaggerated relevance when certain experimental compounds are studied. For example, dietary folate becomes an important covariate when studying contraceptives or anticonvulsants. In rodent cancer studies, low dietary folate increases the risk of a malignant response to colonic carcinogens and depresses the safety and efficacy of chemotherapeutic agents such as cyclophosphamide. In a similar fashion, high dietary Fe can exacerbate aminoglycoside ototoxicity due to the generation of free radicals and depletion of glutathione in the ear, whereas high dietary Ca can affect Zn absorption and metabolism, altering appetite and a variety of other metabolic processes. Phytochemicals become of importance when studies involving the induction or suppression of phase I or phase II drug-metabolizing enzymes are being performed or when the toxicity (as well as safety and/or efficacy) of a drug is dependent on induction or suppression of a particular detoxification enzyme.

Although more attention has been paid to sources of components for dietary formulations in recent years, major variations in dietary concentrations of various bioactive compounds have been observed in past studies, especially in the so-called natural product diets. This variation has resulted in appreciable variations in response in certain species to specific drugs or chemicals both within studies and between studies. This is especially relevant in the context of mycotoxin contamination of dietary components, where minuscule concentrations can cause significant alterations in response or even trigger toxicity in a sensitive species (e.g., aflatoxin in the rat). Common contaminants of experimental diets that have been identified in the past include mycotoxins such as aflatoxin, heavy metals (lead, mercury, cadmium, and arsenic), nitrates, nitrosamines, chlorinated hydrocarbons, and polychlorinated biphenyls. Therefore, it is of prime importance that all dietary components, natural or formulated, be evaluated and analyzed before inclusion in any experimental diet.

SUGGESTED READING

Macronutrients

Becker, D. E., Ullrey, D. E., and Terrill, S. W. (1954). A comparison of carbohydrates in a synthetic milk diet for the baby pig. *Arch. Biochem. Biophys.* **48**, 178–183.

Becker, D. E., Ullrey, D. E., Terrill, S. W., and Notzoid, R. A. (1954). Failure of the newborn pig to utilize sucrose. *Science* **120**, 345–346.

Carpenter, K. J., Harper, A. E., and Olson, R. E. (1997). Experiments that changed nutritional thinking. *J. Nutr.* **127**, 1017S–1053S.

Chandra, R. K. (1997). Nutrition and the immune system: An introduction. *Am. J. Clin. Nutr.* **66**, 460S–463S.

Cori, G. T., Ochoa, S., Slein, M. W., and Cori, C. F. (1951). The metabolism of fructose in liver: Isolation of fructose-1-phosphate and inorganic pyrophosphate. *Biochim. Biophys. Acta* **7**, 304–317.

Henning, S. J. (1981). Postnatal development: Coordination of feeding, digestion and metabolism. *Am. J. Physiol.* **241**, G199–G214.

Vitamins

Bendich, A., and Machlin, I. J. (1988). Safety of oral intake of vitamin E. *Am. J. Clin. Nutr.* **48**, 612–619.

Biesalski, H. K., and Seelert, K., (1989). Vitamin A deficiency: New knowledge on diagnosis, consequences and therapy. *Z. Ernahrungswiss.* **28**, 3–16.

Chen, L. H. (1981). An increase in vitamin E requirement induced by high supplementation of vitamin C in rats. *Am. J. Clin. Nutr.* **34**, 1036–1041.

Hathcock, J. N., Hattan, D. G., Jenkins, M. Y., McDonald, J. T., Sundaresan, P. R., and Wilkening, V. I. (1990). Evaluation of vitamin A toxicity. *Am. J. Clin. Nutr.* **52**(2), 183–202.

Jones, T. C., Hunt, R. J., and King, N. W. (1996) Nutritional Deficiencies. *In* "Veterinary Pathology" (T. C. Jones, R. J. Hunt, and N. W. King, eds.), 6th Ed., Chapter 16, pp. 781–815, Williams & Wilkins, Baltimore.

Kato, Y., Sakamoto, S., Miura, Y., and Takaku, F. (1985). Disorders of cobalamin metabolism. *Crit. Rev. Oncol. Hematol.* **3**, 1–34.

Marks, K. H., Kilav, R., Naveh-Many, T., and Silver, J. (1996). Calcium, phosphate, vitamin D, and the parathyroid. *Pediatr. Nephrol.* **10**, 364–367.

Moore, T. (1965). Vitamin A deficiency and excess. *Proc. Nutr. Soc.* **24**, 129–135.

National Academy of Sciences Subcommittee on Vitamin Tolerance (1987). "Vitamin Tolerance of Animals." National Academy Press, Washington, DC.

Rechcigl, M. (ed.) (1978). *In* "Nutritional Disorders," CRC Handbook Series in Nutrition and Food, Vol. 1, Sec. E. CRC Press, Boca Raton, FL.

Scott, J., and Weir, D. (1994). Folate/vitamin B12 interrelationships. *Essays Biochem.* **28**, 63–72.

Shane, B., and Stokstad, E. L., (1985). Vitamin B12-folate interrelationships. *Ann. Rev. Nutr.* **5**, 115–141.

Smith, J. C., Jr. (1980). The vitamin A-zinc connection: A review. *Ann. N. Y. Acad. Sci.* **355**, 62–75.

Van Vleet, J. F., and Ferrans, V. J., (1992). Etiologic factors and pathologic alterations in selenium-vitamin E deficiency and excess in animals and humans. *Biol. Trace Elem. Res.* **33**, 1–21.

Minerals

Mertz, W. (ed.) (1987). "Trace Elements in Human and Animal Nutrition," 5th Ed., Vols. 1 and 2. Academic Press, San Diego.

National Academy of Sciences Subcommittee on Mineral Tolerance of Animals (1980). "Mineral Tolerance of Domestic Animals." National Academy Press, Washington, DC.

Pais, I., and Benton Jones, J. (1997). "The Handbook of Trace Elements." St. Lucie Press, Boca Raton, FL.

Taylor, A. (1996). Detection and monitoring of disorders of essential trace elements. *Ann. Clin. Biochem.* **33**, 486–510.

Ziegler, E., and Filer, L. (eds.) "Present Knowledge in Nutrition," 7th Ed. ILSI Press, Washington, DC.

Dietary Contaminants

Abelson, P. H. (1995). Exaggerated risks of chemicals. *J. Clin. Epidemiol.* **48**, 173–178.

Ames, B., and Gold, L. S. (1998). The causes and prevention of cancer: The role of environment. *Biotherapy* **11**, 205–220.

Gross, R. L., and Newberne, P. M. (1977). Naturally occuring toxic substances in foods. *Clin. Pharmacol. Ther.* **22**(5 Pt. 2), 680–698.

Karew, W., Akhtar, M. H., and Khan, S. U. (1996). Bioavailability of bound pesticide residues and potential toxicologic consequences: An update. *Proc. Soc. Exp. Biol. Med.* **11**, 62–68.

Lodovici, M., Casalini, C., Briani, C., and Dolara, K. (1997). Oxidative liver DNA damage in rats treated with pesticide mixtures. *Toxicology* **14**, 55–60.

Newberne, P. M., and McConnell, R. G. (1980). Dietary nutrients and contaminants in laboratory animal experimentation. *J. Environ. Pathol. Toxicol.* **4**, 105–122.

Newberne, P. M., and Sotnikov, A. V. (1996). Diet: The neglected variable in chemical safety evaluations. *Toxicol. Pathol.* **24**, 745–756.

Walker, R. (1998). Toxicity testing and derivation of the ADI. *Food Addit. Contam.* **15**(Suppl.), 11–16.

24

Phycotoxins

Philip F. Solter
Department of Veterinary Pathobiology
University of Illinois at Urbana-Champaign
Urbana, Illinois

Val R. Beasley
Department of Veterinary Biosciences
University of Illinois at Urbana-Champaign
Urbana, Illinois

I. Introduction

Phycotoxins are potent organic compounds produced by dinoflagellates, other flagellated phytoplankton, and cyanobacteria that inhabit marine, brackish, or freshwater environments. At least 100 different species of organisms may harbor toxins. In the marine environment, exposure of humans, other mammals, and birds to toxins can occur either from direct contact or consumption of these toxins or by passage of the toxin through the food chain to shellfish or finfish. Large die-offs of fish may also occur. High concentrations of dinoflagellates can color the waters, and some are known as red tides. However, clear water may also harbor toxic levels of phycotoxins as well. Exposure to cyanobacterial toxins in fresh water environments is most frequently through direct consumption of contaminated water. Eutrophication of fresh, estuarine, or marine waters can result in massive blooms of toxic cyanobacteria.

Handbook of Toxicologic Pathology, Second Edition
Volume 1

II. Diarrheic Shellfish Poisoning

Diarrheic shellfish poisoning (DSP) is most commonly caused by the toxin okadaic acid or related analogues known as dinophysistoxins (Fig. 1). The toxins are potent inhibitors of serine/threonine protein phosphatase types 1 (PP1) and 2A (PP2A). Okadaic acid is a more potent inhibitor of PP2A than PP1, with IC_{50} values for PP2A from 0.07 to $0.2\,nM$ and for PP1 of 3.4 to $19\,nM$.

The principal route of exposure of humans to DSP toxins is through consumption of contaminated mussels, scallops, and other shellfish. The toxins accumulate in the hepatopancreas of shellfish. Clinical signs of toxicosis are best described for humans who experience mild to severe diarrhea, vomiting, and abdominal pain. Experimentally, okadaic acid has been shown to be a potent tumor promoter and an inducer of apoptosis. It may also be genotoxic, forming DNA adducts. Effects of experimental exposure of suckling balb/c mice to dinophystoxin-1 were described by Terao and colleagues in 1986. Gross lesions were limited to the small intestine, which contained mucus as well as distension in the upper small intestine. Histopathological

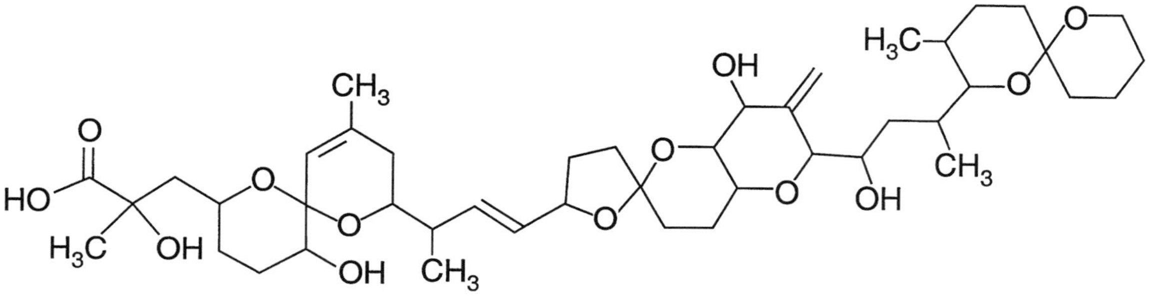

Okadaic Acid

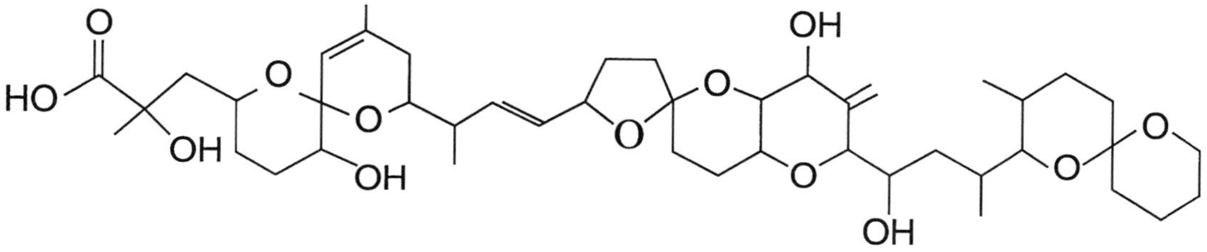

Dinophysistoxin-1

Figure 1. Basic structures of okadaic acid and dinophysistoxin-1, which are causes of diarrheic shellfish poisoning.

findings also included edema of the lamina propria of villi and, at higher doses, vacuolation of mucosal epithelial cells. The villous and submucosal vessels were congested and became severely so at higher doses. Transmission electron microscopy revealed three dose-dependent sequential levels or stages of degenerative change to the intestine. The first stage involved edema and extravasation of serum into the lamina propria. In the second stage, epithelial absorptive cells contained dilated Golgi apparatus cisternae, filled with flocculent material and large vaculoes within the apical portions of the cells. Degeneration of microvilli of epithelial cells was seen at higher dosages. The third stage consisted of detachment of mucosal epithelial cells from the basement membrane, desquamation of perivascular tissues, and focal erosions of the intestinal mucosa.

Okadaic acid and dinophystoxin-1 also cause hepatic damage, including subcapsular hemorrhage, degeneration of hepatic sinusoidal endothelial cells, and dissociation of ribosomes from endoplasmic reticulum as well as autophagic vacuoles within midzonal hepatocytes.

Two other toxins, pectenotoxins and yessotoxin, also have been classified as DSP toxins, despite the fact that they reportedly do not cause diarrhea and produce different histopathologic findings. Neither is as likely as okadaic acid to occur at toxic concentrations in the environment or in food. Pectenotoxins are polyether lactone hepatotoxins (Fig. 2). Lesions include hepatic congestion, necrosis, and vacuolation of periportal hepatocytes that can compress organelles. Yessotoxins are sulfated compounds whose toxic effects include dyspnea and rapid death when administered intraperiton-

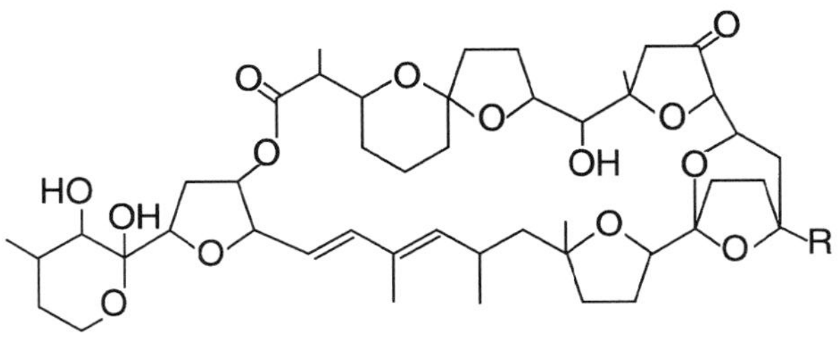

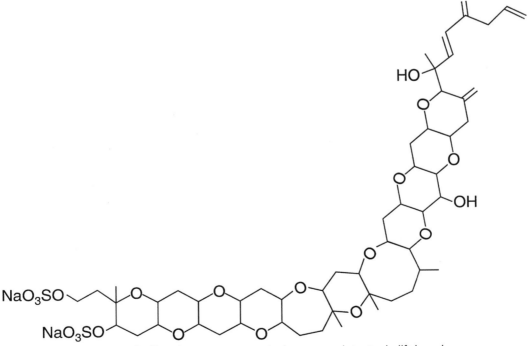

Figure 2. The structure of pectenotoxin-1, a polyether lactone hepatotoxin found in shellfish.

eally to mice (Fig. 3). The target organ appears to be the heart with intracytoplasmic edema present in cardiac muscle cells on electron microscopic examination. With higher doses, swelling occurs in most cardiac muscle cells and degeneration is apparent in endothelial capillaries of the left ventricle. The desulfated form of yessotoxin causes little evidence of heart damage, but instead evidence of hepatic and pancreatic damage, including pale, swollen livers, hepatic fatty degeneration, fat droplets in hepatocytes, swollen mitochondria, and pancreatic acinar cell degeneration.

III. Paralytic Shellfish Poisoning

Paralytic shellfish poisoning (PSP) is caused by several structurally related tricyclic guanidium alkaloids that are found in several species of marine dinoflagellates (Fig. 4). The toxins are concentrated in shellfish, particularly bivalve shellfish, such as mussels, clams, and scallops, the ingestion of which serve as the major cause of PSP. Cases of poisoning have occurred after consumption of reef crabs, some marine gastropods, and, very rarely, finfish. Fish kills from toxic blooms are nevertheless common. The PSP toxins, including saxitoxin, neosaxitoxin, gonyautoxin, and decarbomyl toxin, block voltage-regulated sodium channels in myelinated and nonmyelinated nerves, resulting in relaxation of vascular smooth muscle, depression of cardiac muscle action potentials, and inhibition of axonal impulse transmission to skeletal muscles.

Clinical signs of toxicoses in animals include incoordination, recumbency, and death by

Figure 3. The structure of sulfated yessotoxin, a toxin that accumulates in shellfish and causes cardiac damage.

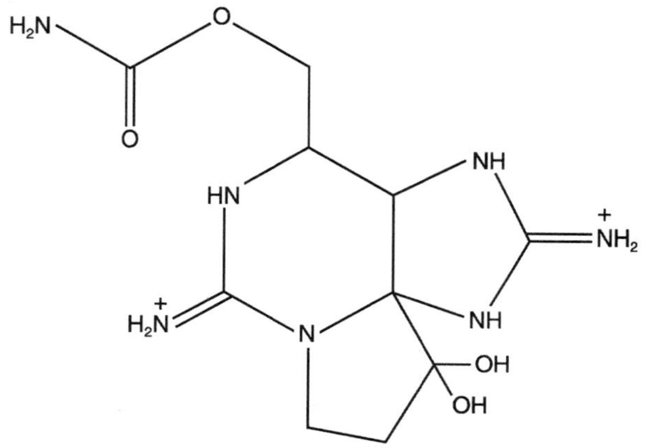

Figure 4. The structure of saxitoxin, one cause of paralytic shellfish poisoning. Its structure is representative of toxins of this group.

respiratory failure. In humans, clinical signs include paresthesia and numbness of the lips and mouth that progress to the face, neck, and extremities. Acute death occurs from respiratory failure. Nausea and vomiting can also occur. There are no specific lesions of PSP, although evidence of cyanosis may be noted.

IV. Amnesic Shellfish Poisoning

Domoic acid and several isomers of domoic acid that are structural analogs of the neuroexcitatory amino acid, glutamate, cause amnesic shellfish poisoning (Fig. 5). The toxins bind to N-methy-D-aspartate (NMDA) receptors and cause neuronal damage by producing

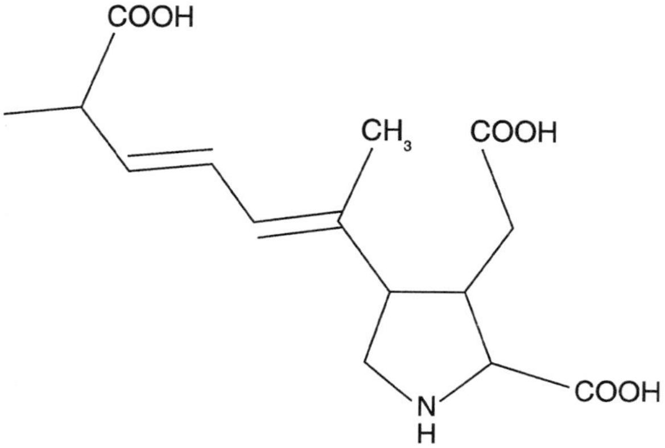

Figure 5. The structure of domoic acid, the cause of amnesic shellfish poisoning.

continuous stimulation. Such receptors are important to synaptic plasticity, which plays a role in formation and acquisition of memory. Domoic acid is produced by diatoms of the genus *Pseudo-nitzschia* and is also found in red algae. Symptoms in humans include abdominal cramps, vomiting, diarrhea, disorientation, and memory loss. Experimental exposure of cynomolgus monkeys causes vomiting, mastication, and yawning. In mice injected with domoic acid, bizarre but distinctive behaviour includes scratching of the shoulders with the hind leg, inactivity, and seizures. Acute deaths in birds, including pelicans, have also occurred. Brain damage is most evident in the limbic system and hippocampus. Mass deaths of California sea lions (*Zalophus californianus*) along the central California coast have been attributed to domoic acid toxicosis. Seizures, depression, head weaving, and ataxia occurred in affected animals. Scratching was also noted, reminiscent of the sign seen in domoic acid-exposed mice and pelicans.

Exposure to domoic acid is principally by the consumption of contaminated mussels, although the sea lion deaths were attributed to planktivorous fish. Experimental toxicoses in cynomolgus monkeys cause degeneration of neuronal bodies and terminals within the hippocampus and other limbic structures, including the entorhinal cortex, the subiculum, the piriform cortex, the lateral septum, and the dorsal lateral nucleus of the thalamus. Neurologic lesions in monkeys also included bilateral vacuolation of the neutropil, astrocytic swelling, and neuronal shrinkage in the area postrema of the medulla oblongata, which contains the vomiting center. Losses of neurons in the CA1, CA3, and CA4 area of the hippocampus have been noted in both humans and rodents. Other histology lesions include edema and neuronal degeneration in the arcuate nucleus and vacuolation and pyknosis of cells in the inner nuclear layer of the retina. Zonal vacuolation involving the neuropil of the hippocampus was seen in the affected sea lions. Several strata were involved, but pathology was most severe in the anterior ventral hippocampus. The lesions were considered similar to those observed in other species suffering from domoic acid toxicosis.

V. Ciguatera Fish Poisoning

Ciguatera fish poisoning (CFP) occurs by consumption of tropical and subtropical coral reef fish. It is the most commonly reported poisoning from consumption of fish. CFP is caused by ciguatoxins, which are lipid-soluble polyethers, structurally similar to brevetoxins and yessotoxin (Fig. 6). Several variants occur; however, the most common and potent is ciguatoxin-1. The toxins originate from *Gambierdiscus toxicus* and possibly other benthic dinoflagellates, including genera *Ostreopsis, Prorocentrum, Amphidinium,* and *Coolia*. The toxins are concentrated through the food chain, and therefore high levels are found most commonly in predatory fish. Water-soluble toxins, such as maitotoxin, coexist with ciguatoxins in *G. toxicus* and can be isolated from the digestive tracts of herbivorous fish; however, they are unlikely to be a major cause of toxicity because they are found in low concentrations in muscle tissues.

Ciguatoxins are agonists at voltage-gated sodium channels of neuromuscular junctions and membranes of sensory neurons and other excitable cells. They have a high affinity for such sodium channels and the opposite effect of tetrodotoxin or saxitoxin, which blocks sodium channels. Both cholinergic and α-andrenergic receptors are affected by ciguatoxins. Contrac-

tion of the ileum and a positive intropic effect on guinea pig cardiac muscle occur *in vitro*.

The clinical manifestations of CFP have been best described in humans and include a combination of gastrointestinal, cardiovascular, and neurological effects. Death is rare. The first symptoms appear within 10 to 30 min postingestion and include paresthesia, marked by the onset of prickling and numbness of the oral and perioral regions that extend to the hands and feet. Nausea, vomiting, watery diarrhea, abdominal cramps, myalgia, arthralgia, and, upon occasion, hypersalivation are also early clinical signs. Effects also may include chills and sweating. Exhaustion, weakness and fatigue, paresthesia, and pruritis can be present for 2 or 3 weeks. Chronic dysthesia, characterized by a reversal of hot and cold sensations, is also evident after exposure. Clinical signs of toxicoses in mice following oral or intraperitoneal exposure to ciguatoxin include hypothermia, diarrhea, lacrimation, hypersalivation, penile erection, dyspnea, cyanosis, convulsions, and death. In cats that have consumed contaminated fish, clinical signs include vomiting, diarrhea, inappetance, hypersalivation, partial tetraparesis, and ataxia.

Gross lesions in mice given ciguatoxin experimentally include large amounts of mucus in the upper colon, similar to that seen with cholera toxin. However, histologic evidence of damage to the intestinal mucosa is not a consistent finding. Ultrastructurally, there is swelling of nerve fibers and synapses in the small intestinal muscle layers and a loss of synaptic

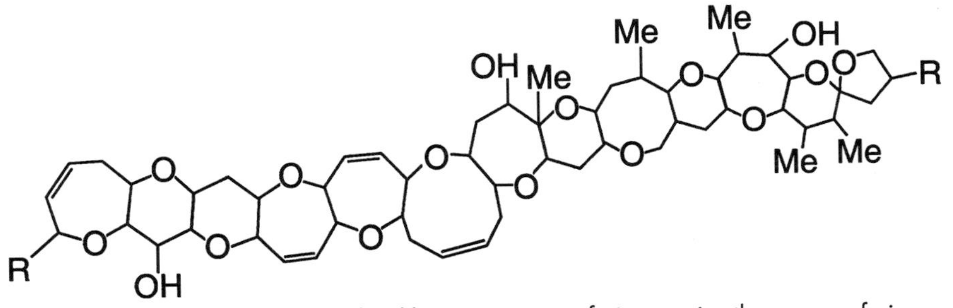

Figure 6. The basic polyether backbone structure of ciguatoxin, the cause of ciguatera fish poisoning.

vesicles. In the heart, histological findings include focal necrosis and swelling of cardiac myocytes and effusion into cardiac interstitial spaces. Capillaries in the heart may exhibit swelling of endothelial cells, narrowing of capillary lumens, and intracapillary platelet accumulation. Diffuse interstitial cardiac fibrosis of the intraventricular septum and ventricles and bilateral ventricular hypertrophy may follow repeated intraperitoneal or oral administration of ciguatoxin. Mice with severe dyspnea may have pulmonary edema and congestion, as well as degeneration of the adrenal medulla.

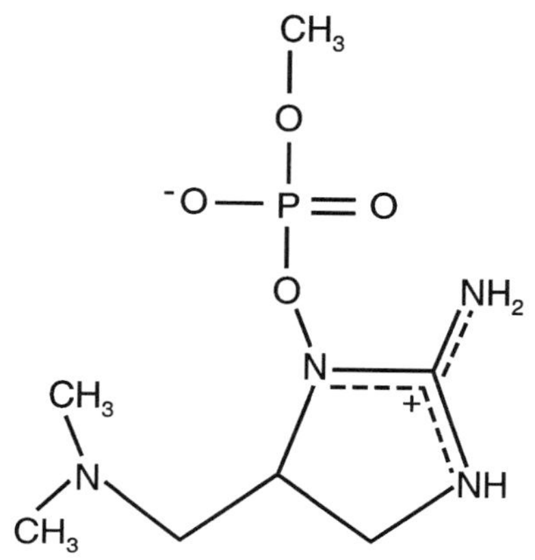

Figure 7. The structure of anatoxin-a(s), which is representative of toxins of this group.

VI. *Pfiesteria* Toxicoses

Exotoxins from the estuarine dinoflagellate *Pfiesteria piscicida* produce mass fish kills. Neurotoxic effects have been observed in laboratory workers and fishermen. The route of exposure is by aerosols or absorption from contaminated water. Clinical signs of toxicosis include neuropsychological symptoms such as reduced verbal and higher cognitive functions, memory loss, and headache. Skin lesions or a burning sensation of the skin on contact with water may also occur. Asthma-like effects and fatigue as well as sensory symptoms, including tingling or numbness of the lips, hands, and feet, also occur. Fish develop necrotic lesions over their surfaces. Histologic findings of *Pfiesteria* toxicoses have not been reported.

VII. Cyanobacterial Toxins

A. NEUROTOXINS

Neurotoxins are produced by several species of principally freshwater cyanobacteria, including *Anabaena* spp., *Oscillatoria* spp., and *Aphanizomenon* spp., and some varieties of *O. aghardii* produce the nicotinic alkaloid, anatoxin-a, which causes depolarization at postsynaptic neuromuscular junctions. *A. flos-aquae* also produces the organophosphorous cholinesterase inhibitor, anatoxin-a(s) (Fig. 7), and may also produce the sodium channel blocking

agents, saxitoxin and neosaxitoxin, which are the cause of paralytic shellfish poisoning.

Toxic exposure to cyanobacterial neurotoxins is by consumption of cyanobacteria-contaminated water supplies. Voluntary consumption is unlikely due to the poor taste of contaminated water, and therefore consumption is more frequent in animals without access to uncontaminated water, from accidental swallowing or inhalation, or consumption of dried algal crusts. Pigs and dogs are extremely sensitive to oral exposure, whereas cattle and rodents are resistant to orally administered anatoxin-a(s). Ducks have intermediate sensitivity.

Signs of anatoxin-a toxicosis include rigidity and muscle tremors, paralysis, cyanosis, and death. Death may occur very rapidly. Clinical signs of toxicosis following the experimental exposure of mice to anatoxin-a can occur within 1 or 2 min, with seizures, characterized by jumping or leaping movements, progressive limb paralysis, labored breathing, and death by respiratory arrest occurring within 15 min. Acute death may be the only thing noted in some toxicoses involving larger animals. In birds, opisthotonos may occur.

Anatoxin-a(s) toxicosis causes signs of cholinesterase inhibition, resulting in excessive salivation, urination, diarrhea, and, in mice, lacrimation, whereas rats produce red-tinged tears, or chromodacryorrhea. If severe, tremors, incoordination, paresis, paralysis, bradycardia, cyanosis, and death from respiratory arrest may occur. Anatoxin-a(s) does not cross the blood–brain or blood–retinal barriers and, as a result, does not inhibit retinal or brain cholinesterase. Anatoxin-a toxicosis is not associated with lesions. Anatoxin-a(s) toxicosis may show evidence of salivation, diarrhea, and possibly mucoid ocular discharge at necropsy.

B. HEPATOTOXINS

Several species of freshwater Cyanobacteria produce hepatotoxins, with three species of the genus *Microcystis, M. aeruginosa, M. viridis*, and *M. wesenbergii* responsible for the majority of reports of toxicoses worldwide (Fig. 8). The principal toxins involved are microcystins, which are cyclic heptapeptides of which over 50 variants have been described (Fig. 9). Microcystins may also be found in *Anabaena spp., Oscillatoria spp.,* and *Nostoc spp.* (Fig. 10). A second important hepatotoxin, nodularin, is a structurally similar cyclic pentapeptide produced by some strains of *Nodularia spumigena* (Fig. 11). *Nodularia* blooms occur in brackish water. At least two species of Cyanobacteria, *Cylindrospermopsis raciborskii* and *Umezaki natans*, produce a small cyclic guanine derivative alkaloid, cylindrospermopsin, that causes a po-

tent form of hepatoenteritis (Fig. 12). Exposure to the cyanobacteria or toxin is most commonly by oral consumption of contaminated water, however, inhalation exposure or exposure via wounds may occur. Both birds and mammals may develop hepatotoxicosis from cyanobacteria.

The mechanism of toxicity of microcystins and nodularin is inhibition of cellular serine/threonine protein phosphatase types 1 and 2A. The toxins are primarily hepatotoxins because they are cleared by bile acid-like receptors on hepatocytes. However, in humans, skin and eye irritation, hay fever symptoms, dizziness, fatigue, and gastroenteritis may all be associated with exposure to cyanobacteria. It can be difficult to say whether these signs are from hepatotoxins or neurotoxins in cyanobacteria as they are frequently found together. In other mammals, clinical signs of toxicosis related to hepatotoxicity have been described following both natural and experimental exposure. Acute fatalities within 24 hr of exposure can occur and have been attributed to hypovolemic shock from intrahepatic hemorrhage, hypoglycemia, and hyperkalemia. Further shock-like symptoms, including mucus membrane pallor,

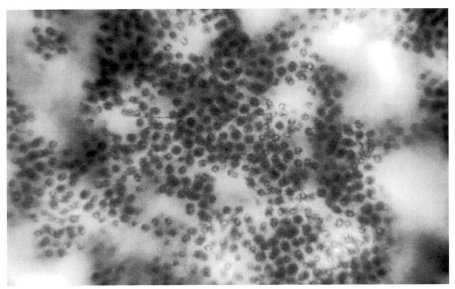

Figure 8. Typical compact colony of *Microcystis spp.* Individual cells generally average 3.0 to 5.5 μm in diameter.

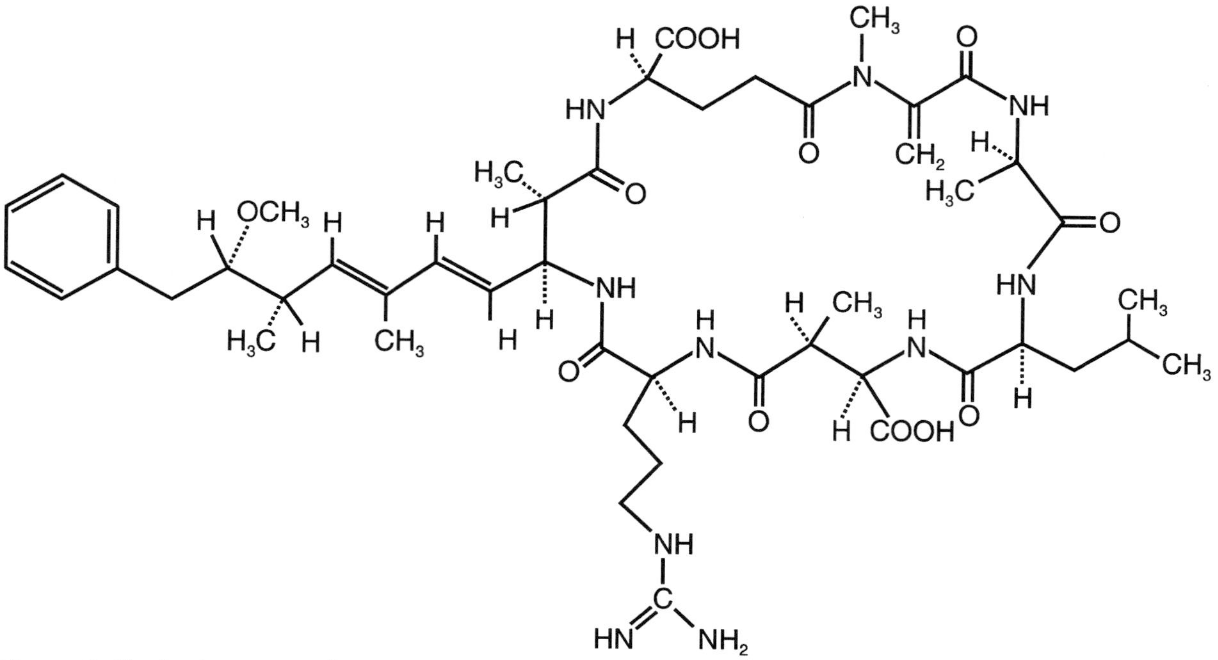

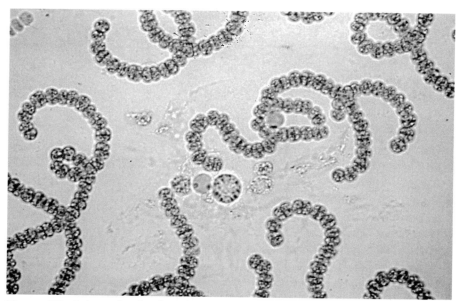

Figure 9. The basic structure of microcystin-LR, a cyclic heptapeptide hepatotoxin found in *Microcystis spp.*

tachycardia, and tachypnea, possibly secondary to acidosis, also occur. Other clinical signs in mammals include abdominal pain, vomiting, diarrhea that can be bloody, anorexia, ataxia, coma, and death. Evidence of other conditions associated with liver failure, such as photosensitivity, may occur in cattle and sheep following sublethal toxicosis. The microcystins have also been shown to have the properties of potent tumor promoters.

Many of the lesions from acute microcystin toxicity can be attributed to the mechanism of

Figure 10. Spherical cells of *Anabaena spiroides* arranged in typical filaments.

638

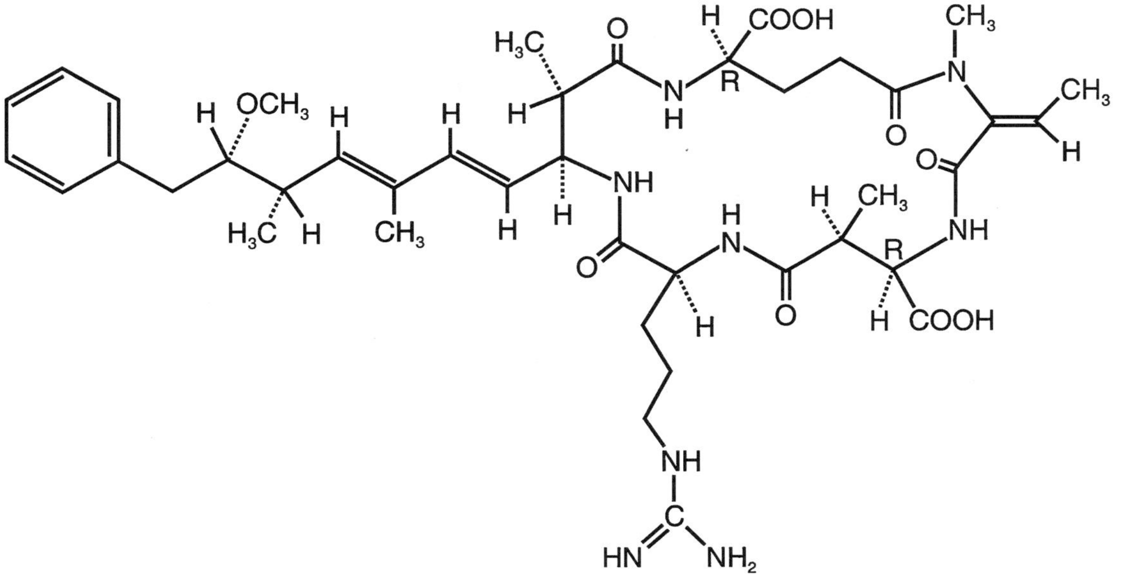

Figure 11. The basic structure of nodularin toxin, a cyclic pentapeptide hepatotoxin produced by some strains of *Nodularia spumigena*.

uptake of the toxin as well as its mechanism of toxicity. The toxin is taken up from the intestine principally in the ileum, which has a concentration of bile acid receptors. The toxin is then cleared by hepatocytes where it inhibits protein phosphatase activity, resulting in hyperphosphorylation of numerous hepatocellular proteins. Hyperphosphorylation of cytoskeletal elements causes hepatocytes to round up and to lose cell-to-cell adhesion. This results in a loss of the normal hepatic architecture, sinusoidal destruction, and intrahepatic hemorrhage. Gross lesions include a large, dark, swollen liver with an accentuated lobular pattern caused by the intrahepatic hemorrhage. There may be

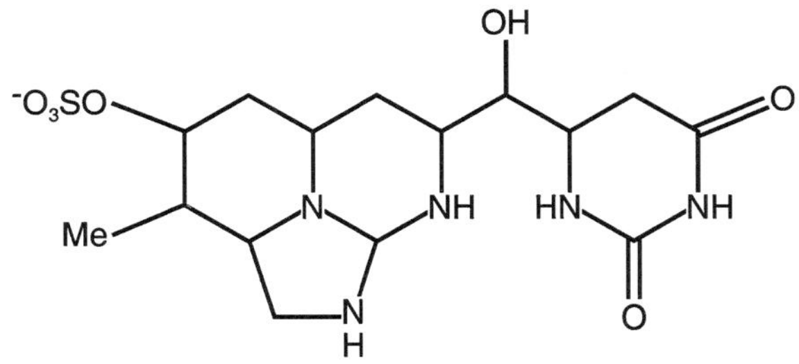

edema in and around the gallbladder wall. Hemorrhagic enteritis and pulmonary edema may also be seen.

Histopathologic examination of the liver reveals separation of hepatocytes from each other and intrahepatic hemorrhage (Fig. 13). Centrilobular apoptosis of hepatocytes and cellular necrosis may extend to periportal regions. Dislodged hepatocytes may be found as emboli in pulmonary and renal vessels (Fig. 14). Chronic toxicosis results in hepatocellular apoptosis, necrosis, fatty degeneration, and hepatic fibrosis and inflammation.

Cylindrospermopsin is a potent inhibitor of protein synthesis that subsequently leads to metabolic disturbances in affected cells. Oxidative damage results from decreased reduced glutathione concentrations and diminished glutathione synthesis. Exposure to cylindrospermopsin is from contaminated water supplies. Clinical signs of toxicosis include bloody diarrhea, lethargy, dehydration, hypovolemia, shock, and acute death. Studies frequently mention the liver as being the most severely affected organ.

Lesions of cylindrospermopsin toxicosis in mice include hepatic, small intestinal and renal

Figure 12. The structure of cylindrospermopsin, a hepatotoxin produced by at least two species of cyanobacteria: *Cylindrospermopsis raciborskii* and *Umezaki natans*.

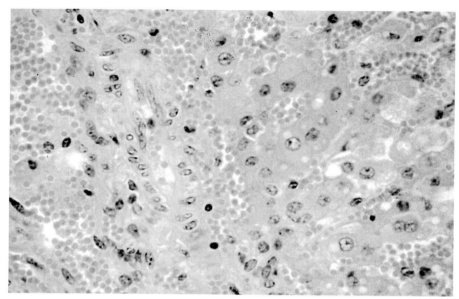

Figure 13. Section of liver from a calf treated experimentally with microcystin-LR showing intrahepatic hemorrhage and dissociation of hepatocyte cords.

hemorrhage and pulmonary congestion. Histopathologic findings include centrilobular hepatic necrosis and lipid accumulation that progress to generalized necrosis at higher dosages, as well as renal tubular epithelial damage. Pathogenesis in the liver occurs in four consecutive phases: (1) inhibition of protein synthesis, (2) membrane proliferation, (3) fat droplet accumulation, and (4) cell death. Necropsy of a calf that died after exposure to *C. raciborskii* revealed abdominal and thoracic hemorrhagic effusion, hyperemia of the mesentery, a pale, swollen liver, and a distended gallbladder. Histopathologic findings included extensive

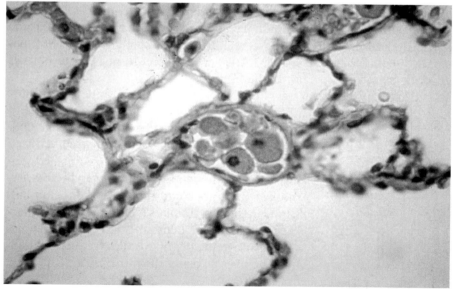

Figure 14. Dislodged hepatocytes in a pulmonary vein of a rat treated experimentally with microcystin-LR.

hepatic fibrosis and bile duct proliferation. Subserosal hemorrhages of the epicardium, small intestine, and omentum were also seen.

SUGGESTED READING

General

Eastaugh, J., and Shepherd, S. (1989). Infectious and toxic syndromes from fish and shellfish consumption: A review. *Arch. Intern. Med.* **149**, 1735–1740.

Falconer, I. R. (1993). "Algal Toxins in Seafood and Drinking Water," p. 224. Academic Press, San Diego.

Glavin, G. B., Pinsky, C., and Bose, R. (1990). Gastrointestinal effects of contaminated mussels and putative antidotes thereof. *Can. Dis. Wkly. Rep.* **16**(Suppl. 1E), 111–115.

Granéli, E., Sundström, B., Edler, L., and Anderson, D. M. (1990). "Toxic Marine Phytoplankton: Proceedings of the Fourth International Conference on Toxic Marine Phytoplankton," p. 554. Elsevier Science, New York.

Sakamoto, Y., Lockey, R. F., and Krzanowski, J. J., Jr. (1987). Shellfish and fish poisoning related to the toxic dinoflagellates. *South Med. J.* **80**, 866–872.

Trevino, S. (1998). Fish and shellfish poisoning. *Clin. Lab. Sci.* **11**, 309–314.

Vecsei, L., Dibo, G., and Kiss, C. (1998). Neurotoxins and neurodegenerative disorders. *Neurotoxicology* **19**, 511–514.

Watters, M. R. (1995). Organic neurotoxins in seafoods. *Clin. Neurol. Neurosurg.* **97**, 119–124.

Diarrheic Shellfish Poisoning

Bialojan, C., and Takai, A. (1988). Inhibitory effect of a marine-sponge toxin, okadaic acid, on protein phosphatases: Specificity and kinetics. *Biochem. J.* **256**, 283–290.

Fujiki, H., Suganuma, M., Suguri, H., Yoshizawa, S., Takagi, K., Uda, N., Wakamatsu, K., Yamada, K., Murata, M., Yasumoto, T., *et al.* (1988). Diarrhetic shellfish toxin, dinophysistoxin-1, is a potent tumor promoter on mouse skin. *Jpn. J. Cancer Res.* **79**, 1089–1093.

Fujiki, H., Suganuma, M., Yoshizawa, S., Nishiwaki, S., Winyar, B., and Sugimura, T. (1991). Mechanisms of action of okadaic acid class tumor promoters on mouse skin. *Environ. Health Perspect.* **93**, 211–214.

Ito, E., and Terao, K. (1994). Injury and recovery process of intestine caused by okadaic acid and related compounds. *Nat. Toxins* **2**, 371–377.

Terao, K., Ito, E., Oarada, M., Murata, M., and Yasumoto, T. (1990). Histopathological studies on experimental marine toxin poisoning, 5. The effects in mice of yessotoxin isolated from *Patinopecten yessoensis* and of a desulfated derivative. *Toxicon* **28**, 1095–1104.

Terao, K., Ito, E., Yanagi, T., and Yasumoto, T. (1986). Histopathological studies on experimental marine toxin poisoning. I. Ultrastructural changes in the small intestine and liver of suckling mice induced by dinophysistoxin-1 and pectenotoxin-1. *Toxicon* **24**, 1141–1151.

Paralytic Shellfish Poisoning

Andrinolo, D., Michea, L. F., and Lagos, N. (1999). Toxic effects, pharmacokinetics and clearance of saxitoxin, a component of paralytic shellfish poison (PSP), in cats. *Toxicon* **37**, 447–464.

de Carvalho, M., Jacinto, J., Ramos, N., de Oliveira, V., Pinho e Melo, T., and de Sa, J. (1998). Paralytic shellfish poisoning: Clinical and electrophysiological observations. *J. Neurol.* **245**, 551–554.

Franz, D. R., and LeClaire, R. D. (1989). Respiratory effects of brevetoxin and saxitoxin in awake guinea pigs. *Toxicon* **27**, 647–654.

Gessner, B. D., and Middaugh, J. P. (1995). Paralytic shellfish poisoning in Alaska: A 20-year retrospective analysis. *Am. J. Epidemiol.* **141**, 766–770.

Morse, E. V. (1977). Paralytic shellfish poisoning: A review. *J. Am. Vet. Med. Assoc.* **171**, 1178–1180.

Amnesic Shellfish Poisoning

Dakshinamurti, K., Sharma, S. K., Sundaram, M., and Watanabe, T. (1993). Hippocampal changes in developing postnatal mice following intrauterine exposure to domoic acid. *J. Neurosci.* **13**, 4486–4495.

Iverson, F., and Truelove, J. (1994). Toxicology and seafood toxins: Domoic acid. *Nat. Toxins* **2**, 334–339.

Iverson, F., Truelove, J., Nera, E., Tryphonas, L., Campbell, J., and Lok, E. (1989). Domoic acid poisoning and mussel-associated intoxication: Preliminary investigations into the response of mice and rats to toxic mussel extract. *Food Chem. Toxicol.* **27**, 377–384.

Nijjar, M. S., and Madhyastha, M. S. (1997). Effect of pH on domoic acid toxicity in mice. *Mol. Cell. Biochem.* **167**, 179–185.

Scholin, C. A., Gulland, F., Doucette, G. J., Benson, S., Busman, M., Chavez, F. P., Cordaro, J., Delong, R., De Vogelaere, A., Harvey, J., Haulena, M., Lefebvre, K., Lipscomb, T., Loscutoff, S., Lowenstine, L. J.,

Marin, R., Miller, P. E., Mclellan, W. A., Moeller, P. D. R., Powell, C. L., Rowles, T., Silvagni, P., Silver, M., Spraker, T., Trainer, V., and Van Dolah, F. M. (2000). Mortality of sea lions along the central California coast linked to a toxic diatom bloom. *Nature* **403**, 80–84.

Strain, S. M., and Tasker, R. A. (1991). Hippocampal damage produced by systemic injections of domoic acid in mice. *Neuroscience* **44**, 343–352.

Sutherland, R. J., Hoesing, J. M., and Whishaw, I. Q. (1990). Domoic acid, an environmental toxin, produces hippocampal damage and severe memory impairment. *Neurosci. Lett.* **120**, 221–223.

Tryphonas, L., Truelove, J., Todd, E., Nera, E., and Iverson, F. (1990). Experimental oral toxicity of domoic acid in cynomolgus monkeys (*Macaca fascicularis*) and rats: Preliminary investigations. *Food Chem. Toxicol.* **28**, 707–715.

Ciguatera Fish Poisoning

Cameron, J., Flowers, A. E., and Capra, M. F. (1991). Effects of ciguatoxin on nerve excitability in rats (Part I). *J. Neurol. Sci.* **101**, 87–92.

Cameron, J., Flowers, A. E., and Capra, M. F. (1991). Electrophysiological studies on ciguatera poisoning in man (Part II). *J. Neurol. Sci.* **101**, 93–97.

Cameron, J., Flowers, A. E., and Capra, M. F. (1993). Modification of the peripheral nerve disturbance in ciguatera poisoning in rats with lidocaine. *Muscle Nerve* **16**, 782–786.

Clark, L., and Whitwell, G. B. (1968). Ciguatera poisoning in cats in Brisbane. *Aust. Vet. J.* **44**, 81.

Dechraoui, M. Y., Naar, J., Pauillac, S., and Legrand, A. M. (1999). Ciguatoxins and brevetoxins, neurotoxic polyether compounds active on sodium channels. *Toxicon* **37**, 125–143.

Fasano, A., Hokama, Y., Russell, R., and Morris, J. G., Jr. (1991). Diarrhea in ciguatera fish poisoning: Preliminary evaluation of pathophysiological mechanisms. *Gastroenterology* **100**, 471–476.

Gillespie, N. C., Lewis, R. J., Pearn, J. H., Bourke, A. T., Holmes, M. J., Bourke, J. B., and Shields, W. J. (1986). Ciguatera in Australia: Occurrence, clinical features, pathophysiology and management. *Med. J. Aust.* **145**, 584–590.

Hashmi, M. A., Sorokin, J. J., and Levine, S. M. (1989). Ciguatera fish poisoning. *N. J. Med.* **86**, 469–471.

Hoffman, P. A., Granade, H. R., and McMillan, J. P. (1983). The mouse ciguatoxin bioassay: A dose-response curve and symptomatology analysis. *Toxicon* **21**, 363–369.

Ito, E., Yasumoto, T., and Terao, K. (1996). Morphological observations of diarrhea in mice caused by experimental ciguatoxicosis. *Toxicon* **34**, 111–122.

Lange, W. R. (1994). Ciguatera fish poisoning. *Am. Fam. Physician* **50**, 579–584.

Legrand, A. M., Galonnier, M., and Bagnis, R. (1982). Studies on the mode of action of ciguateric toxins. *Toxicon* **20**, 311–315.

Levine, D. Z. (1995). Ciguatera: Current concepts. *J. Am. Osteopath. Assoc.* **95**, 193–198.

Lewis, R. J., and Hoy, A. W. (1993). Comparative action of three major ciguatoxins on guinea-pig atria and ilea. *Toxicon* **31**, 437–446.

Lewis, R. J., Hoy, A. W., and Sellin, M. (1993). Ciguatera and mannitol: In vivo and in vitro assessment in mice. *Toxicon* **31**, 1039–1050.

Lewis, R. J., and Sellin, M. (1993). Recovery of ciguatoxin from fish flesh. *Toxicon* **31**, 1333–1336.

Lombet, A., Bidard, J. N., and Lazdunski, M. (1987). Ciguatoxin and brevetoxins share a common receptor site on the neuronal voltage-dependent Na+ channel. *FEBS Lett.* **219**, 355–359.

Morris, J. G., Jr., Lewin, P., Hargrett, N. T., Smith, C. W., Blake, P. A., and Schneider, R. (1982). Clinical features of ciguatera fish poisoning: A study of the disease in the US Virgin Islands. *Arch. Intern. Med.* **142**, 1090–1092.

Poli, M. A., Lewis, R. J., Dickey, R. W., Musser, S. M., Buckner, C. A., and Carpenter, L. G. (1997). Identification of Caribbean ciguatoxins as the cause of an outbreak of fish poisoning among U.S. soldiers in Haiti. *Toxicon* **35**, 733–741.

Strachan, L. C., Lewis, R. J., and Nicholson, G. M. (1999). Differential actions of pacific ciguatoxin-1 on sodium channel subtypes in mammalian sensory neurons. *J. Pharmacol. Exp. Ther.* **288**, 379–388.

Swift, A. E., and Swift, T. R. (1993). Ciguatera. *J. Toxicol. Clin. Toxicol.* **31**, 1–29.

Terao, K., Ito, E., Kakinuma, Y., Igarashi, K., Kobayashi, M., Ohizumi, Y., and Yasumoto, T. (1989). Histopathological studies on experimental marine toxin poisoning, 4. Pathogenesis of experimental maitotoxin poisoning. *Toxicon* **27**, 979–988.

Terao, K., Ito, E., Oarada, M., Ishibashi, Y., Legrand, A. M., and Yasumoto, T. (1991). Light and electron microscopic studies of pathologic changes induced in mice by ciguatoxin poisoning. *Toxicon* **29**, 633–643.

Terao, K., Ito, E., Sakamaki, Y., Igarashi, K., Yokoyama, A., and Yasumoto, T. (1988). Histopathological studies of experimental marine toxin poisoning. II. The acute effects of maitotoxin on the stomach, heart and lymphoid tissues in mice and rats. *Toxicon* **26**, 395–402.

Terao, K., Ito, E., and Yasumoto, T. (1992). Light and electron microscopic studies of the murine heart after repeated administrations of ciguatoxin or ciguatoxin-4c. *Nat. Toxins* **1**, 19–26.

Pfiesteria Toxicoses

Bever, C. T., Jr., Grattan, L., and Morris, J. G. (1998). Neurologic symptoms following *Pfiesteria* exposure: Case report and literature review. *Md. Med. J.* **47**, 120–123.

Fleming, L. E., Easom, J., Baden, D., Rowan, A., and Levin, B. (1999). Emerging harmful algal blooms and human health: *Pfiesteria* and related organisms. *Toxicol. Pathol.* **27**, 573–581.

Levin, E. D., Schmechel, D. E., Burkholder, J. B., Deamer-Melia, N. J., Moser, V. C., and Harry, G. J. (1997). Persisting learning deficits in rats after exposure to *Pfiesteria piscicida. Environ Health. Perspect.* **105**, 1320–1325.

Shoemaker, R. C. (1997). Diagnosis of *Pfiesteria*-human illness syndrome. *Md. Med. J.* **46**, 521–523.

Cyanobacterial Toxins

Beasley, V. R., Dahlem, A. M., Cook, W. O., Valentine, W. M., Lovell, R. A., Hooser, S. B., Harada, K., Suzuki, M., and Carmichael, W. W. (1989). Diagnostic and clinically important aspects of cyanobacterial (blue-green algae) toxicoses. *J. Vet. Diagn. Invest.* **1**, 359–365.

Carmichael, W. W., Eschedor, J. T., Patterson, G. M., and Moore, R. E. (1988). Toxicity and partial structure of a hepatotoxic peptide produced by the cyanobacterium Nodularia spumigena Mertens emend. L575 from New Zealand. *Appl. Environ. Microbiol.* **54**, 2257–2263.

Falconer, I. R., Beresford, A. M., and Runnegar, M. T. (1983). Evidence of liver damage by toxin from a bloom of the blue-green alga, *Microcystis aeruginosa. Med. J. Aust.* **1**, 511–514.

Falconer, I. R., and Buckley, T. H. (1989). Tumour promotion by *Microcystis* sp., a blue-green alga occurring in water supplies. *Med. J. Aust.* **150**, 351.

Falconer, I. R., Dornbusch, M., Moran, G., and Yeung, S. K. (1992). Effect of the cyanobacterial (blue-green algal) toxins from *Microcystis aeruginosa* on isolated enterocytes from the chicken small intestine. *Toxicon* **30**, 790–793.

Falconer, I. R., Smith, J. V., Jackson, A. R., Jones, A., and Runnegar, M. T. (1988). Oral toxicity of a bloom of the cyanobacterium *Microcystis aeruginosa* administered to mice over periods up to 1 year. *J. Toxicol. Environ. Health* **24**, 291–305.

Jackson, A. R., McInnes, A., Falconer, I. R., and Runnegar, M. T. (1984). Clinical and pathological changes in sheep experimentally poisoned by the blue-green alga *Microcystis aeruginosa. Vet. Pathol.* **21**, 102–113.

Negri, A. P., Jones, G. J., and Hindmarsh, M. (1995). Sheep mortality associated with paralytic shellfish poisons from the cyanobacterium *Anabaena circinalis. Toxicon* **33**, 1321–1329.

Runnegar, M. T., Jackson, A. R., and Falconer, I. R. (1988). Toxicity of the cyanobacterium *Nodularia spumigena* Mertens. *Toxicon* **26**, 143–151.

Watanabe, M. F., Harada, K., Carmichael, W. W., and Fujiki, H. (1996). "Toxic Microcystis," p. 262. CRC Press, Boca Raton, FL.

Selected Mycotoxins Affecting Animal and Human Health

Wanda M. Haschek
Department of Veterinary Pathobiology
University of Illinois
at Urbana-Champaign
Urbana, Illinois

Kenneth A. Voss
Agricultural Research Service
U.S. Department of Agriculture
Athens, Georgia

Val R. Beasley
Department of Veterinary
Biosciences
University of Illinois
at Urbana-Champaign
Urbana, Illinois

I. Introduction

Many species of fungi colonize food crops such as rice, corn, wheat, barley, oats, peanuts, cottonseed, and soybeans. These crops are the basic ingredients of many human and animal foods. Mycotoxins are secondary fungal metabolites (i.e., metabolites not essential to the normal growth and reproduction of the fungus) that cause biochemical, physiologic, and/or pathologic changes in other species, including animals, plants, and other microbes. The word mycotoxin is derived from "myco," meaning mold, and toxin, a poison. A great number of fungal metabolites have been identified as mycotoxins. Mycotoxicosis is the term used to denote a syndrome resulting from poisoning of a biological system by a mycotoxin. Conditions that predispose to mycotoxin production by fungi include appropriate moisture (humidity), temperature, aeration, and substrate type and availability.

Temperature and moisture variations affect the growth rate of fungi and also the types and amounts of toxins produced. Individual fungi often produce several different mycotoxins so that combinations of mycotoxins are frequently consumed with the possibility of interactive effects. Fungi are aerobic organisms, but significant differences in oxygen requirements exist among different species. Fungi can be either parasitic or saprophytic. Environmental stress, insect damage, and plant disease predispose to colonization, growth, and toxin production by field fungi. Field fungi invade developing and mature seed grains while still on the plant and the optimal moisture content for growth is 22–25%. Storage fungi invade seed grain after harvest while in storage; and the optimal moisture for growth is 13–18%. Advanced decay fungi typically require moisture of 22–25% but rarely develop and grow on seed grain in the field. Generally, molds grow readily between 20–30°C, but optimal temperature ranges are from below 0°C to above 60°C.

Mycotoxicoses occur worldwide and have been recognized for centuries. Many factors

Handbook of Toxicologic Pathology, Second Edition
Volume 1

contribute to the occurrence of mycotoxicoses in humans, livestock, pets, and wildlife. For example, modern harvesting methods in which corn is handled at higher moisture concentrations, combined with damage caused by harvesting machinery, increase the number of kernels in which fungi can initiate growth. Also the feeding of ground diets prevents food-producing animals from sorting out and avoiding damaged kernels.

A partial listing of mycotoxins is provided in Table I. Our knowledge of many mycotoxins is extremely limited. In many instances, very limited surveys of the frequencies of occurrence have been done. In other instances, the compounds have been investigated in some detail but surveys have not revealed sufficiently frequent occurrence in the United States or other countries for these toxins to be of major concern to animal or human health. For example, T-2 toxin and diacetoxyscirpenol have been studied in some detail. They are encountered only rarely in the United States, with T-2 toxin causing occasional outbreaks of toxicosis in the midwestern United States and Canada. In contrast, T-2 toxin was responsible for severe outbreaks of mycotoxicosis in humans and animals in the Soviet Union. Similarly, the nephrotoxic mycotoxin ochratoxin A is not a major problem in the United States, causing only occasional problems in poultry and swine, whereas it is responsible for widespread outbreaks of toxicosis in swine in Denmark. Four mycotoxin groups account for at least 95% of the confirmed diagnoses of mycotoxicoses in the midwestern United States. These toxins are fumonisins, deoxynivalenol (DON, vomitoxin), zearalenone, and aflatoxins. Another group of mycotoxins, the ergot alkaloids, causes significant losses in livestock production in the United States, as well as Australia, Argentina, and New Zealand. Other common mycotoxins occurring worldwide are ochratoxin A and trichothecenes, such as T-2 toxin. The primary fungal species producing these toxins are listed in Table II.

Interpretation of the significance of mycotoxin residues in animal diets is straightforward

when extremely high concentrations are present. However, when low concentrations are present in foods, the interpretation of the toxicologic significance of mycotoxin residues can be more difficult. This is because experimental

TABLE 1
A Partial Listing of Mycotoxins

Aflatoxins and structurally related mycotoxins
  Aflatoxins B_1, B_2, G_1, G_2, M_1, M_2, Q_1, and aflatoxicol
  Sterigmatocystins
  Versicolorins
  Aspertoxins
  Autocystins
  Sterigmatin
  Bipolarin
  Averufarin
  Curvularin
Rubratoxins A and B
Sporodesmin
Penicillic acid
Ochratoxin series, especially ochratoxin A
Citrinin
Citreoviridin
Cyclosporine
Luteoskyrin
Ergot alkaloids
  Ergotamine
  Ergonovine
  Ergovaline
Tremorgens
  Penitrem A
  Roquefortine
  Paspaline
  Paspalanine
  Paspalitrems A and B
  Verruculogen
  Fumitremorgen
  Fumigaclavine
Slaframine
Patulin
Fusarium toxins
  Trichothecenes
    T-2 toxin
    Diacetoxyscirpenol (DAS)
    Deoxynivalenol (vomitoxin) (DON)
    Verrucarins
    Roridins
    Satratoxins
  Fumonisins
  Zearalenone and zearalenol
  Moniliformin
  Butenolide
  Fusaric acid
  Fusarin A, B, C, and D
  Beauvericin
  Fusaproliferin
  Gliotoxin

TABLE II
Major Mycotoxins and Fungi Producing Them

Fungal species	Mycotoxins produced
Aspergillus parasiticus	Aflatoxins B_1, B_2, G_1, and G_2
A. flavus	Aflatoxins B_1, and B_2
Fusarium sporotrichioides	T-2 toxin
F. roseum (graminearum)	Deoxynivalenol (DON, vomitoxin), zearalenone
F. verticillioides, F. proliferatium	Fumonisins
Penicillium verrucosum, A. ochracoeus	Ochratoxin A
Claviceps spp., *Neotyphodium coenophialum*	Ergot alkaloids

mycotoxicoses cannot always be extrapolated directly to the field situation. There are a number of reasons why experimental and field cases of mycotoxin poisoning are not identical. In mycotoxin poisoning under field conditions, the identified toxin may be consumed along with other related or unrelated mold metabolites, which may include as yet unidentified mycotoxins; mold damaged, stressed grains may be of lower nutrient value and altered palatability; the toxin(s) is distributed unevenly in the diet; the concentration(s) is generally so variable that multiple samples are required to estimate the concentration(s) present; if sufficient moisture and appropriate temperatures occur during transit, additional mold growth and toxin production may occur before analysis, potentially confounding diagnostic efforts; and stressors, such as infectious agents, reproduction, lactation, crowding, and temperature variation, overlap and interact with effects of mycotoxins.

During experimental mycotoxin administration, a single purified toxin is usually administered; the diet is generally balanced and contains undamaged grains; the toxin is mixed evenly in the diet; the toxin concentration is known; the sample is presented to the laboratory without additional mold growth or toxin production occurring; and a controlled, high-quality environment is provided for the experimental animals. However, interpretation of experimental work presented in the mycotoxin literature can be difficult because of the nature of the toxin administered, the route of admin-

istration, the regimen of administration, the numbers and types of animal (species, sex, age, disease status) used, the end points examined, and the interpretations of data. Although purified toxin is the preferred form of toxin for many experimental studies, limitations on the amount of toxin available (especially when working with larger species) often result in the use of naturally contaminated food, culture material inoculated with a known toxin-producing fungal strain, or semipurified toxin. Naturally contaminated food may contain other known or unknown toxins, and determination of the concentration of the toxin of interest may be confounded by binding of the toxin to food components. Culture material may also contain other known or unknown toxins and may have low palatability, which can reduce food intake, especially when it comprises a significant portion of the diet. When food intake is reduced, either due to unpalatability or toxic effects in the exposed animal, nutritional deficiencies may result.

Mycotoxicoses may manifest as acute/subacute, subchronic, or chronic disease. Alternatively, the effects remain subclinical, but there is increased susceptibility to nutritional disorders or infection due to immunosuppression. Mycotoxins may be carcinogenic, mutagenic, or teratogenic. As can be seen in Table III, mycotoxins can affect virtually all organ systems and all species; however, each mycotoxin group has limited toxicological targets such that their syndromes are highly distinctive. Conversely, there is no syndrome consistent

Wanda M. Haschek, Kenneth A. Voss, and Val R. Beasley

TABLE III
Mycotoxins Classified as to Target Organ Toxicity

Specific agent(s)	Species affected[a]	Time of onset	Usual duration (if survive)
Mycotoxins that cause neurotoxicity			
Toxicants associated with central nervous system (CNS) stimulation or seizures			
Tremorgenic mycotoxins (e.g., penitrem, roquefortine, lolitrem B, paspalitrems)	All species, especially dogs, cattle, sheep	Minutes to days	One day to weeks; often lethal in dogs
Toxicants with mixed effects on the CNS			
Ergot alkaloids	Herbivores, humans	Minutes to days	Days to months (with chronic exposure; e.g., from endophyte-infected fescue); sometimes lethal
Fumonisins	Horses	Days to months	Permanent damage likely in survivors; often lethal
Diplodia maydis on corn (South Africa)	Cattle, sheep	2–5 days	Few days, reversible
Muscarinic agonists			
Slaframine	Cattle, horses, sheep	Hours	Up to 3 days; rarely lethal
Mycotoxins that cause paralysis (may eventually include respiratory paralysis)			
Lolitrem B	Sheep, cattle, sometimes horses	Chronic	Chronic; rarely lethal
Citreoviridin	Cattle	Importance in the field is not well established	
Patulin	Cattle	Toxicosis is very rare	
Mycotoxins that cause cardiotoxicity			
Citreoviridin (rare)			
Moniliformin	Poultry		
Fumonisin	Pigs, horses (E)	Days	Acute form lethal
Fusaric acid	Rabbits, rats, cats, dogs, humans		
Nephrotoxic mycotoxins			
Ochratoxins	Swine, poultry, humans	Days to weeks	Days to permanent damage; often lethal in poultry
Citrinin (may potentiate effect of ochratoxins)	Swine		
Fumonisins	Rabbits, sheep, calves, rats and mice (E)	Days to weeks	Days to weeks to permanent damage; potentially lethal in rabbits and ruminants
Cyclosporine	Humans (immunosuppressive use)		
Mycotoxins that affect the liver			
Aflatoxins	Most species, humans; trout, ducklings, and young poultry are highly susceptible	Days to chronic	Weeks to permanent damage, potentially lethal
Sterigmatocystin	Most species	Weeks to chronic	Weeks to months; toxicoses very rare
Rubratoxins A and B	Chickens; possible cattle and swine	Days to chronic	Unknown; toxicoses rare

(Continues)

TABLE III (*Continued*)

Specific agent(s)	Species affected[a]	Time of onset	Usual duration (if survive)
Sporodesmin	Cattle, especially sheep	Chronic	Chronic; primarily Australia, New Zealand
Penicillic acid	Swine	Chronic	Chronic; toxicoses very rare
Fumonisins	All species	Days	Weeks; may be lethal in horses
Cyclopiazonic acid (rare)			
Mycotoxins that affect the lungs			
3-Substituted furans, e.g., ipomeanol	Ruminants	Hours to days	Days; often lethal
Fumonisins	Swine	Days	Usually lethal
Stachybotrys toxins, e.g., satratoxins	Humans, horses, cattle, pigs, sheep, poultry (when inhaled)		
Mycotoxins that cause immunosuppression			
Aflatoxins	All species		
Trichothecenes	All species		
Fumonisins	Pigs, rodents (E)		
Ochratoxin A	Pigs		
Mycotoxins that induce cancer			
Aflatoxins	Most species, trout, humans (liver)		
Ochratoxin A	Mice, rats (kidney and urinary tract) (E)		
Fumonisins	Rat (kidney), mouse (liver) (E)		
Sterigmatocystin	Rat (liver) (E)		
Mycotoxins that affect reproduction and/or mammary gland function			
Toxins with multiple effects			
Ergovaline, an ergot alkaloid	Horses	Oversize, weak foals with overgrown hooves	
Ochratoxin A	Most species, except pig	Teratogen	
Mycotoxins that are estrogenic			
Zearalenone and zearalenol	Swine, cattle, sheep	Days to weeks	Days to weeks, permanent reproductive damage rare
Other mycotoxins that affect reproduction			
Ergot alkaloids	Cattle, horses	Chronic	Chronic
Trichothecenes (E)			
Mycotoxins that affect the mammary gland			
Ergot alkaloids	Cattle, horses	Days to weeks	Days to weeks; rarely lethal
Zearalenone	Swine	Days to weeks	Days to weeks (not lethal)
Mycotoxins that affect the gastrointestinal tract			
Deoxynivalenol (vomitoxin)	Swine, cattle, dogs, and poultry	Hours to days	Days; unlikely to be lethal
T-2 toxin, HT-2 toxin, diacetoxyscirpenol (DAS), and other trichothecenes	Cattle, swine, small animals, poultry, humans	Hours to chronic	Days; potentially lethal

(*Continues*)

TABLE III (*Continued*)

Specific agent(s)	Species affected[a]	Time of onset	Usual duration (if survive)
Mycotoxins that may affect the skin			
Trichothecene mycotoxins (not DON)	All species		
Mycotoxins that affect peripheral circulation (may cause sloughing)			
Ergot alkaloid (gangrenous ergotism)	Cattle, sheep	Days to weeks	Weeks; potentially lethal
Ergot alkaloids in tall fescue	Cattle	Weeks to months	Weeks to months

[a]E, experimental.

with exposure to mycotoxins as an overall group.

Mycotoxins have attracted worldwide attention since the 1970s because of their perceived impacts on human health, because of the economic losses accruing from condemned foods and decreased animal productivity, and because of the serious impact of mycotoxin contamination on internationally traded commodities. Mycotoxins are considered direct-acting agents of food-borne diseases, i.e., toxicoses, and some mycotoxins act via immunosuppression, thereby contributing to a wide range of infectious diseases.

Preharvest control of mycotoxin production is difficult; however, much effort has been expended to develop resistant crop strains by both breeding and direct genetic modification. Biocontrol technology, in which a nontoxigenic organism competes with a toxigenic fungus for a specific ecological niche (competitive exclusion technology) or otherwise inhibits fungal growth, is being developed. Postharvest control of mycotoxin production is aimed primarily at effective drying and storage regimens. However, despite the best efforts of the agricultural community, mycotoxins will continue to be present in a wide range of foods. Approaches utilized to limit exposure, bioavailability, and toxicity of mycotoxins in foodstuffs for animals include the identification and segregation of contaminated material, chemical sorbents used as sequestering agents, and chemical destruction (detoxification). Alternative methods of control are actively being studied because all ap-

proaches available have costs and limitations. Strategies for removal of mycotoxins from food materials also need to be developed.

This chapter addresses selected mycotoxins known to cause disease in animals and humans. Major emphasis is placed on the fumonisins, the most recently identified group of mycotoxins that can cause significant livestock disease.

II. Aflatoxins

A. SOURCE/OCCURRENCE

Aflatoxins are a group of bishydrofurans produced by some *Aspergillus flavus* and *A. parasiticus* isolates. These saprophytic fungi are distributed worldwide. When environmental conditions are favorable, as occurs in warm temperate, subtropical, or tropical climates, such as the southeastern United States, southern Asia, and Africa, fungal growth and toxin production occurs. Aflatoxin production occurs both in the field and in storage. In the field, these fungi reside in the soil but, when conditions are favorable, they invade the host plants by various routes. Heat, drought, and insect damage to the plants are conditions conducive to fungal infection and aflatoxin production in the field. Fungal growth and aflatoxin production may also begin or, if infection was established in the field, continue after harvest if the grain has not been dried properly or is otherwise stored improperly. Aflatoxin can be produced in conditions of 85% relative humidity (e.g., corn moisture content of 15–28%) and

650

temperatures over 25°C that persist for over 48 hr. Increased aflatoxin concentrations while in storage can be extreme, thus grain drying and subsequent handling are of great importance to minimize hazards to animals and associated economic losses.

Corn, peanuts, cottonseed, and treenuts are common aflatoxin sources, however, these mycotoxins also may be found in other foodstuffs such as wheat, rice, copra, figs, some spices, eggs, and milk. Meats and poultry are not considered significant sources; however, aflatoxin residues, mostly aflatoxin M_1, can be found in the muscle of exposed animals. Of greater concern is the presence of aflatoxin M_1 in milk.

Aflatoxins were first identified as the causative agent of an acute and fatal disease in turkeys, called turkey X disease, which occurred in England in 1960 when moldy ground nut (peanut) meal from Brazil was used as a food source. Over 100,000 turkeys died in the outbreak. Since then, the aflatoxins, especially aflatoxin B_1, have become the most thoroughly studied mycotoxins, both in the laboratory and as the subject of epidemiology studies of mycotoxins and human disease. Although classically regarded as hepatotoxins and hepatocarcinogens, aflatoxins also exert adverse affects on other tissues, most notably the kidneys and the hematopoietic and immune systems.

B. TOXICOLOGY

1. Toxin

At least 13 aflatoxins have been identified. Aflatoxins B_1, B_2, G_1, and G_1 [the designation B and G refer to the fact that these aflatoxins can be visualized in commodities, such as peanuts and corn, by the bluish (B) or greenish (G) fluorescence that they emit under ultraviolet light] are the most common, and aflatoxin B_1 is the more studied (Fig. 1). Aflatoxins are potent toxins, mutagens, and carcinogens. Aflatoxin B_1 is a more potent carcinogen than aflatoxins B_2, G_1, and G_2. Aflatoxins M_1 and M_2 are important metabolites of aflatoxins B_1 and B_2. They are considerably less potent than their metabolic precursors, but are nonetheless of concern because they occur in milk and dairy products, thereby posing a hazard to infants and young children.

2. Species Susceptibility

Aflatoxin B_1 is toxic to some degree in all species tested to date, although significant differences in sensitivity occur. Among

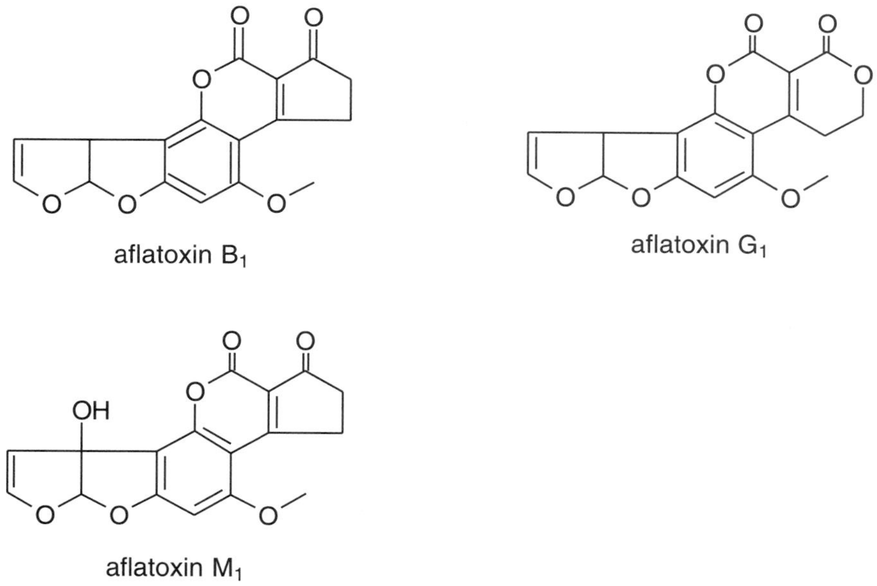

aflatoxin B_1

aflatoxin G_1

aflatoxin M_1

Figure 1. Chemical structures of representative aflatoxins.

agriculturally important mammals, pigs are generally more sensitive than cattle of similar age, which, in turn, are more sensitive than sheep. As a rule, young animals are more susceptible than adults. Ducklings and turkey poults are more sensitive than quail or chicks. Among laboratory species, rats, guinea pigs, and rabbits are significantly more sensitive than mice. Trout are very sensitive to the hepatocarcinogenic effects of aflatoxin.

3. Biodistribution, Metabolism, and Excretion

Aflatoxins, such as aflatoxin B_1 and G_1, are procarcinogens that are subjected to both phase I and phase II metabolism in the liver and other tissues. In mammals, cytochromes P450 (CYP) are responsible for phase I metabolism with CYP 1A2 and 3A4 important for metabolism in humans. Phase I metabolism leads to the formation of both less toxic molecules and more reactive, electrophilic molecules that react readily with cellular macromolecules. The conversion of aflatoxin B_1 to aflatoxin M_1, which is estimated to be 10 times less potent a carcinogen than aflatoxin B_1, is an example of the former, whereas CYP-mediated metabolism of aflatoxin B_1 to aflatoxin B_1-8,9-epoxide is an important example of the latter. Like other bioactive epoxides, aflatoxin epoxides may undergo further reactions, including phase II (glutathione S-transferase mediated) conjugation to glutathione, conversion to dihydrodiols, binding to macromolecules, or adduction to DNA. Aflatoxin–DNA adduction occurs readily. It is clear that the N7 sites of guanine are particularly susceptible to this adduction. The presence of N7 guanine adducts liberated during DNA repair, in blood and urine, serves as a biomarker for aflatoxin exposure.

Differences among species and sexes in susceptibility to aflatoxicosis are explained in part by differences in the rate of metabolism and the amounts and types of metabolites formed. Phase II metabolism also contributes to interspecies differences. For example, the relative insensitivity of mice to hepatocarcinogenicity can be attributed to their significantly higher levels of glutathione S-transferase activity, as compared to more sensitive species like the rat. Cytosolic phase II metabolism of aflatoxin is significantly less efficient in humans than in mice. The importance of phase II metabolism for detoxification of aflatoxin is illustrated further by the protective effects of agents such as Oltipraz and 1,2-dithiole-3-thione, which act as inducers of glutathione S-transferase activity.

4. Mechanism of Action

Aflatoxins are hepatotoxic. The mechanism of this toxicity is the result of widespread and nonspecific interactions between aflatoxins or their activated metabolites and various cell proteins, which can result in the disruption of basic metabolic processes and protein synthesis, and cause cell death.

Aflatoxins are genotoxic. The correlation between aflatoxin exposure and the appearance of N7 guanine–aflatoxin adducts in serum and urine has been demonstrated repeatedly. As a consequence of DNA adduction, mutations occur during DNA repair or replication and, if mutations are located in critical genes, they can alter cell functions significantly. A number of studies suggest a high correlation between aflatoxin exposure and point mutations at a specific location, the third base of codon 249, of the p53 tumor suppressor gene. This mutation, a transversion of guanine to thymidine, has been shown to be present in some Chinese and African patients with liver cancer. The role of this mutation in aflatoxin-induced cancers is still uncertain, as data obtained from other studies suggest that aflatoxin carcinogenesis is independent of p53 mutations.

Although classified as a human carcinogen, there is evidence that aflatoxin requires the presence of other factors to induce liver cancer. In this regard, the role of hepatitis B as a cofactor for aflatoxin has been a matter of some controversy. Hepatitis B infection is common in areas where aflatoxin exposure is high, such as Africa and southeast Asia. Some epidemiological studies, using hepatitis B surface antigen as a biomarker for viral exposure, suggest that carcinogenesis is related to an interaction between hepatitis B virus and aflatoxin. Oxidative damage to DNA and other macromolecules caused by aflatoxin induced lipid peroxidation may also play an important mechanistic role.

C. CLINICAL SIGNS AND PATHOLOGY

1. Overview

The aflatoxin literature is extensive, more so than for any other mycotoxin. A comprehensive treatment of the subject is therefore beyond the scope of this chapter. The reader is referred to the extensive reviews of the toxicity and pathology of aflatoxin, especially the hepatic histopathology, by Newberne and Butler (see Suggested Reading) and by others.

Acute aflatoxin poisoning occurs less commonly than chronic aflatoxicosis. The principal target organ is the liver with fatty change and hepatocyte degeneration and necrosis leading to the loss of liver function. This can result in icterus, decreased synthesis of serum proteins (hypoproteinemia), and coagulopathy, which can lead to extensive hemorrhaging and anemia. Clinical signs of chronic aflatoxicosis are nonspecific. Chronic intoxication is associated with decreased weight gain or weight loss, decreased food consumption and conversion, and decreased reproductive performance, including abortion. Laying hens exhibit reduced egg production and milk production of cows declines. Biochemical evidence of hepatocyte and biliary damage can be obtained from serum. Affected animals have increased susceptibility to infection, presumably due to immunosuppression, because aflatoxins have an adverse effect on cell-mediated immunity, principally by affecting the reticuloendothelial system, macrophages, and T cells.

Although affecting other tissues, aflatoxins usually are thought of in terms of hepatotoxicity and hepatocarcinogenicity. There is a reasonable degree of similarity in the type of liver lesions seen in different species, both on gross and on microscopic levels, and in accompanying clinical pathology changes. However, some variability exists; for example, the distribution of hepatic necrosis tends to be centrilobular in some species (guinea pig, dog, pig, cattle) and more periportal in other (rat, poultry, cat). Qualitatively, lesions caused by the various aflatoxins appear similar, although there is a difference in potency. For example, aflatoxin B_1 is more toxic than aflatoxin G_1 and far more toxic than aflatoxin M_1.

Grossly, the liver has been variably described as enlarged, swollen, or fatty; it tends to be pale with gray to yellow or orange discoloration. Congestion or petechial hemorrhages are sometimes evident. The texture is variable and may be firm, fibrous, friable, or, particularly in chickens, fatty. The gallbladder may be enlarged and turgid with mucosal hemorrhage. Splenic or renal enlargement, hydrothorax, hydropericardium, or ascites may also be found.

Microscopic lesions caused by acute or subchronic exposure in most species include hepatocyte degeneration, necrosis, hepatocellular vacuolation (fatty change), cellular pleomorphism with variability in cell (anisocytosis) and nuclear (anisonucleosis) size, bile duct or oval cell proliferation (Fig. 2), and nodular regeneration, which may progress to cirrhosis or cancer. The predominance of individual findings such as bile duct proliferation, distribution of necrotic hepatocytes, degree of lobular architectural disruption, and time course of lesion development varies by species and mode of exposure.

2. Laboratory Animals

Rats are sensitive to the acute effects of aflatoxin. Guinea pigs are more and mice are less sensitive than rats. Lesions are obvious and progressive in rats given a single LD_{50} dose. Shortly after dosing there is periportal degeneration and necrosis of hepatocytes and biliary and oval cell proliferation. Later, hepatocytes become more pleomorphic with nuclear hyperchromasia and differences in nuclear size and shape. Regeneration becomes more obvious until overt nodular regeneration is present. Fibrosis may not be extensive and hepatocellular tumors, which morphologically resemble those routinely induced by other rodent hepatocarcinogens, develop in the absence of cirrhosis. Similar lesions are found in mice, guinea pigs, and rabbits;

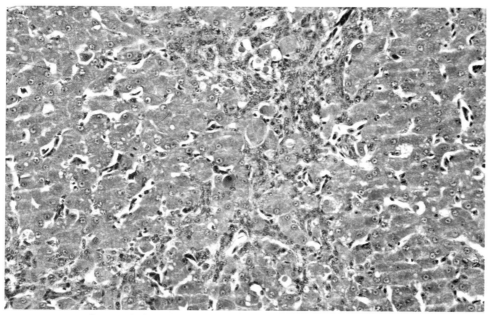

Figure 2. Liver from a duck with aflatoxicosis demonstrating biliary epithelial proliferation as well as mild scattered hepatocyte necrosis and mitosis (H&E × 200).

however, hepatic necrosis in guinea pigs is typically centrilobular and in rabbits is centrilobular to midzonal.

3. Poultry

Poultry, particularly ducklings, are sensitive to aflatoxin. As in mammals, biliary hyperplasia is a predominant feature (Fig. 2). Hepatocellular degeneration and necrosis occur. Necrotic cells may be scattered throughout the hepatic lobules or, more commonly, are found in the periportal zone. In ducklings, periportal hepatocellular necrosis may be accompanied by the development of lesions described in the literature as "lakes of fat." Biliary hyperplasia and nodular regeneration become pronounced, and fibrosis progresses to cirrhosis

4. Livestock

Aflatoxicosis is a problem in livestock, most notably swine and cattle. Young pigs are especially sensitive to acute exposures. Gross lesions include hepatic enlargement, congestion, yellow discoloration, and friability; petechiae or more generalized hemorrhage; and edema and ecchymotic or petechial hemorrhages of the gall blad-der. Microscopic findings depend on the dose and duration of exposure but are typical of aflatoxicosis with hepatocellular degeneration and necrosis in the centrilobular zone.

Cattle are more resistant than pigs, but lesions typical of aflatoxicosis can be found. Fibrosis and bile duct proliferation may be extensive and found together with fibrotic veno-occlusion of the central veins. Sheep are resistant to aflatoxin.

5. Other Species

Other species, including nonhuman primates, have shown varying degrees of sensitivity to aflatoxin and develop lesions of the type described earlier, particularly hepatocellular degeneration and necrosis, and biliary proliferation, which progress to nodular cirrhosis. Dogs are quite sensitive. Acute exposure results in jaundice and liver and gallbladder lesions. Microscopic findings are consistent with those found in other species and include centrilobular hepatocyte degeneration and biliary hyperplasia.

Aflatoxin toxicity is not confined to mammalian and avian species, but extends to fish, with trout being particularly sensitive. The acute and subchronic effects include hemorrhage and hepatocyte necrosis. Biliary proliferation, regenerative nodules, and hepatocellular carcinoma are common chronic findings.

6. Liver Cancer in Laboratory Animals

Lesions associated with aflatoxin hepatocarcinogenesis were studied thoroughly and reported in the late 1960s and early 1970s (see Suggested Reading). These investigations not only brought attention to the carcinogenic potential of aflatoxins, but also established mycotoxins as important environmental toxins. The morphology of hepatic neoplasms induced by aflatoxins is similar to those induced by other well-characterized carcinogens. However, in contrast to tumors induced by some other compounds, aflatoxin-induced hepatomas and hepatocarcinomas can arise in livers that are not cirrhotic.

The sequence of lesions that occur in rats fed aflatoxin B_1 (≤ 1 ppm in the diet) was described in detail by Newberne and Wogen. In the early stages, there is bile duct proliferation and foci of altered hepatocytes consisting of intensely stained cells with small nuclei or, alternatively, larger cells with clear to lightly staining cytoplasm. With continued exposure, hyperplastic nodules, hepatomas, and overt carcinomas develop. Hyperplastic nodules contain well-demarcated collections of hepatocytes undergoing mitosis or fatty change that compress the surrounding parenchyma. Carcinomas range in appearance from well differentiated, with cells arranged in trabeculae, to poorly differentiated types. In the latter, cells display varying degrees of anaplasia and may be arranged in sheets, cords, cysts, or duct-like structures. Tumors invade the adjacent parenchyma and vasculature and frequently metastasize to the lung. Cholangiofibromatous lesions and cholangiocarcinoma are rare.

D. HUMAN RISK

Acute aflatoxicosis following the ingestion of highly contaminated food has been documented in various locations, particularly in Africa and southeastern Asia. Diagnosis of aflatoxicosis in humans is difficult, as symptoms are not specific for aflatoxin. Clinical findings may include anorexia, diarrhea, malaise, or depression. Death may occur. Hepatobiliary involvement is suggested by jaundice, ascites, or tenderness when pressure is applied to the upper abdomen. Detection of aflatoxin B_1 in liver as well as histopathological findings consistent with aflatoxin-induced injury, such as fatty infiltration and centrilobular necrosis, have been reported following acute outbreaks of suspected human aflatoxicosis. In 1972, acute aflatoxicosis from the consumption of contaminated corn caused fatalities in Kenya. In India, many human fatalities occurred in 1974 when unseasonable rain and a scarcity of food resulted in the consumption of corn that was heavily contaminated with aflatoxin.

Aflatoxin is considered a human carcinogen and liver cancer is the major concern. The association between aflatoxin and liver cancer has been a focus of intense epidemiologic investigation in the developing world, particularly in China and various African countries in which high liver cancer rates are found. Significant human exposure to aflatoxin in these regions has been demonstrated unequivocally by the presence of aflatoxin–lysine adducts in serum and aflatoxin B_1–guanine adducts, which result from the removal of aflatoxin-adducted guanine from DNA, in urine. However, a number of nutritional and other conditions frequently exist in affected human populations that confound the situation. Exposure to hepatitis B virus is now recognized as a potentially important cofactor; however, epidemiological and other investigations on aflatoxin and hepatitis B virus in regard to liver cancer have yielded mixed results: some suggest that aflatoxin acts independently, some correlate liver cancer with hepatitis B exposure, and still others show an interaction between the two. Although the issue remains unresolved, studies in China, in which biomarkers were used to assess exposures, indicate the likelihood that both aflatoxin B_1 and hepatitis B virus are involved and that an interaction between the two contributes to risk.

E. DIAGNOSIS, TREATMENT, AND CONTROL

When conditions are favorable for the production of aflatoxin, grain elevators often utilize black light to screen commodities. This test only indicates fungal growth and not toxin presence. All positives should be followed up by a specific test to identify and quantify any aflatoxin actually present. Available ELISA tests (Quik-card, E-Z-Screen, Signal, Agri-Screen Aflatoxin) give a positive or negative result, with the "cut-off" in the United States being 20 ppb, the actionable limit concentration set by the U.S. Food and Drug Administration for aflatoxin B_1 in feed grain for interstate commerce. ELISA tests that can estimate a concentration are also available. Aflatoxin M_1, a hydroxylated metabolite of aflatoxin B_1, is detected readily in the milk of exposed dairy cattle. For the sale of milk, the actionable limit is ≥ 0.5 ppb aflatoxin.

Diagnosis of aflatoxicosis in a clinical or field setting cannot be based on lesions and clinical pathology findings alone. Confirmation of diagnosis requires direct evidence of aflatoxin exposure, such as the identification of aflatoxin–albumin adducts in serum, the presence of aflatoxin–N7 guanine adducts in the urine, or identification of a sufficient concentration of aflatoxin(s) in source materials.

Treatment of affected animals consists of changing the diet to an aflatoxin-free ration, increasing dietary protein, and supplementing the diet with vitamin B_{12}, vitamin K, and selenium. Toxicity can be prevented to some extent by treatment of contaminated food stuffs. NovaSil (hydrated calcium aluminum silicates-HSCAS) binds aflatoxin, thereby decreasing its absorption and toxicity in swine. A similar effect is seen in poultry; however, the efficacy of NovaSil in preventing residues of aflatoxin M_1 in the milk of dairy cows is considerably less than desirable. NovaSil has been approved by FDA only as an anticaking agent at up to 2% of a ration. Ammoniation of corn to reduce its aflatoxin concentration is a last resort only and ammoniated corn turns brown. Ammoniation has been used a great deal to detoxify aflatoxin in cottonseed intended for animal consumption. Both NovaSil and ammoniation can be used only for animal feed.

III. Ochratoxins

A. SOURCE/OCCURRENCE

Ochratoxins are produced by *Aspergillus ochraceous*, *Penicillium verrocusum*, and related species. Ochratoxins A, B, C, D, and their methyl and ethyl esters have been isolated. Ochratoxin A is the most common and, along with ochratoxin C, is among the most toxic homologues. Ochratoxin A contains a phenylalanine moiety attached to a dihydroisocoumarin group via an amide bond (Fig. 3). Ochratoxin A is nephrotoxic to several species and is a renal carcinogen in rodents.

The principal source of ochratoxins is cereal grains, including barley, rye, wheat, corn, sorghum, and oats, but ochratoxins may occur in

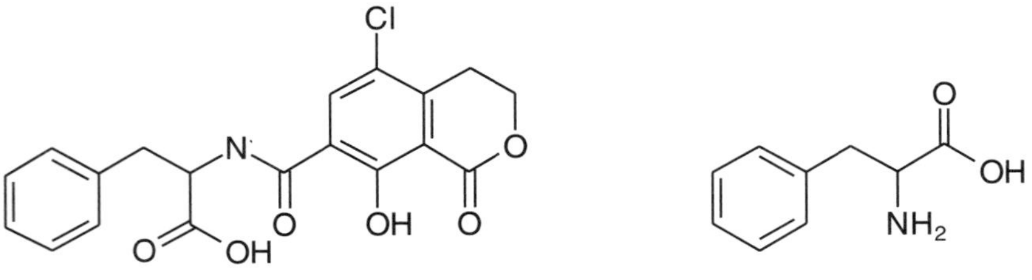

ochratoxin A

phenylalanine

Figure 3. Chemical structures of ochratoxin A and phenylalanine. Ochratoxins compete with phenylalanine for binding sites of enzymes.

other commodities such as cottonseed, nuts, dried beans, and coffee beans. Geographically, ochratoxins occur in regions with temperate climates, with the northern European countries, the Balkans, and Canada being most affected. Ochratoxin concentrations in grains vary, but periodically they can be high enough to cause disease outbreaks, as illustrated by episodic porcine nephropathy. Optimal conditions for ochratoxin A production are a moisture content of 19–22% and a temperature of 24°C.

Humans are exposed via the diet. Cereals and grain products are the main sources; however, ochratoxins are found in animal tissues with the highest residues in the kidneys. Thus, meat products such as sausages, bacon, or ham also contribute to exposure. Human exposure is particularly high within, but not limited to, the Balkans and northern Europe. Ochratoxin A residues have been found in human serum, plasma, and milk from northern European countries, particularly Denmark and Germany, and from Canada.

B. TOXICOLOGY

1. Species Susceptibility

The toxicity of ochratoxin A is approximately equal to that of ochratoxin C, although ochratoxin A is encountered much more commonly. Ochratoxin B is several times less toxic. Synergistic or additive effects occur with aflatoxin, citrinin, or penicillic acid. Ochratoxins are potentially hazardous to livestock, and toxicity has been demonstrated in swine, horses, ducklings, chickens, turkeys, and dogs. Cattle are reportedly resistant to ochratoxin A due to metabolism of the toxin by ruminal microflora, but calves are sensitive until the rumen is developed. In general, young animals are more sensitive than adults. The kidney is the major target organ, particularly in swine, although the liver, immune system, and other organs may also be affected. Ochratoxin A is teratogenic in most species examined, and dose-dependent transfer of ochratoxin A across the placenta has been demonstrated in rodents. Swine are a notable exception, as ochratoxin A is not teratogenic and, in contrast to rodents, does not cross the placenta when given to sows at low levels.

2. Biodistribution, Metabolism, and Excretion

The pharmacokinetics of ochratoxin A in mammals vary somewhat, depending on species and dose. In general, about 60% of orally administered ochratoxin A is absorbed from the gastrointestinal tract of rats and other monogastrics. In rats, significant amounts are bound to albumin in the plasma, with maximum concentrations occurring within 4 hr of dosing. Binding to serum albumin is also high in cattle, pigs, and humans. The $T_{1/2}$ varies from about 8 hr in rabbits to slightly over 500 hr in monkeys. The $T_{1/2}$ in pigs is about 90 hr with the rate of elimination from the kidneys and liver being approximately 100 hr. The high serum binding and greater retention rates in pigs lead to the presence of ochratoxin A residues, especially in the kidneys. Reported Cp_{max} ranges from 0.50 μg/ml or less in mice and monkeys to as high as 87 μg/ml in rats. Biliary excretion and enterohepatic circulation occur, and ochratoxins and their metabolites are excreted in urine and feces. Ochratoxin A accumulates in the kidney. The anionic transporter mechanism plays a major role in its accumulation in kidney and absorption occurs along the entire length of the renal tubule. Ochratoxin A residues of up to 100 ppb have been documented in swine kidney. Similar but much less severe residue problems occur in chickens. Other tissues that accumulate ochratoxin A are liver, skeletal muscle, and fat.

Ochratoxin A is metabolized by carboxypeptidases found in the rumen, intestine, and in enteric bacteria. The hydrolysis product, ochratoxin α, is less toxic. Hepatic and renal metabolic pathways also exist in various species including rat, mouse, rabbit, and monkey. These pathways convert ochratoxin A to ochratoxin B, 4-R- and 4-S-hydroxyochratoxin A, 10-hydroxyochratoxin A, and other, as yet, uncharacterized products. Metabolism varies by species, sex, and strain of animal and is mediated by various cytochrome P450s.

3. Mechanism of Action

As a result of their structural similarity to phenylalanine (Fig. 3), ochratoxins effectively compete with phenylalanine for the binding sites of enzymes that utilize the latter as a substrate. All the results of such metabolic inhibitions, for example, the inhibition of phenylalanine hydroxylase, are not known. It is clear, however, that phenylalanine tRNA synthetase is inhibited by ochratoxin and, as a result, there is a reduction in cellular protein synthesis. Ochratoxin also inhibits mitochondrial respiration, leading to depletion of cellular ATP, interference with cellular calcium homeostasis, lipid peroxidation, and oxidative damage of macromolecules. Phenylalanine and aspartame, which contain phenylalanine, are antagonistic to ochratoxins, presumably by competing with the mycotoxin for phenylalanine-binding sites. Toxicity is influenced by metabolism, as discussed previously.

The carcinogenic mechanism of ochratoxin A remains unresolved. There is no compelling evidence that ochratoxin A reacts directly with DNA and it is therefore generally regarded as a nongenotoxic carcinogen. Ochratoxin A has elicited negative to weakly mutagenic responses in the *Salmonella typhimurium* assay. However, some mammalian cells are susceptible to ochratoxin A-induced genetic damage. DNA adducts have been found in various cell types *in vitro* following ochratoxin A treatment; however, the toxicological significance of these adducts is unknown. They have not been characterized chemically and it is not known if they are formed by ochratoxin metabolites or if they are secondary, indirect events resulting from DNA damage caused by lipid oxidation products or free radicals. In any case, formation of these adducts appears to be correlated with toxicity and carcinogenicity.

Ochratoxin A induces renal tumors in rats. Male Dark Agouti (DA) rats appear to be more sensitive to the renal carcinogenic effect of ochratoxin A than male Lewis rats. The latter appear to be more sensitive than Lewis rats, whereas female DA rats are resistant. Among DA and Lewis rats, sensitivity to tumorigenicity by strain and sex has been correlated with both the formation of uncharacterized renal DNA adducts and the ability of the animals to metabolize debrisoquine to 4-hydroxydebrisoquine (a cytochrome P450-dependent reaction).

C. CLINICAL SIGNS AND PATHOLOGY

1. Swine

Swine are particularly sensitive to ochratoxin, with chronic toxicity occurring after the ingestion of diets containing 0.2 to 4 ppm ochratoxin A. The kidney is the main target organ, although toxic effects following experimental exposure have been reported in the liver, lymphoid organs, and the digestive tract. The disease in swine, referred to as porcine nephropathy, was first described in Denmark. It occurs mostly in northern European countries, but may be found elsewhere, including the United States. Clinically there is a reduced rate of growth and signs of renal tubular dysfunction. The latter includes polyuria, glycosuria, and proteinuria. The earliest indicator is an increase in urinary leucine amino-peptidase, an enzyme present in the brush border of the proximal tubule. This is followed by decreased glomerular filtration rate (GFR), increased blood urea nitrogen (BUN), and decreased osmolality.

Renal involvement is typically bilateral and widespread subcutaneous, mesenteric, and perirenal edema may be present. Grossly, the kidneys may be slightly to markedly enlarged and pale, mottled or gray-white. The texture of the capsule is variable, ranging from smooth to rough, or irregular due to cyst formation. The microscopic pathology is nonspecific but is consistent with the pathology found in other species and humans with Balkan endemic nephropathy (BEN). There is proximal tubular degeneration and atrophy with interstitial fibrosis and mononuclear infiltration. As the disease progresses, cystic dilation of degenerated tubules occurs and, like in BEN, glomerular hyalinization can be present in severe cases. Morphologic findings alone are insufficient to diagnose ochratoxin-induced porcine nephropathy, as other agents, including the mycotoxin citrinin, induce similar histologic changes and clinical signs.

2. Poultry

Poultry are more sensitive to ochratoxin A than to aflatoxin B_1 or T-2 toxin, with growth impairment of young broiler chickens occurring at 2 ppm as compared to 2.5 ppm with aflatoxin B_1 and 4 ppm for T-2 toxin. The principal effect is nephropathy. Neurological and intestinal effects and visceral gout may be observed. There is a decrease in serum carotenoids and carotenoid pigmentation (the loss of yellow color from the fat), which decreases marketability. Hemorrhage, especially in the proventriculus, due to a multifactorial coagulopathy, as well as decreased bone strength, have been reported. Reduced food consumption and egg production with substandard, stained, or rubbery shells may be observed.

3. Laboratory Animals

Ochratoxin A is toxic and carcinogenic to rats and mice. The kidney is the major target organ in both species. Descriptions of the microscopic lesions found in Fischer 344 (F344) rats fed diets containing 70 or 210 µg/kg ochratoxin A or DA and Lewis rats treated by gavage are similar. Males are more sensitive than females. Nephropathy is characterized by the simultaneous presence of degenerative and regenerative changes in the tubules of the inner cortex and outer medulla found adjacent to the corticomedullary junction. Characteristic features include necrosis of single epithelial cells, tubular dilation and formation of cysts, dilated tubules lined by a hyperplastic, multilayered epithelium, tubular atrophy, and karyomegaly and cytomegaly of tubular epithelial cells characterized by eosinophilic, granular cytoplasm (Fig. 4A). If the dose is sufficiently high, nephropathy may develop in several days to weeks.

Neoplastic lesions, including renal tubular adenomas and carcinomas, are found after prolonged exposure and multiple primary tumors may be found in an animal. Adenomas are generally well differentiated and circumscribed (Fig. 4B). They resemble hyperplastic tubules; however, unlike hyperplastic tubules, the lumen and other tubular features may be obliterated by the proliferating adenoma cells. Carcinomas tend to be larger lesions and, in contrast to the adenomas, are not well circumscribed (Fig. 4C). They have a considerable degree of cellular atypia and numerous mitotic figures. Areas of necrosis suggest that these masses expand rapidly, outgrowing their blood supply. Metastases are readily demonstrable. A low incidence of transitional cell carcinomas or benign transitional cell papillomas of the urinary bladder may also be found in rats treated with ochratoxin A.

In both sexes of B6C3F$_1$ mice, diets containing 40 ppm ochratoxins (about 90% ochratoxin A and 10% ochratoxin B) caused nephropathy, characterized by cystic dilation and hyperplasia of tubules. When fed for up to 2 years, renal tubular adenomas and carcinomas were found only in males. Both carcinomas and adenomas contained solid and tubular forms. No metastases were reported.

Neoplastic lesions of tissues other than the urinary tract have also been described in rodents exposed to ochratoxin A for up to 2 years. Ochratoxin A increased the incidence of mammary gland fibroadenomas in female F344 rats and hepatic carcinomas in female B6C3F$_1$ mice.

D. HUMAN RISK

Ochratoxin A and the structurally related mycotoxin, citrinin, are the suspected etiological agents of BEN. As its name implies, BEN is found in a geographical area that includes parts of Serbia, Croatia, Bosnia and Herzegovina, Rumania, and Bulgaria. BEN occurs in distinct foci within this endemic area. These foci are characteristically found in rural areas and are composed of individual households interspersed irregularly among unaffected households. Although unequivocally affecting households, heredity does not appear to play a major role. Rather, most evidence suggests an environmental etiology, including the observation that the

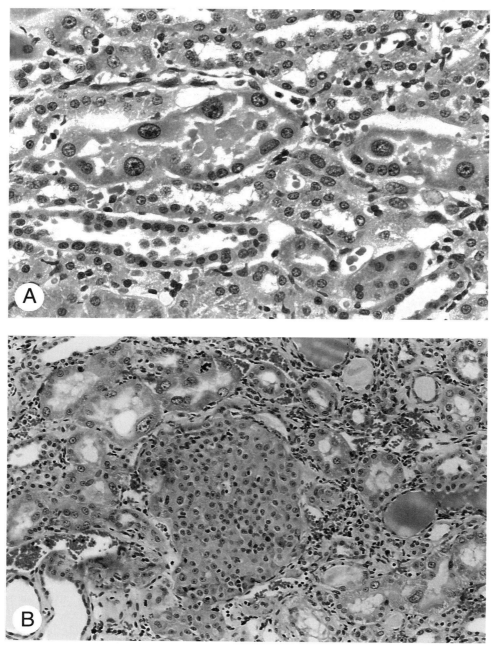

Figure 4. Renal changes induced in F344 rats by chronic oral exposure to 20 or 210 µg/kg body weight of ochratoxin A (H&E). (A) Renal epithelial cell hypertrophy and hyperplasia. Note the presence of enlarged epithelial cells, karyomegaly, and dilation of the tubular lumen (× 100). (B) Renal tubular adenoma. The adenoma has obliterated the tubular structure, but is well circumscribed and displays little cellular atypia (× 50). (C) Renal tubular carcinoma. Carcinomas occurred more frequently in males than females. In contrast to the adenoma, carcinomas are larger, less circumscribed, show cellular atypia, and metastasize (× 3.3). Courtesy of G. A. Boorman, J. Peckham, and M. H. Puccini, National Toxicology Program, Research Triangle Park, NC.

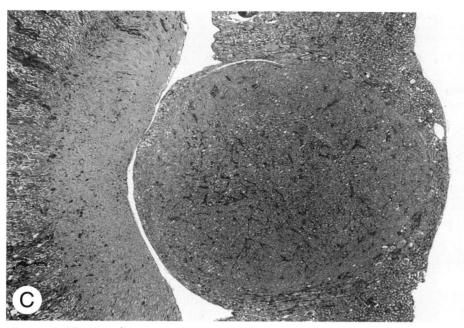

Figure 4. (*Continued*)

disease occurs in outsiders settling into the endemic area.

The microscopic lesions of BEN and porcine nephropathy, which is known to be caused by ochratoxin A-contaminated feeds, are similar. This mycotoxin has a worldwide distribution, however, both ochratoxin A and ochratoxin A-producing fungi are particularly common in the endemic area, and ochratoxin A concentrations of grain and foodstuffs have been shown repeatedly to be high in this region. Furthermore, both the frequency and the concentration of ochratoxin A in blood or urine from BEN patients are significantly higher than those found outside the endemic area.

Clinically, BEN is difficult to diagnose because of its insidious onset and protracted course. Although primarily a kidney disease, liver involvement has been reported in some cases. In the early stages, there may be fatigue, pallor, headache, weight loss, pain in the loins, and proteinuria. The clinical course is one of slowly progressing chronic renal failure with disturbances in urine volume regulation, acid–base and electrolyte balance, and waste product excretion. As the disease progresses, there is azotemia, uremia, and, in some patients, hematuria or hypertension. The nephrotic syndrome of hypoalbuminemia, proteinuria, edema, and hyperlipidemia is not a feature of BEN.

The characteristic finding at autopsy is bilateral atrophy of the kidneys. The histopathology of BEN is variable depending on the stage of the disease. Lesions are found mainly in the cortex, are usually multifocal, and involve the interstitium, vasculature, and renal tubules. More generalized involvement may be found in the end stages of the disease. Specific histological features include interstitial fibrosis, interstitial mononuclear cell infiltrates, multifocal atrophy of the proximal tubules, and vascular hyalinosis and sclerosis. Although considered a tubular disease, segmental or global thickening of the glomerular vascular may be present and, during the end stage of the disease, may progress to overt glomerular sclerosis or hyalinization in some patients. A high incidence of urinary tract cancers, especially urotheliomas and renal cell carcinomas, is associated with BEN and tumors occur in patients independent of clinical signs of renal failure.

661

E. DIAGNOSIS, TREATMENT, AND PREVENTION

In animals, ochratoxicosis may be tentatively diagnosed based on clinical signs of polydipsia and polyuria as well as renal and other lesions. Specific diagnosis is done by the detection of ochratoxin in toxic concentrations in foodstuffs. Experimentally, ochratoxin-α can be detected in kidney, liver, and skeletal muscle, and ochratoxin in urine and feces. No specific treatment is available. Supportive care should be similar to that for other causes of renal failure. Ammoniation of ochratoxin-containing grain is very effective in reducing its toxicity.

IV. Trichothecene Mycotoxins

A. SOURCES/OCCURRENCE

Trichothecene mycotoxins are a family of tetracyclic sesquiterpenoid substances (12,13-epoxy-trichothecenes) comprising over 100 compounds of widely varying toxicity that are produced primarily by field fungi of the genus *Fusarium*. The macrocyclic trichothecenes are produced primarily by *Stachybotrys* and *Myrothecium* spp. Other genera that have been reported to produce trichothecenes include *Trichoderma*, *Trichothecium*, *Cephalosporium*, and *Gliocladium*. Trichothecenes occur worldwide in grains and other commodities grown in cooler climates. Colonization and toxin production by *Fusarium* spp occur in the field; however, some toxin production can also occur in storage. Mild temperatures tend to encourage fungal growth and cool temperatures increase toxin production (0–15°C). Trichothecenes tend to be produced in toxic concentrations in years of wet weather when harvests are delayed and prolonged.

Trichothecenes known to cause problems in livestock include deoxynivalenol (DON, vomitoxin), nivalenol, T-2 toxin, HT-2 toxin, diacetoxyscirpenol (DAS), and macrocyclic trichothecenes (e.g., roridins, verrucarins, satratoxins). In the United States and Canada, deoxynivalenol appears to be the most significant member of the group despite its comparatively low toxicity. T-2 toxin has caused widespread epidemics of alimentary toxic aleukia (ATA) in humans in the Soviet Union and, as with DAS, is an occasional cause of outbreaks of important toxicoses in animals in North America (moldy corn toxicosis) and Japan (bean hull poisoning in horses). T-2 toxin and DAS, along with deoxynivalenol and zearalenone, were detected in specimens of the alleged chemical warfare agent "yellow rain" in southeast Asia.

Deoxynivalenol is produced primarily by *F. roseum* (*Gibberella zeae*, *F. graminearum*), with corn, oats, barleys, and wheat, as well as other small grains, being important sources of exposure to livestock. T-2 toxin is produced primarily by *F. sporotrichioides* and may occur in corn, but highest concentrations generally occur in small grains such as barley and wheat. Forages are sometimes contaminated. Macrocyclic trichothecene toxins can be produced by fungi such as *Stachybotrys chartarum* (*S. atra*), a black fungus growing in wet forages and/or straw as well as in rain-damaged building materials and water-soaked air ducts.

B. TOXICOLOGY

1. Toxin

All trichothecene mycotoxins have a basic tetracyclic sesquiterpene structure with a six-membered oxygen-containing ring, an epoxide group in the 12,13 position, and an olefinic bond in the 9,10 position (Fig. 5). Trichothecenes have been classified into four groups based on their structural characteristics. Group A trichothecenes possess hydroxyl or esterified hydroxyls at the 3, 4, 7, 8, or 15 position and include T-2 toxin, DAS, and monoacetoxyscirpenol. Group B trichothecenes contain a carboxyl group in the 8 position, in addition to other functional groups as in group A, and include DON. Group C trichothecenes bear a bridge of varying length and composition between carbons 4 and 5 and consist of macrocyclic trichothecenes, such as satratoxins, that are not produced by *Fusarium* spp. Group D trichothecenes have a second epoxide at the 7,8 position and include crotocin. While fungi frequently produce several toxins, most species

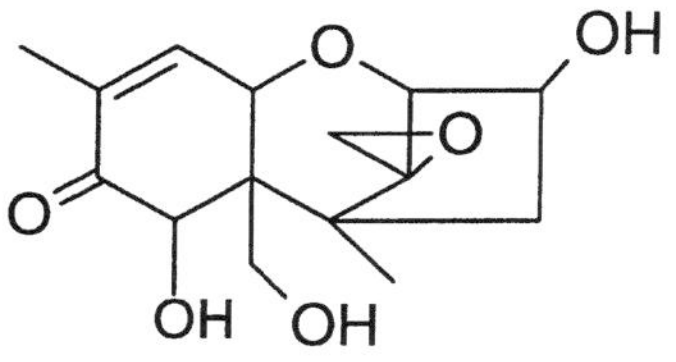

deoxynivalenol

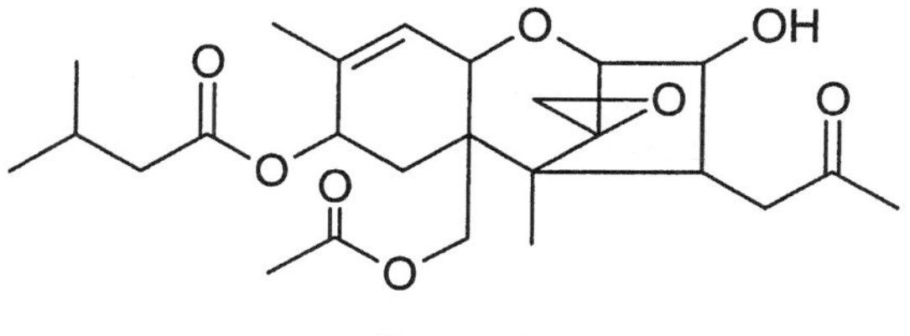

T-2 toxin

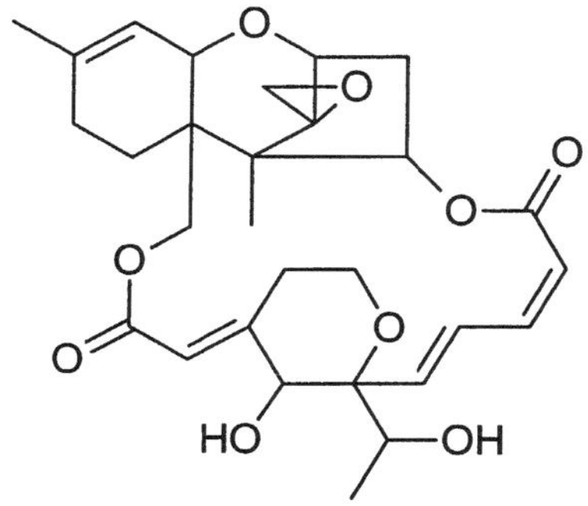

satratoxin H

Figure 5. Chemical structure of trichothecene mycotoxins from groups A (T-2 toxin), B (deoxynivalenol), and C (satratoxin H).

tend to produce either group A or group B toxins. However, several different types of toxins may be produced by a single fungal species. For example, *F. roseum*, a primary producer of zearalenone, can synthesize both group A and B toxins. Although *Fusarium* spp. generally colonize grains or cereals in the field, most toxin production occurs in storage.

2. Biodistribution, Metabolism, and Excretion

Radiolabeled studies with the trichothecene skeleton, as well as individual toxins, indicate rapid absorption, distribution, and excretion following oral or parenteral administration. Trichothecenes do not accumulate in the body to any great extent, and residues are excreted readily within several days after exposure. In contrast, the absorption of T-2 toxin is slow following dermal administration, with skin and subcutaneous fat acting as a reservoir for the toxin, delaying absorption and sustaining metabolism and excretion. Comparison of oral and intravenous routes of administration of the trichothecene skeleton indicate a first-pass effect of the liver. Trichothecenes can undergo phase I (hydrolysis, oxidation, reduction) and II (glucuronide conjugation) metabolism. The hydrolysis of esters appears to be the major pathway in the metabolism of trichothecenes containing esterified side chains such as DAS or T-2 toxin. However, the initial hydrolysis or oxidation pathways cannot be considered to be detoxification reactions because the initial metabolites are often as toxic as the parent compounds. Excretion is via the biliary system and urine. Enterohepatic recirculation may occur, especially in swine, resulting in delayed excretion and ultimately increased toxicity.

3. Mechanism of Action

Although toxicologically important trichothecenes vary in their chemical structure and biological effects, all are potent inhibitors of protein synthesis. Inhibition takes place in the translational stage that occurs in the polysomes of the endoplasmic reticulum. All three translational processes—initiation, elongation, and termination—can be affected by trichothecenes. However, the inihibitory potency and major site of action during translation vary among trichothecenes. Inhibition of DNA synthesis as a secondary event has also been reported. Trichothecenes induce cell death in lymphoid organs, the gastrointestinal tract, and other organs via apoptosis (see Chapter 3). Inhibition of protein synthesis could play a role in the induction of apoptosis. Many of the trichothecene-induced biological effects have not been explained by the impairment of protein synthesis and may be mediated by the reaction of the epoxy groups of trichothecenes with sulfhydryl groups on enzymes and binding of certain trichothecenes to membrane components.

4. Biological Effects and Species Susceptibility

Trichothecene toxicosis is manifested by a broad spectrum of clinical disorders, which vary according to the specific toxin or mixture of toxins present in contaminated feed. Species differences in response are generally related to severity of the response, and young animals are more susceptible than adults. Toxicosis can be acute or chronic, with clinical signs remaining fairly similar.

Reduced feed intake and vomiting (emesis) are associated with most trichothecenes, with swine being the most sensitive species. Decreased feed consumption leads to reduced weight gain. Vomiting is an acute reaction that can occur rapidly after either oral or parenteral administration. It is believed that vomiting is a result of central nervous stimulation, although gastric irritation cannot be ruled out. The more potent trichothecene mycotoxins, T-2 toxin, DAS, and the macrocyclic toxins, are also known for their cytotoxic effects on the skin and oral cavity following direct contact. The local cytotoxic effects of these compounds may result in lesions on the snout, muzzle, lips, and tongue. Deoxynivalenol does not produce dermal or oral effects. T-2 toxin, DAS, and the macrocyclic toxins can also cause hematotox-

icity and immune suppression due to effects on rapidly dividing cells and, in some cases, neurotoxicity. Abortion and retarded growth rate of offspring have been reported at doses toxic to the dam.

Immune suppression may be the most significant effect of low-level trichothecene exposure with increased susceptibility of exposed animals and humans to infectious and other diseases. Trichothecene immunotoxicity is amplified by low levels of Gram-negative bacterial lipopolysaccharide (LPS), a prototypic inflamagen. Exposure to such bacterial toxins may explain some cases of increased individual susceptibility to trichothecenes and other mycotoxins. Trichothecenes lack mutagenic activity and there is no evidence of direct carcinogenic potential.

C. CLINICAL SIGNS AND PATHOLOGY

1. Deoxynivalenol (DON, Vomitoxin)

Among domesticated animals, swine appear to be most susceptible to DON, but cattle, horses, dogs, and poultry are all reported to be susceptible. Although not one of the more acutely toxic trichothecenes, deoxynivalenol has caused great economic loss to the livestock, especially swine, industry due to the well-documented reduction in feed consumption and weight gain. With pure DON, transient effects on feed intake can be observed in swine at concentrations as low as 1–2 ppm, although more permanent effects are not typically noted until >5 ppm. Complete food refusal occurs at >20 ppm. In one study, 4 ppm deoxynivalenol caused a 2% reduction in feed intake, whereas at 40 ppm a 90% reduction was observed. In the field, however, concentrations of DON associated with feed refusal may be as low as 1 ppm. This may be due to the presence of other mycotoxins, known or unknown. Other signs may include soft stools, diarrhea, failure to thrive, and a predisposition to other disease entities and poor nutrition. Vomiting is seen infrequently, therefore, the name vomitoxin seems inappropriate. After prolonged exposure, animals may develop a resistance to deoxynivalenol and make compensatory gains. Although a mild thickening of the squamous mucosa of the stomach has been noted experimentally in swine, specific lesions are not observed under field conditions. DON is not significantly transferred into milk, meat, or eggs.

Chronic dietary studies in mice have shown that DON impairs humoral immunity, cell-mediated immunity, and host resistance. In addition, serum immunoglobulin A (IgA) becomes elevated due to the disruption of regulation of IgA production and IgA accumulates in the mesangium of the kidney. This is similar to IgA nephropathy, the most common form of glomerulonephritis in humans worldwide. In up to 50% of affected individuals, the disease is progressive, resulting in renal failure. The cause of IgA nephropathy in humans is unknown, and the possibility of mycotoxin involvement in the disease process needs to be considered. Similar results have been obtained with nivalenol in mice. In swine, nivalenol produced elevated plasma IgA levels and gross evidence of nephropathy.

2. T-2 Toxin and Diacetoxyscirpenol (DAS)

a. Overview. T-2 toxin and DAS can cause much more serious toxicoses than DON. Toxicoses occur mainly in cattle, swine, and poultry and occasionally in horses, dogs, cats, and humans. Signs most often include reduced feed intake or feed refusal, vomiting and diarrhea, necrosis of skin and oral mucosa, and increased incidence of infection. Because T-2 toxin causes feed refusal and vomiting, severe toxicosis is rarely reported in field situations. However, an extensive literature on the effects of experimental induction of severe toxicosis is available. With severe toxicosis, lesions include hemorrhage and necrosis of gastrointestinal mucosa (high doses), destruction of hemopoietic tissue and lymphoid necrosis (high doses), and meningeal hemorrhage (massive doses). Shock and death can follow (massive doses). Less well-known effects include necrosis of the adrenal cortex, kidney, liver, and, in pigs, myocardium and pancreas. Clotting disorders and reproductive problems have also been reported with T-2

toxin. At doses toxic to the dam, embryotoxicity and fetotoxicity, as well as abortion, may occur. Testicular damage in males may occur with highly toxic levels of exposure.

b. Swine. The LD_{50} values for DAS and T-2 toxin administered intravenously in swine are 0.3 and 1.3 mg/kg, respectively. Acute effects include vomiting, lethargy, frequent defecation, and posterior paralysis. Cytotoxicity occurs on direct contact with skin or oral cavity, resulting in necrotizing lesions. Systemic T-2 toxin toxicosis is similar whether the toxin is given orally or intravenously. In all species, systemic toxicity is manifested by injury to the gastrointestinal tract (especially stomach and small intestine) and the immune and hematopoietic systems. Gastric toxicity is characterized by hemorrhagic ulcerative gastritis (Fig. 6). In the small intestine, there is ulceration of the surface mucosa and selective (apoptotic) necrosis of crypt epithelial cells (Fig. 7). Apoptotic necrosis of lymphocytes in the thymus, lymph nodes, spleen, and other lymphoid tissues occurs, with B lymphocytes affected more severely than T lymphocytes. Cell-mediated and humeral systemic and pulmonary immune responses are depressed. Hematologic effects include a transient leukocytosis due to neutrophilia followed by leukopenia due to lymphopenia. The selective targeting of rapidly dividing cells, such as intestinal crypt epithelial cells, as well as those in immune and hematopoietic systems, is the so-called "radiomimetic effect" ascribed to T-2 toxin and DAS.

Toxicity to the heart (Fig. 8) and pancreas, as well as adrenal cortex, liver, and kidney, has also been reported. Transient interstitial pneumonia occurred following experimental inhalation exposure and severe dermatonecrosis following dermal exposure (Fig. 9), both presumably due to direct cytotoxicity. Most effects following inhalation exposure were similar to those following intravenous exposure. With dermal exposure, local effects were marked but systemic effects were much less severe and limited to the lymphoid system and pancreas.

c. Poultry. Oral necrosis, nervous disorders, hepatic hematoma, and reduced weight gain

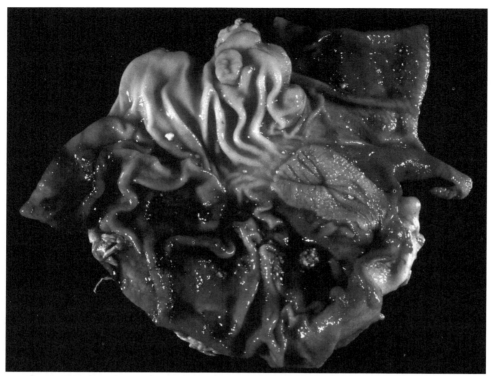

Figure 6. Stomach from a pig given T-2 toxin at approximately 2 mg/kg as a single inhalation exposure 8 hr previously. There is severe necrohemorrhagic gastritis, especially in the fundic portion.

have been reported in broilers fed diets containing 4 ppm T-2 toxin or DAS. At higher exposure concentrations, hematopoietic damage and coagulopathy have been reported. Other signs include abnormal feathering and reduced feed efficiency, as well as decreased egg production, eggshell thickness, and shell strength. Other reported effects include abnormal feces with urate crystals and diarrhea.

d. Dairy Cattle. A field case involving hemorrhagic syndrome was reported in diary cattle fed moldy corn containing T-2 toxin at 1 ppm; however, this syndrome was not reproduced experimentally. T-2 toxin fed to calves at 10 to 50 ppm caused necrosis of the oral mucosa, ruminal and abomasal ulcers, and severe diarrhea. Atrophy of the thymus has also been reported.

3. Macrocyclic Trichothecenes (Stachybotryotoxicosis)

Stachybotryotoxicosis occurs after the consumption of moldy straw or hay. It has been reported in the USSR and adjacent countries, as well as Finland, Hungary, France, and South Africa, in horses, ruminants, swine, and poultry. Fungi causing the disease are *Stachybotrys chartarum (S. atra)* and possibly *Myrothecium* and *Dendrodochium* spp., which produce macrocyclic trichothecenes, including satratoxins, roridin, and verrucarin on straw or hay. These toxins are directly toxic to mucosal membranes causing necrosis and edema of the lips, tongue, and buccal membranes, and later diarrhea due to gastrointestinal toxicity. Similar perioral, pharyngeal, and gastrointestinal effects are seen as with T-2 toxin and DAS. Hematopoietic toxicity follows and is characterized by leukopenia, thrombocytopenia, and coagulopathy, which can result in systemic hemorrhage, septicemia, and death.

The consumption of large amounts of contaminated feed by horses results in nervous signs, circulatory collapse, and death in 1 to 3 days. This has been termed the "shocking"

666

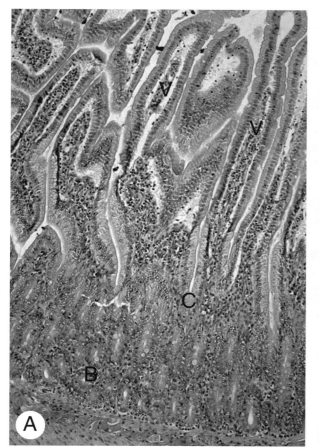

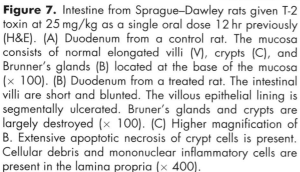

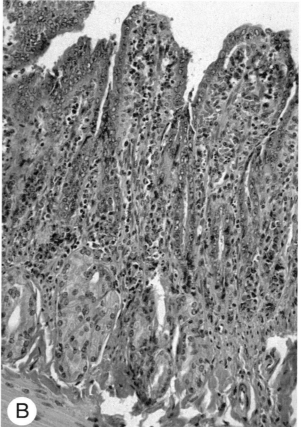

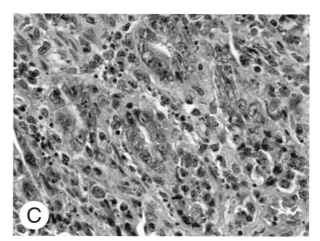

Figure 7. Intestine from Sprague–Dawley rats given T-2 toxin at 25 mg/kg as a single oral dose 12 hr previously (H&E). (A) Duodenum from a control rat. The mucosa consists of normal elongated villi (V), crypts (C), and Brunner's glands (B) located at the base of the mucosa (× 100). (B) Duodenum from a treated rat. The intestinal villi are short and blunted. The villous epithelial lining is segmentally ulcerated. Bruner's glands and crypts are largely destroyed (× 100). (C) Higher magnification of B. Extensive apoptotic necrosis of crypt cells is present. Cellular debris and mononuclear inflammatory cells are present in the lamina propria (× 400).

form of stachybotryotoxicosis. Such horses may experience hyperesthesia, hyperirritability, blindness, stupor, a wide stance, crossed legs, difficulty swallowing, an atonic intestinal tract, diarrhea, shock, and cyanosis. At necropsy, lesions include widespread hemorrhages (evidence of hemorrhagic diathesis), ulceration of mucosa of the alimentary tract, pneumonia, renal infarcts, multifocal hepatic necrosis, bone marrow necrosis, and lymphoid depletion. Some of these latter lesions may be due to secondary infections.

Dermal toxicity, as well as respiratory distress, epistaxis (nose bleeds), and eye irritation,

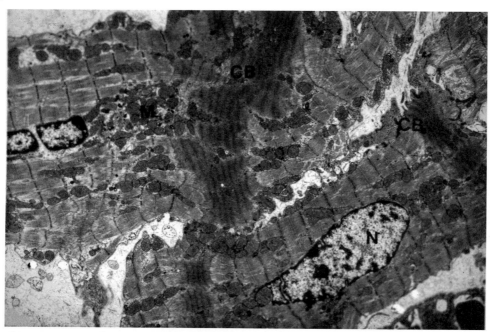

Figure 8. Heart from a pig given T-2 toxin at 2.4 mk/kg iv 4 hr previously. Prominent contraction bands (CB) of electron-dense contractile material with adjacent mitochondrial accumulation (M) are present. Edema is present between myocytes (× 6700).

due to contact with infected material have been reported in humans. When the fungus grows in water-damaged homes or air ducts, people can become chronically affected. This has been called the "sick building" syndrome.

D. HUMAN RISK

T-2 toxin has been implicated in outbreaks of acute human mycotoxicoses. It is believed to be the principal causal toxin of the human disease, alimentary toxic aleukia (ATA), which was recognized since the 19th century in the USSR. During World War II, thousands of people developed ATA and many died after consuming cereals that overwintered in fields. Entire villages were lost. The symptoms of ATA included fever, vomiting, acute inflammation of the entire alimentary tract, anemia, sepsis, circulatory failure, and convulsions. Death often followed.

T-2 toxin, together with DON, nivalenol, and deoxynivalenol monoacetate, was isolated from moldy flour used to make bread that was associated with an outbreak of human illness in Kashmiri, India, in 1987. The major symptoms were abdominal pain, inflammation of the throat, diarrhea, vomiting, and bloody stools.

DON has been implicated in outbreaks of acute human mycotoxicoses occurring in Japan and China. In the 1984–1985 outbreak in China, a large number of people who had ingested moldy maize and wheat containing DON and zearalenone developed symptoms including nausea, vomiting, abdominal pain, diarrhea, dizziness, and headache within 5 to 30 min of ingestion.

Human exposure to trichothecene mycotoxins was also alleged to occur in southeast Asia and Afghanistan from exposure to a chemical warfare agent named "yellow rain." T-2 toxin, DON, nivalenol, and DAS were implicated as components of "yellow rain" and were detected in low concentrations in blood, urine, and tissue samples of alleged victims. Skin rashes, emesis, respiratory difficulties, hemorrhage, and even death were reported.

In the 1970s, DAS (Anguidine) underwent phase I and II clinical trials in humans for the treatment of cancer, but minimal antitumor

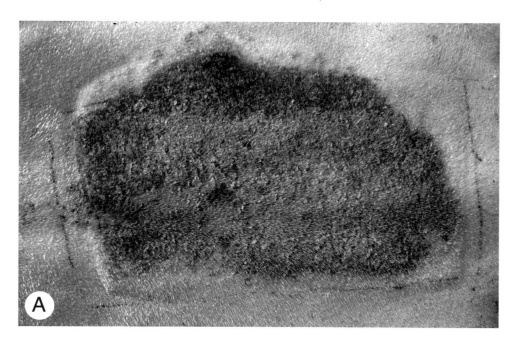

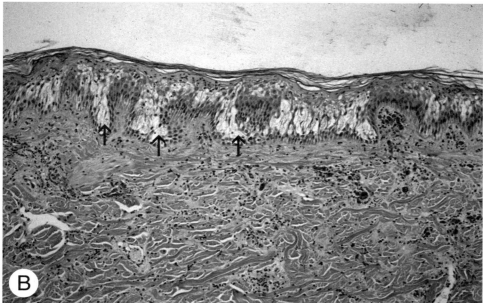

Figure 9. Skin from a pig given T-2 toxin at 15 mg/kg as a single dermal application. (A) At 3 days after application the area was markedly reddened and edematous. (B) At 1 day after application there is multifocal ballooning degeneration (arrows) of the epidermis, as well as edema and mild cellular infiltration around congested vessels in the dermis (H&E × 10).

activity was reported. Toxic signs included nausea and vomiting; less frequently, diarrhea, and hypotension; and, rarely, death.

Stachybotryotoxicosis is well recognized in humans in the USSR and adjacent countries following contact with macrocyclic trichothecenes produced by *S. chartarum* and other non-*Fusarium* spp. on moldy straw or hay. Farm workers in contact with infected litter or feed developed skin rashes, respiratory distress, epistaxis (nose bleeds), and eye irritation. A more recent concern is the growth of fungi producing trichothecenes and other mycotoxins, such as sterigmatocystin, in water-damaged homes or air ducts. Chronic illness in occupants is termed the "sick building syndrome," with irritation of the eyes and nose a common complaint. The possible involvement of exposure to such fungi in asthma is an issue because there is an association between fungal exposure and increased bronchial responsiveness (see Chapter 28). Additionally, idiopathic pulmonary hemorrhage in infants, which can be fatal, has been attributed by some scientists to exposure to fungi, especially *S. chartarum*, growing in water-damaged homes.

E. DIAGNOSIS, TREATMENT, AND PREVENTION

When a history from a clinical case in livestock includes feed refusal and failure to thrive, mycotoxins should be included in the differential diagnosis and feed should be submitted for a mycotoxin screen. Specific quantitative assays are available for a limited number of trichothecenes. In response to increased international concern, Neogen has improved its quantitative ELISA test for T-2 toxin with the sensitivity range being 25–250 ppb. These mycotoxins are not found at very high concentrations in tissues, although stomach contents may contain detectable levels if the animals were eating prior to death. There are no specific antidotes for trichothecene mycotoxins; however, a change of diet and supportive and symptomatic treatment are indicated. Effective therapies for massive doses of trichothecenes have been identified because of concerns regarding possible chemical warfare. Adsorption of toxins with activated charcoal fluids and supportive care are indicated and would likely be of value for the rare case of acute trichothecene toxicosis in the field.

V. Zearalenone

A. SOURCE/OCCURRENCE

Zearalenones are a family of phenolic compounds produced by species of *Fusarium*, primarily *F. roseum; F. avenaceum, F. nivale*, and *F. verticillioides* may also produce zearalenone. Zearalenone and its relatives, such as zearalenol and zearalenone glycoside, cause subacute to chronic toxicosis, but not death. Zearalenones can cause estrogenic effects and infertility in animals. Swine, cattle, and sheep are susceptible, whereas poultry are extremely resistant.

Fusarium spp. have a worldwide distribution and infect corn, wheat, other grains, and occasionally forages. Zearalenone occurs in grasses infected with *Fusarium* spp. in New Zealand. The most frequently contaminated crop is corn. The greatest production of zearalenone by *Fusarium* sp. usually occurs in storage when moisture and temperature conditions are optimal. However, in the field, infection of corn with *F. roseum* (the sexual stage is *Gibberella zeae*) may produce Gibberella rot and toxins, such as deoxynivalenol, simultaneously with zearalenone. The equivalent of Gibberella rot in wheat, barley, and oats is called scab. Irrespective of when colonization occurs (in storage or in the field), growth is optimum at 20–25°C and a high moisture content (greater than 23%). Zearalenone production is stimulated when the temperature drops to about 15°C.

B. TOXICOLOGY

1. Toxin and Mechanism of Action

Zearalenone (also called F-2 toxin) and its derivatives (Fig. 10) are the only known mycotoxins whose effects are primarily estrogenic in nature. A three-dimensional model of the zearalenone molecule can be used to demonstrate the similarity of the configuration of this toxin to estradiol. Thus, zearalenone can occupy and stimulate estrogenic receptors, and the induced estrogenic response is indistinguishable from that caused by estradiol. Uterine and mammary effects are induced by an interaction of zearalenone with estrogenic cytosolic receptors in these organs. In addition, zearalenone also acts on the hypothalamus and pituitary similarly to estrogen.

α-Zearalenol is associated with natural zearalenone occurrence and may have three times

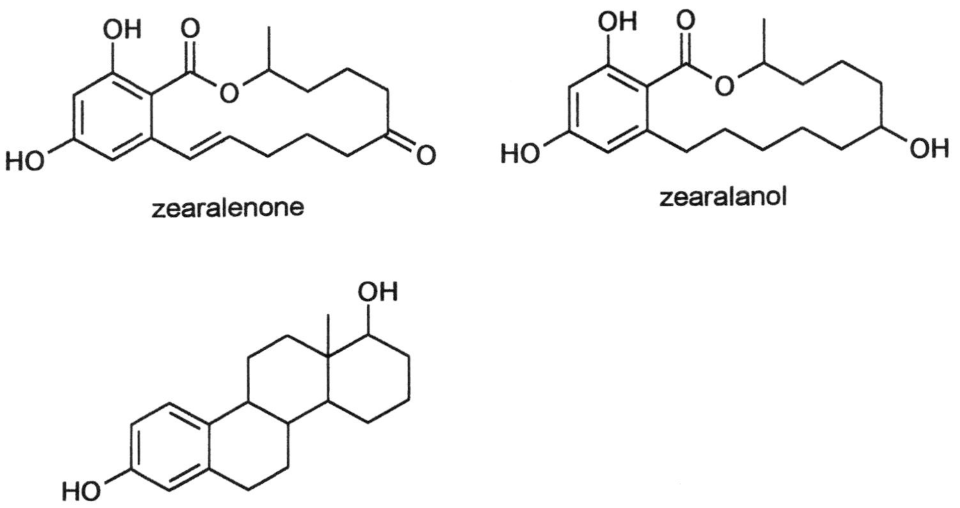

Figure 10. Chemical structures of zearalenone, zearalenol, and estradiol. These compounds induce similar responses due to binding and stimulation of estrogenic receptors.

the estrogenic activity of zearalenone. It is not, however, included routinely in mycotoxin screens by analytical laboratories. Zeranol, a synthetic growth promoter, has a similar structure to zearalenone; however, zeranol and its metabolites can be separated from zearalenone and its metabolites, thus allowing identification of the growth promoter in countries that have banned its use.

2. Biodistribution, Metabolism, and Excretion

Zearalenone is absorbed easily from the gastrointestinal tract. In the liver, metabolic reduction produces two stereoisomers, α- and β-zearalenol. There is significant species variation in the extent of zearalenone metabolism to zearalenol and the proportion of the two isomers, which vary significantly in their estrogenic potency. Zearalenone (as a combination of free and conjugated forms) and zearalenol are excreted relatively quickly in urine, feces, and milk. Considerable enterohepatic recycling of glucuronidated metabolites occurs in swine, extending the half-life of plasma zearalenone and prolonging its estrogenic effects. Zearalenone residues do not persist in animal tissues, although a small amount (less than 1%) of the

dose is excreted in milk; thus, significant contamination of the food chain does not occur.

C. CLINICAL SIGNS AND PATHOLOGY

1. Swine

Swine are the most susceptible species to zearalenone toxicity, with prepubertal animals the most sensitive. In the field, estrogenic effects may occur in swine fed diets containing ≥ 1 ppm zearalenone. In prepubertal gilts, effects include swelling and edema of the vulva, vaginal and rectal prolapse, uterine enlargement and edema, atrophy of the ovaries, enlargement of the mammary glands, and a thin catarrhal exudate from the vulva. Zearalenone in prepubertal boars may reduce libido and plasma testosterone. In castrated or prepubertal males, there is an enlargement of mammary glands and swelling of the prepuce. Testicular atrophy has also been reported.

Experimental exposure of prepubertal gilts to estradiol, zearalenone, and *F. roseum*-inoculated corn was reported by Kurtz to induce similar histological changes (for a detailed description of estrogenic changes in the reproductive tract, see Chapter 43). Cervical changes consisted of epithelial metaplasia; the normal double layer of columnar-type cells was replaced by a stratified squamous cellular layer, which was up to 15 cells thick and irregular in distribution. Similar but more severe changes were seen in the vagina. Interstitial edema, together with this cellular proliferation, accounts for the clinically observed tumefaction (swelling) of the vulva. The uterine horns were grossly enlarged due to edema with cellular proliferation and hypertrophy of all uterine layers. This uterotropic effect is the basis for the rat uterus bioassay, a practical laboratory test for estrogenic effects. Ovarian changes were variable, with the only consistent effect being an irregularity in the size of the developing follicles. The mammary gland and nipples were enlarged. Interstitial edema and ductal hyperplasia were observed in the mammary gland.

Reproductive problems may occur in sows, but higher levels of zearalenone are required. Changes induced by zearalenone depend on the time of administration in relation to the estrus cycle, as well as on the dose administered. Anestrus or nymphomania may be noted. In sows exhibiting nymphomania, ovaries are atrophic and lack corpora lutea and graafian follicles, indicating follicular atresia. The effects of zearalenone on the uterus, cervix, vagina, and mammary gland are similar to the effects in prepubertal gilts. A reduced litter size due to fetal resorption (mummification) and/or implantation failure occurs when the effects of dietary zearalenone are present at 7 to 10 days postmating. Pigs may be weak or stillborn and occasionally exhibit swollen vulvas at or shortly after birth (juvenile hyperestrogenism). Pseudopregnancy may develop with multiple persistent corpora lutea in the ovary, indicating a luteotrophic property of zearalenone. Uterine changes, characterized by both hyperplasia and hypertrophy, are indicative of estrogenic effects from zearalenone as well as a progesterone effect due to the persistent corpora lutea (see Chapter 43). Squamous metaplasia was present in the vagina. Alveolar development and ductular squamous metaplasia were observed in the mammary gland. Field observations of zearalenone-induced abortions are now

thought to be largely erroneous, as estrogens are luteotropic in swine. Instead, it is suspected that implantation failure followed by pseudopregnancy leads to a diagnosis of abortion.

2. Cattle and Sheep

Cattle and sheep are much less sensitive than pigs to the estrogenic effects of zearalenone. Zeranol, in the form of an implant, is widely used as a growth promoter in cattle. In cattle, zearalenone toxicity may be associated with precocious udder development in heifers and reduced fertility in breeding animals. Most animals exposed to zearalenone for brief periods of time will recover normal reproductive function. However, severe toxicosis may be characterized by ovarian fibrosis and changes in the fallopian tube and uterus, which could conceivably have more prolonged effects on reproduction. Ewe infertility with a decrease in ovulation rate and lambing percentage has been reported in New Zealand.

D. HUMAN RISK

Zearalenone in the diet could increase the estrogen burden of humans (see Chapter 21)

E. DIAGNOSIS, TREATMENT, AND PREVENTION

Clinical signs, together with the identification of zearalenone in the diet, form a strong basis for diagnosis. The diagnosis is usually confirmed when normal reproductive function returns after withdrawal of the contaminated feed. Zearalenone can be quantified by high-performance liquid chromatography in foodstuffs at most veterinary diagnostic laboratories. Semiquantitative methods such as thin-layer chromatography (TLC) and ELISA can also be used. Removal of contaminated feed is generally curative.

VI. Fumonisins

A. SOURCE/OCCURRENCE

Fumonisins are mycotoxins produced by *Fusarium verticillioides* (= *F. moniliforme*), *F. proliferatum*, and a few other *Fusarium* species. Both

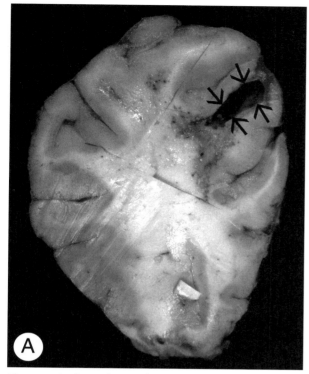

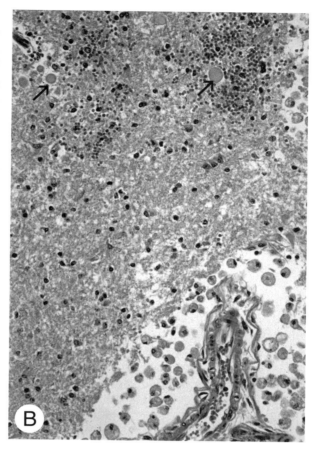

Figure 12. Brain from a horse that died from naturally occurring leukoencephalomalacia due to ingestion of a fumonisin-contaminated diet. (A) Section of left cerebrum. Focal malacia (necrosis, arrows) is confined to the subcortical white matter. (B) Section from the periphery of a malacic area. Extravasated red cells (hemorrhage) and swollen axons (spheroids, arrows) are present (top), as well as perivascular necrosis (malacia), edema, and infiltrating gitter cells (macrophages) (bottom) (H&E × 20).

are reported. Anorexia occurs due to glossopharyngeal paralysis and paralysis of the lips and tongue, with loss of ability to grasp and chew food. Incoordination, circling, ataxia, head pressing, marked stupor, and hyperesthesia are common, as are hyperexcitability, profuse sweating, mania, and convulsions. Acutely affected animals often progress through the manic and depressive stages of the syndrome within 4 to 12 hr of onset and become recumbent and moribund. Death may also occur without clinical signs being noted.

The hepatotoxic syndrome usually takes 5 to 10 days from time of onset to death. Icterus is usually prominent and there may be edema of the head and submandibular space, as well as oral petechia. Elevated serum bilirubin concentration and liver enzyme activities are typically present. Terminal neurologic signs may be noted, possibly due to secondary hepatoencephalopathy. The liver is often small and firm, with an increased lobular pattern. Centrilobular necrosis and moderate to marked periportal fibrosis can be observed histologically.

In the classical neurotoxic form, there is liquefactive necrosis of the white matter, primarily in the cerebrum (Fig. 12A). Liquefactive necrosis, located most commonly in the subcortical white matter, is often evident grossly as cavitation or discoloration. Histologically, necrosis with an influx of gitter cells, edema, and hemorrhage are primary lesions (Fig. 12B). Some cases may only exhibit histologic lesions consisting of perivascular edema and hemorrhage, with infiltration of mononuclear and plasma cells and occasionally eosinophils.

Experimental administration of purified FB_1, either by oral or intravenous route, can induce both neurologic and hepatic disease, with these generally occurring concurrently. Clinical signs and time course of the neurologic disease are similar to that in naturally occurring disease. In recent studies (Constable, personal communication), horses with neurologic disease were found to have increased protein in the cerebrospinal fluid and other changes consistent with vasogenic cerebral edema. Histologic lesions characterized by perivascular edema and hemorrhage, primarily of the white matter, were found in both brain and spinal cord. Serum biochemical evidence of hepatic injury was present in horses with neurologic disease, as well as in those horses given a dose that did not induce neurologic disease. This dose (0.01 mg/kg for 28 days) approximated oral ingestion of FB_1 at 8 ppm. These findings contradict the clinical literature, which suggests that the neurologic form occurs at lower exposure levels, whereas the hepatic form occurs at higher exposure levels. Hepatic lesions were characterized by hepatocellular apoptosis and necrosis (Fig. 13). Sphingosine and sphinganine levels were elevated in serum and tissues such as heart, liver, and kidney, but not in brain. An increase in serum cholesterol concentration was also present. Cardiovascular abnormalities in horses with neurologic disease were similar to those described for swine and included decreased cardiac contractility, heart rate, arterial pulse pressure, and increased systemic vascular resistance. However, histologic lesions were not observed in the heart.

2. Swine

Outbreaks of a fatal disease in swine fed *F. verticillioides*-contaminated corn screenings from the 1989 corn crop in the mid western and south eastern United State led to the identification of FB_1 as the causative agent of porcine pulmonary edema (PPE). Thousands of pigs died in these outbreaks. In Hungary, outbreaks of this disease have been reported since the 1950s. A decline in feed consumption is usually the first sign following fumonisin exposure. If fumonisin consumption is high, acute pulmonary edema and, generally, death follow within 4 to 7 days after onset of feeding the contaminated diet. Typically deaths cease within 48 hr after withdrawal from contaminated food.

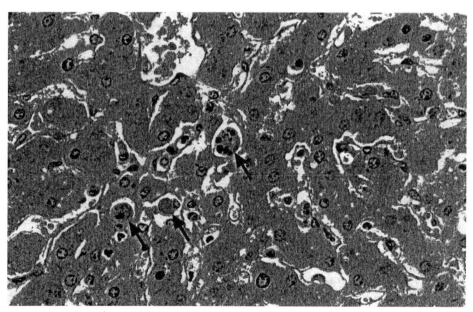

Figure 13. Liver from a horse given intravenous fumonisin B_1 at 0.2 mg/kg. Scattered apoptotic necrosis (arrows) is present (H&E × 400).

Porcine pulmonary edema has been reproduced experimentally in swine by feeding naturally contaminated feed, FB-containing culture material, and purified FB$_1$. Pulmonary edema has not been reported as a consistent finding in any other species. Severe pulmonary edema and hydrothorax occur in the acute form. Edema appears to originate in the interstitium with perivascular edema and markedly dilated lymphatics a prominent feature early in the disease (Fig. 14A). Ultrastructurally, pulmonary capillary endothelial cells contain membranous material in their cytoplasm (Fig. 14B). Liver injury is similar to that found in other species and is characterized by scattered hepatocyte apoptosis, necrosis, and proliferation. Pancreatic necrosis has been reported in some studies. Alterations in clinical pathology reflect hepatic injury, and the serum cholesterol concentration is elevated. Progressive and marked elevations in spinganine and sphingosine are found in serum and in major organs such as kidney, liver, lung, and heart, indicating a major disruption in sphingolipid biosynthesis. Although cardiac lesions have not been documented, FB$_1$ decreases cardiac contractility, mean systemic arterial pressure, heart rate, and cardiac output and increases mean pulmonary artery pressure and pulmonary artery wedge pressure. Therefore, fumonisin-induced pulmonary edema appears to result from acute left-sided heart failure. These changes are compatible with the inhibition of L-type calcium channels due to increased sphingosine and/or sphinganine.

At lower doses, slowly progressive liver disease may occur. Subacute hepatic injury is characterized by hepatocellular cytomegaly, disorganized hepatic cords, and early perilobular fibrosis, whereas chronic injury is characterized by icterus with severe hepatic fibrosis and nodular hyperplasia. Additional findings reported include esophageal plaques and right ventricular hypertrophy due to pulmonary hypertension.

As with other mycotoxins, fumonisin appears to affect the immune system. Effects on both specific and nonspecific immunity have

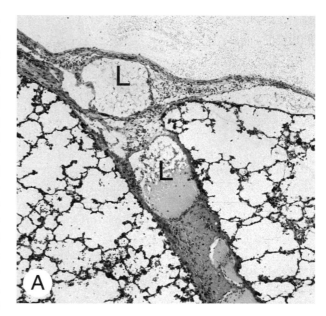

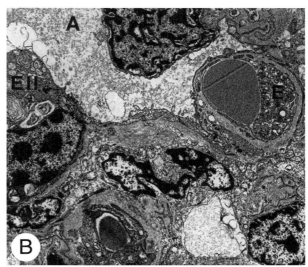

Figure 14. Lung from pigs fed fumonisin B$_1$ at 20 mg/kg/day as culture material in feed. (A) Prominent proteinaceous interstitial edema is present in the interlobular septum and pleura (top). Note the widely dilated lymphatics (L) present in the septum and pleura (H&E × 100). (B) Alveoli (A) contain proteinaceous edema fluid, whereas pulmonary capillary endothelial cells (E) contain abundant cytoplasmic granular material (EI, = type I epithelial cell; EII, type Ii epithelial cell). At higher magnification, this material has a membranous appearance (× 7400).

been reported. FB$_1$ decreased phagocytosis and inhibited sphingolipid biosynthesis in swine pulmonary macrophages and decreased clearance of particulates and bacteria from the pulmonary circulation.

3. Laboratory Animals

a. Rodents. The main target organs in rodents and rabbits are liver and kidney. The pathology has been described variously as "hepatopathy," "hepatosis," "nephropathy," or "nephrosis" and is similar in animals given purified fumonisin B_1, culture material (corn that is infected with a single fungal isolate and then molded under controlled laboratory conditions), or corn naturally contaminated with fumonisins.

In the liver, the earliest finding is hepatocellular apoptosis (previously called "single cell necrosis"). Affected cells are scattered throughout the hepatic lobules. Inflammation is usually absent. With increasing tissue injury, apoptotic cells become more numerous, and cytoplasmic vacuolation, mitotic figures, and hepatocytes undergoing oncotic necrosis are increasingly found. Cytomegaly, anisocytosis, and anisonucleosis occur as injury progresses.

Chronic nonneoplastic lesions consist of bile duct and oval cell proliferation, fibrosis, nodular regeneration (regenerative hyperplasia), foci of cellular alteration, and cholangiomatous lesions. There is loss of parenchyma around and between central veins. Macrophages containing pigment may be present in the centrilobular zone in mice. Inflammation remains minimal; when present, it is usually associated with focal necrosis. γ-Glutamyl transferase (GGT) and glutathione S-transferase (GST)-positive foci are demonstrated readily in rats.

Serum biochemical profiles support microscopic findings. Alanine and aspartate aminotransferase, alkaline phosphatase, and γ-glutamyl transpeptidase activities, as well as bile acids and bilirubin concentrations, are increased. Hypercholesterolemia occurs readily. Leukocytosis and altered differential leukocyte counts, thrombocytopenia, changes in serum immunoglobulin levels, and other evidence suggest that fumonisins exert subtle immunological or hematological effects.

Neoplastic hepatic lesions have been found only in male BD IX rats and female $B6C3F_1$ mice. They have been variously classified as neoplastic nodules, hepatocellular adenomas, or carcinomas. Proliferative biliary lesions, such as cholangiofibrosis, angiofibrosis, and cholangiocarcinoma, occur only in rats. Hepatocellular carcinomas in rats range from well-differentiated to more anaplastic, poorly differentiated types. In female $B6C3F_1$ mice, hepatic tumors ranged from discrete adenomas containing well-differentiated cells to hepatocellular carcinomas with poorly differentiated, anaplastic cells organized in the trabecular or adenoidal patterns commonly found in murine liver carcinomas.

The kidney is the other major target organ in rodents and rabbits. In Sprague–Dawley and Fisher 344 rats, males are more sensitive to nephrotoxic effects than females. Rabbits are also sensitive and display well-developed lesions at relatively low doses. In contrast, mice are relatively resistant to fumonisin-induced nephrotoxicity. Lesions, when found, generally consist of a only a few, scattered apoptotic tubular epithelial cells.

As in liver, apoptosis is the earliest finding in the kidney (Fig. 15). Apoptotic epithelial cells are scattered throughout the tubules of the outer stripe of the outer medulla and inner cortex (or corticomedullary junction). Apoptotic cells are detached from adjacent cells and slough into the tubular lumen. Accelerated apoptosis has been defined as a pivotal feature in the renal toxicity of fumonisin (see Chapter 33). More advanced lesions extend into the adjacent inner cortex and have both regenerative and atrophic components. Regenerative tubules are lined by epithelium that is basophilic and hyperplastic, often cuboidal rather than columnar, and with occasional mitoses. Mitoses are found more readily in advanced cases. Other tubules are atrophic and have flattened, squamous epithelium that make the lumina appear distended. The basement membrane of affected tubules may be amorphously thickened. Interstitial fibrosis is present in the most advanced cases. Inflammation is not a prominent feature.

680

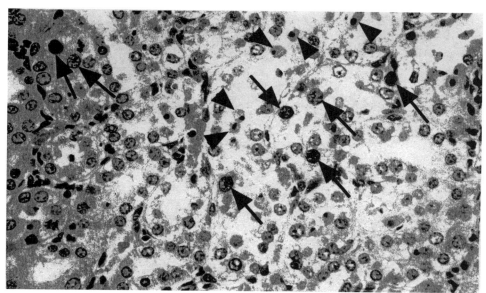

Figure 15. Kidney from a male F344 rat fed 50 ppm fumonisin B₁ for 6 weeks. Proliferating, BrdU-positive cells (arrows) and apoptotic (arrowheads) epithelial cells are present simultaneously in the renal tubules (BrdU immunostain). Similar lesions were found consistently in males fed 50 or 150 ppm FB₁ for up to 26 weeks. Courtesy of P. C. Howard, A. Warbritton, and T. J. Bucci, FDA National Center for Toxicological Research, Jefferson, AR.

Renal lesions are accompanied by decreased kidney weight and clinical signs of tubular dysfunction. The latter includes increased serum creatinine and decreased serum total carbon dioxide. Urine output and water consumption may be increased transiently. Other urinary findings include decreased osmolality, increased enzyme activities of γ-glutamyl transpeptidase, N-acetyl-β-glucosaminidase, and lactate dehydrogenase, inhibition of ρ-aminohippurate and tetraethylammonium transport, and proteinuria. Glomerular involvement is negligible.

Renal tubular adenomas and carcinomas have been found in F344 male rats fed high doses of fumonisins over an extended period (≥ 50 ppm for 2 years) (Fig. 16). Tumor morphology ranged from a clear cell type to a sarcomatous variant composed of spindle-shaped cells. Many of the carcinomas displayed a high degree of anaplasia, numerous mitosis, aggressive infiltration of the surrounding tissue, and metastases to the lung and lymph nodes. Neoplasms arose in kidneys that displayed varying degrees of apoptosis, tubular basophilia, regen-

eration and hyperplasia, and focal tubular atrophy, suggesting that an imbalance between cell loss and replication played a role in tumor induction.

b. Nonhuman Primates. There are no reports on the pathological effects of pure fumonisins in nonhuman primates. However, two of three baboons fed a diet contaminated with a strain of *Fusarium verticillioides*, now known to produce fumonisins, died of acute congestive heart failure after 143 to 248 days of exposure. After 720 days of exposure, the third baboon was found to have cirrhosis. Other findings in nonhuman primates (vervet monkeys) suggesting that fumonisins may have cardiovascular effects, in this case, atherogenic effects, are based on serum chemical findings and include elevated plasma cholesterol, low density lipoprotein C, and apoprotein B, as well as fibrinogen and coagulation factor VIII activation.

South African scientists have conducted a 13.5-year study on the effects of fumonisin-containing diets (varying concentrations) in vervet monkeys. Clinical findings suggestive of

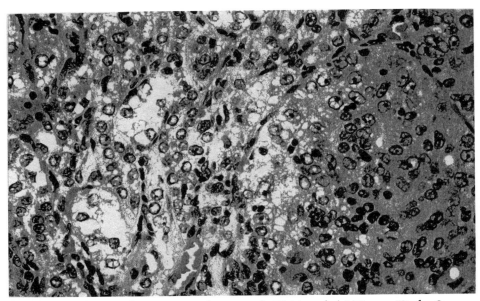

Figure 16. Renal tubular carcinoma from a male F344 rat fed 150 ppm FB$_1$ for 2 years (H&E). Fumonisin B$_1$ induced renal tubular carcinomas in males, but not females, fed 50 to 150 ppm. Courtesy of P. C. Howard, A. Warbritton, and T. J. Bucci, FDA National Center for Toxicological Research, Jefferson, AR.

liver dysfunction included increased alanine and aspartate aminotransaminase, γ-glutamyl transpeptidase, and lactate dehydrogenase activities. As in other species, serum cholesterol concentrations were also elevated. Serum creatinine concentrations were increased and creatinine clearance was decreased, suggesting that fumonisins affected renal function. Descriptions of microscopic lesions were confined to the liver, which was clearly a target organ. Lesions were consistent with those seen in other species and included apoptosis, bile duct proliferation, nodular hyperplasia, and perilobular fibrosis. Mitotic figures and apoptotic cells were present in the nodular structures.

D. HUMAN RISK

The risks to humans posed by fumonisins are at present undetermined. However, there is a correlation between consumption of moldy, "home grown" corn as a dietary staple and high rates of esophageal cancer in the Transkei, southern Africa, and Linxiang, north central China. Esophageal cancer in these regions occurs in both men and women, most often at age 50–60. It is

usually detected late and prognosis is poor. Retrosternal pain and dysphagia are common clinical signs due to the mass causing esophageal stricture. The tumors are located most frequently in the middle third of the esophagus, followed by the lower third and then the upper third. Ulceration is commonly seen. The tumors most often are keratinizing, squamous cell carcinomas. A variety of esophageal cytological changes, including dysplasia, chronic inflammation, basal cell hyperplasia, and hyperkeratosis, have been demonstrated in patients without frank malignancy.

In the Transkei, esophageal cancer tends to occur in clusters, leading to the formation of "high cancer" and "low cancer" areas. Home grown corn from "high cancer areas" is contaminated more frequently with *F. verticillioides* and has higher average fumonisin concentrations than adjacent, "low esophageal cancer areas." Surveys of corn in China have shown either a higher average fumonisin concentration or a higher percentage of contaminated corn in "high cancer areas" compared to low cancer areas. It has been speculated that fumonisins

682

may also be an etiological factor for liver cancer in China, especially in regions where it and aflatoxin occur together. Liver cancer is also one of the more frequently encountered cancers in men from the Transkei. These observations do not conclusively show a link between fumonisins and cancer in man. A number of other factors have been cited as being the cause of, or contributing to, esophageal and other cancers found in these regions. Among these are nitrosamines from food and tobacco, mineral deficiencies in the soil, and poor nutrition. Furthermore, it remains a possibility that other mycotoxins, acting alone or in concert with fumonisins, are the cause of the esophageal cancer that has been associated with *F. verticillioides*. Support for this possibility comes from the lack of data from chronic experimental studies in rodents and nonhuman primates that would implicate the esophagus as a target organ of fumonisins. Perhaps of greater concern for humans is the link between cardiovascular disease and fumonisins documented in swine, horses, and nonhuman primates, and the consistent finding of elevated cholesterol levels in all species exposed to fumonisins.

E. DIAGNOSIS, TREATMENT, AND PREVENTION

Diagnosis is based on a history of ingestion of corn, particularly corn screenings or unscreened corn, together with characteristic clinical signs and lesions. Detection of approximately 10 ppm fumonisin in horse feed or ≥ 50 ppm in swine feed is highly suggestive of toxicosis. Assays [high-pressure liquid chromatography (HPLC), derivatization] are now available for fumonisin at most veterinary diagnostic laboratories. An ELISA-based screening test for fumonisin is available from Neogen. In addition, elevated sphinganine and sphingosine in serum and tissues are considered an excellent biomarker of exposure. There is no known effective therapy.

For equine species, it has been recommended that the total diet contain no more than 1 ppm fumonisin B_1, whereas for swine the total diet

should contain less than 10 ppm fumonisin B_1. For dairy and beef cattle, the total diet should contain no more than 15 and 50 ppm fumonisin B_1 respectively. For nonbreeding poultry, it has been recommended that the total diet contain no more than 50 ppm fumonisin B_1.

VII. Ergot Alkaloids

A. SOURCE/OCCURRENCE

Ergot alkaloids are produced by various fungi, in particular those that parasitize the seed heads of grasses and small grains (*Claviceps* spp.), and the endophyte (*Neotyphodium coenophialum*), which infects grasses such as tall fescue. The term ergot is used in two ways: as the common name for the fungus *Claviceps*, which invades the ovary of grasses and cereals, and in reference to the sclerotium, the hard purple or black mass consisting largely of mycelial hyphae that replaces the seed head of grasses and contains ergot alkaloids. Hence the term ergotism or ergot toxicosis, which is used primarily for poisoning resulting from the ingestion of *Claviceps* spp.-infected grains and grasses. The term fescue toxicosis connotes syndromes that result from the ingestion of tall fescue infected with *N. coenophialum*. This term was well entrenched before the identification of ergot alkaloids, particularly ergovaline, produced by *N. coenophialum* as potential causative agents.

1. Claviceps spp.

Host plants for *C. purpurea* include rye, triticale, barley, oats, wheat, Kentucky bluegrass, brome grass, timothy, and quack grasses. In commercial grain trade, wheat or rye is classified as "ergoty" and rejected for commercial sale if more than 0.3% by weight is composed of infected grain, and oats, triticale, and barley are so graded when they contain more than 0.1%. *C. paspali* grows on grasses of the *Paspalum* spp. In some parts of the world, *Claviceps* fungi have been isolated from *Sorghum* grain that contained ergot alkaloids. The severity of infection by *Claviceps* spp. is of high seasonal variability because the extent of infection depends on many factors, including temperature, humidity, and farming practices.

Ergot toxicosis in livestock can be manifested by hyperthermia (elevated body temperature) and susceptibility to heat stress with an accompanying reduction of feed intake, weight gain, reproductive performance, prolactin secretion, and milk production; dry gangrene of the extremities (gangrenous form); and behavioral effects (convulsive form). These effects are relatively species specific and are modified by the ergot source, amount consumed, period of exposure, and age and stage of production of the animal.

Ergot poisoning in humans, sometimes of epidemic proportions, has occurred due to the ingestion of rye contaminated by *Claviceps* spp. It was first described in the Middle Ages and was characterized by gangrene and intense burning of the extremities, giving rise to the term "Saint Anthony's fire." Behavioral abnormalities, convulsions, and miscarriages were also reported.

2. Neotyphodium coenophialum

Tall fescue (*Festuca arundinacea*) is the major plant host for the endophytic fungus *N. coenophialum*, previously known as *Acremonium coenophianum*, and before that as *Epichloe typhina*. This organism is a Clavicipitaceae fungus that is transmitted in the seed (and not via spores) and can produce ergot alkaloids, especially ergovaline, as well as other mycotoxins. Infection with *N. coenophialum* confers drought and stress tolerance and pest resistance to the plant.

Tall fescue is a major forage grass, grown on an estimated 35 million acres in the United States. The grass is sometimes allowed to "accumulate or stockpile" for winter grazing and is cultivated extensively as hay. Fescue is especially important in the Pacific Northwest, Kentucky, and southeastern sections. It is estimated that over 90% of tall fescue fields in the United States are infected with the endophyte to some extent, with an average of 62% of the plants infected within each field. It is estimated

that ergot alkaloids cause $1 billion in livestock damage each year in the United States alone due to toxic effects after livestock consumption of endophyte-infected plant materials. Fescue toxicosis has also been reported in Argentina, Australia, and New Zealand. The toxicoses can manifest as circulatory and thus thermoregulatory disturbances, culminating in local hypothermia (fescue foot) or generalized hyperthermia (summer fescue toxicosis); altered lipid metabolism (fat necrosis); increased oxidative stress; and reproductive effects.

B. TOXICOLOGY

1. Toxins

Ergot alkaloids can be divided into two structural groups: amino acid alkaloids (e.g., ergotamine) and amine alkaloids and congeners (e.g., lysergic acid and ergonovine) (Fig. 17). Amino acid alkaloids and amine alkaloids are derived from lysergic acid. Amino acid alkaloids are the most physiologically active with ergotamine and ergocristine of greatest importance. Of amine alkaloids, ergonovine is among the most potent. Amino acid alkaloids are potent vasoconstrictors and are highly oxytocic (stimulate uterine smooth muscle) if given intravenously, but not orally. Amino acid alkaloids also inhibit nerves stimulated by sympathomimetic amines. Amine alkaloids are rapid acting, powerful oxytocics and weak vasoconstrictors. Lysergic acid diethylamide (LSD) causes depersonalization or hallucinations and may produce toxic psychosis.

The toxic effects of *Claviceps* spp.-infected grains and grasses are due to numerous ergot alkaloids, such as ergotamine, ergocristine, and ergonovine, that are present in the sclerotia. Most or all of the toxicological problems associated with tall fescue are believed to be caused by endophyte-produced alkaloids, with amino acid alkaloids being primarily responsible. Ergovaline accounts for about 90% of the amino acid alkaloids in endophyte-infected fescue. However, some questions regarding the identity of the toxin(s) causing endophyte-infected fescue toxicity still remain.

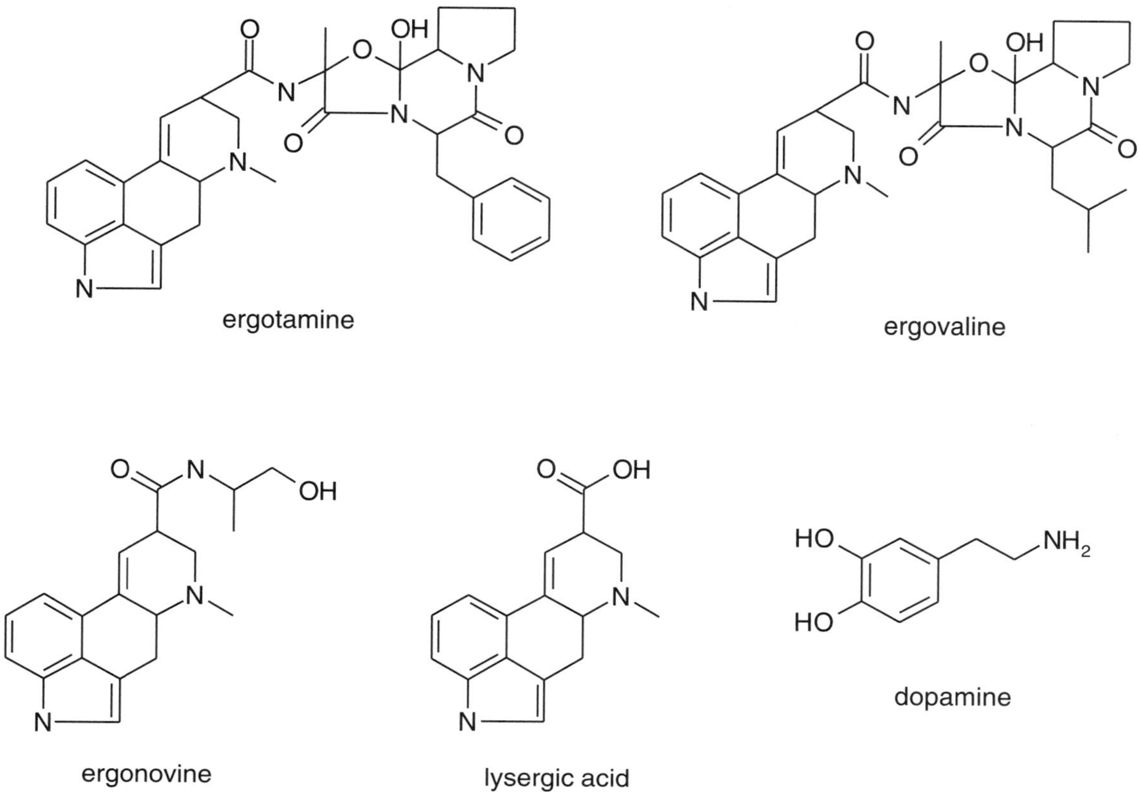

Figure 17. Chemical structures of selected ergot alkaloids and dopamine. The structural similarity of ergot alkaloids to dopamine influences action at the dopamine receptor.

Ergovaline is believed to account for the decrease in prolactin and other major effects of endophyte-infected fescue, most of which are compatible with the effect of ergot alkaloids (vasoconstrictive and dopamine agonist properties). Other ergot alkaloids include ergosine, ergonine, and lysergic acid amide (ergine). Lysergic acid has sedative properties as well as effects on the autonomic nervous system, such as hypersalivation, emesis, dizziness, and diarrhea. Loline alkaloids are another class of alkaloids that originate from the endophyte in tall fescue. These are saturated pyrrolizidine alkaloids. Their role, if any, in fescue toxicoses is considered minor.

2. Biodistribution, Metabolism, and Excretion

Although ergot alkaloids disappear rapidly from blood and tissue, their physiologic effects persist for a long time. For example, ergotamine produces vasoconstriction that lasts for at least 24 hr despite a plasma half-life of about 2 hr. Ergotamine is absorbed poorly and erratically from the upper gastrointestinal tract with a high first-pass clearance by the liver. Ergotamine is metabolized (detoxified) in the liver by cytochrome P450 enzymes with metabolites excreted primarily in the bile. Ergot alkaloids are not transferred in the milk of cows consuming ergot. Meat and milk residues have not been detected in any field outbreaks.

In humans, bioavailability depends on the route of administration, but can also vary widely when given repeatedly to the same patient. Bioavailability is <5% with oral formulations with peak plasma levels occurring at 1 to 3 hr. Absorption is considerably higher with rectal administration (as suppositories). LSD

685

is absorbed rapidly after oral administration and is distributed widely. LSD crosses the blood—barrier easily and enters the brain, its target site of action.

3. Mechanism of Action

The wide spectrum of pharmacological activity of ergot alkaloids is, in general, attributed to their action as partial agonists and antagonists at adrenergic, dopaminergic, and tryptaminergic [also called serotonin or serotonergic, e.g., 5-hydroxytryptamine (5-HT)] receptors. For example, the marked effects of ergotamine on the cardiovascular system are due to simultaneous peripheral vasoconstriction, depression of vasomotor centers, and peripheral adrenergic blockade. The spectrum of effects depends on the agent, species, tissue, and experimental or physiologic conditions.

The primary effects of ergot alkaloids are due to actions on the central nervous system (central/neurohormonal) and direct stimulation of smooth muscle (peripheral). Central neurohormonal effects are due to the structural similarity of ergot alkaloids to biogenic amines. Dopaminergic action, through activation of D2-dopamine receptors in pituitary lactotrophs, can result in a reduction of prolactin secretion by the pituitary, which can reduce milk production. Other neuroendocrine compounds whose secretion is affected include epinephrine and norepinephrine, melatonin (secreted by the pineal gland), and serotonin. The resulting neurotransmitter imbalance affects growth, reproduction, and the ability to respond to seasonal changes in photoperiod and environmental temperature.

Peripheral effects include vasoconstriction, elevated blood pressure, and damage to the capillary endothelium. Contraction of all smooth muscle, vascular and nonvascular, occurs independent of innervation or chemical mediators. Blood vessels in all vascular beds are constricted by the ergot alkaloids, but the larger arteries are most sensitive. Occlusion may be demonstrated by arteriograms. The overall result is ischemia of tissues perfused by

the artery. It is possible for blood flow to be reestablished without permanent damage or the tissue may become gangrenous. The limbs, toes, ears, and tail are often affected, but usually not all in the same animal. Occasionally, scattered areas of the skin may also become gangrenous.

During the third trimester of pregnancy, ergot alkaloids have an oxytocin-like effect on the uterus and can induce labor, as uterine muscle is more sensitive to ergot at this time than other smooth muscle. In early pregnancy, these alkaloids are more stimulatory to the cervix than to the uterus.

Various ergot alkaloids, including LSD, produce hallucinogenic effects. The toxic mechanism of LSD is likely related to perturbations of serotonergic neurotransmission, resulting in profound alterations in perception, mood, and judgement, as well as hallucinogenic effects in humans. This effect appears to be mediated by the activation of 5-HT_{1c} receptors. Catecholaminergic stimulation also occurs, resulting in mydriasis, increased blood pressure, tachycardia, elevated body temperature, tremors, and hyperreflexia.

4. Species Susceptibility

Individual responses vary with the total amount and mixture of individual alkaloids in the feed, frequency of ingestion, climatic conditions (cool, wet weather is associated with apparent increases in the risk of gangrenous lesions), and species. The gangrenous form can affect all domestic animals, birds, and humans. The extremities (nose, ears, tail, and limbs) are affected due to the vasoconstriction of arterioles and damage to capillary endothelium. The convulsive form can occur in cattle, horses, sheep, and humans, is manifested by convulsions and incoordination, and may be accompanied by lameness, difficulty in breathing, excessive salivation, and diarrhea. Reproductive effects are characterized by abortion, high neonatal mortality, and reduced lactation or agalactia.

C. CLINICAL SIGNS AND PATHOLOGY

1. Syndromes Associated Primarily with Claviceps spp. Infection

a. Cattle. The gangrenous form results when animals ingest ergot alkaloids over a period of days or weeks. Clinical signs include reduced feed intake, unthriftiness, lameness, swelling, and sloughing of feet below the fetlocks (generally the hind feet). Less commonly the ears and tail are sloughed. Affected extremities may become inflamed and then cold, with numbness and dry gangrene developing. Usually a line of demarcation separates the proximal viable tissue and the distal dry, cold epidermis. Eventually, there is a loss (sloughing) of distal tissue. Cutaneous ergotism with skin necrosis resembling photosensitization has been reported.

The convulsive form is primarily associated with *C. paspali* infection of *Paspalum* spp. grasses (e.g., dallisgrass). Clinical signs, including nervousness and stamping of the feet, develop in animals kept on contaminated hay after about 1 week. They progress to include hyperexcitability, belligerency, incoordination, convulsions, and opisthotonus (star-gazing posture). Reproductive effects are rarely observed.

b. Swine, Horses, and Poultry. The primary signs in swine with ergotism are agalactia, early parturition, weak or dead piglets, infertility, and reduced rate of gain. Sheep consuming *C. purpurea* ergot have breathing difficulty, excessive salivation, diarrhea, and gastrointestinal bleeding. In addition, necrosis of the tongue, gastroenteritis, abortions, gangrene, and central nervous system involvement have been reported. Horses grazing *C. paspali*-infected grasses may develop convulsive ergotism. Comb gangrene is a major symptom of ergotism in mature poultry.

Hyperthermia and susceptibility to heat stress, as well as agalactia due to a severe reduction in serum prolactin, also occur in livestock consuming ergot alkaloids.

2. Syndromes Associated Primarily with Neotyphodium coenophialum Infection of Tall Fescue

a. Overview. Syndromes associated with the ingestion of endophyte-infected tall fescue include summer syndrome (summer fescue toxicosis, summer slump), fescue foot, and fat necrosis in cattle and reproductive and lactation problems in cattle, sheep, and especially horses. Summer syndrome is the most commonly reported manifestation of fescue toxicoses. Severe hypoprolactemia (serum prolactin as low as 1–2% of normal) is the most dramatic clinical sign. Prolactin influences milk secretion, reproduction, gut motility, appetite, and fat metabolism (lipogenesis).

b. Summer Fescue Toxicosis (Systemic Hyperthermia, Cattle). Summer syndrome in cattle is characterized by hyperthermia (elevated body temperature), poor weight gain, reduced feed intake, reduced conception rates, intolerance to heat, failure to shed the winter hair coat (rough hair), nervousness, and excessive salivation. The vasoconstrictive effects of ergot alkaloids interfere with the normal physiological response to heat stress, which consists of dissipation of heat from the body surface by way of increased blood flow to the periphery where surface blood vessels are dilated. Instead, in fescue toxicosis, there is reduced blood flow to peripheral tissues and heat does not dissipate normally, leading to elevated body temperature.

c. Fescue Foot (Local Hypothermia, Cattle). Fescue foot in cattle is characterized by lameness and gangrene of the extremities, which is identical to classical gangrenous ergotism. This most often follows the onset of cooler or cold weather (below 60°F and especially in the presence of snow or ice) when blood supply to the extremities tends to be reduced. Clinical manifestations are noted from 5 to 15 days, up to weeks, after being on pasture and occasionally where continuously pastured. Signs include slight arching of the back, rough hair coat, soreness in one or both rear limbs, weight shifting, and holding one foot up as well as knuckling and loose stools. In addition, there is swelling of the coronary band (Fig. 18) and redness, swelling, and purple-black discoloration of the tip of the tail. Sloughing of the ear tips, as well as sloughing of the feet, usually at or just above the coronary band and sometimes higher, can occur. In horses, laminitis has been reported following exposure to endophyte-infected tall fescue.

d. Fat Necrosis (Cattle). Fat necrosis or lipomatosis in cattle is characterized by the presence of multiple hard, yellowish or chalky white irregularly shaped masses in the abdominal adipose tissue, most notably in the mesenteries. On cut section, the masses have a dry, hard, cheesy, opaque appearance; calcification occasionally may be present; subcutaneous fat is not affected. Exposure to toxic tall fescue over several seasons is required. Causative factors may be vasoconstriction, either directly or secondary to a febrile condition and increased oxidative stress that can trigger lipolytic processes. Because of its sporadic nature, this condition is of limited economic importance when sizable herds are encountered.

Consequences of fat necrosis include digestive disturbances due to obstruction or intestinal constriction, scanty feces, bloating, and occasionally death. Dystocia, due to hardening of adipose tissue around the birth canal, or urine retention, due to similar deposits along the urinary tract, with associated postrenal uremia, may occur. Other signs associated with fat necrosis include weight loss, poor appetite, listlessness, and rough hair coat. Masses associated with fat necrosis may be detected on rectal exam.

e. Reproductive Effects (Horses, Cattle, Sheep). The effects of endophyte-infected fescue are manifested when mares consume the grass after day 300 of pregnancy. Serum cortisol concentrations do not increase normally near parturition and serum prolactin, progesterone,

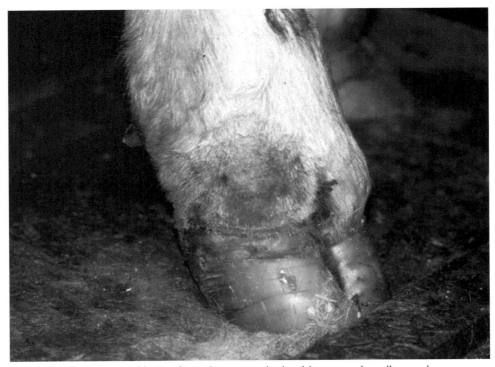

Figure 18. Field case of fescue foot. There is marked reddening and swelling at the coronary band. This is similar to an early case of gangrenous ergotism.

and triiodothyronine levels are extremely low. Mares may abort or, more often, have dystocia after prolonged gestation. A tough, thickened, and edematous placenta may be present that increases the need for assistance during parturition. Placental changes include edema, mucoid degeneration of vessels, and fibrosis. These changes are consistent with anoxia. The low progesterone may contribute to prolonged gestation. Foals may be carried past term and become large and weak and have elongated hooves. Survival of foals is very low and death losses increase in mares, especially if they are not assisted during parturition. Affected mares have low milk production or agalactia attributable to low prolactin levels. Other clinical signs in pregnant mares grazing toxic pastures are intermittent diarrhea and excessive sweating.

Reproductive and lactation problems also occur in cattle and sheep. General reproductive efficiency is impaired, but without the pronounced effects on the fetus and parturition that occur in horses. In cattle, reduced calving rates (a 70–80% calf crop) may be due to altered luteal function and decreased circulating progesterone. Dairy cows may have a marked decrease in milk production due, in part, to depressed prolactin concentrations. In ewes, serum prolactin levels are depressed by the ingestion of affected fescue and there is an increased rate of return to estrus.

D. HUMAN RISK

Epidemics of human ergotism occurred in Europe in the Middle Ages and in France from the 9th to the 14th centuries due to the consumption of ergotized (*Claviceps* spp.-infected) grain. Manifestations of ergotism included itching, numbness, muscle cramps, sustained spasms and convulsions, and extreme pain. A victim's extremities, usually a foot or leg, would feel cold, alternating with a burning sensation (St. Anthony's fire). Numbness and dry gangrene, followed by loss of fingers, hands, or feet, was common. Abortion was a frequent complication of ergot poisoning. A convulsive form of ergotism was also known. It has been suggested by Matossian that the frenzied activities of peasants that culminated in the French Revolution may have been due to ergot alkaloids in rye bread, the staple food of the peasants at that time. With changes in farming practices, such as wheat replacing rye as the major grain crop, the epidemics ceased. A recent report was published following an outbreak of ergotism affecting humans (and animals) in France in 1951, when moldy rye was used to make bread.

The official introduction of ergot into human medicine was early in the 19th century as a means to quicken childbirth. However, the dangers of using ergot in childbirth, including stillbirth, were rapidly recognized and it was recommended that ergot only be used to control postpartum hemorrhage. Current clinical medical use of ergot alkaloids is for the treatment of migraine, Parkinson's disease, and postpartum hemorrhaging.

Human risk from ergot alkaloids in developed countries is primarily from the overdose of therapeutic drugs (ergotamine tartrate, generally in combination with caffeine) used for migraine headaches, from drug abuse, as with ingestion of large amounts of ergotamine to induce abortion, or from use of recreational drugs such as LSD rather than ingestion of contaminated cereal grains. Side effects of therapeutic usage of ergotamine in migraine preparations include nausea and, less commonly, abdominal and muscle cramps of the lower extremities, diarrhea, and vertigo. At high doses, acute effects include vomiting, diarrhea, intense thirst, itching, tingling and cold skin, rapid and weak pulse, confusion, and coma. Death may follow. The most common serious chronic effect reported is ischemia of the extremities due to severe peripheral vasospasms resulting in gangrenous ergotism. Overuse of ergotamine has also been reported to result in encephalopathy, focal motor or sensory symptoms, seizures, and coma. Use of ergotamine for its abortifacient effects frequently led to excessive uterine contraction and often caused ischemic damage to the child.

Lysergic acid diethylamide (lysergide), in humans, causes signs of catecholaminergic stimulation, such as mydriasis, increased blood pressure, tachycardia, elevated body temperature, tremor, and hyperreflexia, as well as severe perceptual distortion and hallucinations. The effects generally disappear over a 12-hr period. Long-term use may precipitate persistent psychosis or posthallucinogenic perceptual disorder.

E. DIAGNOSIS, TREATMENT, AND PREVENTION

1. Toxicoses Associated with Claviceps spp. Infection (Ergotism)

Ergot sclerotia in cereal grains and grasses (ergot does not occur in corn) are generally readily detectable by visual examination. Sclerotia in baled forages can be found by shaking several handfuls over a plastic bag and examining the chaff. However, microscopic examination of ground diets (feed microscopy) may be needed to determine the presence of ergot. Ergot alkaloids may be identified in toxicology laboratories by TLC, HPLC, or gas chromatography–mass spectrometry (GCMS).

Treatment consists of isolating animals from the source and, if appropriate, moving them to a dry, warm environment to avoid aggravation of the vascular insult. An intravenous infusion of sodium nitroprusside, a potent vasodilator, has been used to alleviate the vasoconstriction. In humans, anticoagulants, low molecular weight dextran, and nitroprusside have been used for treatment.

2. Toxicoses Associated with Neotyphodium coenophialum Infection of Tall Fescue (Fescue Toxicity)

Clinical signs are highly suggestive of fescue toxicosis. Foot rot, frost bite, and mechanical injuries such as stone bruising should be ruled out in suspected fescue foot cases. Fescue tillers (large grass shafts cut at the level of the soil) should be submitted to a veterinary diagnostic laboratory for determination of the percentage infection by the endophyte. Also, grass or hay should be analyzed for ergovaline, with HPLC quantification being the predominant method. An ELISA method that detects

nonspecific ergot alkaloids can also be used. Recently, urinary alkaloid excretion has been suggested as a useful diagnostic test. Reduced serum prolactin levels have been used for research purposes.

Prevention is by avoiding or decreasing exposure of animals to endophyte-infected pastures, especially where seeds are present. Ammoniation of hay will reduce toxicity, and detoxification is dependent on ammonia concentrations. Brahman-type cattle are more resistant than European breeds to both heat stress and other aspects of fescue toxicosis. Pregnant mares should be removed from endophyte-infected tall fescue by 300 days of gestation.

VIII. Summary/Conclusion

As this chapter demonstrates, mycotoxins are a structurally and functionally diverse group of organic compounds. They can affect all body systems with some compounds causing primarily acute and highly reversible effects and others causing irreversible organ damage. Recognizing the character of specific body system effects, the usual time course of pathogenesis and reversibility, and linkage to sufficiently contaminated source materials (most often a foodstuff) are essential in the diagnosis of mycotoxicoses. Although mycotoxin-induced diseases were often recognized many years, even centuries, ago, their recognition as specific causes of diseases is a comparatively recent development. As a result, major knowledge gaps remain to be filled through research for many of the known mycotoxins, particularly effects of low-level chronic exposure and mycotoxin interactions.

ACKNOWLEDGMENTS

Thanks to Dr. Shih-Hsuan Hsiao and Sandra Durst for assistance with the illustrations and Jaime Davis for typing the manuscript.

SUGGESTED READING

General

Berry, C. L. (1988). The pathology of mycotoxins. *J. Pathol.* **154**, 301–311.

Bondy, G. S. and Pestka, J. J. (2000). Immunomodulation by fungal toxins. *J. Toxicol. Environ. Health B Crit. Rev.* **3**, 109–143.

Bottalico, A., Logrieco, A., Ritieni, A., Moretti, A., Randazzo, G., and Corda, P. (1995). Beauvericin and fumonisin B₁ in preharvest *Fusarium moniliforme* maize ear rot in Sardinia. *Food Addit. Contam.* **12**, 599–607.

Bray, G. A., and Ryan, D. H. (eds.) (1991). "Mycotoxins, Cancer and Health." Louisiana State University Press, Baton Rouge and London.

Cheeke, P. R. (1998). "Natural Toxicants in Feeds, Forages, and Poisonous Plants." Interstate Publishers, Danville, IL.

Gaultier, P. (1999). Biotransformation and fate of mycotoxins. *J. Toxicol. Toxin Rev.*, **18**, 295–312.

Hollinger, K., and Ekperigin, H. E. (1999). Mycotoxicosis in food producing animals. *Vet. Clin. North Am. Food Anim. Pract*, **15**, 133–165.

Kadis, S., Ciegler, A., and Ajl, S. J. (eds.) "Microbial Toxins: Algal and Fungal Toxins," Vol. 8. Academic Press, New York.

Keeler, R. F., and Tu, A. T. (eds.) (1983). "Handbook of Natural Toxins," Vol. 1. Dekker, New York.

Kurata, H. H., and Ueno, Y. (eds.) (1984). "Toxigenic Fungi: Their Toxins and Health Hazard." Elsevier, New York.

Kuiper-Goodman, T. (1998). Food safety: Mycotoxins and phycotoxins in perspective. *In* "Mycotoxins and Phycotoxins: Developments in Chemistry, Toxicology, and Food Safety" (M. Miraglia, H. van Egmond, C. Brera, and J. Gilbert, eds.). International Union of Pure and Applied Chemistry (IUPAC), Oxford.

Kuiper-Goodman, T. (1995). Mycotoxins: Risk assessment and legislation. *Toxicol Lett.* **82–83**, 853–859.

Leeson, S., Diaz, G., and Summers, J. D. (1995). "Poultry Metabolic Disorders and Mycotoxins." University Books, Guelph, Canada.

Malloy, C. D., and Marr, J. S. (1997). Mycotoxins and public health: A review. *J. Public Health Manag. Prac.* **3**, 61–69.

Matossian, M. A. K. (1989). "Poisons of the Past: Molds, Epidemics and History." Yale Univ. Press, New Haven, CT.

Miller, D., and Trenholm, L. H. (1994). "Mycotoxins in Grain: Compounds Other Than Aflatoxin." Eagan Press, St. Paul, MN.

Mycotoxins: Economic and Health Risks (1989). Task Force Report 116, Council for Agricultural Science and Technology, Ames, IA.

Pier, A. C. (1981). Mycotoxins and animal health. *Adv. Vet. Sci. Comp. Med.* **25**, 185–243.

Peraica, M., Radic, B., Lucic, A., and Pavlovic, M. (1999). Toxic effects of mycotoxins in humans. *Bull. WHO* **77**, 754–766.

Richard, J. L., Bennett, G. A., Ross, P. F., and Nelson, P. E. (1993). Analysis of naturally occurring mycotoxins in feedstuffs and food. *J. Anim. Sci.* **71**, 2563–2574.

Richard, J. L., and Thurston, J. R. (eds.) (1986). "Diagnosis of Mycotoxicosis." Martinus Nijhoff Publishers, Dordrecht.

Scudamore, K. A., Hetmanski, M. T., Nawaz, S., Naylor, J., and Rainbird, S. (1997). Determination of mycotoxins in pet foods sold for domestic pets and wild birds using linked-column immunoassay clean-up and HPLC. *Food Addit. Contam.* **14**, 175–86.

Seawright, A. A. (1989). "Animal Health in Australia," Vol. 2. Australian Government Publishing Service, Canberra.

Selected Mycotoxins: Ochratoxins, Trichothecenes, Ergot. Environmental Health Criteria; 105, United Nations Environmental Programme, International Labour Organization and the World Health Organization, Geneva, 1990.

Sharma, R. P. (1993). Immunotoxicity of mycotoxins. *J. Diary Sci.* **76**, 892–897.

Sudakin, D. L. (1997). Effects of mycotoxins in health and disease. *J. Am. Med. Assoc.* **278**, 1063.

van Egmond, H. P., Visconti, A., Boenke, A., and Speijers, G. J. A. (1995). Mycotoxins and toxic plant components. *Natural Toxins* **3**, 181–341.

Aflatoxins

Adhikari, M., Ramjee, G., and Berjak, P. (1994). Aflatoxin, kwashiorkor, and morbidity. *Natural Toxins* **2**, 1–3.

Carnaghan, R. B. A., and Crawford, M. (1964). Relationship between ingestion of aflatoxin and primary liver cancer. *Br. Vet. J.* **120**, 201–204.

Cysewski, S. J., Pier, A. C., Baetz, A. L., and Cheville, N. F. (1982). Experimental equine aflatoxicosis. *Toxicol. Appl. Pharmacol.* **65**, 354–365.

Dvorackova, I. (1990). "Aflatoxins and Human Health." CRC Press, Boca Raton, FL.

Eaton, D. L., and Groopman, J. D. (eds.) (1994). "The Toxicology of Aflatoxins." Academic Press, San Diego.

Groopman, J. D., Cain, L. G., and Kensler, T. W. (1988). Aflatoxin exposure in human populations: Measurement and relationship to cancer. *Crit. Rev. Toxicol.* **19**, 113–145.

Hoerr, F. J., D'Andrea, G. H., Giambrone, J. J., and Panangala, V. S. (1986). Comparative histopathologic changes in aflatoxicosis. *In* "Diagnosis of Mycotoxicoses" (J. L. Richard, J. R. Thurston, eds.), pp 179–189. Martin Nijhoff Publishers, Boston, MA.

IARC-WHO (1993). Some naturally occurring substances: Food items and constituents, heterocyclic aromatic amines and mycotoxins. *In* "IARC Monographs on the Evaluation of Carcinogenic Risks to Humans," pp. 246–315. International Agency for Research on Cancer, Lyon, France.

Massey, T. E., Stewart, R. K., Daniels, J. M., and Liu, L. (1995). Biochemical and molecular aspects of mammalian susceptibility to aflatoxin B_1 carcinogenicity. *Proc. Soc. Exp. Biol. Med.* **208**, 213–227.

Miller, D. M., Crowell, W. A., and Stuart, B. P. (1982). Acute aflatoxicosis in swine: Clinical pathology, histopathology, and electron microscopy. *Am. J. Vet. Res.* **43**, 273–277.

Newberne, P. M., and Butler, W. H. (1969). Acute and chronic effects of aflatoxin on the liver of domestic and laboratory animals: A review *Cancer Res.* **29**, 236–250.

Newberne, P. M., and Wogan, G. N. (1968). Sequential morphological changes in aflatoxin B_1 carcinogenesis in the rat. *Cancer Res.* **28**, 770–781.

Norred, W. P. (1986). Occurrence and clinical manifestations of aflatoxicosis. *In* "Diagnosis of Mycotoxicosis" (J. R. Thurston and J. L. Richard, eds.), pp. 11–30. Matinus Nijhoff, Dordrecht.

Ramsdell, H. S., and Eaton, D. L. (1990). Species susceptibility to aflatoxin B_1 carcinogenesis: Comparative kinetics of microsomal biotransformation. *Cancer Res.* **50**, 615–620.

Richard, J. L., Pier, A. C., Stubblefield, R. D., Shotwell, O. L., Lyon, R. L., and Cutlip, R. C. (1983). Effect of feeding corn naturally contaminated with aflatoxin on feed efficiency, on physiologic, immunologic, and pathological changes, and on tissue residues in steers. *Am. J. Vet. Res.* **44**, 1294–1299.

Sun, Z., Lu, P., Gail, M. H., Pee, D., Zhang, Q., Ming, L., Wang, J., Wu, Y., Lui, G., Wu, Y., and Zhu, Y. (1999). Increased risk of hepatocellular carcinoma in male hepatitis B surface antigen carriers with chronic hepatitis who have detectable aflatoxin metabolite M_1. *Hepatology* **30**, 379–383.

Wang, J. S., and Groopman, J. D. (1999). DNA damage by mycotoxins. *Mutat. Res.* **424**, 167–181.

Wang, J. S., Shen, X., He, X., Zhu, Y. R., Zhang, B. C., Wang, J. B., Qian, G. S., Kuang, S. Y., Zarba, A., Egner, P. A., Jacobson, L. P., Muñoz, A., Helzlsouer, K. J., Groopman, J. D., Kensler, T. W. (1999). Protective alterations in phase I and phase II metabolism of aflatoxin B_1 by oltipraz in residents of Qidong, People's Republic of China. *J. Natl. Cancer Inst.* **91**, 347–354.

Wild, C. P., Jiang, Y. Z., Allen, S. J., Jansen, L. A. M., Hall, A. J., and Montesano, R. (1990). Aflatoxin-albumin adducts in human sera from different regions of the world. *Carcinogenesis* **12**, 2271–2274.

Wogan, G. N., and Newberne, P. M. (1967). Dose-response characteristics of aflatoxin B_1 carcinogenesis in the rat. *Cancer Res.* **27** (Part I), 2370–2376.

Wogan, G. N. (1992). Aflatoxins as risk factors for hepatocellular carcinoma in humans. *Cancer Res.* **52**(Suppl.), 2114s–2118s.

Wogan, G. N. (1999). Aflatoxins as a human carcinogen. *Hepatology* **30**, 573–575.

Ochratoxins and Citrinin

Adlouni, C. E., Pinelli, E., Azèmar, B., Zauoi, D., Beaune, P., and Pfohl-Leszkowicz, A. (2000). Phenobarbitol increases DNA adduct and metabolites formed by ochratoxin A: Role of CYP 2C9 and microsomal glutathione-S-transferase. *Environ. Mol. Mut.* **35**, 123–131.

Bach, P. H. (1991). A molecular basis for target-cell toxicity and upper urothelial carcinoma in analgesic abusers and patients with Balkan endemic nephropathy. *IARC Sci. Publ.* **115**, 215–227.

Beardall, J. M., and Miller, J. D. (1994). Diseases in humans with mycotoxins as possible causes. *In* "Mycotoxins in Grain, Compounds Other Than Aflatoxin" (J. D. Miller, and H. L. Trenholm, eds.), pp. 487–539. Eagan Press, St. Paul, MN.

Bendele A, Carlton W. W., Krogh P., Lillihoj E. B. Ochratoxin A carcinogenesis in the (C57BL/J6 × C3HD)F_1 mouse. *J. Natl. Cancer Inst.* **75**, 733–742.

Berndt, W. O., Hayes, A. W., and Phillips, R. D. (1980). Effects of mycotoxins on renal function: Mycotoxic nephropathy. *Kidney Int.* **18**, 656–664.

Boorman, G. A., McDonald, M. R., Imoto, S., and Persing, R. (1992). Renal lesions induced by ochratoxin A exposure in the F344 rat. *Toxicol. Pathol.* **20**, 236–245.

Braunberg, R. C., Barton, C. N., Gantt, O. O., and Friedman, L. (1994). Interaction of citrinin and ochratoxin A. *Natural Toxins* **2**, 124–131.

Breitholz-Emanuelsson, A., Fuchs, R., Hult, K., and Appelgren, L. E. (1992). Synthesis of 14C-ochratoxin A and 14C-ochratoxin B and a comparative study of their distribution in rats using whole body autoradiography. *Pharmacol. Toxicol.* **70**, 255–261.

Breithotlz-Emanuelsson, A., Minervini, F., Hult, K., and Visconti, A. (1994). Ochratoxin A in human serum samples collected in southern Italy from healthy individuals and individuals suffering from different kidney disorders. *Natural Toxins* **2**, 366–370.

Carlton, W. W., and Tuite, J (1986). Comparative pathologic changes in ochratoxicosis and citrinin toxicosis.

In "Diagnosis of Mycotoxicoses" (J. L. Richard, J. R. Thurston, eds.), pp 195–204. Martin Nijhoff Publishers, Boston, MA.

Castegnaro, M., Mohr, U., Pfohl-Leszkowicz, A., Estève, J., Steinmann, J., Tillman, T., Michelon, J., and Bartsch, H. (1998). Sex- and strain-specific induction of renal tumors by ochratoxin A in rats correlates with DNA adduction. *Int. J. Cancer* **77**, 70–75.

Castegnaro, M., Plestina, R., Dirheimer, G., Chernozemsky, I. N., and Bartsch, H. (eds.) (1991) "Mycotoxins, Endemic Nephropathy, and Urinary Tract Tumours." Lyon: IARC Sci. Pub. 115; Oxford University Press, UK.

Creppy, E. E., Castegnaro, M., and Dirheimer, G. (eds.) (1993). "Human Ochratoxicosis and Its Pathologies." Bordeaux, France: Colloque INSERM/John Libbey Eurotext Ltd., 231: 129–139.

Cook, W. O., Osweiler, G. D., Anderson, T. D., and Richard, J. L. (1986). Ochratoxicosis in Iowa swine. *J. Am. Vet. Med. Assoc.* **188**, 1399–1402.

Čvorišćec, D., Čeovič, S., and Stavljenič-Rukavina, A. (eds.) (1996). "Endemic Nephropathy in Croatia." Academia Croatica Scientiarum Medicarum, Zagreb.

Di Paolo, N., Guarnieri, A., Garosi, G., Sacchi, G., Mangiarotti, A. M., and Di Paolo, M. (1994). Inhaled mycotoxins lead to acute renal failure. *Nephrol. Dial. Transplant* **9**(Suppl. 4), 116–120.

Dirheimer, G., and Creppy, E. E. (1991). Mechanism of action of ochratoxin A. *IARC Sci. Publ.* **115**, 171–186.

Fink-Gremmels, J., Jahn, A., and Blom, M. J. (1995). Toxicity and metabolism of ochratoxin A. *Natural Toxins* **3**, 214–220.

Gekle, M., Sauvant, C., Schwerdt, G., and Silbernagl, S. (1998). Tubulotoxic mechanisms of ochratoxin A. *Kidney Blood Press. Res.* **21**, 277–279.

Gekle, M., and Silbernagl, S. (1996). Renal toxicodynamics of ochratoxin A: A pathophysiological approach. *Kidney Blood Press. Res.* **19**, 225–235.

Hald, B. (1991). Porcine nephropathy in Europe. *IARC Sci. Publ.* **115**, 49–56.

Hall, P., III, and Batuman, V. (eds.) (1991). Balkan endemic nephropathy. *Kidney Int.* (Suppl. 34).

Hanika, C., Carlton, W. W., and Tuite, J. (1983). Citrinin mycotoxicosis in the rabbit. *Food Chem. Toxicol.* **21**, 487–494.

IARC-WHO (1993) Some naturally occurring substances: Food items and constituents, heterocyclic aromatic amines, and mycotoxins. *In* "IARC Monographs on the Evaluation of Carcinogenic Risks to Humans," pp. 489–521. International Agency for Research on Cancer, Lyon, France.

Jørgensen, K., Rasmussen, G., and Thorup, I. (1996). Ochratoxin A in Danish cereals 1986–1992 and daily intake by the Danish population. *Food Addi. Contam.* **13**, 95–104.

Kanizawa, M., and Suzuki, S. (1978). Induction of hepatic and renal tumors in mice by ochratoxin A, a mycotoxin. *Gann* **69**, 599–600.

Kozaczynski, W. (1994). Experimental ochratoxicosis A in chickens: Histopathological and histochemical study. *Arch. Vet. Pol.* **34**, 205–219.

Kuiper-Goodman, T., and Scott, P. M. (1989). Risk assessment of the mycotoxin ochratoxin A. *Biomed. Environ. Sci.* **2**, 179–248.

Maaroufi, K., Zakhama, A., Baudrimont, I., Achour, A., Abid, S., Ellouz, F., Dhouib, S., Creppy, E. E., and Bacha, H. (1999). Karyomegaly of tubular cells as early stage marker of the nephrotoxicity induced by ochratoxin A in rats. *Hum. Exp. Toxicol.* **18**, 410–415.

Mantle, P. G., McHugh, K. M., Adatia, R., Heaton, J. M., Gray, T., and Turner, D. R. (1991). *Penicillium aurantiogriseum*-induced, persistent renal histopathological changes in rats; an experimental model for Balkan endemic nephropathy competitive with ochratoxin A. *IARC Sci. Publ.* **115**, 119–127.

Mantle, P. G., Milijkovic, A., Udupa, V., and Dobrota, M. (1998). Does apoptosis cause renal atrophy in Balkan endemic nephropathy? *Lancet* **352** (9134), 1118–1119.

Marquardt, R. R., and Frohlich, A. A. (1992). A review of recent advances in understanding ochratoxicosis. *J. Anim. Sci.* **70**, 3968–3988.

National Toxicology Program (1989). Technical Report on the Toxicology and Carcinogenesis Studies of Ochratoxin A (Cas No 303-47-9) in F344 N Rats. NTP Technical Report No. 358. (G. Boorman, ed.). U.S. Department of Health and Human Services, National Institutes of Health, Research Triangle Park, NC.

Omar, R. F., Rahimtula, A. D., and Bartsch, H. (1991). Role of cytochrome P450 in ochratoxin A-stimulated lipid peroxidation. *J. Biochem. Toxicol.* **6**, 203–209.

Pfohl-Leszkowicz, A., Pinelli, E., Bartsch, H., Mohr, U., and Castegnaro, M. (1998). Sex- and strain specific expression of cytochrome P450s in ochratoxin A-induced genotoxicity and carcinogenicity in rats. *Mol. Carcinogen.* **23**, 76–85.

Pohland, A. E., Nesheim, S., and Friedman, L. (1992). Ochratoxin A: A review. *Pure Appl. Chem.* **64**, 1029–1046.

Stoev, S. D. (1998). The role of ochratoxin A as a possible cause of Balkan endemic nephropathy and its risk evaluation. *Vet. Hum. Toxicol.* **40**, 352–360.

Stoev, S. D., Hald, B., and Mantle, P. G. (1998). Porcine nephropathy in Bulgaria: A progressive syndrome of complex or uncertain (mycotoxin) aetiology. *Vet. Rec.* **142**, 190–194.

Szczech, G. M., Carlton, W. W., and Tuite, J. (1973). Ochratoxicosis in beagle dogs. II. Pathology. *Vet. Pathol.* **10**, 219–231.

Szczech, G. M., Carlton, W. W., Tuite, J., and Caldwell, R. (1973). Ochratoxin A toxicosis in swine. *Vet. Pathol.* **16**, 466–475.

Tsuda, M., Sekine, T., Takeda, M., Cha, S. H., Kanai, Y., Kimura, M., and Endou, H. (1999). Transport of ochratoxin A by renal mutispecific organic anion transporter I. *J. Pharmacol. Exp. Ther.* **289**, 1301–1305.

Wei, X., and Sulik, K. K. (1993). Pathogenesis of craniofacial and body wall malformations induced by ochratoxin A in mice. *Am. J. Med. Genet.* **47**, 862–871.

Trichothecene Mycotoxins

General

Beasley, V. R. (ed.) (1989). "Trichothecene Mycotoxicosis: Pathophysiologic Effects." CRC Press, Boca Raton, FL.

IARC-WHO (1993). Some naturally occurring substances: Food items and constituents, heterocyclic aromatic amines and mycotoxins. *In* "IARC Monographs on the Evaluation of Carcinogenic Risks to Humans," vol. 56, 467–488.

Kurtz, H. J. (1986). Comparative pathologic changes in trichothecene toxicosis. *In* "Diagnosis of Mycotoxicoses" (J. L. Richard and J. R. Thurston, eds.) pp 191–194. Martin Nijhoff Publishers, Boston, MA.

Smith, T. K. (1992). Recent advances in the understanding of *Fusarium* trichothecene mycotoxicoses. *J. Anim. Sci.* **79**, 3989–3993.

Deoxynivalenol

Charmley, E., Trenholm, H. L., Thompson, B. K., Vudathala, D., Nicholson, J. W. G., Prelusky, D. B., and Charmley, L. L. (1993). Influence of level of deoxynivalenol in the diet of dairy cows on feed intake, milk production, and its composition. *J. Dairy Sci.* **76**, 3580–3587.

Greene, D. M., Azcona-Olivera, J. I. and Pestka, J. J. (1994). Vomitoxin (deoxynivalenol)-induced IgA nephropathy in the B6C3F1 mouse: Dose response and male predilection. *Toxicology* **92**, 245–260.

Hedman, R., Pettersson, H., Engstrom, B., Elwinger, K., and Fossum, O. (1995). Effects of feeding nivalenol-contaminated diets to male broiler chickens. *Poult. Sci.* **74**, 620–625.

Hedman, R., Thuvander, A., Gadhasson, I., Reverter, M., and Pettersson, H. (1997). Influence of dietary nivalenol exposure on gross pathology and selected immunological parameters in young pigs. *Natural Toxins* **5**, 238–246.

Hinoshita, F., Suzuki., Y., Yokoyama, K., Hara, S., Yamada, A., Ogura, Y., Hashimoto, H., Tomura, S., Marumo, F., and Ueno, Y. (1997). Experimental IgA nephropathy induced by a low-dose environmental mycotoxin, nivalenol. *Nephron* **75**, 469–478.

Iverson, F., Armstrong, C., Nera, E., Truelove, J., Fernie, S., Scott, P., Stapley, R., Hayward, S., and Gunner, S. (1995). Chronic feeding study of deoxynivalenol in B6C3F1 male and female mice. *Teratog. Carcinog. Mutagen.* **15**, 283–306.

Pestka, J. J., Moorman, M. A., and Warner, R. L. (1989). Dysregulation of IgA production and IgA nephropathy induced by the trichothecene vomitoxin. *Food Chem. Toxic.* **27**, 361–368.

Prelusky, D. B. (1997). Effect of intraperitoneal infusion of deoxynivalenol on feed consumption and weight gain in the pig. *Natural Toxins* **5**, 121–125.

Rotter, B. A., Prelusky, D. B., and Pestka, J. J. (1996). Toxicology of deoxynivalenol (vomitoxin). *J. Toxicol. Environ. Health* **48**, 1–34.

Rotter, B. A., Thompson, B. K., and Lessard, M. (1995). Effects of deoxynivalenol-contaminated diet on performance and blood parameters in growing swine. *Can. J. Anim. Sci.* **75**, 297–302.

Trenholm, H. L., Foster, B. C., Charmley, L. L., Thompson, B. K., Hartin, K. E., Coppock, R. W., and Albassam, M. A. (1994). Effects of feeding diets containing *Fusarium* (naturally) contaminated wheat or pure deoxynivalenol (DON) in growing pigs. *Can. J. Anim. Sci.* **74**, 361–369.

Yan, D., Rumbeiha, W. K., and Pestka, J. J. (1998). Experimental murine IgA nephropathy following passive administration of vomitoxin-induced IgA monoclonal antibodies. *Food. Chem. Toxicol.* **36**, 1095–1106.

Zhou, H.-R., Harkema, J. R., Hotchkiss, J. A., Yan, D., Roth, R. A., and Pestka, J. J. (2000). Lipopolysaccharide and the trichothecene vomitoxin (deoxynivalenol) synergistically induce apoptosis in murine lymphoid organs. *Toxicol. Sci.* **53**, 253–263.

T-2 Toxin

Friend, D. W., Thompson, B. K., Trenholm, H. L., Boermans, H. J., Hartin, K. E., and Panich, P. L. (1992). Toxicity of T-2 toxin and its interaction with deoxynivalenol when fed to young pigs. *Can. J. Anim. Sci.* **72**, 703–711.

Ihara, T., Sugamata, M., Sekijima, M., Okumura, H., Yoshino, N., and Ueno, Y. (1997). Apoptotic cellular damage in mice after T-2 toxin-induced acute toxicosis. *Natural Toxins* **5**, 141–145.

Joffe, A. Z. (1983). Food borne diseases: Alimentary toxic aleukia. *In* "CRC Handbook of Food-Borne Diseases of Biological Origin" (M. Recheigl, ed.), pp. 353–495, CRC Press, Boca Raton, FL.

Li, G., Shinozuka, J., Uetsuka, K., Nakayama, H., and Doi, K. (1997). T-2 toxin-induced apoptosis in intestinal crypt epithelial cells of mice. *Exp. Toxicol. Pathol.* **49**, 447–450.

Pang, V. F., Adams, J. H., Beasley, V. R., Buck, W. B., and Haschek, W. M. (1986). Myocardial and pancreatic lesions induced by T-2 toxin, a trichothecene mycotoxin, in swine. *Vet. Pathol.* **23**, 310–319.

Pang, V. F., Felsburg, P. J., Beasley, V. R., Buck, W. B., and Haschek, W. M. (1987). The toxicity of T-2 toxin in swine following topical application. II. Effects on hematology, serum biochemistry, and immune response. *Fundam. Appl. Toxicol.* **9**, 50–59.

Rafai, P., Bata, A., Vanyi, A., Papp, Z., Brydl, E., Jakab, L., Tuboly, S., and Tury, E. (1995). Effect of various levels of T-2 toxin on the clinical status, performance and metabolism of growing pigs. *Vet. Rec.* **136**, 485–489.

Rafai, P., Tubolu, S., Bata, A., Tilly, P., Vanyi, A., Papp, Z., Jakab, L., and Tury, E. (1995). Effect of various levels of T-2 toxin in the immune system of growing pigs. *Vet. Rec.* **136**, 511–514.

Shinozuka, J., Li, G., Kiattipattanasakul, W., Uetsuka, K., Nakayama, H., and Doi, K. (1997). T-2 toxin-induced apoptosis in lymphoid organs of mice. *Exp. Toxicol. Pathol.* **49**, 387–392.

Smith, B. J., Holladay, S. D., and Blaylock, B. L. (1994). Hematopoietic alterations after exposure to T-2 mycotoxin. *Toxicon* **32**, 1115–1123.

Stachybotrys Toxins

Andersson, M. A., Nikulin, M., Koljalg, U., Andersson, M. C., Rainey, F., Reijula, K., Hintikka, E. L., and Salkinoja-Salonen, M. (1997). Bacteria, molds, and toxins in water-damaged building materials. *Appl. Environ. Microbiol.* **63**, 387–393.

Etzel, R. A., Montaña, E., Sorenson, W. G., Kullman, G. J., Allan, T. M., Dearborn, D. G., Olson, D. R., Jarvis, B. B., and Miller, J. D. (1998). Acute pulmonary hemorrhage in infants associated with exposure to Stachybotrys atra and other fungi. *Arch. Pediatr. Adolesc. Med.* **152**, 757–762.

Fung, F., Clark, R., and Williams, S. (1998). Stachybotrys, a mycotoxin-producing fungus of increasing toxicologic importance. *J. Toxicol. Clin. Toxicol.* **36**, 629–631.

Harrach, B., Bata, A., Bajmocy, E., and Benko, M. (1983). Isolation of satratoxins from the bedding straw of a sheep flock with fatal stachybotryotoxicosis. *Appl. Environ. Microbiol.* **45**, 1419–1422.

Jarvis, B. B., Salemme, J., and Morais, A. (1995). Stachybotrys, toxins 1. *Natural Toxins* **3**, 10–16.

Johanning, E., Biagini, R., Hull, D., Morey, P., Jarvis, B., and Landsbergis, P. (1996). Health and immunology study following exposure to toxigenic fungi (*Stachybotrys chartarum*) in water-damaged office environment. *Int. Arch. Occup. Environ. Health* **68**, 207–218.

Mahmoudi, M., and Gershwin, M. E. (2000). Sick building syndrome. III. *Stachybotrys chartarum. J. Asthma* **37**, 191–198.

Nikulin, M., Reijula, K., Jarvis, B. B., and Hintikka, E. L. (1996). Experimental lung mycotoxicosis in mice induced by *Stachybotrys Atra. Int. J. Exp. Pathol.* **77**, 213–218.

Nikulin, M. Reijula, K., Jarvis, B. B., Veijalainen, P., and Hintikka, E. L. (1997). Effects of intranasal exposure to spores of *Stachybotrys atra* in mice. *Fundam. Appl. Toxicol.* **35**, 182–188.

Rotter, B. A., Prelusky, D. B., and Pestka, J. J. (1996). Toxicology of deoxynivalenol (vomitoxin). *J. Toxicol. Environ. Health* **48**, 1–34.

Tuomi, T., Reijula, K., Johnsson, T., Hemminki, K., Hintikka, E. L., Lindroos, O., Kalso, S., Koukila-Kahkola, P., Mussalo-Rauhamaa, H., and Haahtela, T. (2000). Mycotoxins in crude building materials from water-damaged buildings. *Appl. Environ. Microbiol.* **66**, 1899–1904.

Zearalenone

Biehl, M. L., Prelusky, D. B., Koritz, G. D., Hartin, K. E., Buck, W. B., and Trenholm, H. L. (1993). Biliary excretion and enterohepatic cycling of zearalenone in immature pigs. *Toxicol. Appl. Pharmacol.* **121**, 152–159.

Chang, K., Kurtz, H. J., and Mirocha, C. J. (1979). Effects of the mycotoxin zearalenone on swine reproduction. *Am. J. Vet. Res.* **40**, 1260–1267.

Dacasto, M., Rolando, P., Nachtmann, C., Ceppa, L., and Nebbia, C. (1995). Zearalenone mycotoxicosis in piglets suckling sows fed contaminated grain. *Vet. Hum. Toxicol.* **37**, 359–361.

Eienne, M., and Dourmad, J. Y. (1994). Effects of zearalenone or glucosinolates in the diet on reproduction in sows: A review. *Livestock Prod. Sci.* **40**, 99–113.

Haschek, W. M., and Haliburton, J. C. (1986). *Fusarium moniliforme* and zearalenone toxicoses in domestic animals: A review. In "Diagnosis of Mycotoxicoses" (J. L. Richard and J. R. Thurston, eds.), pp. 213–235. Martin Nijhoff Publishers, Boston, MA.

Kordic, B., Pribicevic, S., Muntanola-Cvetkovic, M., Nikolic, P., and Nikolic, B. (1992). Experimental study of the effects of known quantities of zearalenone on swine reproduction. *J. Environ. Pathol. Toxicol. Oncol.* **11**, 53–55.

Kurtz, H. J., Nairn, M. E., Nelson, G. H., Christensen, C. M., and Mirocha, C. J. (1969). Histologic changes in the genital tracts of swine fed estrogenic mycotoxin. *Am. J. Vet. Res.* **30**, 551–556.

Long, G. G., Diekman, M. A., Tuite, J. F., Shannon, G. M., and Vesonder, R. F. (1983). Effect of *Fusarium roseum (Gibberella zea)* on pregnancy and the estrus cycle in gilts fed molded corn on days 7–17 post estrous. *Vet. Res. Commun.* **6**, 199–204.

Marasas, W. F. O. (1991). Toxigenic *Fusaria*. *In* "Mycotoxins and Animal Foods" (J. E. Smith and R. S. Henderson, eds.), pp. 119–139. CRC Press, Boca Raton, FL.

Palyusik, M., Harrach, B., Horvath, G., and Mirocha, C. J. (1990). Experimental fusariotoxicosis of swine produced by zearalenone and T-2 toxins. *J. Environ. Pathol. Toxicol. Oncol.* **10**, 52–55.

Perez-Martinez, C., Garcia-Iglesias, M. J., Bravo-Moral, A. M., Ferreras-Estrada, M. C., Martinez-Rodriguez, J. M., and Escudero-Diez, A. (1995). Effect of diethylstilbestrol or zeranol on fetal development, gestation duration, and number of offspring in NMRI mice. *Am. J. Vet. Res.* **56**, 1615–1619.

Smith, J. F., DiMenna, M. E., and McGowan, L. T. (1990). Reproductive performance of Coopworth ewes following oral doses of zearalenone before and after mating. *J. Reprod. Fert.* **89**, 99–106.

Yang, H. H., Aulerich, R. J., Helferich, W., Yamini, B., Chou, K. C., Miller, E. R., and Bursian, S. J. (1995). Effects of zearalenone and/or tamoxifen on swine and mink reproduction. *J. Appl. Toxicol.* **15**, 223–232.

Young, L. G., Ping, H., and King, G. J. (1990). Effects of feeding zearalenone to sows on rebreeding and pregnancy. *J. Anim. Sci.* **68**, 15–20.

Fumonisins

Allaben, W. T., Bucher, J. R., and Howard, P. C., (eds.) (2001). Toxicology of fumonisin. *Environ. Health Persp.* **109**,(Suppl.2), 235–342.

Bhat, R. V., Shetty, P. H., Amruth, R. P., and Sudershan, R. V. (1997). A foodborne disease outbreak due to the consumption of moldy sorghum and maize containing fumonisin mycotoxins. *J. Toxicol. Clin. Toxicol.* **35**, 249–255.

Dombrink-Kurtzmann, M. A., Dvorak, T. J., Barron, M. E., and Rooney, L. W. (2000). Effect of nixtamalization (alkaline cooking) on fumonisin-contaminated corn for production of masa and tortillas. *J. Agric. Food Chem.* **48**, 5781–5786.

Dragan, Y. P., Bidlack, W. R., Cohen, S. M., Goldsworthy, T. L., Hard, G. C., Howard, P. C., Riley, R. T., and Voss, K. A. (2001). Implications of apoptosis for toxicity, carcinogenicity and risk assessment: Fumonisin B$_1$ as an example. *Toxicol. Sci.* **61**, 6–17.

Dutton, M. F. (1996). Fumonisins, mycotoxins of increasing importance: Their nature and their effects. *Pharmacol. Ther.* **70**, 137–161.

Fincham, J. E., Marasas, W. F., Taljaard, J. J., Kriek, N. P., Badenhorst, C. J., Gelderblom, W. C., Seier, J. V., Smuts, C. M., Faber, M., Weight, M. J., Slazus, W., Woodroof, C. W., van Wyk, M. J., Kruger, M., and Thiel, P. G. (1992). Atherogenic effects in a nonhuman primate of *Fusarium moniliforme* cultures added to a carbohydrate diet [published erratum appears in *Atherosclerosis* **96**(1), 87 (1992)] *Atherosclerosis* **94**, 13–25.

Fumonisin B$_1$. Environmental Health Criteria 219. (2000). United Nations Environmental Programme, International Labour Organization and the World Health Organization, Geneva.

Gelderblom, W. C. A., Jaskiewicz, K., Marasas, W. F. O., Thiel, P. G., Horak, R. M., Vllaggar, R., and Kriek, N. P. J. (1988). Fumonisins-novel mycotoxins with cancer promoting activity produced by *Fusarium moniliforme*. *Appl. Environ. Microbiol.* **54**, 1806–1811.

Gelderblom, W. C. A., Kriek, N. P. J., Marasas, W. F. O. and Thiel, P. G. (1991). Toxicity and carcinogenecitiy of the *Fusarium moniliforme* metabolite, fumonisin B$_1$ in rats. *Carcinogenesis* **12**, 1247–1251.

Gelderblom, W. C. A., Seier, J. V., Snijman, P. W., Van Schalkwyk, D. J., Shephard, G. S., and Marasas, W. F. O. (2001). Toxicity of culture material of *Fusarium verticillioides* strain MRC 826 to nonhuman primates. *Environ. Health Persp.* **109**(Suppl. 2), 267–276.

Goel, S., Schumacher, J., Lenz, S. D., and Kemppainen, B. (1996). Effects of *Fusarium moniliforme* isolates on tissue and serum sphingolipid concentrations in horses. *Vet. Hum. Toxicol.* **38**, 265–270.

Gumprecht, L. A., Beasley, V. R., Weigel, R. M., Parker, H. M., Tumbleson, M. E., Bacon, C. W., Meredith, F. I., and Haschek, W. M. (1998). Development of fumonisin-induced hepatotoxicity and pulmonary edema in orally dosed swine: Morphological and biochemical alterations. *Toxicol. Pathol.* **26**, 777–789.

Harrison, L. R., Colvin, B. M., Greene, J. T., Newman, L. E., and Cole, J. R. (1990). Pulmonary edema and hydrothorax in swine produced by fumonisin B$_1$, a toxic metabolite of *Fusarium moniliforme*. *J. Vet. Diag. Invest.* **2**, 217–221.

Hard, G. C., Howard, P. C., Kovatch, R. M., and Bucci, T. J. (2001). Rat kidney pathology induced by chronic exposure to fumonisin B$_1$ includes rare variants of renal tubular tumor. *Toxicol. Pathol.* (in press).

Haschek, W. M., Gumprecht, L. A., Smith, G., Tumbleson, M. E., and Constable, P. D. (2001). Fumonisin toxicosis in swine: An overview of porcine pulmonary edema and current perspectives. *Environ. Health Persp.* **109**(Suppl. 2), 251–257.

Haschek, W. M., and Haliburton, J. C. (1986). *Fusarium moniliforme* and zearalenone toxicoses in domestic animals: A review. *In* "Diagnosis of Mycotoxicoses" (J. L. Richard and J. R. Thurston, eds.) pp. 213–235. Martin Nijhoff Publishers, Boston, MA.

Haschek, W. M., Motelin, G., Ness, D. K., Harlin, K. S., Hall, W. F., Vesonder, R. F., Peterson, R. E., and Beasley VR. (1992). Characterization of fumonisin toxicity in orally and intravenously dosed swine. *Mycopathologia* **117**, 83–96.

Howard, P. C., Eppley, R. M., Stack, M. E., Warbritton, A., Voss, K. A., Lorentzen, R. J., Kovach, R., and Bucci, T. J. (1999). Carcinogenicity of fumonisin B_1 in a two-year bioassay with Fischer 344 rats and B6C3F$_1$ mice. *Mycotoxins* (Suppl. 99), 45–54.

Hwan-soo, Y., Norred, W. P., Showker, J., and Riley, R. T. (1996). Elevated sphingoid bases and complex sphingolipid depletion as contributing factors in fumonisin-induced cytotoxicity. *Toxicol. Appl. Pharmacol.* **138**, 211–218.

Jackson, L. S., DeVries, J. W., and Bullerman, L. B. (eds.) (1996). "Fumonisins in Food," Plenum Press, New York.

Kellerman, T. S., Marasas, W. F., Thiel, P. G., Gelderblom, W. C., Cawood, M., and Coetzer, J. A. (1990). Leukoencephalomalacia in two horses induced by oral dosing of fumonisin B_1. *Onderstepoort. J. Vet. Res.* **57**, 269–275.

Kuiper-Goodman, T., Scott, P. M., McEwen, N. P., Lombaert, G. A., and Ng, W. (1996). Approaches to the risk assessment of fumonisins in corn-based foods in Canada. *In* "Fumonisins in Food" (L. S. Jackson, J. W. DeVries, and L. B. Bullerman, eds.), pp. 369–393. Plenum Press, New York.

Lazarus, C., and Ventor, T. H. (1986). Carcinoma of the oesophagus in Ciskei. *S. Afr. Med. J.* **69**, 747–748.

Ledoux, D. R., Brown, T. P., Weibking, T. S., and Rottinghaus, G. E. (1992). Fumonisin toxicity in broiler chicks. *J. Vet. Diag. Invest.* **4**, 330–333.

Li, Y. C., Ledoux, D. R., Bermudez, A. J., Fritsche, K. L., and Rottinghaus, G. E. (2000). The individual and combined effects of fumonisin B_1 and moniliformin on performance and selected immune parameters in turkey poults. *Poult. Sci.* **79**, 871–878.

Lim, C. W., Parker, H. M., Vesonder, R. F., and Haschek, W. M. (1996). Intravenous fumonisin B_1 induces cell proliferation and apoptosis in the rat. *Natural Toxins* **4**, 34–41.

Marasas, W. F. O. (1996). Fumonisins: History, worldwide occurrence and impact. *In* "Fumonisins in Food" (L. S. Jackson, J. W. DeVries, and L. B. Bullerman, eds.), pp. 1–17. Plenum Press, New York.

Marasas, W. F. O. (1995). Fumonisins: Their implications for human and animal health. *Natural Toxins* **3**, 193–198.

Merrill, A. H., Jr., Wang, E., Gilchrist, D. G., and Riley, R. T. (1993). Fumonisins and other inhibitors of *de novo* sphingolipid biosynthesis. *Adv. Lipid Res.* **26**, 215–234.

Miller, A., Honstead, J. P., and Lovell, R. A. (1996). Regulatory aspects of fumonisins with respect to animal feed: Animal derived residues in foods. *In* "Fumonisins in Food" (L. S. Jackson, J. W. DeVries, and L. B. Bullerman, eds.), pp. 363–368. Plenum Press, New York.

Murphy, P. A., Hendrich, S., Hopmans, E. C., Hauck, C. C., Lu, Z., Buseman, G., and Munkvold, G. (1996). Effect of processing on fumonisin content of corn. *In* "Fumonisins in Food" (L. S. Jackson, J. W. DeVries, and L. B. Bullerman, eds.), pp. 323–334. Plenum Press, New York.

Norred, W. P., Plattner, R. D., and Chamberlain, W. J., (1993). Distribution and excretion of [^{14}C]FB$_1$ in male Sprague-Dawley rats. *Natural Toxins* **1**, 341–346.

Pohland, A. E. (1996). Occurrence of fumonisins in the U. S. food supply, *In* "Fumonisins in Food" (L. S. Jackson, J. W. DeVries, and L. B. Bullerman, eds), pp. 19–26. Plenum Press, New York.

Prelusky, D. B., Trenholm, H. L., Rotter, B. A., Miller, J. D., Savard, M. E., Yeung, J. M., and Scott, P. M. (1996). Biological fate of fumonisin B_1 in food-producing animals. *In* "Fumonisins in Food" (L. S. Jackson, J. W. DeVeries, and L. B. Bullerman, eds.), pp. 265–278. Plenum Press, New York.

Rheeder, J. P., Marasas, W. F. O., Thiel, P. G., Sydenham, E. W., Shephard, G. S., and van Schalkwyk, D. J. (1992). *Fusarium moniliforme* and fumonisins in corn in relation to human esophageal cancer in Transkei. *Phytopathology* **82**, 353–357.

Shephard, G. S., Thiel, P. G., Sydenham, E. W., and Snijman, P. W. (1995). Toxicokinetics of the mycotoxin fumonisin B_2 in rats. *Food Chem. Toxicol.* **33**, 591–595.

Smith, G. W., Constable, P. D., Bacon, C. W., Meredith, F. I., and Haschek, W. M. (1996). Cardiovascular effects of fumonisins in swine. *Fundam. Appl. Toxicol.* **31**, 169–172.

Smith, G. W., Constable, P. D., Eppley, R. M., Tumbleson, M. E., Gumprecht, L. A., and Haschek, W. M. (2000). Purified fumonisin B_1 decreases cardiovascular function but does not alter pulmonary capillary permeability in swine. *Toxicol. Sci.* **56**, 240–249.

Sumeruk, R., Segal, I., Te Winkel, W., and van der Merwe, C. F. (1992). Oesophageal cancer in three regions of South Africa. *S. Afr. Med. J.* **81**, 91–93.

Voss, K. A., Chamberlain, W. J., Bacon, C. W., Herbert, R. A., Walters, D. B., and Norred, W. P. (1995). Subchronic feeding study of the mycotoxin fumonisin B_1 in B6C3F$_1$ mice and Fischer 344 rats. *Fundam. Appl. Toxicol.* **24**, 102–110.

Voss, K. A., Chamberlain, W. J., Bacon, C. W., and Norred, W. P. (1993). A preliminary investigation on renal and hepatic toxicity in rats fed purified fumonisin B_1. *Natural Toxins* **1**, 222–228.

Wang, E., Norred, W. P., Bacon, C. W., Riley, R. T., and Merrill, A. H. (1991). Inhibition of sphingolipid biosynthesis by fumonisins. *J. Biol. Chem.* **266**, 14486–14490.

Yoshizawa, T., Yamashita, A., and Luo, Y. (1994). Fumonisin occurrence in corn from high-and low-risk areas for human esophageal cancer in China. *Appl. Environ. Microbiol.* **60**, 1626–1629.

Ergot Alkaloids

General

Ball, S. E., Maurer, G., Zollinger, M., Ladona, M., and Vickers, A. E. M. (1996). Characterization of the cytochrome P-450 gene family responsible for the *N*-dealkylation of the ergot alkaloid CQA 206–291 in humans. *Drug Metab. Disp.* **20**, 56–63.

Coppock, R. W., Mostrom, M. S., Simon, J., Mckenna, D. J., Jacobsen, B., and Szlachta, H. L. (1989). Cutaneous ergotism in a herd of dairy calves. *J. Am. Vet. Med. Assoc.* **194**, 549–551.

Porter, J. K., Bacon, C. W., Plattner, R. D., and Arrendale, R. F. (1987). Ergot peptide alkaloid spectra of *Claviceps*-infected tall fescue, wheat, and barley. *J. Agric. Food Chem.* **35**, 359–361.

Ross, A. D., Bryden, W. L., Bakau, W. and Burgess, L. W. (1989). Induction of heat stress in beef cattle by feeding the ergots of *Claviceps pupurea*. *Aust. Vet. J.* **66**, 247–249.

Tall Fescue Toxicoses

Bacon, C. W. (1995). Toxic endophyte-infected tall fescue and range grasses: Historic perspectives. *J. Anim. Sci.* **73**, 861–870.

Ball, D. M., Pedersen, J. F. and Lacefield, G. D. (1993). The tall-fescue endophyte. *Am. Sci.* **81**, 370–379.

Boosinger, T. R., Brendemuehl, J. P., Bransby, D. L., Wright, J. C., Kemppainen, R. J., and Kee, D. D. (1995). Prolonged gestation, decreased triiodothyronine concentration, and thyroid gland histomorphologic features in newborn foals of mares grazing *Acremonion coenophialum*-infected fescue. *Am. J. Vet. Res.* **56**, 66–69.

Cross, D. L., Redmond, L. M., and Strickland, J. R. (1995). Equine fescue toxicosis: Signs and solutions. *J. Anim. Sci.* **73**, 899–908.

Gould, L. S., and Hohenboken, W. D. (1993). Differences between progeny of beef sires in susceptibility to fescue toxicosis. *J. Anim. Sci.* **71**, 3025–3032.

Hammond A. C., Bond, J., and Strand, B. (1982). Tall fescue summer toxicosis in the cattle. *Bov. Pract.* **17**, 137–142.

Hemken, R. W., Jackson, J. A. and Bolin, J. A. (1984). Toxic factors in tall fescue. *J. Anim. Sci,* **58**, 1011–1016.

Ireland, F. A., Loch, W. E., Worthy, K., and Anthony, R. V. (1991). Effects of bromocriptine and perphenazine on prolactin and progesterone concentrations in pregnant pony mares during late gestation. *J. Reprod. Fert.* **92**, 179–186.

Lyons, P. C., Plattner, R. D., and Bacon, C. W. (1986). Occurrence of peptide and clavine ergot alkaloids in tall fescue grass. *Science* **232**, 487–489.

McCann, J. S., Caudle, A. B., Thompson, F. N., Stuedemann, J. A., Heusner, G. L., and Thompson, D. L., Jr. (1992). Influence of endophyte-infected tall fescue on serum prolactin and progesterone in gravid mares. *J. Anim. Sci.* **70**, 217–223.

Merriam, A. E. (2000). Lysergide. *In* "Experimental and Clinical Neurotoxicology" (P. S. Spencer, H. H. Schaumberg, and A. L. Ludolph, eds.), 2nd Ed., pp. 535–537. Oxford Univ. Press, Oxford.

Newman, L. C., and Lipton, R. B. (2000). Ergot alkaloids. *In* "Experimental and Clinical Neurotoxicology" (P. S. Spencer, H. H. Schaumberg, and A. L. Ludolph, eds.), 2nd Ed., pp. 535–537. Oxford Univ. Press, Oxford.

Oliver, J. W., Abney, L. K., Strickland, J. R., and Linnabary, R. D. (1993). Vasoconstriction in bovine vasculature induced by the tall fescue alkaloid lysergamide. *J. Anim. Sci.* **71**, 2708–2713.

Paterson, J., Forcherio, C., Larson, B., Samford, M., and Kerley, M. (1995). The effects of fescue toxicosis on beef cattle productivity. *J. Anim. Sci.* **73**, 889–898.

Peet, R. L., McCarthy, M. R., and Barbetti, M. J. (1991). Hyperthermia and death in feedlot cattle associated with the ingestion of *Claviceps purpurea*. *Aust. Vet. J.* **68**, 121.

Poppenga, R. H., Mostrom, M. S., Haschek, W. M., Lock, T. F., Buck, W. B., and Beasley, V. R. (1984). Mare agalactia, placental thickening, and high foal mortality associated with the grazing of tall fescue: A case report. Am. Assoc. Vet. Lab. Diag. 27th Ann. Proc, 325–336.

Porter, J. K., Stuedemann, J. A., Thompson, F. N. Buckanan, B. A., and Tucker, H. A. (1994). Melatonin and pineal neurochemicals in steers grazed on endophyte-infected tall fescue: Effects of metoclopramide. *J. Anim. Sci.* **71**, 1526–1531.

Porter, J. K., Stuedemann, J. A., Thompson, F. N., Jr., and Lipham, L. B. (1990). Neuroendocrine measurements in steers grazed on endophyte-infected fescue. *J. Anim. Sci.* **68**, 3285–3292.

Porter, J. K., and Thompson, F. N., Jr. (1992). Effects of fescue toxicosis on reproduction in livestock. *J. Anim. Sci.* **70**, 1594–1603.

Putnam, M. R., Bransby, D. I., Schumacher, J., Boosinger, T. R., Bush, L., Shelby, R. A., Vaughan, J. T., Ball, D. and Brendemuehl, J. P. (1991). Effects of the fungal endophyte *Acremonium coenophialum* in fescue on pregnant mares and foal viability. *Am. J. Vet. Res.* **52**, 2071–2074.

Rhodes, M. T., Paterson, J. A., Kerley, M. S., Garner, H. E. and Laughlin, M. H. (1991). Reduced blood flow to peripheral and core body tissues in sheep and cattle induced by endophyte-infected all fescue. *J. Anim. Sci.* **69**, 2033–2043.

Riet-Correa, F., Mendez, M. C., Schild, A. L., Bergamo, P. N. and Flores, W. N. (1988). Agalactica, reproductive problems and neonatal mortality in horses associated with the ingestion of *Claviceps purpurea*. *Aust. Vet. J.* **65**, 192–193.

Rohrback, B. W., Green, E. M., Oliver, J. W., and Schneider, J. F. (1995). Aggregate risk study of exposure to endophyte-infected (*Acremonium coenophialum*) tall fescue as a risk factor for laminitis in horses. *Am. J. Vet. Res.* **56**, 22–26.

Rottinghaus, G. E., Garner, G. B., Cornell, C. N., and Ellis, J. L. (1991). HPLC method for quantitating ergovaline in endophyte-infected tall fescue: Seasonal variation of ergovaline levels in stems with leaf sheaths, leaf blades, and seed heads. *J. Agric. Food Chem.* **39**, 112–115.

Roylance, J. T., Hill, N. S., and Agee, C. S. (1994). Ergovaline and peramine production in endophyte-infected tall fescue: Independent regulation and effects of plant and endophyte genotype. *J. Chem. Ecol.* **20**, 2171–2183.

Rumsey, T. S., Stuedemann, J. A., Wilkinson, S. R., and Williams, D. J. (1979). Chemical composition of necrotic fat lesions in beef cows grazing fertilized "Kentucky 31" tall fescue. *J. Anim. Sci.* **48**, 673–682.

Stamm, M. M., DelCurto, T., Horney, M. R., Brandyberry, S. D., and Barton, R. K. (1994). Influence of alkaloid concentration of tall fescue straw on the nutrition, physiology and subsequent performance of beef steers. *J. Anim. Sci.* **72**, 1068–1075.

Strickland, J. R., Cross, D. L., Birrenkott, G. P. and Grimes, L. W. (1994). Effect of ergovaline, loline, and dopamine antagonists on rat pituitary cell prolactin release *in vitro*. *Am. J. Vet. Res.* **55**, 716–721.

Strickland, J. R., Oliver, J. W., and Cross, D. L. (1993). Fescue toxicosis and its impact on animal agriculture. *Vet. Hum. Toxicol.* **35**, 454–464.

26

Heavy Metals

Sharon M. Gwaltney-Brant
ASPCA/National Animal Poison Control Center
Urbana, Illinois

I. Introduction

Less than half of the known metals have the potential for toxicity to humans and animals. The toxicities of some metals, such as lead and arsenic, have been recognized for hundreds of years, whereas the hazards of other metals, such as cadmium and beryllium, have only more recently been acknowledged. Contamination of the environment by some metals, such as mercury, is of continuing medical and political concern. The ability of wildlife to accumulate and concentrate toxic metals such as mercury increases the threat of toxicity to those further up the food chain. Because metals are so widely utilized in everyday life, they have the potential to pose a continuous risk for human and animal health.

Although the clinical presentations of toxicities of the different metals may be quite varied, most metals induce damage through similar mechanisms, either by binding of the metals to vital enzymes or by substitution of the metals

for other elements in biochemical reactions (Table I). Differences in clinical disease induced by metals more often reflect differences in absorption, distribution, or metabolism rather than differences in toxic mechanism. Because of this, discussion of the toxicologic pathology of heavy metals must include pertinent kinetic information, for by knowing the fate of a given metal within the body one can then understand the pathogenesis of the signs and lesions induced by that particular metal.

II. Cadmium

A. SOURCES AND EXPOSURE

Cadmium has become of increasing industrial importance since the early 1900s. The largest use of cadmium is in the electroplating and galvanizing industries, although it also has wide use in color pigments for paints, pigments and stabilizers for plastics, cathode materials for nickel–cadmium batteries, and as alloys that lend temperature and pressure stability to industrial equipment. Cadmium is a by-product of zinc and lead mining, refining and smelting, and it is sometimes present in large

Handbook of Toxicologic Pathology, Second Edition
Volume 1
Copyright © 2002 by Academic Press
All rights of reproduction in any form reserved.

TABLE I
Toxicity of Metals

Metal	Mechanism	Primary organ(s)/system(s) affected
Antimony	Enzyme inhibition through binding of sulfhydryl groups	Gastrointestinal tract
Arsenic	Impairment of cellular respiration through binding to sulfhydryl groups on cellular enzymes	*Inorganic arsenic*: gastrointestinal tract, vascular endothelium (acute); skin, peripheral nerves, liver (chronic)
		Phenylarsonics: brain, spinal cord, peripheral nerves
		Arsine: red blood cells
Beryllium	Corrosive tissue injury (acute)	Gastrointestinal tract, respiratory tract
	Type IV hypersensitivity	Respiratory tract
Bismuth	Alteration of fluid and electrolyte transport; interference with sulfur-containing enzymes	Kidney (acute), gastrointestinal (chronic), central nervous system
Cadmium	Enzyme inhibition through replacement of zinc in metallo-enzyme systems	Gastrointestinal tract, respiratory tract (actue)
	Competitive replacement of calcium in metabolic systems	Kidney, bone, testicle (chronic)
Lead	Impairment of cellular metabolic pathways through binding to sulfhydryl groups; glutathione depletion	Central nervous system, gastrointestinal tract, kidney, red blood cells
	Competition with calcium ions	Bone, nerve, muscle
Mercury	Enzyme inhibition through binding to sulfhydryl groups; alteration of membrane transport channels; glutathione depletion	*Elemental mercury*: respiratory tract, kidney (acute); gastrointestinal tract, central nervous system (chronic)
		Inorganic mercury: gastrointestinal tract (acute), kidney (subacute), central nervous system (chronic)
		Organic mercury: central nervous system
Plutonium	Enzyme inhibition and membrane damage through binding to cellular proteins and phospholipids	Kidney, bone marrow
Thallium	Replacement of potassium in potassium-dependent processes, binding to sulfhydryl groups on enzymes and structural proteins	Gastrointestinal tract, kidney, skin
Uranium	Enzyme inhibition and membrane damage through binding to cellular proteins and phospholipids	Kidney

quantities in sewage sludge used as fertilizer. Cadmium has been used in the past as a fungicide for turf, although cadmium-based fungicides have largely been replaced by less toxic products.

The main sources of exposure to cadmium are through contamination of food, water, and air. Ingestion of contaminated food serves as the most significant nonoccupational source of cadmium in humans and animals. Cadmium in soil is taken up by plants, which tend to contain higher levels than animal food products. Animals grazing cadmium-contaminated plants will concentrate the element in the liver and kidney, and shellfish from contaminated water may also accumulate high levels of cadmium. Inhalational exposure sources include industry, fossil fuel combustion, and cigarette smoking. Cigarettes serve as one of the major non-occupational sources of inhaled cadmium in humans.

B. KINETICS

Ingested cadmium salts are poorly absorbed from the gastrointestinal tract, with approximately 95% or more being excreted in the feces without being absorbed systemically. Cadmium absorption is enhanced by poor nutritional status, including dietary deficiencies of calcium, zinc, iron, or protein. Young children and animals have a higher capacity to absorb cadmium than adults.

Absorption of inhaled cadmium is dependent on the particulate size of the inhaled agent. Particles greater than 2 μm will be deposited in the upper airways and removed through the mucociliary escalator. Up to 30% of inhaled cadmium may reach the lungs, where it enters the bloodstream readily, binds to red blood cells, albumin, or metallothionein, and accumulates primarily in the kidney.

In the gastrointestinal tract, ingested cadmium enters enterocytes and binds with metallothionein, an approximately 6800 molecular weight, cysteine-rich protein. Metallothionein is present in most tissues, but is in highest concentrations in the liver and kidney, where its production can be induced in the presence of cadmium, zinc, and other metals. Zinc exposure can induce metallothionein synthesis and thus increase cellular tolerance for cadmium. Conversely, zinc deficiency may alter the distribution of cadmium within the body and enhance cadmium toxicity. In the intestine, much of the cadmium–metallothionein complex is eliminated in the feces, as enterocytes are desquamated during the normal process of mucosal cell turnover. Ingested cadmium that is absorbed is transported within the bloodstream bound to plasma albumin, red blood cells, or metallothionein and enters the liver via the portal vein. In the liver, cadmium binds to and induces the further production of metallothionein by hepatocytes. The cadmium–metallothionein complexes are excreted into the bile and eliminated via the feces, but some of the complexes are released by the liver into the general circulation where they distribute widely throughout the tissues. Circulating complexes are filtered through the renal glomerulus and taken up by the proximal tubular cells, resulting in concentration within the renal tubular cells.

Liver and kidney cells have the largest capacity for metallothionein synthesis—up to 75% of the total body burden of cadmium ultimately accumulates in the liver and kidneys. In the proximal renal tubular epithelium, the cadmium–metallothionein complex is broken down by lysosomes to release free cadmium. This free cadmium stimulates the *de novo* synthesis of additional metallothionein within the cell. If the rate of cadmium release from metallothionein exceeds the ability of the cell to produce metallothionein, the cadmium attaches to other proteins within the cell, interfering with cellular metabolism and damaging organelle membranes.

Once in tissues, cadmium has an extremely long biological half-life—estimates of the half-life of cadmium in human kidneys range from 15 to 30 years. Cadmium is eliminated slowly through the urine under normal circumstances; in cases of cadmium-induced nephropathy, the elimination of cadmium through the urine is increased. In addition to the liver and kidney, cadmium may also be stored in the lung and pancreas.

C. MECHANISM OF ACTION

The mechanism of cadmium toxicity is due largely to its replacement of and competition with zinc in biologic systems, resulting in the disruption of intracellular metallo-enzyme systems. Other mechanisms of cadmium-induced cellular injury include alterations of calcium metabolism by direct competition in calcium-dependent pathways, direct membrane damage from cadmium binding to cellular membrane constituents, and interference with signal transduction pathways within cells, resulting in altered cellular homeostasis.

There are marked differences in susceptibility to cadmium-induced tissue injury, both within and between species. Compared to other domestic animal species, horses appear to be able to accumulate higher tissue cadmium levels without showing signs of toxicosis. Inbred mouse strains vary in their susceptibility to cadmium toxicity, and in some cases there are significant sex-related differences as well (Table II).

The increased susceptibility of transgenic metallothionein-null mice to cadmium-induced nephrotoxicity demonstrates the importance of

TABLE II
Species and Strain Differences in Susceptibility to Cadmium-Induced Injury

Toxicologic effect	Relative susceptibility	
	Sensitive	Resistant
Hepatotoxicity	C3H/HEJ mice	DBA/2J mice
Nephrotoxicity	MT-null mice	MT-competent mice
Testicular necrosis	129/J mice	A/J mice
Ectrodactyly (teratogenic)	C57BL/6N mice	SWV mice
Lung cancer	Wistar–Furth rats	Mice (most strains) Syrian hamsters

the cadmium–metallothionein complex in protecting the renal tubular epithelium against cadmium-associated injury. However, other cadmium-sensitive strains of mice develop cadmium-induced injury in the presence of tissue metallothionein levels similar to those of more resistant strains, suggesting that other factors are involved in cytoprotection from cadmium toxicity.

Cadmium-sensitive 129/J mice accumulate significantly more cadmium within the testicle, brain, and epididymis following parenteral cadmium chloride administration than A/J mice (a cadmium-resistant strain). This difference is attributed to a transport system that regulates the passage of cadmium across vascular barriers and that appears to be attenuated in cadmium-resistant mouse strains. Other factors, such as differences in inflammatory response to injury and differences in antioxidant systems, have been demonstrated between cadmium-sensitive and resistant animals.

D. ACUTE TOXICITY

The primary target organs for acute cadmium toxicity are dependent on the route of exposure. In general, acute oral exposure leads to gastrointestinal disturbances, and acute cadmium inhalation results in pulmonary dysfunction. Oral exposure to high levels of cadmium causes vomiting, diarrhea, abdominal pain, and tenesmus. Depending on the dose ingested, effects of acute oral cadmium toxicity may range from mild, self-limiting gastritis to severe, ful-

minating hemorrhagic gastroenteritis. Sequelae such as renal necrosis, hepatic necrosis, cardiomyopathy, and metabolic acidosis may occur in a dose-dependent manner. Microscopic gastrointestinal lesions of acute cadmium toxicity range from broadening of intestinal villi with mild to moderate submucosal edema and inflammation to extensive necrosis and denudation of absorptive cells with submucosal hemorrhage, inflammation, and vascular thrombosis.

Acute exposure to significant levels of cadmium by inhalation may result in acute tracheobronchitis, pneumonitis, and/or pulmonary edema. The primary lesions are necrosis of type I pneumocytes with denudation of the alveolar basement membranes and vascular endothelial degeneration and necrosis. Alveoli may contain varying amounts of edema fluid and fibrin, and alveolar macrophages are increased in number. The inflammatory cell response to pneumocyte necrosis may lead to further oxidative damage to alveoli and bronchioles and, ultimately, fibrosis of pulmonary interstitium. In the human lung, subacute-to-chronic exposure to inhaled cadmium results in bronchitis with progressive alveolar injury and lower airway fibrosis secondary to emphysema. The level of damage correlates to the duration and degree of cadmium exposure. Much of the damage is due to the necrosis of alveolar macrophages, with the release of lysosomal enzymes causing alveolar damage and fibrosis. In early lesions, fibrosis is restricted to the alveolar interstitium. More progressive lesions include peribronchiolar fibrosis and bronchiectasis, alveolar interstitial and intraluminal fibrosis, and emphysema. Similar pulmonary lesions have been produced experimentally in rats injected with cadmium sulfide and in mice and rats exposed to inhaled cadmium over periods of several weeks.

E. CHRONIC TOXICITY

Cadmium-induced nephropathy is one of the more common manifestations of chronic cadmium toxicity. Renal damage from cadmium exposure occurs when the levels of cadmium within the proximal tubular epithelium exceed

Acute metal fume fever due to the inhalation of mercury is rarely nowadays because of tighter regulations that reflect the increased knowledge of the toxic potential of mercury. Acute mercury inhalation causes severe bronchial irritation and coughing followed by fever, dyspnea, nausea, stomatitis, vomiting, diarrhea, confusion dehydration, and shock. Death may occur within a few hours of massive exposure. Those surviving the initial onset may develop progressive pulmonary dysfunction, ulcerative colitis, oliguria, or azotemia. Lesions include erosive bronchitis and bronchiolitis with acute pneumonitis and edema. Progressive fibrosis of the lungs has been reported in human exposure to mercury vapor. Renal damage is characterized by hydropic degeneration and necrosis of tubular epithelium, epithelial desquamation, and albuminous lumenal casts; those surviving 7–10 days will have evidence of regeneration of tubular epithelial cells. Experimentally, signs and lesions consistent with metal fume fever have been reproduced in rabbits and rats exposed to moderate-to-high levels of mercury vapor.

Chronic elemental mercury toxicity, while still quite uncommon, is seen more frequently than acute toxicity. Gastrointestinal disturbances such as hypersalivation, gingivitis, and stomatitis occur, accompanied by neurological manifestations such as fine muscle tremors that worsen with emotional stress, hyperexcitibility, irritability, aggression, or anxiety. Other signs include lethargy, weakness, diaphoresis, ataxia, hemiplegia, and lens opacities. Glomerulonephritis resembling that seen with inorganic mercury toxicosis (see later) has been described occasionally in humans but has not been reproduced in laboratory animals exposed to mercury fumes.

D. INORGANIC MERCURY

Because of their uses as topical and oral medications in the past, the monovalent and divalent salts of inorganic mercury have historical significance. The use of mercury-based medicinals is currently banned in many countries, but some countries still find use for these products as medicinal agents. In the United States, the most common source of inorganic exposure is through the occupational inhalation of elemental mercury with *in vivo* conversion to inorganic mercury.

Less than 15% of ingested inorganic mercury salts are absorbed by the gastrointestinal tract. Significant absorption of topically applied inorganic mercurial compounds may occur, however. Once absorbed, inorganic mercury is transported by plasma proteins and accumulates in the kidneys. Although the blood–brain barrier serves to keep most inorganic mercury from the nervous system, with chronic administration significant levels of mercury may accumulate in cerebellar and cerebral cortices. Poor passage of mercuric ions through the placenta results in little risk of fetotoxicity. Inorganic mercury is oxidized by catalase to divalent mercury, which localizes within lysosomes of renal tubular epithelium. Elimination of mercury is through the urine; however, renal excretion is inefficient, resulting in an accumulation of mercury within the kidneys.

Many inorganic mercurial salts are corrosive, and ingestion can lead to necrosis of oral, pharyngeal, esophageal, and gastrointestinal mucosa. Vomiting, oral pain, abdominal pain, and gastrointestinal bleeding may occur. In severe cases, gastrointestinal corrosion may lead to severe gastrointestinal hemorrhage, luminal pooling of fluids, hypovolemia, electrolyte imbalance, shock, and death. Acute renal failure may occur in those surviving beyond 24 hr. Lesions include hemorrhagic and ulcerative lesions throughout the gastrointestinal tract and necrosis of renal tubular epithelium, beginning in the pars recta and ultimately spreading throughout all regions of the renal tubules.

Chronic inorganic mercury poisoning may result in renal failure, dementia, and acrodynia ("pink disease"). Renal damage is due to renal tubular necrosis and is similar to that seen with acute elemental mercury toxicity. Experimentally, autoimmune-mediated glomerulonephritis has been produced in mice and rats following the administration of inorganic mercurial salts. Early antibasement membrane glomerulonephritis is followed by IgM-mediated immune complex glomerulonephritis with transient elevations of circulating immune complexes. Eventually, an interstitial immune complex nephritis may develop. Dementia and tremors similar to those seen in elemental mercury toxicity may occur with chronic inorganic mercury toxicity. Acrodynia is described in humans as erythema and edema of hands and feet, hyperkeratosis, skin rash, tachycardia, hypertension, photophobia, irritability, and decreased muscle tone. Splenomegaly and lymphadenopathy are described in children, who are more disposed to developing acrodynia. The mechanisms of acrodynia are unknown, but it is postulated to be a manifestation of a hypersensitivity reaction.

E. ORGANIC MERCURY

Organic mercury toxicity usually occurs through the ingestion of contaminated food products, especially fish and seafood products due to the bioaccumulation of mercury from contaminated water. Minamata disease was a neurological syndrome described in humans, birds, and cats that were exposed to methylmercury-contaminated fish in the Minamata area of Japan in the 1960s. Organomercurials are also used as fungicides for seeds and plants. In humans, sporadic outbreaks of neurological diseases related to the ingestion of flour made from ethylmercury-treated seed grain were reported in Iraq in the 1950s through 1970s.

Organomercurials are well absorbed by inhalation or ingestion. Dermal absorption, although slow, can be sufficient to cause toxicity. Absorbed organomercurials are transported bound to red blood cells and are widely distributed throughout the body. Organomercurials cross the blood–brain barrier and placenta readily, where fetal blood levels can exceed maternal blood levels by up to 20%. Organomercurials are also secreted into milk. The biological half-life of organic mercury in humans is approximately 65 days.

Alkyl mercury compounds have stable mercury–carbon bonds that are slowly cleaved after absorption, making these products more persistent and more toxic. Aryl and alkoxyalkyl mercury compounds have mercury–carbon bonds that are cleaved more readily and these compounds are subsequently catabolized to free mercury ions, which are then eliminated. Methylmercury is the most toxic of organomercurials. Methylmercury is demethylated and primarily excreted in the feces as inorganic mercury.

The primary target organ for organomercurials is the nervous system. Signs may begin days to weeks following exposure, depending on the amount and type of organic mercury involved. Neurological signs include visual disturbances, ataxia, paresthesia, hearing loss, dysarthria, mental deterioration, muscle tremor, sensory dysfunction, movement disorders, behavioral changes, and death. Pigs tend to develop a paralytic disease, whereas in cattle, the syndrome resembles lead toxicity. Rats and monkeys (*Macaca fasicularis*) develop ataxia, impaired motor function, and gait abnormalities upon exposure to dietary organomercurials. Neurologic lesions include cortical neuronal loss that may be manifested grossly as laminar cortical necrosis, with or without cerebellar or cerebral edema.

Histopathologic nervous system lesions in organomercury toxicity have been described in humans, cats, swine, laboratory rodents, mink, nonhuman primates, and several other species. There is atrophy of folia in the sulci of the lateral lobes of the cerebellum, most evident in the granular cell layers. Purkinje cell degeneration may be quite pronounced in mice and cats. Bilateral cortical atrophy in the anterior calcarine fissure may be present. Areas of neuronal degeneration and necrosis with neuronophagia are present within the hypothalamus, thalamus, midbrain, and basal ganglia. Neuronal lesions are accompanied by multifocal to extensive areas of gliosis and spongiosis. Fibrinoid necrosis of cerebral arterioles has been reported in several species, and cattle and pigs may have fibrinoid necrosis of the leptomeningeal arteries. Axonal lesions include Wallerian degeneration and demyelination of sensory nerve fibers, dorsal nerve roots, and peripheral nerves; in humans, demyelination of the lateral columns of the spinal cord has been associated with toxicity to aryl mercury compounds.

Nonneurologic lesions of organomercury toxicity are reported less commonly. Renal lesions described in rats, cattle, and pigs include grossly swollen, wet, pale kidneys. Histopathologically, there is hypertrophy and dilatation of proximal convoluted tubules, with epithelial degeneration and necrosis (Fig. 1). Chronically, mononuclear interstitial inflammation and fibrosis occur. In organomercurial toxicity of cattle, pigs, rats, and humans, myocardial injury may result in cardiac arrhythmias and failure. Grossly, cardiac lesions are minimal, although hydropericardium has been described in pigs. Histologically, Purkinje fiber degeneration, myocarditis, and myocardial mineralization have been described; cardiac lesions may be minimal to absent in pigs. Gastrointestinal signs (vomiting, abdominal pain, and diarrhea) have been reported occasionally in humans, but specific gross or histopathologic gastrointestinal lesions are not reported.

Organomercurials cross the placenta readily and may result in spontaneous abortions, severe cerebellar and cerebral deformities, cleft palate, and limb deformities in mice, hamsters, and rats. Significant strain and species variation in sensitivity to organomercurial teratogenesis exists. In studies using guinea pigs, rats, mice, and monkeys, organomercurials administered during gestation frequently resulted in alterations in learning and behavioral abnormalities in offspring. Behavioral alterations were associated with decreased numbers of muscarinic receptors in the brains of young Sprague–Dawley rats exposed prenatally to methylmercury, although no specific neurologic histopathologic lesions were noted.

F. CARCINOGENICITY

Exposure of male Fischer 344 rats to inorganic mercuric chloride for 2 years resulted in an increased incidence of forestomach squamous cell papillomas and thryoid follicular cell carcinomas. Wistar rats exposed to phenylmercuric acetate in the drinking water at 4.2 mg/kg/day for 2 years had significant increases in renal cell adenomas. Dietary exposure of ICR mice and B6C3F₁ mice to dietary organomercurials resulted in the development of renal epithelial

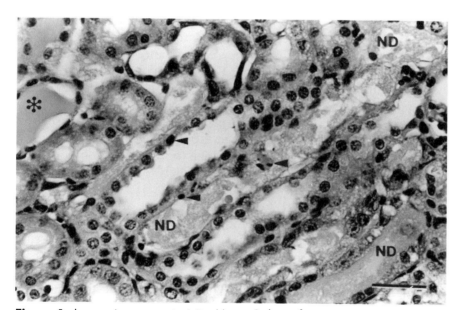

Figure 1. Inorganic mercury toxicity. Mouse 3 days after receiving an intraperitoneal injection of 3 mg/kg mercuric chloride. Tubular epithelial necrosis (arrowhead) and dilatation, intralumenal necrotic debris (ND), and hyaline casts (*). Hematoxylin and eosin. Bar: 50 μm.

cell adenomas and carcinomas. Although the International Agency for Research on Cancer (IARC) has not classified mercury as to its human carcinogenicity, the Environmental Protection Agency categorizes mercury chloride and methylmercury as potential human carcinogens.

IV. Lead

A. SOURCES AND EXPOSURE

Lead is one of the most ubiquitous and useful metals known to humans and has been widely utilized throughout history for a variety of purposes. Historically, lead was used in everyday products such as food utensils and was also added to wine to smooth out the flavor and color. Because of the well-recognized health hazards with such uses, lead is now rarely used in products associated with food or food preparation However, lead continues to be used for a variety of products, and lead contamination of the environment remains a concern.

Up to 50% of lead usage today is in the production of lead storage batteries; remaining uses for lead and lead alloys include solders, electrical and telephone line shieldings, and paints (use in residential paints was banned in the United States in 1977, but outdoor and agricultural use of lead-based paints is still common). In human children, ingestion of lead-based paint flakes and chips from older buildings remains a medical and political concern. Improperly glazed cooking bowls have on occasion been sources of lead toxicity in humans. Tetraethyl lead used in gasolines has been associated with elevated lead levels in humans and animals in urban areas; however, with the banning of leaded gasolines, a reduction in lead levels due to urban exposure has been reported.

In cattle, lead toxicity is associated most commonly with the ingestion of discarded batteries, farm machinery grease or oil, lead-based paints, putties and caulks, or roofing felt. The curious nature of cattle coupled with the unfortunate habit of some people to use pastures as junk piles has made lead toxicity in cattle a relatively common occurrence. Horses and sheep are exposed most commonly when grazing on pastures contaminated by airborne emission from nearby smelters. Other sources of lead for livestock include water from lead-lined water pipes, lead in drinking or feeding utensils, and lead arsenate pesticides (although acute arsenic toxicity is the more common manifestation). Swine are considered to be relatively resistant to the effects of lead, and reports of lead toxicity in swine are rare. Household pets may be exposed to lead through the ingestion of leaded paints in old houses, leaded artists paints, linoleum, and lead toys, weights, or ornaments. Lead toxicity in waterfowl due to the ingestion of spent lead shot is a serious concern (as few as eight No. 6 lead short can cause fatal lead toxicosis in waterfowl) and has been partially alleviated through the requirement that steel shot be used when hunting waterfowl.

B. KINETICS

Lead fumes or fine particles less than 0.5 μm are absorbed readily across the lungs; larger particles may be coughed up and swallowed, causing oral exposure. Ingested lead is poorly absorbed in adults, but the young can absorb up to 50% of ingested lead, making them more susceptible to lead toxicity. Calcium, zinc, or iron deficiency can enhance the absorption of ingested lead. Due to the poor bioavailability of nonionized lead, lead embedded in soft tissues is not absorbed appreciably and does not cause toxicity. Conversely, tetraethyl lead is absorbed readily through the skin.

Absorbed lead is bound to red blood cells and distributed widely throughout tissues, with the highest concentrations in bone, teeth, liver, lung, kidney, brain, and spleen. Lead crosses the blood–brain barrier and concentrates in the gray matter of the brain. Lead crosses the placenta readily, and alterations in calcium metabolism during pregnancy may result in significant amounts of lead being released from maternal bone and transferred to the developing fetus. Over time, most absorbed lead will be found in the bone, where it is substituted for calcium in the bone matrix. Bone serves as a long-term storage depot for lead, allowing the accumulation of large bone stores that may result in continued toxicity long after exposure has ceased. Metabolic processes that enhance bone remodeling may release stored lead and precipitate signs of toxicity. Absorbed lead is excreted slowly through the kidneys, primarily through glomerular filtration, and a significant loss of lead can occur through sloughing of renal tubular epithelium, where lead tends to concentrate. Chelation therapy can enhance the urinary excretion of lead greatly.

C. MECHANISM OF ACTION

Lead exerts its effects through the binding of sulfhydryl groups, competition with calcium ions, inhibition of membrane-associated enzymes, and altered metabolism of vitamin D. Lead has high affinity for sulfhydryl groups and can thereby inactivate enzymes, especially those involved in heme synthesis, such as δ-aminolevulinic acid dehydratase and ferrochelatase (Fig. 2). By competing with calcium, lead becomes stored in bone, alters nerve and muscle transmission, and displaces calcium in the activity of essential calcium-binding proteins such as calmodulin. Lead inhibits membrane-associated enzymes such as sodium–potassium pumps, causing increased red blood cell fragility, renal tubular damage, and, in humans, hypertension. Interference with vitamin D metabolism results in derangements in calcium

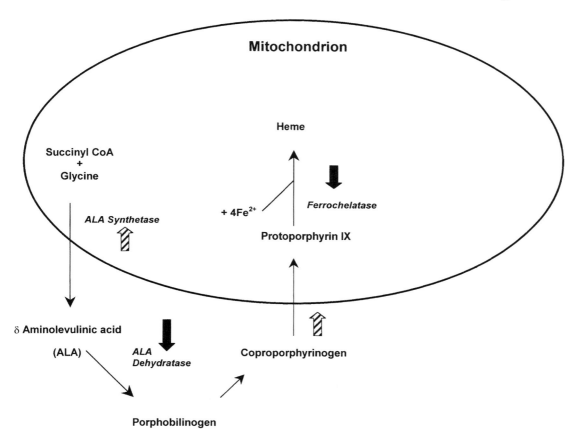

Figure 2. Effect of lead on heme synthesis. Lead inhibits δ-aminolevulinic acid dehydratase and indirectly stimulates δ-aminolevulinic acid synthetase, resulting in accumulation of δ-aminolevulinic acid and decreased formation of porphobilinogen. Lead-mediated inhibition of ferrochelatase decreases the incorporation of iron into protoporphyrin, which leads to decreased formation of heme. Lead also stimulates the activation of coproporphyrinogen to coproporphyrin. Large black arrows designate lead-mediated inhibition, whereas large striped arrows designate lead-mediated stimulation.

absorption. Lead may also interfere with zinc in some enzymes and, at high concentrations, may interfere with GABA production or activity in the central nervous system.

D. ACUTE TOXICITY

Acute lead toxicity in humans is less common than the chronic form, and it usually manifests as nephropathy characterized by acute renal failure, oliguria, aminoaciduria, glucosuria, and altered tubular ion transport. Specific lesions may be absent in acute lead toxicity, or renal lesions may be present. Degeneration and necrosis of tubular cells are often accompanied by the presence of dense, eosinophilic, and homogeneous intranuclear inclusion bodies that represent lead complexed with nonhistone nuclear proteins (Fig. 3). These inclusions are seen more commonly in chronic lead exposure and should not be considered pathognomonic, as similar inclusions can occur with exposure to other metals such as bismuth and neptunium. Other signs of acute lead toxicity in humans include nausea, abdominal pain, vomiting, shock, paresthesia, and muscle weakness. Acute hemolysis resulting in anemia and hemoglobinuria has been reported. Death can occur

within 1 to 2 days or the patient may survive to develop signs of chronic lead poisoning.

Acute lead toxicity in animals occurs most often in cattle and is usually manifested by neurological signs. Affected cattle develop hyperesthesia, ataxia, and muscle tremors followed quickly by recumbency and intermittent convulsions. Death generally occurs within 12 to 24 hr. Adult cattle may show less tendency to become recumbent and instead may develop dementia, head pressing, and blindness prior to terminal convulsions. Those animals surviving 4–5 days become apathetic, anorexic, and may appear blind. Cattle may display salivation, hyperesthesia, tenesmus, and severe depression. Sheep display similar signs as cattle. Horses may develop acute paralytic disease upon exposure to large amounts of lead. Signs begin as depression and progress to general paralysis, sometimes with clonic convulsions and abdominal pain. Acute lead poisoning in dogs and cats is again neurologic in nature, with signs including anorexia, agitation, muscle tremors, ataxia, and intermittent convulsions. Waterfowl may die acutely without prior signs or they may display weakness, ataxia, and lethargy prior to death. Specific lesions may be

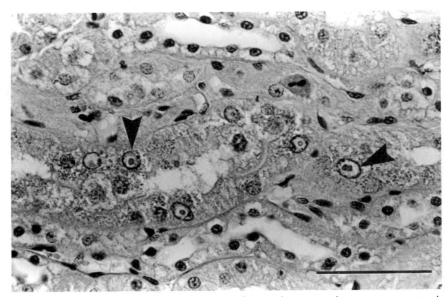

Figure 3. Lead nephropathy, civet. Intranuclear inclusions in degenerate proximal renal epithelial cells (arrows). Hematoxylin and eosin. Bar: 50 μm.

absent in animals dying of acute lead intoxication. Intranuclear inclusions in liver and kidney cells have been reported in dogs with lead toxicity, although these are seen more commonly with chronic toxicity.

E. CHRONIC TOXICITY

Chronic lead toxicity (plumbism) in humans is often divided into separate categories based on the organ system involved: gastrointestinal, neuromuscular, central nervous system, renal, and hematological. These syndromes may occur separately or in combination. In the United States, the central nervous system syndrome (lead encephalopathy) is seen more commonly in children and the gastrointestinal syndrome is more prevalent in adults. In children, lead encephalopathy is characterized by lethargy, mental dullness, vomiting, irritability, anorexia, and dizziness that may progress to ataxia, stupor, and possibly death. Sequelae in those recovering may include epilepsy, mental deficits, and optic neuropathy with blindness. In some cases, progressive decreases in cognitive function and increases in behavior disorders, especially aggression and hyperactivity, may be overlooked for many months or even years. Lesions include prominence of cerebral and cerebellar capillaries with endothelial cell swelling and necrosis, resulting in severe cerebral edema due to enhanced capillary leakage. There is gliosis and loss of neuronal cells most prominent in the middle to deep layers within the cerebral sulci. Degeneration and necrosis of cerebellar Purkinje cells may be present. Radiologic evaluation of growing bones may show heavy, multiple bands of increased density in the epiphyseal margins (lead lines). "Lead lines" may also be seen as blue-black discoloration of the gingiva in cases of lead encephalopathy.

The gastrointestinal syndrome of lead toxicity usually begins insidiously with anorexia, myalgia, malaise, headache, and a metallic taste in the mouth. Early diarrhea may occur, but constipation eventually develops and may become quite severe. Severe abdominal cramping ("lead colic") develops over time—attacks of colic are intermittent and severe. There are no specific lesions associated with the gastrointestinal syndrome.

The neuromuscular syndrome or "lead palsy" is an uncommon manifestation of advanced lead toxicity. Signs begin as muscle weakness and fatigue that may progress to paralysis. The muscles involved tend to be the most actively used muscles, especially the extensors of the forearm, wrist, fingers, and extraocular muscles. The result is an inability to extend the hand or foot, resulting in "wrist drop" or "foot drop," which, when they occur, are considered almost pathognomonic for lead toxicity in humans. Motor nerves appear to be selectively involved, as no sensory nerve deficits have been reported. Lesions include segmental demyelination and axonal degeneration of peripheral nerves.

Hematological manifestations of lead toxicity relate to the interference of lead with normal heme synthesis and to increased erythrocyte membrane fragility due to lead-induced alterations in membrane associated enzymes (see Table V). These abnormalities result in microcytic–hypochromic anemia. Inhibition of pyrimidine-5-nucleosidase results in the production of reticulocytes with basophilic stippling.

The renal syndrome of chronic lead toxicity is often subclinical, although renal function tests will detect asymptomatic renal azotemia and a decreased glomerular filtration rate. Eventually chronic renal failure develops. Lesions begin as tubular degeneration similar to that seen in the acute disease. Eventually, damage to tubular epithelium progresses to tubular atrophy and interstitial fibrosis. Intranuclear inclusions may be found in renal tubular epithelial cells and, occasionally, hepatocytes.

Chronic lead toxicity in cattle generally presents with nervous signs similar to those of acute toxicity, but of lesser severity and longer duration. There is, as well decreased rumen motility, emaciation, diarrhea, colic, and anorexia. Significant microscopic lesions include laminar cortical necrosis with swelling of cerebral capillary endothelium (Fig. 4). Some cattle may have evidence of renal tubular epithelial cell

TABLE V
Mechanisms of Lead-Induced Anemia

Enzyme inhibited	Mechanism	Effect
δ-Aminolevulinic acid dehydratase (ALA)	Decreased conversion of ALA to porphobilinogen	Accumulation of ALA, decreased heme synthesis
Ferrochelatase	Decreased incorporation of iron into protoporphyrin IX to form heme	Accumulation of protoporphyrin IX, decreased heme synthesis
Red blood cell (RBC) sodium/potassium ATPase	Alteration of cellular energy metabolism	Increased RBC membrane fragility
Pyrimidine-5-nucleosidase	Accumulation of pyrimidine nucleotides within RBC or reticulocyte	RBC basophilic stippling

degeneration, with or without fibrosis; these lesions are seen more commonly in calves. Basophilic stippling of erythrocytes, considered a diagnostic aid in humans and dogs, is not diagnostic of lead toxicity in cattle, which may normally have stippled erythrocytes. In horses, chronic lead toxicity manifests as "roaring," an abnormal breathing noise secondary to laryngeal and pharyngeal paralysis; other cranial nerve deficits may also be present. Lesions include segmental myelin and axonal degeneration of motor neurons and are similar to those seen in the peripheral neuropathy in humans. In dog and cats, chronic lead toxicity often presents with a combination of vague signs of gastrointestinal upset and neurological dysfunction, including personality changes, seizures, lethargy, and ataxia. Prolonged anorexia, vomiting, and diarrhea may result in severe emaciation. Significant lesions are found in the nervous tissue and include edema of white matter of the brain and spinal cord, myelin degeneration within the cerebellum and cerebrum, and spongy degeneration in the subthalamus, head of the caudate nucleus, and deep cortical laminae. Vascular lesions similar to those seen in the nervous systems of cattle and human may be noted, but are not found consistently. Mild astrogliosis may be present. The liver and kidney of dogs with lead toxicity may show degenerative changes accompanied by intranuclear inclusions similar to those seen in the kidneys of humans with lead toxicity.

Chronic lead toxicity in waterfowl and other wildlife most often results in chronic weight loss, emaciation, and death. Lead shot may be present in the gizzard. Atrophy of breast muscles results in a "razor keel" appearance. Pale streaks may be seen within the myocardium, corresponding to patchy areas of myocardial necrosis associated with the fibrinoid necrosis of arterioles. Other microscopic lesions include hepatocellular necrosis, renal tubular degeneration, and necrosis with occasional intranuclear inclusions in the proximal tubules, edema of brain and meninges, myelin degeneration in peripheral nerves, patchy necrosis of muscle of gizzard, and anemia with abnormalities in erythrocyte size and shape.

Reproductive effects of lead include decreased fertility in males and females and increased fetal deaths. Defects in cognitive ability in infants exposed to lead *in utero* have been reported.

F. CARCINOGENICITY

Lead has been reported to cause renal tumors, specifically renal adenocarcinomas in rats and mice. Evidence for lead-induced tumors in humans is not conclusive, although lead is classified as a probable human carcinogen.

V. Arsenic

A. CHEMICAL FORMS

Arsenic has a complex chemical structure, being present in elemental, trivalent (+3, arsenite), and pentavalent (+5, arsenate) inorganic forms and trivalent and pentavalent organic forms. Inorganic arsenicals of interest include the

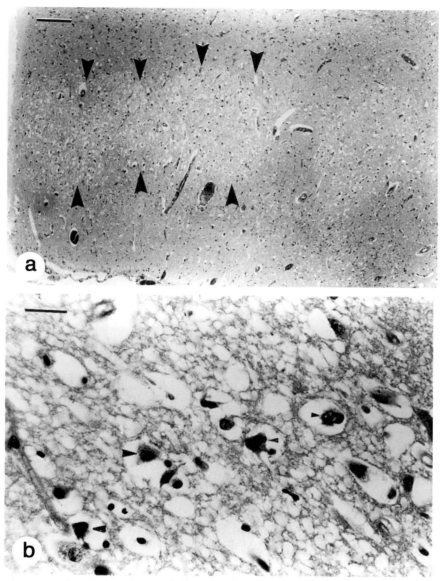

Figure 4. Lead-induced encephalopathy, bovine. (a) Focus of laminar cortical necrosis of cerebrum (arrows ➤) and (b) higher magnification of lesion showing shrunken, necrotic neurons (large arrows), and neuronophagia (small arrows). Hematoxylin and eosin. Bar: 100μm (a), 25 μm (b).

trivalent arsenic trioxide, sodium arsenite and arsenic trichloride, and the pentavalent arsenic pentoxide, arsenic acid, arsenates (lead arsenate, calcium arsenate, etc). Organic arsenic compounds may also be trivalent and pentavalent; these organic arsenicals may also be methylated. Trivalent arsenic compounds are more soluble, and therefore more toxic, than

pentavalent arsenic compounds. Phenylarsonics and arsine gas are addressed separately.

B. INORGANIC ARSENIC

1. Sources and Exposure

Sources of exposure to inorganic arsenicals include air and water contamination from glass and chemical manufacturers and from copper, zinc, and lead smelters (where arsenic is a by-product). In some areas, naturally occurring arsenic in bedrock may contaminate drinking water. The use of arsenic compounds as herbicides, pesticides, and fungicides are other sources of environmental arsenic contamination. Shellfish may accumulate relatively high levels of arsenic from contaminated water. Historically, arsenic was used medicinally, and arsenic-based pharmaceuticals were a significant source of arsenic; currently, the pharmacologic use of arsenicals in the United States is now almost exclusively limited to veterinary medicine.

2. Kinetics

Inhaled arsenic, usually in the form of trivalent arsenic oxide, is deposited in the respiratory tract and absorbed from the lung in a manner that is dependent on particulate size. Oral arsenic is well absorbed from the gastrointestinal tract. Absorption of arsenic through the skin is minimal; however, loss of dermal integrity may result in enhanced transdermal arsenic absorption. Once absorbed, 95% of arsenic is bound to red blood cells, where it is widely distributed throughout the body. In acute exposures, highest tissue levels are present within liver, kidney, heart, and lungs. Arsenic has a predilection for sulfhydryl-rich keratin, and in chronic exposures, arsenic tends to concentrate in the skin, nails, hooves, sweat glands, and hair. Arsenic can also deposit in bones and teeth in chronic cases. Inorganic arsenic does not cross the blood–brain barrier readily. The passage of arsenic through the placenta can result in arsenic levels in fetal cord blood that approximate maternal blood levels.

Elimination of absorbed inorganic arsenic requires *in vivo* transformation of inorganic arsenic to methylated organic forms. Pentavalent inorganic arsenicals must be reduced to the more soluble (and more toxic) arsenic trioxide prior to transformation to dimethylarsenate, which is excreted rapidly via the kidneys. Exposures to levels of inorganic arsenic that exceed the rate of biotransformation can result in toxicity.

3. Mechanism of Action

The mechanism of arsenic toxicity is related to its effects on enzyme systems within the cell, primarily by binding to sulfhydryl groups on enzymes and other cellular proteins. The accumulation of arsenic in mitochondria results in the inhibition of pyruvate oxidases and phosphatases, interference with NAD-linked substrates within mitochondria, inhibition of succinate dehydrogenase activity, and uncoupling of oxidative phosphorylation by replacing phosphates in high-energy phosphorylated substrates (arsenolysis). The consequences of these effects are functional and morphological cellular abnormalities secondary to the impairment of cellular respiration and depletion of energy stores. Tissues affected most severely by arsenic toxicity are those rich in oxidative enzymes, i.e., alimentary tract, liver, kidney, lung, endothelium, and epidermis.

4. Actue Toxicity

Peracute respiratory failure and aysytole may occur within hours following the ingestion of large amounts of arsenic. Some victims may display profound depression prior to death; alternatively, no antemortem signs may be noted. In cases causing death within 24 hr of exposure, lesions may be few and are generally limited to mild splanchnic congestion and edema.

A latent period of up to 48 hr may precede the development of signs in acute arsenic toxicity. The initial signs are an acute onset of profuse vomiting, diarrhea, colic, and salivation. Extensive inflammation and necrosis of gastrointestinal mucosa lead to severe hemorrhagic gastroenteritis. Increased vascular permeability due to endothelial damage results in fluid loss to the interstitium, which, coupled with intestinal blood loss, contributes to intravascular volume depletion, dehydration, hypotension, and hypovolemic shock. Damage to pulmonary capillary endothelium may initiate fulminant pulmonary edema. Hepatic and renal failure may result from the direct effects of arsenic on these organs or may be due to multi-organ failure secondary to acute cardiovascular collapse. Cardiac arrhythmias, skeletal muscle fasiculations, and weakness may occur, especially in cases surviving longer than 48 hr. Terminally, there may be delerium, dementia, or seizures. Inhalational exposure may result in cough, dyspnea, chest pain, and pulmonary edema with acute respiratory distress syndrome (ARDS) and respiratory failure. Cutaneous erythema ("flushing") may occur in acute arsenic exposures.

Subacute arsenic toxicity may result in milder manifestations of the signs just described as well as lethargy, anorexia, fever, hepatomegaly, polyuria progressing to anuria, weakness, paresis, tremor, hypothermia, stupor, cardiovascular failure, and death. Those surviving may later develop polyneuropathy, bone marrow depression, encephalopathy, cardiac arrhythmias, and visual disturbances.

5. Chronic Toxicity

Chronic arsenic toxicity is well documented in humans, although it is recognized less commonly in domestic animals. The effects of chronic arsenic exposure include dermal, gastrointestinal, bone marrow, and hepatic manifestations. Mee's lines (semilunar white bands on nails) may develop along with hyperkeratosis of skin on the extremities, acrocyanosis, cutaneous vesiculation edema, and ulceration. In extreme cases, gangrene of the feet may occur. Brick red discoloration of mucous membranes, ulcerative stomatitis, anorexia, chronic diarrhea, and cachexia may develop. Reversible bone marrow suppression may lead to leukopenia and anemia. Generalized hepatomegaly associated with elevations in liver enzymes may progress to cirrhosis, icterus, and ascites. Peripheral neuropathy with neural pain and weakness and dementia due to encephalopathy has been described in humans. Periarticular fibrosis resulting in stiff gait and asymmetrical joint enlargements has been reported in cattle exposed chronically to arsenic. Abortions may occur in pregnant humans and animals.

Many of the lesions of arsenic toxicity are secondary to severe vascular injury, leading to congestion, edema, and hemorrhage. Gastrointestinal lesions of arsenic poisoning include generalized reddening of gastrointestinal mucosa, mucosal hemorrhage and necrosis, and gastric ulceration. Extensive thickening of stomach or abomasal walls due to edema fluid may occur. Gastrointestinal contents are fluid, have a foul odor, and frequently contain blood and tags of shredded intestinal mucosa. In humans, pseudomembranous enteritis has been described. Histopathologic lesions in the gastrointestinal tract include severe congestion, denudation of mucosal epithelium, submucosal hemorrhage and edema, and thrombosis of submucosal vessels with multifocal infarction. The liver is soft and yellow. Histopathologically there is generalized hepatocellular swelling, severe fatty change, glycogen depletion, and focal necrosis; ultrastructurally, severe swelling of mitochondria is present. In rats, enlargement of the common bile duct up to 10 times the normal diameter has been described as a specific lesion of arsenic toxicity. Fatty change in heart and kidney and cerebral edema with petechiation may occur in those surviving several days. Dermal lesions range from erythema, necrosis, and ulceration to hyperkeratosis with hyperpigmentation. Histologically, dermal blood vessels may show evidence of endothelial swelling, necrosis, and thrombosis. Degeneration of myelin and axons occurs in those cases where peripheral neuropathy is evident. Degeneration of the ganglion cell layers of the retina has been reported in humans from the use of pentavalent arsenicals in the treatment of syphilis.

Arsenic can cause fetal deaths and resorptions in humans and animals. Experimentally, exposure to arsenic in utero has resulted in genitourinary deformities in animals, but no teratogenic effects have been attributed to arsenic exposure in humans.

6. Carcinogenicity

Arsenic is considered to be carcinogenic with increased incidence of basal cell tumors and squamous cell carcinomas in chronically exposed humans. Other neoplasms associated with arsenic exposure in humans include epidermoid bronchogenic carcinoma, hepatic hemangiosarcoma, lymphomas and leukemias, and cancers of the nasopharynx, kidney, and bladder. In rats and mice, increased incidences of pulmonary adenomas, papillomas, and adenomatoid lesions have been produced by arsenic trioxide; however, the development of malignant neoplasms through oral, dermal, or inhalational exposure to arsenic has not been reported.

C. PHENYLARSONICS

1. Sources and Exposure

Phenylarsonics are used in animal feeds as growth promoters and to control blood parasites and other infectious diseases. Significant human exposures are rare, and phenylarsonic toxicity in animals usually occurs when mixing errors result in overdosage or when these products are fed to dehydrated animals (dehydration appears to lower the resistance to toxicity). Phenylarsonics include arsanilic acid, 3-nitro-4-hydroxyphenylarsonic acid, 4-nitro-phenylarsonic acid, and p-ureidobenzenearsonic acid.

2. Kinetics and Mechanism of Action

Phenylarsonics are well absorbed through the skin and gastrointestinal tract and are excreted in the urine largely unchanged. Some storage occurs within nervous tissues. Phenylarsonics are not used in ruminant animals, as rumen fermentation may break them down, releasing arsenic and resulting in a syndrome consistent with inorganic arsenic toxicosis (see previous discussion). The proposed mechanism of action of phenylarsonic toxicity is through the impairment of vitamin B function, resulting in neuropathy rather than binding of sulfhydryl groups as with inorganic arsenic toxicity.

3. Toxicity

Signs and lesions of acute phenylarsonic toxicity do not develop for at least 10 days following overexposure. In swine, the most commonly affected species, the syndromes of toxicity differ depending on the type of phenylarsonic involved. Arsanilic acid toxicity presents as acute

dermal erythema, hyperesthesia, vestibular dysfunction, blindness, muscle weakness, and severe ataxia progressing to paraparesis or paralysis. Histologically, there is edema of the white matter of the brain and spinal cord. Neuronal degeneration is present within the brain stem. Wallerian degeneration and demyelination of axons of the optic and peripheral nerves, as well as necrosis of myelin-supporting cells, may be present. In contrast, 3-nitro-4-hydroxyphenylarsonic acid toxicity in swine is manifested as exercise-induced tremors and seizures, mild paraparesis or paralysis, and involuntary urination and defecation. Unlike arsanilic acid toxicity, blindness is not a feature of 3-nitro-4-hydroxyphenylarsonic acid toxicity. Histologic lesions are present within the dorsal proprioceptive and spinocerebellar tracts of the cervical spinal cord and the peripheral regions of the ventral and lateral funiculi of the posterior spinal cord; lesions consist of Wallerian degeneration of axons with mild myelin changes. Mild optic and peripheral nerve Wallerian degeneration may be present but is not a consistent finding. Chronic overdoses of phenylarsonics may manifest as a gradual onset of ataxia, proprioceptive deficits, and poor growth. Lesions are similar to those seen in the acute disease.

D. ARSINE

Arsine is a highly toxic gas that is generated upon exposure of arsenic-containing ores to acids, and it is a by-product of refining of nonferrous metals. Arsine is used extensively in the manufacture of microchips. Exposure to arsine gas results in the severe depletion of erythrocyte glutathione, causing red blood cell membrane instability and rapid, massive intravascular hemolysis. Onset of signs occurs within 30–60 min of exposure. Severe abdominal pain, vomiting, dyspnea, icterus, hemoglobinuria, hematuria, anemia, and death occur due to rapid intravascular hemolysis. Those surviving the acute episode may develop renal failure, bone marrow depression, or conditions associated with chronic arsenic exposure.

nels in the myocardium resulting in altered myocardial contractility and altered nervous stimulation due to vagus nerve damage. Multifocal necrosis of both myocardial and skeletal muscle fibers has been described in thallium intoxication in animals. Other lesions of thallium toxicity include renal tubular degeneration and necrosis, pulmonary edema, reticuloendothelial hyperplasia, lymphoid depletion, and secondary bronchopneumonia. Hepatic necrosis and bone marrow suppression have been described in cats with thallium intoxication. Chronic thallotoxicosis may lead to progressive debilitation, secondary infections, and death.

Adult male Wistar rats exposed chronically to 10 ppm of thallium sulfate in drinking water developed testicular lesions characterized by degenerative changes of Sertoli cells and seminiferous tubules.

In chick embryos, thallium causes achondroplasia, bone and beak deformities, microencephaly, and growth retardation, but similar lesions have not been described in mammals. Alopecia and nail abnormalities have been described in a human fetus exposed to thallium in the last trimester.

E. CARCINOGENICITY

Thallium can induce DNA damage and is mutagenic *in vitro*. Rats exposed chronically to thallium developed proliferative gastric lesions and gastric papillomas. However, due to insufficient data, thallium has not been classified as a carcinogen in animals or humans.

VIII. Bismuth

A. SOURCES AND EXPOSURE

Bismuth salts, both organic and inorganic, have been used medicinally to treat a variety of infectious diseases, gastrointestinal disorders, and dermatological conditions. Bismuth-based radiocontrast media are used in diagnostic medicine. Bismuth is also used in alloys in the manufacture of dental devices, steel, and some forms of shot used in hunting game. Some bismuth salts have been used in cosmetic prepara-

tions such as dusting powders and hair dyes. Because many bismuth compounds are poorly soluble and poorly absorbed, significant exposure is primarily through the pharmaceutical use of bismuth-based formulations.

B. KINETICS

Bismuth is not absorbed appreciably via inhalation or by cutaneous exposure; minimal absorption of bismuth occurs from bismuth tin shot embedded in the muscles of waterfowl. Gastrointestinal absorption is also relatively poor, with the total absorption of ingested bismuth being approximately 1%. Absorbed bismuth is transported in the blood bound to a plasma metallothionein (MW 50,000) and distributes widely throughout tissues. Bismuth accumulates in kidney, liver, spleen, bone (metaphysis), lung, heart, and muscle. Bismuth in bone is turned over very slowly, with a half-life of months to years. Protein-bound bismuth also concentrates in the placenta and can cross the placenta into the amniotic fluid and the fetus. Bismuth is excreted primarily by the kidney, which contains the highest bismuth concentrations; lesser amounts of bismuth are excreted via saliva, milk, and bile.

C. MECHANISM OF ACTION

Bismuth has an affinity for epithelial cells, and many of the manifestations of bismuth toxicity are the result of alterations of fluid and electrolyte transport within epithelial tissues. Bismuth also interferes with thiol-containing enzymes, resulting in altered cellular oxidation and metabolism. In humans, the main syndromes described in bismuth intoxication involve the kidney, alimentary tract, brain, and bone; natural bismuth toxicity in animals is rare.

D. TOXICITY

Acute renal failure may result from either acute or chronic bismuth toxicity. The concentration of bismuth in the epithelium of proximal tubules causes epithelial swelling, necrosis, and mineralization. Affected epithelial cells may contain intranuclear inclusion bodies resembling those seen in lead toxicity. The inclusions are composed of bismuth bound to nonhistone nuclear proteins. In addition to the renal tubular changes, bismuth may cause damage to glomeruli, resulting in proteinuria. The glomerular injury is secondary to capillary endothelial damage and microthrombosis.

Oral ulcers, anorexia, vomiting, hypersalivation, colic, and diarrhea may occur in acute bismuth toxicity, although massive oral overdosage is required to produce acute toxicity. Gastrointestinal signs and lesions are seen more commonly with chronic oral overdosage of bismuth compounds. The deposition of bismuth in the mucosa of the oral cavity, colon, and vagina results in blue-black pigmentation to these areas; lesions in the oral cavity tend to occur on the gums and are termed "metal lines." Alimentary lesions associated with bismuth toxicity include ulcerative stomatitis, ulcerative colitis, and cervicovaginitis, all with blue-black mucosal pigmentation. In addition to the alimentary syndrome, bismuth toxicity has been associated with hepatic failure, icterus, and clotting disorders secondary to multifocal hepatocellular degeneration and necrosis.

In the 1970s and 1980s, incidents of bismuth-induced encephalopathy were reported in Europe and Australia in association with the ingestion of bismuth-containing medications. The syndrome resembled Creutzfeldt–Jakob disease and was characterized by postural instability, ataxia, dementia, memory disorders, multifocal myoclonic jerks, coarse postural tremors, coma, and rare deaths. A similar syndrome has been produced in mice given large intraperitoneal doses of bismuth subnitrate. Lesions of murine bismuth encephalopathy include hydrocephalus and swelling of axons within the spinal cord. Both human and murine encephalopathies are reversible, and cessation of bismuth administration generally results in complete recovery.

Storage of bismuth in the bone may lead to osteoporosis and osteomalacia, manifested clinically as bony deformities, increased bone fragility, and bone pain. Osteoarthropathy has also been reported in humans with bismuth-induced encephalopathy; skeletal abnormalities in these patients were suspected of being secondary to microfractures that occurred during repetitive episodes of severe myoclonis. An exfoliative dermatitis has been reported in humans with bismuth toxicity.

E. TERATOGENICITY AND CARCINOGENICITY

Bismuth is not considered to be teratogenic, and although some mutagenic assays have reported DNA damage from certain bismuth compounds, bismuth is not currently classified as a carcinogen.

IX. Antimony

A. SOURCES AND EXPOSURE

Antimony is in the same periodic group as arsenic and has similar chemical and metabolic properties. Like arsenic, antimony exists in trivalent and pentavalent forms. Antimony is used in the metals industry and in the production of fireproofing materials, ceramics, glassware, and pigments. Antimony is used as an insecticide, and the inclusion of antimony in rodenticides serves as an emetic in the case of accidental ingestion by pets and humans. Medicinally, antimony is used to treat parasitic diseases such as schistosomiasis and leishmaniasis.

B. KINETICS AND MECHANISM OF ACTION

Antimony is absorbed slowly via the gastrointestinal tract. Because it is such a potent gastrointestinal irritant, vomiting of ingested antimony often limits exposure. Inhaled antimony is absorbed poorly, with most inhaled particles remaining in the lung. Absorbed trivalent antimony concentrates in the red blood cells and liver, whereas pentavalent forms are carried primarily by plasma proteins. Antimony is excreted rapidly through the urine and feces, and no appreciable metabolism or storage occurs, although inhalation may result in concentration of antimony within the interstitium of the lungs.

Like several other heavy metals, the mechanism of toxicity of antimony is due to the binding of sulfhydryl groups with subsequent enzyme

726

inhibition. Enzymes involved in cellular respiration and carbohydrate or protein metabolism are particularly susceptible to inactivation by antimony.

C. TOXICITY

Antimony is a potent emetic, and because it is actively secreted into the gastric lumen following absorption, it can cause profuse vomiting even when administered parenterally. In addition to severe vomiting, corrosive injury to the alimentary tract may occur following antimony ingestion, resulting in ulcerative stomatitis, esophagitis, hemorrhagic gastroenteritis, and colitis. Severe acute exposures may lead to hypovolemia, cardiac insufficiency, shock, and multiorgan failure. Dermatologic lesions have been reported in acute antimony exposures and are characterized by acute onset of a nonallergic dermatitis with pustules, eczema, and alopecia. Alterations in cardiac function may lead to arrhythmias that can contribute to cardiovascular compromise in acute antimony toxicity. Inhalation of antimony can result in rhinitis and bronchitis, and high levels of inhalation exposure may cause acute pulmonary edema. More commonly, inhalational exposure is chronic, resulting in chronic rhinits, tracheitis, bronchitis, and pneumoconiosis that may progress to obstructive lung disease and emphysema. A chronic oral exposure of rats of 0.35 mg/kg/day of antimony resulted in alterations in blood glucose and cholesterol levels.

Lesions of acute antimony toxicity include multifocal ulceration of gastrointestinal mucosa with submucosal edema and hemorrhage. There may be extensive centrilobular hepatocellular necrosis in severe cases. Myocardial degeneration, renal glomerular congestion, proximal renal tubular degeneration, and necrosis may also be present. Chronic changes include pneumoconiosis, pulmonary interstitial and peribronchiolar fibrosis, emphysema, and myocardial necrosis with fibrosis and mineralization. Degeneration of hair and supporting cells within the organ of Corti has been reported in rats and guinea pigs administered therapeutic doses of antimonial antibilharzial

agents; cochlear damage was enhanced in a dose-dependent fashion when the dose was increased to twice the recommended therapeutic dose. Chronic inhalation of antimony trioxide increased the incidence of cataract and corneal irregularities in rats.

Female laboratory rats exposed to chronic levels of inhaled antimony have reduced litter sizes, uterine metaplasia, and ovarian abnormalities. Similarly, reproductive abnormalities have been reported in women working in antimony plants, although questions regarding study methodology make interpretation of the results difficult. No specific reproductive or developmental lesions have been described.

D. CARCINOGENICITY

In Fischer and Wistar rats, chronic inhalation of antimony trioxide has resulted in an increase in lung tumors in some studies, but other studies failed to establish a link between antimony exposure and lung tumors. Similarly, conflicting results of human epidemiologic studies have failed to firmly establish antimony as carcinogenic, and it currently has not been classified as a human carcinogen by the Environmental Protection Agency or the International Agency for Research on Cancer.

X. Beryllium

A. SOURCES AND EXPOSURE

As beryllium has become of increasing industrial importance since the 1940s, its effects on human health have become recognized to the point that "beryllium disease" is a well-described entity resulting from occupational exposure to beryllium compounds. Beryllium is a by-product of coal combustion, and it is produced in alloys used in a variety of manufacturing industries, including aerospace, electronics, computers, nuclear, weapons, dental, welding, plating, and lighting manufacturing. Environmental sources, primarily through exposure to combustion products from coal and oil, account for the bulk of nonoccupational exposure.

B. KINETICS

Beryllium is absorbed poorly by oral exposure, and although cutaneous exposure may result in dermatitis, no significant dermal absorption occurs. The most significant route of exposure is via inhalation of beryllium fumes or dusts. Particulate size determines the degree of penetration of inhaled beryllium into the lung—particles with diameters of less than 1–2 μm are deposited deep within the lung. Many of these particles are cleared by phagocytosis and transported either to the airways, where they are coughed up, swallowed, and eliminated via the feces, or to the pulmonary interstitium or lymph nodes where immunologic responses are triggered. Beryllium that is absorbed into the blood is carried on plasma proteins and distributes to bone, liver, and kidney. Approximately 50% of inhaled beryllium is cleared within 2 weeks via the pulmonary mucociliary escalator; the remainder is largely sequestered within fibrotic granulomata or translocated to tracheobronchial lymph nodes, where it persists. Excretion of solubilized beryllium in the blood is via tubular secretion into the urine.

C. ACUTE TOXICITY

Although beryllium can be directly cytotoxic to tissues, the primary lesions of acute beryllium toxicity are usually related to the intense inflammatory response that the metal induces. Acute oral exposure to beryllium causes mild to moderate gastrointestinal irritation and inflammation. Cutaneous exposure may cause dermatitis, ulceration, and may delay wound healing. Ocular exposure may result in conjunctivitis. Acute inhalation of beryllium salts or fumes may result in a dose-related inflammation of the respiratory tract from the nares to the lungs. Signs associated with acute berylliosis include dyspnea, productive cough, hemoptysis, fever, tachycardia, tachypnea, rales, and cyanosis. Severe acute fulminating pneumonitis may occur at higher levels of exposure; in humans this process has occasionally been fatal, largely due to severe pulmonary edema. Lesions of acute pulmonary berylliosis include severe bronchitis and alveolitis with acute intraalveolar inflammation and edema. Radiographic examination may show diffuse alveolar infiltrates and/or pulmonary edema. Subacutely, bronchiectasis has been reported in humans as a sequela of acute berylliosis. Nonlethal cases resolve over periods of weeks or months, and approximately 17% of humans surviving the acute episode will develop chronic beryllium disease.

D. CHRONIC TOXICITY

Chronic beryllium disease has been recognized in humans since the early 20th century. Unlike acute berylliosis, the ultimate severity of the chronic form does not appear to be dependent on the magnitude of exposure. In humans, there is a variable latency period between initial beryllium exposure and onset of clinical disease; the latent period ranges from several months to 30 years or more, averaging 6–10 years. Chronic beryllium disease is a type IV hypersensitivity, with beryllium acting as an antigen or hapten (Fig. 5). The susceptibility to and extent and nature of the chronic response to beryllium are species and individual specific. A specific histocompatability antigen gene mutation has been associated with chronic beryllium disease in humans. The human leukocyte antigen class II marker HLA-DP Glu69 has been found to play a direct role in the immunopathogenesis of chronic berylliosis by altering the shape of the HLA-binding peptide pocket, thereby altering antigen specificity.

In the lung, beryllium combines with tissue proteins, and the beryllium–protein complexes are phagocytosed and processed by antigen-presenting cells. Presentation of beryllium antigen to T lymphocytes results in their stimulation, mediated by cytokines such as interleukin-1 and interleukin-6, which serve to amplify the immune response. T-helper (CD4[+]) cells proliferate in the presence of processed beryllium; this response is further amplified by cytokines such as interleukin-2, interleukin-4, interleukin-6, and interferon-γ The end result is a massive mononuclear cell infiltration that leads to the formation of granulomas containing a preponderance of CD4[+] cells.

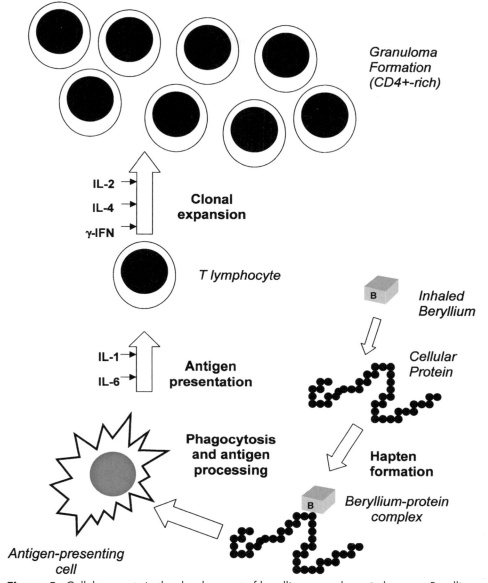

Figure 5. Cellular events in the development of beryllium granuloma in humans. Beryllium binds to cellular proteins, forming a hapten. Phagocytosis, antigen processing, and presentation of antigen to T lymphocytes by antigen-presenting cells stimulate the proliferation of CD4$^+$ cells. Recruitment of additional lymphocytes, macrophages, and giant cells results in the formation of granulomas containing a preponderance of CD4$^+$ lymphocytes. Lymphocyte stimulation and proliferation are mediated by cytokines such as interleukins -1, -2, -4, and -6 and interferon-γ.

Lesions of chronic beryllium disease include the formation of granulomas and fibrogranulomas within the lungs and often in other organs, such as liver, spleen, lymph nodes, myocardium, kidney, salivary gland, skeletal muscle, bone, and skin. Cutaneous granulomas may form due to direct contact, but can also occur via inhalation exposure. Lesions range from diffuse mononuclear cell infiltration of the pulmonary interstitium to multifocal, noncaseating lymphogranulomas. Granulomas induced by beryllium in humans differ from those

---

formed in rats, which are more of typical foreign body reactions containing large numbers of macrophages, monocytes, and small populations of lymphocytes. In contrast, the human beryllium granuloma is characterized by large numbers beryllium-specific CD4$^+$ lymphocytes with smaller numbers of macrophages and monocytes.

Mice exposed to inhaled beryllium develop pulmonary granulomas similar in appearance to those in humans, but these lesions tend to take longer to develop and usually resolve following cessation of beryllium exposure; additionally, mouse granulomas tend to have significant numbers of B lymphocytes. Guinea pigs exposed to intratracheal injections of beryllium oxide have developed pulmonary granulomas, although attempts to reproduce the lesions under inhalation exposure have not been successful. Dogs exposed to inhaled beryllium develop granulomas similar to those seen in humans.

Oral exposure to beryllium has resulted in "beryllium rickets" in rats, thought to be due to beryllium-induced interference with phosphorus absorption from the gastrointestinal tract and resulting in altered systemic calcium: phosphorus ratios. Oral dosing of beryllium in dogs has resulted in bone marrow erythroid hypoplasia and erosive and inflammatory lesions of the gastrointestinal tract. Gastrointestinal lesions are most severe in the small intestine and include desquamation and necrosis of mucosal epithelium, focal ulceration, mucosal and submucosal edema, fibrin thrombi in submucosal capillaries, and infiltration of neutrophils (early) and mononuclear cells (late). Rat and mouse studies using the same beryllium dose as in dogs failed to produce significant gastrointestinal lesions.

No information is available on the reproductive or developmental effects of beryllium in humans or animals following inhalation exposure.

E. CARCINOGENICITY

Intratracheal instillation of beryllium has been shown to cause lung cancers (adenocarcinomas, bronchiolar alveolar cell tumors, anaplastic sarcomas, squamous cell carcinomas, and malignant lymphomas) in rats and monkeys (*M. mulatta*). Intramedullary and intravenous administration of beryllium has produced osteosarcomas in rabbits. Human epidemiologic studies have not been conclusive as to the carcinogenicity of beryllium, although beryllium has been classified as a probable human carcinogen of medium carcinogenic hazard based on animal studies.

XI. Summary and Conclusions

As should be apparent from this discussion, although our knowledge regarding the signs and lesions of heavy metal intoxication might be quite broad, in many cases, the exact mechanism of action of the metal is still not fully elucidated. For example, lead is a metal that has been utilized for centuries, yet we are only now beginning to grasp the biochemical mechanisms surrounding the development of lesions of lead toxicity, and it may be quite some time before the full nature of cellular damage induced by lead is comprehended. In other cases, such as chronic beryllium disease, much of the biochemistry has been determined to the point that it is now possible to detect those people who possess the genetic mutation that puts them at risk for the hypersensitivity caused by beryllium exposure. Because metals will continue to be present in every aspect of human life, further research into mechanisms of metal-induced toxicity may prove the key to reducing environmental contamination, minimizing risk of toxicity, and improving the available treatment modalities.

SUGGESTED READING

General

Boulahdour, H., and Berry, J. P. (1996). Intranuclear dense bodies after metal intoxication: A review of ultrastructural and microanalytical findings. *Cell Mol. Biol.* **42**, 421–429.

Cheville, N. (1994). Cytopathology of toxic disease. *In* "Ultrastructural Pathology," pp. 840–845. Iowa State Univ. Press, Ames, IA.

Fowler, B. A. (1993). Mechanisms of kidney cell injury from metals. *Environ. Health Perspect.* **100**, 57–63.

Goyer, R. A. (1996). Toxic effects of metals. *In* "Casarett and Doull's Toxicology" (C. D. Klaassen, ed.), 5th Ed.,) pp. 691–736. McGraw-Hill, New York.

Quig, D. (1998). Cysteine metabolism and metal toxicity. *Altern. Med. Rev.* **3**, 262–270.

Venugopal, B., and T. D. Luckey. (1978). "Metal Toxicity in Mammals," 2nd Ed. Plenum Press, New York.

Cadmium

Clarkson, T. W. (1991). Inorganic and organometal pesticides. *In* "Handbook of Pesticide Toxicology". (J. Hayes and E. Laws, eds.), Vol 2, pp. 508–512. Iowa State Univ. Press, Ames, IA.

Dunnick, J., and Fowler, B. (1988). Cadmium. *In* "Handbook on Toxicity of Inorganic Compounds" (H. Seiler and H. Sigel, eds.), pp. 55–79. Drekker, New York.

Farina, J., Ribas, B., Fernandez-Acenero, M. J., and Gascon, C. (1996). Pulmonary toxicity of cadmium in rats: A histological and ultrasound study. *Gen. Diagn. Pathol.* **141**, 365–369.

Hamada, T., Nakano, S., Iwai, S., Taniomoto, A. Ariyoshi, K., and Koide, O. (1991). Pathological study on beagles after long-term oral administration of cadmium. *Toxicol. Pathol.* **19**, 138–147.

Klaassen, C. D., and Liu, J. (1997). Role of metallothionein in cadmium-induced hepatotoxicity and nephrotoxicity. *Drug Metab. Rev.* **29**, 79–102.

Noda, M., and Kitagawa, M. (1990). A quantitative study of iliac bone histopathology on 62 cases with itai-itai disease. *Calcif. Tissue Int.* **47**, 66–74.

Nordberg, M., Jin, T., and Nordberg, G. F. (1992). Cadmium, metallothionein and renal tubular toxicity. *IARC Sci. Publ.* **118**, 293–297.

Phillpotts, C. J. (1986). Histopathological changes in the epithelial cells of rat duodenum following chronic dietary exposure to cadmium, with particular reference to Paneth cells. *Br. J. Exp. Pathol.* **67**, 505–516.

Richardson, M. E. (1974). Dietary cadmium and enteropathy in the Japanese quail: Histochemical and ultrastructural studies. *Lab. Invest.* **31**, 722–731.

Shannon, M. (1998) The toxicology of other heavy metals. *In* "Clinical Management of Poisonings and Drug Overdosage" (L., Haddad, M., Shannon, and J., Winchester, eds.), 3rd Ed., pp. 793–794. Saunders, Philadelphia.

Taylor, J., DeWoskin, R., and Ennever, F. K. (1999) "Toxicological Profile for Cadmium," pp. 15–165. Department of Health and Human Services, Washington, DC.

Valberg, L. S., Haist, J., Cherian, M. G., Delaquerriere-Richardson, L., and Goyer, R. A. (1977). Cadmium-induced enteropathy: Comparative toxicity of cadmium chloride and cadmium-thionein *J. Toxicol. Environ. Health* **2**, 963–975.

Wallkes, M. P., Wahba, Z., and Rodriguez, R. (1992). Cadmium. *In* "Hazardous Materials Toxicology" (J. Sullivan and G. Krieger, eds.), pp. 845–852. William and Wilkins, Baltimore.

Mercury

Bigazzi, P. E. (1994). Autoimmunity and heavy metals. *Lupus* **3**, 449–453.

Chang, L. W. (1990). The neurotoxicology and pathology of organomercury, organolead, and organotin. *J. Toxicol. Sci.* **4**, 125–151.

Campbell, D., Gonzales, M., and Sullivan, J. (1992). Mercury. *In* "Hazardous Materials Toxicology" (J. Sullivan and G. Krieger, eds.), pp. 845–852. William and Wilkins, Baltimore.

Clarkson, T. W. (1991). Inorganic and organometal pesticides. *In* "Handbook of Pesticide Toxicology" (J. Hayes and E. Laws, eds.), Vol. 2, pp. 512–525. Iowa State Univ. Press, Ames, IA.

Clarkson, T. W. (1997). The toxicology of mercury. *Crit. Rev. Clin. Lab. Sci.* **34**, 369–403.

Davies, T. S., and Nielsen, S. W. (1977). Pathology of subacute methylmercurialism in cats. *Am. J. Vet. Res.* **38**, 59–67.

Davies, T. S., Nielsen, S. W., and Kircher, C. H. (1976). The pathology of subacute methylmercurialism in swine. *Cornell Vet.* **66**, 32–55.

Diamond, G, and Zalups, R. (1998). Understanding renal toxicity of heavy metals. *Toxicol. Pathol.* **26**, 92–103.

Heinz, G. H. (1996). Mercury poisoning in wildlife. *In* "Non Infectious Diseases of Wildlife" (A. Fairbrother, L. Locke, and G. Hoff, eds.), pp. 118–126. Iowa State Uni. Press, Ames, IA.

Hua, J., Brun, A., and Berlin, M. (1995). Pathological changes in the Brown Norway rat cerebellum after mercury vapour exposure. *Toxicology* **104**, 83–90.

Magos, L. (1988). Mercury. *In* "Handbook on Toxicity of Inorganic Compounds" (H. Seiler and H. Sigel, eds.), pp. 419–436. Drekker, New York.

Moszczynski, P. (1997). Mercury compounds and the immune system: A review. *Int. J. Occup. Med. Environ. Health* **10**, 247–258.

Nagashima, K. (1997). A review of experimental methylmercury toxicity in rats: Neuropathology and evidence for apoptosis. *Toxicol. Pathol.* **25**, 624–631.

Risher, J., and DeWoskin, R. (1999). "Toxicological Profile for Mercury," pp. 29–220. Department of Health and Human Services, Washington, DC.

Lead

Abadin, H., and Llados, F. (1999) "Toxicological Profile for Lead," pp. 19–257. Department of Health and Human Services, Washington, DC.

Clarkson, T. W. (1991). Inorganic and organometal pesticides. *In* "Handbook of Pesticide Toxicology" (J. Hayes and E. Laws, eds.), Vol. 2, pp. 530–537. Iowa State Univ. Press, Ames, IA.

Goyer, R. A. (1988). Lead. *In* "Handbook on Toxicity of Inorganic Compounds" (H. Seiler and H. Sigel, eds.), pp. 359–382. Drekker, New York.

Kane, A. B., and Kumar, V. (1999) Environmental and nutritional pathology. *In* "Robbins' Pathologic Basis of Disease" (R. S. Cotran, V. Kumar, and T. Collins, eds.), 6th Ed., pp. 420–421. Saunders, Philadelphia.

Keogh, J. (1992). Lead. *In* "Hazardous Materials Toxicology" (J. Sullivan and G. Krieger, eds.), pp. 834–844. William and Wilkins, Baltimore.

Locke, L. N., and Thomas, N. J. (1996) Lead poisoning of waterfowl and raptors. *In* "Non Infectious Diseases of Wildlife" (A. Fairbrother, L. Locke, and G. Hoff, eds.), pp. 108–115. Iowa State Univ. Press, Ames, IA.

Papaioannou, N., Vlemmas, I., Balaskas, N., and Tsangaris, T. (1998). Histopathological lesions in lead intoxicated dogs. *Vet. Hum. Toxicol.* **40**, 203–207.

Arsenic

Arnold, W. (1988). Arsenic. *In* "Handbook on Toxicity of Inorganic Compounds" (H. Seiler, A. Sigel, and H. Sigel, eds.), pp. 79–93. Drekker, New York.

Chou, S., and George, J. (1998). "Toxicological Profile for Arsenic (Update)," pp. 13–132. Department of Health and Human Services, Washington, DC.

Clarkson, T. W. (1991). Inorganic and organometal pesticides. *In* "Handbook of Pesticide Toxicology" (J. Hayes and E. Laws, eds.), Vol. 2, pp. 545–552. Iowa State Univ. Press, Ames, IA.

Dart, R. (1992). Arsenic. *In* "Hazardous Materials Toxicology" (J. Sullivan and G. Krieger, eds.), pp. 818–823. William and Wilkins, Baltimore.

El Bahri, L., and Ben Romdane, S. (1991). Arsenic poisoning in livestock. *Vet. Hum. Toxicol.* **33**, 259–264.

Kennedy, S., Rice, D. A., and Cush, P. F. (1986). Neuropathology of experimental 3-nitro-4-hydroxyphenylarsonic acid toxicosis in pigs. *Vet. Pathol.* **23**, 454–461.

Tsukamoto, H., Parker, H. R., Gribble, D. H., Mariassy, A., and Peoples, S. A. (1983). Nephrotoxicity of sodium arsenate in dogs. *Am. J. Vet. Res.* **44**, 2324–2330.

Uranium and Plutonium

Fisher, D. R. (1988). Uranium. *In* "Handbook on Toxicity of Inorganic Compounds" (H. Seiler and H. Sigel, eds.), pp. 739–748. Drekker, New York.

Gilman, A. P., Moss, M. A., Villeneuve, D. C., Secours, V. E., Yagminas, A. P., Tracy, B. L., Quinn, J. M., Long, G., and Valli, V. E. (1998). Uranyl nitrate: 91-day exposure and recovery studies in the male New Zealand white rabbit. *Toxicol. Sci.* **41**, 138–151.

Gilman, A. P., Villeneuve, D. C., Secours, V. E., Yagminas, A. P., Tracy, B. L., Quinn, J. M., Long, G., Valli, V. E., Willes, R. J., and Moss, M. A. (1998). Uranyl nitrate: 28-day and 91-day toxicity studies in the Sprague-Dawley rat. *Toxicol. Sci.* **41**, 117–128.

Haley, D. P., Bulger, R. E., and Doyban, D. C. (1982). The long-term effects of uranyl nitrate on the structure and function of the rat kidney. *Virch. Arch. B Cell. Pathol. Incl. Mol. Pathol.* **41**, 181–192.

Keith, S., Spoo, W., and Corcoran, J. (1999) "Toxicological Profile for Uranium." Department of Health and Human Services, Washington, DC.

McDonald-Taylor, C. K., Singh, A., and Gilman, A.(1997). Uranyl nitrate-induced proximal tubule alterations in rabbits: A quantitative analysis. *Toxicol. Pathol.* **25**, 381–389.

Pavlakis, N., Pollock, C. A., McLean, G., and Bartrop, R. (1996). Deliberate overdose of uranium: Toxicity and treatment. *Nephron* **72**, 313–317.

Sullivan, J. (1992). Organometals and reactive metals. *In* "Hazardous Materials Toxicology" (J. Sullivan and G. Krieger, eds.), pp. 933–935. William and Wilkins, Baltimore.

Tannoo, D. R., and Paquet, F. (1996). Early ultrastructural alterations in rats after administration of ^{239}Pu-citrate. *Cell Mol. Biol.* **42**, 431–438.

Voelz, G. L. (1992). Uranium. *In* "Hazardous Materials Toxicology" (J. Sullivan and G. Krieger, eds.), pp. 1155–1160. William and Wilkins, Baltimore.

Zamora, M. L., Tracy, B. L., Zielinski, J. M., Myerhof, D. P., and Moss, M. A. (1998). Chronic ingestion of uranium in drinking water: A study of kidney bioeffects in humans. *Toxicol. Sci.* **43**, 68–77.

Thallium

Clarkson, T. W. (1991). Inorganic and organometal pesticides. *In* "Handbook of Pesticide Toxicology" (J. Hayes and E. Laws, eds.), Vol. 2, pp. 525–530. Iowa State Univ. Press, Ames.

Galvan-Arzate, S., and Santamaria, A. (1998). Thallium toxicity. *Toxicol. Lett.* **99**, 1–13.

Manzo, L., and Sabbioni, E. (1988). Thallium. *In* "Handbook on Toxicity of Inorganic Compounds" (H. Seiler and H. Sigel, eds.), pp. 677–696. Drekker, New York.

Mulkey, J. P., and Oheme, F. W. (1993). A. review of thallium toxicity. *Vet. Human. Toxicol.* **35**, 445–452.

Sullivan, J. (1992). Thallium. *In* "Hazardous Materials Toxicology" (J. Sullivan and G. Krieger, eds.), pp. 845–852. William and Wilkins, Baltimore.

Bismuth

Clarkson, T. W. (1991). Inorganic and organometal pesticides. *In* "Handbook of Pesticide Toxicology" (J. Hayes and E. Laws, eds.), Vol. 2, pp. 541–543. Iowa State Univ. Press, Ames, IA.

Emile, J., De Bray, J. M., Bernat, M., Morer, T., and Allain, P. (1981). Osteoarticular complications in bismuth encephalopathy. *Clin. Toxicol.* **18**, 1285–1290.

Ross, J. F., Sahenk, Z., Hyser, C., Mendell, J. R. and Alden, C. L. (1988). Characterization of a murine model for human bismuth encephalopathy. *Neurotoxicology* **9**, 81–86.

Sanderson, G. C., Anderson, W. L., Foley, G. L., Havera, S. P., Skowron, L. M. Brawn, J. W. Taylor, G. D., and Seets, J. W. (1998). Effects of lead, iron, and bismuth alloy shot embedded in the breast muscles of game-farm mallards. *J. Wildl. Dis.* **34**, 688–697.

Slikkerveer, A., and de Wolff, F. A. (1989). Pharmacokinetics and toxicity of bismuth compounds. *Med. Toxicol. Adverse Drug Exp.* **4**, 303–323.

Thomas, D. W., Hartley, T. F., Coyle, P., and Sobecki, S. (1988). Bismuth. *In* "Handbook on Toxicity of Inorganic Compounds" (H. Seiler, A. Sigel, and H. Sigel, eds.), pp. 115–127. Drekker, New York.

Antimony

Clarkson, T. W. (1991). Inorganic and organometal pesticides. *In* "Handbook of Pesticide Toxicology" (J. Hayes and E. Laws, eds.), Vol. 2, pp. 543–545. Iowa State Univ. Press, Ames, IA.

Gebel, T. (1997). Arsenic and antimony: Comparative approach on mechanistic toxicology. *Chem. Biol. Interact.* **107**, 131–144.

Hashash, M., Serafy, A., and State, F. (1981). Histopathological cochlear changes induced by antimonial antibilharzial drugs. *J. Laryngol. Otol.* **95**, 455–459.

Iffland, R. (1988). Antimony. *In* "Handbook on Toxicity of Inorganic Compounds" (H. Seiler, Sigel, H., and A. Sigel, eds.), pp. 67–76. Drekker, New York.

Poon, R., Chu, I., Lecavalier, P., Valli, V. E., Foster, W., Gipta, S., and Thomas, B. (1998). Effects of antimony on rats following 90-day exposure via drinking water. *Food Chem. Toxicol.* **36**, 21–35.

Beryllium

Shannon, M. (1998) The toxicology of other heavy metals. *In* "Clinical Management of Poisonings and Drug Overdosage" (L. Haddad, M. Shannon, and J. Winchester, eds.), 3rd Ed., pp. 793–794. Saunders, Philadelphia.

Fontenot, A. P., Falta, M. T., Freed, B. M., Newman, L. S., and Kotzin, B. L. (1999). Identification of pathogenic T cells with patients with beryllium-induced lung disease. *J. Immunol.* **163**, 1019–1026.

Haley, P. J. (1991). Mechanisms of granulomatous lung disease from inhaled beryllium: The role of antigenicity in granuloma formation. *Toxicol. Pathol.* **19**, 514–525.

Inoue, Y., Barker, E., Daniloff, E., Kohno, N., Hiwada, K., and Newman, L. S. (1997). Pulmonary epithelial cell injury and alveolar-capillary permeability in berylliosis. *Am. J. Respir. Crit. Care Med.* **15**, 109–115.

Jones, W. W. (1988). Beryllium Disease. *Postgrad. Med. J.* **64**, 511–516.

Newman, L. (1992). Beryllium. *In* "Hazardous Materials Toxicology" (J. Sullivan and G. Krieger, eds.), pp. 882–890. William and Wilkins, Baltimore.

Richeldi, L., Sorrentino, R., and Saltini, C. (1993). HLA-DPB1 glutamate 69: A genetic marker of beryllium disease. *Science* **262**, 197–198.

Tinkle, S. S., Schwitters, P. W., and Newman, L. S. (1996). Cytokine production by bronchoalveolar lavage cells in chronic beryllium disease. *Environ. Health Perspect.* **104**, 969–971.

Zorn, H. R., Stiefel, T. W., Buers, J., and Schlegelmilch, R. (1988). *In* "Handbook on Toxicity of Inorganic Compounds" (H. Seiler, Sigel, H., and A. Sigel, eds.), pp. 105–113. Drekker, New York.